Clinical Practice
of the **Dental Hygienist**

Ninth Edition

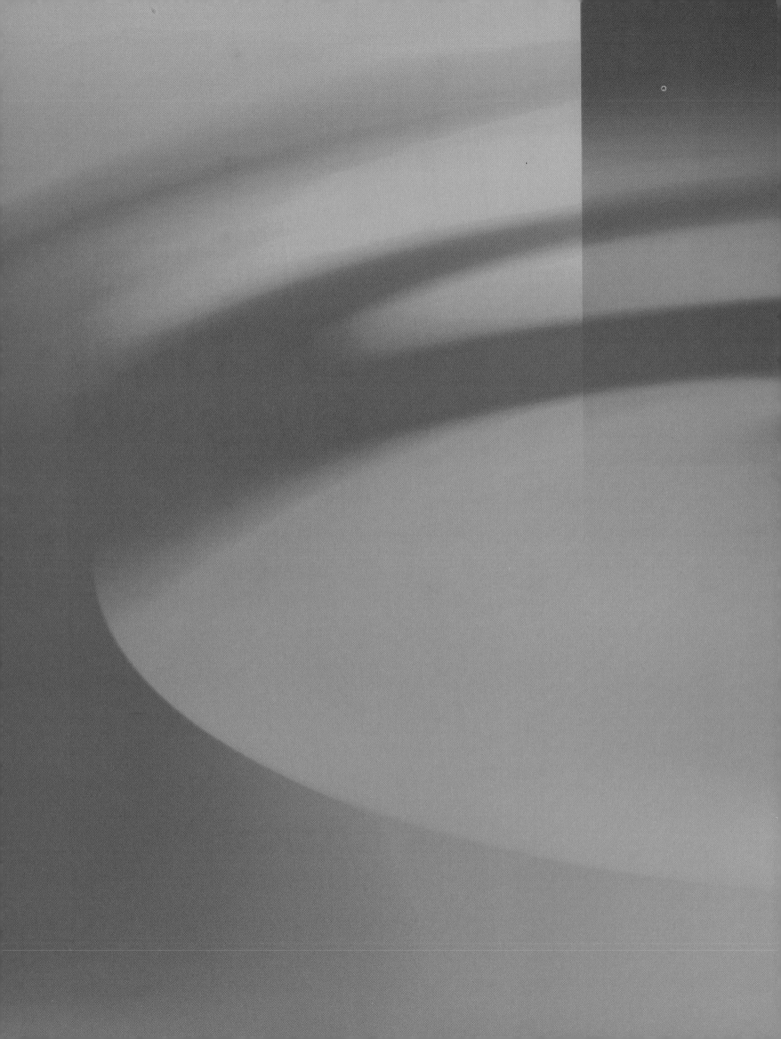

Clinical Practice
of the
Dental Hygienist

Ninth Edition

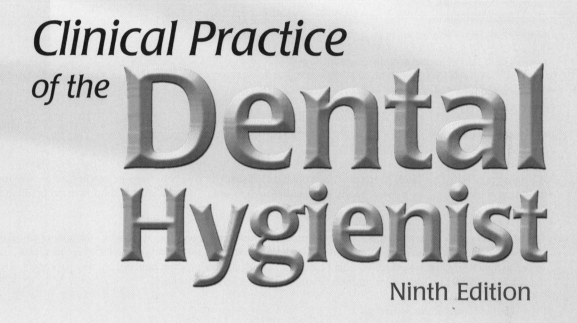

Esther M. Wilkins, BS, RDH, DMD
Department of Periodontology
Tufts University, School of Dental Medicine
Boston, Massachusetts

LIPPINCOTT WILLIAMS & WILKINS
A **Wolters Kluwer** Company

Philadelphia • Baltimore • New York • London
Buenos Aires • Hong Kong • Sydney • Tokyo

Senior Acquisitions Editor: John Goucher
Managing Editor: Kevin C. Dietz
Marketing Manager: Hilary Henderson
Production Editor: Caroline Define
Designer: Doug Smock
Compositor: TechBooks
Printer: R.R. Donnelley

Library of Congress Cataloging-in-Publication Data

Wilkins, Esther M.
   Clinical practice of the dental hygienist / Esther M. Wilkins.–9th ed.
      p. ; cm.
   Includes bibliographical references and index.
   ISBN 0-7817-4090-8
     1. Dental hygiene.   I. Title.
   [DNLM: 1. Dental Prophylaxis–Outlines.   2. Dental Hygienists–Outlines. WU 18.2
W684c 2004]
RK60.5.W5 2004
617.6'01–dc22

                                                                2003071031

The ninth edition of Clinical Practice of the Dental Hygienist is dedicated to all past and present students who have studied from the eight preceding editions. Also to their teachers in the many different dental hygiene programs around the world, for their leadership in, and devotion to, dental hygiene education.

A very special recognition goes to the students of the first ten classes in dental hygiene at the University of Washington in Seattle for whom the original "mimeographed" syllabus was created. They are remembered with much appreciation because their need for text study material made this book possible in the first place.

Esther Wilkins

Contributors

Caren M. Barnes, RDH, BS, MEd
Clinical Research and Department of Dental Hygiene
University of Nebraska Medical Center
College of Dentistry
Lincoln, Nebraska

Su-yan L. Barrow, RDH, BS, MA, MPH
Dental Hygiene Program
New York University College of Dentistry
New York, New York

Cynthia R. Biron, RDH, EMT, MA
The Dental Hygiene Program
Tallahassee Community College
Tallahassee, Florida

Patricia A. Cohen, RDH, BS, MS
Department of Periodontology
Tufts University School of Dental Medicine
Boston, Massachusetts

Marilyn Cortell, RDH, MS
Dental Hygiene Program
New York University College of Dentistry
New York, New York
and
Department of Dental Hygiene
New York City college of Technology
Brooklyn, New York

Ann Overton Dickinson, RDH, MS
Dental Technologies Department
St. Louis Community College
St. Louis, Missouri

Dorathea L. Foote, RDH, MEd
Department of Dental Hygiene
Springfield Technical Community College
Springfield, Massachusetts

Joan C. Gibson-Howell, RDH, BS, MSEd, EdD
Division of Dental Hygiene
West Virginia University School of Dentistry
Morgantown, West Virginia

Marylou Gutmann, BSDH, MA
Department of Dental Hygiene
Baylor College of Dentistry

Texas A&M University System Health Science Center
Dallas, Texas

Donna F. Homenko, RDH, MEd, PhD
Department of Dental Hygiene/Bioethics
Cuyahoga Community College
Cleveland, Ohio

Carol A. Jahn, RDH, MS
Educational Programs
Waterpik Technologies
Fort Collins, Colorado

Janis G. Keating, RDH, MA
Department of Dental Hygiene
University of Colorado School of Dentistry,
Denver, Colorado

Nancy Sisty LePeau, RDH, MS, MA
Child Health Clinic
Johnson County Public Health
Iowa City, Iowa

Deborah Mancinelli Lyle, RDH, BS, MS
Professional Marketing and Education
Waterpik Technologies
Fort Collins Colorado

Stacy A. Matsuda, RDH, BS
Department of Periodontology
School of Dentistry
Oregon Health and Science University
Portland, Oregon

Durinda J. Mattana, RDH, MS
Department of Periodontology and Dental Hygiene
University of Detroit Mercy School of Dentistry
Detroit, Michigan

Joan M. McGowan, RDH, MPH,PhD
Periodontics/Prevention/Geriatrics Department
University of Michigan School of Dentistry
Ann Arbor, Michigan

Laura Mueller-Joseph, RDH, MS, EdD
Department of Dental Hygiene
Farmingdale State University of New York
Farmingdale, New York

Kathleen M. Nace, RDH, AA
Dental Hygiene Department
Harrisburg Area Community College
Harrisburg, Pennsylvania

Luisa Nappo-Dattoma, RDH, RD, EdD
Dental Hygiene Program
New York University, College of Dentistry
New York, New York

Anna Matsuishi Pattison, RDH, MS
Department of Dental Hygiene
Division of Primary Health Care
School of Dentistry
University of Southern California
Los Angeles, California

Kathryn Ragalis, RDH, MS, DMD
Department of General Dentistry
Tufts University School of Dental Medicine
Boston, Massachusetts

Tonya S. Ray, RDH, MA
Professional Education
Oral-B Laboratories
Boston, Massachusetts

Janet B. Selwitz-Segal, RDH, CDA, MS
Forsyth Dental Hygiene Program
Massachusetts College of Pharmacy and Health Sciences
Boston, Massachusetts

Donna Stach, BS, RDH, MEd
Department of Dental Hygiene
University of Colorado School of Dentistry
Denver, Colorado

Lisa B. Stefanou, RDH, BS, MPH
Dental Hygiene Department
New York University College of Dentistry
New York, New York

Terri S.I. Tilliss, RDH, MS, MA
Department of Dental Hygiene
University of Colorado School of Dentistry,
Denver, Colorado

Janet H. Towle, RN, RDH, BS, MEd
Forsyth Dental Hygiene Program
Massachusetts College of Pharmacy and Health
Sciences
Boston, Massachusetts

Nancy L. J. Williams, RDH, MS, EdD
Department of Dental Hygiene
College of Allied Health Sciences
University of Tennessee
Memphis, Tennessee

Charlotte J. Wyche, RDH, MS
Department of Periodontology and Dental Hygiene
University of Detroit Mercy School of Dentistry
Detroit, Michigan

Preface

During the 45 years since the original publication of *Clinical Practice of the Dental Hygienist*, many changes have influenced what constitutes adequate clinical practice and the significance of the role of the dental hygienist in oral disease prevention and health promotion. Extensions in scientific knowledge and technical inventions have had major impact on the profession of dental hygiene.

The new research on dental biofilm clarifies the need to treat dental caries and periodontal diseases as infectious and communicable. Emphasis on a patient's personal risk factors and the interwoven effects of oral health and systemic conditions finally brings to the front that needed medical-dental tie. New requirements for standard infection control during clinical practice have introduced improved levels for the safety of patients and dental healthcare personnel. Identification and treatment of early periodontal conditions and the determination of prognosis and outcomes from dental hygiene therapy show the significant role of dental hygienists in total patient oral care.

OBJECTIVES

The preface of the first edition of the book opened with: *"The major purpose of this book is to provide the dental hygienist with a comprehensive outline of the principles and techniques of dental hygiene care and instruction for the individual patient. It is hoped that through greater understanding of the patient's oral and general health needs, more complete and effective service may be rendered. It is expected that the book will be useful as a textbook for preclinical and clinical theory and practice courses for students, as a reference and guide for practicing dental hygienists, and as a source of review material for temporarily retired dental hygienists with plans for returning to practice."*

As the ninth edition comes into use, the same basic objectives hold true. To be sure, the knowledge and skills needed to reach the competency required for contemporary practice have greatly widened. Evidence-based practice provides security in the realization that the patient is receiving the best possible service to meet individual needs.

THE NEW EDITION

Many chapters were extensively revised, while others required minimal change.

The new chapters are Chapter 24, Protocols for the Prevention and Control of Dental Caries; Chapter 46, Pediatric Oral Health Care: Infancy Through Age 5; Chapter 57, Family Abuse and Neglect; and Chapter 62, The Patient with a Respiratory Disease.

Other chapters have been combined, namely, Chapter 6, Records and Charting, and Chapter 28, The Patient with Orthodontic Appliances. Two chapters have been divided, Chapter 21, Planning Dental Hygiene Care, and Chapter 22, The Dental Hygiene Care Plan, and Chapter 26, Interdental Care, and Chapter 27, Chemotherapeutics and Topical Delivery Systems.

TEXTBOOK SECTIONS

Clinical Practice of the Dental Hygienist is divided into seven sections. Section I includes an orientation to the profession of dental hygiene with a detailed explanation of the Dental Hygiene Process of Care. Sections II through VI have their foundation on the Dental Hygiene Process of Care to include assessment, dental hygiene diagnosis, care planning, implementation, and evaluation. Section VII describes a variety of patients needing special care because of age, systemic health problems, or disability.

Section I. Orientation to Clinical Dental Hygiene Practice
Section II. Preparation for Dental Hygiene Appointments
Section III. Patient Assessment
Section IV. Care Planning
Section V. Prevention
Section VI. Treatment
Section VII. Patients with Special Needs

Supplementary information is available in the added section on Prefixes, Suffixes, and Combining Forms. Appendices provide the Codes of Ethics of both the American Dental Hygienists' Association and the Canadian Dental Hygienists' Association, and the Recommendations from the *Guidelines for Infection Control in Dental Health-Care Settings—2003*, Centers for Disease Control and Prevention of the U.S. Department of Health and Human Services.

DENTAL HYGIENE ETHICS

A special new feature of the ninth edition is the introduction of a theme of dental hygiene ethics throughout the text, which has been prepared by Donna Homenko. The text portion starts with the introductory material in Chapter 1 and continues in each of the introductions to the Sections. With the knowledge that each dental hygiene program may have a full credit course in ethics, the objective here is to provide integration with the clinical textbook and experiences.

Each chapter has, near the end of the chapter, a short case titled Everyday Ethics, which presents either an ethical issue or a dilemma, with questions for consideration to open a discussion of possible solutions. Opportunities for use of the Everyday Ethics appear in both the Student Workbook and the Instructors' Website.

STUDENT WORKBOOK

The first workbook of its kind for dental hygiene accompanies the main text of *Clinical Practice of the Dental Hygienist*. The workbook, authored by Charlotte Wyche, provides a variety of experiences to help students learn the important concepts that are the basis for dental hygiene practice.

Exercises are designed to take students from basic *knowledge* (ability to recall and identify concepts from the text) through *competency* (being able to use information in the text to think critically and make decisions regarding patient care) and on to *discovery* (being able to use what was learned in the text to gather new, relevant information from sources other than in the text).

INSTRUCTORS' WEBSITE

The first Instructors' Website to accompany *Clinical Practice of the Dental Hygienist* has been planned by Rhoda Gladstone and Cheryl Westphal. New information not included in the text is included and more may be added at a later time. The website will make available case studies, quiz questions, power point slides that provide lecture notes and slide images, and active learning exercises. Hyperlinks to websites and resources for each chapter can

provide relevant material. A feature will be using evidence-based learning to facilitate critical thinking.

ACKNOWLEDGEMENTS

Ideas and recommendations come from many teachers, students, and practitioners from around the world. Any suggestion, whether for a whole new chapter or a simple word change, is considered and activated whenever possible. It is hoped that this new edition will bring forth comments and requests as in the past.

First, thanks go to all our contributors for their new or revised chapters. Dr. Donna Homenko, our contributor for the new ethics theme, has earned particular recognition for producing this new feature and presenting the Everyday Ethics appropriate to each chapter.

Much appreciation goes to Charlotte Wyche, who, through the Student Workbook, has added a new dimension to the teaching/learning capacity of the textbook. The Teachers' Website will provide a special means of communication with the devoted teachers around the world. To Rhoda Gladstone and Cheryl Westphal and their faculty at the New York University, we owe a debt of gratitude.

The illustrations for this and two previous editions have been the work of the talented artist Marcia Williams of Newton Highlands, Massachusetts. Her personal interest and patience in preparing the new artwork and adding color for selected previously used art is very sincerely appreciated. Many thanks to Emily Williams who has done such skillful work in producing the computerized copies of many chapters that they required practically no changes when they came through production.

As stated in the first edition, the author and contributors will feel amply rewarded if *Clinical Practice of the Dental Hygienist* helps dental hygienists to understand and meet more completely the oral health needs of their patients.

Esther M. Wilkins

Contents

Orientation to Clinical Dental Hygiene Practice

CHAPTER 1

The Professional Dental Hygienist

Laura Mueller-Joseph, RDH, MS, EdD
Donna F. Homenko, RDH, MEd, PhD
Esther M. Wilkins, BS, RDH, DMD

CHAPTER OUTLINE

The dental hygienist is a licensed primary healthcare professional, oral health educator, and clinician who provides preventive, educational, and therapeutic services supporting total health for the control of oral diseases and the promotion of oral health. Dental hygiene services are available for general and specialty dental practices, programs for research, professional education, community health, and hospital and institutional care of disabled persons, as well as for federal programs, the armed services, and dental product promotion. Key words relating to dental hygienists and their practice are defined in Box 1-1.

Within the wide span of dental hygiene practice areas, dental hygienists may serve in a variety of capacities. With the challenges brought about by the advances in scientific research and the changes in healthcare systems, the scope of practice has widened. Dental hygienists are found serving in several interrelated roles, including clinicians, health promoters, educators, consumer advocates, change agents, administrators, managers, and researchers. Areas of responsibility in this variety of roles are defined in Box 1-2.

Dental Hygiene Care

The term *dental hygiene care* is used to denote all integrated preventive and treatment services administered to a patient by a dental hygienist. This term is parallel to the commonly used term *dental care*, which refers to the services provided by the dentist.

Clinical services, both dental and dental hygiene, have limited long-range probability of success if the patient does not understand the need for cooperation in daily procedures of personal care and diet and for regular appointments for professional care. Educational and clinical services, therefore, are mutually dependent and inseparable in the total dental hygiene care of the patient.

BOX 1-1 KEY WORDS AND ABBREVIATIONS: Professional Dental Hygienist

ADHA: American Dental Hygienists' Association.

CDHA: Canadian Dental Hygienists' Association.

CEU: continuing education unit; 1 unit commonly refers to 1 clock hour of instruction.

Competency: the skills, understanding, and professional values of an individual ready for beginning dental hygiene practice.

Continuing education: postlicensure short-term educational experiences for refresher, updating, and renewal; continuing education units may be required for relicensure.

Cotherapist: term used to describe the relationships between patient, dentist, and dental hygienist when coordinating the efforts to attain and maintain the oral health of the patient.

Dental hygiene care: the science and practice of the prevention of oral diseases; the integrated preventive and treatment services administered for a patient by a dental hygienist.

Dental hygiene care plan: the services within the framework of the total treatment plan to be carried out by the dental hygienist.

Dental hygiene diagnosis: identification of an existing or potential oral health problem that a dental hygienist is qualified and licensed to treat.

Dental hygiene process of care: an organized systematic group of activities that provides the framework for delivering quality dental hygiene care.

Dental hygienist: dental health specialist whose primary concern is the maintenance of oral health and the prevention of oral disease (see also opening paragraph, page 3).

Dentistry: the evaluation, diagnosis, prevention, and/or treatment (nonsurgical, surgical, or related procedures) of diseases, disorders, and/or conditions of the oral cavity, maxillofacial area, and/or the adjacent and associated structures and their impact on the human body, provided by a dentist, within the scope of his/her education, training, and experience, in accordance with the ethics of the profession and applicable law (American Dental Association).

Health: state of physical, mental, and social well-being, not only the absence of disease.

Health promotion: the process of enabling people to increase control and improve their health through self-care, mutual aid, and the creation of healthy environments.

Hygiene: the science of health and its preservation; a condition or practice, such as cleanliness, that is conducive to the preservation of health.

Oral hygiene: procedures for preservation of health of the oral cavity; personal maintenance of cleanliness and other measures recommended by dental professionals.

Intervention: an action taken by a dental hygienist to maintain or restore a patient's optimal oral health.

License by credential: acceptance for licensure by a regulatory body (state, province) on the evidence from a license obtained in another state where equivalent standards and requirements are required; also called reciprocity, a mutual or cooperative exchange.

Primary healthcare: employs the techniques and agents to abort the onset of disease, to reverse the progress of the initial stages of disease, or to arrest the disease process before treatment becomes necessary.

Profession: occupation or calling that requires specialized knowledge, methods, and skills, as well as preparation, from an institution of higher learning, in the scholarly, scientific, and historic principles underlying such methods and skills; a profession continuously enlarges its body of knowledge, functions autonomously in formulation of policy, and maintains high standards of achievement and conduct; members of a profession are committed to continuing study, place service above personal gain, and are committed to providing practical services vital to human and social welfare.

KEY WORDS AND ABBREVIATIONS: Professional Dental Hygienist, continued

Prognosis: a forecast of the probable course and outcome of the treatment of a condition or disease.

Supervision: term applied to a legal relationship between dentist and dental team members in practice. Each practice act defines the type of supervision required.

Collaborative Practice of Dental Hygiene: the science of the prevention and treatment of oral disease through the provision of educational, assessment, preventive, clinical, and other therapeutic services in a collaborative working relationship with a consulting dentist, but without general supervision.

Direct supervision: means that the dentist has diagnosed and authorized the condition to be treated, remains on the premises while the procedure is performed, and approves the work performed before dismissal of the patient.

General supervision: means that the dentist has authorized the procedure for a patient of record but need not be present when the authorized procedure is carried out by a licensed dental hygienist. The procedure is carried out in accordance with the dentist's diagnosis and treatment plan.

Personal supervision: means that while the dentist is personally treating a patient, the dental hygienist is authorized to aid in the treatment by concurrently performing a supportive procedure.

Dr. Alfred C. Fones, the "father of dental hygiene," emphasized the important role of education. In the first textbook for dental hygienists, he wrote:

"It is primarily to this important work of public education that the dental hygienist is called. She must regard herself as the channel through which dentistry's knowledge of mouth hygiene is to be disseminated. The greatest service she can perform is the persistent education of the public in mouth hygiene and the allied branches of general hygiene."[1]

Dental hygiene has been studied and the scope of practice has developed from Dr. Fones' original concept.

BOX 1-2 The Six Roles of Dental Hygienists

CLINICIAN
Assesses, diagnoses, plans, implements, and evaluates treatment for prevention, intervention, and control of oral diseases while practicing in collaboration with other professionals.

EDUCATOR/HEALTH PROMOTER
Uses educational theory and methodology to analyze health needs, develops health promotion strategies, and delivers and evaluates the results of attaining or maintaining oral health for individuals or groups.

CONSUMER ADVOCATE
Influences legislators, health agencies, and other organizations to bring existing health problems and available resources together to resolve problems and improve access to care.

ADMINISTRATOR/MANAGER
Applies organizational skills, communicates objectives, identifies and manages resources, and evaluates and modifies programs of health, education, or healthcare.

CHANGE AGENT
Analyzes barriers to change; develops mechanisms to effect change; implements processes and evaluates the success of programs that promote health for individuals, families, or communities; and promotes lifestyle changes for individual patients.

RESEARCHER
Applies the scientific method to select appropriate therapies, educational methods, or content; interprets and applies findings and solves problems.

Scientific information about the prevention of oral diseases has been advancing steadily. The public has become increasingly aware of the need for dental hygiene care and the importance of oral health instruction. The clinical practice of the dental hygienist integrates specific care with instructional services required by the individual patient.

▪ Types of Services

The clinical and educational responsibilities of the dental hygienist are divided into preventive and therapeutic services. Clinical and educational activities are inseparable and overlap as patient care is planned and accomplished.

Preventive Services

Preventive services are the methods employed by the clinician and/or patient to promote and maintain oral health. Preventive services fall into three groups: primary, secondary, and tertiary.
- *Primary prevention* refers to measures carried out so that disease does not occur and is truly prevented.

Example: An example of primary prevention is the use of fluorides.
- *Secondary prevention* involves the treatment of early disease to prevent further progress of potentially irreversible conditions that, if not arrested, can lead eventually to extensive rehabilitative treatment or even loss of teeth.

Example: Removal of all calculus and dental biofilm while debriding a root surface in a relatively shallow periodontal pocket is an example of secondary prevention in that the treatment contributes to the prevention of continued attachment loss and the formation of a deep pocket.
- *Tertiary prevention* uses methods to replace lost tissues and to rehabilitate the oral cavity to a level where function is as near normal as possible after secondary prevention has not been successful.

Example: An example of tertiary prevention is the replacement of a missing tooth using a fixed partial denture or implant and therefore restoring function.

Educational Services

Educational services are the strategies developed for an individual or a group to elicit behaviors directed toward health. Educational aspects of dental hygiene service permeate the entire patient care system. The preparation for clinical treatment, the outcomes of treatment, and the long-term success of both preventive and therapeutic services depend on the patient's understanding of each procedure and on the daily care of the oral cavity.

Therapeutic Services

Therapeutic services are clinical treatments designed to arrest or control disease and maintain oral tissues in health. Dental hygiene treatment services are an integral part of the total treatment procedures. All scaling and root debridement, along with the steps in posttreatment care are parts of the therapeutic phase in the treatment of periodontal infections. Placement of a pit and fissure sealant is an example of both a preventive and a therapeutic service.

▪ Dental Hygiene Process of Care

The dental hygiene process of care includes assessment, dental hygiene diagnosis, planning, implementation, and evaluation.[2] As a process, the procedures performed are continual in nature and may overlap or occur simultaneously (Figure 1-1).

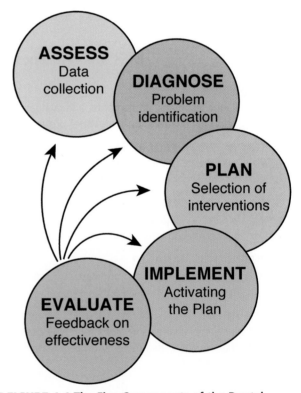

▪ **FIGURE 1-1 The Five Components of the Dental Hygiene Process of Care.** All components are interrelated and depend upon evaluation to determine the need for change in the care plan.

Purposes of the Dental Hygiene Process of Care

- To provide a framework within which individualized needs of the patient can be met.
- To identify the causative or influencing factors of a condition that can be reduced, eliminated, or prevented by the dental hygienist.

I. ASSESSMENT

- First phase of the dental hygiene process.[3]
- A systematic collection of comprehensive data relative to the health status of the individual.
- Provides a foundation for patient care.
- Documented in the patient's record.

A. Subjective Data

- Obtained by observation and interaction with the patient.
- Includes chief complaint, perception of healthcare, and the value placed on oral health.

B. Objective Data

- Includes physical and oral assessment.
- Records clinical and radiographic findings to show evidence of disease in teeth and periodontal tissues, including probing depths, loss of periodontal attachment, dental carious lesions, and defective restorations.

II. DENTAL HYGIENE DIAGNOSIS

- Identifies the health behaviors of individuals as well as the actual or potential health problems that dental hygienists are licensed to treat.[4]
- Provides the basis on which the dental hygiene treatment plan is designed, implemented, and evaluated.
- Justifies the treatment proposed to the patient.
- Challenges the dental hygienist to assume responsibility for patient care and to move beyond a rote system of clinical practice.

A. Data Processing

- Uses critical thinking skills to collect and interpret information.
- Includes the classification, interpretation, and validation of information collected during the assessment phase.
1. *Classification.* Classification of data involves the sorting of information into specific categories such as general systemic, oral soft tissue, peri-
odontal, dental, and oral hygiene. As information is organized, pertinent data are interpreted according to the patient's needs.
2. *Interpretation.* Data interpretation relies upon critical thinking to identify significance. The cognitive processes of analysis, synthesis, inductive reasoning, and deductive reasoning are the bases for determining a diagnosis.
   - Compare findings with standards or norms.
   - Recognize deviations or abnormalities.
   - Analyze abnormalities with respect to significance.
3. *Validation.* Validation is an attempt to verify the accuracy of data interpretation. Validation can assist in recognizing errors, isolating discrepancies, and identifying the need for additional information.
   - Direct interaction with the patient.
   - Consultation with other healthcare professionals.
   - Comparison of data with an authoritative reference.

B. Diagnosis Formulation

- Focuses on the patient's individual needs.
- Determines potential or actual problems that can be prevented, minimized, or resolved by independent or interdependent interventions.
- Identifies the patient's condition or potential for risk.
- Specifies the causative and contributing factors, such as environmental, psychological, sociocultural, and physiological factors, believed to be related to the health condition.
- Expresses the problem and cause, for example, "Generalized brown tooth stains related to use of cigars."
- Sample diagnostic statements are provided in Table 1-1.

III. DENTAL HYGIENE CARE PLANNING[5]

- Strategies are developed to meet the individual needs of the patient as identified by the dental hygiene diagnosis.
- Steps include establishing priorities, setting goals, determining interventions, and defining expected outcomes.

A. Establishing Priorities

- Priorities are determined by the immediacy of the condition, the severity of the problem, and available resources.

■ TABLE 1-1 EXAMPLES OF DENTAL HYGIENE DIAGNOSTIC STATEMENTS

PROBLEM		CAUSE (RISK FACTORS AND ETIOLOGY)
Halitosis	*Related to*	Dental biofilm accumulation on the tongue
Cervical abrasion	*Related to*	Incorrect toothbrushing
Potential for dental caries	*Related to*	Deep occlusal pits and fissures
Bleeding on probing	*Related to*	Marginal dental biofilm accumulation
Anxiety	*Related to*	Dental phobia

- Patients are active participants in the identification of priorities.

B. Setting Goals

- Each problem is accompanied by a goal.
- Goals are directly related to the problem and represent the anticipated level of achievement.

C. Determining Interventions

- Interventions are dental hygiene therapies or patient educational activities that reduce, eliminate, or prevent the cause of the problem.

Example: For the prevention of halitosis, dental hygiene interventions may include tongue cleaning and patient instruction about the papillae on the tongue that trap biofilm.

D. Identifying Expected Outcomes (Prognosis)

- Expected outcomes represent measurable criteria for each intervention.
- Selected according to the anticipated effectiveness of the interventions.
- Provide a way to evaluate the results of the intervention.

Example: An expected outcome following a patient education intervention about tongue anatomy might be that the patient is now able to perform a self-evaluation of tongue cleanliness.

E. Presenting the Dental Hygiene Care Plan

1. To the dentist: for integration with the total treatment plan.
2. To the patient: for complete understanding of the interventions needed and the appointment requirements.

F. Obtaining Informed Consent (page 370)

1. To show that the care plan has been thoroughly explained to the patient.
2. To show the willing participation of the patient.

IV. IMPLEMENTATION

- Phase in which the care plan is put into action.
- Identified activities to be performed by the patient, dental hygienist, or others are carried out at this time.

V. EVALUATION

- Compare current health status with baseline data.
- Assess progress or lack thereof toward the stated goal.
- Determine change or modification of the care plan.

At this point, the process comes full circle. The evaluation phase is used to determine if the patient should be re-treated, referred, or placed on maintenance.

- The maintenance phase of care has also been termed "continuing care" or "supportive therapy" and may be scheduled at intervals of 3, 4, or 6 months depending on the patient's health status and adherence to personal care.
- All patients need to be placed on a maintenance program to prevent progression or recurrence of disease and to maintain their current level of health.

VI. APPLICATIONS FOR THE PROCESS OF CARE

The five components of the dental hygiene process of care serve as the foundation for clinical practice of the dental hygienist. Chapter 22, *The Dental Hygiene Care Plan*, further illustrates the process through the utilization of the Patient-Specific Dental Hygiene Care Plan (Figure 22-1). The plan provides a framework for completing and recording the details of the various components of the process.

■ Dental Hygiene Ethics

The ethics of a profession provide the general standards of right and wrong that guide the behavior of the members in that profession. Key words relating to ethics and ethical principles are defined in Box 1-3.

BOX 1-3 KEY WORDS: Ethics

Autonomy: the act of self-determination by persons with the ability to make a choice or decision. Autonomy exists for both the dental hygienist and the patient.

Beneficence: doing good for a benefit or enhanced welfare.

Confidentiality: involves the rights of patients to privacy; a duty of dental hygienists is to protect privileged communication.

Core values: basic values of a profession; guide to choices or actions by implying a preference for what is deemed to be acceptable in the profession.

Ethical dilemma: a problem that involves two morally correct choices or courses of action. There may not be a single answer and, depending on the choice, the outcomes can differ.

Ethical issue: a common problem wherein a solution is readily grounded in the governing practice act, recognized laws, or acceptable standards of care. Decisions involving ethical issues are generally more clearly defined than are dilemmas.

Ethics: a sense of moral obligation; a system of moral principles that govern the conduct of a professional group, planned by them for the common good of people; principles of morality.

Justice/fairness: fair treatment according to an equitable distribution of benefits and burdens; impartiality; a core value.

Moral: a principle or habit with respect to right or wrong behavior.

Nonmaleficence: avoidance of harm to others; a core value.

Rights: expectations by the patient that correlate with the duties of a professional person when providing care.

Societal trust: maintaining a bond of trust in the relationships between the dental hygienist and patients, other professional persons, and the public.

Veracity: a duty to tell the truth when information is disclosed to patients about treatment.

Virtue: character trait; one must intend to act virtuously as a professional. Examples include honesty, compassion, care, and wisdom.

The members of a profession:
- Have extensive specialized education.
- Possess an intellectual body of knowledge from study and research.
- Provide services important for the common good of society; dental hygienists provide preventive, educational, and therapeutic services.
- Maintain an organization of members that sets professional standards.
- Exercise autonomy and judgment.
- Prepare their own code of ethics.

■ The Code of Ethics

- Describes professional conduct.
- Outlines responsibilities and duties of each member toward patients, colleagues, and society in general.

Purposes of the Code of Ethics

- To define a standard of conduct that will give each individual a strong sense of ethical consciousness not only in professional practice but in all phases of life.
- To increase the awareness of, and sensitivity to, ethical situations in practice.

Dental Hygiene Codes

- The Code of the American Dental Hygienists' Association and the Code of the Canadian Dental Hygienists' Association can be read in Appendices I and II (pages 1124 and 1128).
- Each dental hygienist studies and applies the code of the particular association in which membership is held.

■ TABLE 1-2 A FRAMEWORK FOR MAKING DECISIONS IN THE DENTAL SETTING

Step 1. Dental Hygiene Situation	Step 2. Individual Preferences

• Is this situation an ethical issue or a dilemma?
• What is the chief concern/problem?
• Summarize the history of the patient or situation.
• List all the facts in the case.
• Who is involved in making this decision?
• What guidelines exist that apply to this situation?
	• What are the rights of the individuals involved in the case?
	• What are the duties of the dental hygienist?
	• In a clinical case:
	  • Has informed consent been obtained?
	  • How has the choice for care been communicated by the patient and explained by dental professionals?

Step 3. Choices vs. Alternatives	**Step 4. Case Parameters**
• Which core ethical values apply to the case? • What are the benefits of care? • Are there short-term vs. long-term options for this situation/treatment? • Describe the realistic alternatives that exist. • Has patient education been provided? • Explain benefits and burdens to the patient or the dental professional.	• Does the "scope of practice" apply to this situation? If so, explain. • What financial, legal, or cultural factors need consideration? • Is there a conflict of interest between a patient, dental providers, or other individuals? • Should an outside source be consulted in this case?

■ Core Values

"Core Values" are selected principles of ethical behavior that can be considered the heart of the code of a profession.

Core Values in Dental Hygiene

- Individual autonomy and respect for human beings.
- Confidentiality.
- Societal trust.
- Nonmaleficence.
- Beneficence.
- Justice and fairness.
- Veracity.

Personal Values

- A dental hygienist develops character traits and virtues consistent with the care provided for each patient.

- Value development begins at an early age and is influenced by familial, social, and economic factors.
- Life experiences, grounded in previous successes and failures, serve as a foundation for professional virtues.
- Members of a health profession can benefit from periodic self-assessment of individual values, attitudes, and responsibilities. The questions for thought in Box 1-4 can provide a personal review or may be used in a group discussion.

The Patient First

- The responsibility to put the patient first is foremost.
- Dental hygienists are ethically, morally, and legally responsible to provide oral care for all patients without discrimination.
- Ethical decision making and professional behavior are reflected in every aspect of dental hygiene practice.

BOX 1-4 Value Self-Assessment

1. When do you first remember learning the meaning of right and wrong?

2. Which individuals have been role models in your life and why?

3. Explain any rules that taught you to be a "morally good" adult in society.

4. Which character traits are important to provide patient care and/or be a member of a dental team?

5. Describe what you value most in life, and why.

Lifelong Learning: An Ethical Duty

- To ensure optimal care for each patient.
- To maintain competency.
- To learn scientific advances from new research.
- To provide patient care that is evidence based.
- To apply consistent ethical reasoning.
- To ensure fulfillment of each patient's rights.

■ Ethical Applications

A dental hygienist may be involved in a variety of moral, ethical, and legal situations as part of the daily routine. In ethics, a problem situation is considered either an *ethical issue* or an *ethical dilemma*.

Ethical Issue

- More clearly defined than a dilemma.
- A common problem wherein a solution is grounded in the governing practice act, recognized laws, or accepted standards of care.
- May be resolved on decisions based on the standard rules of practice.

Ethical Dilemma

- A problem that involves two morally correct choices or courses of action.
- May not have a single answer and, depending on the choice, the outcomes can differ.
- To resolve a dilemma, the facts are gathered, ethical principles and theories are applied, and options are explored.

When a dilemma or an issue arises, the four steps in Table 1-2 provide a reasonable approach. Consider each step in a logical sequence.

- Identify the problem and the individuals involved.
- Gather the facts from all persons concerned.
- Determine which ethical principles may apply.
- List alternative solutions or outcomes as they are proposed by each participant.
- Consider the benefits and disadvantages of all possible outcomes.
- Compare the anticipated action with acceptable professional standards.

SUMMARY: The Final Decision

Only after addressing the items in each box of the decision framework can the dental hygienist take action and make a decision. Many factors can be used to solve a dilemma. All dental healthcare providers involved in the decision process can participate in a follow-up evaluation of the action taken.

Once a decision has been made, the concluding assessment should be: Is the decision/action that is selected morally defensible? In essence, can the choice be defended to solve the dilemma? A professional person may need to defend it to the patient, the dentist, members of the dental team, a state board, or even a court of law. Most importantly, the decision must be defensible based on standards of practice established for the dental hygiene profession.

Applications

Various ethical issues and dilemmas are presented throughout this book for discussion and consideration. The examples usually appear at the end of the chapter where the problem may apply.

■ Legal Factors in Practice

The law must be studied and respected by each dental hygienist practicing within the state, province, or country. Although the various practice acts have certain basic similarities, differences in scope and definition exist. Terminology varies, but each practice act regulates the patient services that may be practiced by the licensed dental hygienist. Changes may be made from time to time. Frequent review of the practice acts and/or regulations is recommended to keep dental health professionals up to date.

■ Personal Factors in Practice

Each dental hygienist represents the entire profession to the patient being served. The dental hygienist's expressed or demonstrated attitudes toward dentistry, dental hygiene, and other health professions, as well as toward health services and preventive measures, will affect the subsequent attitude of the patient toward other dental hygienists and dental hygiene care in general.

Members of health professions must exemplify the traits they hold as objectives for others if response and cooperation are to be expected. Many personal factors of general physical health, oral health, cleanliness, appearance, and mental health are to be considered. A few of these are mentioned as follows:

- *General Physical Health.* Optimum physical health depends to a great extent on a well-planned diet, a sufficient amount of sleep, and an adequate amount of exercise.

  Because of the occupational hazards of dental personnel, routine examinations at least annually should include tests for hearing, sight, urinary mercury, and certain communicable diseases. Immunizations are described on page 51.

Everyday Ethics

The first term of the dental hygiene curriculum has just finished. The instructor asks for student volunteers to help at the college's health fair to provide basic routine brushing and flossing directions to people who stop at the dental hygiene information table. Three students, Alice, Annette, and Josephine, sign up to volunteer for this community service. The day before the health fair, which takes place on a Saturday, Annette is asked to work in the dental office where she is employed part-time. Since she really needs the money, she decides not to attend the health fair and instead goes to work without telling anyone.

Questions for Consideration

1. In general, would this situation be described as a professional issue or an ethical dilemma? Why?

2. Discuss Annette's actions in terms of the core ethical values.

3. What aspects of the Dental Hygiene Code of Ethics can you use to support your choice of action?

- *Oral Health.* The maintenance of a clean, healthy mouth demonstrates by example that the dental hygienist follows the teachings of the dental and dental hygiene professions relative to prevention and control of oral disease.
- *Mental Health.* The mental health of the dental hygienist is reflected in interpersonal relationships and the ability to inspire confidence through a display of professional and emotional maturity. Adequate physical health, recreation, and participation in professional and community activities contribute to optimum mental health.

■ Special Practice Areas

A wide range of settings is available for the practice of a dental hygienist. Likewise, a wide range of patient problems requires specialized knowledge and skills.

Dental Specialties

There are nine areas of dentistry in which a dentist may conduct an ethical limited practice. They are the following[6]:
- Dental Public Health
- Endodontics
- Oral and Maxillofacial Pathology
- Oral and Maxillofacial Surgery
- Orthodontics and Dentofacial Orthopedics
- Pediatric Dentistry
- Periodontics
- Prosthodontics
- Oral and Maxillofacial Radiology

Education and training for certification in the dental specialties require a minimum of 2 or 3 years of graduate or postdoctoral study and the successful completion of written and practical examinations. Masters and postdoctoral specialty degrees require 3 or more years beyond basic dental education.

Dental Hygiene Specialties

Although licensure is not required for dental hygienists to practice within a specialty, educational curricula exist for certain areas. For example, advanced degree programs to prepare for dental hygiene education and public health have been available for many years. Other dental hygienists with masters or doctoral degrees have majored in nutrition and dietetics, business and administration, law, as well as a variety of sciences.

In other special areas, short-term courses have been developed, such as for instruction in the care of patients with disabilities. In-service training may be available in long-term care institutions, hospitals, and skilled nursing facilities. Other dental hygienists have learned to practice in a specialty through private study, special conferences, and personal experience.

Dental hygienists are needed to practice with dentists in specialty areas, particularly orthodontics, pediatric dentistry, and periodontics. Others are involved in special clinics with a variety of health specialists, where patients with dental deformities such as cleft lip and/or palate or with oral cancer are under care. In other facilities, dental hygienists serve with a combined medical and dental team in the treatment of patients with severe systemic diseases; patients with physical, mental, or emotional handicapping conditions; or patients with combinations of any of the problems mentioned.

■ Objectives for Professional Practice

A dental hygienist's self-assessment is essential in attaining goals of perfection for service to each patient and in collaboration with the dentist in a total dental and dental hygiene care program. Personal objectives should be outlined and reviewed frequently in a plan for continued self-improvement.

The overall professional goals of the dental hygiene profession relate to health promotion and disease prevention. The goal of each dental hygienist with respect to patient care is *to aid individuals and groups in attaining and maintaining optimum oral health.* Other personal objectives are related to this primary one.

The professional dental hygienist will:
- Strive toward the highest degree of professional ethics and conduct.
- Plan and carry out effectively the dental hygiene services essential to the total care program for each individual patient.
- Apply evidenced-based knowledge and understanding of the basic and clinical sciences in the recognition of oral conditions and the prevention of oral diseases.
- Apply evidenced-based scientific knowledge and skill to all clinical and instructional procedures.
- Recognize each patient as an individual and adapt care planning and interventions accordingly.
- Identify and care for the needs of patients who have unusual general health problems that affect dental hygiene procedures.
- Demonstrate interpersonal relationships that permit attending the patient with assurance and presenting dental health information effectively.
- Provide a complete and personalized instructional service to help each patient become motivated toward changes in oral health behavioral practices.
- Practice safe and efficient clinical routines for the application of standard precautions for infection control.
- Apply a continuing process of self-evaluation in clinical practice throughout professional life.
- Recognize the need for lifelong learning to acquire updated knowledge through reading professional literature and enrolling in continuing education programs.
- Maintain membership and participate actively in the local, national, and international dental hygiene professional associations.

✔ Factors To Teach The Patient

- The role of the dental hygienist as a cotherapist with each patient and with members of the dental profession.

- The moral and ethical nature of becoming a dental hygiene professional person.

- The scope of service of the dental hygienist as defined by various practice acts.

- The interrelationship of instructional and clinical services in dental hygiene patient care.

- The patient's potential state of oral health and how it can be improved and maintained.

REFERENCES

1. **Fones**, A.C., ed.: *Mouth Hygiene*, 4th ed. Philadelphia, Lea & Febiger, 1934, p. 248.
2. **Mueller-Joseph**, L. and Petersen, M.: *Dental Hygiene Process: Diagnosis and Care Planning.* Albany, Delmar, 1995, pp. 9–14.
3. Ibid., pp. 20–25.
4. Ibid., pp. 46–55.
5. Ibid., pp. 89–104.
6. **American Dental Association**: *Principles of Ethics and Code of Professional Conduct.* Revised January, 2002.

SUGGESTED READINGS

Brutvan, E.L.: Current Trends in Dental Hygiene Education and Practice, *J. Dent. Hyg., 72,* 44, Fall, 1998.

Chichester, S.R., Wilder, R.S., Mann, G.B., and Neal, E.: Incorporation of Evidence-based Principles in Baccalaureate and Nonbaccalaureate Dental Hygiene Programs, *J. Dent. Hyg., 76,* 60, Winter, 2002.

Gaston, M.A.: Managing Change, (Editorial), *J. Dent. Hyg., 71,* 179, Fall, 1997.

Gaston, M.A.: What Will the Future Hold? (Editorial), *J. Dent. Hyg., 74,* 2, Winter, 2000.

Gluch, J.I.: Are Hygienists Ready for a New Challenge? *Contemporary Oral Hyg., 2,* 23, March/April, 2002.

Jevack, J.E., Wilder, R.S., Mann, G., and Hunt, R.J.: Career Satisfaction and Job Characteristics of Dental Hygiene Master's Degree Graduates, *J. Dent. Hyg., 74,* 219, Summer, 2000.

King, C.C. and Craig, B.J.: The Role of the Dental Hygienist as Change Agent, *Canad. Dent. Hyg. Assoc./Probe, 31,* 81, May/June, 1997.

Luxmore, J.S., Mattana, D., Wyche, C., Zager, S., and Zarkowski, P.: Learning the Process of Collaborative Clinical Research, *J. Dent. Hyg., 71,* 207, Fall, 1997.

Pack, A.R.C.: Hygienists and Their Role in Dental Practice, *N. Zeal. Dent. J., 91,* 57, June, 1995.

Sisty-LePeau, N.: Life-long Learning, (Editorial), *J. Dent. Hyg., 66,* 331, October, 1992.

Sisty-LePeau, N.: What's in a Name? (Editorial), *J. Dent. Hyg., 71,* 3, January–February, 1997.

Professionalism and Ethics

Beemsterboer, P.L.: *Ethics and Law in Dental Hygiene,* Philadelphia, W.B. Saunders, 2001, pp. 3–50, 81–91.

Chally, P.S. and Loriz, L. Decision Making in Practice: A Practical Model for Resolving the Types of Ethical Dilemmas You Face Daily, *Am. J. Nurs., 98,* 17, June, 1998.

Devore, C.H.: Legal Risk Management for the Dental Hygienist, *J. Pract. Hyg., 6,* 59, July/August, 1997.

Fleming, W.C.: The Attributes of a Profession and Its Members, *J. Am. Dent. Assoc., 69,* 390, September, 1964.

Gaston, M.A., Brown, D.M., and Waring, M.B.: Survey of Ethical Issues in Dental Hygiene, *J. Dent. Hyg., 64,* 217, June, 1990.

Hine, M.K.: The Professional Concept—Its History and Meaning to Health Service, *J. Am. Coll. Dent., 37,* 19, January, 1970.

Homenko, D.F.: Use of an Inventory for Ethical Awareness in Dental Hygiene, *J. Am. Coll. Dent., 69,* 31, Winter, 2002.

Jenson, L.: My Way or the Highway: Do Dental Patients Really Have Autonomy?, *J. Am. Coll. Dent., 70,* 26, Spring, 2003.

Kimbrough, V.J. and Lauter, C.J.: *Ethics, Jurisprudence, and Practice Management in Dental Hygiene.* New Jersey, Prentice Hall, 2003, pp. 19–66.

Lautar, C.: Is Dental Hygiene a Profession? A Literature Review, *Canad. Dent. Hyg. Assoc./Probe, 29,* 127, July/August, 1995.

MacQuarrie, E.E.: Factors in the Development of Professional Attitude, *J. Am. Dent. Hyg. Assoc., 45,* 86, March–April, 1971.

Motley, W.E.: *Ethics, Jurisprudence and History for the Dental Hygienist,* 3rd ed. Philadelphia, Lea & Febiger, 1983, 217 pp.

Wynia, M.K., Latham, S.R., Kao, A.C., Berg, J.W., and Emanuel, L.L.: Medical Professionalism in Society, *N. Engl. J. Med., 341,* 1612, November 18, 1999.

Zarkowski, P. and Graham, B.: A Four-year Curriculum in Professional Ethics and Law for Dental Students, *J Am. Coll. Dent., 68,* 22, Number 2, 2001.

Preparation for Dental Hygiene Appointments

INTRODUCTION

Preparation for a dental hygiene appointment centers on the standard precautions for infection control for the safety of the patients and the clinician. Chapter 2 provides specific information about the chain of infection and the microorganisms that can be transmitted in the dental setting when standard precautions are not observed.

In Chapters 3 and 4, specific materials and procedures are described that are necessary for safe clinical practice. Chapter 5 deals with the reception and seating of the patient. Special emphasis is placed on the ergonomic factors of body posture and hand, wrist, and arm positions for prevention of musculoskeletal problems.

In oral healthcare practice, an objective is to protect patients, dental personnel, and others who may be exposed from acquiring infection in the environment of the clinic or office. Health services facilities, including dental facilities, must be places for cure and prevention, not for dissemination of disease due to inadequate precautionary measures and habits of the professional personnel.

The first responsibility of the entire team is to organize and maintain a system for the sterilization and care of instruments and equipment. The second step is to develop and maintain work practices for all appointments that will prevent direct or indirect cross-infections between dental personnel and patients and from one patient to another.

▪ ETHICAL APPLICATIONS

A dental hygienist may be involved in a variety of moral, ethical, and legal situations during practice. All professional actions related to the process of care must apply the principles of ethics. The goal is to increase the awareness of, and sensitivity to, ethical situations during practice.

Ethical applications of the basic core values and principles as outlined in the Dental Hygiene Code of Ethics are identified in every phase of the dental hygiene appointment. The Code and the basic core values in dental hygiene are identified on page 10 as selected principles of ethical behavior that can be considered the heart of the Code of a profession. An overview of the core values with definitions and applications are found in Table II-1.

Ethical principles contained in most codes of ethics clarify the standards of judgment that professionals must follow. Principles by themselves cannot be prioritized in order of importance. They must be combined with philosophical theories when making a decision.

▪ TABLE II-1 DENTAL HYGIENE CORE VALUES		
ETHICAL PRINCIPLE/CORE VALUE	**EXPLANATION**	**APPLICATIONS**
Autonomy	Patient's right to self-determination and making choices for care	Educating the patient prior to obtaining informed consent
Beneficence	Performing services for the good of the patient	Universal precautions for all patients
Nonmaleficence	Removing or preventing harm during treatment	Individualize plaque control recommendations and perform subgingival debridement
Justice	Fair treatment for all patients	Following acceptable standards of and access to care
Confidentiality	Protection of sensitive information	Securing patient files in locked cabinets
Veracity	Truth-telling	Trust in the provider-patient relationship when obtaining the medical history
Fidelity	Keeping promises	Helping a fearful patient be comfortable by using local anesthesia or nitrous oxide
"Ethical Applications" is prepared by Donna Homenko, Ethics Editor.		

CHAPTER 2

Infection Control: Transmissible Diseases

CHAPTER OUTLINE

For dental health-care personnel (DHCP), infection and communicable disease can lead to illness, disability, and loss of work time. In addition, patients, family members, and community contacts can become exposed and may become ill and lose productive time or suffer permanent after-effects.

In oral health-care practice, the objective is to protect patients, dental personnel, and others who may become exposed by acquiring infection in the environment of the office or clinic. Health services facilities, including dental facilities, must be places for cure and prevention, not for dissemination of disease due to inadequate precautionary measures and habits of the professional personnel.

The first responsibility of the entire dental team is to organize and maintain a system for the sterilization, disinfection, and care of instruments and equipment. The second step is to develop and maintain work practices for all appointments that will prevent direct or indirect cross-infections between dental personnel and patients and from one patient to another. Box 2-1 lists and defines terms that apply to the transmission of infectious agents.

▪ STANDARD PRECAUTIONS[1]

Previous infection control recommendations from the United States Centers for Disease Control and Prevention were focused on the risk of transfer of the blood-borne pathogens, and the term **universal precautions** was used. With recognition that other body fluids besides blood carry infectious agents, the new concepts have been enclosed within the all inclusive term **standard precautions**.

A. STANDARD PRECAUTIONS

- Integrate and expand the elements of universal precautions.
- Represent a standard of care which protects DHCP and their patients from pathogens that can be spread by blood or any other body fluid, excretion, or secretion.
- Apply to contact with:
    1. blood

    2. all body fluids, secretions, and excretions (except sweat), regardless of whether they contain blood
    3. nonintact skin
    4. mucous membranes

B. OTHER PRECAUTIONS

- Transmission-based precautions (examples: tuberculosis, influenza, varicella)
- Diseases transmitted through airborne, droplet (sneezing, coughing)
- Skin contact transmission

▪ MICROORGANISMS OF THE ORAL CAVITY

In utero the oral cavity is sterile, but after birth within a few hours to 1 day a simple oral flora develops.[2] As the infant grows there is continuing introduction of microorganisms normal for an adult oral cavity. The microbiota of the adult is very complex.

Most of the salivary bacteria come from the dorsum of the tongue, but some are from other mucous membranes. Much higher counts of total microorganisms are found in dental biofilm, periodontal pockets, and carious lesions than in saliva.

The intact mucous membrane of the oral cavity protects against infection to a degree. However, when the gingival tissues are inflamed and are manipulated during instrumentation, microorganisms can be introduced into the underlying tissues by way of the gingival sulcus or periodontal pocket.

Pathogenic (disease-producing), potentially pathogenic, or nonpathogenic microorganisms may be present in the oral cavity of each patient. Pathogenic organisms may be transient. Patients may be carriers of certain diseases. Inadvertent transmission to subsequent susceptible patients or to dental personnel may occur as a result of inappropriate work practices, such as careless handwashing, unhygienic personal habits, or inadequate sterilization and handling of sterile instruments and materials.

Cross-contamination refers to the spread of microorganisms from one source to another: person to person, or

BOX 2-1 KEY WORDS AND ABBREVIATIONS: Disease Transmission

Aerosol: an artificially generated collection of particles suspended in air.

Microbial aerosol: suspension of particles in the air that consists partially or wholly of microorganisms; it may be capable of causing an infection.

Anergy: diminished reactivity to specific antigen(s); inability to react to skin-test antigen (even if person is infected with the organism tested) because of immunosuppression.

Antibody: a soluble protein molecule produced and secreted by body cells in response to an antigen; it is capable of binding to that specific antigen.

Antigen: a substance that is capable, under appropriate conditions, of inducing a specific immune response and of reacting with the products of that response, that is, with the specific antibody.

Carrier: a person who harbors a specific infectious agent in the absence of discernible clinical disease and serves as a potential source of infection. The carrier state may be temporary, transient, or chronic.

Asymptomatic carrier: an individual who harbors pathogenic organisms without clinically recognizable symptoms; a carrier may infect those he/she contacts.

CDCP: United States Centers for Disease Control and Prevention, Department of Health and Human Services, Public Health Service, Atlanta, GA 30333.

Communicable period of a disease: the time during which an infectious agent may be transferred directly or indirectly from an infected person to another person; the communicable period may include or overlap the incubation period.

Droplet: diminutive drop, such as the particles of moisture expelled while coughing, sneezing, or speaking, that may carry infectious agents.

ELISA or EIA: an enzyme-linked immunosorbent assay; a laboratory test to detect antibody in the blood serum.

Western blot (WB): a laboratory test for antibody that is more specific than EIA and is used to validate seropositive reactions to the EIA.

Endemic: the constant presence of a disease or infectious agent within a geographic area.

Epidemic: widespread occurrence of cases of an illness in a community or region; greater than the expected number of cases for the particular population.

Fomite or fomes: an inanimate object or material on which disease-producing agents (microorganisms) may be conveyed.

HCP: health-care personnel; **DHCP:** dental health-care personnel.

Immunity: the resistance that a person has against disease; it may be natural or acquired.

Passive immunity: short-duration immunity either naturally attained by transplacental transfer from the mother or artificially acquired by inoculation of specific protective antibodies.

Active immunity: immunity either naturally attained by infection, with or without clinical manifestations, or artificially acquired by inoculation of the agent in a killed, modified, or variant form; in response, the body produces its own antibodies; usually lasts for years.

Incubation period: the time interval between the initial contact with an infectious agent and the appearance of the first clinical sign or symptom of the disease.

Infection: a state caused by the invasion, development, or multiplication of an infectious agent into the body.

Primary infection: first time; no preexisting antibodies.

Latent infection: persistent infection following a primary infection in which the causative agent remains inactive within certain cells.

Recurrent infection: symptomatic reactivation of a latent infection.

KEY WORDS AND ABBREVIATIONS: Disease Transmission, continued

Infectious agent: organism capable of producing an infection.

Jaundice: yellowness of skin, sclerae, mucous membranes, and excretions due to hyperbilirubinemia and deposition of bile pigments. Also called *icterus.*

Microbiota: the microscopic living organisms of a region.

Pandemic: widespread epidemic usually affecting the population of an extensive region, several countries, or sometimes the entire globe.

Parenteral: injection by a route other than the alimentary tract, such as subcutaneous, intramuscular, or intravenous.

Parotitis: inflammation of the parotid gland.

Pathogen: a virus, microorganism, or other substance that causes disease.

> **Opportunistic pathogen:** capable of causing disease only when the host's resistance is lowered.

Percutaneous: by way of, or through, the skin.

Permucosal: by way of, or through, a mucous membrane.

Prodrome: early or premonitory symptom (adj: prodromal).

Replication: process by which viruses reproduce and multiply.

Retrovirus: virus with RNA as its core genetic material; requires the enzyme reverse transcriptase to convert its RNA into proviral DNA.

Serologic diagnosis: the identification of a disease by serum markers of that specific condition.

Seroconversion: after exposure to the etiologic agent of a disease, the blood changes from negative ("seronegative") to positive ("seropositive") for the serum marker for that disease; the time interval for conversion is specific for each disease.

Serum marker: a specific finding (such as an antibody or antigen) by laboratory blood analysis that identifies an existing disease state.

Shedding (viral): presence of virus in body secretions, in excretions, or in body surface lesions with potential for transmission.

Standard precautions: an approach to infection control to protect DHCP and patients from pathogens that can be spread by blood or any other body fluid, secretion, or excretion (except sweat), regardless of whether they contain blood.

STD: sexually transmitted disease.

Surveillance (of disease): continuing scrutiny of all aspects of occurrence and spread of a disease that are pertinent to effective control.

Susceptible host: host not possessing resistance against an infectious agent.

Transmission (horizontal): passage of an infectious agent from one individual to another.

> **Vertical transmission:** passage of an infectious agent from one generation to another by breast milk or across the placenta.

Universal precautions: an approach to infection control in which all human blood and certain human body fluids are treated as if known to be infectious for HIV, HBV, and other blood-borne pathogens.

Vector: a carrier that transfers an infectious microorganism from one host to another.

> **Biologic vector:** an arthropod, insect, or other living carrier in whose body the infecting organism multiplies before becoming infective to the recipient.

Vehicle: a substance or object that serves as an intermediate means by which an infectious agent is transported and introduced into a susceptible host through a suitable portal of entry.

KEY WORDS AND ABBREVIATIONS: Disease Transmission, continued

Virion: complete virus particle made up of the **nucleoid** (the genetic material) and **capsid** (the shell of protein that protects the nucleoid).

Virulence: the degree of pathogenicity or disease-evoking power of an infectious agent.

Virus: a subcellular genetic entity capable of gaining entrance into a limited range of living cells and capable of replication only within such cells; a virus contains either DNA or RNA but not both. (DNA and RNA are defined in Box 2-2, page 37.)

Window period: the time between exposure resulting in infection and the presence of detectable serum antibody; antibody test is negative but infectious agent is transmissible during the window period.

person to an inanimate object and then to another person. Recognition of the many possibilities for the transfer of infection in a dental office or clinic provides a basis for planning the system of sterilization, disinfection, and handling of instruments and equipment.

▪ THE INFECTIOUS PROCESS

A chain of events is required for the spread of an infectious agent. The six essential links are shown in Figure 2-1.

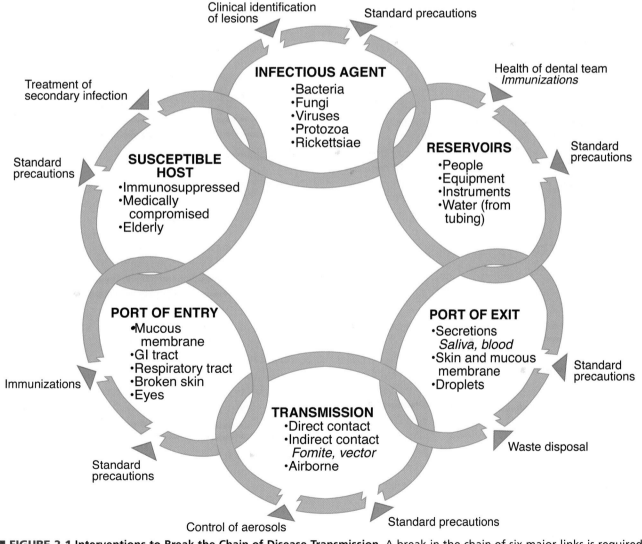

▪ **FIGURE 2-1 Interventions to Break the Chain of Disease Transmission**. A break in the chain of six major links is required for the spread of an infectious agent. Standard precautions are applied to interrupt the chain.

I. ESSENTIAL FEATURES FOR DISEASE TRANSMISSION

A. An *infectious agent*, the *invading organism* (bacterium, virus, fungus, rickettsia, or protozoa). Each organism has its own specific reaction in an infected host.

B. A *reservoir* where the invading organisms live and multiply. The infectious agent has its own essential environment, which may be inanimate matter, an insect, or human cells or blood. For example, soil is the reservoir for tetanus, and humans are reservoirs for herpetic infections.

C. A *mode of escape*, the port of exit from the reservoir. Organisms exit through various body systems, such as the respiratory tract, or through skin lesions. Escape from the blood stream may be through skin abrasions, hypodermic needles, or dental instruments.

D. A *mode of transmission*, which may be direct, person to person, or indirect by way of an intermediate vehicle, such as contaminated hands or a hypodermic needle. Transmission by a droplet may be direct from the respiratory tract of one person to the oral cavity of the receiving host. Droplets also may pass indirectly to hands or inanimate objects to be transferred indirectly to the susceptible host.

E. A *mode of entry*, the port of entry of the infectious agent into the new host. Modes of entry may be similar to modes of escape, such as the respiratory tract, mucous membranes, or a break in the skin.

F. A *susceptible host* that does not have immunity to the invading infectious agent.

II. FACTORS THAT INFLUENCE THE DEVELOPMENT OF INFECTION

The presence of an infectious agent does not lead inevitably to infection or disease. Factors involved include, but are not limited to, the following:

A. Number of organisms and duration of exposure.

B. Virulence of the organisms: their ability to survive interim exposure.

C. Immune status of the host; antibody response; defense cell reaction.

D. General physical health and nutritional status of the host. In health, disease is resisted, whereas in a deprived state, the body can be susceptible to infection.

III. FACTORS THAT ALTER NORMAL DEFENSES

The patient's complete medical and dental history must be reviewed to identify specific problems and take necessary precautions. Examples of situations that alter the normal defenses are included under the following topics.

A. Abnormal Physical Conditions

A heart valve may be defective as a result of a congenital or acquired condition. Such a valve may be susceptible to infective endocarditis resulting from a bacteremia created during dental or dental hygiene instrumentation.

B. Systemic Diseases

Examples of systemic conditions in which susceptibility to infection is increased are diabetes mellitus, alcoholism, leukemia, glomerulonephritis, acquired immunodeficiency syndrome, and all causes of immunosuppression.

C. Drug Therapy

Certain drugs used in the treatment of systemic disease alter the body's defenses. Examples are steroids and chemotherapeutic agents that are immunosuppressive. Special precautions, such as prophylactic antibiotics, may be indicated to prevent infection.

D. Prostheses and Transplants

A patient with, for example, a joint replacement, a cardiac prosthesis, a ventriculoatrial shunt for hydrocephalus, or an organ transplant may require antibiotic premedication.

▪ AIRBORNE INFECTION

I. DUST-BORNE ORGANISMS

Clostridium tetani (tetanus bacillus), *Staphylococcus aureus,* and enteric bacteria are among the organisms that may travel in the dust brought in from outside and that moves in and about dental treatment areas. When doors are opened and closed and people pass in and out, dust is set into motion that can settle on instruments, other objects, or people.

Infectious microorganisms also reach dust from the oral cavities of patients by way of large airborne particles. Dust-borne organisms can be sources of contamination for dental instruments and the hands of dental personnel.

Surface disinfection of all equipment contacted during an appointment contributes to control of dust-borne pathogens. Procedures for surface disinfection are described on page 77.

II. AEROSOL PRODUCTION[3]

Airborne particles are usually classified by size as either aerosols or *spatter.* They are constantly being produced.

A. Aerosols

A particle of a true aerosol is less than 50 μm in diameter, and nearly all are less than 5 μm. Aerosols are biologic contaminants that occur in solid or liquid form, are invisible, and remain suspended in air for long periods.

Aerosol particles that are 5 μm or smaller may be breathed deep into the lungs. Larger particles get trapped higher in the respiratory tree. The tiny particles may contain respiratory disease–producing organisms or traces of mercury or amalgam that collect in the lung because they are not biodegradable.

B. Spatter

Heavier, larger particles may remain airborne a relatively short time because of their own size and weight. They drop or spatter on objects, people, and the floor. The spatter is composed of particles greater than 50 μm in diameter.

In contrast to aerosols, spatter may be visible, particularly after it has landed on skin, hair, clothing, or environmental surfaces where gross contamination can result.

C. Origin

Aerosols and spatter are created during breathing, speaking, coughing, or sneezing. They are produced during all intraoral procedures, including examination and manual scaling. When produced by air spray, air–water spray, handpiece activity, or ultrasonic scaling, the number of aerosols increases to tremendous proportions.[3-5]

D. Contents

1. *Microorganisms.* An aerosol may contain a single organism or a clump of microorganisms adhered to a dust or debris particle. The organisms may be contained within a liquid droplet.
2. *Particles From Cavity Preparation.* Tooth fragments; microorganisms from saliva, biofilm, and/or oropharynx/nasopharynx; oil from a handpiece; and water from the cooling equipment may be in aerosols following cavity preparation.
3. *Ultrasonic Scaling.* The many microorganisms found in the aerosols from ultrasonic scalers include *Staphylococcus aureus, albus,* and *pyogenes, Streptococcus viridans,* lactobacilli, actinomyces, pneumococci, and diphtheroids.[4,5] Viruses also may be spread by ultrasonic instruments.

E. Concentration

Bacteria-laden aerosols and spatter are in greater concentration close to the scene of instrumentation; the quantity decreases with distance. The aerosols travel with air currents and, therefore, move from room to room.

III. PREVENTION OF TRANSMISSION

The control of airborne infection depends on elimination or limitation of the organisms at their source, interruption of transmission, and protection of the potentially susceptible recipient.

Carefully monitored procedures are necessary for all patients with or without a known serious communicable disease.

A. Preprocedural Oral Hygiene Measures

Toothbrushing and using an antiseptic mouthrinse reduce the numbers of bacteria contained in aerosols.

B. Interruption of Transmission

1. Use rubber dam, high-volume evacuation, and manual instrumentation as much as possible.
2. Install air-control methods to supply adequate ventilation, filtration, and relative humidity.
3. Employ vacuum cleaning to remove dirt and microorganisms rather than dust-arousing housekeeping methods. The cleaner must have a filter to prevent the escape of organisms after they are suctioned.[6]

C. Clean Water

Run water through all tubings to handpieces, ultrasonic scalers, and air–water spray for at least 2 minutes at the start of the day and at least 30 seconds after each appointment during the day. Contamination by spatter and aerosols is reduced by this method.[7]

D. Protection of the Clinician

The use of masks and protective eyewear can prevent direct contact of spatter and aerosols with the faces of the dental team.

■ PATHOGENS TRANSMISSIBLE BY THE ORAL CAVITY

Selected pathogens that may be transmitted by way of the oral cavity and their disease manifestations, mode of transfer, and incubation and communicability periods are listed in Table 2-1.

TABLE 2-1 INFECTIOUS DISEASES

INFECTIOUS AGENT	DISEASE OR CONDITION	ROUTE OR MODE OF TRANSMISSION	INCUBATION PERIOD	COMMUNICABLE PERIOD	VACCINE
Human immuno-deficiency virus (HIV)	Acquired immunodeficiency syndrome (AIDS) HIV infection	Blood and blood products (infected IV needles) Sexual contact Transplacental and perinatal	To detectable antibodies: 1 to 3 months To disease diagnosis: less than 1 to 15 years or more	From asymptomatic through life	*
Hepatitis A virus (HAV)	Type A hepatitis "Infectious" hepatitis	Fecal–oral Food, water, shellfish	15 to 50 days (average 28 to 30 days)	2 to 3 weeks before onset (jaundice) through 8 days after	Yes
Hepatitis B virus (HBV)	Type B hepatitis "Serum" hepatitis	Blood Saliva and all body fluids Sexual contact Perinatal	2 to 6 months (average 60 to 90 days)	Before, during, and after clinical signs Carrier state: indefinite	Yes
Hepatitis C virus (HCV) PT-NANB	Type C hepatitis Parenterally transmitted non-A, non-B	Percutaneous Blood Needles	2 weeks to 6 months (6 to 9 weeks)	1 week before onset of symptoms Carrier state: indefinite	No
Delta hepatitis virus (HDV) Delta agent	Delta hepatitis	Coinfection with HBV Blood Sexual contacts Perinatal	2 to 8 weeks	All phases	HBV vaccine
Hepatitis E virus (HEV) ET-NANB	Type E hepatitis Enterically transmitted non-A, non-B	Fecal–oral Contaminated water	15 to 64 days	Not known	No
Herpes simplex virus Type 1 (HSV-1) Type 2 (HSV-2)	Acute herpetic gingivostomatitis Herpes labialis Ocular herpetic infections Herpetic whitlow	Saliva Direct contact (lip, hand) Indirect contact (on objects, limited survival) Sexual contact	2 to 12 days	Labialis: 1 day before onset until lesions are crusted Acute stomatitis: 7 weeks after recovery Asymptomatic infection: with viral shedding Reactivation period: with viral shedding	No
Varicella-zoster virus (VZV)	Chickenpox Herpes zoster (shingles)	Direct contact Indirect contact Airborne droplet	2 to 3 weeks	5 days prior to onset of rash until crusting of vesicles	Yes
Epstein-Barr virus (EBV)	Infectious mononucleosis	Direct contact Saliva	4 to 6 weeks	Prolonged Pharyngeal excretion 1 year after infection	No
Cytomegalovirus (CMV)	Neonatal cytomegalovirus infection Cytomegaloviral disease	Perinatal Direct contact (most body secretions) Blood transfusion Saliva	3 to 12 weeks after delivery 3 to 8 weeks after transfusion	Months to years	No

TABLE 2-1 INFECTIOUS DISEASES (Continued)

INFECTIOUS AGENT	DISEASE OR CONDITION	ROUTE OR MODE OF TRANSMISSION	INCUBATION PERIOD	COMMUNICABLE PERIOD	VACCINE
Mycobacterium tuberculosis	Tuberculosis	Droplet nuclei Sputum Saliva	2 to 10 weeks	As long as viable bacilli are discharged in sputum	B.C.G. (Bacille Calmette-Guérin)
Treponema pallidum	Syphilis Congenital syphilis	Direct contact Transplacental	10 days to 3 months	Variable and indefinite May be 2 to 4 years	No
Neisseria gonorrhoeae	Gonorrhea Gonococcal pharyngitis	Direct contact Indirect (short survival of organisms)	2 to 7 days	During incubation Continued for months and years if untreated	No
Bordetella pertussis	Whooping cough Pertussis	Direct contact with discharges	7 to 20 days	Not treated: from early catarrhal stage to 3 weeks after paroxysmal cough	Yes
Mumps virus (paramyxovirus)	Infectious parotitis (mumps)	Direct contact (saliva) Airborne droplet	12 to 25 days (average 18 days)	12 to 25 days after exposure From 6 to 7 days before symptoms until 9 days after swelling	Yes
Poliovirus types 1, 2, 3	Poliomyelitis	Direct contact (saliva) Droplet Fecal–oral	7 to 14 days	Probably most infectious 7 to 10 days before and after onset of symptoms	Yes
Influenza viruses (A, B, C)	Influenza	Nasal discharge Respiratory droplets	1 to 3 days	3 to 5 days from clinical onset	Yes
Measles virus (Morbillivirus)	Rubeola (measles)	Direct contact Saliva Airborne droplet	7 to 18 days to fever, 14 days to rash	Few days before fever to 4 days after rash appears	Yes
Rubella virus (togavirus)	Rubella (German measles) Congenital rubella syndrome	Nasopharyngeal secretions Direct contact Airborne droplets Maternal infection first trimester	16 to 23 days	From 1 week before to at least 4 days after rash appears Highly communicable Infants shed virus for months after birth	Yes
Group A streptococci (beta-hemolytic) *Streptococcus pyogenes*	Streptococcal sore throat Scarlet fever Impetigo Erysipelas	Respiratory droplets Direct contact	1 to 3 days	10 to 21 days, untreated Many nasal oropharyngeal carriers	No
Staphylococcus aureus Staphylococcus epidermidis	Abscesses Boils (furuncle) Impetigo Bacterial pneumonia	Saliva Exudates Nasal discharge	4 to 10 days Variable and indefinite	While lesions drain and carrier state persists	No
Candida albicans	Candidiasis	Secretions Excretions (oral, skin, vagina)	Variable 2 to 5 days for "thrush" in children	While lesions are present	No
Streptococcus pneumoniae	Pneumonia Pneumococcal pneumonia	Droplet Direct contact Indirect	1 to 3 days Not well determined	While virulent organisms are discharged	Yes

*Vaccine progress.

Tuberculosis, viral hepatitis, acquired immunodeficiency syndrome, and herpetic infections are described in detail in this chapter because of the special problems they create in personal and patient care. The general preventive measures described for these diseases should be applied during all appointments.

The etiologic agents of many communicable diseases enter the body by way of the oral cavity. Many infectious diseases have specific oral manifestations from which the disease can be identified. Pathogens are often present within the oral cavity without producing oral signs or symptoms, a fact of particular importance to the total consideration of prevention of disease transmission.

▪ TUBERCULOSIS[8]

Mycobacterium tuberculosis, the etiologic agent in tuberculosis, is a resistant organism that requires special consideration when sterilization and disinfection methods are selected and administered. Tuberculosis is a serious disease that can involve many months and years of lost time during the active stages of illness and the following convalescence. Clinical procedures must be planned to prevent exposure and infection from this debilitating disease.

Tuberculosis is a common communicable disease throughout the world and a major public health problem. The incidence has increased in population groups with a high prevalence of HIV infection. Tuberculosis is an AIDS-defining illness.[9]

I. TRANSMISSION

A. Inhalation

Tuberculosis is contracted by the inhalation of fresh droplets containing tubercle bacilli. The organisms are disseminated from sputum and saliva of the infected individual by coughing, breathing heavily, or sneezing (Figure 2-2). During the use of ultrasonic and other handpieces, and of air–water spray, aerosols are created that can carry the bacilli.

When the organisms are in tiny aerosols, they can pass readily into the lungs and the respiratory bronchioles. There, they can invade the tissue and establish an infection.

B. Factors Affecting Transmission

Transmission of tuberculosis is dependent on the following: (1) the degree to which the infected person produces infectious droplets, (2) the amount and duration of exposure, and (3) the susceptibility of the recipient. Some patients are more contagious than are others. Maximum communicability is usu-

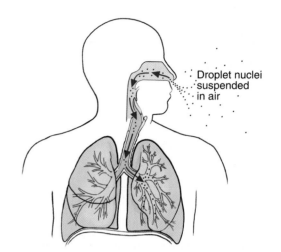

▪ **FIGURE 2-2 Droplet Nuclei.** Many potentially pathogenic microorganisms are disseminated by aerosols and spatter. The primary mode of transmission of tubercle bacilli is by droplet nuclei breathed directly into the lung. (Adapted from McInnes, M.E.: *Essentials of Communicable Disease,* 2nd ed. St. Louis, The C.V. Mosby Co., 1975.)

ally just before the disease is diagnosed, when the person may have a severe cough and other respiratory symptoms.

C. Other Modes of Transmission

The tubercle bacillus may enter the body by ingestion or direct inoculation, as well as by inhalation. Infection of the lungs is most common, but the tubercle bacillus also infects lymph nodes, meninges (tuberculous meningitis), kidneys, bone, skin, and the oral cavity.[8]

II. DISEASE PROCESS

A. Predisposing Factors

Any debilitating or immunosuppressive condition can predispose a person to invasion by the tubercle bacillus. Systemic conditions that may be related to lowered resistance to infection include diabetes, congenital heart disease, chronic lung disease, alcoholism, and the acquired immunodeficiency syndrome.

B. Incubation Period

As shown in Table 2-1, the incubation period may be as long as 10 weeks. After such an extended period, the origin of the disease can be difficult or impossible to trace.

C. Early Symptoms

In the early stages before marked symptoms appear, the patient may have a low-grade fever, loss of appetite, and weight loss and may tire easily. There may be a slight cough, and eventually sputum, indicating the possible presence of tubercle bacilli in the throat and saliva.

D. Later Symptoms

Definite temperature elevation, particularly in the afternoon, night sweats, weakness, and a persistent cough become apparent. Diagnosis is by chest radiograph and tuberculin testing.

E. Reactivation Tuberculosis

A focus of an infection may remain inactive and later produce a recurrence. Treatment of a primary infection may have been incomplete. Reactivity may be related to a debilitating condition or immunosuppression.

Reactivation of latent tuberculous infection may occur after many years. Usually a patient with a healthy immune system is asymptomatic and cannot spread the disease to others. The infection can be eliminated with antituberculosis drugs.

F. Multidrug-Resistant Tuberculosis

Multiple antituberculosis drugs are taken daily or several times a week for 6 months to treat active tuberculosis (TB). Three of the principal drugs used are isoniazid, pyrazinamide, and rifampin.

If medications are not prescribed properly or are not taken by the patient regularly, the tubercle bacilli can become resistant. The drug-resistant organisms can be transmitted and can cause disease in the recipient. Multidrug-resistant TB is difficult and expensive to treat.

The first line of prevention for multidrug-resistant TB is supervision of treatment so the medication is used properly. The second approach is to locate and treat persons with latent TB, particularly those at a high risk of reactivation. Direct supervision to ensure completion of the full course of treatment is required.

III. CLINICAL MANAGEMENT

A. Official Recommendations (CDC)[10]

1. *Periodic Risk Assessment.*
2. *Medical History.* Routine questioning of patients about a history of tuberculosis and symptoms suggestive of disease; updating history regularly.
3. *Referral.* Prompt referral of patients with symptoms or a history suggestive of tuberculosis for medical evaluation.
4. *Deferral of Elective Dental Treatment.* Obtain a physician's confirmation of the state of the patient's health. If the patient is diagnosed as

having active tuberculosis, elective treatment should be deferred until the patient is no longer infectious.
5. *Urgent Dental Care.* For a patient suspected of having infectious tuberculosis, use of a facility that can offer isolation and optimal ventilation and wearing respiratory protection (highest filtration level mask) are needed.
6. *Dental Health-Care Personnel.* Prompt medical evaluation for a dental team member with a persistent cough (3 weeks), especially if with weight loss, fever, and other symptoms.
7. *Separation of Suspected or Confirmed Tuberculosis Patients.* A separate reception area where the patient can wait may be indicated. Appointments arranged to prevent a waiting period are preferred.

B. Extraoral and Intraoral Examination

Tuberculosis is primarily a lesion of the lungs, but any organ or tissue may be involved.
1. *Lymphadenopathy.* Regional lymph nodes may be enlarged.
2. *Oral Lesions.*[11] Oral lesions are relatively rare, but when they occur, they are usually ulcers. They may be located on the soft or hard palate and, occasionally, on the tongue.

C. Patient Under Treatment

Chemotherapy can control the patient's contagious condition. Isoniazid, rifampin, and pyrazinamide are used, sometimes in combinations. After a few weeks from the beginning of therapy, bacilli in the sputum, the cough, and the infectivity are decreased.

■ VIRAL HEPATITIS

Hepatitis means inflammation of the liver. Viruses cause a variety of types of hepatitis. Some of the viruses have been specifically identified, and hepatitis A, hepatitis B, hepatitis C, hepatitis D (delta), and hepatitis E are described in this section. New viruses designated non-ABCDE and HGV have emerged from viral hepatitis in posttransfusion patients or injection-drug users.[12-14]

The incidence of hepatitis B has increased significantly during the past 20 years. It has been a serious occupational hazard for health-care personnel. Among professional personnel, both medical and dental, the use of strict sterilization of equipment and materials, aseptic techniques, and self-protection measures is mandatory.

Table 2-2 lists the hepatitis terminology with abbreviations and significance.

TABLE 2-2 VIRAL HEPATITIS: ABBREVIATIONS

ABBREVIATION	TERM	SIGNIFICANCE
Hepatitis A		
HAV	Hepatitis A virus	Etiologic agent for hepatitis A
anti-HAV	Antibody to hepatitis A virus	Acute or resolved infection
		Protective immune response to infection
		Passively acquired antibody
		Response to vaccination
IgM anti-HAV	IgM antibody to hepatitis A virus	Recent HAV infection
HAV-RNA	RNA of HAV	Detected by nucleic acid amplification and/or hybridization
Hepatitis B		
HBV	Hepatitis B virus (Dane particle)	Etiologic agent for hepatitis B
		Current HBV infection
HBsAg	Hepatitis B surface antigen	Surface marker in acute disease and carrier state
		Antigen used in hepatitis B vaccine
anti-HBs	Antibody to hepatitis B surface antigen	Indicates
		(1) Active immunity to HBV (past infection)
		(2) Passive immunity from HBIG
		(3) Immune response from HB vaccine
HBeAg	Hepatitis B e antigen	High titer HBV in serum indicates high infectivity
		Persists into carrier state
anti-HBe	Antibody to hepatitis B e antigen	Low titer HBV
		Low degree infectivity
HBcAg	Hepatitis B core antigen	Indicates acute, chronic, or resolved HBV infection
		Not elicited by vaccination
anti-HBc	Antibody to hepatitis B core antigen	Indicates prior HBV infection
IgM anti-HBc	IgM class antibody to hepatitis B core antigen	Indicates recent HBc infection
HBV-DNA	DNA of HBV	Detected by nucleic acid amplification and/or hybridization
Hepatitis C		
HCV	Hepatitis C virus (formerly parentally transmitted non-A, non-B)	Etiologic agent for hepatitis C
anti-HCV	Antibody to hepatitis C virus	Indicates acute disease and chronic state
		Resembles hepatitis B
HCV-RNA	RNA of HCV	Defines viremia; detected by nucleic acid amplification
Hepatitis D		
HDV	Hepatitis delta virus	Etiologic agent for hepatitis D
		Only infectious in presence of acute or chronic HBV infection
HDV-Ag	Delta antigen	Detectable during early acute HDV infection
anti-HDV	Antibody to hepatitis D virus	Indicates acute, resolved, or chronic infection
IgM anti-HDV	IgM-class antibody to HDV	Indicates either acute or chronic infection with active viral replication
HDV-RNA	RNA of HDV	Detected by nucleic acid amplification or hybridization
Hepatitis E		
HEV	Hepatitis E virus (formerly enterically transmitted non-A, non-B)	Etiologic agent for hepatitis E
anti-HEV	Antibody to hepatitis E virus	Indicates acute or resolved infection
IgM anti-HEV	IgM-class antibody to hepatitis E virus	Indicates acute infection
Non-ABCDE		
Parenterally transmitted	Diagnosis of exclusion	Epidemiologic evidence of parenteral or sexual transmission
Enterically transmitted	Diagnosis of exclusion	Epidemiologic evidence of fecal–oral transmission
Immune globulins		
IG	Immune globulin	Contains antibodies to HAV and low–titer HBV antibodies
HBIG	Hepatitis B immune globulin	Contains high-titer antibodies to HBV

■ HEPATITIS A[15]

Hepatitis A occurs much more frequently in children and young adults than in older adults. It is more severe in adults. Early immunization is indicated.

I. TRANSMISSION

A. Fecal–Oral Route

The most common transmission is through close contact in unsanitary conditions. Unwashed hands of an infected person can contaminate anything touched.

B. Water-borne and Food-borne

Epidemics may occur when sanitation is inadequate. Contaminated water may carry hepatitis A virus directly to those using the water, or it may contaminate shellfish grown in the water.

Infected food handlers can contaminate uncooked food or food handled after cooking.

C. Blood

In the earliest days of active disease, the blood contains transient hepatitis A viruses; however, transmission by blood transfusion is rare.

II. DISEASE PROCESS

A. Incubation and Communicability

The incubation period is 15 to 50 days, with an average of 28 to 30 days. During the 2- to 3-week period before the onset of jaundice, the infection is communicable. Shortly after jaundice appears, the communicability begins to diminish. A carrier state has not been demonstrated.

B. Signs and Symptoms

The stages are defined by the incidence of jaundice as preicteric (before jaundice appears) and icteric (while jaundice is present). Hepatitis A without jaundice (anicteric) is two to three times more prevalent than the icteric form. A diagnosis of hepatitis is not always made because without jaundice, symptoms may resemble influenza or other diseases.
1. *Preicteric Phase.* Typically, there is an abrupt onset of an influenza-like illness, with fever, headache, fatigue, nausea, vomiting, and abdominal pain. The liver may be enlarged and tender to palpation.
2. *Icteric Phase.* Jaundice may appear in adults, but rarely in children. Other symptoms become prolonged, and the patient may be ill for a few days to a month. Occasionally, chronic hepatitis follows, but 85% to 90% of patients recover completely.

III. IMMUNITY

Anti-HAV is usually detectable in the serum within 2 weeks of onset. Immunity to reinfection follows with recovery.

In addition to those who are known to have had the disease, many more people acquire immunity from undetected disease.

Vaccines for active immunization are available.

IV. PREVENTION

A. Sanitation and Personal Hygiene

Because the principal means of transmission is by way of the feces, prevention on that level is indicated.
1. Public health control of food handlers and of water contamination.
2. Personal hygiene control through scrupulous handwashing by a patient and all contacts, as well as by all health-care personnel involved in patient care.

B. Application in Dental Setting

Instrument sterilization, use of disposable materials, and all related precautions for persons and objects contacted by the patient.

■ HEPATITIS B[15]

Hepatitis B differs in many respects from hepatitis A, particularly in mode of transmission, the length of the incubation period, the onset, and the existence of a chronic carrier state. Hepatitis B occurs at any age. Figure 2-3 shows a diagram of the hepatitis B virus.

I. TRANSMISSION

A. Blood and Other Body Fluids

Nearly all body fluids carry the virus, but only blood, saliva, semen, and vaginal fluids have been shown to be infectious. Hepatitis B viruses also have been found in gingival sulcus fluid, menstrual blood, tears, urine, perspiration, and nasopharyngeal secretions.

B. Modes of Transmission

Hepatitis B is transmitted by percutaneous and permucosal exposure.
1. Percutaneous (intravenous, intramuscular, subcutaneous).
2. Accidents with needle stick or other sharp instruments.

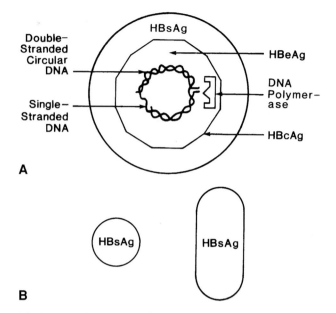

■ **FIGURE 2-3 Diagram of the Hepatitis B Virus. (A)** The virus is composed of an outer component of HBsAg and an inner component of HBcAg. Inside the core particle is a single molecule of circular, partially double-stranded DNA, an endogenous DNA polymerase, and HBeAg. **(B)** Spherical and tubular particles of HBsAg circulate in infected blood in great numbers. (Redrawn from Hoofnagle, J.H. and Schafer, D.F.: Serologic Markers of Hepatitis B Virus Infection, *Semin. Liver Dis., 6,* 1, No. 1, 1986.)

3. Perinatal exposure.
4. Exchanging of contaminated needles, syringes, and other paraphernalia by users of intravenous drugs.
5. Sexual exposure.
6. Infection from blood transfusion and blood products (extremely rare because all donors are screened and all blood has been tested since 1985).

C. Perinatal Transmission

During pregnancy, transmission of the hepatitis virus to the fetus can occur, and the newborn may be exposed during birth. An infant infected perinatally is at a high risk for chronic infection, which can lead to chronic liver disease or cancer of the liver later in life. Preventive measures are possible when pregnant women are tested for HBsAg and HBeAg.

II. INDIVIDUALS AT RISK OR WITH RISK BEHAVIORS FOR HEPATITIS B[15]

Risk populations are those that have an increased prevalence of infection, increased chances or likelihood of infection, and increased prevalence of disease carriers. High risk in HBV infection can be related to a variety of factors, including occupation, place of residence, lifestyle, confinement to an institution, other diseases and their treatments, and parenteral drug abuse. A person may belong to more than one of the risk groups listed here.

Health-care personnel are included in the list; however, when they adhere to standard precautions with the use of protective barriers (gloves, masks, eyewear) and follow essential precautions for blood and other body fluid infection control, as well as have immunity following vaccination or acquired antibody to hepatitis B, they are really at a low risk.

A. Infants born to HIV-infected mothers.
B. Users of parenteral drugs (swapping contaminated needles).
C. Homosexually active men not practicing safe sex.*
D. Heterosexually active persons with multiple partners, including prostitutes, not practicing safe sex.*
E. Persons who have repeatedly contracted sexually transmitted diseases.
F. Patients and staff in institutions for the mentally retarded and current or former residents, particularly individuals with Down's syndrome.
G. Patients and staff in hemodialysis units.
H. Recipients of blood products used for treating clotting disorders, particularly before all blood was screened (prior to 1985).
I. Patients with active or chronic liver diseases.
J. Health-care personnel with frequent blood contact are at a higher risk than are other health-care personnel who have no or infrequent blood contact. Included are emergency room staff, hospital surgical staff, dental hygienists, dentists, and blood bank and plasma fractionation workers.
K. Household contacts of HBV carriers.
L. Male prisoners.
M. Military populations stationed in countries with high endemic HBV.
N. Returned travelers from areas of endemic HBV who stayed longer than 3 months or who were treated medically by transfusion while there.
O. Morticians and embalmers.
P. Immigrants and refugees from areas of high endemic HBV.

III. DISEASE PROCESS

A. Incubation and Communicability

The incubation period is longer than that for hepatitis A and ranges from 2 to 6 months, with an average of 60 to 90 days. The period of communicability varies,

---

*"Practice safe sex" is meant to include barrier protection and no exchange of body fluids (saliva, semen, vaginal secretions), in accord with recommended guidelines.

but HBsAg may be detected in the blood as early as 30 days after exposure to the disease.

The presence of serum HBsAg indicates communicability. HBsAg may no longer be detected in the blood from a few days to 3 months after the icteric or jaundice stage of illness.

B. Transient Subclinical Infection

The majority of patients do not have an icteric stage but have subclinical disease. Many remain undiagnosed for hepatitis but develop antibodies and permanent immunity.

The infection is transient because the individual has a rapid, strong immune response to the hepatitis virus, and the HBV is cleared before it can become established.

C. Acute Type B Hepatitis

Hepatitis B cannot be distinguished from other viral hepatitis infections on the basis of the clinical signs and symptoms. The onset or preicteric stage with fever, malaise, and influenza-like symptoms is typical of all types of acute viral hepatitis. The onset may be slower and more insidious for hepatitis B and may include skin rash, itching, and joint pains.

The period of illness extends from 4 to 6 weeks for hepatitis A and usually longer for hepatitis B.

Convalescence begins with the disappearance of jaundice. During this period, serum antibody (anti-HBs) rises except in those who become permanent carriers.

D. Carrier State

A chronic carrier of HBV is defined as an individual with the HBsAg marker in the blood serum for more than 6 months. From 5% to 10% of infected persons develop a chronic carrier state.

A carrier state may also result following a subclinical undiagnosed exposure and, therefore, may be unknown to the individual. Many carriers eventually develop cirrhosis or cancer of the liver.

E. Immunity

The presence of anti-HBs in the serum shows that the person had a previous exposure to hepatitis B and is, therefore, immune to reinfection. The anti-HBs may be present, although unknown, because immunity may have been acquired following a subclinical, anicteric, or otherwise unrecognized case of hepatitis B. Pretesting for anti-HBs prior to vaccination for hepatitis may be indicated.

▪ PREVENTION OF HEPATITIS B

Hepatitis B viruses cause serious illness, including acute and chronic hepatitis, cirrhosis, and liver cancer, that sometimes leads to disability and death. Hepatitis is a critical occupational hazard for dental personnel because of their close association with the potentially infected body fluids of patients. Every health-care individual should be immunized so that the possibilities of disease acquisition and transmission can be minimized.

I. COMPREHENSIVE PREVENTIVE PROGRAM[15,16]

A. Eliminate Transmission During Infancy and Childhood

1. Prenatal testing of all pregnant women for HBsAg.
   a. To locate newborns who require immunoprophylaxis to prevent perinatal infection.
   b. To identify household contacts who should be vaccinated.
2. Universal immunization of infants and children to be accomplished during routine health-care visits when vaccinations are usually administered. Hepatitis vaccine can be combined with diphtheria-tetanus-pertussis (DTP) or with influenza vaccine to reduce the number of injections.
3. Immunization of uninfected children in special education classes.
4. Immunization of adolescents and adults, particularly those at high risk. Eventually, as the universal vaccination of children continues, adult requirements will be lessened.

B. Enforce Blood Bank Control Measures[16]

1. Screening of donors; rejection of individuals who have a history of viral hepatitis, who show evidence of drug addiction, or who have received a blood transfusion or tattoo within the preceding 6 months.
2. Strict testing for all donated blood.

C. Enforce Sterilization or Use of Disposable Syringes and Needles

1. For acupuncture, skin testing, parenteral inoculations, body piercing, and all types of clinic treatments available to the public.
2. Education of public to expect certain standards.

II. ACTIVE IMMUNIZATION: THE VACCINES[15]

Hepatitis B vaccines are available for preexposure and postexposure prophylaxis. They are administered intramuscularly in three doses, the first at the outset, then at 1 and 6 months.

The vaccine should be given only in the deltoid muscle for adults and children and in the anterolateral thigh muscle for infants and neonates.

A. Plasma-Derived HB Vaccine[†]

The original vaccine was prepared using purified and formalin-treated HBsAg from the plasma of chronic HBsAg carriers. In its preparation, the treatment steps inactivated all classes of viruses so that transmission of any other disease became impossible.

B. Recombinant DNA HB Vaccine[‡]

Recombinant DNA technology has been used to synthesize HBsAg in a culture of *Saccharomyces cerevisiae*, a yeast. The HBsAg is purified and sterilized.

C. Effectiveness

1. Both vaccines act in a comparable manner to stimulate antibody, and both convey the same degree of immunity.
2. In healthy 20- to 39-year-old adults, immunity is conferred in more than 95%. In children, protective antibodies are shown in 99%.
3. Postvaccination testing for anti-HBs within 1 to 6 months is recommended for a hemodialysis patient or other at-risk person having frequent exposure, including dental personnel.
4. Lower responses have been noted in older people, in hemodialysis patients, and in people receiving the injection in the buttock rather than in the deltoid muscle.[17]
5. The vaccines have no effect on a person who is already a carrier and no effect on a person who already has antibodies.
6. Immunization is not contraindicated during pregnancy. An HBV infection during pregnancy can be severe, and the newborn can become a permanent carrier.

D. Booster

1. The higher initial peak of response usually means longer persistence of antibody. Even when the antibody level drops there can still be protection.
2. Immunity against HBV is believed to persist for at least 15 years after successful immunization.

[†]Heptavax, Merck Sharp & Dohme.
[‡]Recombivax HB, Merck Sharp & Dohme; (Engerix B, Smith Kline Biologicals).

3. For certain at-risk patients, particularly hemodialysis patients, annual antibody testing has been recommended.

III. POSTEXPOSURE PROPHYLAXIS

A. Indications for Prophylaxis

1. Newborn of HBsAg-positive mother.
2. Significant hepatitis B exposure to HBsAg-positive blood.

B. Hepatitis B Immune Globulin (HBIG)

High-titer anti-HBs immune globulin (HBIG) is available. Its primary use is for postexposure prophylaxis.

IG contains low-titer anti-HBs of varying amounts. It is effective against HBV to a lesser degree than is HBIG, but it should be used when HBIG is not available. IG is recommended when protection for exposure to hepatitis C and E is needed.

C. Procedure for Newborn of HBsAg-Positive Mother

1. *Immediate Treatment.* HBIG and HBV vaccine intramuscularly within 12 hours of birth and subsequently as recommended for a specific vaccine.
2. *Effect.* The combined treatment prevents up to 94% of infants from developing a carrier state.
3. *Risk.* Breast-feeding poses no risk of infection when prophylaxis has been started.

D. Procedure for Percutaneous Exposure or Wound From a Contaminated Instrument

▪ HEPATITIS C[15,18]

Hepatitis that developed as a result of transfusion but could not be classified with hepatitis A or B was originally called hepatitis non-A, non-B. When studied over time, two patterns of non-A, non-B hepatitis were recognized. The first, associated with blood transfusion and the use of contaminated needles, became hepatitis C. The second type was associated with waterborne epidemics and is now called hepatitis E.

Hepatitis C, caused by the hepatitis C virus (HCV), has been recognized as the former chief cause of transfusion-associated non-A, non-B hepatitis. HCV also has a role in many cases of chronic liver disease. Now, a serologic test for antibody to HCV has been developed and is an established test for blood donors. This advance in making blood transfusion safe is highly significant.

I. TRANSMISSION

Hepatitis C can be acquired by percutaneous exposure to contaminated blood and plasma derivatives, contaminated needles and syringes, transfusion, or accidental needle stick. HCV has been demonstrated in saliva. Nonpercutaneous routes include sexual transmission and perinatal exposure.

II. DISEASE PROCESS

The onset of viral hepatitis C can be insidious, with no clinical symptoms, or the patient can have abdominal discomfort, nausea, and vomiting and can progress to jaundice. Chronic liver disease is more common than with hepatitis B.

III. PREVENTION AND CONTROL

Measures recommended for hepatitis B can be applied to hepatitis C. Testing of all donated blood is basic to control.

■ HEPATITIS D[15,18]

The delta hepatitis virus, also called the delta agent, cannot cause infection except in the presence of HBV infection. The diagram in Figure 2-4 shows the delta antigen surrounded by HBsAg.

I. TRANSMISSION

Most frequently, the delta infection is superimposed on HBsAg carriers. It occurs primarily in persons who have multiple exposures to HBV, particularly patients with hemophilia and intravenous drug users.

Transmission is similar to that of HBV, that is, by direct exposure to contaminated blood and serous body fluids, contaminated needles and syringes, sexual contacts, and perinatal transfer.

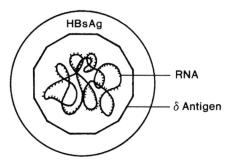

■ **FIGURE 2-4 Diagram of the Hepatitis Delta Virus. The delta agent antigen is surrounded by the hepatitis B surface antigen.** (Redrawn from Hoofnagle, J.H.: Type D Hepatitis and the Hepatitis Delta Virus, in Thomas, H.C. and Jones, E.A.: *Recent Advances in Hepatology.* Edinburgh, Churchill Livingstone, 1986.)

II. DISEASE PROCESS

Delta hepatitis is more severe and the mortality rate is greater than with hepatitis B alone. The onset is abrupt, and signs and symptoms resemble hepatitis B. Infection can occur in the following ways.

A. Coinfection

Acute delta hepatitis occurring with acute HBV infection may lead to resolution of both types. Clearance of HBV may lead to clearance of delta virus.

B. Superinfection

Acute delta hepatitis is superimposed on an existing carrier HBV state. The HBV carrier state remains unchanged, and a delta carrier state may develop in addition.

C. Superimposition

Chronic delta hepatitis superimposes on the chronic HBsAg carrier.

III. PREVENTION

All measures used to prevent hepatitis B prevent delta hepatitis because HDV is dependent on the presence of HBV. Immunization with hepatitis B vaccine also protects the recipient from delta hepatitis infection.

■ HEPATITIS E[15,18]

Hepatitis E (HEV) was formerly known as enterically transmitted non-A, non-B hepatitis. The clinical course and distribution are like those of hepatitis A.

I. TRANSMISSION

Hepatitis E is transmitted by contaminated water, as well as person-to-person by the fecal–oral route. Reported large outbreaks have been associated with fecally contaminated water sources after heavy rains where sewage disposal was inadequate. Adults have been affected more than children. The mortality rate in pregnant women has been high.

II. PREVENTION AND CONTROL

  A. Sanitary disposal of wastes.
  B. Handwashing, especially before handling food.

■ HERPESVIRUS DISEASES

The herpesvirus infections represent a wide variety of disease entities that are highly infectious. Each virus is

TABLE 2-3 HERPESVIRUSES

ABBREVIATION	NAME OF VIRUS	INFECTIONS
VZV	Varicella-zoster	Varicella (chickenpox) Herpes zoster (shingles)
EBV	Epstein-Barr	EBV mononucleosis
HCMV	Human cytomegalovirus	Cytomegalovirus disease Fetal infection
HSV-1 HSV-2	Herpes simplex virus, types 1 and 2	Herpes labialis Herpetic gingivostomatitis Herpetic kerato- conjunctivitis Herpetic whitlow Encephalitis Neonatal herpes
HHV-6	Human herpesvirus 6	Mononucleosis-like rash
HHV-7	Human herpesvirus 7	Febrile illnesses
KSHV HHV-8	Kaposi's sarcoma herpesvirus	Kaposi's sarcoma

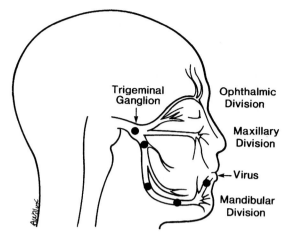

▪ **FIGURE 2-5 Latent Infection of Herpes Simplex Virus.** Path of the virus traced from point of viral penetration on lip to establishment of latent infection in the trigeminal ganglion.

antigenically distinct. Herpesviruses produce diseases with latent, recurrent, and sometimes malignant tendencies. For example, herpes simplex type 2 has been implicated in cervical cancer and herpes simplex type 1 in oral cancer.

Immunosuppressed patients have more frequent and severe herpes infections. Herpesviruses are among the opportunistic organisms in acquired immunodeficiency syndrome (AIDS). Gingival infection with herpesviruses (notably EBV-1 and HCMV) decreases the resistance of periodontal tissues, thereby permitting subgingival overgrowth of periodontal pathogens.[19]

Table 2-3 lists herpesviruses, their abbreviations, and some of the infections they cause.

▪ VIRAL LATENCY

I. GANGLIA

The herpesviruses have the ability to travel along sensory nerve pathways to specific ganglia. The specific ganglia are usually the following:
  A. Herpes simplex type 1 (HSV-1) travels to the trigeminal nerve ganglion (Figure 2-5).
  B. Herpes simplex type 2 (HSV-2) goes to the thoracic, lumbar, and sacral dorsal root ganglia.
  C. Varicella-zoster virus (VZV) goes to the sensory ganglia of the vagal, spinal, or cranial nerves.

II. PRIMARY INFECTION: SEQUENCE OF EVENTS

  A. Exposure of person to the virus at the mucosal surface or abraded skin.
  B. Replication begins in the cells of the dermis and epidermis.
  C. Infection of sensory or autonomic nerve endings.
  D. Virus travels along the nerve to the ganglion.
  E. After primary disease resolves, the virus becomes latent in the ganglion.
  F. Reactivation at a later date is precipitated by a stimulus, such as sunlight, immunosuppression, infection, or stress (physical or emotional).
  G. Virus transports along the nerve to the body surface where replication takes place and a lesion forms, usually in the same spot as the previous activation.

▪ VARICELLA-ZOSTER VIRUS (VZV)[20]

Chickenpox (varicella) and shingles (herpes zoster) are caused by the same virus, the varicella-zoster virus.

I. CHICKENPOX

A. Transmission

Chickenpox is a highly contagious disease transmitted by direct contact, by droplet (possibly airborne), or by indirect contact with articles soiled by discharges from the vesicles and the respiratory tract.

B. Disease Process

Primarily a disease of children, chickenpox is occasionally found in adults not previously exposed. Chickenpox can be life threatening in children who are immunocompromised, such as children with HIV infection.

When primary maternal VZV occurs during pregnancy or during the peripartum period, fetal infection may result in congenital malformations.

The disease is characterized by a maculopapular rash that becomes vesicular in a few days and then scabs. When oral lesions occur, they may spread into the upper respiratory tract.

If the itchy, crusted lesions of the skin are scratched, a secondary bacterial infection can result.

II. SHINGLES

A. Recurrent Infection

Chickenpox leaves a lasting immunity, but the VZV remains latent in the dorsal root ganglia. Reactivation in adulthood may result from immunosuppression, such as from drug therapy or from HIV infection, and in people with advanced neoplastic disease.

B. Disease Process

Shingles consists of localized unilateral eruptions associated with the nerve endings of the area innervated by the infected sensory nerves. When the second division of the trigeminal nerve is involved, intraoral lesions may occur.

■ EPSTEIN-BARR VIRUS (EBV)[21]

One type of infectious mononucleosis is caused by infection with the EBV. It has also been shown that the EBV replicates within the epithelial cells in hairy leukoplakia, the lesion associated with subsequent development of the acquired immunodeficiency syndrome. EBV is also a factor in the development of certain lymphomas.

Infectious mononucleosis is generally a disease of adolescents and young adults. It is characterized by fever, lymphadenopathy, and sore throat and is identified by specific atypical lymphocytes called mononucleosis cells.

The disease is transmitted orally by direct contact and by droplet. Viruses are excreted through the saliva even when the patient has no symptoms of disease, so there may be a long period of communicability or a lasting carrier state. EBV can remain latent and become reactivated, particularly when the immune system is compromised by disease or drug therapy.

■ CYTOMEGALOVIRUS (HCMV)[22]

Cytomegalovirus infections appear in various forms. The most affected age groups are from 1 to 2 years and from 16 to 50 years. The infections are sometimes latent or subclinical in adults.

I. TRANSMISSION

A. Congenital and Neonatal

The virus from the mother's primary or recurrent infection may infect the infant *in utero,* in the birth canal, or through breast milk.

B. Direct Infections

The virus is excreted in urine, saliva, cervical secretions, and semen. Infection can result from the following:
1. Blood transfusion.
2. Graft transplant from a donor with latent infection.
3. Sexual transmission through semen, vaginal fluid, or saliva.
4. Respiratory droplet, especially among children. Children attending day-care centers have a high prevalence of HCMV infection.

II. DISEASE PROCESS

A. Infants

Cytomegalic inclusion disease in a fetus is the most severe form of the infection. Survivors may be premature, anemic, and have mental retardation, microcephaly, motor disabilities, deafness, and chronic liver disease.

B. Adult Infection

Symptomatic infection is relatively rare, but infectious mononucleosis, pneumonitis, and other infections may be caused by HCMV.

C. Immunosuppression and Debilitation

HCMV, an opportunistic agent, is a common cause of both primary and reactivated infections in immunodeficient or immunosuppressed patients. Infection with HCMV is a serious complication of the acquired immunodeficiency syndrome.

III. PREVENTION

A. Personal hygiene: handwashing.
B. Standard precautions by health-care personnel.
C. Seropositivity of donor checked before organ transplant.

■ HERPES SIMPLEX VIRUS INFECTIONS[19,23]

Primary infection usually occurs in children but may occur at any age. Antibodies (anti-HSV) are produced but do not guarantee immunity to recurrent herpes or to other herpesvirus infections.

Sulcular epithelium serves as a reservoir for the viruses.[24] Anti-HSV is present in the gingival sulcus fluid. The possibility exists that trauma to the oral area during a dental or dental hygiene appointment may bring about herpetic recurrence.

Acyclovir, an antiviral drug, has been used in topical, oral, and intravenous forms. Acyclovir is a selective inhibitor of replication of HSV and VZV. It is established as the drug of choice for treatment of a wide range of infections caused by HSV and VZV.

I. PRIMARY HERPETIC GINGIVOSTOMATITIS

The primary infection may be asymptomatic. When clinical disease is evident, gingivostomatitis and pharyngitis are the most frequent manifestations, with fever, malaise, inability to eat, and lymphadenopathy for 2 to 7 days. Painful oral vesicular lesions may occur on the gingiva, mucosa, tongue, and lips. Both first-episode HSV-1 and HSV-2 can cause pharyngitis.

A patient may be a subclinical carrier, and reactivation from the trigeminal ganglia (Figure 2-5) may be followed by asymptomatic excretion of the viruses in the saliva. On the other hand, reactivation may lead to herpetic ulcerations of the lip, the typical "cold sore."

II. HERPES LABIALIS (COLD SORE, FEVER BLISTER)

Both HSV-1 and HSV-2 cause genital and oral–facial infections that cannot be distinguished clinically. Reactivations of oral–facial HSV-1 infections are more frequent than of oral–facial HSV-2 infections. Reactivations of genital HSV-2 are more frequent than of genital HSV-1 infections.

Recurrent (HSV) lesions occur at or near the primary lesion at indefinite intervals. They are usually triggered by stress, sunlight, illness, or trauma. Not infrequently, they relate to the patient's dental appointment, when emotional stress and oral trauma may be involved.

A. Prodrome

Before the local lesion appears, there may be burning or slight stinging sensations with slight swelling as a forewarning or prodrome. Most frequently, the recurrent lesion is at the vermilion border of the lower lip, although less commonly, the lesions may occur intraorally on the gingiva or the hard palate.

B. Clinical Characteristics

A group of vesicles forms and eventually ruptures and coalesces. Crusting follows, and healing may take up to 10 days. The lesions are infectious, with viral shedding. Care must be taken by the patient because autoinfection (to the eye, nose, or genitals, for example) is possible, as is infection of others.

III. HERPETIC WHITLOW

Herpetic whitlow is the herpes simplex infection of the fingers that results from the virus entering through minor skin abrasions. The most frequent location is around a fingernail, where cracks in the skin often occur.

A. Transmission

A whitlow may be a primary or recurrent infection of HSV-1 or HSV-2. Transmission results from direct contact with a vesicular lesion on a patient's lip or with saliva that contains the viruses.

Members of the dental team who do not wear protective gloves can have whitlow on the index fingers and thumbs that are in close contact with the patient's saliva where instrumentation and retraction are performed.

Autoinfection from a lip or intraoral herpetic lesion is possible while nail biting.

B. Disease Process

The whitlow usually starts suddenly as an area of irritation that becomes tender and painful. Groups of vesicles coalesce, and the whole healing process may last up to 2 weeks. The lesions are infectious and transmissible even before the whitlow appears and is diagnosed. Recurrences are not unusual.

IV. OCULAR HERPES[19]

Herpes simplex lesions in the eye can be a primary or recurrent infection of HSV-1 or HSV-2.

A. Transmission

1. Splashing saliva or fluid from a vesicular lesion directly into an unprotected eye.
2. Extension of infection from a facial lesion.
3. Infection of an infant's eye *in utero* or during birth.

B. Disease Process

Symptoms include fever, pain, blurring of vision, swelling, excess tears, and secondary bacterial infection. Herpes keratoconjunctivitis can cause deep inflammation and, when left untreated, is a leading cause of loss of sight.

▪ CLINICAL MANAGEMENT

I. PATIENT HISTORY

All patient histories need questions to determine experiences with herpesviruses. Terminology may be a problem, so such terms as "fever blisters" or "cold sores" need to be used to ensure patient understanding.

II. POSTPONE APPOINTMENT WITH PATIENT WITH ACTIVE LESION

A. Problems of Transmission

Explain the following to the patient:
1. Contagiousness, with possible transmission to other patients.
2. Autoinoculation possible from instrumentation that can splash viruses to the patient's eye or extend the lesion to the nose.

B. Irritation to Lesions

Irritation to the lesions can prolong the course and increase the severity of the infection.

C. Prodromal State May Be the Most Contagious

The patient should be requested to call ahead to change an appointment when it is known that a lesion is developing.

▪ HIV-1 INFECTION[25]

The acquired immunodeficiency syndrome (AIDS) is a severe condition caused by infection with the *human immunodeficiency virus* (HIV-1). A second virus, HIV-2, isolated in West Africa and later in Europe and North America, has been shown to have similar characteristics and transmission as the original HIV-1. Both are slow, progressive, often lethal diseases and have the ability to persist within cells such as macrophages for long periods of time.

HIV-1–infected patients may present with manifestations that range from mild abnormalities in immune response without apparent signs and symptoms to profound immunosuppression associated with a variety of life-threatening infections and rare malignant conditions. Box 2-2 provides abbreviations and terminology relating to HIV-1 infection and AIDS.

BOX 2-2 KEY ABBREVIATIONS: HIV and AIDS

AIDS: acquired immunodeficiency syndrome.

AZT (ZDV): zidovudine, retrovir; drug used for the treatment of HIV infection and AIDS; first antiviral drug approved by the United States Food and Drug Administration (FDA).

CD4+: T-helper lymphocyte; primary target cell for HIV infection; CD4+ count decreases with the severity of HIV-related illness.

DNA: deoxyribonucleic acid; a nucleic acid found in a cell nucleus; a carrier of genetic information.

HIV: human immunodeficiency virus; causes AIDS.

HIV-1 antibody: antibody to human immunodeficiency virus type 1; antibody can be detected in the blood 6 to 8 weeks after infection.

HL: hairy leukoplakia.

IDU: injection-drug user.

KS: Kaposi's sarcoma; a malignant vascular tumor; an opportunistic neoplasm that may occur in people with HIV infection.

LAV: lymphadenopathy-associated virus; one of the former names for HIV.

MMWR: *Morbidity and Mortality Weekly Report;* publication of the United States Centers for Disease Control and Prevention **(CDCP),** Atlanta, GA.

PCP: pneumocystis pneumonia; caused by *Pneumocystis carinii;* an opportunistic infection that occurs in people with HIV infection.

PGL: persistent generalized lymphadenopathy.

PWA: person with AIDS.

RNA: ribonucleic acid; a nucleic acid found in cytoplasm and in the nuclei of certain cells; RNA directs the synthesis of proteins and replaces DNA as a carrier of genetic codes in some viruses.

▪ TRANSMISSION

The HIV-1 virus has been found in most body fluids. Transmission has been demonstrated by way of blood, semen, vaginal secretions, and breast milk.

I. ROUTES OF TRANSMISSION

A. Sexual Contact (Heterosexual or Homosexual)

The virus from an infected person's blood, semen, or vaginal secretions enters the blood circulation through tiny breaks in the rectum, vagina, or penis.

B. Blood and Blood Products

1. Injection drug users: contaminated, shared needles carry the infection.
2. Transfusion and use of blood products by patients with blood disorders. The serologic testing of all donor blood has nearly eliminated the threat of infection from transfusion or blood products.
3. Occupational accidental injuries: low risk of infection.

C. Perinatal

1. Placenta: viruses can be transmitted across the placenta.
2. During delivery: exposure during passage through infected genital tract.
3. Postnatally: through breast-feeding.

II. INDIVIDUALS AT HIGH RISK OF INFECTION

A. Sexually active homosexual and bisexual men having multiple partners without practicing safe sex.[§]
B. Users or former users of intravenous drugs, particularly when contaminated needles are shared.
C. Recipients of blood transfusions or blood products prior to mandatory testing for HIV-1 antibodies in 1985. People with hemophilia or other coagulation disorders are included.
D. Male and female prostitutes who do not practice safe sex.[§]
E. Health-care workers who do not adhere to strict barrier procedures and do not follow essential blood and other body fluid precautions for infection control.
F. Females artificially inseminated with HIV-1–infected semen.

G. Recipients of HIV-1–infected organ transplants.
H. Steady sexual partners of all those previously listed who do not practice safe sex.[§]
I. Steady sexual partners of those infected with AIDS or at high risk of AIDS who do not practice safe sex.[§]
J. Infants born to HIV-1-infected mothers.
K. Infants fed breast milk from HIV-1-infected mothers.

▪ LIFE CYCLE OF THE HIV-1[26]

HIV-1 is a retrovirus, and in a retrovirus, RNA is the core genetic material. The enzyme reverse transcriptase is essential for replication. A diagram of the HIV-1 virus is shown in Figure 2-6.

The complex life cycle of the HIV-1 can be divided into two general phases: the establishment of infection and the production of new virus particles.

I. ESTABLISHMENT OF INFECTION

A. Binding to a Target/Host Cell

1. HIV-1 enters the body and passes by way of the blood to a target cell surface, where it binds to a specific cellular receptor, CD4+.
2. Target cells that have CD4+ receptors include T-helper lymphocytes, monocytes, macrophages, and certain neurons and glial cells of the brain tissue.

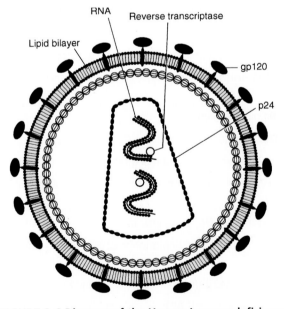

▪ **FIGURE 2-6 Diagram of the Human Immunodeficiency Virus (HIV-1).** The envelope of the virion is composed of the lipid bilayer with glycoproteins (gp120). The core contains two strands of RNA, enzymes, and core proteins (p24).

[§]"Practice safe sex" is meant to include barrier protection and no exchange of body fluids (saliva, semen, vaginal secretions) in accord with recommended guidelines.

B. Entry Through Wall of the Target/Host Cell

Fusion occurs between the virion and the target cell membrane, and the virus becomes uncoated. Only the viral RNA and the enzymes enter the cell.

C. Reverse Transcription

1. Viral RNA is changed into single-stranded DNA by the enzyme *reverse transcriptase.* Another enzyme, *ribonuclease,* destroys the RNA, which is no longer needed. Single-stranded DNA is then translated to a double-stranded DNA, which is called the *provirus.*
2. The provirus migrates to the nucleus of the host cell, enters the nucleus, and becomes permanently integrated with host DNA.

D. Infection Is Established

Once the viral DNA enters the host nucleus, infection is established. Succeeding progeny of the host cell are HIV-1 infected.

E. Latent Period

The integrated proviral DNA stays latent indefinitely.

II. PRODUCTION OF NEW VIRUS

A. Activation of the Host Cell

1. Stimulation causes activation. The DNA of the infected host cell can form new viral RNA and protein.
2. Viral proteins are broken down to form "building blocks" for progeny viral particles.
3. DNA is transcribed into RNA for the new virus.

B. Budding From Host Cell: Release

1. Host cell membrane is used to make a new viral envelope.
2. Free new virion is released into the bloodstream; it proceeds to find another CD4+ for attachment.

C. Host Cell Outcome

1. Loss of normal function.
2. Destruction; reduced numbers of host CD4+ cells lead to immune suppression.
3. The CD4+, or T-helper lymphocyte, is the primary target cell for HIV-1 infection. A decrease in the number of the CD4+ cells correlates with the risk and severity of HIV-1-related illnesses.

■ HIV-1 CLASSIFICATION SYSTEM FOR ADOLESCENTS AND ADULTS[27]

The CDC classification system emphasizes the importance of the CD4+ lymphocyte count in the clinical management of HIV-1–infected individuals. Measures of CD4+ counts are used to guide clinical and/or therapeutic treatment using antimicrobial prophylaxis and antiretroviral therapies.

The AIDS surveillance case definition includes all HIV-1–infected persons with less than 200 CD4+ lymphocytes/mm^3.[27] The system, charted in Table 2-4, is based on **3 laboratory** categories, numbered (1), (2), and (3), and **3 clinical** categories, lettered (A), (B), and (C).

I. LABORATORY CATEGORIES

Category 1: ≥ 500 CD4+ lymphocytes/mm^3
Category 2: 200 to 499 CD4+ lymphocytes/mm^3
Category 3: < 200 CD4+ lymphocytes/mm^3

TABLE 2-4 1992 REVISED CLASSIFICATION SYSTEM FOR HIV INFECTION AND EXPANDED AIDS SURVEILLANCE CASE DEFINITION FOR ADOLESCENTS AND ADULTS*

LABORATORY CD4+ CELL CATEGORIES	CLINICAL CATEGORIES		
	(A) ASYMPTOMATIC, OR PGL[†]	**(B)** SYMPTOMATIC, NOT (A) OR (C)	**(C)** AIDS-INDICATOR CONDITIONS[‡]
(1) ≥500 mm^3	A1	B1	C1
(2) 200–499 mm^3	A2	B2	C2
(3) <200–499 mm^3 AIDS-indicator cell count	A3	B3	C3

*The shaded boxes illustrate the expansion of the AIDS surveillance case definition. Persons with AIDS-indicator conditions (category C) are currently reportable to the health department in every state and U.S. territory. In addition to persons with clinical category C conditions (categories C1, C2, and C3), persons with CD4+ lymphocyte counts of less than 200/mm³ (categories A3 or B3) also have been reportable as AIDS cases in the United States and its territories since April 1, 1992.
†PGL = persistent generalized lymphadenopathy. Clinical category A includes acute (primary) HIV infection.
‡See text.

II. CLINICAL CATEGORIES

Category A: Asymptomatic (acute primary) HIV-1 or PGL
One or more of the following conditions. (Conditions in categories B and C must not have occurred.)

- Asymptomatic HIV-1 infection.
- Persistent generalized lymphadenopathy (PGL).
- Acute (primary) HIV-1 infection or history of acute HIV-1 infection.

Category B: Symptomatic (not A or C)
Examples of conditions in category B follow. They must be attributed to HIV-1 infection, indicative of a defect in cell-mediated immunity, and not listed under category C.

- Bacillary angiomatosis.
- Candidiasis, oropharyngeal (thrush).
- Candidiasis, vulvovaginal: persistent, frequent, or poorly responsive to therapy.
- Cervical dysplasia (moderate or severe)/cervical carcinoma in situ.
- Constitutional symptoms, such as fever (38.5° C) or diarrhea lasting >1 month.
- Hairy leukoplakia, oral.
- Herpes zoster (shingles), involving at least two distinct episodes or more than one dermatome.
- Idiopathic thrombocytopenic purpura.
- Listeriosis.
- Pelvic inflammatory disease, particularly if complicated by tubo-ovarian abscess.
- Peripheral neuropathy.

Category C: AIDS-Indicator Conditions
Conditions that follow in category C are strongly associated with severe immunodeficiency, occur frequently in HIV-1–infected individuals, and cause serious morbidity or mortality.

- Candidiasis of bronchi, trachea, or lungs.
- Candidiasis, esophageal.
- Cervical cancer, invasive.**
- Coccidioidomycosis, disseminated or extrapulmonary.
- Cryptococcosis, extrapulmonary.
- Cryptosporidiosis, chronic intestinal (duration >1 month).
- Cytomegalovirus disease (other than liver, spleen, or nodes).
- Cytomegalovirus retinitis (with loss of vision).
- Encephalopathy, HIV-1 related.
- Herpes simplex: chronic ulcer(s) (duration >1 month); or bronchitis, pneumonitis, or esophagitis.
- Histoplasmosis, disseminated or extrapulmonary.
- Isosporiasis, chronic intestinal (duration >1 month).

- Kaposi's sarcoma.
- Lymphoma, Burkitt's (or equivalent term).
- Lymphoma, immunoblastic (or equivalent term).
- Lymphoma, primary, of brain.
- *Mycobacterium avium* complex of *M. kansasii,* disseminated or extrapulmonary.
- *Mycobacterium tuberculosis,* any site (pulmonary** or extrapulmonary).
- *Mycobacterium,* other species or unidentified species, disseminated or extrapulmonary.
- *Pneumocystis carinii* pneumonia.
- Pneumonia, recurrent.††
- Progressive multifocal leukoencephalopathy.
- *Salmonella* septicemia, recurrent.
- Toxoplasmosis of brain.
- Wasting syndrome caused by HIV-1.

■ CLINICAL COURSE OF HIV-1 INFECTION[28]

A detectable antibody level usually can be detected within 1 to 3 months after exposure to the HIV-1 virus. Antibody presence indicates infection. Viral production is high throughout all stages of infection.

I. INCUBATION PERIOD

The incubation period ranges from the time of infection until the time when symptoms of AIDS are evident, which may be 15 years or longer.

II. THE ACUTE SEROCONVERSION SYNDROME

A. Initial Infection

After exposure, approximately one-half of those infected will have flulike or mononucleosis-like symptoms within 2 to 6 weeks. They are often unsuspected as associated with HIV-1 infection.

1. *Symptoms.* A wide variety of possible symptoms have been experienced, especially fever, lymphadenopathy, pharyngitis, fatigue, muscle pain, and a skin rash.
2. *Viremia.* Within 2 to 4 weeks after the initial infection, high levels of virus occur related to dissemination and development of antibody.

III. EARLY HIV-1 DISEASE

A. CD4+ Count: greater than 500 cells/mm³.
B. Symptoms: with CD4+ count high, no symptoms usually, but if any, lymphadenopathy and dermatologic lesions.

**Added in the 1993 expansion of the AIDS surveillance case definition.

††Added in the 1993 expansion of the AIDS surveillance case definition.

C. Oral Lesions: more common in later stages.
   1. Aphthous ulcers, herpes simplex labialis.
   2. Hairy leukoplakia: pathognomonic for underlying HIV-1 infection; when occurring in early HIV-1 disease, it is considered an indicator of disease progression.

IV. INTERMEDIATE STAGE OF HIV-1 DISEASE

A. CD4+ Count: 200 to 500 cells/mm^3.
B. Symptoms: skin and oral lesions become more common; recurrent herpes simplex, varicella-zoster, fever, weight loss, candidiasis (oropharyngeal or vaginal), myalgias, headaches, fatigue.
C. Oral Lesions: more common; candidiasis is considered a predictor for *Pneumocystis carinii* pneumonia.

V. LATE-STAGE DISEASE: AIDS

A. CD4+ Count: 50 to 200 cells/mm^3.
B. Symptoms: AIDS-indicator conditions (Table 2-4).
   1. *Opportunistic Infections.* An opportunistic infection is caused by a microorganism that is capable of taking advantage of a compromised immune system as an opportunity to develop in a person in whom the disease would not otherwise develop. When the immune reactions of the person with HIV-1 infection decrease, as monitored by the lowered CD4+ lymphocyte count, opportunistic infections can become more frequent, extensive, and severe.
   2. *Constitutional Disease: HIV-1 Wasting Syndrome.* Long-term fever, severe weight loss, anemia, chronic diarrhea, and chronic weakness are all effects of loss of immune response and repeated opportunistic diseases. The wasting syndrome symptoms, along with organic mental disorders (HIV-1 dementia), contribute to the severe degeneration during the terminal AIDS illness.
   3. *Encephalopathy: Organic Mental Disorders.* Disabling cognitive and/or motor dysfunction may develop with symptoms of apathy, inability to concentrate, poor memory, and depression.
   4. *Neoplasms.* Several neoplasms, related to the underlying immunodeficiency, are common indicators of HIV-1 infection and AIDS. These include Kaposi's sarcoma, primary B-cell lymphoma of the brain, and non-Hodgkin's lymphoma.

■ ORAL MANIFESTATIONS OF HIV-1 INFECTION

Many HIV-1–infected patients have head and/or neck manifestations. Certain oral findings have been identified as indicators of HIV-1 infection.

Oral symptoms can be integrated with information from the patient's medical history. From the complete assessment, an early recognition by dental clinicians, or at least a suspicion, of HIV-1 infection may result. Referral for medical evaluation and testing can be recommended.

Early recognition of an HIV-1-seropositive condition is important because drugs available for treatment can slow down the process of the disease. With early intervention, severe complications may be prevented, and the long-term quality of life can be improved.

Table 2-5 lists oral lesions according to whether the condition is strongly associated, less commonly associated, or possibly associated with HIV-1 infection.

I. EXTRAORAL EXAMINATION

A careful extraoral assessment is essential and must be conducted at each appointment.

A. Lymphadenopathy

Palpation for enlarged lymph nodes is a routine part of every extraoral examination.

B. Skin Lesions

Several conditions listed in Table 2-5 develop in the skin. Examples are Kaposi's sarcoma, purpura, and herpetic lesions.

II. INTRAORAL EXAMINATION

Of the intraoral lesions listed as strongly associated with HIV-1 infection (group I in Table 2-5), candidiasis, Kaposi's sarcoma, and hairy leukoplakia have been highly correlated with the subsequent development of advanced HIV-1 infection. All three lesions are readily observable during an oral examination.

A. Fungal Infections[29]

Oral candidiasis, the most frequently occurring oral infection, appears in various forms. They are listed in Table 2-5.

Although usually recognized by clinical examination, the dentist may request the use of exfoliative cytology for differential distinction.

TABLE 2-5 ORAL LESIONS ASSOCIATED WITH HIV INFECTION CLASSIFICATION

GROUP I. LESIONS STRONGLY ASSOCIATED WITH HIV INFECTION	GROUP III. LESIONS SEEN WITH HIV INFECTION

Candidiasis
  Erythematous
  Pseudomembranous
Hairy leukoplakia
Kaposi's sarcoma
Non-Hodgkin's lymphoma
Periodontal disease
  Linear gingival erythema
  Necrotizing (ulcerative) gingivitis
  Necrotizing (ulcerative) periodontitis
	Bacterial infections
	  Actinomyces israelii
	  Escherichia coli
	  Klebsiella pneumoniae
	Cat-scratch disease
	Drug reactions (ulcerative erythema multiforme,
	  lichenoid, toxic epidermolysis)
	Epithelioid (bacillary) angiomatosis
	Fungal infection other than candidiasis
	  Cryptococcus neoformans
	  Geotrichum candidum
	  Histoplasma capsulatum
	  Mucoraceae (mucormycosis/zygomycosis)
	  Aspergillus flavus

GROUP II. LESIONS LESS COMMONLY ASSOCIATED WITH HIV INFECTION	Neurologic disturbances
	  Facial palsy
	  Trigeminal neuralgia
	Recurrent aphthous stomatitis
	Viral infections
	  Cytomegalovirus
	  Molluscum contagiosum

Bacterial infections
  Mycobacterium avium-intracellulare
  Mycobacterium tuberculosis
Melanotic hyperpigmentation
Necrotizing (ulcerative) stomatitis
Salivary gland disease
  Dry mouth due to decreased salivary flow rate
  Unilateral or bilateral swelling of major salivary
    glands
Thrombocytopenic purpura
Ulceration NOS (not otherwise specified)
Viral infections
  Herpes simplex virus
  Human papillomavirus
    (warty-like lesions)
    Condyloma acuminatum
    Focal epithelial hyperplasia
    Verruca vulgaris
  Varicella-zoster virus
    Herpes zoster
    Varicella	

(From European Commission Clearinghouse on Oral Problems Related to HIV Infection and World Health Organization Collaborating Centre on Oral Manifestations of the Human Immunodeficiency Virus, 1990, with revisions, 1992.)

B. Viral Infections[29]

Herpes simplex, hairy leukoplakia, oral lesions of chickenpox, verruca vulgaris, condyloma acuminatum, and cytomegalovirus ulcer are all examples of lesions that may be seen.

C. Bacterial Infections: Gingival and Periodontal Infections

As with other oral manifestations, gingival changes may be an initial indicator of undiagnosed HIV-1 infection. On the other hand, there may not be any unusual gingival or periodontal changes that can be associated with HIV-1 infection, especially when the patient maintains a high level of personal and professional oral care.

The general clinical sequelae are that periodontal infections associated with HIV-1 infection tend to show more severe symptoms and to progress more rapidly than do periodontal conditions in people who are not immunosuppressed.

1. *Gingivitis: Linear Gingival Erythema.* Unusual degrees of severity of gingivitis may be observed. A 2- to 3-mm red band may appear along the gingival margin with petechia-like and/or diffuse red lesions of the attached gingiva. Spontaneous bleeding and bleeding on gentle probing occur. Scaling, root planing, and an increased dental biofilm control effort on a frequent maintenance plan are necessary but may not reach the degree of health usually expected.

2. *Necrotizing Ulcerative Gingivitis (NUG).* An increased incidence of NUG has been observed in HIV-1–positive patients. Ulceration and destruction of interdental papillae with spontaneous bleeding and pain may develop rapidly.

3. *Periodontal Infection.* A range of severity of periodontal involvement may be observed in HIV-1–infected patients. Severe soft tissue necrosis and rapid destruction of periodontal attachment characteristic of a rapidly progressive periodontitis can occur in a few months. In extreme cases, loss of crestal alveolar bone has led to bone exposure and sequestration.

　　Severe pain and difficulty in mastication contribute to patient discomfort and malnutrition.

D. Dental Assessment

Dental caries and dental erosion can be problems for patients medicated with zidovudine (AZT) or retrovir. Common side effects of AZT are nausea and vomiting. The patient who uses the medication several times each day and vomits each time could have dissolution of the enamel in the form of dental erosion. Personal daily and periodic professional fluoride applications must be included in the preventive oral hygiene program.

E. Xerostomia

Xerostomia, as a result of salivary gland diseases (Table 2-5, group II) or as a side effect of medications, can contribute to dental caries and discomfort from dry mucosa. In addition to fluoride therapy for dental caries control, the patient's diet should be reviewed and instruction given in the selection of noncariogenic foods and snack items.

■ HIV-1 INFECTION IN CHILDREN[30]

An increasing number of patients with HIV-1 infection are children younger than 13 years of age. Children older than 13 years are diagnosed and treated as adults.

I. CHILDREN AT RISK

A. Perinatal Transmission

Infants born to mothers infected with HIV-1; approximately 25% to 40% of infants born to HIV-1-seropositive mothers become infected.

B. Breast-fed Infants

HIV-1 has been demonstrated in human milk, and postpartum transmission does occur. Human milk contains components, such as immunoglobulins and leukocytes, that could reduce the infectivity of the HIV-1. Many questions remain unanswered. The World Health Organization has recommended that women in developing countries whose water supplies are unsafe for preparation of infant formulas continue to breast-feed their infants.[31]

C. Infected Blood and Blood Products

Infants or children who received transfusions or treatments with infected blood or blood products are at risk. This mode of transfer is under control in countries where blood donors are screened and all donated blood is tested.

D. Sexual Abuse

Children who have been sexually abused by an infected perpetrator.[32]

II. CLASSIFICATION

The classification system for HIV-1 infection in children younger than 13 years has been developed by the United States Centers for Disease Control and Prevention. In the revised 1994 system, infected children are classified by three parameters: the infection status, the clinical status, and the immunologic status.[33]

III. CLINICAL MANIFESTATIONS

A. Incubation or Latent Period

The progression of HIV-1 in infants is more severe and faster than in adults due to the immature immune system, which provides less resistance to infection. The time before clinical symptoms appear is variable and may range from months after birth to several years.

B. Diagnosis

Initial diagnosis is based on blood screening for the presence of virus or HIV-1 antibody. Diagnosis of HIV-1 infection in the neonate during the first year is complicated by the persistence of maternal antibody, which has been passively transferred across the placenta to the fetus.

　　When the mother is without symptoms and has never been tested for HIV-1, the child's diagnosis may be the index case in the family. Testing of family members and parental counseling is indicated.

C. Systemic Findings[30]

The wide range of symptoms includes disorders of nearly every body organ system. Oral lesions are common clinical signs of HIV-1 infection in children. Bacterial infections tend to be more frequent and more severe than those in adults. Following is a partial list of frequently found conditions:

1. Failure to thrive; developmental delay.
2. Hepatomegaly; splenomegaly.
3. Generalized lymphadenopathy.
4. Chronic pneumonitis.
5. Progressive encephalopathy.

D. Oral Findings[34]

Oral lesions are common clinical signs of HIV-1 infection in children. They are frequently among the earliest symptoms to appear and may be used to diagnose HIV-1.

1. Persistent oral candidiasis; *Candida* esophagitis.
2. Parotiditis; swelling of the parotid glands.
3. Herpetic gingivostomatitis; sore mouth and poor oral intake lead to malnutrition and dehydration.
4. Aphthous ulcers.
5. Hairy leukoplakia.
6. Linear gingival erythema.
7. Necrotizing ulcerative gingivitis and periodontitis (less frequently).

IV. TREATMENT/MANAGEMENT

A. Counseling

Family counseling can be essential to the patient's care. Family and caregivers of the child need to watch for symptoms that are significant to disease progression. They also need to understand the reasons for frequent follow-up for testing and to attend faithfully to the medications program.

Counseling for oral health becomes an important part of the child's care. The healthy mouth, free from pain, can allow comfort during eating and thereby contribute to the nutritional status and the overall welfare and quality of life.

B. Medications: Threat to Dental Caries[35,36]

Children with HIV-1 infection or AIDS take many types of medications. Many children's medications have a base with a high percentage of sucrose, some of which may be taken by the child several times each day. They may be prepared for the children as an elixir, in a sweet, sticky form to disguise an unpleasant flavor.

Other children's preparations with high sucrose are nutritional supplements. Multivitamins, given as drops for infants and toddlers, contain high quantities of sucrose. Mycostatin (for oral candidiasis) may be recommended for several applications a day and may have a sucrose content as great as 50%.[36]

All these preparations can contribute to the initiation of dental caries. Infants and toddlers with HIV-1 infection can be at great risk for early childhood caries. When a parent is counseled concerning oral care, recommendations must be given relative to the nursing bottle and pacifiers, as well as to cleaning the mouth immediately after giving the various medications.

▪ PREVENTION OF HIV-1 INFECTION

Until a vaccine is available, prevention depends to a large degree on community education for attitudinal and behavioral changes. People need to understand the modes of transmission of the HIV-1 and the preventive measures necessary to halt its transmission. Dental

Everyday Ethics

(?) Mr. Sands, a patient returning for his regular maintenance appointment, is scheduled with Jenny, one of the two dental hygienists available that day. Mr. Sands has a history of hepatitis C. When Jenny reviewed the history prior to seating the patient, she immediately makes up an excuse and asks Marilyn, the other hygienist, to treat this patient while she attends to the two pedodontic patients in a different treatment room.

Questions for Consideration

1. What should Jenny understand about refusing to treat the patient with hepatitis C history?

2. Using the decision framework in Chapter 1, list alternative solutions or outcomes that apply to this situation.

3. How is the principle of justice related to the actions of the dental hygienist?

Factors To Teach The Patient

- Reasons for postponing an appointment when a herpes lesion ("fever blister" or "cold sore") is present on the lip or in the oral cavity.

  - Importance of not touching or scratching the lesion because of self-infection to fingers or eyes, for example.

- How the viruses can survive on objects and transfer infection to other people.

- How to help by keeping the medical history up-to-date by informing of additional exposures and immunizations to communicable diseases for self and family members.

- Preparation for a dental or dental hygiene appointment by thorough mouth cleaning with toothbrush and dental floss to lower the bacterial count and thus lessen aerosol contamination in the treatment room.

personnel must keep well informed with accurate, current information that can be applied in practice and give support to community health programs.

The goal of *primary prevention* (for those not infected) is to lower the rate at which new cases of HIV-1 infection appear. Programs for women, particularly of childbearing age; intravenous drug users who share needles; and teenagers are focused to reach the most vulnerable groups. HIV-1 testing should be offered for all pregnant women, and all newborns should be tested in the attempt to control the increasing numbers of children with HIV-1 infection.

The goals of *secondary prevention* (for seropositive individuals) are to reduce the rate of transmission and to introduce treatment early. Early intervention may postpone severe clinical manifestations of advanced illness. A leading part of the program is to counsel the HIV-1–infected individuals to practice safe sex[§§] and to cooperate with the program to screen and counsel their sexual contacts and families.

Ongoing programs include strict testing for blood donors and all tissue organ donors, as well as identification and counseling of recipients of blood transfusions before 1985 and their sexual partners. The incubation period has been shown to be much longer than was originally thought. With early diagnosis and medical inter-

vention, people with HIV-1 infection can be symptom free and healthy and can live longer than was possible earlier in the epidemic.

REFERENCES

1. **United States Department of Health and Human Services, Centers for Disease Control and Prevention:** Guidelines for Infection Control in Dental Health-care Settings–2003, *MMWR, 52,* 2, RR-17, December 19, 2003.
2. **Socransky,** S.S. and Manganiello, S.D.: The Oral Microbiota of Man From Birth to Senility, *J. Periodontol., 42,* 485, August, 1971.
3. **Miller,** R.L. and Micik, R.E.: Air Pollution and Its Control in the Dental Office, *Dent. Clin. North Am., 22,* 453, July, 1978.
4. **Larato,** D.C., Ruskin, P.F., and Martin, A.: Effect of an Ultrasonic Scaler on Bacterial Counts in Air, *J. Periodontol., 38,* 550, November–December, 1967.
5. **Holbrook,** W.P., Muir, K.F., MacPhee, I.T., and Ross, P.W.: Bacteriological Investigation of the Aerosol from Ultrasonic Scalers, *Br. Dent. J., 144,* 245, April 18, 1978.
6. **Pokowitz,** W. and Hoffman, H.: Dental Aerobiology, *N.Y. State Dent. J., 37,* 337, June–July, 1971.
7. **Gross,** A., Devine, M.J., and Cutright, D.E.: Microbial Contamination of Dental Units and Ultrasonic Scalers, *J. Periodontol., 47,* 670, November, 1976.
8. **Benenson,** A.S., ed.: *Control of Communicable Diseases in Man,* 16th ed. Washington, D.C., American Public Health Association, 1995, pp. 488–499.
9. **United States Centers for Disease Control:** Revised Classification System for HIV Infection and Expanded Surveillance Case Definition for AIDS Among Adolescents and Adults, *MMWR, 41,* 1–19, RR-17, December 18, 1992.
10. **United States Centers for Disease Control and Prevention:** Guidelines for Preventing the Transmission of *Mycobacterium tuberculosis* in Health-care Facilities, 1994, *MMWR, 43,* 52, October 28, 1994.
11. **Robinson,** H.B.G. and Miller, A.S.: *Colby, Kerr, and Robinson's Color Atlas of Oral Pathology,* 5th ed. Philadelphia, J.B. Lippincott Co., 1990, p. 91.
12. **Miyakawa,** Y. and Mayumi, M.: Hepatitis G Virus—A True Hepatitis or an Accidental Tourist? (Editorial), *N. Engl. J. Med., 336,* 795, March 13, 1997.
13. **Alter,** H.J., Nakatsuji, Y., Melpolder, J., Wages, J., Wesley, R., Shih, J.W.-K., and Kim, J.P.: The Incidence of Transfusion-associated Hepatitis G Virus Infection and Its Relation to Liver Disease, *N. Engl. J. Med., 336,* 747, March 13, 1997.
14. **Alter,** M.J., Gallagher, M., Morris, T.T., Moyer, L.A., Meeks, E.L., Krawczynski, K., Kim, J.P., and Margolis, H.S.: Acute Non-A-E Hepatitis in the United States and the Role of Hepatitis G Virus Infection, *N. Engl. J. Med., 336,* 741, March 13, 1997.
15. **Benenson:** op. cit., pp. 217–233.
16. **United States Centers for Disease Control:** Hepatitis B Virus: A Comprehensive Strategy for Eliminating Transmission in the United States Through Universal Childhood Vaccination, *MMWR, 40,* 1–25, RR-13, November 22, 1991.
17. **United States Centers for Disease Control:** Suboptimal Response to Hepatitis B Vaccine Given by Injection Into the Buttock, *MMWR, 34,* 105, March 1, 1985.
18. **Porter,** S., Scully, C., and Samaranayake, L.: Viral Hepatitis: Current Concepts for Dental Practice, *Oral Surg. Oral Med. Oral Pathol., 78,* 682, December, 1994.
19. **Yapar,** M., Saygun, I., Ozdemir, A., Kubar, A., and Sahin, S.: Prevalence of Human Herpesviruses in Patients with Aggressive Periodontitis, *J. Periodontol., 74,* 1634, November, 2003.

[§§]"Practice safe sex" is meant to include barrier protection and no exchange of body fluids (saliva, semen, vaginal secretions) in accord with recommended guidelines.

20. **Benenson:** op. cit., pp. 87–91.

21. **Benenson:** op. cit., pp. 312–314.

22. **Cheeseman,** S.H.: Cytomegalovirus, in Gorbach, S.L., Bartlett, J.G., and Blacklow, N.R.: *Infectious Diseases.* Philadelphia, W.B. Saunders Co., 1992, pp. 1715–1720.

23. **Benenson:** op. cit., pp. 233–236.

24. **Amit,** R., Morag, A., Ravid, Z., Hochman, N., Ehrlich, J., and Zakay-Rones, Z.: Detection of Herpes Simplex Virus in Gingival Tissue, *J. Periodontol., 63,* 502, June, 1992.

25. **Benenson:** op. cit., p. 1–8.

26. **Folks,** T.M. and Hart, C.E.: The Life Cycle of Human Immunodeficiency Virus Type I, in DeVita, V.T., Hellman, S., and Rosenberg, S.A., eds.: *AIDS: Etiology, Diagnosis, Treatment and Prevention,* 4th ed. Philadelphia, Lippincott-Raven, 1997, pp. 29–39.

27. **United States Centers for Disease Control and Prevention:** 1993 Revised Classification System for HIV Infection and Expanded Surveillance Case Definition for AIDS Among Adolescents and Adults, *MMWR, 41,* 1–19, No. RR-17, December 18, 1992.

28. **Saag,** M.S.: Clinical Spectrum of Human Immunodeficiency Virus Diseases, in DeVita, V.T., Hellman, S., and Rosenberg, S.A., eds.: *AIDS: Etiology, Diagnosis, Treatment and Prevention,* 4th ed. Philadelphia, Lippincott-Raven, 1997, pp. 203–213.

29. **Greenspan,** D., Greenspan, J.S., Schiødt, M., and Pindborg, J.J.: *AIDS and the Mouth: Diagnosis and Management of Oral Lesions.* Copenhagen, Munksgaard, 1990, pp. 91–102, 113–134.

30. **Mueller,** B.U. and Pizzo, P.A.: Pediatric Human Immunodeficiency Virus Infections, in DeVita, V.T., Hellman, S., and Rosenberg, S.A., eds.: *AIDS: Etiology, Diagnosis, Treatment and Prevention,* 4th ed. Philadelphia, Lippincott-Raven, 1997, pp. 443–464.

31. **World Health Organization:** Global Program on AIDS: Consensus Statement From WHO/UNICEF Consultation on HIV Transmission and Breast-feeding, *Weekly Epidemiol. Rec., 67,* 177, 1992.

32. **Gutman,** L.T., St. Claire, K.K., Weedy, C., Herman-Giddens, M.E., Lane, B.A., Niemeyer, J.C., and McKinney, R.E.: Human Immunodeficiency Virus Transmission by Sexual Abuse, *Am. J. Dis. Child., 145,* 137, February, 1991.

33. **United States Centers for Disease Control and Prevention:** 1994 Revised Classification System for Human Immunodeficiency Virus Infection in Children Less Than 13 Years of Age, *MMWR, 43,* 1–19, No. RR-12, September 30, 1994.

34. **Chigurupati,** R., Raghavan, S.S., and Studen-Pavlovich, D.A.: Pediatric HIV Infection and Its Oral Manifestations: A Review, *Pediatr. Dent., 18,* 106, March/April, 1996.

35. **Gehrke,** F.S. and Johnsen, D.S.: Bottle Caries Associated With Anti-HIV Therapy (Letter), *Pediatr. Dent., 13,* 73, January/February, 1991.

36. **Howell,** R.B. and Houpt, M.: More Than One Factor Can Influence Caries Development in HIV-Positive Children (Letter), *Pediatr. Dent., 13,* 247, July/August, 1991.

SUGGESTED READINGS

Bagg, J.: Common Infectious Diseases, *Dent. Clin. North Am., 40,* 385, April, 1996.

Bentley, C.D., Burkhart, N.W., and Crawford, J.J.: Evaluating Spatter and Aerosol Contamination During Dental Procedures, *J. Am. Dent. Assoc., 125,* 579, May, 1994.

Harfst, S.: Infection Control Update: Vaccinations, *J. Pract. Hyg., 5,* 43, July/August, 1996.

Laskaris, G.: Oral Manifestations of Infectious Diseases, *Dent. Clin. North Am., 40,* 395, April, 1996.

Slavkin, H.C.: First Encounters: Transmission of Infectious Oral Diseases From Mother to Child, *J. Am. Dent. Assoc., 128,* 773, June, 1997.

Tuberculosis

Abou-Shala, N. and Mauldin, G.: Tuberculosis: An Old Nemesis Returns, *Am. Acad. Phys. Assist., 6,* 639, October, 1993.

Bagg, J.: Tuberculosis: A Re-emerging Problem for Health Care Workers, *Br. Dent. J., 180,* 376, May 25, 1996.

Bednarsh, H.S. and Eklund, K.J.: TB Prevention Through Screening and Therapy, *Access, 10,* 4, July, 1995.

Brown, B.S.: Oral Manifestations of Tuberculosis, *Pros and Contra Angles, 20,* 5, April, 1998.

Harlow, R.F. and Rutkauskas, J.S.: Tuberculosis Risk in the Hospital Dental Practice, *Spec. Care Dent., 15,* 50, March/April, 1995.

Iseman, M.D.: Treatment of Multidrug-resistant Tuberculosis, *N. Engl. J. Med., 329,* 784, September 9, 1993.

Molinari, J.A.: Tuberculosis Infection Control: A Reasonable Approach for Dentistry, *Compend. Cont. Educ. Dent., 16,* 1080, November, 1995.

Phelan, J.A., Jimenez, V., and Tompkins, D.C.: Tuberculosis, *Dent. Clin. North Am., 40,* 327, April, 1996.

Shearer, B.G.: MDR-TB. Another Challenge From the Microbial World, *J. Am. Dent. Assoc., 125,* 43, January, 1994.

Villanueva, A.V. and Chandrasekar, P.H.: Emergence of Antimicrobial-Resistant Pathogens: A Growing Concern, *J. Pract. Hyg., 6,* 37, September/October, 1997.

Woods, R.G., Amerena, V., David, P., Fan, P.L., Heydt, H., and Marianos, D.: Additional Precautions for Tuberculosis and a Self Assessment Checklist, *FDI World, 6,* 10, May/June, 1997.

Hepatitis

Hoofnagle, J.H. and Lau, D.: Chronic Viral Hepatitis: Benefits of Current Therapies, *N. Engl. J. Med., 334,* 1470, May 30, 1996.

Hoofnagle, J.H. and DiBisceglie, A.M.: The Treatment of Chronic Viral Hepatitis, *N. Engl. J. Med., 336,* 347, January 30, 1997.

Lee, W.M.: Hepatitis B Virus Infection, *N. Engl. J. Med., 337,* 1733, December 11, 1997.

Lemon, S.M. and Thomas, D.L.: Vaccines to Prevent Viral Hepatitis, *N. Engl. J. Med., 336,* 196, January 16, 1997.

Molinari, J.A.: Hepatitis. Vaccination Information, *DentalHygienist-News, 9,* 15, Number 3, 1996.

Najm, W.: Viral Hepatitis: How to Manage Type C and D Infections, *Geriatrics, 52,* 28, May, 1997.

Reddi, S. and Garg, A.K.: Patients With Chronic Hepatitis: Potential Risks When Undergoing Dental Surgery: Review and Case Report, *Spec. Care Dentist., 14,* 241, November/December, 1994.

Slavkin, H.G.: The A,B,C,D, and E of Viral Hepatitis, *J. Am. Dent. Assoc., 127,* 1667, November, 1996.

Szmuness, W., Stevens, C.E., Harley, E.J., Zang, E.A., Oleszko, W.R., William, D.C., Sadovsky, R., Morrison, J.M., and Kellner, A.: Hepatitis B Vaccine: Demonstration of Efficacy in a Controlled Clinical Trial in a High-Risk Population in the United States, *N. Engl. J. Med., 303,* 833, October 9, 1980.

Hepatitis C

Alter, M.J., Margolis, H.S., Krawczynski, K., Judson, F.N., Mares, A., Alexander, W.J., Hu, P.Y., Miller, J.K., Gerber, M.A., Sampliner, R.E., Meeks, E.L., and Beach, M.J.: The Natural History of Community-Acquired Hepatitis C in the United States, *N. Engl. J. Med., 327,* 1899, December 31, 1992.

Donahue, J.G., Muñoz, A., Ness, P.M., Brown, D.E., Yawn, D.H., McAllister, H.A., Reitz, B.A., and Nelson, K.E.: The Declining Risk of Post-transfusion Hepatitis C Virus Infection, *N. Engl. J. Med., 327,* 369, August 6, 1992.

Kelen, G.D., Green, G.B., Purcell, R.H., Chan, D.W., Qaquish, B.F., Sivertson, K.T., and Quinn, T.C.: Hepatitis B and Hepatitis C in Emergency Department Patients, *N. Engl. J. Med., 326,* 1399, May 21, 1992.

Pereira, B.J.G., Milford, E.L., Kirkman, R.L., Quan, S., Sayre, K.R., Johnson, P.J., Wilber, J.C., and Levey, A.S.: Prevalence of Hepatitis C Virus RNA in Organ Donors Positive for Hepatitis C Antibody and in the Recipients of Their Organs, *N. Engl. J. Med., 327,* 910, September 24, 1992.

Pereira, B.J.G., Milford, E.L., Kirkman, R.L., and Levey, A.S.: Transmission of Hepatitis C Virus by Organ Transplantation, *N. Engl. J. Med., 325,* 454, August 15, 1991.

Weintrub, P.S., Veereman-Wauters, G., Cowan, M.J., and Thaler, M.M.: Hepatitis C Virus Infection in Infants Whose Mothers Took Street Drugs Intravenously, *J. Pediatr., 119,* 869, December, 1991.

Herpesvirus

Fons, M.P., Flaitz, C.M., Moore, B., Prabhakar, B.S., Nichols, C.M., and Albrecht, T.: Multiple Herpesviruses in Saliva of HIV-Infected Individuals, *J. Am. Dent. Assoc., 125,* 713, June, 1994.

Foreman, K.E., Friborg, J., Kong, W.-P., Woffendin, C., Polverini, P.J., Nickoloff, B.J., and Nabel, G.J.: Propagation of a Human Herpesvirus From AIDS-Associated Kaposi's Sarcoma, *N. Engl. J. Med., 336,* 163, January 16, 1997.

Gibbs, R.S. and Mead, P.B.: Preventing Neonatal Herpes—Current Strategies (Editorial), *N. Engl. J. Med., 326,* 946, April 2, 1992.

Gilden, D.H.: Herpes Zoster With Postherpetic Neuralgia—Persisting Pain and Frustration, (Editorial), *N. Engl. J. Med., 330,* 932, March 31, 1994.

Greenberg, M.S.: Herpesvirus Infections, *Dent. Clin. North Am., 40,* 359, April, 1996.

Manzella, J.P., McConville, J.H., Valenti, W., Menegus, M.A., Swirkosz, E.M., and Arens, M.: An Outbreak of Herpes Simplex Virus Type I Gingivostomatitis in a Dental Hygiene Practice, *JAMA, 252,* 2019, October 19, 1984.

Martin, J.N., Ganem, D.E., Osmond, D.H., Page-Shafer, K.A., Macrae, D., and Kedes, D.H.: Sexual Transmission and the Natural History of Human Herpesvirus 8 Infection, *N. Engl. J. Med., 338,* 948, April 2, 1998.

Poland, J.M.: Current Therapeutic Management of Recurrent Herpes Labialis, *Gen. Dent., 42,* 46, January–February, 1994.

Pruksananonda, P., Hall, C.B., Insel, R.A., McIntyre, K., Pellett, P.E., Long, C.E., Schnabel, K.C., Pincus, P.H., Stamey, B.A., Dambaugh, T.R., and Stewart, J.A.: Primary Human Herpesvirus 6 Infection in Young Children, *N. Engl. J. Med., 326,* 1446, May 28, 1992.

Robbins, D.L.: Human Herpesviruses: Research and Threats to Health Professionals, *Gen. Dent., 42,* 418, September–October, 1994.

Scott, D.A., Coulter, W.A., and Lamey, P.J.: Oral Shedding of Herpes Simplex Virus Type I: A Review, *J. Oral Pathol. Med., 26,* 441, November, 1997.

HIV: General

American Dental Association, Health Foundation: Dental Management of the HIV-Infected Patient, Chicago, *J. Am. Dent. Assoc., Supplement,* 1995.

Cao, Y., Qin, L., Zhang, L., Safrit, J., and Ho, D.D.: Virologic and Immunologic Characterization of Long-term Survivors of Human Immunodeficiency Virus Type I Infection, *N. Engl. J. Med., 332,* 201, January 26, 1995.

Chaisson, R.E., Keruly, J.C., and Moore, R.D.: Race, Sex, Drug Use, and Progression of Human Immunodeficiency Virus Disease, *N. Engl. J. Med., 333,* 751, September 21, 1995.

de Vincenzi, I., for the European Study Group on Heterosexual Transmission of HIV: A Longitudinal Study of Human Immunodeficiency Virus Transmission by Heterosexual Partners, *N. Engl. J. Med., 331,* 341, August 11, 1994.

Johnson, A.M.: Condoms and HIV Transmission, *N. Engl. J. Med., 331,* 391, August 11, 1994.

Katz, M.H. and Gerberding, J.L.: Postexposure Treatment of People Exposed to the Human Immunodeficiency Virus Through Sexual Contact or Injection-drug Use, *N. Engl. J. Med., 336,* 1097, April 10, 1997.

Levy, J.A.: Infection by Human Immunodeficiency Virus—CD4 Is Not Enough, *N. Engl. J. Med., 335,* 1528, November 14, 1996.

Lipton, S.A. and Gendelman, H.E.: Dementia Associated With the Acquired Immunodeficiency Syndrome, *N. Engl. J. Med., 332,* 934, April 6, 1995.

Pantaleo, G., Graziosi, C., and Fauci, A.S.: The Immunopathogenesis of Human Immunodeficiency Virus Infection, *N. Engl. J. Med., 328,* 327, February 4, 1993.

Phillips, K.A., Flatt, S.J., Morrison, K.R., and Coates, T.J.: Potential Use of Home HIV Testing, *N. Engl. J. Med., 332,* 1308, May 11, 1995.

Royce, R.A., Sena, A., Cates, W., and Cohen, M.S.: Sexual Transmission of HIV, *N. Engl. J. Med., 336,* 1072, April 10, 1997.

Waddell, C.: Perception of HIV Risk and Reported Compliance With Universal Precautions: A Comparison of Australian Dental Hygienists and Dentists, *J. Dent. Hyg., 71,* 17, January–February, 1997.

HIV: Oral Complications

Begg, M.D., Panageas, K.S., Mitchell-Lewis, D., Bucklan, R.S., Phelan, J.A., and Lamster, I.B.: Oral Lesions as Markers of Severe Immunosuppression in HIV-Infected Homosexual Men and Injection Drug Users, *Oral Surg. Oral Med. Oral Pathol. Oral Radiol. Endod., 82,* 276, September, 1996.

Brady, L.J., Walker, C., Oxford, G.E., Stewart, C., Magnusson, I., and McArthur, W.: Oral Diseases, Mycology and Periodontal Microbiology of HIV-I-infected Women, *Oral Microbiol. Immunol., 11,* 371, December, 1996.

Glick, M., Abel, S.N., Muzyka, B.C., and Delorenzo, M.: Dental Complications After Treating Patients With AIDS, *J. Am. Dent. Assoc., 125,* 296, March, 1994.

Glick, M., Muzyka, B.C., Lurie, D., and Salkin, L.M.: Oral Manifestations Associated With HIV-Related Disease as Markers for Immune Suppression and AIDS, *Oral Surg. Oral Med. Oral Pathol., 77,* 344, April, 1994.

Grbic, J.T., Lamster, I.B., and Mitchell-Lewis, D.: Inflammatory and Immune Mediators in Crevicular Fluid From HIV-Infected Injecting Drug Users, *J. Periodontol., 68,* 249, March, 1997.

Tillis, T.S.I. and Vojir, C.P.: Identification of HIV/AIDS-Associated Oral Lesions, *J. Dent. Hyg., 67,* 30, January, 1993.

HIV Children

Asher, R.S., McDowell, J., Acs, G., and Belanger, G.: Pediatric Infection With the Human Immunodeficiency Virus (HIV): Head, Neck, and Oral Manifestations, *Spec. Care Dentist., 13,* 113, May/June, 1993.

Bryson, Y.J., Pang, S., Wei, L.S., Dickover, R., Diagne, A., and Chen, I.S.Y.: Clearance of HIV Infection in a Perinatally Infected Infant, *N. Engl. J. Med., 332,* 833, March 30, 1995.

Cohen, F.L. and Nehring, W.M.: Foster Care of HIV-Positive Children in the United States, *Public Health Rep., 109,* 60, January–February, 1994.

Howell, R.B., Jandinski, J.J., Palumbo, P., Shey, Z., and Houpt, M.I.: Oral Soft Tissue Manifestations and CD4 Lymphocyte Counts in HIV-Infected Children, *Pediatr. Dent., 18,* 117, March/April, 1996.

Laskaris, G., Laskaris, M., and Theodoridou, M.: Oral Hairy Leukoplakia in a Child With AIDS, *Oral Surg. Oral Med. Oral Pathol., 79,* 570, May, 1995.

Madigan, A., Murray, P.A., Houpt, M., Catalanotto, F., and Feuerman, M.: Caries Experience and Cariogenic Markers in HIV-Positive Children and Their Siblings, *Pediatr. Dent., 18,* 129, March/April, 1996.

Moniaci, D., Cavallari, M., Greco, D., Bruatto, M., Raiteri, R., Palomba, E., Tovo, P.A., and Sinicco, A.: Oral Lesions in Children

Born to HIV-I Positive Women, *J. Oral Pathol. Med., 22,* 8, January, 1993.

Valdez, I.H., Pizzo, P.A., and Atkinson, J.C.: Oral Health of Pediatric AIDS Patients: A Hospital-Based Study, *ASDC J. Dent. Child., 61,* 114, March–April, 1994.

Ethics

Bayer, R.: AIDS Prevention: Sexual Ethics and Responsibility, *N. Engl. J. Med., 334,* 1540, June 6, 1996.

Chiodo, G.T. and Tolle, S.W.: The Ethical Foundations of a Duty to Treat HIV-Positive Patients, *Gen. Dent., 45,* 14, January–February, 1997.

Keyes, G.G. and Waithe, M.E.: HIV Infection in Dentistry: Ethical and Legal Issues, in Weinstein, B.D.: *Dental Ethics.* Philadelphia, Lea & Febiger, 1993, pp. 81–100.

Romano, J.E.: AIDS Social Policy Education for the Dental Hygienist, Thesis submitted in partial fulfillment for the Master of Arts, State University of New York, Empire State College, Saratoga, New York, 1997.

Exposure Control: Barriers for Patient and Clinician

Exposure control refers to all procedures during clinical care necessary to provide top-level protection from exposure to infectious agents for members of the dental team and their patients. Dental health-care personnel (DHCP) have a professional obligation to serve *all* patients with comprehensive oral care, including patients with known or unknown communicable diseases. The practice of *standard precautions* means that the body fluids of all patients are treated as if they were infectious.

An organized system for exposure control is needed. First, a written exposure control plan is prepared to serve as a guide for the entire team.[1] Consistency between DHCPs is necessary to maintain standards of asepsis and to prevent cross-contamination. The written plan can be the basis for training new personnel. As new research and commercial products become available, the written protocol must be revised.

Using the protocol and transferring the objectives and overall aims to the clinical setting are the responsibilities of each member of the dental team. It should be realized that physical barriers and other requirements of the protocol provide safety for both the DHCP and the patient. Selected terms for the application of exposure control and immunizations are defined in Box 3-1. Refer to Appendix III page 1133 to review specific recommendations from the U.S. Department of Health and Human Services.

BOX 3-1 KEY WORDS AND ABBREVIATIONS: Exposure Control

Allergen: substance, protein or nonprotein, capable of inducing allergy or specific hypersensitivity; can enter the body by being inhaled, swallowed, touched, or injected.

Hypoallergenic: property of a substance that indicates it does not create a hypersensitive reaction; may apply to various chemicals; not specified on manufacturer's labels.

Antimicrobial soap: a soap containing an active ingredient against skin microorganisms.

Atopy: clinical hypersensitivity state or allergy with a hereditary predisposition; includes hay fever, eczema, and asthma.

Barrier protection: refers to placing a physical barrier between the patient's body fluids (such as blood and saliva) and the health-care personnel (HCP) to prevent disease transmission.

Barriers for HCP: include gloves, mask, protective eyewear, and protective clothing (gown).

Barriers for patient: include protective eyewear, headcover during surgeries, and rubber dam during restorative and sealant procedures.

Booster dose: amount of immunogen (vaccine, toxoid, or other antigen preparation), usually smaller than the original amount, injected at an appropriate interval after the primary immunization to sustain the immune response to that immunogen.

Exposure incident: a specific eye, mouth, mucous membrane, nonintact skin, or parenteral contact with blood or other potentially infectious material that results from the performance of one's usual professional duties.

Immunization: the process of rendering a subject immune to a particular disease by stimulation with a specific antigen to promote antibody formation in the body.

Inoculation: introduction of antigenic material or vaccine; more frequently used to refer to introduction of material into a culture medium.

Latex allergy: an acquired hypersensitivity reaction to the proteins found in natural rubber latex (NRL).

Occupational exposure: reasonably anticipated skin, eye, mucous membrane, or parenteral contact with blood or other potentially infectious materials that may result from the performance of one's usual duties.

PPD: purified protein derivative for tuberculin intracutaneous skin test for tuberculosis; positive reaction means previous infection with *Mycobacterium tuberculosis.*

Rhinitis: inflammation of the mucous membrane of the nose; may result from infection by bacteria or virus, or may be a seasonal (hay fever) or nonseasonal allergic reaction.

Toxoid: toxin treated by heat or chemical agent to destroy its deleterious properties without destroying its ability to combine with, or stimulate the formation of, antitoxin; examples of toxoids used for active immunization are tetanus and diphtheria.

Tuberculin test (Mantoux): a test for the presence of active or inactive tuberculosis; a positive test is denoted by redness and induration at the injection site by 48 to 72 hours after injection.

Vaccination: process of introducing a vaccine into the body to produce immunity to a specific disease.

Vaccine: a suspension of attenuated or killed microorganisms administered for the prevention or treatment of an infectious disease.

▪ PERSONAL PROTECTION OF THE DENTAL TEAM

The continuing health and productivity of dental health personnel depend to a large degree on the control of cross-contamination. Loss of work time, personal suffering, long-term systemic effects, and even exclusion from continued practice are possible results from communicable diseases. The only safe procedure is to practice defensively at all times, with specific precautions for personal protection.

In this section, topics include immunizations and periodic tests; clothing; barriers to infectious microorganisms, such as face mask and protective eyewear; personal hygiene; handwashing; gloves; and habits.

▪ IMMUNIZATIONS AND PERIODIC TESTS

Dental personnel in a hospital setting are subject to the rules and regulations for all hospital employees. Policies usually require certain immunizations for new employees if written proof of immunizations is not available and tests for antibodies prove to be negative.

In private dental practices, individual initiative is required to maintain standards of safety for all dental team members. All staff members should be well aware of the signs and symptoms of diseases that are occupational hazards. All must be encouraged to seek early diagnosis and treatment of a seemingly minor condition that could be the initial symptom of a more serious communicable disease.

At the time of employment, it is reasonable for a dentist-employer to request of employees a record of current immunizations and their most recent updating, as well as specific tests, such as for tuberculosis. Immunization for rubella is particularly important for female employees of childbearing age.

I. IMMUNIZATIONS

A. Basic Schedule[2,3]

The immunization schedule for infants and children includes protection against poliomyelitis, diphtheria, tetanus, pertussis (whooping cough), measles, mumps, rubella (German measles), influenza, and hepatitis B.

Immunization is required for children either at school entry or at entry into middle or junior high school (at 5 to 6 years or 11 to 12 years of age) if not immunized previously.

For adolescents aged 11 to 21 years, which includes college students, planned immunizations aim to vaccinate those who have not previously been vaccinated, provide booster shots, and promote preventive health services.[3]

B. Booster and Reimmunization

Each agent requires booster or reimmunization on a specific plan, which may range from 1 to 10 years, or reimmunization only upon intimate contact or exposure. The needs differ in different climates, countries, and locations. Persons moving or traveling need to become aware of specific precautions.

For tetanus boosters, intervals of 10 years are indicated. If an injury occurs, however, a booster should be given on the day of the injury.[4]

C. Adult Immunizations

The Advisory Committee on Immunization Practices (ACIP) revises the schedule for adults, and another for children, periodically in keeping with new research findings and the release of new vaccines and toxoids. The adult recommendations are divided into two components by age and medical conditions. All immunizations are recommended for all dental healthcare personnel.

The current recommendations are as follows[5]:

- **Tetanus & Diphtheria** (Td): Primary series for adults is 3 doses; 1 dose booster every 10 years
- **Influenza:** 1 dose annually
- **Pneumococcal** (polysaccharide): 1 dose
- **Hepatitis B:** 3 doses (0, 1-2, 4-6 months)
- **Hepatitis A:** 2 doses (0, 6-12 months)
- **Measles, Mumps, Rubella (MMR):** (1 dose if MMR vaccination history is unreliable; 2 doses for persons with occupational or other indications); catch-up on childhood vaccinations
- **Varicella** (chicken pox): 2 doses (0, 4-8 weeks) for persons who are susceptible; catch-up on childhood vaccinations
- **Meningococcal** (polysaccharide): 1 dose

II. MANAGEMENT PROGRAM

A. Recommended Tests

1. Annual tuberculin test (Mantoux); chest radiograph as indicated.
2. Periodic throat culture for possible hemolytic streptococcus carrier.

B. Obtaining Tests

Obtain tests promptly when exposed to certain infectious diseases and seek prophylactic immunization as indicated and available.

C. Written Records

Keep confidential written records of immunizations, boosters, and reimmunizations; plan for regular follow-up. When the status of current immunizations is known, time is saved by not needing a susceptibility test prior to initiating passive immunizations when accidental exposure occurs.

▪ CLINICAL ATTIRE

The wearing apparel of clinicians and their assistants is vulnerable to contamination from splash, spatter, aerosols, and patient contact. The gown or uniform should be designed and cared for in a manner that minimizes cross-contamination.

I. GOWN OR UNIFORM

Gowns or uniforms are expected to be clean and maintained as free as possible from contamination. Wearing clinic coats over street clothes is not recommended because of the exposure of the street clothes to infectious material.

A. Solid, Closed Front

The garment should be closed at the neck and tie in back, preferably. The fabric should be disposable or able to be washed commercially and withstand washing with bleach.

B. No Pockets

Pockets are too readily available for placing contaminated objects, such as writing implements or keys. Gloved hands, prepared for patient treatment, must be kept from touching objects or being placed in pockets.

C. Long Garment to Cover Lap When Seated for Patient Treatment

Long sleeves with fitted cuffs permit protective gloves to extend over the cuffs.

II. HAIR AND HEAD COVERING

A. Hair must be worn off the shoulders and fastened back away from the face. When longer, it should be held within a head cover. Because the hair is exposed to much contamination, an appropriate head cover is advised when using handpieces and ultrasonic or air-powder polishing instruments.

B. Facial hair should be covered with a face mask and face shield.

III. PROTECTION OF UNIFORM

A plastic washable or a disposable apron may be used when clinical services are performed that usually involve blood, spatter, or aerosols.

IV. OUTSIDE WEAR

Clinic uniforms and shoes should not be worn outside the clinic practice setting.[6] When clinical clothing is worn outside, contamination can be carried from, and brought into, the treatment area.

Commercial laundry services are preferred. When laundered at home, the items from a dental office or clinic should be kept separate and treated with household bleach for disinfection.

▪ USE OF FACE MASK: RESPIRATORY PROTECTION

Basic personal barrier protection is composed of face mask, protective eyewear, and gloves. The use of the face mask is described first because it should be positioned first when preparing for clinical care procedures. The protective eyewear is placed second. After that, the hands can be washed prior to gloving.

Dispersion of particles of debris, polishing agents, calculus, and water, all of which are contaminated by the patient's oral flora, occurs regularly during instrumentation. The greatest aerosols are created following the use of a handpiece, prophylaxis angle, or power-driven scaler. Evidence of the spread of particles appears on the splashed face, protective eyewear, and uniform and on the coverall placed over the patient for protection from the spray.

I. MASK EFFICIENCY

A. Criteria: Essential Characteristics (Box 3-2)

1. *Filtration* (measured in BFE = bacterial filtration efficiency). Standard masks block filtration of particles as small as 3 μm with a filter efficiency greater than 95%. Particles of 3 μm and smaller can penetrate to the alveoli of the lower respiratory tract, where their infectivity is increased. Droplet nuclei (*Mycobacterium tuberculosis*) range from 0.5 to 1 μm and are a risk in health-care settings.[7]
2. *Fit.* Proper fit over face is vital to protect against inhaling droplet nuclei from aerosols.

BOX 3-2 Characteristics of an ideal mask

1. No contact with the wearer's nostrils or lips

2. Has a high bacterial filtration efficiency rate

3. Fits snugly around the entire edges of the mask

4. No fogging of eyewear

5. Convenient to put on and remove

6. Made of material that does not irritate skin or induce allergic reaction

7. Does not collapse during wear or when wet

(Adapted from Molinari, J.A.: Face Masks: Effective Personal Protection, *Compend. Cont. Educ. Dent., 17*, 818, September, 1996.)

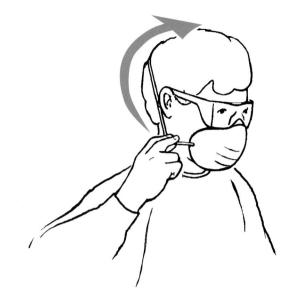

■ **FIGURE 3-1 Removal of Mask.** Handle only by the elastic or tie strings, carefully avoiding the contaminated mask.

3. *Moisture Absorption.* Soak through is an important factor. Lining should be impervious. Mask must be changed for each patient and not worn longer than 1 hour.
4. *Comfort.* Degree of comfort should encourage compliance in wearing.

B. Materials

Various materials have been used for masks, including gauze and other cloth, plastic foam, fiberglass, synthetic fiber mat, and paper. In research studies, foam, paper, and cloth were found to be the least adequate filters of aerosols, whereas glass fiber and synthetic fiber mat were shown to be the most effective.[8,9]

II. USE OF A MASK

A. Adjust the mask and position eyewear before a handwash.
B. Use a fresh mask for each patient.
   1. Change mask each hour or more frequently when it becomes wet.
   2. Chin-cover face shield needs to be supplemented with fitted mask.
C. Keep the mask on after completing a procedure while still in the presence of aerosols. Particles smaller than 5 µm remain suspended longer (up to 24 hours) than do larger particles and can be inhaled directly into terminal lung alveoli. Removal of a mask in the treatment room immediately following the use of aerosol-producing procedures permits direct exposure to airborne organisms.

D. Mask Removal
   1. Grasp side elastic or tie strings to remove (Figure 3-1).
   2. Never handle the outside of a contaminated mask with gloved or bare hands. Never place the mask under the chin.

■ USE OF PROTECTIVE EYEWEAR

Eye protection for the dental team members and patients is necessary to prevent physical injuries and infections of the eyes.

Severe and disabling eye accidents and infections have been reported.[10-12] Eye involvement may lead to pain, discomfort, loss of work time, and, in certain instances, permanent injury. Accidents can occur at any time, and as with most accidents, they occur when least prepared for or expected.

Eye infections can follow the accidental dropping of an instrument on the face or the splashing of various materials from a patient's oral cavity into the eye. Contamination can be introduced from saliva, biofilm, carious material, pieces of old restorative materials during cavity preparation, bacteria-laden calculus during scaling, and any other microorganisms contained in aerosols or spatter. An aerosol created by a power-driven scaler can be heavily contaminated with oral microorganisms.

Careful, deliberate techniques and instrument management, with evacuation and other procedures for the control of oral fluids, contribute to the prevention of accidents and infections of the eyes. All measures described for prevention of airborne disease transmission by aerosols and spatter apply to eye protection. The most effective defense is the use of protective eyewear by all involved, dental team members and patients.

I. INDICATIONS FOR USE OF PROTECTIVE EYEWEAR

A. Dental Team Members

Protective eyewear should be worn for all procedures. For dental personnel who do not require a corrective lens for vision, protective eyewear with a clear lens should be a routine part of clinical dress.

B. Patients

Protective eyewear is essential for each patient at each appointment. The patient's medical history should reflect types of eye surgery, implants, or other special concerns.

Patients with their own prescription lenses may prefer to wear them, but for the safety of the patient's glasses, the use of the protective eyewear provided in the office or clinic may be advisable.

II. PROTECTIVE EYEWEAR

A. General Features of Acceptable Eyewear

1. Wide coverage, with side shields, to protect around the eye.
2. Shatterproof; made of strong, sturdy plastic.
3. Lightweight.
4. Flexible and with rounded smooth edges to prevent discomfort if pressed against the nose or ears.
5. Easily disinfected.
    a. Surface areas should be smooth to prevent accumulation of infectious material.
    b. Frames and lens should not be damaged or distorted by the disinfectant used.
6. A clear or lightly tinted lens, rather than a very dark lens, permits the dental team members to watch the patient's reactions and maintain contact and response.
7. Protection against glare. Certain patients may request tinted lenses or prefer to wear their own sunglasses when their eyes are especially sensitive to the dental light.

B. Types of Eyewear

Many styles, including regular eyeglass shapes and those described as follows, have been used.
1. *Goggles* (Figure 3-2A). Shielding on all sides of the glasses may give the best protection, pro-

vided they fit closely around the edges. Goggle-style coverage is especially necessary for protection during laboratory work.
2. *Eyewear With Side Shields* (Figure 3-2B and C). A side shield can provide added protection. For the member of the dental team who depends on a prescription lens, separate side shields are available that can be connected to the bows.
3. *Eyewear With Curved Frames.* When the sides of the eyewear are curved back, they may provide a protection somewhat similar to that offered by those with the side shield.
4. *Postmydriatic Spectacles Used by Ophthalmologist.* Disposable glasses are available that are made of flexible plastic.

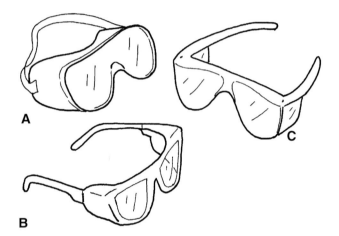

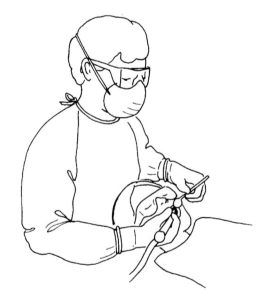

■ **FIGURE 3-2 Protective Eyewear.** Protective cover for both patient and clinician may be goggles-style **(A)** or glasses with side shields **(B and C)**.

5. *Child-Sized.* Child-sized sunglasses and children's play spectacles have been used.

C. Face Shield

Clinician needs to wear a face shield over a regular mask when aerosol-producing handpiece, power scaler, or power polishing equipment is used.

III. SUGGESTIONS FOR CLINICAL APPLICATION

A. Patient Instruction

A patient who has not been asked to wear protective eyewear at previous appointments will appreciate a simple explanation of the reasons for doing so.

B. Contact Lenses

Dental team members and patients who wear contact lenses should always wear protective eyewear over them during dental and dental hygiene procedures.

C. Care of Protective Eyewear

1. Run eyewear under water stream to remove abrasive particles. Rubbing an abrasive agent over the plastic lens can create scratches.
2. Materials used for protective lens may be damaged by some disinfectants. Clean with detergent and rinse thoroughly.[13] Air dry.
3. Check periodically for scratches on the lens, and replace appropriately.

D. Eye Wash Station

The eye wash station equipment should not be connected to a sink used by clinicians for patient preparation. It must not be connected to the regular faucets unless the hot water source is turned off permanently.

■ HAND CARE

In the infectious process of disease transmission, the hands may serve as a *means of transmission* of the blood, saliva, and dental biofilm from a patient, and the hands, especially under the fingernails, may serve as a *reservoir* for microorganisms. Skin breaks in the hands may serve as a *port of entry* for potentially pathogenic microorganisms.

By caring properly for the hands, using effective washing procedures, and following the basic rules for gloving, primary cross-contamination can be controlled. A conscious effort must be made to keep the gloved hands from touching objects other than the instruments and

disinfected parts of the equipment prepared for the immediate patient.

I. BACTERIOLOGY OF THE SKIN[14]

A. Resident Bacteria

Many relatively stable bacteria inhabit the surface epithelium or deeper areas in the ducts of skin glands or depths of hair follicles; they are ultimately shed with the exfoliated surface cells, or with excretions of the skin glands. The flora may be altered by newly introduced pathogens or reduced by washing. Resident bacteria tend to be less susceptible to destruction by disinfection procedures.

B. Transient Bacteria

Transient bacteria reflect continuous contamination by routine contacts; some bacteria are pathogens and may act temporarily as residents. They may be washed away or, in the event that a skin break exists, may cause an autogenous infection. Most transients can be removed with soap and water by washing thoroughly.

II. HAND CARE

A. Fingernails

1. Maintain clean, smoothly trimmed, short fingernails with well-cared-for cuticles to prevent breaks where microorganisms can enter.
2. Effects of short nails.[15]
   a. Make handwashing more effective because of fewer microorganisms harbored under the nails.[16]
   b. Prevent cuts from nail in disposable gloves.
   c. Permit selection of a closer fit of glove; longer glove fingers may be required to protect nails.
   d. Allow greater dexterity during instrumentation.
   e. Decrease chance of patient discomfort.

B. Wristwatch and Jewelry

Remove hand and wrist jewelry at the beginning of the day. Microorganisms can become lodged in crevices of rings, watchbands, and watches, where scrubbing is impossible.

C. Gloves

1. After handwashing, don gloves. Never expose open skin lesions or abrasions to a patient's oral tissues and fluids.

2. After glove removal, wash hands to remove microorganisms.

■ HANDWASHING PRINCIPLES

I. RATIONALE

Effective and frequent handwashing can reduce the overall bacterial flora of the skin and prevent the organisms acquired from a patient from becoming skin residents. It is impossible to sterilize the skin, but every attempt must be made to reduce the bacterial flora to a minimum.

II. PURPOSES

The objective of all handwashing is to reduce the bacterial flora of the hands to an absolute minimum. An effective handwash procedure can be expected to accomplish the following:
  A. Remove surface dirt and transient bacteria.
  B. Dissolve the normal greasy film on the skin.
  C. Rinse and remove all loosened debris and microorganisms.
  D. Provide disinfection with a long-acting antiseptic.

III. FACILITIES

A. Sink

1. Use a sink with a foot pedal or electronic control for water-flow control to avoid contamination to/from faucet handles.
2. For regular sink, turn on water at the beginning and leave on through the entire procedure. Turn faucets off with the towel after drying hands.
3. Clean around brim of sink with disinfectant. The sink must be of sufficient size so that contact with the inside of the wash basin can be avoided easily. A sink cannot be sterilized and can be highly contaminated.
4. Prevent contamination of clothing by not leaning against the sink.
5. Use a separate area and sink reserved for instrument washing. Contaminated instruments must be removed from the treatment room prior to preparation for the next patient.

B. Soap

1. Use a liquid surgical scrub containing an antimicrobial agent. Povidone-iodine (iodophore) has a broad spectrum of action. Chlorhexidine preparations are used extensively to provide rapid disinfection and a cumulative, persistent (residual) action.
2. Apply from a foot- or knee-activated or electronically controlled dispenser to avoid contamina-

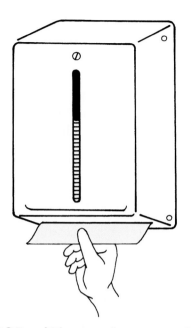

■ **FIGURE 3-3 Towel Dispenser.** Correct type of dispenser that requires no contact except with the towel itself, which hangs down from the container.

tion to and from a hand-operated dispenser or cake soap.
3. Rinsing is a very important part of the handwashing procedure.

C. Scrub Brushes

1. Avoid overvigorous use of a brush to minimize skin abrasion. Skin irritation and abrasion can leave openings for additional cross-contamination.
2. Disposable sponges are available commercially and may be preferred when a scrub brush is traumatic to the skin.

D. Towels

1. Obtain disposable towel from a dispenser that requires no contact except with the towel itself, which hangs down (Figure 3-3).
2. Cloth towels are not recommended.

■ METHODS OF HANDWASHING

Handwashing is considered the most important single procedure for the prevention of cross-contamination.

I. INDICATIONS

- Before and after treating each patient (before glove placement and after glove removal)
- Before regloving after removing gloves that are torn, cut, or punctured

- After barehanded touching inanimate objects that may be contaminated with blood or saliva
- When hands are visibly soiled
- Before leaving the treatment room

II. DEFINITIONS[17]

A. Routine Handwash

- Water and nonantimicrobial soap (plain soap)
- To remove soil and transient microorganisms

B. Antiseptic Handwash

- Water and antimicrobial liquid soap (eg, chlorhexidine, iodine and iodophors, chloroxylenol [PCMX], triclosan)
- To remove or destroy transient microorganisms and reduce resident flora

C. Antiseptic Hand Rub

- Alcohol-based hand rub (contains 60-95% ethanol or isopropanol)
- To remove or destroy transient microorganisms and reduce resident flora

D. Surgical Antisepsis (also called Surgical Scrub)

- Water and antimicrobial liquid soap (eg, chlorhexidine, iodine and iodophores, chloroxylenol [PCMX], triclosan)
- To remove or destroy transient microorganisms and reduce resident flora with a persistent or prolonged effect that inhibits proliferation or survival of microorganisms

III. ROUTINE HANDWASH

- Wet hands, apply soap; avoid hot water.
- Rub hands together for at least 15 seconds; cover all surfaces of fingers, hands, and wrists.
- Interlace fingers and rub to cover all sides.
- Rinse under running water; dry thoroughly with disposable towels.
- Turn off faucet with the towel.
- Bar soap harbors microorganisms; keep on soap rack where drainage and drying is possible.

IV. ANTISEPTIC HANDWASH

A. Preliminary Steps

- Remove watch and jewelry from hands
- Fasten hair back securely

- Don protective eyewear and mask before handwashing to prevent contamination of washed hands ready for gloving
- Use cool water

B. Handwashing Procedure

- Lather hands, wrists, and forearms quickly with liquid antimicrobial soap.
- Rub all surfaces vigorously; interlace fingers and rub back and forth with pressure.
- Rinse thoroughly, running the water from fingertips down the hands. Keep water running.
- Repeat two more times. One lathering for 3 minutes is less effective than are 3 short latherings and 3 rinses in 30 seconds. The latherings serve to loosen the debris and microorganisms and the rinsings wash them away.
- Use paper towels for drying, taking care not to recontaminate.

V. ANTISEPTIC HAND RUB

- Decontaminate hands with an alcohol-based hand rub
- Apply the product (follow manufacturer's directions for amount to use) to the palm of one hand, and rub hands together
- Rub hands vigorously, covering all surfaces of fingers and hands, until the hands are dry.

VI. SURGICAL ANTISEPSIS

Each hospital or oral surgery clinic has rules and regulations for surgical antisepsis. These should be posted over the scrub sinks.

A surgical antisepsis performed as the first of a day should be 10 minutes and subsequent ones may be 3 to 5 minutes. Following treatment of a contagious or isolated patient, the procedure should take at least 5 minutes.

A. Preliminary Steps

1. Remove watch and jewelry. Place hair and beard coverings and make sure hair is completely covered. Don protective eyewear and mask.
2. Open sterile brush package to have ready.
3. Wash hands and arms, using surgical liquid antimicrobial soap to remove gross surface dirt before using the scrub brush. Lather vigorously with strong rubbing motions, 10 on each side of hands, wrists, and arms. Interlace the fingers and thumbs to clean the proximal surfaces.
4. Rinse thoroughly from fingertips across hands and wrists. Hold hands higher than elbows throughout the procedure. Leave water running.

5. Use orangewood stick from the sterile package to clean nails. Rinse.

B. First Hand

1. Lather the hands and arms and leave the lather on to increase the exposure time to the antimicrobial ingredient.
2. Apply surgical liquid antimicrobial soap, and begin the brush procedure. Scrub in an orderly sequence without returning to areas previously scrubbed.
3. First hand and arm.
   a. Brush back and forth across nails and fingertips, passing the brush under the nails.
   b. Fingers and hand. Use small circular strokes on all sides of the thumb and each finger, overlapping strokes for complete coverage.
   c. Continue to wrist. Apply more soap to maintain a good lather.
   d. When arm is completed, leave lather on.

C. Second Hand

1. Repeat on other arm. Some systems require the use of a second sterile brush for the second hand. When this is so, discard the first brush into the proper container and obtain the second brush.
2. At one-half of scrub time, rinse hands and arms thoroughly, first one and then the other, starting at the fingertips and letting water pass down over the arm.
3. Lather and repeat.
4. At end of time (or counts), rinse thoroughly, each arm separately, from fingertips. Apply towel from fingertips to elbow without reapplying to hand area.
5. Hold hands up and clasped together. Proceed to dressing area for gowning and gloving.

■ GLOVES AND GLOVING

Wearing gloves is standard practice to protect both the patient and the clinician from cross-contamination.

I. CRITERIA FOR SELECTION OF TREATMENT/EXAMINATION GLOVES

A. Safety Factors

1. Effective barrier; evidence from manufacturer of quality control standards.
2. Impermeable to patient's saliva, blood, and bacteria.
3. Strength and durability to resist tears and punctures.
4. Impervious to materials routinely used during clinical procedures.
5. Nonirritating or harmful to skin; use nonlatex gloves when patient or clinician is allergic.

B. Comfort Factors

1. Fit hand well; no interference with motion; glove cuff extends to provide coverage over cuff of long sleeve.
2. Tactile sense minimally decreased.
3. Taste and odor not unpleasant for patient.

II. TYPES OF GLOVES

A. Material

1. Latex.
2. Nonlatex: neoprene, block copolymer, vinyl, N-nitrile.

B. For Patient Care

1. *Nonsterile Single-Use Examination/Treatment.* Latex, nonlatex.
2. *Presterilized Single-Use Surgical.* Latex, nonlatex.

C. Utility Gloves

1. *Heavy duty.* Latex, nonlatex (puncture resistant for clinic cleanup).
2. *Plastic.* Food handler's glove to wear as overglove.

D. Dermal Underglove: To Reduce Irritation from Latex or Nonlatex.

III. PROCEDURES FOR USE OF GLOVES

A. Mask and Eyewear Placement

Place mask and protective eyewear prior to handwashing and gloving to prevent the need for manipulating the mask around the face and hair after washing the hands.

B. Pregloving Handwash

1. Use an antiseptic handwash prior to gloving.
2. Hands must be dried thoroughly to control moisture inside glove and thus discourage growth of bacteria.

C. Glove Placement

1. Always glove and deglove in front of the patient; a patient may need assurance that gloves are new and used only for that appointment.
2. Place gloves over the cuff of long-sleeved clinic wear to provide complete protection of arms from exposure to contamination.

D. Avoiding Contamination

Keep gloved hands away from face, hair, clothing (pockets), telephone, patient records, clinician's stool, and all parts of the dental equipment that have not been predisinfected and covered with a barrier material.

E. Torn, Cut, or Punctured Glove

Remove immediately, wash hands thoroughly, and don new gloves.

F. Removal of Gloves

1. Develop a procedure whereby gloves can be removed without contaminating the hands from the exposed external surfaces of the gloves. Figure 3-4 illustrates one system for glove removal.
2. Wash hands promptly after glove removal. Organisms on the hands multiply rapidly inside the warm, moist environment of the glove, even when no external contamination has occurred.

IV. FACTORS AFFECTING GLOVE INTEGRITY

A. Length of Time Worn

New pair for each patient is the basic requirement; total time worn should be no longer than 1 hour; when gloves develop a sticky surface, remove, wash hands, and reglove with a fresh pair.

B. Complexity of the Procedure

Certain procedures are more likely to promote perforations, especially when sharp instruments must be changed frequently.

C. Packaging of the Gloves

Top gloves of a new package are tightly packed and can be torn when removed; must be handled carefully until pressure is relieved.

D. Size of Glove

When too long, the extra material at the fingertips can get caught, torn, or in the way; picking up small objects is difficult, especially sharp instruments.

E. Pressure of Time

Stress; working too fast increases the risk of glove damage.

F. Storage of Gloves

Keep in cool, dark place; exposure to heat, sun, or fluorescent light increases potential for deterioration and perforations.

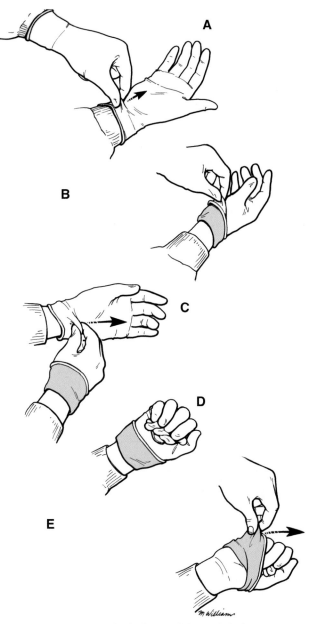

■ **FIGURE 3-4 Removal of Gloves. (A)** Use left fingers to pinch right glove near edge to fold back. **(B)** Fold edge back without contact with clean inside surface. **(C)** Use right fingers to contact outside of left glove at the wrist to invert and remove. **(D)** Bunch glove into the palm. **(E)** With ungloved left hand, grasp inner noncontaminated portion of the right glove to peel it off, enclosing other glove as it is inverted.

G. Agents Used

Certain chemicals react with the glove material; for example, petroleum jelly, alcohol, and products made with alcohol tend to break down the glove integrity.

H. Hazards From the Hands

Long fingernails and rings worn inside gloves.

▪ LATEX HYPERSENSITIVITY

Patients and clinicians may have or may develop a sensitivity to natural rubber latex. Symptoms of a hypersensitive reaction range from a dermatitis to a life-threatening anaphylactic shock. The only available treatment for latex allergy is avoiding all contact.

Latex sensitivity is due to the protein allergens and to additives used when the commercial latex is prepared. Latex allergens occur in any equipment or product used that contains natural rubber latex. Box 3-3 lists a few of the possible sources. Gloves are the most frequently used, and when powdered (cornstarch), the allergen can become airborne and be dispersed throughout the clinical area and on the personnel.

Equipment listed in Box 3-3 may contain NRL. However, many of the items also are made of alternative materials. When the label on a product does not list the contents, the manufacturer should be contacted to identify latex-free items.

I. CLINICAL MANIFESTATIONS

A. Methods of Exposure

1. Aeroallergen inhalation (from powdered gloves).
2. Donning gloves.
3. Mucosal contact.

B. Type I Hypersensitivity (immediate reaction)

1. Urticaria: hives.
2. Dermatitis: rash, itching.
3. Nasal problems: sneezing, itchy nose, runny nose.

BOX 3-3 Equipment that may contain latex

Gloves	Stopper in anesthesia carpule
Masks (elastic head band)	
Goggles	Orthodontic elastics
Rubber dam	Bite blocks
Nitrous oxide nosepiece and tubing	Mixing bowl
O ring (on ultrasonic insert)	Suction adapter
Lead apron cover	Blood pressure cuff
Rubber polishing cup	Stethoscope

---

4. Respiratory reaction: breathing difficulty, asthmalike wheezing, coughing.
5. Eyes: watery, itchy.
6. Drop in blood pressure: shock.
7. Anaphylaxis.

C. Type IV Hypersensitivity (delayed reaction)

Contact dermatitis develops 6 to 72 hours after contact.

II. INDIVIDUALS AT HIGH RISK OF LATEX SENSITIVITY

A. Have Had Frequent Exposure to Latex Products

1. Occupational exposure: health-care personnel who wear latex gloves regularly for patient care.
2. Multiple medical surgeries or treatments requiring placement of rubber tubes or drains. Examples: genitourinary anomalies, spina bifida.

Everyday Ethics

? After Mr. Green's dental hygiene treatment is completed, the dentist, Dr. Root, is notified so that the final examination can be made. Dr. Root comes in shortly and sits down next to the patient. He browses through the notations made in the patient's chart and then picks up the mirror and explorer to proceed with a clinical examination. It is apparent that he has not washed his hands or donned a new pair of gloves. This situation has happened occasionally before.

Questions for Consideration

1. Mabel, the dental hygienist, notes that the dentist did not change his gloves or wash his hands. What choices of action are there to take in such a situation?

2. As the situation is analyzed, would this be considered an ethical issue or an ethical dilemma? Why?

3. How is beneficence for this patient threatened?

Factors To Teach The Patient

- Importance of the patient's complete history for the protection of both the patient and the professional person.
- Necessity for use of barriers (face mask, protective eyewear, and gloves) by the clinician for the benefit of the patient.
- Importance of eye protection.

B. Have Other Documented Allergies

Examples: food allergies (avocado, banana, kiwi fruit, chestnuts, papaya).

C. Worker in a Rubber-Manufacturing Plant

III. MANAGEMENT

A. Medical History

1. Questions in history should reveal all allergies.
2. Questions directed to latex may not suffice. Questions about other specific products should be asked.
3. Advise allergic patients to obtain and wear an alert badge (bracelet).

B. Document

All information should be carefully recorded for continuing reference.

C. Appointment Planning for Allergic Patient

1. *Early in the Day*. Meet before glove powder contaminates the air throughout the facility. Outerwear of clinical attire becomes laden with airborne latex.
2. *Clean Clinical Areas*
   a. Person preparing room must wear nonlatex gloves.
   b. Wipe all surfaces to remove allergen.
3. *No Latex in the Treatment Room*. Use nonlatex products for high-risk patients (whether or not specific latex sensitivity has been known and reported in the history).
4. *Prepare Latex-Free Carts*.[18] Materials and gloves, for use when seeing high-risk patients, can be readied in advance.

E. Emergency Treatment Equipment and Drugs Ready

1. Inform the entire dental team of appointment.
2. Have a latex-free emergency cart available.[18]
3. Alert for emergency.

REFERENCES

1. **United States Department of Labor**, Occupational Safety and Health Administration: Controlling Occupational Exposure to Bloodborne Pathogens in Dentistry, OSHA 3129, 1992. United States Government Printing Office: 1992–312-410/64790.
2. **United States Centers for Disease Control and Prevention, Advisory Committee on Immunization Practices (ACIP)**: Recommended Childhood Immunization Schedule—United States, 1998, *MMWR, 47*, 8, January 16, 1998.
3. **United States Centers for Disease Control and Prevention**: Immunization of Adolescents, *MMWR, 45*, 1–13, No. RR-13, November 22, 1996.
4. **Benenson**, A.S., ed.: *Control of Communicable Disease in Man*, 16th ed. Washington, D.C., American Public Health Association, 1995, p. 464.
5. **United States Centers for Disease Control and Prevention**: Recommended Adult Immunization Schedule—United States, 2003-2004, *MMWR, 52,* 965, October 10, 2003.
6. **Federation Dentaire Internationale**, Commission on Dental Practice: Technical Report: Recommendations for Hygiene in Dental Practice, *Int. Dent. J., 29*, 72, March, 1979.
7. **United States Centers for Disease Control**: Guidelines for Preventing the Transmission of *Mycobacterium tuberculosis* in Health-care Facilities, *MMWR, 43*, 1–132, No. RR-13, October 28, 1994.
8. **Micik**, R.E., Miller, R.L., and Leong, A.C.: Studies on Dental Aerobiology: III. Efficacy of Surgical Masks in Protecting Dental Personnel from Airborne Bacterial Particles, *J. Dent. Res., 50*, 626, May–June, 1971.
9. **Miller**, R.L. and Micik, R.E.: Air Pollution and Its Control in the Dental Office, *Dent. Clin. North Am., 22*, 453, July, 1978.
10. **Cooley**, R.L., Cottingham, A.J., Abrams, H., and Barkmeier, W.W.: Ocular Injuries Sustained in the Dental Office: Methods of Detection, Treatment, and Prevention, *J. Am. Dent. Assoc., 97*, 985, December, 1978.
11. **Wesson**, M.D. and Thornton, J.B.: Eye Protection and Ocular Complications in the Dental Office, *Gen. Dent., 37*, 19, January–February, 1989.
12. **Roberts-Harry**, T.J., Cass, A.E., and Jagger, J.D.: Ocular Injury and Infection in Dental Practice: A Survey and a Review of the Literature, *Br. Dent. J., 170*, 20, January 5, 1991.
13. **Office of Safety and Asepsis Procedures Research Foundation**: The Dental Infection Control Program, *OSAP Monthly Focus*, Focus no. 2, p. 2, 1998.
14. **Gröschel**, D.H.M. and Pruett, T.L.: Surgical Antisepsis, in Block, S.S.: *Disinfection, Sterilization, and Preservation*, 4th ed. Philadelphia, Lea & Febiger, 1991, pp. 642–648.
15. **Harfst**, S.A.: Personal Barrier Protection, *Dent. Clin. North Am., 35*, 357, April, 1991.
16. **Allen**, A.L. and Organ, R.J.: Occult Blood Accumulation Under the Fingernails: A Mechanism for the Spread of Blood-borne Infection, *J. Am. Dent. Assoc., 105*, 455, September, 1982.
17. **United States Department of Health and Human Services, Centers for Disease Control and Prevention**: Guidelines for Infection Control in Dental Health-care Settings–2003, *MMWR, 52*, 15, RR-17, December 19, 2003.

18. **Falcone**, K.J. and Powers, D.O.: Latex Allergy: Implications for Oral Health Care Professionals, *J. Dent. Hyg., 72,* 25, Summer, 1998.

SUGGESTED READINGS

Cottone, J.A., Terezhalmy, G.T., and Molinari, J.A.: *Practical Infection Control in Dentistry,* 2nd ed. Philadelphia, Williams & Wilkins, 1996, pp. 127–145.

Fedson, D.S.: Adult Immunization: Summary of the National Vaccine Advisory Committee Report, *JAMA, 272,* 1133, October 12, 1994.

Foley, E.S.: Update on Clinical Attire Requirements in Dental Hygiene Programs, *J. Dent. Hyg., 68,* 131, May–June, 1994.

Harfst, S.: Infection Control Update: Vaccinations, *J. Pract. Hyg., 5,* 43, July/August, 1996.

Hill, J.G., Grimwood, R.E., Hermesch, C.B., and Marks, J.G.: Prevalence of Occupationally Related Hand Dermatitis in Dental Workers, *J. Am. Dent. Assoc., 129,* 212, February, 1998.

McDonnell, W.M. and Askari, F.K.: Molecular Medicine: DNA Vaccines, *N. Engl. J. Med., 334,* 42, January 4, 1996.

Miller, C.H. and Palenik, C.J.: *Infection Control and Management of Hazardous Materials for the Dental Team.* St. Louis, Mosby, 1994, pp. 106–131.

Molinari, J.A.: Dermatitis in Dental Professionals: Causes, Treatment, and Prevention, *J. Pract. Hyg., 5,* 13, July/August, 1996.

Eye Protection

Christensen, R.P., Robison, R.A., Robinson, D.F., Ploeger, B.J., and Leavitt, R.W.: Efficiency of 42 Brands of Face Masks and Two Face Shields in Preventing Inhalation of Airborne Debris, *Gen. Dent., 39,* 414, November/December, 1991.

Ing, E., Ing, H.C., Ing, M., Fusco, D., and Ing, T.G.E.: Diagnosing Oral Diseases That Affect the Eyes, *J. Am. Dent. Assoc., 125,* 608, May, 1994.

Miller, C.: Make Eye Protection a Priority to Prevent Contamination and Injury, *RDH, 15,* 40, October, 1995.

Pacak-Carroll, D.: Remember Eye Protection is Necessary for Patients Too, *RDH, 12,* 14, June, 1992.

Shingleton, B.J.: Eye Injuries, *N. Engl. J. Med., 325,* 408, August 8, 1991.

Stokes, A.N., Burton, J.F., and Beale, R.P.: Eye Protection in Dental Practice, *N.Z. Dent. J., 86,* 14, January, 1990.

Gloves

Boyer, E.M.: The Effectiveness of a Low-Chemical, Low-Protein Medical Glove to Prevent or Reduce Dermatological Problems, *J. Dent. Hyg., 69,* 67, March–April, 1995.

Brownson, K.M. and Gobetti, J.P.: Fluorescein Dye Evaluation of Double-Gloving, *Gen. Dent., 38,* 362, September–October, 1990.

Brunick, A.L., Burns, S., Gross, K., Tishk, M., and Feil, P.: A Comparative Study: The Effects of Latex and Vinyl Gloves on the Tactile Discrimination of First Year Dental Hygiene Students, *Clin. Prev. Dent., 12,* 21, June–July, 1990.

Burke, F.J.T. and Wilson, N.H.F.: The Incidence of Undiagnosed Punctures in Non-sterile Gloves, *Br. Dent. J., 168,* 67, January 20, 1990.

Chua, K.L., Taylor, G.S., and Bagg, J.: A Clinical and Laboratory Evaluation of Three Types of Operating Gloves for Use in Orthodontic Practice, *Br. J. Orthod., 23,* 115, May, 1996.

European Panel for Infection Control in Dentistry (EPICD): Hand Hygiene, Hand Care and Hand Protection for Clinical Dental Practice, *Br. Dent. J., 176,* 129, February 19, 1994.

Molinari, J.A.: Handwashing and Hand Care: Fundamental Asepsis Requirements, *Compend. Cont. Educ. Dent., 16,* 834, September, 1995.

Munksgaard, E.C.: Permeability of Protective Gloves to (di)Methacrylates in Resinous Dental Materials, *Scand. J. Dent. Res., 100,* 189, June, 1992.

Patton, L.L., Campbell, T.L., and Evers, S.P.: Prevalence of Glove Perforations During Double-Gloving for Dental Procedures, *Gen. Dent., 43,* 22, January–February, 1995.

Powell, B.J., Winkley, G.P., Brown, J.O., and Etersque, S.: Evaluating the Fit of Ambidextrous and Fitted Gloves: Implications for Hand Discomfort, *J. Am. Dent. Assoc., 125,* 1235, September, 1994.

Schwimmer, A., Massoumi, M., and Barr, C.E.: Efficacy of Double Gloving to Prevent Inner Glove Perforation During Outpatient Oral Surgical Procedures, *J. Am. Dent. Assoc., 125,* 196, February, 1994.

Shah, M., Lewis, F.M., and Gawkrodger, D.J.: Delayed and Immediate Orofacial Reactions Following Contact With Rubber Gloves During Treatment, *Br. Dent. J., 181,* 137, August 24, 1996.

Tinsley, D. and Chadwick, R.G.: The Permeability of Dental Gloves Following Exposure to Certain Dental Materials, *J. Dent., 25,* 65, January, 1997.

Latex Hypersensitivity

Brick, P. and Berthold, M.: Latex Allergies: The Hidden Occupational Hazard, *Access, 10,* 17, December, 1996.

Field, E.A. and Fay, M.F.: Issues of Latex Safety in Dentistry, *Br. Dent. J., 179,* 247, October 7, 1995.

Haman, C.P., Turjanmaa, K., Rietschel, R., Siew, C., Owensby, D., Gruninger, S.E., and Sullivan, K.M.: Natural Rubber Latex Hypersensitivity: Incidence and Prevalence of Type I Allergy in the Dental Professional, *J. Am. Dent. Assoc., 129,* 43, January, 1998.

Miller, C.: Offices Manage Allergies to Latex Material by Understanding Risks, Reducing Exposure, *RDH, 17,* 43, May, 1997.

Roy, A., Epstein, J., and Onno, E.: Latex Allergies in Dentistry: Recognition and Recommendations, *J. Can. Dent. Assoc., 63,* 297, April, 1997.

Safadi, G.S., Safadi, T.J., Terezhalmy, G.T., Taylor, J.S., Battisto, J.R., and Melton, A.L.: Latex Hypersensitivity: Its Prevalence Among Dental Professionals, *J. Am. Dent. Assoc., 127,* 83, January, 1996.

Spina Bifida

Engibous, P.J., Kittle, P.E., Jones, H.L., and Vance, B.J.: Latex Allergy in Patients With Spina Bifida, *Pediatr. Dent., 15,* 364, September/October, 1993.

Nelson, L.P., Soporowski, N.J., and Shusterman, S.: Latex Allergies in Children With Spina Bifida: Relevance for the Pediatric Dentist, *Pediatr. Dent., 16,* 18, January/February, 1994.

Peters, H.C.: Latex Allergy and Spina Bifida, (Letter), *J. Can. Dent. Assoc., 60,* 177, March, 1994.

Infection Control: Clinical Procedures

The success of a planned system for control of disease transmission depends on the cooperative effort of each member of the dental health team. The aim is to provide the highest level of infection control possible and practical that will ensure a safe environment for both patients and clinicians.

The presence of specific disease-producing organisms is rarely known; therefore, application of protective, preventive procedures is needed prior to, during, and following *all* patient appointments. Definitions and abbreviations related to infection control are provided in Box 4-1.

I. OBJECTIVES OF INFECTION CONTROL

The following are necessary to prevent the transmission of infectious agents and eliminate cross-contamination:

A. Reduction of available pathogenic microorganisms to a level at which the normal resistance mechanisms of the body may prevent infection.

B. Elimination of cross-contamination by breaking the chain of infection.

C. Application of standard precautions by treating each patient as if all human blood and body fluids are known to be infectious for HIV, HBV, HCV, and other blood-borne pathogens.

II. BASIC CONSIDERATIONS FOR SAFE PRACTICE

Basic factors involved in the conduct of safe practice include the following, to be described in this chapter:

A. Treatment room features.

B. Instrument management.
  1. Precleaning.
  2. Sterilization and disinfection.

C. Preparation for appointment.

D. Unit water lines.

E. Environmental surfaces.

F. Care of sterile instruments.

G. Patient preparation.

H. Summary of procedures for the prevention of disease transmission.

I. Disposal of waste.

▪ TREATMENT ROOM FEATURES

The design of many treatment rooms may not be conducive to ideal planning for infection control. Changes can be made in routines so that updated, preferred systems can be adapted. When renovations or a new dental office or clinic are anticipated, plans must reflect the most advanced knowledge available relative to safety and disease control.

A partial list of notable features is included here and illustrated in Figure 4-1. The objective is to have materials, shapes, and surface textures that facilitate the effective use of infection control measures.

1. UNIT
   • Designed for easy cleaning and disinfection, with smooth, uncluttered surfaces.
   • Removable hoses that can be cleaned and disinfected.
   • Hoses that are not mechanically retractable, but are straight, not coiled, with round smooth outer surfaces.
   • Syringes with autoclavable tips or fitted with disposable tips.
   • Handpieces with anti-retraction valves.
   • Handpieces that can be autoclaved.

2. DENTAL CHAIR
   • Controls all foot operated. If manually operated, need disposable barrier cover for buttons (switches).
   • Surface and seamless finish of easily cleaned plastic material that withstands chemical disinfection without damage or discoloring; cloth upholstery to be avoided.

3. LIGHT
   • Foot-activated switches.
   • Removable handle for sterilization or disposable barrier cover.

4. CLINICIAN'S STOOL
   • Smooth, plastic material that is easily disinfected and has a minimum of seams and creases.
   • Foot-operated controls. If manually operated, must have a barrier cover for the control.

BOX 4-1 KEY WORDS AND ABBREVIATIONS: Infection Control

ADA: American Dental Association, 211 E. Chicago Ave., Chicago, IL 60611.

Antimicrobial agent: any agent that kills or suppresses the growth of microorganisms.

Antiseptic: a substance that prevents or arrests the growth or action of microorganisms either by inhibiting their activity or by destroying them; term used especially for preparations applied topically to living tissue.

Asepsis: free from contamination with microorganisms; includes sterile conditions in tissues and on materials, as obtained by exclusion, removing, or killing organisms.

> **Chain of asepsis:** a procedure that avoids transfer of infection. The "chain" implies that each step, related to the previous one, continues to be carried out without contamination.

Aseptic technique: procedures carried out in the absence of pathogenic microorganisms.

Bioburden: a microbiologic load, that is, the number of contaminating organisms present on a surface prior to sterilization or disinfection.

Biofilm: the surface film that contains microorganisms and other biologic substances.

Biohazard: a substance that poses a biologic risk because it is contaminated with biomaterial with a potential for transmitting infection.

Biologic indicator: a preparation of nonpathogenic microorganisms, usually bacterial spores, carried by an ampule or a specially impregnated paper enclosed within a package during sterilization and subsequently incubated to verify that sterilization has occurred.

Broad spectrum: indicates a range of activity of a drug or chemical substance against a wide variety of microorganisms.

Chemical indicator: a color change stripe or other mark, often on autoclave tape or bag, used to monitor the process of sterilization; color change indicates that the package has been brought to a specific temperature, but it is not an indicator of sterilization.

Contamination: introduction of microorganisms, blood, or other potentially infectious material or agent onto a surface or into tissue.

Decontamination: disinfection; use of physical or chemical means to remove, inactivate, or destroy pathogenic microorganisms on a surface or item to the extent that they are no longer capable of transmitting infectious disease; the surface or item is rendered safe for handling, use, or disposal.

Disinfectant: an agent, usually a chemical, but may be a physical agent, such as x rays or ultraviolet light, that destroys microorganisms but may not kill bacterial spores; refers to substances applied to inanimate objects.

EPA: United States Environmental Protection Agency, Washington, DC.

> **EPA registered:** number on a label indicates that the product has the acceptance of EPA.

FDA: United States Food and Drug Administration, 5600 Fishers Lane, Rockville, MD 20857; regulates food, drugs, biologic products, medical devices, radiologic products.

Infection control: the selection and use of procedures and products to prevent the spread of infectious disease.

Infectious waste: contaminated with blood, saliva, or other substances; potentially or actually infected with pathogenic material; officially called "regulated" waste.

Invasive procedure: entry into tissues during which bleeding occurs or the potential for bleeding exists.

Nosocomial infection: an infection occurring in a patient while in a health-care facility that was not present at the time of admission; includes infections acquired in the health-care facility but appearing after dismissal.

OSAP: Organization for Safety and Asepsis Procedures Research Foundation, P.O. Box 6297, Annapolis, MD 21401.

KEY WORDS AND ABBREVIATIONS: Infection Control, continued

OSHA: United States Occupational Safety and Health Administration, Department of Labor, Washington, DC 20210.

PEP: postexposure prophylaxis.

PPE: personal protective equipment.

Sanitation: the process by which the number of organisms on inanimate objects is reduced to a safe level. It does not imply freedom from microorganisms and generally refers to a cleaning process.

Shelf life: stability of an item after it has been prepared; length of time a substance or preparation can be kept without changes occurring in its chemical structure or other properties.

Sporicide: substance that kills spores.

Sterilization: process by which all forms of life, including bacterial spores, are destroyed by physical or chemical means.

Synergism: the joint action of agents so that their combined effect is greater than the sum of their individual parts.

Waste:

    Infectious waste: capable of causing an infectious disease.

    Contaminated waste: items that have contacted blood or other body secretions.

    Hazardous waste: poses a risk to humans or the environment.

    Toxic waste: capable of having a poisonous effect.

    Regulated waste: liquid blood or saliva, sharps contaminated with blood or saliva, and nonsharp solid waste saturated with or caked with liquid or semisolid blood or saliva or tissue including teeth (OSHA).

5. FLOOR
   - Carpeting should be avoided.
   - Floor covering should be smooth, easily cleaned, nonabsorbent.
6. SINK
   - Smooth material (stainless steel).
   - Wide and deep enough for effective hand-washing without splashing.
   - Water faucets and soap dispensers with electronic, "knee," or foot-operated controls.
   - Separate room or area for contaminated instrument care.
7. SUPPLIES
   - All sterilizable or disposable.
8. WASTE
   - Receptacle with opening large enough to prevent contact with sides when material is dropped in; heavy-duty plastic bag liner to be sealed tightly for disposal.
   - Sharps disposal.
   - Small biohazard receptacle near treatment area to receive contaminated sponges and other waste, for disposal in large waste container clearly marked for contaminated waste.

▪ INSTRUMENT PROCESSING CENTER

The successful practice of standard precautions to prevent cross-contamination depends on the development of, and strict adherence to, a planned program for instrument management. A good rule is to learn the most effective, safe system and then to follow that method without exception. A specific routine is easier for the entire dental team to follow, and peer review is built-in.

The basic steps in the recirculation of instruments from the time an appointment procedure is completed until the instruments are sterilized and ready for use in the next clinical appointment are shown in the flowchart in Figure 4-2. Each of the steps is described in the following sections.

▪ CLEANING STEP[1]

Ideally the instruments are contained within a cassette so that little or no handling is required. When instruments are not in a cassette, transfer forceps are used for transferring contaminated instruments.

OPTIMAL TREATMENT ROOM FEATURES

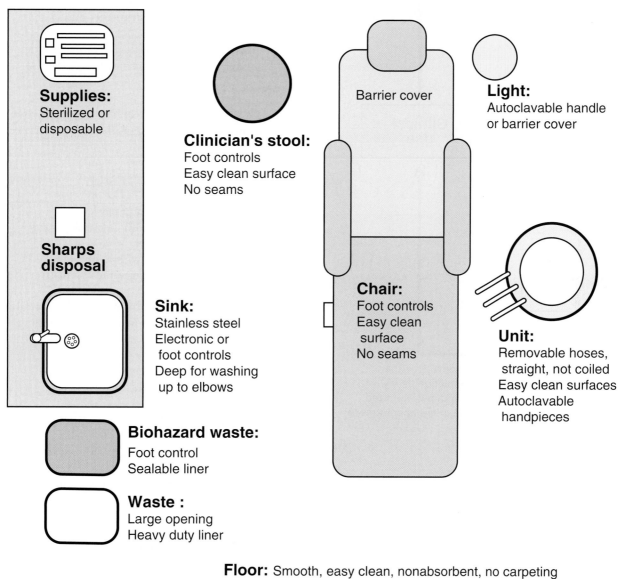

■ **FIGURE 4-1 Optimal Treatment Room Features.**

For all cleaning processes, heavy-duty, puncture-resistant gloves must be used, and a face mask and protective eyewear must be worn. The three methods for cleaning instruments are ultrasonic processing, washer-disinfector, and manual cleaning.

I. ULTRASONIC PROCESSING

Ultrasonic cleaning prior to sterilization is safer than manual cleaning. Manual cleaning of instruments is a dangerous, difficult, and time-consuming procedure.

Ultrasonic equipment is maintained and used according to manufacturer's guidelines. *Ultrasonic processing*

is not a substitute for sterilization; it is only a cleaning process.

A. Advantages

Benefits from the use of ultrasonic cleaning include the following:
- Increased efficiency in obtaining a high degree of cleanliness.
- Reduced danger to clinician from direct contact with potentially pathogenic microorganisms.
- Improved effectiveness for disinfection.

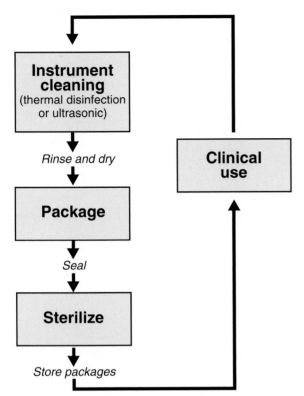

■ **FIGURE 4-2 Recirculation of Instruments.** Flowchart shows step-by-step process. At the completion of treatment, instruments are cleaned, packaged, sterilized, and stored. They are kept sealed until patient appointment begins.

- Elimination of possible dissemination of microorganisms through release of aerosols and droplets, which can occur during the scrubbing process.
- Penetration into areas of the instruments where the bristles of a brush may be unable to contact.
- Removal of tarnish.

B. Procedure

1. Guard against overloading; the solution must contact all surfaces. Instruments must be completely immersed.
2. Dismantle instruments with detachable parts, such as the mirror from the handle. Open jointed instruments.
3. Time accurately by manufacturer's guide.
4. Drain, rinse, and air dry.
5. Indications for thorough drying:
   a. When sterilizing by dry heat, chemical vapor, or ethylene oxide.

b. Nonstainless steel instruments require predip in rust inhibitor before steam autoclaving; water on instruments dilutes the antirust solution.
   c. Instruments to be packaged in paper wrap.

II. MANUAL CLEANING

Ultrasonics and washer-disinfector are the methods of choice, but when manual cleaning is the only alternative, precautions must be taken.

A. Procedure

1. Wear heavy-duty gloves and mask.
2. Dismantle instruments with detachable parts. Open jointed instruments.
3. Use detergent and scrub with a long-handled brush under running water; hold the instruments low in the sink.
4. Brush with strokes away from the body; use care not to splash and contaminate the surrounding area.
5. Rinse thoroughly.
6. Dry on paper towels (same reasons as those listed for ultrasonic processing).

B. Care of Brushes

1. Color code brushes to distinguish from handwash brushes.
2. Soak and wash contaminated brushes in detergent; rinse thoroughly and sterilize.

■ PACKAGING STEP[1]

I. PURPOSES

A. To prevent contamination of newly sterilized instruments as soon as they are removed from the sterilizer.
B. To provide a means of storing instruments to keep them in sets for individual appointment use and sterilized and ready for immediate use on opening.

II. INSTRUMENT ARRANGEMENT

A. Preset cassettes, trays, or packages can be preplanned to contain all the items usually needed for a particular appointment.
B. Each tray or package should be dated and marked for identification of contents: for

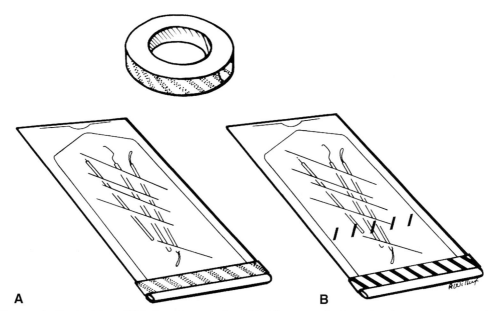

▪ **FIGURE 4-3 Process Indicator Tape (A)** Before autoclaving. **(B)** After autoclaving. The change of color in the stripes indicates that the package has been subjected to the proper temperature for sterilization but does not show sterilization. A biologic indicator is also needed for periodic monitoring to determine that the autoclave is functioning properly and that sterilization is actually taking place.

example, *Adult Scaling and Root Planing; Examination.*

C. Clear packages with self-seal permit instrument identification without special labeling. Figure 4-3 shows clear, "see-through" packages for easy identification of package contents.

III. PREPARATION

A. Materials

Each method of sterilization has specific requirements, and the manufacturer's recommendations must be reviewed. Sturdy wrapping is necessary to prevent punctures or tears that break the chain of asepsis and require a repeat of the process. The wrap must permit the steam or chemical vapor to pass through the contents.

B. Seal

Indicator tape is used. Pins, paper clips, or other types of metal fasteners are not used because they provide holes for the entry of microorganisms.

IV. CHEMICAL INDICATOR FOR CYCLE MONITORING

Chemical indicator tape is used to seal all packages, except when the wrap has built-in indicators. The chemical, usually in the form of a series of stripes, changes color during the sterilization process. The change of color means that the autoclave reached a designated temperature required for penetration and that does not designate sterilization (Figure 4-3). Distinct black stripes should appear. A lighter color change may be a warning signal that the autoclave function should be checked.

Indicator tape does not serve to test for true sterilization. A biologic indicator in the form of microbial spores must be used to test each sterilizer routinely.

The striped indicator tape is left on the sealed package and thereby serves to identify those packages ready for use. Packages are kept completely sealed until unwrapped in front of the patient.

▪ STERILIZATION

I. APPROVED METHODS

Each of the methods listed here is described in detail in the sections following. Table 4-1 summarizes the operating requirements of each.

A. Moist heat: steam under pressure.
B. Dry heat.
C. Chemical vapor.
D. Ethylene oxide.

II. SELECTION OF METHOD

All materials and items cannot be treated by the same system of sterilization. It is necessary to supplement with

■ TABLE 4-1 METHODS OF STERILIZATION

METHOD	STERILIZING REQUIREMENT		
	TIME	TEMPERATURE	PRESSURE
Moist heat Steam under pressure (steam autoclave)	15–30 min	250°F 121°C	15 psi
Dry heat oven	120 min	320°F 160°C	
Unsaturated chemical vapor	20 min	270°F 132°C	20–40 psi
Ethylene oxide gas	10–16 hr	75°F 25°C	

disposable single-use products when sterilization is not possible.

The method for sterilization that is selected must provide complete destruction of all microorganisms, viruses, and spores and yet must not damage the instruments and other materials. In addition, the procedures must not be overly complex, or many errors in the processing can occur.

Careful, specific use of sterilizing equipment in accord with the manufacturer's specifications is necessary. Incomplete sterilization most frequently results from inadequate preparation of the materials to be sterilized (cleaning, packaging), misuse of the equipment (overloading, timing, temperature selection), or inadequate maintenance.

III. TESTS FOR STERILIZATION

Sterilization is the process by which all forms of life are destroyed. That definition provides the rationale for testing whether a sterilizer is working properly. The testing system requires the use of selected test microorganisms that are put through a regular cycle of sterilization and then are cultured. When no growth occurs, the sterilizer has performed with maximum efficiency.

A. Microorganisms Used

- *Steam Autoclave.* Bacillus stearothermophilus vials, ampules, or strips.
- *Dry Heat Oven.* Bacillus subtilis strips.
- *Chemical Vapor.* Bacillus stearothermophilus strips.
- *Ethylene Oxide.* Bacillus subtilis strips.

B. Procedures

The ampule, vial, or strip is placed in the center of a package, which in turn is placed in the middle of the load of packages to be sterilized. After the cycle has been completed at the customary time and temperature, the ampule or strip is incubated. Ampules and vials show the color change associated with no living microorganisms, whereas the strip organisms are cultured and show no growth if the sterilizer has performed properly.

Table 4-2 shows indications for performing spore tests in dental settings. Records that are kept should show dates and outcomes.

C. Frequency

At least weekly testing is recommended. Equipment can be obtained for performing the testing, or commercial mail-in services are available.

IV. THE CHEMICAL INDICATOR

In contrast to spore testing, the chemical indicator is related only to the temperature to which the autoclave was heated. A chemical indicator is used routinely when packaging instruments (Figure 4-3).

■ MOIST HEAT: STEAM UNDER PRESSURE

Destruction of microorganisms by heat takes place as a result of inactivation of essential cellular proteins or enzymes. Moist heat causes coagulation of protein.

I. USE

Moist heat may be used for all materials except oils, waxes, and powders that are impervious to steam or for materials that cannot be subjected to high temperatures.

II. PRINCIPLES OF ACTION

A. Sterilization is achieved by action of heat and moisture; pressure serves only to attain high temperature.

B. Sterilization depends on the penetrating ability of steam.
   1. Air must be excluded, otherwise steam penetration and heat transfer are prevented.
   2. Space between objects is essential to ensure access for the steam.
   3. Materials must be thoroughly cleaned and air dried; adherent material can provide a barrier to the steam.
   4. Air discharge occurs in a downward direction; load must be arranged for free passage of steam toward bottom of autoclave.

▪ TABLE 4-2 SPORE TESTING

WHEN	WHY
Once per week	To verify proper use and functioning
Whenever a new type of packaging material or tray is used	To ensure that the sterilizing agent is getting inside to the surface of the instruments
After training of new sterilization personnel	To verify proper use of the sterilizer
During initial uses of a new sterilizer	To make sure unfamiliar operating instructions are being followed
First run after repair of a sterilizer	To make sure that the sterilizer is functioning properly
With every implantable device and hold device until results of test are known	Extra precaution for sterilization of item to be implanted into tissues
After any other change in the sterilizing procedure	To make sure change does not prevent sterilization

Adapted from Miller, C.H. and Palenik, C.J.: Sterilization, Disinfection, and Asepsis in Dentistry, in Block, S.S.: *Disinfection, Sterilization, and Preservation,* 4th ed. Philadelphia, Lea & Febiger, 1991, p. 680.

III. OPERATION

A. Packing Autoclave

Pack loosely to permit steam to reach all instruments in all packages; place jars and tall vessels on their sides to permit air to leave as steam enters.

B. Standard Procedure

The temperature must remain at 121°C (250°F) at 15 pounds pressure for 15 minutes after the meters show that proper pressure and temperature have been reached. Use 30 minutes for heavy loads to ensure penetration.

C. Cooling

1. *Dry Materials.* Release steam pressure, turn operating valve, and open the door; required time for drying is about 15 minutes.
2. *Liquids.* Reduce chamber pressure slowly at an even rate over 10 to 12 minutes to prevent boiling or escape of fluids into the chamber; it is preferable to turn off the autoclave and let the pressure fall before opening the door. Check

heat sensitivity of each solution and avoid prolonged exposure, as indicated.

IV. CARE OF AUTOCLAVE

Manufacturer's instructions must be followed.

A. Daily

Maintain proper level of distilled water; wash trays and interior surfaces of chamber with water and a mild detergent; clean removable plug, screen, or strainer.

B. Weekly

Flush chamber discharge system with an appropriate cleaning solution, such as hot trisodium phosphate or a commercial cleaner.

V. EVALUATION OF STEAM UNDER PRESSURE

A. Advantages

- All microorganisms, spores, and viruses are destroyed quickly and efficiently.
- Wide variety of materials may be treated; most economical method of sterilization.

B. Disadvantages

- May corrode carbon steel instruments if precautions are not taken.
- Unsuitable for oils or powders that are impervious to heat.

▪ DRY HEAT

The action of dry heat is oxidation.

I. USE

- A. Primarily for materials that cannot safely be sterilized with steam under pressure.
- B. For oils and powders when they are thermostabile at the required temperatures.
- C. For small metal instruments enclosed in special containers or that might be corroded or rusted by moisture.

II. PRINCIPLES OF ACTION

- A. Sterilization is achieved by heat that is conducted from the exterior surface to the interior of the object; the time required to penetrate varies among materials.
- B. Sterilization can result when the whole material is treated for a sufficient length of time at the required temperature; therefore, timing for

sterilization must start when the entire contents of the sterilizer have reached the peak temperature needed for that load.

C. Oil, grease, or organic debris on instruments insulates and protects microorganisms from the sterilizing effect.

III. OPERATION

A. Temperature

A temperature of 160°C (320°F) maintained for 2 hours; 170°C (340°F) for 1 hour. Timing must start after the desired temperature has been reached.

B. Penetration Time

Heat penetration varies with different materials, and the nature and properties of various materials must be considered.

C. Care

Care must be taken not to overheat because certain materials can be affected. Temperatures over 160°C (320°F) may destroy the sharp edges of cutting instruments.

IV. EVALUATION OF DRY HEAT

A. Advantages

- Useful for materials that cannot be subjected to steam under pressure.
- When maintained at correct temperature, it is well suited for sharp instruments.
- No corrosion compared with steam under pressure.

B. Disadvantages

- Long exposure time required; penetration slow and uneven.
- High temperature critical to certain materials.

▪ CHEMICAL VAPOR STERILIZER

A combination of alcohols, formaldehyde, ketone, water, and acetone heated under pressure produces a gas that is effective as a sterilizing agent.

I. USE

Chemical vapor sterilization cannot be used for materials or objects that can be altered by the chemicals that make the vapor or that cannot withstand the high temperature. Examples are low-melting plastics, liquids, or heat-sensitive handpieces.

II. PRINCIPLES OF ACTION

Microbial and viral destruction results from the permeation of the heated formaldehyde and alcohol. Heavy, tightly wrapped, or sealed packages would not permit the penetration of the vapors.

III. OPERATION

A. Temperature

From 127° to 132°C (260° to 270°F) with 20 to 40 pounds pressure in accord with the manufacturer's directions.

B. Time

Minimum of 20 minutes after the correct temperature and pressure have been attained. Time should be extended for a large load or a heavy wrap.

C. Cooling at the Completion of the Cycle

Instruments are dry. Instruments need a short period for cooling.

IV. CARE OF STERILIZER

Depending on the amount of use, refilling is needed by at least every 30 cycles. In accord with manufacturer's instructions, the condensate tray is removed, the exhausted solution emptied, and the tray cleaned.

V. EVALUATION OF CHEMICAL VAPOR STERILIZER

A. Advantages

- Corrosion- and rust-free operation for carbon steel instruments.
- Ability to sterilize in a relatively short total cycle.
- Ease of operation and care of the equipment.

B. Disadvantages

- Adequate ventilation is needed; cannot use in a small room.
- Slight odor, which is rarely objectionable.

▪ ETHYLENE OXIDE[2]

Gaseous sterilization using ethylene oxide is not commonly found in a private dental office or clinic but rather in hospitals and larger clinics.

I. USE

Nearly all materials, whether metal, plastic, rubber, or cloth, can be sterilized in ethylene oxide with little or no damage to the material.

II. PRINCIPLES OF ACTION

Ethylene oxide vapor is effective against all types and forms of microorganisms provided sufficient time is allowed.

III. OPERATION

Specific operation is related to the type of equipment. Operation in a well-ventilated room is necessary. Overnight processing is usually the most practical.

A. Time and Temperature

The time may vary from 10 to 16 hours, depending on both the temperature and the concentration of ethylene oxide used.

B. Aeration After Completion of the Cycle

Plastic and rubber products need to be aerated for at least 24 hours. Metal instruments are ready for immediate use.

IV. EVALUATION OF ETHYLENE OXIDE

A. Advantages

- Many types of materials (including plastic and rubber items) can be sterilized with minimum or no damage to the material itself.
- Low temperature for operation.

B. Disadvantages

- High cost of the equipment.
- Problems of dispersement of gaseous exhaust. Need for planned and tested ventilation system.
- Increased time of operation.
- Gas absorption requires airing of plastic, rubber, and cloth goods for several hours.

■ CARE OF STERILE INSTRUMENTS

Instruments stored without sealed wrappers are only momentarily sterile because of airborne contamination.

Labeled, sterilized, and sealed packages are stored unopened in clean, dry cabinets or drawers. Paper-wrapped packages must be handled carefully to prevent tearing. All stored packages should be dated and used in rotation.

Packages wrapped and sealed in paper usually do not need resterilizing for several months to 1 year.[3] Plastic or nylon wrap with a tape or heat seal may be expected to remain sterile longer. However, the expected shelf life before resterilizing depends on the area surrounding the stored packages. A closed, protected area without exposure, such as a cabinet or drawer that can be disinfected routinely, is preferred.

■ CHEMICAL DISINFECTANTS

Chemical disinfectants are used in several forms, including the surface disinfectants, immersion disinfectants, immersion sterilants, and hand antimicrobials. Each variety has specific chemicals, dilutions, and directions for application.

I. CATEGORIES[4]

Disinfectants are categorized by their biocidal activity as high level, intermediate level, or low level. Biocidal activity refers to the ability of the chemical disinfectant to destroy or inactivate living organisms.

A. High Level

High-level disinfectants inactivate spores and all forms of bacteria, fungi, and viruses. Applied at different time schedules, the high-level chemical is either a disinfectant or a sterilant.

B. Intermediate Level

Intermediate-level disinfectants inactivate all forms of microorganisms but do not destroy spores.

C. Low Level

Low-level disinfectants inactivate vegetative bacteria and certain lipid-type viruses but do not destroy spores, tubercle bacilli, or nonlipid viruses.

II. USES

A. Environmental Surfaces Disinfection

Following each appointment, the treatment area is cleaned and disinfected.

B. Dental Laboratory Impressions and Prostheses

Impressions can be carriers of infectious material to a dental laboratory, and completed prostheses must be disinfected before delivery to a patient.

III. PRINCIPLES OF ACTION

A. Disinfection is achieved by coagulation, precipitation, or oxidation of protein of microbial cells or denaturation of the enzymes of the cells.

B. Disinfection depends on the contact of the solution at the known effective concentration for the optimum period of time.

C. Items must be thoroughly cleaned and dried because action of the agent is altered by foreign matter and dilution.

D. A solution has a specific shelf life, use life, and reuse life. Some may be altered by changes in pH, or the active ingredient may decrease in potency. Check manufacturer's directions.

IV. CRITERIA FOR SELECTION OF A CHEMICAL AGENT

The objective is to select a product that is effective in the control of microorganisms and practical to use. Properties of an ideal disinfectant are shown in Table 4-3.

▪ TABLE 4-3 PROPERTIES OF AN IDEAL DISINFECTANT

1. Broad spectrum:
   Should always have the widest possible antimicrobial spectrum.

2. Fast acting:
   Should always have a rapidly lethal action on all vegetative forms and spores of bacteria and fungi, protozoa, and viruses.

3. Not affected by physical factors:
   Active in the presence of organic matter, such as blood, sputum, and feces.
   Should be compatible with soaps, detergents, and other chemicals encountered in use.

4. Nontoxic

5. Surface compatibility:
   Should not corrode instruments and other metallic surfaces.
   Should not cause the disintegration of cloth, rubber, plastics, or other materials.

6. Residual effect on treated surfaces

7. Easy to use

8. Odorless:
   An inoffensive odor would facilitate its routine use.

9. Economical:
   Cost should not be prohibitively high.

From Molinari, J.A., Gleason, M.J., Cottone, J.A., and Barrett, E.D.: Comparison of Dental Surface Disinfectants, *Gen. Dent., 35,* 171, May–June, 1987.

The manufacturer's informational literature and container labels must provide facts about the product that ensure its effectiveness. After the product has been selected, it is the responsibility of the dental personnel to use it as directed to obtain the best possible infection control. When the label has insufficient information, the manufacturer should be contacted and instructions obtained.

The criteria should include at least the following:

A. EPA approval.

B. Chemicals must be tuberculocidal, bacteriocidal, virucidal, and fungicidal.

C. Label must state:

1. Effectiveness and stability expressed by
   a. *Shelf life*: the expiration date indicating the termination of effectiveness of the unopened container.
   b. *Use life*: the life expectancy for the solution once it has been activated but not actually put to use with contaminated items.
   c. *Reuse life*: the amount of time a solution can be used and reused while being challenged with instruments that are wet or coated with bioburden.

2. Directions for activation (mixing proportions).

3. Type of container for storage and place (conditions such as heat and light).

4. Directions for use
   a. Precleaning and drying of items to be submerged.
   b. Time/temperature ratio.

5. Instructions for disposal of used solution.

6. Warnings
   a. Toxic effects (on eyes, skin).
   b. Specific directions for emergency care in the event of an accident (for example, splash in eye).
   c. Keep manufacturer's *Materials Safety Data Sheets* for reference.

▪ RECOMMENDED CHEMICAL DISINFECTANTS[5]

The agents that have been shown adequate for use in dentistry are glutaraldehydes, chlorine compounds, iodophores, and complex phenolics. These are listed in Table 4-4 and are described in sections that follow.

Alcohols are not approved for instrument or environmental surface disinfection. The alcohols, ethanol and isopropanol, have been widely accepted and used for the preparation of the skin prior to injections or blood-taking procedures. The use of alcohol for this purpose is as a cleansing agent; the length of time involved is not enough for antibacterial effect.

■ **TABLE 4-4 CHEMICAL DISINFECTING AGENTS**

GLUTARALDEHYDES
Glutaraldehyde, 2% neutral
Glutaraldehyde, 2% alkaline
Glutaraldehyde, 2% alkaline with phenolic buffer
Glutaraldehyde, 2% acidic

CHLORINES
Chlorine dioxide
Sodium hypochlorite, 5.25% household bleach

IODOPHORS
Iodophor (1% available iodine)

PHENOLICS
o-phenylphenyl 9% with o-benzyl-p-chlorophenol 1%

I. GLUTARALDEHYDES

As shown in Table 4-4, the three types of glutaraldehydes are the alkaline, acidic, and neutral preparations.

A. Action

At the designated time exposure, they are high-level disinfectants and act to kill microorganisms by damaging their proteins and nucleic acids.

B. Preparation

The solutions become activated when the components of the two containers are mixed. The manufacturers' labels must show shelf life and reuse life because the various preparations differ.

C. Limitations

- Caustic to skin; use forceps and wear gloves.
- Irritating to eyes; need protective eyewear.
- Corrosive to some metal instruments.
- Items must be rinsed in sterile water after removal from immersion bath.
- Not used as a surface disinfectant because of toxic effects of fumes; surfaces wiped with glutaraldehyde should have residual film wiped off with sterile water.

II. CHLORINE COMPOUNDS

A. Action

Chlorine compounds have been used in a variety of ways for disinfection. Their use in water purification is well known. Solutions of sodium hypochlorite are used in cleaning dentures. Microorganisms are destroyed primarily by oxidation of microbial enzymes and cell wall components.

B. Chlorine Dioxide

The use life of chlorine dioxide is only 1 day. The preparation is economical and generally nontoxic but is corrosive to nonstainless steel instruments.

C. Sodium Hypochlorite

Daily fresh solutions are needed because sodium hypochlorite tends to be unstable. Use distilled water for mixing to improve the stability. The solutions can harm the eyes, skin, and clothing, and can corrode certain instruments; the strong odor may be offensive. In spite of certain disadvantages, it is widely used and economical.

III. IODOPHORS

A. Action

Iodine is released slowly from the iodophor compound and creates a disinfecting action as a broad-spectrum antimicrobial.

Povidone-iodine preparations are widely used in the forms for surgical antisepsis, liquid soaps, mouthrinses, and surface antiseptics prior to hypodermic injection.

B. Environmental Surface Disinfectant

Concentrated solutions of iodophor contain less free iodine; therefore, the correct dilution for hard-surface disinfection is 1 part iodophor concentrate to 213 parts soft or distilled water. Hard water inactivates iodophors. The solution changes from amber to clear as it loses its activity.

IV. COMBINATION PHENOLICS (SYNTHETIC)

Phenolics may be water-based or alcohol-based.[5]

A. Action

High-concentration phenols act as protoplasmic poisons that destroy the cell wall and precipitate the protein. The lower concentrations used as surface disinfectants inactivate enzyme systems.

B. Use

As with iodophores, the synthetic phenolic disinfectants are broad spectrum, with residual biocidal activity.

■ CHEMICAL STERILANTS (IMMERSION)

Immersion in a chemical sterilant is used only for items that cannot be sterilized by heat. Because the immersion chemicals cannot be verified by spore testing, their use is limited. When ethylene oxide sterilizers are available, many of the items may be treated by that method.

A chemical that may require only 10 to 30 minutes for disinfection requires as many as 10 hours for sterilization at the same or different concentrations. Temperature may also be a factor. Manufacturer's instructions must be followed explicitly.

Instruments cannot be packaged, so maintenance of strict asepsis is not possible after chemical sterilization. Also, because of toxic effects to skin and mucosa, the chemical must be rinsed away with sterile water and the instruments dried before clinical use.

■ PREPARATION OF THE TREATMENT ROOM

The cleanliness and neatness of the treatment room reflect the character and conscientiousness of the dental personnel. The patient, with limited knowledge of dental science, may judge the ability of the dental personnel by the appearance of the office or clinic. Other patients may inquire about sterilization and infection control.

The patient's attitude is important, but more important is the relationship of cleanliness to the presence of microorganisms. The need is to provide clinical services in an environment that minimizes cross-contamination.

The orderliness and immaculate cleanliness of the treatment rooms result from continuing care. An excellent test for the effects of care and any minor oversights is for each dental team member to sit in the dental chair occasionally and look around at what the patient sees from that vantage point.

I. OBJECTIVES

Effective care of instruments and equipment contributes to the following:
- Control of disease transmitted by way of environmental surfaces.
- An increase in the working efficiency of the office personnel.
- An atmosphere of cleanliness and orderliness that contributes to the patient's and the clinician's well-being.
- An increase in the patient's confidence in the ability of the dental personnel.
- The maintenance of the working efficiency of office equipment and instruments.
  - To prolong their span of usefulness.
  - To contribute to patient safety.
- A decrease in the occurrence of unpleasant odors in the office.

II. PRELIMINARY PLANNING

Preparation of the treatment room when time between appointments is limited requires an efficient procedural system. The classification of inanimate objects (Table 4-5) provides a guide for analysis.[4]

First, all surfaces and items that will be used or contacted during the appointment can be categorized and listed as critical, semicritical, or noncritical. The most logical and scientific sequence for preparation for the appointment can then be outlined.

A. Hand Contacts

Only contacts essential to the service to be performed should be made. Planning ahead to have materials

■ TABLE 4-5 CLASSIFICATION OF INANIMATE OBJECTS[4]

SURFACE CATEGORY	DEFINITION	STERILIZATION/DISINFECTION	EXAMPLES
Critical	Penetrate soft tissue or bone	Sterilize or disposable	Needles Curets Explorers Probes
Semicritical	Touch intact mucous membrane, oral fluids Does not penetrate	Sterilize after each use High level disinfection when sterilization cannot be used	Radiographic biteblock Ultrasonic handpiece Amalgam condenser Mirror
Noncritical	Do not touch mucous membranes (only contact unbroken epithelium)	Cleaning and tuberculocidal intermediate-level disinfection	Light handles Certain x-ray machine parts Safety eyewear
Environmental surfaces	No contact with patient (or only intact skin)	Cleaning and intermediate to low disinfection	Counter tops Equipment surfaces Housekeeping surface

ready so that cabinet knobs or drawer handles do not have to be contacted is an example.

B. Sterilizable Items

Critical and semicritical items are sterilized or are disposable.

C. Disposable Items

Disposable items should be used wherever possible.

D. Items That May Be Covered

Barrier coverings prevent contamination from reaching surfaces. Covers for light handles, counter tops, x-ray machine parts, and water faucets are examples. Care must be taken when removing the covers not to contaminate the object beneath.

E. Items That Require Chemical Disinfection

Objects and surfaces that cannot be included in one of the preceding categories must be treated with a chemical disinfectant. If the material is not compatible with the chemical action of the disinfectant, a substitute item, which is either disposable or coverable, will be needed.

III. CLEAN AND DISINFECT ENVIRONMENTAL SURFACES

A. Agent

1. Approved effective agents are iodophors, sodium hypochlorite, or complex phenols (Table 4-4).
2. The effectiveness of the disinfection procedure is the result of two actions:
   a. The physical rubbing and removal of contaminated material.
   b. The chemical inactivation of the living microorganisms.
3. Do not store gauze sponges in the solution. Use a spray bottle to dispense the disinfectant.

B. Procedure

1. Wear heavy-duty household gloves and mask.
2. Use several large gauze sponges or paper towels. The use of small sponges wastes time. A disinfectant-soaked sponge in each hand can decrease the time of cleaning certain objects, and contaminated objects, such as tubings, can be held with one sponge while scrubbing with the other sponge.

   Spraying of a disinfectant must be followed by vigorous scrubbing for cleaning. When applied only by spray without scrubbing, the agent does not penetrate or remove the film of microorganisms.
3. Scrub the disinfectant over the entire surface, with attention to irregularities where contaminated material can aggregate.
4. Spray and leave the surfaces wet.

▪ UNIT WATER LINES

A biofilm of microorganisms forms on the inside of the water line tubings after overnight standing. Tests have been made on tubings to handpieces, water syringes, and ultrasonic scalers. When the lines were flushed for 2 minutes, the microbial counts were reduced.[6]

Contaminated water should not be used for surgical purposes or during the irrigation of pocket areas because infective microorganisms can be introduced. If contaminated water is directed forcefully into a pocket, microorganisms can enter the tissue and infection or bacteremia can result. Refer to Appendix III (page 1139) for the recommendations from the United States Department of Health and Human Services.

I. PROCEDURES FOR CLINICAL USE

A. Flush all water lines at least 2 minutes at the beginning of each day.
B. Run water through water syringes for 30 seconds before and 30 seconds after each patient appointment.

II. WATER RETRACTION SYSTEM

To correct saliva and debris suck-back in the water line of a handpiece, the water retraction valve should be removed and a check valve or antiretractor valve installed.[7] Originally, handpieces were made with a retraction valve to prevent dripping when the instrument was turned off. Material sucked into the line, possibly filled with microorganisms, including hepatitis viruses, tubercle bacilli, and other pathogens, then was discharged when the handpiece was used for the next patient.

▪ PATIENT PREPARATION

The use of preprocedural rinsing and toothbrushing has been shown to lower the numbers of oral bacteria and, therefore, to lower the numbers of infected aerosols created during instrumentation.

Oral procedures that require penetration of tissues, such as giving anesthesia by injection or scaling subgingival pocket surfaces, can introduce bacteria into the tissues and hence into the bloodstream. Organisms injected into the tissue could multiply and create an abscess.

Because of natural resistance, the body can handle and destroy invading microorganisms, provided the numbers can be kept to a minimum.

Practical procedures for the preparation of a patient include preprocedural oral hygiene measures and rinsing with an antimicrobial mouthrinse. These contribute to the prevention of disease transmission.

I. PREPROCEDURAL ORAL HYGIENE MEASURES

A. Toothbrushing

Toothbrushing disturbs and removes microorganisms. When a patient is being trained in dental biofilm control measures and needs supervision at each appointment, a double purpose can be accomplished. Demonstration of biofilm removal from the teeth, tongue, and gingiva contributes to lowering the microbial count prior to treatment procedures.

B. Rinsing

The numbers of bacteria on the gingival or mucosal surfaces can be reduced by the use of a preprocedural antiseptic mouthrinse.[8]

The substantivity of 0.12% chlorhexidine provides a lowered bacterial count for more than 60 minutes. Preprocedural rinsing before injections is advised.

II. APPLICATION OF A SURFACE ANTISEPTIC

A. Prior to Injection of Anesthetic[9,10]

As a needle is introduced into the mucosa for penetration to deeper tissues, microorganisms on the surface can be carried into the tissue. During positioning of the instrument for injection, the needle might accidentally contact a tooth surface and pick up some biofilm, which could be carried to and into the injection site.

An antiseptic applied prior to the injection can decrease the risk of introducing septic material into the soft tissue.
1. Dry the surface (gauze square).
2. Apply antiseptic (swab).
3. Apply topical anesthetic (swab).

B. Prior to Scaling and Other Dental Hygiene Instrumentation[11]

1. *Instrumentation* in a sulcus or pocket and around the gingival margin can create breaks in the tissue where bacteria can enter. Subgingival instrumentation in a pocket with broken down sulcular epithelium contributes to the entrance of bacteria into the underlying tissues and bacteremia.
2. *Procedure.* Dry the surface and swab the area prior to instrumentation. Use an antiseptic solution to irrigate the sulci and pockets carefully.

■ SUMMARY OF STANDARD PROCEDURES FOR THE PREVENTION OF DISEASE TRANSMISSION

Basic procedures for clinical management are listed here.

I. PATIENT FACTORS

A. Prepare a comprehensive patient history. Refer patients suspected of carrying infectious disease for medical evaluation.
B. Avoid elective procedures for a patient who is suffering from a communicable condition, such as a respiratory infection, or who has an open lesion on or about the lips or oral tissues, for the benefit of all who would be subjected to exposure.
C. Ask the patient to rinse with an antimicrobial mouthrinse to reduce the numbers of oral microorganisms.
D. Provide protective eyewear.

II. CLINIC PREPARATION

A. Run water through all water lines, including the air–water syringe, handpieces, and ultrasonic unit, for 2 minutes at the start of the day and for at least 30 seconds before and after each use during the day.
B. Disinfect all environmental surfaces that may be touched during the appointment. Make an orderly sequence for surface disinfection. Apply barrier covers as indicated.
C. Sterilize instruments and all other equipment that can be sterilized by one of the methods for complete sterilization.

III. FACTORS FOR THE DENTAL TEAM

A. Have medical examinations; keep immunizations up to date; have appropriate testing on a periodic basis.
B. Always use mask, protective eyewear, gloves, and a clean closed-front gown with fitted wrist cuffs.

C. Wash hands and dry thoroughly at the start of the day and handwashes with three latherings and thorough rinsings before donning and after removal of gloves. Use antimicrobial soap.

D. Develop habits that minimize contacts with switches and other parts of the dental unit, dental chair, light, and clinician's stool, and avoid all environmental contacts unrelated to the procedure at hand.

IV. TREATMENT FACTORS

A. Hypodermic Needles

- Use a safe recapping method to prevent accidental penetration or self-inoculation.
- Place used needles into a puncture-resistant sharps container.
- Dispose of all partially emptied carpules of anesthetics.

B. Removable Oral Prostheses

Routinely, gloves should be worn to receive a septic prosthesis from a patient. Place the prosthesis in a disposable cup and cover with a disinfectant. Use a fresh solution of 0.05% iodophor in water, or a 1:5 dilution of 5% sodium hypochlorite. Clean by ultrasonics.

When a lathe is used for cleaning the denture, wear goggles and a mask and use a sterile ragwheel and fresh pumice. Pumice is used only once and caught on a disposable paper liner in the dustbin and discarded.

V. POSTTREATMENT

A. Use heavy puncture-resistant gloves to handle used instruments.

B. Follow routines to disinfect, clean in ultrasonic cleaner, and prepare the instruments for sterilization.

C. Contaminated waste is secured in plastic disposal bags.

D. Disinfect safety eyewear for patient and dental team members.

■ OCCUPATIONAL ACCIDENTAL EXPOSURE MANAGEMENT

Accidents happen even to the most skillful clinician. Accidental percutaneous (laceration, needle stick) or permucosal (splash to eye or mucosa) exposure to blood or other body fluids requires prompt action.

A. Significant Exposures

1. Percutaneous or permucosal stick or wound with needle or sharp instrument contaminated with blood, saliva, or other body fluids.

2. Contamination of any obviously open wound, nonintact skin, or mucous membrane with blood, saliva, or a combination.

3. Exposure of patient's body fluids to unbroken skin is not considered a significant exposure.

B. Procedure Following Exposure

1. Immediately wash the wound with soap and water; rinse well.

2. Flush nose, mouth, eyes, or skin with clear water, saline, or a sterile irrigant.

3. Report to designated official.

4. Complete an incident report as required.

5. Follow the required predetermined, posted, procedures of the clinic, institution or other workplace.

6. Postexposure policies must follow the most recent guidelines provided by the United States Public Health Service.[12,13]

C. Follow-up

1. Report signs and symptoms associated with HIV seroconversion.

2. Obtain medical evaluation of any illness involving fever, rash, lymphadenopathy.

3. Pursue counseling and further testing.

■ DISPOSAL OF WASTE[14]

Types of waste are defined in Box 4-1. Each type of waste requires special handling.

I. REGULATIONS

Investigate the regulations of each town or city sanitation division for rules concerning disposal of contaminated waste.

Figure 4-4 illustrates the universal label required by OSHA. The labels must be attached to containers used to store or transport hazardous waste materials.

II. GUIDELINES

A. Disposable materials, such as gloves, masks, wipes, paper drapes, or surface covers, that are contaminated with blood or body fluids should be carefully handled and discarded in sturdy, impervious plastic bags to minimize human contact.

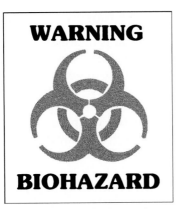

▪ **FIGURE 4-4 Universal Label for Hazardous Material.** A hazard-warning label should be fluorescent orange or orange-red with lettering or a symbol in a contrasting color. The label must be attached to containers used to store or transport waste. A label is not required for regulated waste that has been decontaminated (such as dental waste that has been autoclaved).

B. Blood, suctioned fluids, or other liquid waste may be carefully poured into a drain that is connected to a sanitary sewer system in compliance with applicable local regulations.

C. Sharp items, such as needles and scalpel blades, should be placed intact into a puncture-resistant, leak-proof container.

D. Human tissue and contaminated solid wastes can be disposed of according to the requirements established by local or state environmental regulatory agencies and published recommendations.

E. Infectious medical waste, including tissues and culture media, should be handled in a manner consistent with local regulations before disposal.

F. Liquid chemicals should be carefully poured into a drain connected to a sewer while flushing with copious amounts of water unless labeling or local regulations prohibit such a practice. Disposal methods for solid chemicals vary with the type of chemical and local regulations governing waste-management practices.

▪ SUPPLEMENTAL RECOMMENDATIONS

I. CLEANING THE FACE

Check and clean the exposed parts of the face not covered by mask or protective eyewear, where spatter collects, as an aid to disease control as well as for general sanitation. The face should be cleaned several times each day and washed before eating. When washing the face, an effort should be made not to spread spatter material into the eyes or the mouth.

II. SMOKING AND EATING

Neither smoking nor eating should be permitted in treatment areas.

III. TOYS

Select toys and other reception area items that can be cleaned and disinfected.

IV. HANDPIECE MAINTENANCE

Keep records of handpiece purchase, maintenance, and other information pertinent to longevity and effectiveness. Maintain a sufficient number of handpieces to permit rotation and routine sterilization.

V. STERILIZATION MONITORING

Keep a written record of dates when processing tests and biologic monitor tests were performed for each sterilizer.

Everyday Ethics

Kimberly, the dental hygienist, begins to scale and then notices that the indicator tape on the sterilizing cassette had not changed color. She excuses herself and finds out from the receptionist that a call to the repair service has been made because the autoclave has been shutting down prior to completion of the cycle. It is after 1:00 PM and patients are scheduled all afternoon.

Questions for Consideration

1. When proper sterile technique is not followed, what ethical principles and core values are involved? Explain Kimberly's duty to her patients.

2. Offer possible solutions for this situation. Describe how it could be defended to the patient, the dentist, and other dental team members.

3. What role can a dental hygienist play to ensure that it does not happen again?

✔ **Factors To Teach The Patient**

- The meaning of "standard precautions" and what is included under the term; how these precautions protect the patient and the dental team members.

- The contribution of the accurately completed medical and dental personal history to the provision of the best, safest treatment possible.

- Methods for sterilization of instruments, including handpieces; how the autoclave or other sterilizer is tested daily or weekly.

- Facts about the normal oral flora and the factors that influence an increased number of bacteria on the tongue, mucosa, and in the dental biofilm on the teeth.

- Methods for personal daily control of the oral bacteria through biofilm control and tongue brushing.

- Reasons for preprocedural rinsing.

- Method for thorough rinsing.

Indicate advance dates for the next testing clearly on a calendar or other reference point. Tests made weekly should be performed on the same day to simplify remembering.

VI. OFFICE POLICY MANUAL

Include in the clinic or office policy manual outlines of procedures to follow for standard precautions. Addresses for sources of various materials can be kept in a special reference section of the manual. Emergency procedures to follow when accidentally exposed should also be defined clearly.

REFERENCES

1. **Office Safety and Asepsis Procedures Research Foundation:** The Sterilization Process, *OSAP Monthly Focus*, 1–3, Number 5, 1997.
2. **Parisi,** A.N. and Young, W.E.: Sterilization With Ethylene Oxide and Other Gases, in Block, S.S.: *Disinfection, Sterilization, and Preservation,* 4th ed. Philadelphia, Lea & Febiger, 1991, pp. 580–595.
3. **Butt,** W.E., Bradley, D.V., Mayhew, R.B., and Schwartz, R.S.: Evaluation of the Shelf Life of Sterile Instrument Packs, *Oral Surg. Oral Med. Oral Pathol., 72,* 650, December, 1991.
4. **United States Centers for Disease Control and Prevention:** Recommended Infection-Control Practices for Dentistry, 1993, *MMWR, 42,* 1–10, RR-8, May 28, 1993.
5. **Miller,** C.H.: Infection Control Strategies for the Dental Office, in American Dental Association: *ADA Guide to Dental Therapeutics.* Chicago, ADA Publishing Co., 1998, pp. 489–504.
6. **Gross,** A., Devine, M.J., and Cutright, D.E.: Microbial Contamination of Dental Units and Ultrasonic Scalers, *J. Periodontol., 47,* 670, November, 1976.
7. **Bagga,** B.S.R., Murphy, R.A., Anderson, A.W., and Punwani, I.: Contamination of Dental Unit Cooling Water With Oral Microorganisms and Its Prevention, *J. Am. Dent. Assoc., 109,* 712, November, 1984.
8. **Veksler,** A.E., Kayrouz, G.A., and Newman, M.G.: Reduction of Salivary Bacteria by Pre-procedural Rinses With Chlorhexidine 0.12%, *J. Periodontol., 62,* 649, November, 1991.
9. **Malamed,** S.F.: *Handbook of Local Anesthesia,* 4th ed. St. Louis, Mosby, 1996, p. 134.
10. **Connor,** J.P. and Edelson, J.G.: Needle Tract Infection, *Oral Surg. Oral Med. Oral Pathol., 65,* 401, April, 1988.
11. **Fine,** D.H., Korik, I., Furgang, D., Myers, R., Olshan, A., Barnett, M.L., and Vincent, J.: Assessing Preprocedural Subgingival Irrigation and Rinsing With an Antiseptic Mouthrinse to Reduce Bacteremia, *J. Am. Dent. Assoc., 127,* 641, May, 1996.
12. **United States Centers for Disease Control and Prevention:** Updated U. S. Public Health Service Guidelines for the Management of Occupational Exposures to HBV, HCV, and HIV and Recommendations for Postexposure Prophylaxis, *MMWR, 50,* 1-52, Supplement, No. RR-11, June 29, 2001.
13. **United States Centers for Disease Control and Prevention:** Revised Guidelines for HIV Counseling, Testing, and Referral and Revised Recommendations for HIV Screening of Pregnant Women, *MMWR, 50,* 1-85, Supplement, November 9, 2001.
14. **Miller,** C.H. and Palenik, C.J.: *Infection Control and Management of Hazardous Materials for the Dental Team.* St. Louis, Mosby, 1994, pp. 210–219.

SUGGESTED READINGS

American Dental Association Council on Scientific Affairs and Council on Dental Practice: Infection Control Recommendations for the Dental Office and the Dental Laboratory, *J. Am. Dent. Assoc., 127,* 672, May, 1996.

Harte, J., Davis, R., Plamondon, T., and Richardson, B.: The Influence of Dental Unit Design on Percutaneous Injury, *J. Am. Dent. Assoc., 129,* 1725, December, 1998.

Legnani, P., Cheechi, L., Pelliccioni, G.A., and D'Achille, C.: Atmospheric Contamination During Dental Procedures, *Quintessence Int., 25,* 435, June, 1994.

Miller, C.H.: Infection Control, *Dent. Clin. North Am., 40,* 437, April, 1996.

Wooten, R.K. and Barata, M.-C.: Procedure-specific Infection Control Recommendations for Dentistry, *Compend. Cont. Educ. Dent., 14,* 332, March, 1993.

Occupational Exposure

Beekman, S.E. and Henderson, D.K.: Managing Occupational Risks in the Dental Office: HIV and the Dental Professional, *J. Am. Dent. Assoc., 125,* 847, July, 1994.

Chenoweth, C.E. and Gobetti, J.P.: Postexposure Chemoprophylaxis for Occupational Exposure to HIV in the Dental Office, *J. Am. Dent. Assoc., 128,* 1135, August, 1997.

Ramos-Gomez, F., Ellison, J., Greenspan, D., Bird, W., Lowe, S., and Gerberding, J.L.: Accidental Exposures to Blood and Body Fluids Among Health Care Workers in Dental Teaching Clinics: A Prospective Study, *J. Am. Dent. Assoc., 128,* 1253, September, 1997.

Dental Unit Water

Andrews, N.: Management of Biofilm and Water Quality in Dental Devices, *J. Pract. Hyg., 5,* 33, July/August, 1996.

Bednarsh, H.S., Eklund, K.J., and Mills, S.: Check Your Dental Unit Water IQ, *Access, 10,* 37, November, 1996.

Challacombe, S.J. and Fernandes, L.L.: Detecting *Legionella pneumophila* in Water Systems: A Comparison of Various Dental Units, *J. Am. Dent. Assoc., 126,* 603, May, 1995.

Karpay, R.I., Plamondon, T.J., Mills, S.E., and Dove, S.B.: Validation of an In-office Dental Unit Water Monitoring Technique, *J. Am. Dent. Assoc., 129,* 207, February, 1998.

Murdoch-Kinch, C.A., Andrews, N.L., Atwan, S., Jude, R., Gleason, M.J., and Molinari, J.A.: Comparison of Dental Water Quality Management Procedures, *J. Am. Dent. Assoc., 128,* 1235, September, 1997.

Williams, J.F., Molinari, J.A., and Andrews, N.: Microbial Contamination of Dental Unit Waterlines: Origins and Characteristics, *Compend. Cont. Educ. Dent., 17,* 538, June, 1996.

Sterilization and Disinfection

Andrés, M.T., Tejerina, J.M., and Fierro, J.F.: Reliability of Biologic Indicators in a Mail-Return Sterilization-Monitoring Service: A Review of 3 Years, *Quintessence Int., 26,* 865, December, 1995.

Burkhart, N.W. and Crawford, J.: Critical Steps in Instrument Cleaning: Removing Debris After Sonication, *J. Am. Dent. Assoc., 128,* 456, April, 1997.

Chau, V.B., Saunders, T.R., Pimsler, M., and Elfring, D.R.: In-depth Disinfection of Acrylic Resins, *J. Prosthet. Dent., 74,* 309, September, 1995.

Larsen, T., Andersen, H.-K., and Fiehn, N.-E.: Evaluation of a New Device for Sterilizing Dental High-Speed Handpieces, *Oral Surg. Oral Med. Oral Pathol. Oral Radiol. Endod., 84,* 513, November, 1997.

McGivern, T.: The Use of Glutaraldehyde for Disinfection and Sterilization, *J. Pract. Hyg., 6,* 1, Supplement, September/October, 1997.

Miller, C.H.: Update on Heat Sterilization and Sterilization Monitoring, *Compend. Cont. Educ. Dent., 14,* 304, March, 1993.

Molinari, J.A., Gleason, M.J., and Merchant, V.A.: The Evolution of Sterilization Monitoring Services, *Compend. Cont. Educ. Dent., 15,* 1422–1487 (8 articles), Special Issue, 1994.

Sheldrake, M.A., Majors, C.D., Gaines, D.J., and Palenik, C.J.: Effectiveness of Three Types of Sterilization on the Contents of Sharps Containers, *Quintessence Int., 26,* 771, November, 1995.

Young, J.M.: Dental Air-Powered Handpieces: Selection, Use, and Sterilization, *Compend. Cont. Educ. Dent., 14,* 358, March, 1993.

Preprocedural Rinse

Buckner, R.Y., Kayrour, G.A., and Briner, W.: Reduction of Oral Microbes by a Single Chlorhexidine Rinse, *Compend. Cont. Educ. Dent., 15,* 512, April, 1994.

Logothetis, D.D. and Martinez-Welles, J.M.: Reducing Bacterial Aerosol Contamination with a Chlorhexidine Gluconate Pre-rinse, *J. Am. Dent. Assoc., 126,* 1634, December, 1995.

Rahn, R., Schneider, S., Diehl, O., Schafer, V., and Shah, P.M.: Preventing Post-treatment Bacteremia: Comparing Topical Povidone-Iodine and Chlorhexidine, *J. Am. Dent. Assoc., 126,* 1145, August, 1995.

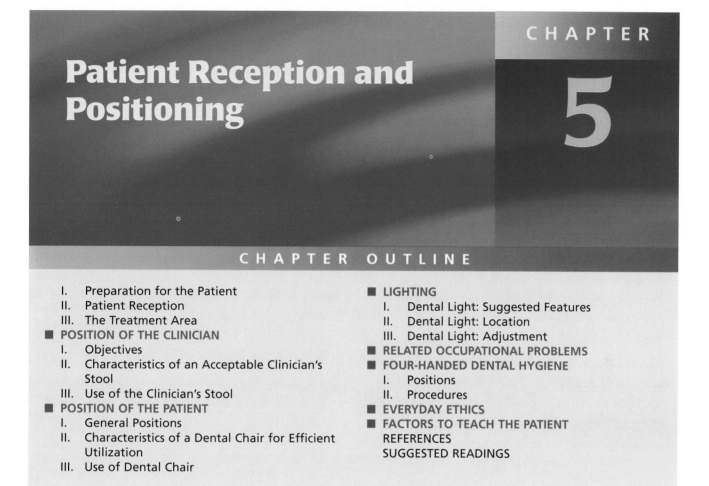

The patient's well-being is the all-important consideration throughout the appointment. At the same time, the clinician must function effectively and efficiently in a manner that minimizes stress and fatigue.

The physical arrangement and interpersonal relationships provide the setting for specific services to be performed. Key words related to the positioning of patient and clinician are defined in Box 5-1.

The patient's presence in the office or clinic is an expression of confidence in the dentist and the dental hygienist. The confidence is inspired by the reputation for professional knowledge and skill, the appearance of the office, and the actions of the workers in it.

I. PREPARATION FOR THE PATIENT

A. Treatment Area

The procedures for the prevention of disease transmission are described elsewhere. The requirements are standard precautions for all patients whether or not the presence of a communicable disease is known.

1. *Environmental Surfaces.* All contact areas must be thoroughly disinfected or covered to control cross-contamination.

2. *Instruments.* Sterile packaged instruments remain sealed until the start of the appointment.

3. *Equipment.* Prepare and make ready other materials that will be used, such as for the determination of blood pressure and patient instruction. Anticipate specific needs for assessment procedures.

B. Records

By leaving the record open for reference, the need for handling the record after handwashing and gloving may be avoided. Radiographs can be placed on the viewbox and the light left on.

1. Review the patient's medical and dental history for pertinent appointment information and need for updating.

2. Read previous appointment case records to focus the current treatment needs.

3. Anticipate examination procedures and new record making for a new patient.

C. Position Chair

1. Upright, in low position.
2. Chair arm adjusted for access.

BOX 5-1 KEY WORDS: Chair Positioning

Body language: a set of nonverbal signals, including body movements, postures, gestures, and facial expressions, that gives expression to various physical, mental, and emotional states.

Body mechanics: the field of physiology that studies muscular actions and functions in the maintenance of the posture of the body.

Cumulative trauma: disorders of the musculoskeletal, autonomic, and peripheral nervous system caused by repeated, forceful, and awkward movements of the human body, as well as by exposure to mechanical stress, vibration, and cold temperatures.

Ergonomics: a branch of ecology dealing with human factors in the design and operation of machines and the physical environment; in dentistry, the science encompassing all factors that relate to quality and quantity of dental care delivered in comparison to the physical and mental fatigue generated.

Postural hypotension: also called orthostatic hypotension; a fall in blood pressure associated with dizziness, syncope, and blurred vision that occurs upon standing or when standing motionless in a fixed position.

Supine: flat position with head and feet on the same level.

Trendelenburg: the modified supine position when the head is lower than the heart.

Work simplification: application to clinical procedure of time and motion studies, analysis of instruments and equipment, and body mechanics to provide the patient with a smooth, systematic, simplified approach for comprehensive dental hygiene therapy.

---

3. Clear pathway to chair of obstacles: rheostat, clinician's stool.

II. PATIENT RECEPTION

A. Introductions

1. The dental assistant or the dentist may introduce the new patient to the dental hygienist, but more frequently, a self-introduction is in order. The patient is greeted by name, and the hygienist's name is clearly stated, for example, "Good morning, Mrs. Smith; I am Miss Jones, the dental hygienist." Wearing a name tag for the patient's convenient observation is helpful.
2. Procedure for introducing the patient to others:
   a. A lady's name always precedes a gentleman's.
   b. An older person's name precedes the younger person's (when of the same sex and when the difference in age is obvious).
   c. In general, the patient's name precedes that of a member of the dental personnel.
3. An older patient is not called by the first name except at the patient's request.

B. Escort Patient to Dental Chair

1. Invite patient to be seated.
   a. For the average patient, stand ready to adjust the chair.

   b. Assist the elderly, the infirm, or very small children; guide into the chair by supporting the patient's arm.
2. Assist with wheelchair. Bring wheelchair adjacent to the dental chair and provide assistance when indicated.
3. Place handbag in a safe place, if possible within the patient's view.
4. Apply drape and napkin. Stabilization aids for patients with disabilities are described elsewhere.
5. Receive removable prostheses and cover with water in a protective container.
6. Provide protective eyewear. When a patient removes personal corrective eyeglasses to substitute those provided by the office or clinic, make sure the personal glasses are placed in their case in a safe place.

III. THE TREATMENT AREA

The treatment area centers around the patient's oral cavity. The entire "work area" refers to the dental chair with patient, the unit, and the instrument tray as they are positioned for the convenience and accessibility of the clinician on the clinician's stool.

Patient and clinician positioning is described in detail in this chapter. In summary, the general features of an appropriate work area include the following:

A. Unit and instruments positioned for visibility and convenient selection by the clinician, and for ready access without stretching or reaching over the patient.

B. Clinician's shoulders, elbows, and wrists are comfortably in neutral position.

C. The patient is in supine position adjusted so that the oral cavity is at the elbow height of the clinician.

D. The dental light is directed from a height that illuminates as large an area as possible, yet allows the clinician to adjust conveniently.

■ POSITION OF THE CLINICIAN

The position of the patient is contingent upon the position of the clinician. Attention to the patient's comfort must always be foremost, but when the working arrangement is considered, it is realistic to remember that the patient's position will be assumed for a relatively short time compared with that of the clinician.

Neutral positions are described in conjunction with instrumentation on page 620. The patient is positioned so that a thorough, biologically oriented service may be performed conveniently and efficiently within a reasonable length of time.

I. OBJECTIVES

Objectives concern the health of the clinician, the service to be performed, and the effect on the patient. The *preferred* neutral positions attempt to accomplish the following:

- Contribute to, rather than detract from, the health of the clinician.
- Provide physical comfort and mental tranquility that reduce stress.
- Apply principles of body mechanics that reduce fatigue and maintain stamina for prolonged periods of peak efficiency.
- Contribute to ease and efficiency of performance.
- Transmit to the patient a sense of well-being, security, and confidence, as well as a need for cooperation with dental personnel.
- Develop better patient–clinician relationships because of greater comfort, lessened physical stress, and reduced appointment time.
- Be flexible in relation to individual needs of physically challenged patients with special health problems, where limitations of physiologic or pathologic conditions require variations in chair positions.

II. CHARACTERISTICS OF AN ACCEPTABLE CLINICIAN'S STOOL[1,2]

A. Base

Broad and heavy for stability, with no fewer than four casters. A stool with five casters has greater stability.

B. Mobility

Completely mobile; not connected to other dental equipment; built with free-rolling casters; allows free movement around the patient's head for instrumentation from either side.

C. Seat

Relatively large to provide complete body support; padded firmly, yet not too hard; without a welt on the leaning edge that could dig into the upper part of the thigh.

D. Height

Adjustable to provide exactly the correct level for the individual so that feet can be flat on the floor and thighs parallel with the floor.

E. Adjustment

In accord with standard precautions, the stool is adjusted by a foot control mechanism.

F. Assistant's Stool

Needs additional support at the base, with at least five casters recommended for maximum stability; should be freely adjustable for height. A footrest is needed at the base of the chair because the assistant is positioned 4 to 6 inches higher than the clinician, and generally, the feet cannot reach the floor.

III. USE OF THE CLINICIAN'S STOOL

Once the stool is adjusted for the individual, it does not need changing, unless other personnel also use it. Once adjusted, the height remains constant, and other dental equipment is arranged to accommodate for optimum usage. Positioning that incorporates principles of good body mechanics benefits both the clinician and the patient. Basic positioning includes the following features related to posture and the treatment area to incorporate a neutral position.

A. Feet are flat on the floor; thighs parallel with the floor (Figure 5-1A).

B. Back is straight; head is relatively erect; shoulders are relaxed and parallel with floor.

C. Body weight is completely supported by the chair; balancing on the edge of the stool should be avoided (Figure 5-1B).

D. Eyes are directed downward in a manner that prevents neck strain and eye strain; it is not necessary to bend the head.

E. Distance from the patient's mouth to the eyes of the clinician should be 14 to 16 inches (Figure 5-2).

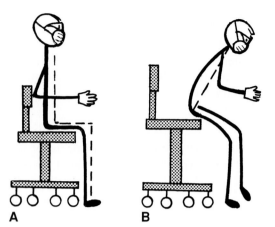

▪ **FIGURE 5-1 Clinician's Use of Stool. (A)** Correct position, with feet flat on the floor, thighs parallel with floor, and body weight supported by the stool. **(B)** Incorrect position, with seat high, body balanced on the edge of the stool, and back bent forward.

    F. With elbows close to the sides, the treatment area (patient's mouth) is adjusted to elbow height.
    G. Neutral forearm and wrist are in a straight line.

▪ POSITION OF THE PATIENT

I. GENERAL POSITIONS

Four commonly used body positions are shown in Figure 5-3. Body positions are of extreme importance during emergency care.

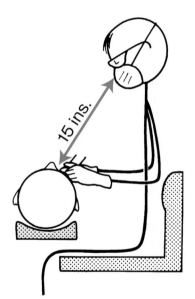

▪ **FIGURE 5-2 Distance From Clinician to Patient.** Acceptable positioning shows the patient at the clinician's elbow level and the oral cavity of the patient approximately 15 inches from the clinician's eyes.

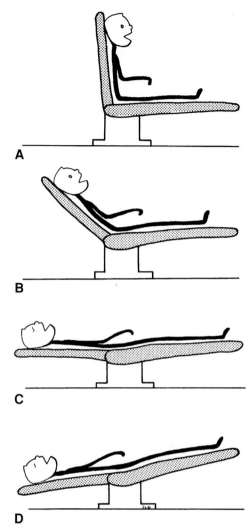

▪ **FIGURE 5-3 Basic Patient Positions. (A)** Upright. **(B)** Semi-upright. **(C)** Supine or horizontal, with the brain on the same level as the heart. **(D)** Trendelenburg, with the brain lower than the heart and the feet slightly elevated.

A. Upright

This is the initial position from which chair adjustments are made.

B. Semi-upright

A patient with certain types of cardiovascular or respiratory problems may need to be in a semi-upright position during treatment.

C. Supine

The patient is flat, with the head and feet on the same level.

D. Trendelenburg

The patient is in the supine position and tipped back and down 35° to 45° so that the heart is higher than the head (Figure 5-3D).

II. CHARACTERISTICS OF A DENTAL CHAIR FOR EFFICIENT UTILIZATION

A dental chair provides complete body support for the patient, which increases patient relaxation. The clinician can be in a comfortable working position with good access, light, and visibility, which in turn contribute to an efficient performance.

In a supine position, a patient is ideally situated for support of the circulation. Rarely could a patient faint while lying in a supine position.

- A. Provides complete body support.
- B. Seat and leg support moves as a unit; back and headrest move as a unit; both are power controlled.
- C. Has a thin back without protruding adjustment devices so that the chair may be lowered close to the clinician's elbow height.
- D. Has supports that hold the patient's arms as the chair is lowered into the supine position; otherwise the hands hang down or the patient must hold them up forcibly.
- E. Chair base should be shallow to permit the chair to be lowered as close to the floor as needed for correct treatment position.
- F. Foot controls for the back and seat should be readily available to both the assistant and clinician.

III. USE OF DENTAL CHAIR

A. Prepositioning for Patient Reception

1. Chair at low level; back upright.
2. Chair arm raised on side of approach.

B. Adjustment Steps

1. Patient is seated first with back upright.
2. Chair seat and foot portion are raised first to help the patient settle back.
3. Backrest is lowered until the patient reaches the supine position for maxillary instrumentation. For mandibular teeth, chair back is adjusted to a 20° angle with the floor.
4. Patient is requested to slide up until the head is at the upper edge of the backrest and on the side next to the clinician. Note patient's head position in Figure 5-5.

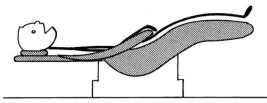

▪ **FIGURE 5-4 Dental Chair in Supine Position.** For instrumentation in the maxillary arch, the patient is in supine position, with the back of the chair nearly parallel with the floor and the feet slightly higher than the head. For mandibular teeth, adjust the chair back to a 20° angle with the floor.

C. Final Adjustment

Lower or raise the total chair until the patient's mouth is at the clinician's elbow level when the shoulder is relaxed.

D. Position of Clinician

Clinician's positions can be designated by the hours of a clock around the patient's head. Noon, or 12:00, is at the top, over the patient's forehead, as shown in Figure 5-5.

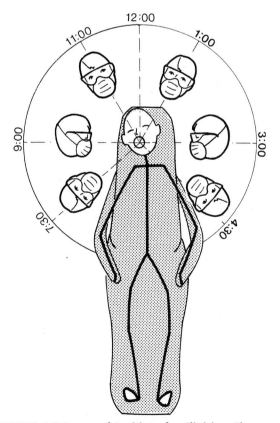

▪ **FIGURE 5-5 Range of Positions for Clinician.** The patient's head is placed at the upper edge of the backrest or headrest at the convenience of the clinician.

E. Flexibility of Clinician's Position

Traditionally, right-handed clinicians treated primarily from the right side of the patient and left-handed clinicians from the left side. However, flexibility of position around the patient's head is made possible by the easy movement of the clinician's stool and turning the patient's head. Visibility and accessibility contribute to a more thorough treatment.

F. Conclusion of Appointment

1. Raise backrest slowly.
2. Tilt chair forward.
3. Request that the patient sit in an upright position briefly to avoid effects of postural hypotension.

G. Contraindications for Supine Position

Most patients can be treated in the standard supine position described. Examples of conditions that may contraindicate the use of a supine position include congestive heart disease and any condition associated with breathing difficulty, such as emphysema, severe asthma, or sinusitis. During the third trimester of pregnancy, some women would be uncomfortable.

Usually when positioning is questionable, the patient volunteers a request for position variation. Questions on the patient's history may reveal the need for adaptation.

▪ LIGHTING

During treatment, visibility in the oral cavity is prerequisite to thoroughness without undue trauma to the tissues. With inadequate light, inefficiency increases and leads to prolonged treatment time, which reduces patient cooperation.

The position of the dental light or lights and the intensity of the beam affect the illumination. A study of the treatment room can be made that includes measurement of the total light at the patient's face in working position. Selection of a light that meets certain standards can ensure intensity sufficient for good visibility and yet safe for the eyes.

I. DENTAL LIGHT: SUGGESTED FEATURES

A. The light should be readily adjustable both vertically and horizontally and the beam capable of being focused.
B. The size must be small enough so that it may be brought close to the treatment area without being in the way, blocking the room light, or being a hazard for movement of people in its vicinity.

C. Intensity of room light should be sufficient to prevent a marked contrast between it and the illuminating beam of the dental light. An all-luminous ceiling contributes to evenly distributed room lighting.

II. DENTAL LIGHT: LOCATION

A. *Attachment.* The most versatile arrangement is a ceiling-mounted light on a track, which permits the light to move over a range from behind a supine patient's head to a position in front of the patient's chin.
B. *Dual Lighting.* With a supine patient position in a contoured chair, advantages to the use of two operating lights have been demonstrated. One light directed from the front of the patient may be attached to the dental unit; the other light is mounted on a ceiling track as just described.

III. DENTAL LIGHT: ADJUSTMENT

A. The area being treated should be seen clearly without having to assume body positions that are harmful if held over long periods.
B. Direct the light first on the napkin under the patient's chin, then rotate the light up to the mouth to avoid flashing light in the patient's eyes.

▪ RELATED OCCUPATIONAL PROBLEMS

Dental hygienists are at risk of developing a variety of physical ailments when inappropriate chair positioning and instrument handling continue over a long period of time. Many of the problems come under the category of cumulative trauma.

Prevention of occupational problems of the back, shoulders, and conditions related to cumulative trauma is based on following good principles and practices of posture and stretching exercises to counteract the repetitive activities used during dental hygiene instrumentation. A few of the exercises that can be used during practice hours are shown in Figure 5-6. Other exercises, particularly for the hands and shoulders are shown in Figure 36-20, on page 630.

▪ FOUR-HANDED DENTAL HYGIENE

I. POSITIONS

A. Assistant is seated with eye level 4 to 6 inches above the clinician's eye level and facing toward the head of the dental chair (Figure 5-7).

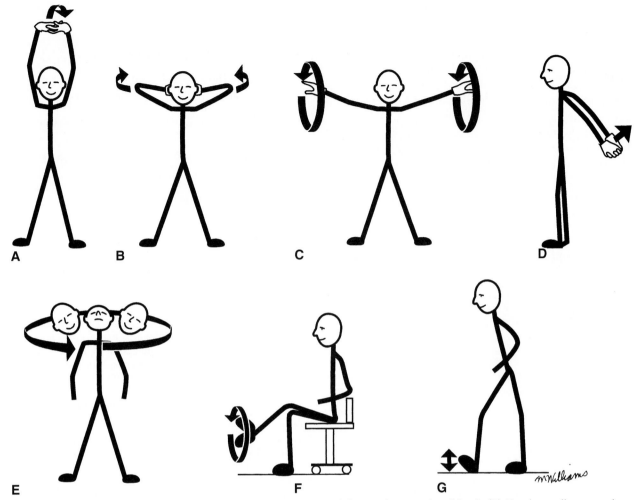

■ **FIGURE 5-6 Exercises to Relieve Tension and Improve Posture. (A)** Stretch up and pull back. **(B)** Head up, elbows push back. **(C)** Circle from the shoulders. Small circles, then gradually larger. **(D)** Clasp hands, pull back, head up. **(E)** Hang the arms and shoulders loose. Circle head to right, then left, 5 to 10 times each. **(F)** Cross leg and circle ankle: right 10 times, then left. Other leg too. **(G)** Foot up and down, heel on ground. Pull the muscles in the back of the leg. Next, the other foot.

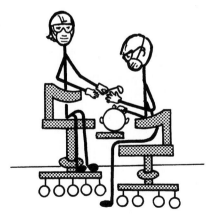

■ **FIGURE 5-7 Clinician With Assistant.** The dental assistant is seated with eye level 4 to 6 inches higher than that of the clinician. The sterile tray is placed on a portable cabinet in front of the assistant within easy reach for passing instruments.

B. When an assistant participates, the patient's oral cavity must be accessible and visible to both clinician and dental assistant.

C. Instruments and other essential materials are kept within arm's length, and the portable cabinet with sterilized prepared tray is in front of the dental assistant.

II. PROCEDURES

A. Four-handed dentistry procedures are practiced with instrument transfers and evacuation.[3,4]

B. Benefits to a dental hygiene practice are multiplied when a dental hygiene assistant is trained to participate in the patient activities that do not require a dental hygiene license.[5,6]

Everyday Ethics

? Recently, several patients have complained to the dentist that Linda, the newest dental hygienist in the practice, lowers the back of the dental chair almost to the ground. Overhearing this, she begins to compensate by raising the clinician's stool and the dental chair. By doing so, she has begun to have some physical discomfort in her shoulders and lower back.

Questions for Consideration

1. Discuss the right of a patient to define how a dental hygienist delivers dental hygiene services.

2. Given this situation, what can Linda do to prepare her patients?

3. Explain alternative solutions that Linda could incorporate into her practice protocol.

✔ Factors To Teach The Patient

- Specific instruction on the components of a dental chair or other equipment that will be of concern to the patient to prevent embarrassment or adverse reactions.

- How certain chair positions needed during scaling relate to the sites around the teeth where more calculus forms.

REFERENCES

1. **Sinnett**, G.M. and Wuehrmann, A.H.: The Dental Operatory of the Future, in Peterson, S., ed.: *The Dentist and His Assistant,* 3rd ed. St. Louis, C.V. Mosby Co., 1972, pp. 392–401.

2. **Tatro**, D.E.: Ergonomics for the Dental Hygienist, *J. Pract. Hyg., 6,* 35, January/February, 1997.

3. **Sinnett**, G.M., McDevitt, E.J., Robinson, G.E., and Wuehrmann, A.H.: Four-Handed Dentistry: A New Mobile Dental Cabinet Design, *J. Am. Dent. Assoc., 78,* 305, February, 1969.

4. **Torres**, H.O., Ehrlich, A., Bird, D., and Dietz, E.: *Modern Dental Assisting,* 5th ed. Philadelphia, W.B. Saunders, 1995, pp. 279–292.

5. **Blitz**, P. and Wright, V.: It Takes Two, *RDH, 14,* 18, September, 1994.

6. **Quinn**, C.: The DHA, *RDH, 17,* 36, February, 1997.

SUGGESTED READINGS

Cunningham, M.A., Sharp, J.D., and Field, H.M.: Teaching Dental Students a Proper Way of Introducing Patients to Instructors, *J. Dent. Educ., 48,* 518, September, 1984.

Ettinger, R.: Office Design for Geriatric Patients, *DentalHygienistNews, 3,* 12, Fall, 1990.

Nield-Gehrig, J.S. and Houseman, G.A.: *Fundamentals of Periodontal Instrumentation,* 3rd ed. Baltimore, Williams & Wilkins, 1996, pp. 15–25.

Nunn, P.J. and Nunn T.D.: Perfect Posture, *RDH, 13,* 14, September, 1993.

Schoen, D.H. and Dean, M.-C.: *Contemporary Periodontal Instrumentation.* Philadelphia, W.B. Saunders Co., 1996, pp. 3–6.

Sunnell, S. and Maschak, L.: Preventing Back, Neck and Shoulder Pain, *Can. Dent. Hyg. (Probe), 30,* 216, November/December, 1996.

Occupational Problems

Barry, R.M., Woodall, W.R., and Mahan, J.M.: Postural Changes in Dental Hygienists: Four Year Longitudinal Study, *J. Dent. Hyg., 66,* 147, March–April, 1992.

Bramson, J.B., Smith, S., and Romagnoli, G.: Evaluating Dental Office Ergonomic Risk Factors and Hazards, *J. Am. Dent. Assoc., 129,* 174, February, 1998.

Liskiewicz, S.T. and Kerschbaum, W.E.: Cumulative Trauma Disorders: An Ergonomic Approach for Prevention, *J. Dent. Hyg., 71,* 162, Summer, 1997.

Seradge, H., Jia, Y.-C., and Owens, W.: *In Vivo* Measurement of Carpal Tunnel Pressure in the Functioning Hand, *J. Hand Surg., 20A,* 855, September, 1995.

Shevach, A., Berg, R.G., Berkey, D.B., and Mann, J.: Ergonomics and Health Considerations at Chairside: Team Members Must Deal With Occupational Risks, *Dent. Teamwork, 9,* 10, November–December, 1996.

Stevens, M.M.: Harmony in Hygiene: The Right Balance to Nutrition and Exercise Can Prolong Your Career, *RDH, 16,* 27, December, 1996.

ASSESSMENT

INTRODUCTION

The dental hygiene process of care is described in Chapter 1. Figure III-1 shows the key position that assessment holds in the subsequent dental hygiene diagnosis, identification of the individual needs of the patient, selection of the interventions to treat and bring health to oral tissues, and carrying out of the clinical treatment needed.

After treatment, when the outcome is evaluated, reassessment reveals the success thus far and the continuing care needed. The process of care makes a full cycle.

Assessment includes the gathering, organizing, and analyzing of all data from observations, patient questioning, and clinical and radiographic examinations. Basically, it is a collection of all pertinent facts and materials to use during care planning and during all treatment as a guide. The chapters in this section, "Assessment," include descriptions for the preparation and assembling of materials for the care plan.

I. PARTS OF THE ASSESSMENT

A. Basic Procedures

1. Patient histories (personal, dental, and medical).
2. Determination of vital signs.
3. Extraoral and intraoral examination.
4. Radiographic survey.

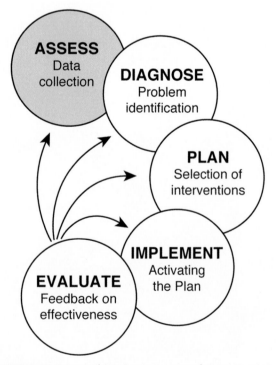

5. Study casts.
6. Examination of the gingival and periodontal tissues, including clinical signs of disease involvement, probing depths and charting, and mobility evaluation.
7. Examination of the teeth to determine and record deposits, restorations, sealants, carious lesions, structural defects, pulp vitality, and occlusal factors.

B. Supplementary Procedures

In addition to the basic assessments, other procedures are selected because of the individual needs of a patient and may be influenced by the age group to which the patient belongs.

Certain procedures may be for an emergency examination. For example, if during the intraoral examination of the oral mucosa a suspicious lesion was found for which a biopsy was indicated, such a diagnostic procedure would take precedence over any other.

Assessment may include photographs, referrals for biopsy when a significant lesion is noted, or laboratory tests to provide essential information before treatment can be undertaken. Special consultations with or referrals to medical specialists are sometimes needed.

C. Assessment for the Preventive Care Plan

Built into the sequence of clinical procedures is the initiation of steps for arresting the disease processes and control of etiologic factors. The patient must learn methods to prevent episodes of recurrence of disease.

Assessment for the preventive care plan will include analysis of the patient's history of dental caries and periodontal infections, and the measures used for self-care. Assessment includes learning about the attitudes of the patient and the values placed on maintenance of oral health and the prevention of disease. Assessment will include gathering information about personal daily care for removal of dental biofilm, use of tobacco, dietary habits, fluoride history and current use, and the regularity of continuing care and the frequency of maintenance appointments.

II. PURPOSES

An efficiently conducted assessment can benefit the patient and provide an overall perspective from which a patient-oriented dental hygiene care program can be formulated. Basic objectives are to:

▪ **FIGURE III-1** Dental Hygiene Process of Care. Section III Assessment.

A. Organize information and materials for use while making the diagnosis and outlining the treatment plan for the patient.
B. Aid in:
- Planning dental hygiene preventive care and instruction for the patient.
- Guiding instrumentation during dental hygiene appointments.
- Correlating dental hygiene care with dental care.
C. Provide a permanent, documented, continuing record of the patient's oral and general health for
- Evaluating the response to treatment, which may be compared with future observations at maintenance appointments.
- Protecting the practice in case of misunderstandings or evidence in legal matters should questions arise.

D. Increase the scope of contribution of the dental hygienist to comprehensive patient care by the dental health team.

▪ ETHICAL APPLICATIONS

An ethical theory offers a general view or approach to an ethical problem. In health care, theories are often based on norms or rules that ask which type of action is morally correct. A dental professional may consider the desired outcome of a particular situation, what guidelines to follow, or whether to rely on personal and professional virtues when making a judgment. There are many philosophical theories that apply to the delivery of dental care. A few key theories and corresponding definitions are referenced in Table III-1.

TABLE III-1 SOME ETHICAL THEORIES

THEORY	DEFINITION	EXAMPLE
Deontology	A study of rules by following the proper duties or obligations pertaining to one's role.	The dental hygienist must complete accurate and detailed documentation of the services rendered for every patient.
Rights Theory	The other side of duties, focusing on maintaining the rights of both patients and providers.	A patient has a right to be informed of what treatment the dental hygienist will perform.
Teleology	Concerned with the consequences or usefulness of one's actions, goal-driven.	A dental hygienist that stays on schedule even if some procedures have to be shortened or eliminated.
Utilitarianism	A form of teleology that says an action is good if it brings about the greatest pleasure for the greatest number of people.	Dental insurance companies set limits of reimbursement based on how a procedure is coded.
Virtue Ethics	A moral theory that is concerned with the virtuous qualities of a professional's character (compassion, empathy, respect, wisdom, patience).	Always being honest and offering the best care to every patient.

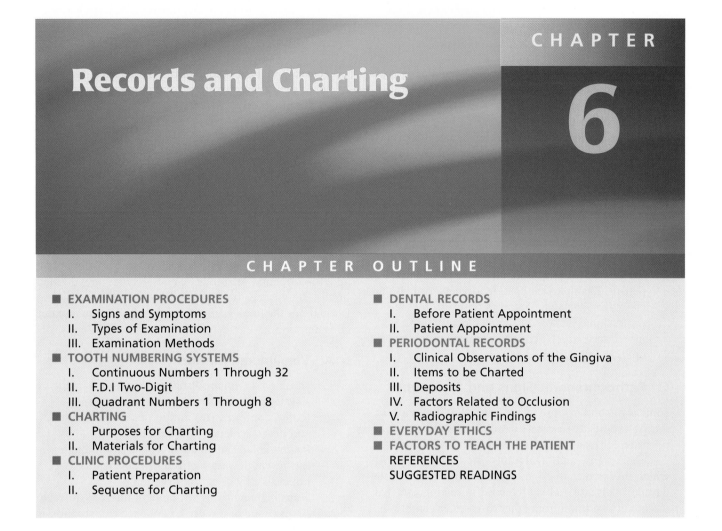

Records and Charting

CHAPTER 6

CHAPTER OUTLINE

Patient health records provide a means of communication between the members of the health team themselves, as well as with their patients. Coordinated planning and continuity of care can be facilitated. The records serve as a basis for the evaluation of the quality of care and aid when a review is made of the effectiveness of patient care practices. Data from health records are utilized in research and education.

Comprehensive health histories, informed consent forms, and accurate documentation are essential to a safe, thorough, and caring practice. They are both business and legal documents for the protection of health-care workers.

Historically, dental health-care personnel have maintained the individual patient's records by long hand. It was essential to write legibly and clearly in ink for a legal permanent record. The personal record was, in reality, a diary of the person's oral health and care over many years for regular patients. Records have also been dictated into a machine to be typewritten into the permanent record later.

Most recently, computerized records have provided a convenient mode of information gathering and preserving. A variety of custom software programs are available. Some provide documentation methods for dental and periodontal assessments with automation, voice-activated recordings, and other systems that include printing off hard copies for the patient when indicated. In all systems, the privacy of personal records must be respected.

■ EXAMINATION PROCEDURES

A specific objective of patient examination as a part of the total assessment is the recognition of deviations from normal that may be signs and symptoms of disease. The importance of careful, thorough examination cannot be overstressed. Concentration and attention to detail are necessary in order that each slight deviation from normal may be entered on the record. Signs and symptoms of disease are the deviations from normal that must be recorded.

I.   SIGNS AND SYMPTOMS

A. Sign

A *sign* is any abnormality that may be indicative of a deviation from normal or of disease that is discovered by a professional person while examining a patient. A sign is an objective symptom.

Examples of signs are changes in color, shape, or consistency of a tissue not observable by the patient. Other signs are findings revealed by the use of a probe, explorer, radiograph, or vitality tester of the dental pulp.

B. Symptom

A *symptom* is also any departure from the normal that may be indicative of disease. Symptoms may be subjective or objective.

1. *Subjective Symptom.* Symptom observed by the patient. Examples are pain, tenderness, or itching.
2. *Objective Symptom.* Symptom observed by the professional person during an examination. As just described, objective symptoms are frequently called *signs*.

C. Pathognomonic Signs and Symptoms

Some signs and symptoms are general and may occur during various disease states. An increase in body temperature, for example, accompanies many infections.

Other signs and symptoms are *pathognomonic*, which means that the sign or symptom is unique to a particular disease and can be used to distinguish that disease or condition from other diseases or conditions.

II. TYPES OF EXAMINATION

A. Complete

A complete examination means that a thorough, comprehensive study is made with all the parts listed on page 92.

B. Screening

Screening implies a brief examination. Screening may be used for initial assessment and classification. In a community health program, a survey of a population made to single out people with a particular condition is called screening.

C. Limited

A limited examination is usually made for an emergency. It may be used in the management of acute conditions.

D. Follow-up

A follow-up examination is a type of limited examination. It is used to observe the effects of treatment after a period of time during which the tissue or lesion can recover and heal. Indications of the need for additional or alternate treatment are apparent at a follow-up examination.

E. Maintenance

An examination is made after a specified period of time following the completion of treatment and the restoration to health. A maintenance examination is a complete reassessment from which a new care plan is derived.

III. EXAMINATION METHODS

A patient is examined by various visual, tactile, manual, and instrumental methods. General types are defined briefly here, and other specific methods are found throughout the book as they apply to a certain area under consideration.

A. Visual Examination

1. *Direct Observation.* Visual examination is made in a systematic order to note surface appearance (color, contour, size) and to observe movement and other evidence of function.
2. *Radiographic Examination.* The use of radiographs can reveal deviations from the normal not noticeable by direct observation.
3. *Transillumination.* A strong light directed through a soft tissue or a tooth to enhance examination is especially useful for detecting irregularities of the teeth and locating calculus.

B. Palpation

Palpation is examination using the sense of touch through tissue manipulation or pressure on an area with the fingers or hand. The method used depends on the area to be investigated. Types of palpation are described on page 176.

C. Instrumentation

Examination instruments, such as the explorer and probe, are used for specific examination of the teeth and periodontal tissues. They are described in detail on pages 225 to 228 and 235 to 237.

D. Percussion

Percussion is the act of tapping or striking a surface or tooth with the fingers or an instrument. Information about the status of health of the part is determined either by the response of the patient or by the sound. For example, a metal mirror handle may be used to tap each tooth successively. When a tooth is known to be painful to movement, percussion should be avoided.

E. Electrical Test

An electrical pulp vitality tester is used to detect the presence or absence of vital pulp tissue. The technique for use is described on pages 273 to 276.

F. Auscultation

Auscultation is the use of sound. An example is the sound of clicking or snapping of the temporomandibular joint when the jaw is moved.

■ TOOTH NUMBERING SYSTEMS

The three tooth designation systems in general use are the *Universal* or *Continuous Numbers 1 Through 32,* adopted by the American Dental Association[1]; the *F.D.I. Two-Digit,* adopted by the Fédération Dentaire Internationale[2]; and the *Palmer* or *Quadrant Numbers 1 Through 8.*[3,4] Because different systems are used in dental offices and clinics, it is necessary to be familiar with all of them.

I. CONTINUOUS NUMBERS 1 THROUGH 32

This tooth numbering method is referred to as the *universal* or *ADA* system.

A. Permanent Teeth

Start with the right maxillary third molar (number 1) and follow around the arch to the left maxillary third molar (16); descend to the left mandibular third molar (17); and follow around to the right mandibular third molar (32). Figure 6-1 shows the crowns of the teeth with the corresponding numbers.

B. Primary or Deciduous Teeth

Use continuous upper case letters A through T in the same order as described for the permanent teeth: right maxillary second molar (A) around to left maxillary second molar (J); descend to left mandibular second molar (K); and around to the right mandibular second molar (T).

II. F.D.I. TWO-DIGIT

The *F.D.I.* system is also called the *International.*

A. Permanent Teeth

Each tooth is numbered by the quadrant (1 to 4) and by the tooth within the quadrant (1 to 8).
1. *Quadrant Numbers*
   1 = Maxillary right
   2 = Maxillary left
   3 = Mandibular left
   4 = Mandibular right
2. *Tooth Numbers Within Each Quadrant.* Start with number 1 at the midline (central incisor) to number 8, third molar. Figure 6-2 shows each tooth number in the four quadrants.
3. *Designation.* The digits are pronounced separately. For example, "two-five" (25) is

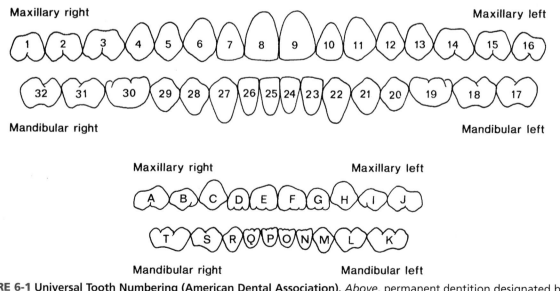

■ **FIGURE 6-1 Universal Tooth Numbering (American Dental Association).** *Above,* permanent dentition designated by numbers 1 through 32, starting at the maxillary right with 1 and following around to the maxillary left third molar (number 16) to the left mandibular third molar (number 17) and around to the right mandibular third molar (number 32). *Below,* primary teeth are designated by letters in the same sequence.

PERMANENT TEETH

Q-1 Maxillary right								Q-2 Maxillary left							
18	17	16	15	14	13	12	11	21	22	23	24	25	26	27	28
48	47	46	45	44	43	42	41	31	32	33	34	35	36	37	38

Mandibular right
Q-4

Mandibular left
Q-3

PRIMARY TEETH

Q-5 Maxillary right					Q-6 Maxillary left				
55	54	53	52	51	61	62	63	64	65
85	84	83	82	81	71	72	73	74	75

Mandibular right
Q-8

Mandibular left
Q-7

■ **FIGURE 6-2 International Tooth Numbering (Fédération Dentaire Internationale).** Each quadrant is numbered 1 through 4, with number 1 on the maxillary right, number 2 on the maxillary left, number 3 on the mandibular left, and number 4 on the mandibular right. Each tooth in a quadrant is numbered 1 through 8 from the central incisor. Quadrants of the primary dentition are numbered from 5 through 8. It is a 2-digit system.

the maxillary left second premolar, and "four-two" (42) is the mandibular right lateral incisor.

B. Primary or Deciduous Teeth

Each tooth is numbered by quadrant (5 to 8) to continue with the permanent quadrant numbers. The teeth are numbered within each quadrant (1 to 5).

1. *Quadrant Numbers*
   5 = Maxillary right
   6 = Maxillary left
   7 = Mandibular left
   8 = Mandibular right
2. *Tooth Numbers Within Each Quadrant.* Number 1 is the central incisor, and number 5 is the second primary molar.
3. *Designation.* The digits are pronounced separately. For example, "eight-three" (83) is the mandibular right primary canine, and "six-five" (65) is the maxillary left second primary molar.

III. QUADRANT NUMBERS 1 THROUGH 8

Names to identify this method are the *Palmer System* or *Set-square*.

A. Permanent Teeth

With number 1 for each central incisor, the teeth in each quadrant are numbered to 8, the third molar (Figure 6-3). To identify individual teeth, horizontal and vertical lines are drawn to indicate the quadrant. For example, the left maxillary first premolar is |4, the right mandibular first and second molars are 76|. An entire quadrant may

be represented by the use of the letter Q, for example, the maxillary right quadrant is Q|.

B. Primary or Deciduous Teeth

Upper case letters A through E are used instead of the numbers. Examples are the mandibular left canine |C and the maxillary right first primary molar D|.

■ CHARTING

Complete and accurate examinations with proper documentation by records and chartings are basic to all patient care. All findings from the comprehensive assessment are recorded. Some systems of recording involve the completion of forms with topics and spaces to check or fill in the information, whereas others call for a prose-style summary.

Radiographs, study casts, photographs, and all other materials collected during the initial examination and during continuing patient appointments are official parts of the permanent records. Each part must be dated.

A filing system is needed that has accessibility to the health records by authorized personnel only. The privacy of records must be maintained.

Computerized systems have many advantages for integration of the records into the total practice. Appointment schedules, medical alerts, and financial aspects all can be part of the data management by the computer.

I. PURPOSES FOR CHARTING

The purpose of each type of charting is defined by its title: the dental charting includes diagrammatic representation

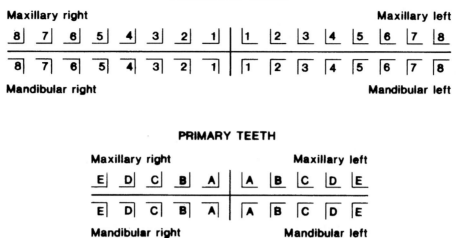

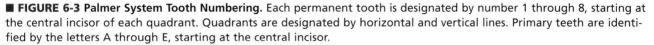

■ **FIGURE 6-3 Palmer System Tooth Numbering.** Each permanent tooth is designated by number 1 through 8, starting at the central incisor of each quadrant. Quadrants are designated by horizontal and vertical lines. Primary teeth are identified by the letters A through E, starting at the central incisor.

of existing conditions of the teeth, whereas the periodontal charting indicates clinical features of the periodontium. Separate types of chart forms may be used to record the special features of each, or the two may be combined on one chart. Neatness in the markings of symbols, drawings, and labels goes hand in hand with the accuracy of the examination itself.

An accurate, detailed, and carefully recorded charting is used as follows:

A. For Care Planning

The charting is a graphic representation of the existing condition of the patient's teeth and periodontium from which needed treatment procedures can be organized into a treatment plan.

B. For Counseling Treatment

During dental and dental hygiene appointments, the charting is useful for guiding specific procedures.

C. For Evaluation

The outcome and degree of lasting effects of treatment are determined by comparing the findings of the initially recorded examination with periodic follow-up examinations.

D. For Protection

In the event of misunderstanding by a patient, or if legal questions should arise, the records and chartings are realistic evidence.

E. For Identification

In the event of emergency, accident, or disaster, a patient may be identified by the teeth for which a record has been maintained.

II. MATERIALS FOR CHARTING

A. Instruments

1. Probe.
2. Explorers.
3. Clear and unscratched mouth mirror.
4. Dental floss.
5. Gauze sponges.
6. Air tip and saliva ejector.
7. Topical anesthetic if probing proves discomforting to the patient.

B. Study Casts

C. Radiographs

1. Advanced preparation of the radiographic survey facilitates coordination between clinical and radiographic examinations. The completely processed and mounted radiographs provide greater assurance of a thorough analysis.
2. A bitewing survey may be sufficient for the charting of dental caries, but a periapical survey is essential for periodontal evaluation.

D. Form for Manual Charting

Many variations of chart forms are in current use, some available commercially, some designed by the individual practitioner to meet particular needs. Specifications for an adequate form include ample space to chart neatly, accurately, and completely; to label as needed for clarity; and to record in a manner that can be interpreted by all who use it. Three types of forms are described here.

1. *Anatomic Drawings of the Crowns of Teeth Only*. Difficult to chart adequately the periodontal findings; designed primarily for charting dental caries.

2. *Geometric*. A diagrammatic representation for each tooth with space for each surface; generally does not include the roots. Without roots, the diagram would not be useful for periodontal charting.

Each tooth in the geometric chart shown in Figure 6-4 includes two circles. The inner circle represents the occlusal surface, and the outer circle, divided into four parts, represents the mesial, facial, distal, and lingual. The individual tooth diagrams may be arranged in a linear format (Figure 6-4A) or in arches to simulate the oral cavity (Figure 6-4B).

3. *Anatomic Tooth Drawings of the Complete Teeth*. Such a chart form lends itself to combined dental and periodontal charting. Figure 6-5 is an example of this type of chart form.

E. Computerized Systems

Voice-operated or mouse-controlled computer systems aid greatly in saving time and solving the problem of cross-contamination by way of chart forms and utensils.

■ CLINIC PROCEDURES

I. PATIENT PREPARATION

A. Patient Position

Position for optimum visibility and accessibility.

B. Illumination

Maximum illumination is important. Use direct or indirect (mirror) light or transillumination.

II. SEQUENCE FOR CHARTING

A. Basic Entries

1. *Name, Birth Date*
2. *Date*. Every entry must be dated.
3. *Missing Teeth*. When radiographs are available in advance, missing teeth can be charted before the clinic appointment. Whether dental or periodontal charting is completed first, marking the missing teeth will be necessary.

B. Systematic Procedure

The use of a set routine is prerequisite to accomplishing a complete and accurate charting, not only for the tooth surface-to-surface pattern, but also for the parts of the charting itself.

Charting of all of one kind of item for the entire mouth, rather than complete chartings of one tooth, helps to obtain accuracy because only one train of thought is required at a time. For example, in the dental charting, record all the restorations first. Then start again at the first tooth and chart all the deviations from normal. Charting all restorations and deviations for each tooth separately is a less efficient method.

■ DENTAL RECORDS

The patient's permanent records include the itemized findings of the clinical and radiographic examinations along with subjective symptoms reported by the patient. Material for the dental records is included in Chapter 15 and for occlusion in Chapter 16. Mobility of teeth has been included with the periodontal examination because the causes of mobility are periodontally oriented.

After initial entries are recorded, additions are made to show the progress of treatment. At each periodic maintenance visit, new and comparative records and chartings must be prepared.

The need for meticulous examination and recording cannot be overemphasized. Finding and recording a carious lesion may mean saving a tooth for the patient's lifetime; inadvertent neglect of a tooth may lead eventually to a need for endodontic therapy or even extraction.

I. BEFORE PATIENT APPOINTMENT

Radiographs and study casts prepared at an initial appointment before clinical examination for charting help to conserve patient chair time.

A. Radiographic Charting

The following may be charted without the presence of the patient: missing, unerupted, impacted teeth; endodontic restorations; overhanging margins of existing restorations; proximal surface carious lesions;

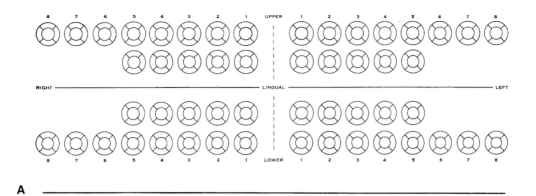

A

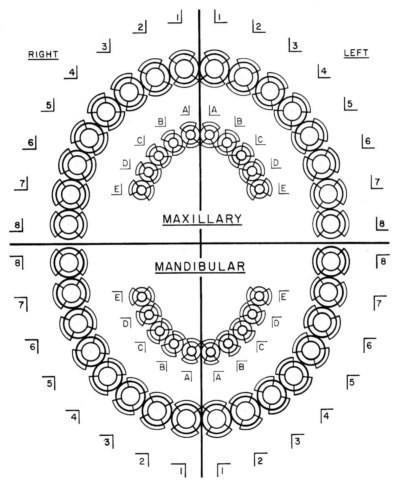

B

■ **FIGURE 6-4 Geometric Charting Form. (A)** Linear format with primary teeth between the permanent teeth. **(B)** Permanent teeth in arch form with primary teeth inside. Teeth are numbered by quadrant numbers 1 through 8.

and any other deviation from normal evident from the radiographs.

Supplemental and confirmational observations and checks are made during the clinical examination with the patient. For example, when an overhanging restoration is noted but dental caries is not visible on the radiograph, examination by exploration is required because the restoration may be superimposed over the carious lesion.

B. Study Casts

Record the classification of occlusion (pages 282 to 284).

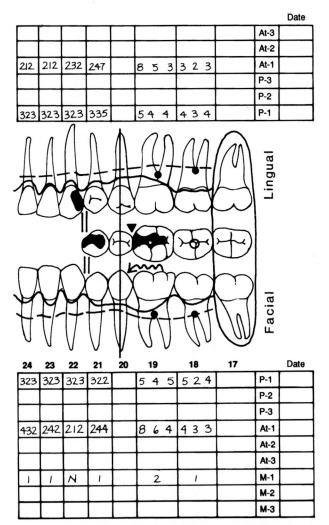

									Date
								At-3	
								At-2	
212	212	232	247		8 5 3	3 2 3		At-1	
								P-3	
								P-2	
323	323	323	335		5 4 4	4 3 4		P-1	

Key

Missing Tooth: | or X
Unerupted or impacted: Encircle tooth
Drift and Migration: ⤳
Open Contact: ‖
Food Impaction: ↓ (at occlusal)

Periodental Chart

Gingival Margin: Black line
Mucogingival Junction: Dashed line
Furca involved: ● (in furcation)
Probing depths: (mm) P-1, P-2, P-3
Clinical attachment level: (mm) At-1, At-2, At-3

Dental Chart

Dental Caries: red
Restorations: blue
Defective Restoration: circle with red
Overhang: ▼ (at occlusal)
Mobility: (+, N, 1, 2, 3) M-1, M-2, M-3
Fremitus: F-1 (recorded on maxillary only)

24	23	22	21	20	19	18	17	Date	
323	323	323	322		5 4 5	5 2 4		P-1	
								P-2	
								P-3	
432	242	212	244		8 6 4	4 3 3		At-1	
								At-2	
								At-3	
I	I	N	I		2	1		M-1	
								M-2	
								M-3	

■ **FIGURE 6-5 Periodontal and Dental Charting.** Section of a charting (mandibular left quadrant) shows combined dental and periodontal charting. Dental caries and restorations are usually marked with colored pencils, such as blue for restorations and red for dental caries, on the anatomic crowns or roots. The gingival margin is clearly drawn to show areas of recession. Boxes at the apices of each tooth provide spaces for probing depths and clinical attachment level recordings, as well as for mobility notations.

II. PATIENT APPOINTMENT

Figure 6-5 is an example of a quadrant of dental charting using anatomic tooth drawings. Dental findings can also be charted on a geometric form, such as that shown in Figure 6-4.

A. Chart missing teeth.
B. Chart existing restorations, including fixed and removable prostheses.
C. Chart sealants.
D. Chart apparent carious lesions and other deviations from normal.
E. Coordinate clinical and radiographic findings.
F. Use dental floss. Chart inadequate contact areas and observe proximal surface roughness. Fraying of dental floss as it is passed over a rough proximal surface may mean the defective margin of a restoration, a sharp cavity margin, or dental calculus.

G. Chart pulp vitality. Record numbers in the permanent record. Chart forms sometimes include a specific place for the recording of such data. Procedures are described on pages 273 to 276.

H. Chart tooth sensitivity. The patient may report hypersensitive areas, or they may be discovered during instrumentation. Record the tooth number and surface for reference during the treatment phase.

Everyday Ethics

? The current protocol in Dr. Grain's office utilizes a medical history form that is slightly larger than a postcard to gather all the patient data. As a fairly recent dental hygiene graduate, the inadequacy of the questions on the history form have bothered Hanna. Hanna, who practices there full-time, has brought up this issue with Dr. Grain personally and also at a recent staff meeting. Dr. Grain has been practicing for 30 years with a perfect record free of violations or lawsuits and boldly states this fact to the entire dental team. Hanna feels she has hit a major roadblock and ponders keeping a separate more thorough history form on each patient in her own treatment room.

Questions for Consideration

1. What benefits vs. burdens should Hanna consider if she decides to begin taking a separate medical history on each patient who presents for dental hygiene appointments?

2. Does the length of the history form directly affect the quality of care delivered to patients? Explain your rationale.

3. How is the autonomy of both the hygienist and the patients she treats being compromised by Dr. Grain's reluctance to change to a more comprehensive history taking protocol?

▪ PERIODONTAL RECORDS

The patient's permanent records include the itemized findings of all the clinical and radiographic examinations. Material for the periodontal charting is described on pages 234 to 235. Entries should be clear and easily understood by all who read them and use them in continuing treatment.

Additions to the records are made to show the progress of treatment and comparative observations throughout the series of treatment appointments. After the mouth has been brought to a state of health, a maintenance plan is outlined. At each succeeding appointment, new and comparative records and chartings are made.

Basic periodontal recordings are listed here.

I. CLINICAL OBSERVATIONS OF THE GINGIVA

A. Describe Gingiva

Color, size, position, shape, consistency, and surface texture; extent of bleeding when probed; and areas where there is minimal attached gingiva (pages 212, 233, and Table 12-1, page 216).

B. Describe Distribution of Gingival Changes

Localized or generalized; specify the areas of severest disease involvement. Use tooth numbers to identify adjacent gingival tissue.

C. Describe Degree of Severity of Disease

Periodontal case type (Table 14-1, page 247).

II. ITEMS TO BE CHARTED

A. Missing teeth.
B. Gingival line (margin) and mucogingival lines (junctions).
C. Probing depths.
D. Areas of suspected mucogingival involvement.
E. Furcation involvement.

✔ Factors To Teach The Patient

- Interpretation of all recordings; meaning of all numbers used, such as for probing depths.

- The importance of making a complete study of the patient's oral problems before beginning treatment.

- Advantages of cooperation and patience in furnishing information that will help dental personnel to interpret observations accurately so that the correct diagnosis and appropriate treatment plan can be made.

- Assurance that all information received is completely confidential and that the records are locked when the office is closed.

F. Abnormal frenal attachments.

G. Mobility and fremitus of teeth.

III. DEPOSITS

A. Stains

1. *Extrinsic*. Record type of stain, color, distribution; specific location by tooth number; whether slight, moderate, or heavy.

2. *Intrinsic*. Record separately from extrinsic and identify by type when known.

B. Calculus

Record distribution and amount of supragingival and subgingival calculus separately for treatment planning purposes.

C. Soft Deposits

1. *Food Debris*. Distribution and amount. Record location by teeth when the biofilm control instruction requires special emphasis on a particular area.

2. *Dental Biofilm*
    a. Record direct observations with or without disclosing agent; include distribution and degree or amount.
    b. Biofilm index recorded (pages 328 to 333).

IV. FACTORS RELATED TO OCCLUSION

Clinical signs of trauma from occlusion are described on pages 287 to 288. The following list is for consideration with other records for the treatment planning.

A. Mobility of Teeth

Record degree for each tooth (pages 240 to 241). In Figure 6-5, an example of a method for recording mobility is shown.

B. Fremitus (page 241)

C. Possible Food Impaction Areas

1. Inquire of patient where fibrous foods usually catch between the teeth.

2. Use dental floss to identify inadequate contact areas that may contribute to food impaction. An example of one method for recording an open contact is shown by the vertical parallel lines between teeth numbered 21 and 22 in Figure 6-5.

D. Occlusion-Related Habits

1. Observe for evidence of, and question patient concerning, such parafunctional habits as bruxism or clenching.

2. Note wear patterns and facets on study cast.

3. Note attrition.

E. Tooth Migration (pages 285 to 286)

F. Sensitivity to Percussion

G. Radiographic Evidences

Related to trauma from occlusion (page 288).

V. RADIOGRAPHIC FINDINGS

Specific notes should be made to correlate the radiographic findings with the clinical observations just listed. Details of radiographic findings in periodontal disease are described on pages 241 to 244. The following should be noted in particular:

A. Height of bone as related to the cementoenamel junction.

B. Horizontal or angular shape of remaining bone.

C. Intact, broken, or missing crestal lamina dura.

D. Furcation involvement.

E. Widening of periodontal ligament space.

F. Overhanging fillings, large carious lesions, and other dental biofilm–retention factors.

REFERENCES

1. **American Dental Association:** System of Tooth Numbering and Radiograph Mounting, Approved by the American Dental Association House of Delegates, October, 1968.

2. **Fédération Dentaire Internationale:** Two-digit System of Designating Teeth, *Int. Dent. J., 21,* 104, March, 1971.

3. **American Dental Association:** Proceedings of Dental Societies, *Dent. Cosmos, 12,* 522, October, 1870.

4. **Palmer,** C.: Palmer's Dental Notation, *Dent. Cosmos, 33,* 194, 1891.

SUGGESTED READINGS

American Academy of Periodontology: *Current Procedural Terminology for Periodontics and Insurance Reporting Manual,* 7th ed. Chicago, American Academy of Periodontology, 1995, 64 pp.

Carranza, F.A. and Newman, M.G.: *Clinical Periodontology,* 8th ed. Philadelphia, W.B. Saunders Co., 1996, pp. 344-361.

Peck, S. and Peck, L.: A Time for Change of Tooth Numbering Systems, *J. Dent. Educ., 57,* 643, August, 1993.

Peck, S. and Peck, L.: Tooth Numbering Progress, *Angle Orthodont., 66,* 83, Number 2, 1996.

Villa Vigil, M.A., Arenal, A.A., and Gonzalez, M.A.R.: Notation of Numerical Abnormalities by an Addition to the F.D.I. System, *Quintessence Int., 20,* 299, April, 1989.

Records

Ekstein, E.C.: Dental Office Record Keeping and Its Impact on Anticipated Litigation, *Compend. Cont. Educ. Dent., 14,* 590, May, 1993.

Eubanks, S.: The Dental Assistant's Role in Risk Management. Patient Records, *Dent. Assist., 61,* 18, Second Quarter, 1992.

Keselyak, N. and Maschak, L.: The Problem-Oriented Dental Record: A Key to Dental Hygiene Treatment Planning and the Problem-Solving Model for Dental Hygiene Practice, *Can. Dent. Hyg./Probe, 27,* 15, January/February, 1993.

McCullough, C.: Clinical Applications of Voice Chart Computer Technology in the Practice of Dental Hygiene, *J. Pract. Hyg., 4,* 29, November/December, 1995.

Nunn, P.: SOAP for Whiter, Brighter Notes! *Access, 8,* 26, February, 1994.

Sfikas, P.M.: Guarding the Files: Your Role in Maintaining the Confidentiality of Patient Records, *J. Am. Dent. Assoc., 127,* 1248, August, 1996.

Stach, D.J.: The Complete Dental Record, in Woodall, I.R.: *Comprehensive Dental Hygiene Care,* 4th ed. St. Louis, Mosby, 1993, pp. 70-77.

Summers, C.J., Gooch, B.F., Marianos, D.W., Malvitz, D.M., and Bond, W.W.: Practical Infection Control in Oral Health Surveys and Screenings, *J. Am. Dent. Assoc., 125,* 1213, September, 1994.

Williams, V.: Getting the Required Information in 10 Minutes, *Access, 8,* 38, January, 1994.

Woodward, B.: Sounding Board. The Computer-based Patient Record and Confidentiality, *N. Engl. J. Med., 333,* 1419, November 23, 1995.

Forensic Identification

Beale, D.R.: The Importance of Dental Records for Identification, *N. Z. Dent. J., 87,* 84, July, 1991.

Clark, D.H., ed.: *Practical Forensic Odontology.* Oxford, Wright, 1992, pp. 101-109 (Dental Record Interpretation).

Parker, L.S.: Dental Detectives, *RDH, 10,* 14, February, 1990.

CHAPTER 7

Personal, Dental, and Medical Histories

For safe, scientific dental and dental hygiene care, a meaningful, complete patient history is an essential part of the complete assessment. The history directs and guides steps to be taken in preparation for, during, and following appointments.

The history is needed before oral examination procedures with periodontal probe and explorer are carried out. The use of instruments that would manipulate the soft tissue around the teeth is contraindicated until after it has been determined whether antibiotic premedication is required.

When a question exists about the medical history as described by the patient, or when an unusual or abnormal condition is observed, consultation with the patient's physician or referral for examination of the patient who does not have a physician is mandatory. Even emergency treatment, such as for the relief of pain, should be postponed tentatively or kept to a minimum until the patient's status is determined.

I. SIGNIFICANCE

The significance of the history cannot be overestimated. Oral conditions reflect the general health of the patient. Dental procedures may complicate or be complicated by existing pathologic or physiologic conditions elsewhere in the body. General health factors influence response to treatment, such as tissue healing, and thereby influence the outcomes that may be expected from oral care.

The state of the patient's health is constantly changing. Therefore, the history represents only the period in the patient's life during which the history was made. With successive appointments, the history must be reviewed and considered along with other new findings. Key words relating to the preparation and use of the histories are defined in Box 7-1.

II. PURPOSES OF THE HISTORY

Carefully prepared personal, medical, and dental histories are used in comprehensive patient care to
- Provide information pertinent to the etiology and diagnosis of oral conditions and the total patient care plan.
- Reveal conditions that necessitate precautions, modifications, or adaptations during appointments to ensure that dental and dental hygiene procedures will not harm the patient and that emergency situations will be prevented.
- Aid in the identification of possible unrecognized conditions for which the patient should be referred for further diagnosis and treatment.
- Permit appraisal of the general health and nutritional status, which, in turn, contributes to the prognosis of success in patient care and instruction.
- Give insight into emotional and psychological factors, attitudes, and prejudices that may affect present appointments as well as continuing care.
- Document records for reference and comparison over a series of appointments for periodic follow-up.
- Furnish evidence in legal matters should questions arise.[1]

■ HISTORY PREPARATION

The general methods in current use for obtaining a health history are the *interview*, the *questionnaire*, or a combination of the two. There are several systems for obtaining the history.

BOX 7-1 KEY WORDS AND ABBREVIATIONS: Personal, Medical, and Dental Histories

Allergy: state of abnormal and individual hypersensitivity acquired through exposure to a particular allergen.

Antibiotic premedication: provision of an effective antibiotic before invasive clinical procedures that can create a transient bacteremia, which, in turn, can cause infective endocarditis or other serious infection.

Bacteremia: presence of microorganisms in the bloodstream.

Drug interaction: a change in the effect of one drug when a second drug is introduced concomitantly; the change may be desirable, adverse, or inconsequential.

Forensic: pertaining to or applied in legal proceedings.

Forensic dentistry: dentolegal science; the relation and application of dental facts to legal problems, as in using the teeth for identifying the dead.

Hematogenous: produced or derived from blood; disseminated through the bloodstream.

Immunocompromised: when the immune response is attenuated by administration of immunosuppressive drugs, by irradiation, by malnutrition, or by certain disease processes.

Informed consent: a medicolegal document that holds providers responsible for ensuring that patients understand the risks and benefits of a procedure or medication before it is administered.

OTC: over the counter; nonprescription drug; pertains to distribution of drugs directly to the public without prescription.

PDR: *Physicans' Desk Reference*; contains current information about the actions, side effects, and interactions of drugs; a new edition is published annually.

Premedication: preliminary medication; may be for the purpose of allaying apprehension, preventing bacteremia, or otherwise facilitating the clinical procedure.

SBE: subacute bacterial endocarditis, now called infective endocarditis.

I. SYSTEMS

A. Preappointment Information

Basic information obtained prior to the initial assessment appointment can save time and facilitate the process. A brief telephone screening interview can help determine potential medical problems and need for premedication, and it can identify medically compromised or physically challenged patients for whom modifications in routine care may be needed.

B. Brief History

A brief history of vital items is obtained at the initial visit; a complete history is obtained at a succeeding appointment.

1. Purposes of brief history are to prepare for emergency care and to learn of any condition that may contraindicate instrumentation.
2. Brief history may be in the form of a questionnaire; an interview for follow-up provides opportunity for individual evaluation.

C. Self-history

Because a self-history can be prepared at home, the history form may be mailed to the patient in advance or given at the first appointment to complete and bring in at the second appointment. Such a form might include some checking, as in a questionnaire, and some space to allow free expression by the patient.

D. Complete History

Complete history is made at the initial visit and may be a combination of interview and questionnaire.

II. RECORD FORMS

A. Basic History Forms

Many varying forms are in current use. Forms are available commercially or from the American Dental Association (ADA),[2] but many dentists and dental hygienists prefer to develop their own and have a form printed to their specifications.

B. Characteristics of an Adequate Form

The number of items or questions included is not necessarily indicative of the value of the form. The extensive and involved form may be as practical or impractical as the brief checklist that permits no detailed description. Success in use depends on function and a clear common understanding of the meaning of the recorded information to all who refer to it.

Some characteristics of an adequate form are that it should

- Provide for conventional notation of important details in a logical sequence.
- Permit quick identification of special needs of a patient when the history is reviewed prior to each appointment.
- Allow ample space to record the patient's own words whenever possible in the interview method, or for self-expression by the patient on a questionnaire.
- Have space for notes concerning attitudes and knowledge as stated or displayed by the patient during the history-taking or other later appointments.
- Be of a size consistent with the complete patient record forms for filing and ready availability.

C. Supplementary Forms

A second questionnaire for specialized topics is needed to determine details. The basic questionnaire reveals whether the topic applies to the individual, and if the answer is positive, additional information is requested.

For example, simple questions may appear on the basic questionnaire to show the use of tobacco. Completion of another questionnaire provides details of the type of tobacco used and frequency.

III. INTRODUCTION TO THE PATIENT

The patient needs to realize why the information requested in the histories is essential before treatment can be undertaken. Dental personnel must convey the idea that oral health and general health are interrelated, without creating undue alarm concerning potential ill effects or harmful sequelae from required treatment.

For building rapport, children may participate in their history preparation, but most of the information will need to be supplied by a parent. The signature of the responsible adult on the record is needed.

IV. LIMITATIONS OF A HISTORY

Many patients cannot or will not provide complete or, in certain cases, correct information when answering medical or dental history questions. There may be problems related to the method of obtaining the histories, how the questions are worded, or an inadvertent lack of neutrality in the attitude of the person preparing the history. Some patients may have difficulty in comprehending a self-administered test, or there may be a language barrier.

Where the questionnaire is completed may influence answers. A crowded reception area where other patients can see the form and the checks made does not provide sufficient privacy.

Another reason for inaccuracy or incompleteness is that patients may not understand the relationship between certain diseases or conditions and dental treatment. Information may seem irrelevant, so it is withheld. Occasionally, a patient will not want to tell about a condition that may be embarrassing to discuss. The patient may fear refusal of treatment, particularly if such had been a previous experience in other dental practices.

■ THE QUESTIONNAIRE

Positive findings on a completed questionnaire need supplementation in a personal interview. A questionnaire by itself cannot be expected to satisfy the overall purposes of the history, but it can be adapted best to phases of the personal history, some aspects of the dental history, and factual information in the medical history.

I. TYPES OF QUESTIONS

The health questionnaire available from the American Dental Association (Figure 7-1) provides useful examples of questions essential to patient evaluation.[2]

A. System Oriented

Direct questions or topics that check whether the patient has had a disease of, for example, the digestive system, respiratory system, or urinary system may be used. The questions may contain references to body parts, for example, the stomach, lungs, kidneys. Questions can then be directed to the specific disease state and the dates and duration.

B. Disease Oriented

A typical set of questions for the patient to check may start with "Do you have, or have you had, any of the following diseases or problems?" A listing under that question contains such items as diabetes, asthma, or rheumatic fever arranged alphabetically or grouped by systems or body organs.

Follow-up questions can determine dates of illness, severity, and outcome.

C. Symptom Oriented

In the absence of previous or current disease states, questions may lead to a suspicion of a condition, which, in turn, can provide an opportunity to recommend and encourage the patient to schedule an examination by a physician. Examples of the symptom-oriented questions are "Are you thirsty much of the time?" "Does your mouth frequently become dry?" or "Do you have to urinate (pass water) more than six times a day?" Positive answers could lead to tests for diabetes detection.

II. ADVANTAGES OF A QUESTIONNAIRE

- Broad in scope; useful during the interview to identify positive areas that need additional clarification.
- Time-saving.
- Consistent; all selected questions are included, and none is omitted because of time or other factors.
- Patient has time to think over the answers; not under pressure, nor under the eyes of the interviewer.
- Patient may write information that might not be expressed directly in an interview.
- Legal aspects of a written record with patient's signature.

III. DISADVANTAGES OF A QUESTIONNAIRE (IF USED ALONE WITHOUT A FOLLOW-UP INTERVIEW)

- Impersonal; no opportunity to develop rapport.
- Inflexible; no provision for additional questioning in areas of specific importance to an individual patient.

■ THE INTERVIEW

In long-range planning for the patient's health, much more is involved than asking questions and receiving answers. The rapport established at the time of the interview contributes to the continued cooperation of the patient.

I. PARTICIPANTS

The interviewer is alone with the patient or parent of the child patient. The history should never be taken in a reception area when other patients are present.

II. SETTING

A. A consultation room or office is preferred; the patient should be away from the atmosphere of the treatment room, where thoughts may be on the techniques to be performed.
B. Treatment room may be the only available place where privacy is afforded.
   1. Seat patient comfortably in upright position.

ADA. American Dental Association
www.ada.org

Medical Alert:	Condition:	Premedication:	Allergies:	Anesthesia:	Date:

HEALTH HISTORY FORM

Name: _____   Home Phone: (   )   Business Phone: (   )
    LAST   FIRST   MIDDLE

Address: _____   City: _____   State: _____   Zip Code: _____
    P.O. BOX or Mailing Address

Occupation: _____   Height: ____   Weight: ____   Date of Birth: ____   Sex: M ❏ F ❏

SS#: _____   Emergency Contact: _____   Relationship: _____   Phone: (   )

If you are completing this form for another person, what is your relationship to that person?
_____
    NAME   RELATIONSHIP

For the following questions, please (X) whichever applies, your answers are for our records only and will be kept confidential in accordance with applicable laws. Please note that during your initial visit you will be asked some questions about your responses to this questionnaire and there may be additional questions concerning your health. This information is vital to allow us to provide appropriate care for you. This office does not use this information to discriminate.

DENTAL INFORMATION

	Yes	No	Don't Know
Do your gums bleed when you brush?	❏	❏	❏
Have you ever had orthodontic (braces) treatment?	❏	❏	❏
Are your teeth sensitive to cold, hot, sweets or pressure?	❏	❏	❏
Do you have earaches or neck pains?	❏	❏	❏
Have you had any periodontal (gum) treatments?	❏	❏	❏
Do you wear removable dental appliances?	❏	❏	❏
Have you had a serious/difficult problem associated with any previous dental treatment?	❏	❏	❏
If yes, explain:			

How would you describe your current dental problem? _____

Date of your last dental exam: _____

Date of last dental x-rays: _____

What was done at that time? _____

How do you feel about the appearance of your teeth? _____

MEDICAL INFORMATION

	Yes	No	Don't Know
If you answer yes to any of the 3 items below, please stop and return this form to the receptionist.			
Have you had any of the following diseases or problems?			
Active Tuberculosis	❏	❏	❏
Persistent cough greater than a 3 week duration	❏	❏	❏
Cough that produces blood	❏	❏	❏
Are you in good health?	❏	❏	❏
Has there been any change in your general health within the past year?	❏	❏	❏
Are you now under the care of a physician?	❏	❏	❏
If yes, what is/are the condition(s) being treated?			

Date of last physical examination: _____

Physician:

NAME		PHONE	
ADDRESS	CITY/STATE		ZIP

NAME		PHONE	
ADDRESS	CITY/STATE		ZIP

	Yes	No	Don't Know
Have you had any serious illness, operation, or been hospitalized in the past 5 years?	❏	❏	❏
If yes, what was the illness or problem?			

_____

	Yes	No	Don't Know
Are you taking or have you recently taken any medicine(s) including non-prescription medicine?	❏	❏	❏
If yes, what medicine(s) are you taking?			
Prescribed:			

Over the counter: _____

Vitamins, natural or herbal preparations and/or diet supplements: _____

	Yes	No	Don't Know
Are you taking, or have you taken, any diet drugs such Pondimin (fenfluramine), Redux (dexphenfluramine) or phen-fen (fenfluramine-phentermine combination)?	❏	❏	❏
Do you drink alcoholic beverages?	❏	❏	❏
If yes, how much alcohol did you drink in the last 24 hours?			
In the past week?			
Are you alcohol and/or drug dependent?	❏	❏	❏
If yes, have you received treatment? (circle one) Yes / No			
Do you use drugs or other substances for recreational purposes?	❏	❏	❏
If yes, please list:			
Frequency of use (daily, weekly, etc.):			
Number of years of recreational drug use:			
Do you use tobacco (smoking, snuff, chew)?	❏	❏	❏
If yes, how interested are you in stopping? (circle one) Very / Somewhat / Not interested			
Do you wear contact lenses?	❏	❏	❏

PLEASE COMPLETE BOTH SIDES

■ **FIGURE 7-1 Health History Form.** Reprinted with permission. ADA Health History Form, Copyright American Dental Association.

Are you allergic to or have you had a reaction to?	Yes	No	Don't Know
Local anesthetics	☐	☐	☐
Aspirin	☐	☐	☐
Penicillin or other antibiotics	☐	☐	☐
Barbiturates, sedatives, or sleeping pills	☐	☐	☐
Sulfa drugs	☐	☐	☐
Codeine or other narcotics	☐	☐	☐
Latex	☐	☐	☐
Iodine	☐	☐	☐
Hay fever/seasonal	☐	☐	☐
Animals	☐	☐	☐
Food (specify) _____	☐	☐	☐
Other (specify)_____	☐	☐	☐
Metals (specify)_____	☐	☐	☐

To yes responses, specify type of reaction.

_____
_____
_____

	Yes	No	Don't Know
Have you had an orthopedic total joint (hip, knee, elbow, finger) replacement?	☐	☐	☐

If yes, when was this operation done? _____

If you answered yes to the above question, have you had any complications or difficulties with your prosthetic joint?

_____
_____

	Yes	No	Don't Know
Has a physician or previous dentist recommended that you take antibiotics prior to your dental treatment?	☐	☐	☐

If yes, what antibiotic and dose? _____

Name of physician or dentist*: _____

Phone: _____

WOMEN ONLY

	Yes	No	Don't Know
Are you or could you be pregnant?	☐	☐	☐
Nursing?	☐	☐	☐
Taking birth control pills or hormonal replacement?	☐	☐	☐

Please (X) a response to indicate if you have or have not had any of the following diseases or problems.

	Yes	No	Don't Know
Abnormal bleeding	☐	☐	☐
AIDS or HIV infection	☐	☐	☐
Anemia	☐	☐	☐
Arthritis	☐	☐	☐
Rheumatoid arthritis	☐	☐	☐
Asthma	☐	☐	☐
Blood transfusion. If yes, date: _____	☐	☐	☐
Cancer/ Chemotherapy/Radiation Treatment	☐	☐	☐
Cardiovascular disease. If yes, specify below:	☐	☐	☐

____ Angina	____ Heart murmur
____ Arteriosclerosis	____ High blood pressure
____ Artificial heart valves	____ Low blood pressure
____ Congenital heart defects	____ Mitral valve prolapse
____ Congestive heart failure	____ Pacemaker
____ Coronary artery disease	____ Rheumatic heart
____ Damaged heart valves	disease/Rheumatic fever
____ Heart attack	

	Yes	No	Don't Know
Chest pain upon exertion	☐	☐	☐
Chronic pain	☐	☐	☐
Disease, drug, or radiation-induced immunosurpression	☐	☐	☐
Diabetes. If yes, specify below:	☐	☐	☐
____ Type I (Insulin dependent) ____Type II			
Dry Mouth	☐	☐	☐
Eating disorder. If yes, specify: _____	☐	☐	☐
Epilepsy	☐	☐	☐
Fainting spells or seizures	☐	☐	☐
Gastrointestinal disease	☐	☐	☐
G.E. Reflux/persistent heartburn	☐	☐	☐
Glaucoma	☐	☐	☐

	Yes	No	Don't Know
Hemophilia	☐	☐	☐
Hepatitis, jaundice or liver disease	☐	☐	☐
Recurrent Infections	☐	☐	☐
If yes, indicate type of infection: _____			
Kidney problems	☐	☐	☐
Mental health disorders. If yes, specify: _____	☐	☐	☐
Malnutrition	☐	☐	☐
Night sweats	☐	☐	☐
Neurological disorders. If yes, specify: _____	☐	☐	☐
Osteoporosis	☐	☐	☐
Persistent swollen glands in neck			
Respiratory problems. If yes, specify below:	☐	☐	☐
____ Emphysema ____ Bronchitis, etc.			
Severe headaches/migraines	☐	☐	☐
Severe or rapid weight loss	☐	☐	☐
Sexually transmitted disease	☐	☐	☐
Sinus trouble	☐	☐	☐
Sleep disorder	☐	☐	☐
Sores or ulcers in the mouth	☐	☐	☐
Stroke	☐	☐	☐
Systemic lupus erythematosus	☐	☐	☐
Tuberculosis	☐	☐	☐
Thyroid problems	☐	☐	☐
Ulcers	☐	☐	☐
Excessive urination	☐	☐	☐
Do you have any disease, condition, or problem not listed above that you think I should know about?	☐	☐	☐
Please explain:			

NOTE: Both Doctor and patient are encouraged to discuss any and all relevant patient health issues prior to treatment.

I certify that I have read and understand the above. I acknowledge that my questions, if any, about inquiries set forth above have been answered to my satisfaction. I will not hold my dentist, or any other member of his/her staff, responsible for any action they take or do not take because of errors or omissions that I may have made in the completion of this form.

_____   _____
SIGNATURE OF PATIENT/LEGAL GUARDIAN   DATE

FOR COMPLETION BY DENTIST

Comments on patient interview concerning health history: _____
_____

Significant findings from questionnaire or oral interview: _____
_____

Dental management considerations: _____
_____

Health History Update: On a regular basis the patient should be questioned about any medical history changes, date and comments notated, along with signature.

Date	Comments	Signature of patient and dentist
_____	_____	_____

S500

▪ **FIGURE 7-1** Health History Form (Continued).

2. Turn off running water and dental light, and close the door.
3. Sit on clinician's stool to be at eye level with the patient.

III. POINTERS FOR THE INTERVIEW

Interviewing involves communication between individuals. Communication implies the transmission or interchange of facts, attitudes, opinions, or thoughts, through words, gestures, or other means. Through tactful but direct questioning, communication can be successful, and the patient will give such information as is known. Frequently, the patient is unaware of a health problem.

The attitude of the dental personnel should be one of friendly understanding, reassurance, and acceptance. Genuine interest and willingness to listen when a patient wishes to describe symptoms or complaints not only aids in establishing the rapport needed but frequently provides insight into the patient's real attitudes and prejudices. By asking simple questions at first and more personal questions later after rapport has developed, the patient will be more relaxed and frank in answering.

Self-confidence and gentle efficiency on the part of the interviewer help give the patient a feeling of confidence. Skill is required because tact, ingenuity, and judgment are taxed to the fullest in the attempt to obtain both accurate and complete information from the patient.

IV. INTERVIEW FORM

The interviewer may use a structured form with places to check and fill in. Another method is to record on blank sheets from questions created from a guide list of essential topics. Either may involve reference to the positive or negative answers on a previously completed questionnaire.

Familiarity with the items on the history permits the interviewer to be direct and informal without reading from a fixed list of topics, a method that may lack the personal touch necessary to gain the patient's confidence. When appropriate, the patient's own words are recorded.

V. ADVANTAGES OF THE INTERVIEW

- Personal contact contributes to development of rapport for future appointments.
- Flexibility for individual needs; details obtained can be adapted for supplementary questioning.

VI. DISADVANTAGES OF THE INTERVIEW

- Time-consuming when not prefaced with questionnaire.
- Unless a list is consulted, items of importance may be omitted.

- Patient may be embarrassed to talk about personal conditions and may hold back significant information.

▪ ITEMS INCLUDED IN THE HISTORY

Information obtained by means of the history is directly related to how the goals for patient care can and will be accomplished. In Tables 7-1, 7-2, and 7-3, items are listed with possible medications and other treatments the patient may have or has had, along with suggested considerations for appointment procedures.

In specialized practices, objectives may require increased emphasis on certain aspects. The age group most frequently served would influence the material needed. Parental history and prenatal and postnatal information may take on particular significance for the treatment of a small child; in a pedodontist's practice, a special form could be devised to include all essential items.

Insight and awareness shown while preparing the patient history depend on background knowledge of the manifestations of systemic diseases and the medications for various conditions. Objectives for the items to include in the various parts of the history are listed here.

I. PERSONAL HISTORY (TABLE 7-1)

The basic objectives in gathering personal information about the patient are
A. Data essential for appointment planning and business aspects.
B. Approval of care of a minor and other legal aspects.
C. For consultation with the patient's physician relative to interrelations between general and oral health.

II. DENTAL HISTORY (TABLE 7-2)

The dental history should contribute to knowledge of
A. The immediate problem, chief complaint, cause of present pain, or discomfort of any kind in the oral cavity.
B. The previous dental hygiene and dental care as described by the patient, including preventive care, periodontal treatments, and the extent of restorative and prosthetic replacement, as well as any adverse effects.
C. The attitude of the patient toward oral health and care of the mouth as may be indicated by previous periodic dental and dental hygiene treatments and family history of oral care.
D. The personal daily care exercised by the patient as evidence of knowledge of the purposes of continuing care and of the value placed on the teeth and their supporting structures.

TABLE 7-1 ITEMS FOR THE PERSONAL HISTORY

ITEMS TO RECORD IN PATIENT HISTORY	RECORD NOTES	CONSIDERATIONS FOR APPOINTMENT PROCEDURES

1. Name
   Addresses: residence and business
   Telephone numbers
   Sex
   Marital status
   For child: name of parent or guardian
   For parent: age and sex of children
	Accurate recording necessary for business aspects of dental practice	Aids in establishing rapport
		Instruction applicable to entire family
		Advice concerning fluorides for children

2. Birthdate	Whether of age or a minor Oral conditions related to age changes; diseases, healing, and other possible characteristics	Informed consent of parent or guardian necessary for care of minor or person with a mental handicap; signature must be obtained Approach to patient instruction
3. Birthplace and residence in early years	Presence of fluoride in drinking water Food and eating patterns Conditions endemic to certain areas	Effects of fluoride on teeth Instruction in dietary needs adapted to cultural practices
4. Occupation: present and former Spouse's occupation For children: parent's occupation	May be a factor in etiology of certain diseases, dental stains, occlusal wear May affect diet, oral habits, general health	Instruction applied to specific needs Dexterity in use of self-care devices related to dexterity gained from occupation Influence on oral care of entire family For child: which parent will supervise and assist child in oral care
5. Physician	Name, address, and telephone number For consultation	Consultation indicated: (1) when disease symptoms are suspected but patient does not state (2) in an emergency (3) Medication/premedication
6. Referred by and address	To whom to send referral acknowledgment and appreciation	Contribution to rapport with patient Patient referred by another patient may have concept of the office procedures

III. MEDICAL HISTORY (TABLE 7-3)

Objectives of the medical history are to determine whether the patient has or has had any conditions in the following categories:

A. Conditions That May Complicate Certain Kinds of Dental and Dental Hygiene Treatment

Examples. Lowered resistance to infection; uncontrolled hypertension; or systemic disease that requires treatment before stressful dental procedures, particularly surgery, can be carried out.

B. Diseases That Require Special Precautions or Premedication Prior to Treatment

Example. Antibiotic coverage for the patient with a history of rheumatic fever or congenital heart defect to prevent infective endocarditis.

C. Conditions Under Treatment by a Physician That Require Medicating Drugs That May Influence or Contraindicate Certain Procedures

Examples. Anticoagulant therapy requires consultation with physician; antihypertensive drugs may alter the choice of local anesthetic used.

TABLE 7-2 ITEMS FOR THE DENTAL HISTORY

ITEMS TO RECORD IN THE HISTORY	RECORD NOTES	CONSIDERATIONS FOR APPOINTMENT PROCEDURES
1. Reason for present appointment	Chief complaint in patient's own words Pain or discomfort Onset, symptoms, duration of an acute condition	Need for immediate treatment Attitude toward dentistry and preventive care
2. Previous dental appointments	Date of last treatment Services performed Regularity	Patient knowledge concerning regular dental care Cooperation anticipated
3. Anesthetics used	Local, general Adverse reactions	Choice of anesthetic
4. Radiation history	Type, number, dates of dental and medical radiographs Therapeutic radiation Availability of dental radiographs from previous dentist Amount of exposure considered with exposure for medical purposes	Amount of exposure; limitations Patient's appreciation for need and use of radiographs
5. Family dental history	Parental tooth loss or maintenance	Attitude toward saving teeth and preventive dentistry
6. Previous treatment a. periodontal b. orthodontic c. endodontic d. prosthodontic e. other	Type of treatment; frequency of maintenance appointments Whether referred to specialist History of acute infection (necrotizing ulcerative gingivitis) Surgery; posttreatment healing Age during treatment; completion date Previous problem Habit correction Dates, etiology Types of prostheses Extent of restorations Tooth loss Implants	Attitude toward specialized care Previous familiarity with role of dental hygienist Attitude toward self-care and disease control For current treatment, consultation with orthodontist needed to determine instructions Periodic recheck Care of prostheses and abutment teeth Understanding prevention
7. Injuries to face or teeth	Causes and extent Fractured teeth or jaws	Limitation of opening Special care during healing
8. Temporomandibular joint	History of injury, discomfort, disease, dislocation Previous treatment	Effect on opening; accessibility during instrumentation
9. Habits	Clenching, bruxism Mouth breathing Biting objects; fingernails, pipe stem, thread, other Cheek or lip biting Patient awareness of habits	Tension of patient Instruction relative to effects of habits
10. Tobacco use	Form of tobacco, amount used Frequency Knowledge of effects on oral tissues	Instruction concerning oral effects Tobacco cessation program Periodontal risk Dental stains; dentifrice selection

(continued)

TABLE 7-2 ITEMS FOR THE DENTAL HISTORY (Continued)

ITEMS TO RECORD IN THE HISTORY	RECORD NOTES	CONSIDERATIONS FOR APPOINTMENT PROCEDURES
11. Fluorides	Systemic, topical, dates Residence during tooth development years Amount of fluoride in drinking water	Current preventive procedures and need for reevaluation
12. Biofilm control procedures	Toothbrushing: current procedures 　type of brush (manual or powered) 　texture of filaments 　frequency of use 　age of brush; frequency of having a new brush Dentifrice 　name 　how selected; reason Additional cleansing devices and frequency of use 　dental floss 　water irrigation 　implants care Mouthrinse or other agents: frequency, purpose Source of instruction in care of oral cavity	Present practice and previous instruction New instruction needed; reception by patient Relation of techniques to prevention of dental caries and periodontal infections Supervision of child by parent: current practices Problems of habit change

D. Allergic or Untoward Reactions

Examples. Latex hypersensitivity; medication or material for which there was a previous adverse reaction.

E. Diseases and Drugs With Manifestations in the Mouth

Examples. Hematologic disorders; phenytoin-induced gingival overgrowth; infectious diseases such as herpesvirus.

F. Communicable Diseases That Endanger the Dental Personnel

Examples. Active tuberculosis; viral hepatitis; herpes; syphilis.

G. Physiologic State of the Patient

Examples. Pregnancy; puberty; menopause; birth control pills.

■ REVIEW OF HISTORY

Updating the history at each maintenance appointment is essential. Changes in health status revealed by interim medical examinations or evidenced by reported illness or hospitalizations must be recorded and considered during continuing treatment.

Following a review of the previously recorded history, questions can be directed to the patient to compare the present condition with the previous one and to determine at least the following:

- Interim illnesses; changes in health.
- Visits to physician; reasons and results.
- Laboratory tests performed and the results; blood, urine, or other analyses.
- Current medications.
- Changes in the oral soft tissues and the teeth observed by the patient.

■ IMMEDIATE APPLICATIONS OF PATIENT HISTORIES

Together with information from all other parts of the diagnostic work-up, the patient histories are essential for the preparation of the dental hygiene care plan.

Immediate evaluation of the histories is necessary before proceeding to complete the assessment.

The list that follows is not intended to be exhaustive but rather suggestive. From these items, the dental personnel should be alerted to precautions that may be needed.

(*text continues on page* 122)

TABLE 7-3 ITEMS FOR THE MEDICAL HISTORY

ITEM TO RECORD IN HISTORY	RECORD NOTES	MEDICATIONS AND TREATMENT MODALITIES	CONSIDERATIONS FOR APPOINTMENT PROCEDURES
1. General health and appearance	Disabilities Overall impression of well-being Patient's appraisal of own health		Response, cooperation, and attitude to expect during appointments
2. Medical examination	Date most recent examination Reason for the examination Tests performed; results Anticipated surgery	New prescriptions received Previous prescriptions continued	Verification with physician for added information Need for superior state of oral health in advance of surgery 1. When long recovery is expected and patient may miss maintenance appointments 2. Prior to transplant, heart surgery, or prosthesis
3. Major illnesses, hospitalizations, surgeries	Causes of illness Type and duration of treatment Anesthetics used Convalescence Course of healing: normal, not normal	Medications, treatments	Influence of illnesses on health and care of the oral cavity Anesthetic choice Expected outcome from gingival treatment
4. Age factors	Problems of health in different age groups Geriatric: multiple disease entities; patient may need to bring the containers for identification of medications	See individual medical problem Update drug regimen at each appointment	Effects on dental and dental hygiene procedures and personal care
5. Height and weight	Weight changes over past years or months Obesity Undernourishment Child growth pattern	Diet pills Substance abuse	Marked weight change may be a symptom of undiagnosed disease; suggest referral for medical examination Influence on dietary instructions for oral health
6. Medications prescribed by physician	Reasons: relation to dental care Frequency Patient's regularity of taking Sugar content of liquid medicines, effect on dental caries (also true of over-the-counter [OTC] items)	List all drugs by name Ask patient for drugs, medicine, injections, tonics, vitamins, patches, pills, capsules, to get a complete answer Dosage; route of administration	Consultation with physician concerning adjustments in dosage for dental or dental hygiene appointments Indications for premedication Side effects of drugs

(continued)

TABLE 7-3 ITEMS FOR THE MEDICAL HISTORY (Continued)

ITEM TO RECORD IN HISTORY	RECORD NOTES	MEDICATIONS AND TREATMENT MODALITIES	CONSIDERATIONS FOR APPOINTMENT PROCEDURES
7. Self-medication	Type, frequency OTC preparations Substance abuse	Pain relievers Sleeping tablets Cough syrup Antacids Cathartics Vitamins Diet pills	Information not revealed by patient could complicate treatment Lack of interest in oral health, only pain relief Drug side effects
8. Family medical history	Predisposition to certain diseases (example: diabetes) History of diseases that occur in the family	Cultural beliefs about medications	May help patient seek medical examination when symptom suggests possible disease
9. Daily diet	Recommendations of patient's physicians, past and present Vitamin supplements Appetite Regularity of meals Food likes and dislikes	Vitamin supplements	Instructions to be given relative to oral health Prognosis for healing after treatment Need for dietary review and analysis
10. Alcohol consumption	Frequency Amount Substance abuse	Recovering alcoholic: May be taking disulfiram, Must avoid all alcohol-containing preparations, including commercial mouthrinses	Excessive use: effect on anesthesia; increased healing time Poor nutritional state is common; lack of oral care Avoid alcohol-containing mouthrinse May result in poor patient cooperation

11. Allergies	Determine substances to which the patient is allergic
	    Latex
	    Anesthetics
	    Penicillin
	    Medicaments
	    Foods
	    Iodine
		Antihistamines
		Inhalers
		Decongestants
		Steroids
			Preparation for emergency
			Xerostomia
			Avoid use of substances to which the patient is allergic
			Consider allergies when planning dietary recommendations

12. Arthritis	Joint pain Immobility Temporomandibular joint involvement	Aspirin Nonsteroidal anti-inflammatory drugs Corticosteroids Total joint replacements	Antibiotic premedication: consult physician if treated with chemotherapeutic agent Dental chair adjustment
13. Blood disorder	Type and duration of disease Leukemia: remission, thrombocytopenia	Vitamins Minerals: iron (iron-deficiency anemia) Folic acid supplement (sickle cell anemia) Antineoplastic drugs	Consultation with physician Need for high level of oral health Antibiotic premedication Immunosuppression Increased bleeding Oral lesions

TABLE 7-3 ITEMS FOR THE MEDICAL HISTORY (Continued)

ITEM TO RECORD IN HISTORY	RECORD NOTES	MEDICATIONS AND TREATMENT MODALITIES	CONSIDERATIONS FOR APPOINTMENT PROCEDURES
14. Bleeding	Bleeding associated with previous dental appointments History of disorder with coagulation problem History of transfusions or other blood products Check use of aspirin (relation to bleeding tendency) Laboratory tests for bleeding time, coagulation may be needed	Anticoagulant medication Hemophilia factor replacement	Emergency prevention through preappointment precautions May need to apply direct pressure or hemostatic agent after scaling Special measures for hemophilia
15. Cancer	Head and neck radiation effects on oral cavity, salivary glands Dental and dental hygiene therapy updated before start of surgery, radiation therapy, or immunosuppression Blood count prior to dental and dental hygiene therapy	Radiation therapy Fluoride therapy: daily topical application Antineoplastic drugs, alkylating agents, antimetabolites, antibiotics, plant alkaloids, steroids	Antibiotic premedication Bleeding; infection; poor healing response Avoid trauma to tissues Effect on oral radiographic survey: prevention of overexposure Dental caries: preventive measures Xerostomia: substitute saliva
16. Cardiovascular diseases	Consultation with physician Refer for examination when patient seems unsure of problem	Cardiac glycosides Antiarrhythmics Antianginals Antihypertensives Anticoagulants	Minimize stress Premedication for stress Ascertain that medications have been taken Monitor vital signs
Congenital heart disease Rheumatic heart disease	Susceptibility to infective endocarditis Type of problem; date of rheumatic fever	Antibiotic (prevent recurrence of rheumatic fever)	Antibiotic premedication required
Hypertension	Symptom of other disease state Monitoring blood pressure for each appointment Anesthesia: limit epinephrine or omit as recommended by physician	Diuretics Antiadrenergic agents Vasodilators Angiotensin-converting enzyme inhibitors Calcium channel–blocking agent	Postural hypotension (raise dental chair slowly) Xerostomia: saliva substitute and fluoride rinse may be needed Gingival enlargement (drug side effect)
Angina pectoris	Prepare for symptoms; have ready amyl nitrite inhalant or nitroglycerin tablets or spray	Amyl nitrite, nitroglycerin, or other antianginal drugs	Allay fears and prevent stress Morning appointment

(continued)

TABLE 7-3 ITEMS FOR THE MEDICAL HISTORY (Continued)

ITEM TO RECORD IN HISTORY	RECORD NOTES	MEDICATIONS AND TREATMENT MODALITIES	CONSIDERATIONS FOR APPOINTMENT PROCEDURES
Heart diseases	History of disease symptoms of fatigue, shortness of breath or cough Consult with physician	Glycosides (digitalis) Anticoagulants Antiarrhythmic drugs Pacemaker	Monitor vital signs Short, more frequent appointments Change dental chair slowly Patient with breathing problem (sleeps with two or more pillows) may need semi-upright position Bleeding tendency associated with anticoagulant Check use of ultrasonic (pacemaker)
Surgically corrected cardiovascular lesions	Type, date of surgery Consultation with physician Before surgical procedure, when possible: the patient needs complete oral evaluation and corrective dental work done, with motivation to high level of oral personal care daily	No tobacco use Anticoagulants Cyclosporine Nifedipine	Antibiotic premedication vital for synthetic valves or other replacements, indefinitely Gingival bleeding can be expected Gingival enlargement
Cerebrovascular accident (stroke)	Date of onset; residual disabilities Speech, vision, mental function	No tobacco; low-salt diet Anticoagulants Antihypertensives Vasodilator Steroid Anticonvulsant	Gingival bleeding likely when anticoagulants are used Adapt procedures for physical disability
17. Communicable diseases	History of diseases; immunizations Present disease; communicability Residence or extended trips in countries with high endemic incidence of certain diseases Risk group factor	Immunizations Drug therapy for current infection	Appointment postponement
Hepatitis B	Jaundice history Clarification of type of hepatitis Laboratory clearance	Vaccine of HBV	Precautions against percutaneous injury
Tuberculosis	Active or passive Cough Duration of disease	Isoniazid Rifampin Pyrazinamide	Length of treatment; infectivity diminished after few months of treatment

TABLE 7-3 ITEMS FOR THE MEDICAL HISTORY (Continued)			
ITEM TO RECORD IN HISTORY	RECORD NOTES	MEDICATIONS AND TREATMENT MODALITIES	CONSIDERATIONS FOR APPOINTMENT PROCEDURES
Sexually transmitted Infections (STIs)	May not obtain history of STIs Oral and pharyngeal lesions may be indicators of disease	Antibiotics	Infectiousness diminishes with antibiotic therapy for gonorrhea and syphilis Refer to physician and postpone treatment when lesions or other signs suggest infection Caution for risk from previously treated diseases
Herpes	Lesions can be transmitted readily	Nondefinitive; symptomatic and palliative treatment Acyclovir	Postpone routine care when oral lesions are present
HIV infection AIDS	Risk group identification Oral manifestations	Wide variety of opportunistic infections and complications require variety of drugs	Oral lesions Complete sterilization and barrier procedures as for all patients
18. Diabetes Mellitus	Uncontrolled: requires antibiotic premedication Undiagnosed: excess thirst, appetite, and urination Family incidence: help in finding susceptible undiagnosed Severe advanced diabetes: complications (vision, kidney, cardiovascular, nervous system)	Insulin Diet control Hypoglycemics	Prepare for emergency; insulin; apple juice; frosting Appointment time related to insulin therapy and mealtime Need frequent maintenance appointments Periodontal disease accelerated Referral for tests for suspected undiagnosed
19. Ears	Deafness or degree of hearing impairment Infections, ringing, dizziness, balance	Treatment for infection Hearing aid	Adaptations for communication and biofilm control instruction
20. Endocrine	Age-group relations to certain conditions Growth, development Menstruation, menopause	Thyroid hormone supplement Antithyroid Estrogen/progestin Oral contraceptives Corticosteroids	Emphasis on high level of biofilm control Any patient taking steroids may need antibiotic premedication for appointments Monitor blood pressure
21. Epilepsy	Type, frequency of seizures precipitating factors Preparation for emergency seizure	Anticonvulsant Sedative	Minimize stress Medications make patient drowsy, less alert Valproic acid requires bleeding time before treatment

TABLE 7-3 ITEMS FOR THE MEDICAL HISTORY (Continued)

ITEM TO RECORD IN HISTORY	RECORD NOTES	MEDICATIONS AND TREATMENT MODALITIES	CONSIDERATIONS FOR APPOINTMENT PROCEDURES
22. Eyes	Disturbance of vision Purpose for corrective eyeglasses or contact lenses Manifestations of systemic disease	Eyedrops (for example, glaucoma)	Avoid epinephrine if glaucoma Protective eyewear during appointment Adaptations for communication with limited sight
23. Gastrointestinal	Nature and treatment of the disease Diet restriction prescribed by physician	Antacids Antidiarrheal Laxatives Antispasmodics	Patient instruction in accord with prescribed diet and medication Xerostomia
24. Kidney	Renal disease; kidney stones Hemodialysis: hypertension, anemia, hepatitis carrier Transplant: hypertension, hepatitis	Salt restriction Many drugs are nephrotoxic Immunosuppressive drugs (cyclosporine)	Antibiotic premedication Monitor blood pressure Bleeding tendency Poor healing Susceptibility to infection Limited stress tolerance
25. Liver	History of jaundice, hepatitis Impaired drug metabolism Cirrhosis: history of alcoholism	 Nutritional emphasis Abstinence from alcohol	Laboratory test for hepatitis Bleeding problems
26. Mental, psychiatric	Emotional problems hinder oral care	Antipsychotic drugs Antianxiety drugs Tranquilizers Antidepressants Antiparkinsonism drugs	Limited stress tolerance Xerostomia (side effect) Avoid mouthrinse containing alcohol
27. Physical activity	Overall health consciousness	Good health habits Regular exercise	Contribute to cooperative attitude in maintaining oral health
28. Physical disabilities	Extent, cause, duration Type of treatment related to individual condition Consultation with physician or medical specialist	Pain reliever Muscle relaxant Anticonvulsant	Adjustment of physical arrangements Wheelchair accessibility and transfer Adaptations of techniques and instruction Consult for antibiotic premedication for certain conditions: for example: prosthetic joint replacement, shunt
29. Pregnancy	Month, parturition date Possible oral manifestations History of previous pregnancies Iron deficiency anemia	Iron Folic acid Multivitamins	Adjust physical position for comfort Frequent appointments for maintaining high level of oral hygiene
30. Respiration	Breathing problems Persistent cough Cough up blood Chest pain Precipitation of asthmatic attack	Codeine cough syrup Antihistamine Bronchial dilator Expectorant Decongestant Steroid	Dental chair position Ultrasonic and air-powder polisher contraindicated Anesthesia choice: nitrous oxide contraindicated No aerosol agents

I. MEDICAL CONSULTATION

Dentist and physician need to consult relative to the patient's current therapy and medications or to elements of the patient's past health status that could influence present dental treatment needs.[3]

A. Telephone or Personal Contact

Immediate consultation may be needed so that urgent treatment may proceed. Follow-up in writing is essential because without legal record of the advice or decision, a misunderstanding could result.

B. Written Request

A letter of formal request is the preferred procedure. A prepared form can be developed with spaces for filling in the specific questions and with space in the lower half for the physician or the assistant completing confidential information from the patient's medical record to provide the necessary directions.

C. Referrals

1. Patient should be referred for medical examination when signs of a possible disease condition are apparent.

2. Patient should be referred for laboratory tests when recent test results are not available or follow-up tests are needed.

II. RADIATION

When a patient is receiving radiation therapy or has had recent radiation for other purposes, a conference with the physician or oncologist involved is recommended to discuss the quantity of radiation to be received from any necessary dental radiographs. No apparent rationale exists for precluding a properly justified dental radiographic examination because of a history of radiation therapy.[4]

III. PROPHYLACTIC PREMEDICATION

Patients at risk of infective endocarditis must have antibiotic premedication prior to any tissue manipulation that could create a bacteremia. All tissue manipulation, particularly the use of instruments subgingivally, must be withheld until the risk has been determined, the condition has been discussed with the patient's physician, and the prescription has been obtained and taken appropriately.

Table 7-4 shows the specific regimen for antibiotic selection and prescription. The timing objective is to have adequate concentrations in the blood during, and immediately following, the actual instrumentation.

TABLE 7-4 PROPHYLACTIC REGIMENS FOR DENTAL, ORAL, RESPIRATORY TRACT, OR ESOPHAGEAL PROCEDURES

SITUATION	AGENT	REGIMEN ADULT	REGIMEN CHILD*
Standard general prophylaxis	Amoxicillin	2.0 g orally 1 hour before procedure	50 mg/kg orally 1 hour before procedure
Unable to take oral medications	Ampicillin	2.0 g IM or IV[†] within 30 minutes before procedure	50 mg/kg IM or IV within 30 minutes before procedure
Allergic to penicillin	Clindamycin or Cephalexin[‡] or Cefadroxil or Azithromycin or Clarithromycin	600 mg orally 1 hour before procedure 2.0 g orally 1 hour before procedure 500 mg orally 1 hour before procedure	20 mg/kg orally 1 hour before procedure 50 mg/kg orally 1 hour before procedure 15 mg/kg orally 1 hour before procedure
Allergic to penicillin and unable to take oral medications	Clindamycin or Cefazolin[‡]	600 mg IV within 30 minutes before procedure 1.0 g IM or IV within 30 minutes before procedure	20 mg/kg IV within 30 minutes before procedure 25 mg/kg IM or IV within 30 minutes before procedure

*Total children's dose should not exceed adult dose.
[†]IM = intramuscularly; IV = intravenously.
[‡]Cephalosporins should not be used in individuals with immediate-type hypersensitivity reaction (urticaria, angioedema, or anaphylaxis) to penicillin.

At-risk patients already taking an antibiotic for other health conditions require additional antibiotic prophylaxis prior to dental and dental hygiene instrumentation. The recommendation is to administer a different class of antibiotic rather than to increase the dose of the current antibiotic.[5]

■ AMERICAN HEART ASSOCIATION GUIDELINES

The American Heart Association and the American Dental Association recommend that certain risk patients have antibiotic premedication for all dental hygiene procedures likely to induce gingival bleeding.[5] The list below specifies the cardiac conditions involved, which includes mitral valve prolapse. The flowchart in Figure 7-2 shows a clinical approach for selecting the patients with mitral valve prolapse who will need antibiotic premedication. Medical evaluation is needed to confirm whether there is mitral regurgitation and therefore a need for premedication.

I. CARDIAC-RELATED CONDITIONS WHERE PROPHYLAXIS IS RECOMMENDED

High Risk Category
Prosthetic cardiac valves, including bioprosthetic and homograft valves

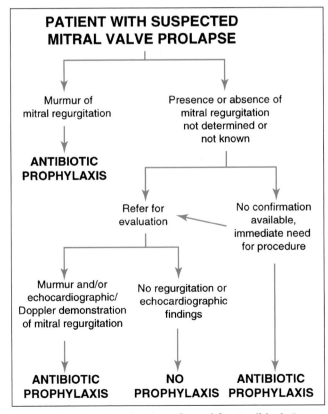

Previous infective endocarditis
Complex cyanotic congenital heart disease
Surgically constructed systemic pulmonary shunts or conduits
Moderate Risk Category
Most other congenital cardiac malformations
Acquired valvular dysfunction (eg, rheumatic heart disease)
Hypertrophic cardiomyopathy
Mitral valve prolapse with valvular regurgitation and/or thickened leaflets

II. CARDIAC CONDITIONS WHERE PROPHYLAXIS IS NOT RECOMMENDED

Negligible Risk Category: (Individuals with these conditions are at no greater risk for infective endocarditis than the general population.)
Isolated ostium secundum atrial septal defect
Surgical repair of atrial septal defect, ventricular septal defect, or patent ductus arteriosus (without residua beyond 6 months)
Previous coronary artery bypass graft surgery
Mitral valve prolapse without valvular dysfunction
Previous Kawasaki disease without valvular dysfunction
Previous rheumatic fever without valvular dysfunction
Cardiac pacemaker (intravascular and epicardial) and implanted defibrillators

III. INDIVIDUALS WITH TOTAL JOINT REPLACEMENT[6]

The risk of endocarditis is much greater in mouths with ongoing periodontal infection than when the periodontal tissues are healthy. When it is known that a person will have surgery for total joint arthroplasty, all possible effort should be made to complete the treatment necessary to bring periodontal tissues to a healthy, maintainable state before the joint replacement.

Patients listed below must be considered for antibiotic prophylaxis. The most critical period for bacteremias to cause hematogenous seeding is up to 2 years following the surgery for joint replacement. Other patients, such as those with pins, plates, or screws, do not require antibiotic prophylaxis for reason of the pin, plate, or screw, but other health factors must always be considered for all patients.

A. Patients at Potential Increased Risk of Hematogenous Total Joint Infection

All patients during first 2 years following joint replacement.
1. *Immunocompromised/immunosuppressed patients*
   a. Inflammatory arthropathies; rheumatic arthritis; systemic lupus erythematosus

■ **FIGURE 7-2 Determination of Need for Antibiotic Prophylaxis in the Patient With Mitral Valve Prolapse.**

b. Disease-, drug-, or radiation-induced immunosuppression

2. *Other Patients*
   a. Type I diabetes (insulin-dependent)
   b. First 2 years following joint replacement
   c. Previous prosthetic joint infections
   d. Malnourishment
   e. Hemophilia

B. Suggested Antibiotic Prophylaxis Regimens

1. *Standard Prophylaxis: patients Not Allergic to Penicillin*

   Cephalexin, cephradine, or amoxicillin: 2 g orally 1 hour before procedure.

2. *Patients Not Allergic to Penicillin and Unable to Take Oral Medications*

   Cefazolin: 1 g, or ampicillin: 2 g, intramuscularly or intravenously 1 hour before procedure.

3. *Patients Allergic to Penicillin*

   Clindamycin: 600 mg orally 1 hour before procedure.

4. *Patients Allergic to Penicillin and Unable to Take Oral Medications*

   Clindamycin: 600 mg intravenously 1 hour before procedure.

IV. OTHER SYSTEMIC CONSIDERATIONS

Specific recommendations are impossible to define for all patients who may require antibiotic premedication. Each patient must be considered individually. Consultation with the patient's physician and the use of intelligent clinical judgment are necessary for the selection of patients who will benefit from antibiotics.

Routine use of antibiotic premedication is never indicated. In certain instances the patient is less at risk from the dental procedure than from the potential side effects of an antibiotic. Overuse of antibiotics can induce microbial resistance and, rarely, allergy or toxicity to the drug used.[7]

The following is a partial list of patients requiring antibiotic premedication:

A. Reduced Capacity to Resist Infection

1. Corticosteroid or other immunosuppressive therapy.
2. Chemotherapy (cancer treatments; certain treatments for arthritis).
3. Blood diseases (acute leukemia, agranulocytosis, sickle-cell anemia).
4. Human immunodeficiency virus infection.[8]

B. Uncontrolled, Unstable Diabetes

Controlled stable diabetes can be treated as normal.

C. Facial Injuries

Grossly contaminated, traumatic facial injuries and compound fractures.

D. Renal Disorders

Renal transplant and hemodialysis, glomerulonephritis, or other renal disorder.[9]

E. Valvular Dysfunction

1. Cardiac transplant with valvular dysfunction.[7]
2. Valvular heart disease resulting from use of fenfluramine and phentermine (appetite suppressants).[10,11]

F. Shunt

Ventriculoatrial shunt.[12]

■ PROPHYLAXIS FOR DENTAL AND DENTAL HYGIENE PROCEDURES

Partial lists of procedures requiring and not requiring antibiotic prophylaxis are provided within the American Heart Association recommendations included here. The incidence and extent of a bacteremia is directly proportional to the degree of infection and inflammation in the tissues as well as the trauma produced by the clinical procedure.

Maintenance of healthy tissues by the patient through personal daily care and routine professional supervision are first in the prevention of bacteremias. Preprocedural rinsing with antimicrobial mouthrinse helps to reduce the incidence and severity of the bacteremias produced.

I. PROCEDURES FOR WHICH PROPHYLAXIS IS RECOMMENDED[5]

Dental extractions
Periodontal procedures, including surgery, scaling and root planing, probing, recall maintenance
Dental implant placement and reimplantation of avulsed teeth
Endodontic (root canal) instrumentation or surgery beyond the apex
Subgingival placement of antibiotic fibers or strips
Initial placement of orthodontic bands but not brackets
Intraligamentary local anesthetic injections

Prophylactic cleaning of teeth or implants where bleeding is anticipated

II. PROCEDURES FOR WHICH PROPHYLAXIS IS NOT DEEMED NECESSARY

In all cases mentioned here, when bleeding is expected, prophylaxis is advised for susceptible individuals. Clinical judgment must be applied.

Restorative dentistry, including restoration of carious teeth and replacement of missing teeth (with or without retraction cords)

Local anesthetic injections (non-intraligamentary)

Intracanal endodontic treatment; postplacement build-up

Postsurgical suture removal

Placement of rubber dams

Placement of removable prosthodontic or orthodontic appliances

Taking of oral impressions

Fluoride treatments

Taking of oral radiographs

Orthodontic appliance adjustment

Shedding of primary teeth

▪ ASA DETERMINATION

With the completion of the patient histories, an overall estimate of medical risk of a patient can be made. The **ASA Physical Status Classification System** was adopted by the American Society of Anesthesiologists in 1962[13] and describes five categories as follows:

ASA I: A patient without apparent systemic disease: a normal healthy patient.

ASA II: A patient with mild systemic disease.

ASA III: A patient with severe systemic disease that limits activity but is not incapacitating.

ASA IV: A patient with an incapacitating systemic disease that is a constant threat to life.

ASA V: A moribund patient not expected to survive 24 hours with or without care.

ASA E: Emergency of any variety: precede the ASA number with E to indicate the patient's physical status (for example, ASA E-III).

In a typical dental setting, the ASA V category is omitted.

▪ RECORDS

- Date all records.
- Keep permanent records in ink.
- Provide a specific line on a health history form for the signature of the patient.[1] The completed history for a minor should be signed by a parent or guardian. A signature is also needed on the informed consent form.
- All information obtained for a patient history must be maintained in strictest privacy.
- For patients with special health problems that require premedication, some type of coded tab can be used to alert all dental personnel to check the medical history prior to each appointment.

Everyday Ethics

Chris is updating the medical history of Irina, a long-time patient originally from Russia who speaks and understands English pretty well. This visit, she indicates that she has a heart murmur. Chris attempts to ask the necessary questions, including when was it diagnosed and has it been evaluated with an echocardiogram.

Irina grabs Chris's arm and firmly requests, "Want teeth cleaned." Chris attempts to explain why he is asking the questions about her heart murmur and the serious, life-threatening illness that may occur if she is not premedicated with an antibiotic prior to her dental hygiene therapy. Chris asks permission to call the physician to obtain the information. Irina just becomes more agitated and keeps repeating "Want teeth cleaned" and refuses to give approval to call her doctor.

Questions for Consideration

1. Professionally and ethically, what are a dental hygienist's responsibilities to ensure that a patient understands the seriousness of an illness?

2. In light of the possible language barrier between Chris and Irina, what actions can Chris take to prepare this patient for the dental hygiene appointment? Are there procedures that do not require premedication that could be accomplished?

3. Which of the dental hygiene core values apply to Chris's actions for the patient's benefit?

✔ **Factors To Teach The Patient**

- The need for obtaining the personal, medical, and dental history prior to performance of dental and dental hygiene procedures, and the need for keeping the histories up to date.

- The assurance that recorded histories are kept in strict professional confidence.

- The relationship between oral health and general physical health.

- The interrelationship of medical and dental care.

- All patients who require antibiotic premedication need special attention paid to (1) the importance of preventive dentistry, (2) the imperative need for regular dental care, and (3) the necessity for taking the prescribed prescription 1 hour before the appointment starts.

- Analyze the usefulness of items on the patient history form periodically, and plan for revision as scientific research reveals new information that must be applied.
- A medical history update wall plaque is available for posting in an appropriate place in a dental office or clinic. It reads: *Please Advise Us of Any Change in Your Medical History Since Your Last Visit.* It is available from the American Dental Association, Department of Salable Materials, 211 East Chicago Avenue, Chicago, Illinois 60611.

REFERENCES

1. **Robbins**, K.S.: Medicolegal Considerations, in Malamed, S.F.: *Medical Emergencies in the Dental Office*, 4th ed. St. Louis, The C.V. Mosby Co., 1993, pp. 91–101.
2. **American Dental Association**: Medical History Form (S-500), ADA Department of Salable Materials, 211 East Chicago Avenue, Chicago, IL 60611-2678.
3. **Chiodo**, G.T. and Rosenstein, D.I.: Consultation Between Dentists and Physicians, *Gen. Dent., 32*, 19, January–February, 1984.
4. **United States Department of Health and Human Services**, Food and Drug Administration, Center for Devices and Radiological Health: *Selection of Patients for X-Ray Examinations: Dental Radiographic Examinations.* Washington, D.C., Superintendent of Documents, HHS Publication FDA 88-8274, 1988, p. 10.
5. **Dajani**, A.S., Taubert, K.A., Wilson, W., Bolger, A.F., Bayer, A., Ferrieri, P., Gewitz, M.H., Shulman, S.T., Nouri, S., Newburger, J.W., Hutto, C., Pallasch, T.J., Gage, T.W., Levison, M.E., Peter, G., and Zuccaro, G.: Prevention of Bacterial Endocarditis. Recommendations by the American Heart Association, *JAMA, 277*, 1794, June 11, 1997.
6. **American Dental Association and American Academy of Orthopaedic Surgeons**: Advisory Statement: Antibiotic Prophylaxis for Dental Patients With Total Joint Replacements, in *ADA Guide to Dental Therapeutics*, Chicago, ADA Publishing Co., 1998, pp. 547–551.
7. **Pallasch**, T.J. and Slots, J.: Antibiotic Prophylaxis and the Medically Compromised Patient, *Periodontol. 2000, 10*,107, 1996.
8. **Lockhart**, P.B. and Schmidtke, M.A.: Antibiotic Considerations in Medically Compromised Patients, *Dent. Clin. North Am., 38*, 381, July, 1994.
9. **DeRossi**, S.S. and Glick, M.: Dental Considerations for the Patient With Renal Disease Receiving Hemodialysis, *J. Am. Dent. Assoc.,127*, 211, February, 1996.
10. **Connolly**, H.M., Crary, J.L., McGoon, M.D., Hensrud, D.D., Edwards, B.S., Edwards, W.D., and Schaff, H.V.: Valvular Heart Disease Associated With Fenfluramine-Phentermine, *N. Eng. J. Med., 337*, 581, August 28, 1997.
11. **United State Centers for Disease Control and Prevention**: Cardiac Valvulopathy Associated With Exposure to Fenfluramine or Dexfenfluramine: U.S. Department of Health and Human Services Interim Public Health Recommendations, November, 1997, *MMWR, 46*, 1061, November 14, 1997.
12. **Little**, J.W., Falace, D.A., Miller, C.S., and Rhodus, N.L.: *Dental Management of the Medically Compromised Patient*, 5th ed. St. Louis, C.V. Mosby Co., 1997, pp. 74, 605.
13. **American Society of Anesthesiologists**: New Classification of Physical Status, *Anesthesiology, 24*, 111, January–February, 1963.

SUGGESTED READINGS

Biron, C.: Patients With Thyroid Dysfunctions Require Risk Management Before Dental Procedures, *RDH, 16*, 42, April, 1996.

DeRossi, S.S. and Glick, M.: Dental Considerations in Asplenic Patients, *J. Am. Dent. Assoc., 127*, 1359, September, 1996.

Drinnan, A.J.: Medical Conditions of Importance in Dental Practice, *Int. Dent. J., 40*, 206, August, 1990.

McClain, D.L., Bader, J.D., Daniel, S.J., and Sams, D.H.: Gingival Effects of Prescription Medications Among Adult Dental Patients, *Spec.Care Dentist., 11*, 15, January/February, 1991.

Miller, C.S., Kaplan, A.L., Guest, G.F., and Cottone, J.A.: Documenting Medication Use in Adult Dental Patients: 1987–1991, *J. Am. Dent. Assoc., 123*, 41, November, 1992.

Naylor, G.D., Hall, E.H., and Terezhalmy, G.T.: The Patient With Chronic Renal Failure Who Is Undergoing Dialysis or Renal Transplantation: Another Consideration for Antimicrobial Prophylaxis, *Oral Surg. Oral Med. Oral Pathol., 65*, 116, January, 1988.

Pyle, M.A., Faddoul, F.F., and Terezhalmy, G.T.: Clinical Implications of Drugs Taken By Our Patients, *Dent. Clin. North. Am., 37*, 73, January, 1993.

Schow, S.R.: Organ Transplant Patients and Immunosuppression, *DentalHygienistNews, 8*, 23, Number 3, 1995.

Smith, R.G. and Burtner, A.P.: Oral Side-Effects of the Most Frequently Prescribed Drugs, *Spec. Care Dentist., 14*, 96, May/June, 1994.

Spolarich, A.E.: The Pharmacologic History, *Access, 9*, 33, March, 1995.

Spolarich, A.E.: Understanding Pharmacology: Basic Principles, *Access, 9*, 25, July, 1995.

Wynn, R.L.: The Top 20 Medications Prescribed in 1993, *Gen. Dent., 43*, 114, March–April, 1995.

History Forms

Cooper, M.D. and Winans, G.J.: Basics of a Good Medical History Form: How to Protect the Patient and Prepare the Staff, *Dent. Teamwork, 5*, 19, January–February, 1992.

deJong, K.J.M., Abraham-Inpijn, L., Oomen, H.A.P.C., and Oosting, J.: Clinical Relevance of a Medical History in Dental Practice: Comparison Between a Questionnaire and a Dialogue, *Community Dent. Oral Epidemiol.*, *19*, 310, October, 1991.

deJong, K.J.M., Borgmeijer-Hoelen, A., and Abraham-Inpijn, L.: Validity of a Risk-Related Patient-Administered Medical Questionnaire for Dental Patients, *Oral Surg. Oral Med. Oral Pathol.*,*72*, 527, November, 1991.

Fenlon, M.R. and McCartan, B.E.: Validity of a Patient Self-completed Health Questionnaire in a Primary Care Dental Practice, *Community Dent. Oral Epidemiol.*, *20*, 130, June, 1992.

Fine, J.I. and Kopriva, K.H.: The Health History: Interview and Communication Skills, *DentalHygienistNews*, *7*, 7, Fall, 1994.

Flaitz, C.M., Vojir, C.P., Bradley, K.A., Casamassimo, P.S., and Kaplan D.W.: A Comparison of Parent and Adolescent Responses From Independent Health Histories, *Pediatr. Dent.*, *13*, 27, January/February, 1991.

Frese, P.A. and Scaramucci, M.K.: Medical History Update, *DentalHygienistnews*, *4* 9, Spring, 1991.

Jolly, D.E.: Evaluation of the Medical History, *Anesth. Prog.*, *42*, 84, Numbers 3/4, 1995.

Levy, S.M. and Jakobsen, J.R.: A Comparison of Medical Histories Reported by Dental Patients and Their Physicians, *Spec. Care Dentist.*, *11*, 26, January/February, 1991.

McDaniel, T.F., Miller, D., Jones, R., and Davis, M.: Assessing Patient Willingness to Reveal Health History Information, *J. Am. Dent. Assoc.*, *126*, 375, March, 1995.

Miller, D.L.: Medical History Evaluation and Alterations for Care, in Hodges, K.O., ed.: *Concepts in Nonsurgical Periodontal Therapy*. Albany, N.Y., Delmar, 1998., pp. 29–48.

Minden, N.J. and Fast, T.B.: Evaluation of Health History Forms Used in U.S. Dental Schools, *Oral Surg. Oral Med. Oral Pathol.*, *77*, 105, January, 1994.

Minden, N.J. and Fast, T.B.: The Patient's Health History Form: How Healthy Is It? *J. Am. Dent. Assoc.*, *124*, 95, August, 1993.

Prisant, L.M. and Doll, N.C.: Hypertension: The Rediscovery of Combination Therapy, *Geriatrics*, *52*,28, November, 1997.

Thibodeau, E.A. and Rossomando, K.J.: Survey of the Medical History Questionnaire, *Oral Surg. Oral Med. Oral Pathol.*, *74*, 400, September, 1992.

Woolley, R.J., Klein, H.G., and Eisenman, D.: Value of Routine Inquiry About Blood Donation (Correspondence), *N. Engl. J. Med.*, *322*, 132, January 11, 1990.

Prophylactic Antibiotics

Barco, C.T.: Prevention of Infective Endocarditis: A Review of the Medical and Dental Literature, *J. Periodontol.*, *62*, 510, August, 1991.

Bender, I.B. and Barkan, M.J.: Dental Bacteremia and Its Relationship to Bacterial Endocarditis: Preventive Measures, *Compend. Cont. Educ. Dent.*, *10*, 472, September, 1989.

Biron, C.R.: Despite Diligent Staff, Infective Endocarditis Surfaces During Periodontal Treatment, *RDH*, *17*, 42, March, 1997.

Carroll, G.C. and Sebor, R.J.: Dental Flossing and Its Relationship to Transient Bacteremia, *J. Peridontol.*, *51*, 691, December, 1980.

Felder, R.S., Nardone, D., and Palac, R.: Prevalence of Predisposing Factors for Endocarditis Among an Elderly Institutionalized Population, *Oral Surg. Oral Med. Oral Pathol.*, *73*, 30, January, 1992.

Friedlander, A.H. and Yoshikawa, T.T.: Pathogenesis, Management, and Prevention of Infective Endocarditis in the Elderly Dental Patient, *Oral Surg. Oral Med. Oral Pathol.*, *69*, 177, February, 1990.

Glick, M.: Intravenous Drug Users: A Consideration for Infective Endocarditis in Dentistry? (Editorial) *Oral Surg. Oral Med. Oral Pathol.*, *80*, 125, August, 1995.

Hobson, R.S. and Clark, J.D.: Management of the Orthodontic Patient At Risk From Infective Endocarditis, *Brit. Dent. J.*,*178*, 289, April 22, 1995.

Luce, E.B., Presti, C.F., Montemayor, I., and Crawford, M.H.: Detecting Cardiac Valvular Pathology in Patients With Systemic Lupus Erythematosus, *Spec. Care Dentist.*, *12*, 193, September/October, 1992.

McLaughlin, J.O.: The Incidence of Bacteremia After Orthodontic Banding, *Am. J. Orthod. Dentofac. Orthop.*, *109*, 639, June, 1996.

Tzukert, A.A., Leviner, E., and Sela, M.: Prevention of Infective Endocarditis: Not By Antibiotics Alone, *Oral Surg. Oral Med. Oral Pathol.*, *62*, 385, October, 1986.

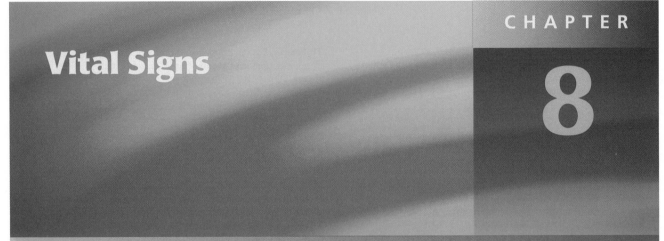

Vital Signs

CHAPTER

8

CHAPTER OUTLINE

I. Patient Preparation and Instruction
II. Dental Hygiene Treatment Planning
- BODY TEMPERATURE
  I. Indications for Taking the Temperature
  II. Maintenance of Body Temperature
  III. Methods of Determining Temperature
  IV. Care of Patient With Temperature Elevation
- PULSE
  I. Maintenance of Normal Pulse
  II. Procedure for Determining Pulse Rate
- RESPIRATION
  I. Maintenance of Normal Respirations
  II. Procedures for Observing Respirations

- BLOOD PRESSURE
  I. Components of Blood Pressure
  II. Factors That Influence Blood Pressure
  III. Equipment for Determining Blood Pressure
  IV. Procedure for Determining Blood Pressure
  V. Blood Pressure Follow-up Criteria
- EVERYDAY ETHICS
- FACTORS TO TEACH THE PATIENT
  REFERENCES
  SUGGESTED READINGS

Determination of four vital signs—*body temperature, pulse and respiratory rates,* and *blood pressure*—is considered standard procedure in patient care. Table 8-1 summarizes the normal values of the four basic vital signs for adolescents and adults.

Adding a fifth new vital sign—*smoking status*—gives the opportunity to introduce early in the encounter with the patient the significance of smoking to general and oral health. The fact that smoking is the number one preventable cause of illness and death more than justifies including smoking status as a vital sign.[1] Figure 8-1 illustrates a vital sign stamp to use for convenient recording of all five signs.

I. PATIENT PREPARATION AND INSTRUCTION

- Seat patient in upright position, at eye level for instruction.
- Explain the vital signs and obtain consent.
- Explain how vital signs can affect dental hygiene and dental treatment.
- Teach the patient to refrain from eating, drinking, or smoking before the vital signs are taken.

- During the process, explain each step as needed by the individual patient.

II. DENTAL HYGIENE TREATMENT PLANNING

- Recording vital signs contributes to the proper systemic evaluation of a patient in conjunction with the complete medical history.
- Dental hygiene care planning and appointment sequencing are directly influenced by the findings.
- When vital signs are not within normal, advise the patient to check with the physician.
- Referral for medical evaluation and treatment is indicated.
- Key words related to the vital signs are defined in Box 8-1.

BODY TEMPERATURE

While preparing the patient history and making the extraoral and intraoral examinations, the need for taking the temperature may become apparent, or the dentist may have requested the procedure in conjunction with current oral disease.

■ TABLE 8-1 ADULT VITAL SIGNS

VITAL SIGN	VALUES OF SIGNIFICANCE IN DENTAL AND DENTAL HYGIENE APPOINTMENTS	
Body temperature (oral)	Normal 37.0°C (98.6°F) Normal range 35.5° to 37.5°C (96.0° to 99.5°F)	
Pulse rate	Normal range 60 to 100 per minute	
Respiration	Normal range 14 to 20 per minute	
BLOOD PRESSURE CATEGORY	**SYSTOLIC mmHg**	**DIASTOLIC mmHg**
Normal	<120	<80
Prehypertension	120–139	80–89
Hypertension		
Stage 1	140–159	90–99
Stage 2	>160	>100

*Data from *The Seventh Report of the Joint National Committee on Prevention, Detection, Evaluation, and Treatment of High Blood Pressure.* National Institutes of Health, National Heart, Lung, and Blood Institute, Publication 03-5233, May, 2003.

I. INDICATIONS FOR TAKING THE TEMPERATURE

A. For the new patient's initial permanent record along with all vital signs.
B. For complete examination during a maintenance appointment.
C. When oral infection is known to be present.
   • Necrotizing ulcerative gingivitis or periodontitis.
   • Apical or periodontal abscess.
   • Acute pericoronitis.
D. With other vital signs prior to administration of local anesthetic.

```
                   VITAL SIGNS

NAME_____ DATE_____
Blood Pressure _____
Pulse _____
Temperature _____
Respiratory Rate _____
Smoking Status  Current  Former  Never
(please circle)
```

■ **FIGURE 8-1 Vital Signs Stamp for a Patient's Record.** (Adapted from Fiore, M.C.: The New Vital Sign. Assessing and Documenting Smoking Status, *JAMA, 266,* 3183, December 11, 1991.)

E. At any appointment when the patient reports illness or there is a suspected infection.
   • Protection of the health of the healthcare personnel and patients or families who may be exposed secondarily.
   • Special significance during epidemics when community exposures are at risk.
   • For patient's referral for medical care when indicated.

II. MAINTENANCE OF BODY TEMPERATURE

A. Normal

1. *Adults.* The normal average temperature is 37.0°C (98.6°F), as illustrated in Figure 8-2. The normal range is from 35.5° to 37.5°C (96.0° to 99.5°F).
2. *Older Adults.* Over 70 years of age, the average temperature is slightly lower (36.0°C, 96.8°F).
3. *Children.* There is no appreciable difference between boys and girls. Average temperatures are as follows:
   • First year: 37.3°C (99.1°F).
   • Fourth year: 37.5°C (99.4°F).
   • Fifth year: 37°C (98.6°F).
   • Twelfth year: 36.7°C (98.0°F).

B. Temperature Variations

1. *Fever (pyrexia).* Values over 37.5°C (99.5°F).
2. *Hyperthermia.* Values over 41.0°C (105.8°F).
3. *Hypothermia.* Values below 35.5°C (96.0°F).

C. Factors That Alter Body Temperature

1. *Time of Day.* Highest in late afternoon and early evening; lowest during sleep and early morning.
2. *Temporary Increase.* Exercise, hot drinks, smoking, or application of external heat.
3. *Pathologic States.* Infection, dehydration, hyperthyroidism, myocardial infarction, or tissue injury from trauma.
4. *Decrease.* Starvation, hemorrhage, or physiologic shock.

III. METHODS OF DETERMINING TEMPERATURE

A. Locations for Measurement

• Oral: most commonly used; patient needs to be able to breathe through the nose and hold lips

BOX 8-1 KEY WORDS: Vital Signs

Anoxia: oxygen deficiency; a reduction of oxygen in the tissues can lead to deep respirations, cyanosis, increased pulse rate, and impairment of coordination.

Apnea: temporary cessation of breathing; absence of spontaneous respirations.

Auscultation: listening for sounds produced within the body; may be performed directly or with a stethoscope.

Bradycardia: unusually slow heartbeat evidenced by slowing of the pulse rate.

Core temperature: the temperature of the deep tissues of the body; remains relatively constant; contrasts with body surface temperature, which rises and falls in response to environment.

Diastole: the phase of the cardiac cycle in which the heart relaxes between contractions and the two ventricles are dilated by the blood flowing into them; diastolic pressure is the lowest blood pressure.

Diurnal: pertaining to or occurring during the daytime or period of light.

Hypertension: systolic blood pressure of 140 mmHg or greater and diastolic blood pressure of 90 mmHg or greater.

Hyperthermia: higher-than-normal body temperature.

Hypothermia: lower-than-normal body temperature.

Korotkoff sounds: the sounds heard during the determination of blood pressure; sounds originating within the blood passing through the vessel or produced by vibratory motion of the arterial wall.

Normotensive: normal tension or tone; of or pertaining to having normal blood pressure.

Pulse pressure: the difference between systolic and diastolic blood pressure; normally 40 mmHg.

Pyrexia: an abnormal elevation of the body temperature above 37.0°C (98.6°F).

Stethoscope: instrument used to hear and amplify the sounds produced by the heart, lungs, and other internal organs.

Systole: the contraction, or period of contraction, of the heart, especially the ventricles, during which blood is forced into the aorta and the pulmonary artery; systolic pressure is the highest, or greatest, pressure.

Tachycardia: unusually fast heartbeat; at a rate greater than 100 beats per minute.

---

closed; must not have sore mouth, very dry mouth, or recent oral surgery.
- Forehead: for disposable thermometer.
- Ear: with a tympanic device.

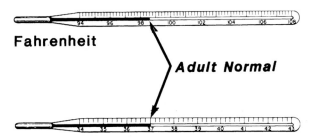

Fahrenheit

Adult Normal

Centigrade

■ **FIGURE 8-2 Thermometers.** Centigrade and Fahrenheit thermometers compared. Adult normal temperature is shown at 37.0° Centigrade and 98.6° Fahrenheit.

- Medical /hospital applications: also use axilla or rectum for assessment.

B. Types of Thermometers

1. *Electronic* with digital readout
   - Cover with disposable protective sheath.
   - Place under tongue; short time required.
   - Read on the digital display.
2. *Tympanic*
   - Cover with protective sheath.
   - Insert gently into ear canal.
   - Short exposure (2-5 seconds) before record appears on digital unit.
3. *Mercury in glass:* oral, blue tip; rectal, red tip
   - Used less because of danger for breakage with mercury spill that must be cleaned up using specified procedures.
   - Sheath cover used for infection protection.

- Takes longer time before reading than other types.
- More difficult to see and read mercury column.
4. *Disposable* single-use chemical strip
   - Apply to appropriate skin area, usually the forehead.
   - Color changes denote temperature.

IV. CARE OF PATIENT WITH TEMPERATURE ELEVATION

A. Temperature Over 41.0°C (105.8°F)

1. Treat as a medical emergency.
2. Transport to a hospital for medical care.

B. Temperature 37.6° to 41.0°C (99.6°C to 105.8°F)

1. Check possible temporary or factitious cause, such as hot beverage or smoking, and observe patient while repeating the determination.
2. Review the dental and medical history.
3. Postpone elective oral care when there are signs of respiratory infection or other possible communicable disease.

▪ PULSE

The pulse is the intermittent throbbing sensation felt when the fingers are pressed against an artery. It is the result of the alternate expansion and contraction of an artery as a wave of blood is forced out from the heart. The pulse rate or heart rate is the count of the heartbeats. Irregularities of strength, rhythm, and quality of the pulse should be noted while counting the pulse rate.

I. MAINTENANCE OF NORMAL PULSE

A. Normal Pulse Rates

1. *Adults.* There is no absolute normal. The adult range is 60 to 100 beats per minute, slightly higher for women than for men.
2. *Children.* The pulse or heart rate falls steadily during childhood.
   a. *In utero*—150 beats per minute (bpm).
   b. At birth—130 bpm.
   c. Second year—105 bpm.
   d. Fourth year—90 bpm.
   e. Tenth year—70 bpm.

B. Factors That Influence Pulse Rate

An unusually fast heartbeat (over 100 beats per minute in an adult) is called *tachycardia;* an unusually slow heartbeat (below 50) is *bradycardia.*
1. *Increased Pulse.* Caused by exercise, stimulants, eating, strong emotions, extremes of heat and cold, and some forms of heart disease.
2. *Decreased Pulse.* Caused by sleep, depressants, fasting, quieting emotions, and low vitality from prolonged illness.
3. *Emergency Situations.* Listed in Tables 66-4 and 66-5.

II. PROCEDURE FOR DETERMINING PULSE RATE

A. Sequence

The pulse rate is obtained following the body temperature. When the mercury in glass thermometer is used, the pulse can be counted while the thermometer is in the mouth.

B. Sites

The pulse may be felt at several points over the body.
- Radial pulse: at the wrist (Figure 8-3).

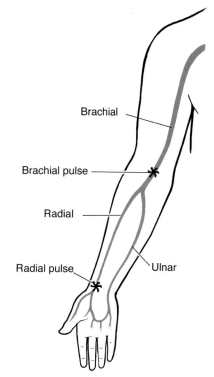

▪ **FIGURE 8-3 Arteries of the Arm.** Note the location of the radial pulse. The brachial pulse may be felt just before the brachial artery branches into the radial and ulnar arteries.

- Other sites convenient for use in a dental office or clinic are the *temporal* artery on the side of the head in front of the ear, or the *facial* artery at the border of the mandible.
- Carotid pulse: used during cardiopulmonary resuscitation (see Figure 66-8) for an adult.
- Brachial pulse: used for an infant.

C. Prepare the Patient

1. Tell the patient what is to be done.
2. Have the patient in a comfortable position with arm and hand supported, palm down.
3. Locate the radial pulse on the thumb side of the wrist with the tips of the first three fingers (Figure 8-4). Do not use the thumb because it contains a pulse that may be confused with the patient's pulse.

D. Count and Record

1. When the pulse is felt, exert light pressure and count for 1 clocked minute. Use the second hand of a watch or clock. Check with a repeat count.
2. While taking the pulse, observe the following:
   - Rhythm: regular, regularly irregular, irregularly irregular.
   - Volume and strength: full, strong, poor, weak, thready.
3. Record on patient's record the date, pulse rate, other characteristics.
4. A pulse rate over 100 should be considered abnormal for an adult.

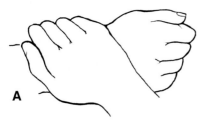

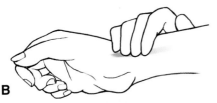

▪ **FIGURE 8-4 Determination of Pulse Rate. (A)** Correct position of hands. **(B)** The tips of the first three fingers are placed over the radial pulse located on the thumb side of the ventral surface of the wrist.

▪ RESPIRATION

The function of respiration is to supply oxygen to the tissues and to eliminate carbon dioxide. Variations in normal respirations may be shown by such characteristics as the rate, rhythm, depth, and quality and may be symptomatic of disease or emergency states.

I. MAINTENANCE OF NORMAL RESPIRATIONS

A respiration is one breath taken in and let out.

A. Normal Respiratory Rate

1. *Adults.* The adult range is from 14 to 20 per minute, slightly higher for women.
2. *Children.* The respiratory rate decreases steadily during childhood. Averages are
   a. First year—30 per minute.
   b. Second year—25 per minute.
   c. Eighth year—20 per minute.
   d. Fifteenth year—18 per minute.

B. Factors That Influence Respirations

Many of the same factors that influence pulse rate also influence the number of respirations. A rate of 12 per minute or fewer is considered subnormal for an adult; over 28 is accelerated; and rates over 60 are extremely rapid and dangerous.

1. *Increased Respiration.* Caused by work and exercise, excitement, nervousness, strong emotions, pain, hemorrhage, shock.
2. *Decreased Respiration.* Caused by sleep, certain drugs, pulmonary insufficiency.
3. *Emergency Situations.* Listed in Tables 66-4 and 66-5.

II. PROCEDURES FOR OBSERVING RESPIRATIONS

A. Determine Rate

1. Make the count of respirations immediately after counting the pulse.
2. Maintain the fingers over the radial pulse.
3. Respirations must be counted so that the patient is not aware, as the rate may be voluntarily altered.
4. Count the number of times the chest rises in 1 clocked minute. It is not necessary to count both inspirations and expirations.

B. Factors to Observe

1. *Depth.* Describe as shallow, normal, or deep.

2. *Rhythm.* Describe as regular (evenly spaced) or irregular (with pauses of irregular lengths between).
3. *Quality.* Describe as strong, easy, weak, or labored (noisy). Poor quality may have an effect on body color; for example, a bluish tinge of the face or nailbeds may mean an insufficiency of oxygen.
4. *Sounds.* Describe deviant sounds made during inspiration, expiration, or both.
5. *Position of Patient.* When the patient assumes an unusual position to secure comfort during breathing or prefers to remain seated upright, mark records accordingly.

C. Record

Record all findings in the patient's record.

■ BLOOD PRESSURE

Information about the patient's blood pressure is essential during dental and dental hygiene appointments because special adaptations may be needed. Blood pressure readings most usually are recorded with the medical history and other assessment data. Readings taken at the start of an appointment can be significantly higher than at the end of treatment.[2]

To establish a baseline reading and determine the need for patient referral for medical attention, several readings are needed, especially at the close of appointments when the patient is relaxed.

Screening for blood pressure in dental offices has been shown to be an effective health service for all ages since many patients are unaware that they have hypertension. Cardiovascular diseases are described in Chapter 63. That information can be a helpful introduction and is recommended for reading in conjunction with this section on the techniques for obtaining blood pressure.

I. COMPONENTS OF BLOOD PRESSURE

Blood pressure is the force exerted by the blood on the blood vessel walls. When the left ventricle of the heart contracts, blood is forced out into the aorta and travels through the large arteries to the smaller arteries, arterioles, and capillaries. The pulsations extend from the heart through the arteries and disappear in the arterioles. During the course of the cardiac cycle, the blood pressure is changing constantly.

A. Systolic Pressure

Systolic pressure is the peak or the highest pressure. It is caused by ventricular contraction. The normal systolic pressure is less than 120 mmHg.

B. Diastolic Pressure

Diastolic pressure is the lowest pressure. It is the effect of ventricular relaxation. The normal diastolic pressure is less than 80 mmHg.

C. Pulse Pressure

The pulse pressure is the difference between the systolic and diastolic pressures. The normal or safe difference is less than 40 mmHg.

II. FACTORS THAT INFLUENCE BLOOD PRESSURE

A. Maintenance of Blood Pressure

Blood pressure depends on
1. Force of the heartbeat (energy of the heart).
2. Peripheral resistance; condition of the arteries; changes in elasticity of vessels, which may occur with age and disease.
3. Volume of blood in the circulatory system.

B. Factors That Increase Blood Pressure

1. Exercise, eating, stimulants, and emotional disturbance.
2. Use of oral contraceptives; blood pressure increases with age and length of use.

C. Factors That Decrease Blood Pressure

1. Fasting, rest, depressants, and quiet emotions.
2. Such emergencies as fainting, blood loss, shock (see Tables 66-4 and 66-5).

III. EQUIPMENT FOR DETERMINING BLOOD PRESSURE

The mercury sphygmomanometer is the preferred instrument. A recently calibrated aneroid manometer or a validated electronic device can be used and are practical for home use. Finger monitors have been shown to be inaccurate.

A. Sphygmomanometer (blood pressure machine)

Consists of an *inflatable cuff* and *two tubes*, one connected to the *pressure hand control bulb* and the other to the *pressure gauge*.
1. *Cuff*
   • Material. The cuff is made of a nonelastic material and is fastened by a Velcro overlap. The inflatable bladder is located within the material of the cuff.

- Size. The diameter of the arm, not the age of the patient, determines the size of the cuff selected. The four cuff sizes available are child size, regular adult, large adult, and thigh. The thigh size is needed for grossly obese persons.
- Dimension. The cuff width that is used should be 20% greater than the diameter of the arm to which it is applied (Figure 8-5). It should cover approximately two-thirds of the upper arm.

  When a cuff is too narrow, the blood pressure reading is too high; when the cuff is too wide, the reading is too low.[3]

2. *Mercury Manometer*
   - Gauges are marked with long lines at each 10 mmHg, with shorter lines at 2-mm intervals between each long line.
   - The level of the column of mercury of the manometer should be at eye level for accurate reading and must not be tilted.

B. Stethoscope (a listening aid that magnifies sound)

Consists of an *endpiece* that is connected by tubes to carry the sound to the *earpieces*.
1. *Types of Endpieces.* Bell-shaped or flat (diaphragm); the bell shape is used for medical examinations, particularly for chest examination.
2. *Care of Earpieces.* Clean by rubbing with gauze sponge moistened in disinfectant.

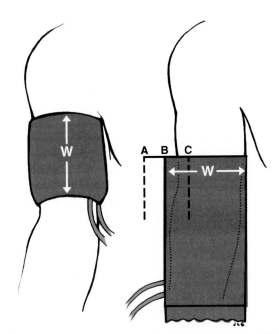

▪ **FIGURE 8-5 Selection of Cuff Size.** The correct width (W) is 20% greater than the diameter of the arm where applied. **(A)** Too wide. **(B)** Correct width. **(C)** Too narrow.

IV. PROCEDURE FOR DETERMINING BLOOD PRESSURE

A. Prepare Patient

1. Tell patient briefly what is to be done. Detailed explanations should be avoided because they may excite the patient and change the blood pressure.

Everyday Ethics

Gracie was having a very busy day and at 10:15 was already late for the 10:00 patient, Mr. McElroy , who had arrived early and was waiting in the reception area. While completing his history, to save time, she copied over the blood pressure recording from his previous appointment just two weeks ago. It had been 130/83, only slightly into the prehypertension level.

The appointment was planned for the maxillary left quadrant with anesthesia. After the scaling was complete and Mr. McElroy was climbing out of the dental chair, looking a bit unsteady as he stood up, he casually remarked: "I just remembered while you were working that my Doc gave me a new prescription—I suppose I should have told you before. But it is only one pill a day—for keeping the blood pressure down. I don't have any trouble anyway, he just wanted to be sure."

Questions for Consideration

1. Explain how the principles of beneficence and maleficence apply to Gracie's actions with Mr. McElroy's examination and charting procedures.

2. Has Gracie placed the office at risk for a possible medical emergency given Mr. McElroy's physical status? Answer by describing the rights and duties of both the hygienist and the patient.

3. Who is responsible for ensuring that accurate documentation has been completed on all patients—from an ethical and a quality assurance perspective?

2. Seat patient comfortably, with the arm slightly flexed, with palm up, and with the whole fore-arm supported on a level surface at the level of the heart.

3. Use either arm unless otherwise indicated, for example, by a handicap. Repeat blood pressure determinations should be made on the same arm, because the difference between arms may be as much as 10 mmHg.

4. Take pressure on bare arm, not over clothing. A tight sleeve should be loosened.

B. Apply Cuff

1. Apply the completely deflated cuff to the patient's arm, supported at the level of the heart. It has been shown that when the arm rests on the arm of a dental chair, higher than the heart, the diastolic pressure shows a small but significant increase.[4]

2. Place the portion of the cuff that contains the inflatable bladder directly over the brachial artery. The cuff may have an arrow to show the point that should be placed over the artery. The lower edge of the cuff is placed 1 inch above the antecubital fossa (Figure 8-6). Fasten the cuff evenly and snugly.

3. Adjust the position of the gauge for convenient reading but so that the patient cannot see the mercury.

4. Palpate 1 inch below the antecubital fossa to locate the brachial artery pulse (Figure 8-3). The stethoscope endpiece is placed over the spot where the brachial pulse is felt.

5. Position the stethoscope earpieces in the ears, with the tips directed forward.

C. Locate the Radial Pulse (Figures 8-3 and 8-4)

Hold the fingers on the pulse.

D. Inflate the Cuff

1. Close the needle valve (air lock) attached to the hand control bulb firmly but so it may be released readily.

2. Pump to inflate the cuff until the radial pulse stops. Note the mercury level at which the pulse disappears.

3. Look at the dial, and pump to 20 or 30 mmHg beyond where the radial pulse was no longer felt. This is the maximum inflation level (MIL). It means that the brachial artery is collapsed by the pressure of the cuff and no blood is flowing through.

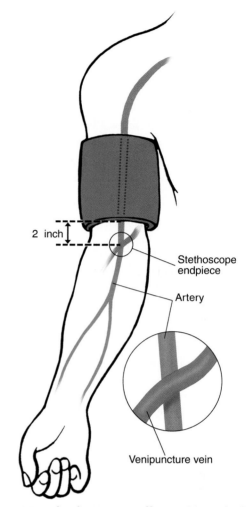

2 inch

Stethoscope endpiece

Artery

Venipuncture vein

■ **FIGURE 8-6 Blood Pressure Cuff in Position.** The lower edge of the cuff is placed approximately 1 inch above the antecubital fossa. The stethoscope endpiece is placed over the palpated brachial artery pulse point approximately 1 inch below the antecubital fossa and slightly toward the inner side of the arm.

Unless the MIL is determined, the level to which the cuff is inflated will be arbitrary. Excess pressure can be very uncomfortable for the patient.

E. Position the Stethoscope Endpiece

Place the endpiece over the palpated brachial artery, 1 inch below the antecubital fossa, and slightly toward the inner side of the arm (Figure 8-6). Hold lightly in place.

F. Deflate the Cuff Gradually

1. Release the air lock slowly (2 to 3 mm per second) so that the dial drops very gradually and steadily.

Factors To Teach The Patient

- How vital signs can influence dental and dental hygiene appointments.

- The importance of having a blood pressure determination at regular intervals.

- For the patient diagnosed as hypertensive, encourage regular continuing use of prescription drugs for control of high blood pressure.

2. Listen for the first sound: *systole* ("tap tap"). Note the number on the dial that is the *systolic pressure*. This is the beginning of the flow of blood past the cuff.

3. Continue to release the pressure slowly. The sound will continue, first becoming louder, then diminishing and becoming muffled, until finally disappearing. Note the number on the dial where the last distinct tap was heard. That number is the *diastolic pressure*.

4. Release further (about 10 mm) until all sounds cease. That is the second diastolic point. In some clinics and hospitals, the last sound is taken as the diastolic pressure.

5. Let the rest of the air out rapidly.

G. Repeat for Confirmation

Wait 30 seconds before inflating the cuff again. More than one reading is needed within a few minutes to determine an average and ensure a correct reading.

H. Record

- Write date and arm used.
- Record blood pressure as a fraction, for example, 120/80. When both diastolic points are recorded, they can be written as 120/80/72.

V. BLOOD PRESSURE FOLLOW-UP CRITERIA

Dental personnel have an obligation to advise and *refer for further evaluation*. Diagnosis of hypertension would never be made or treatment started on the basis of an isolated reading.

When the blood pressure is within the normal range (120/80), it should be rechecked within 2 years. Rechecking within 1 year is recommended for persons at increased risk for hypertension, such as family history, weight gain, obesity, African American, use of oral contraceptives, smoking, and excessive alcohol consumption.

Lifestyle modifications are indicated for all levels of blood pressure classification.[5] Consultation with a patient's physician is indicated prior to dental or dental hygiene treatment when either reading is ≥180/110. (Table 8-1).

REFERENCES

1. **Fiore**, M.C.: The New Vital Sign. Assessing and Documenting Smoking Status, *JAMA, 266,* 3183, December 11, 1991.
2. **Nichols**, C.: Dentistry and Hypertension, *J. Am. Dent. Assoc., 128,* 1557, November, 1997.
3. **Geddes**, L.A. and Whistler, S.J.: The Error in Indirect Blood Pressure Measurement with the Incorrect Size of Cuff, *Am. Heart J., 96,* 4, July, 1978.
4. **Beck**, F.M., Weaver, J.M., Blozis, G.G., and Unverferth, D.V.: Effect of Arm Position and Arm Support on Indirect Blood Pressure Measurements Made in a Dental Chair, *J. Am. Dent. Assoc., 106,* 645, May, 1983.
5. **United States National High Blood Pressure Education Program:** *The Seventh Report of the Joint National Committee on Prevention, Detection, Evaluation, and Treatment of High Blood Pressure.* Washington, D.C., National Institutes of Health, National Heart, Lung, and Blood Institute, N.I.H. Publication No. 03-5233, May, 2003, 52 pp.

SUGGESTED READINGS

Cline, N.V. and Springstead, M.C.: Monitoring Blood Pressure. Five Minutes Critical to Quality Patient Care, *J. Dent. Hyg., 66,* 363, October, 1992.

Fast, T.B.: Physical Evaluation and Monitoring Devices in Dental Practice, *Gen. Dent., 41,* 242, June, 1993.

Martin, C., Moore, D., Templin, K., and Moore, J.: Electronic Blood Pressure Screening: Fast, Easy, and Essential, *Access, 12,* 33, January, 1998.

Nesselroad, J.M., Flacco, V.A., Phillips, D.M., and Kruse, J.: Accuracy of Automated Finger Blood Pressure Devices, *Fam. Med., 28,* 189, March, 1996.

Nunn, P.J.: The Life You Save May Be Your Patient's, *RDH, 14,* 44, April, 1994.

Pyle, M.A., Sawyer, D.R., Jasinevicius, T.R., and Ballard, R.: Blood Pressure Measurement by Community Dentists, *Spec. Care Dentist., 19,* 230, September/October, 1999.

Raab, F.J., Schaffer, E.M., Guillaume-Cornelissen, G., and Halberg, F.: Interpreting Vital Sign Profiles for Maximizing Patient Safety During Dental Visits, *J. Am. Dent. Assoc., 129,* 461, April, 1998.

Yeatts, D.E., Wood, A.J., and McCarter, W.J.: Fevers in Children, *ASDC J. Dent. Child, 61,* 249, July–August, 1994.

Dental Radiographic Imaging

Dorathea Foote, RDH, MEd

Radiographic images are integral assessment components useful when planning comprehensive care for a patient. They provide the clinician with important diagnostic tools that can be used to detect lesions, diseases, and conditions of teeth and supporting structures; to localize foreign objects; to assess growth and development; and to document changes in, and progress of, a condition over time.[1]

The dentist is responsible for determining the need for radiographs. Designation of the number and types of dental exposures must be made selectively only after a review of the patient's health history and a complete clinical examination.[2] A history of oral and body exposures to radiation is recommended. Excessive dental exposure to low levels of ionizing radiation cannot be justified.[3]

The objective in radiography is to use procedures that expose the patient to the least amount of radiation possible to produce radiographs of the greatest interpretive value. The first consideration is to limit the number of exposures to those that have been deemed necessary.

This chapter provides a summary of terminology and fundamentals of x-ray production. Procedures are included for film exposure and processing, safety factors, analysis of the completed radiographs, and suggestions for patient instruction.

Selected terms used in the study of radiography are listed and defined in Box 9-1. Box 9-2 provides a list of universally used abbreviations.

▪ HOW X-RAYS ARE PRODUCED

X-ray energy is electromagnetic ionizing radiation of very short wavelengths, resulting from the bombardment of a target made of tungsten by highly accelerated electrons in a high vacuum. Electric and magnetic fields positioned at right angles to one another produce the electromagnetic energy.

The various types of energy in the electromagnetic spectrum have similar attributes. The properties of x-rays are listed in Table 9-1.

Essential to x-ray production are (1) a source of electrons, (2) a high voltage to accelerate the electrons, and (3) a target to stop the electrons. The parts of the tube and the circuits within the machine are designed to provide these elements.

I. THE X-RAY TUBE (FIGURE 9-1)

A. Protective Tube Housing

Heavy metal enclosure that houses the x-ray tube and reduces the primary radiation to permissible exposure levels.

B. X-Ray Tube

A highly evacuated leaded-glass tube composed of a cathode and anode and surrounded by a specially refined oil with high insulating powers.

BOX 9-1 KEY WORDS: Radiography

Ammeter: an instrument for measuring electric current in amperes.

Attenuation: the process by which a beam of radiation is reduced in intensity when passing through some material; the combination of absorption and scattering processes leads to a decrease in flux density of the beam when projected through matter.

Cassette: a light-tight container in which x-ray films are placed for exposure to x-radiation; usually backed with lead to reduce the effect of backscatter radiation; may be made of cardboard or of metal with an exposure side of bakelite, aluminum, or magnesium and containing an intensifying screen(s).

Impulse: the burst of radiation generated during a half cycle of alternating current; film exposure time is measured in impulses.

Intensifying screen: a card or plastic sheet coated with fluorescent material positioned singly or in pairs in a cassette. When the cassette is exposed to x-radiation, the visible light from the fluorescent image on the screen adds to the latent image produced directly by x-radiation.

Irradiation: exposure to radiation; one speaks of radiation therapy and of irradiation of a body part.

Latent image: the invisible change produced in an x-ray film emulsion by the action of x-radiation or light from which the visible image is subsequently developed and fixed chemically.

Penumbra: the secondary shadow that surrounds the periphery of the primary shadow; in radiography, it is the blurred margin of an image detail (geometric unsharpness).

Photoelectric effect: the ejection of bound electrons by an incident photon such that the whole energy of the photon is absorbed and transitional or characteristic x-ray emissions are produced.

Photon: a finite bundle of energy of visible light or electromagnetic radiation.

Radiation: the emission and propagation of energy through space or a material medium in the form of waves or particles. Types of radiation are defined in Box 9-3.

Radiograph: a visible image on a radiation-sensitive film emulsion produced by chemical processing after exposure of the film emulsion to ionizing radiation that has passed through an area, region, or substance of interest.

Radiography: the art and science of making radiographs.

Radiologic health: the art and science of protecting human beings from injury by radiation, as well as of promoting better health through beneficial applications of radiation.

Radiology: that branch of science that deals with the use of radiant energy in the diagnosis and treatment of disease.

Radiolucency: the appearance of dark images on a radiograph as a result of the greater amount of radiation that penetrates low-density objects and reaches the film.

Radiopacity: the appearance of light (white) images on a radiograph as a result of the lesser amount of radiation that is absorbed by dense objects and does not reach the film.

Rare earth: commonly used to refer to intensifying screens that contain rare earth elements; it may also refer to a screen-film system used for x-ray imaging; the systems are considered "fast" exposure systems.

Rectification: conversion of alternating current (AC) to direct current (DC); a **rectifier** changes AC to DC.

Soma: the entire body with the exclusion of germ cells. Somatic: adj.

BOX 9-2 Abbreviations Used in Radiography*

ALARA	As Low as Reasonably Achievable
Gy	gray
HVL	half value layer
kVp	kilovolt peak
mA	milliampere
mAi	milliampere impulse
mAs	milliampere second
mGy	milligray
MPD	maximum permissible dose
mSv	millisievert
PID	position-indicating device
R	roentgen
rad	radiation absorbed dose
rem	roentgen equivalent man
Sv	sievert
XCP	extension cone paralleling

*Definitions in this chapter are taken from or adapted from and in accord with the *Glossary of Maxillofacial Radiology,* 3rd ed., prepared by the American Academy of Oral and Maxillofacial Radiology, 1990.

▪ TABLE 9-1 PROPERTIES OF X-RAYS

Characteristic
• Invisible
• No mass
• No weight
Travel
• In straight line; can be scattered
• At the speed of light
Wavelengths
• Have short wavelengths, high frequency
• Hard x-rays: short wavelengths, high penetration
• Soft x-rays: relatively longer wavelengths; relatively less penetrating; more likely to be absorbed into the tissue
Penetration
• Pass through matter, or
• Absorbed by matter, depending on atomic structure of matter
Causes
• Ionization
• Fluorescence of certain crystals
• Biologic changes in living cells
Produces
• An image on photographic film

C. Cathode (−)

1. Tungsten filament, which is a coiled wire heated to generate a cloud of electrons. It is a component of the low-voltage circuit.
2. Molybdenum cup around the filament to focus the electrons toward the anode.

D. Anode (+)

A tungsten target embedded in a copper stem, positioned at an angle to the electron beam.

E. Aperture

The window where the useful beam emerges from the tube; covered with a permanent seal of glass.

F. Aluminum Disks

Thin (0.5-mm) sheets of aluminum placed over the aperture to filter out longer-wavelength x-rays.

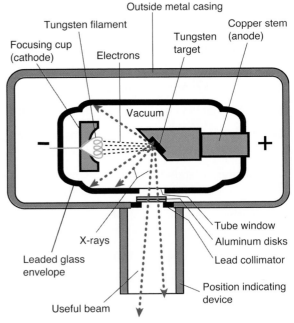

▪ **FIGURE 9-1 X-Ray Tube.** High-speed electrons flowing from cathode to anode hit the tungsten target, create x-ray photons. X-rays exit through the tube window and position-indicating device.

G. Lead Diaphragm

A lead collimator with a hole to restrict the size of the x-ray beam.

H. Position-Indicating Device (PID)

Open-ended cylinder that shapes and aims the x-ray beam.

II. CIRCUITS

A circuit is the complete path over which an electrical current may flow. Two circuits are used to produce x-rays. Refer to Figure 9-2 to examine the electrical circuits in a dental x-ray machine.

A. Low-Voltage Filament Circuit

B. High-Voltage Cathode-Anode Circuit

III. TRANSFORMERS

A transformer increases or decreases the incoming voltage.

A. Autotransformer

A voltage compensator that corrects minor variations in line voltage.

B. Filament Step-down Transformer

Decreases the line voltage to approximately 3 volts to heat the filament and form the electron cloud.

C. High-Voltage Step-up Transformer

Increases the current from 110 volts to 60 to 90 kVp (kilovoltage peak) to give electrons the required energy necessary to produce x-ray photons.

IV. MACHINE CONTROL DEVICES

Machines vary, but, in general, when operating an x-ray machine, there are four factors to control: the power switch (to the electrical outlet), the kilovoltage, the milliamperage, and the time.

A. Voltage Control

Voltage is the unit of measurement used to describe the force that pushes an electric current through a circuit.

1. *Circuit Voltmeter.* Registers line voltage before voltage is stepped up by the transformer (with alternating current, this is 110 volts), or may register the kilovoltage that results after step-up.

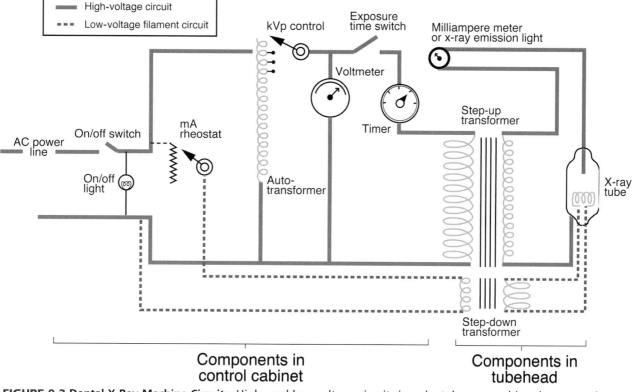

■ **FIGURE 9-2 Dental X-Ray Machine Circuits.** High- and low-voltage circuits in a dental x-ray machine demonstrating flow of electricity from the on/off switch to the x-ray tube head. (Adapted from Olson, S.S.: *Dental Radiography Laboratory Manual.* Philadelphia, W.B. Saunders, 1995, p. 40.)

2. *kVp (Kilovoltage Peak) Selector.* Used to change the line voltage to a selected kilovoltage (60 to 90 kVp).

B. Milliamperage Control

1. *Ampere.* The unit of intensity of an electrical current produced by 1 volt acting through a resistance of 1 ohm. A milliampere (mA) is 1/1000 of an ampere.
2. *Milliammeter.* Instrument used to select the actual current through the tube circuit during the time of exposure.

C. Time Control

1. *X-Ray Timer.* A time switch mechanism used to control the length of the exposure time.
2. *Time-Delay Switch.* Mechanism that applies power to the high-voltage circuit once the filament is heated.

3. *Electronic Timer.* Vacuum tube device; resets itself automatically to the last-used exposure time. The timer is calibrated in seconds or in impulses, with 60 *impulses* in each second (in a 60-cycle AC current).

V. STEPS IN THE PRODUCTION OF X-RAYS

X-rays are produced when high-speed electrons are slowed down or stopped suddenly. The many types of radiation produced are defined in Box 9-3.

A. Tungsten filament is heated, and a cloud of electrons is produced.
B. Difference in electrical potential is developed between the anode and the cathode.
C. Electrons traveling at a high speed are attracted to the anode from the cathode when the anode is charged positive and the cathode negative. When alternating current is used with a self-rectifying tube, the electrons are attracted back into the tungsten filament.

BOX 9-3 KEY WORDS: Types of Radiation

Bremsstrahlung radiation (white radiation): a distribution of x-rays from very-low-energy photons to those produced by the peak kilovoltage applied across an x-ray tube; Bremsstrahlung means "braking radiation" and refers to the sudden deceleration of electrons (cathode rays) as they interact with highly positively charged nuclei, such as tungsten.

Characteristic radiation: the radiation produced by electron transitions from higher energy orbitals to replace ejected electrons of inner electron orbitals; the energy of the electromagnetic radiation emitted is unique or "characteristic" of the emitting atom.

Electromagnetic radiation: forms of energy propagated by wave motion as photons; the radiations differ widely in wavelength, frequency, and photo energy; examples are infrared waves, visible light, ultraviolet radiation, x-rays, gamma rays, and cosmic radiation.

Gamma radiation: short-wavelength electromagnetic radiation of nuclear origin similar to x-rays but usually of higher energy.

Leakage radiation: the radiation that escapes through the protective shielding of the x-ray unit tube head; it may be detected at the sides, top, bottom, or back of the tube head.

Primary radiation: all radiation coming directly from the target of the anode of an x-ray tube.

Scatter radiation: a form of secondary radiation that, during passage through a substance, has been deviated in direction; it may also have been modified by an increase in wavelength.

Backscatter: radiation deflected by scattering processes at angles greater than 90° to the original direction of the beam of radiation.

Coherent scattering (Thompson or unmodified): scattering of relatively low-energy x-rays by elastic collisions without loss of photon energy.

Compton scatter radiation: the incident radiation that has sufficient energy to dislodge a bound electron but attacks a loosely bound electron; the remaining radiation energy proceeds in a different direction as scatter radiation.

Secondary radiation: particles or photons produced by the interaction of primary radiation with matter.

Stray radiation: radiation that serves no useful purpose; it includes leakage, secondary, and scatter radiation.

D. Curvature of the molybdenum cup controls the direction of the electrons and causes them to be projected toward the focal spot.

E. Reaction of the electrons as they strike the tungsten target results in loss of energy.
   1. Approximately 1% of the energy of electrons is converted to x-ray energy (greater percent at higher kilovoltages).
   2. Approximately 99% of the energy is converted to heat and is dissipated through the copper anode and oil of the protective tube housing.

F. *General (Bremsstrahlung, or braking) radiation* occurs when speeding electrons stop, "brake," or slow down near the tungsten target in the anode. When an electron hits the nucleus of the tungsten atom, all of its kinetic energy is converted into a high-energy x-ray photon. When an electron comes close to but misses the nucleus, an x-ray photon of lower energy is created. General radiation produces x-rays of many different energies.[4]

G. *Characteristic radiation* results when a bombarding electron, at 70 kVp or above, displaces an electron from a shell of the target atom, ionizing the atom. Another electron in an outer shell replaces the missing electron, causing a cascading effect. When the displaced electron is replaced, a photon is emitted, resulting in characteristic radiation.

H. X-rays leave the tube through the aperture to form the useful beam.
   1. *Useful Beam.* The part of the primary radiation that is permitted to emerge from the tube head aperture and the accessory collimating devices.
   2. *Central Beam* (central ray). The center of the beam of x-rays emitted from the tube.

■ DIGITAL RADIOGRAPHY

Computerized digital radiography is also called dental digital radiographic imaging. Digital systems include intraoral, panoramic, and cephalometric imaging. Terminology for digital radiography is listed and defined in Box 9-4. Figure 9-3 shows the steps in the system of production. Starting with Figure 9-3A, the dental x-ray machine interfaces with the computer to digitize the radiographic image into pixels so that it can be displayed quickly on the computer's monitor. A sensor,

---

BOX 9-4 KEY WORDS: Digital Radiography

Charge-coupled device (CCD): a solid-state detector used as an image receptor in an intraoral sensor that converts x-rays to electrons and stores the electrons in electron wells.

Complementary-metal-oxide semiconductor (CMOS): a detector that has the same characteristics as a CCD, except the individual pixels can be made smaller.

Digital radiography: a filmless imaging system; a method of capturing a radiographic image using a sensor, breaking it into small electronic pieces, and presenting and storing the image using a computer.

Digital subtraction: a method of reversing the gray-scale as an image is viewed; radiolucent (normally black) images appear white and radiopaque (normally white) images appear black.

Digitize: to convert an image into a digital form that can be used by the computer using a grid of pixels.

Direct digital imaging: a filmless method of obtaining a digital image in which an intraoral sensor is directly exposed to x-rays to capture a radiographic image that can be viewed on a computer monitor.

Indirect digital imaging: a method of obtaining a digital image in which an existing radiograph is scanned and converted into a digital form using a CCD camera.

Pixel: a discrete unit of information. In digital electronic images, digital information is contained in, and presented as, discrete units of information.

Sensor: a small detector that is placed intraorally to capture a radiographic image.

Storage phosphor imaging: a method of obtaining a digital image in which the image is recorded on phosphor-coated plates and then placed into an electronic processor where a laser scans the plate and produces an image on a computer screen.

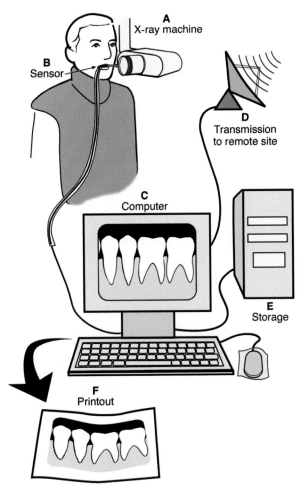

A
X-ray machine

B
Sensor

D
Transmission
to remote site

C
Computer

E
Storage

F
Printout

■ **FIGURE 9-3 Digital Imaging System. (A)** The image is exposed by an x-ray machine, **(B)** captured on a CCD or CMOS sensor in the patient's mouth. **(C)** The signal is transmitted via a cable to the computer, where it is digitized into 256 gray levels. The image is displayed on the computer's monitor, **(D)** transmitted electronically to a remote site, **(E)** stored on a file server, or **(F)** printed on paper.

as shown in Figure 9-4, is placed in the patient's mouth (Figure 9-6) in the usual positions for routine clinical radiography. The image is transmitted via a cable or wireless technology to a computer and possibly a file server (Figure 9-3E), where it is stored. It can be viewed on a monitor, transmitted electronically to a remote site (Figure 9-3D), or printed on paper (Figure 9-3F).

I. STEPS IN THE PRODUCTION OF A DIGITAL RADIOGRAPH

A. The sensor (Figure 9-4), encased in a plastic sleeve (Figure 9-5), is placed in the patient's mouth (Figure 9-6) and held by a sensor holder.

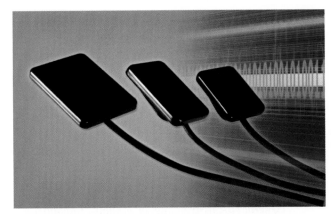

■ **FIGURE 9-4 Digital Sensors. Three sensor sizes are shown.** CCD or CMOS sensors have integrated circuits made up of a grid of small transistor elements that convert x-rays to electrons in electron wells. Each element represents one pixel in the final image. This information is passed through a cable to the computer for processing.

B. An electronic charge, produced on the surface of the sensor, is digitized or converted into digital form.
C. A computer converts the image information from analog form to digital form so that it can be read by the computer.
D. Within seconds, the image is displayed on the monitor and is stored on the computer's hard drive for future reference.

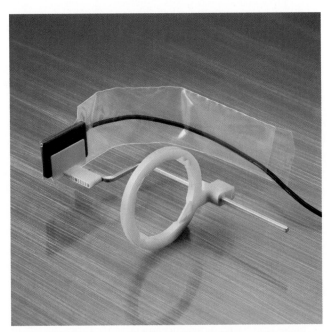

■ **FIGURE 9-5 Sensor Holder in Plastic Sleeve.** The sensor holder is encased in a plastic sleeve for infection control purposes.

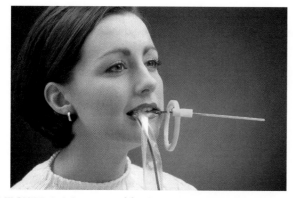

■ FIGURE 9-6 Sensor Holder in Patient's Mouth. The sensor holder and sensor are placed in the patient's mouth using the same criteria for placement as with conventional radiography.

II. TYPES OF SENSORS

A. Charged-coupled device detector (CCD)
B. Complementary-metal-oxide semiconductor detector (CMOS)
C. Charged injection device (CID)

III. TYPES OF DIGITAL IMAGING

A. Direct Digital Imaging

The sensor, placed in the patient's mouth, captures the image and transmits it to the computer. The computer digitizes the image into 256 gray levels. Within seconds, the image appears on the monitor, where it can be enhanced by varying the density and contrast (Figure 9-3).

B. Indirect Digital Imaging

A CCD camera and computer are used to digitize an existing radiographic film by scanning the image with the camera, digitizing it, and displaying it on the monitor.

C. Storage Phosphor Imaging

A reusable phosphor imaging plate is used instead of a sensor with a cable. The phosphor-coated plates are flexible and fit into the mouth similar to the way an intraoral film does. The imaging plate stores the data until a high-speed laser scanner converts the information into a digitized image and displays it on the monitor. This method is less efficient than the direct digital imaging method.[5,6]

IV. EVALUATION

A. Advantages of Digital Radiography

1. Reduced exposure to x-radiation
2. Filmless radiography
3. No darkroom or processing chemistry
4. Immediate feedback for diagnosis
5. Enhancement of diagnostic image
6. Effective patient education tool

B. Disadvantages of Digital Radiography

1. Initial setup costs
2. Sensor may be uncomfortable
3. Infection control of sensor: must be covered by plastic sleeves (Figure 9-5); cannot be heat sterilized.

■ CHARACTERISTICS OF AN ACCEPTABLE RADIOGRAPHIC IMAGE

A *radiographic image* is the visible image on a radiation-sensitive film or a digitized image created by the computer. The image is produced after exposure to ionizing radiation that has passed through an area, or specifically for dentistry, through teeth or a part of the oral cavity. A *radiographic survey* refers to a series of radiographic images.

Before making a radiographic image, it is important to know the characteristics that are expected to result in a radiograph of maximum diagnostic value. The basic essentials are the appearance of the image itself, the area covered, and the quality of the processed radiograph. Table 9-2 provides a list of characteristics of an acceptable radiograph.

■ TABLE 9-2 CHARACTERISTICS OF AN ACCEPTABLE RADIOGRAPH

CHARACTERISTIC	APPEARANCE
Image	All parts of teeth of interest must be shown close to natural size, with minimal overlap and minimal distortion
Area covered	Sufficient tissue surrounding tooth for diagnostic purposes
Density	Proper density for diagnosis
Contrast	Proper contrast for diagnosis
Definition and sharpness	Clear outline of objects; minimal penumbra

I. RADIOLUCENCY AND RADIOPACITY

A radiographic image has gradations from white to black that are referred to as radiopaque or radiolucent. For example, a dense material, such as a metallic restoration, prevents the passage of x-rays and appears white on the processed radiograph. Soft tissue does not resist passage of x-rays and, thus, appears black to gray.

II. RADIOPACITY

The appearance of light (white) images on a radiograph is a result of the lesser amount of radiation that penetrates the structures and reaches the film. A radiopaque structure inhibits the passage of x-rays. Examples include:

- Enamel
- Dentin
- Metallic restorations
- Implants

III. RADIOLUCENCY

The appearance of dark images on a radiograph is a result of the greater amount of radiation that penetrates the structures and reaches the film. A *radiolucent* structure permits the passage of radiation with relatively little attenuation by absorption. Examples include:

- Pulp
- Cysts
- Dental caries
- Periodontal ligament

■ FACTORS THAT INFLUENCE THE FINISHED RADIOGRAPH

As the beam leaves the x-ray tube (Figure 9-1) it is collimated, filtered, and allowed to travel a designated source–film (or focal spot–film) distance before reaching the film of a selected speed. The quality or diagnostic usefulness of the finished radiograph, as well as the total exposure of the patient and clinician, are influenced by the *kilovoltage, milliampere seconds, time, collimation, filtration, target–film distance, object-film distance,* and *film speed,* as outlined in Box 9-5.

Film processing (pages 167 to 169) also directly influences the quality of the radiograph and indirectly the total exposure. Reexposure would be necessary should the film be rendered inadequate during processing.

I. COLLIMATION

Collimation is the technique for controlling the size and shape of the beam of radiation emitted. A *collimator* is a diaphragm or system of diaphragms made of an absorbing material designed to define the dimensions and direction of a beam of radiation.

A. Purposes

1. Eliminate peripheral or more divergent radiation.
2. Minimize exposure to patient's face.
3. Minimize secondary radiation, which can fog the film and expose the bodies of patient and clinician.

B. Methods

1. *Lead diaphragm located between the x-ray tube and the position-indicating device (PID).* A diaphragm usually is made of lead with a central aperture of the smallest practical diameter for making radiographic exposure; it is located between the x-ray tube and the PID.
   a. Recommended thickness of lead: $^1/_8$ inch.
   b. Recommended size of aperture: to permit a diameter of the beam of radiation equal to 2.75 inches or 7 cm at the end of the PID next to the patient's face.
2. *Rectangular Collimation.* As shown in Figure 9-7, a patient receives far less unnecessary radiation with the use of a rectangular PID because the size of the beam is greatly reduced. When a rectangular collimator is used, it should be approximately $1^1/_2 \times 2$ inches at the skin. A rectangular collimator must be rotated to accommodate films positioned horizontally or vertically.
3. *Lead-Lined Cylindrical PID.* The PID must be an open-ended cylinder to reduce secondary radiation.

C. Relation to Techniques

The dimensions of the largest periapical film are $1^1/_4 \times 1^5/_8$ inches.[2] Precise angulation techniques are required to eliminate "cone-cut" of film, particularly when rectangular collimation is used. "Cone-cut" refers to an error of technique that results when the PID is not angled for the beam of radiation to cover completely the film being exposed.

II. FILTRATION

Filtration is the insertion of absorbers or filters for the preferential attenuation of radiation from a primary beam of x-radiation. Two different types of filters provide filtration in the dental x-ray machine.

A. Types of Filters

1. *Aluminum filters* remove low-energy x-ray photons from the x-ray beam.

BOX 9-5 Factors That Influence the Radiographic Image

Kilovoltage Peak
- Affects contrast and density
- Low kVp yields high (long scale) contrast
- High kVp yields low (short scale) contrast

Milliamperage
- Affects density
- High mA yields high density
- Low mA yields low density

Time
- Affects density
- Long time yields high density
- Short time yields low density

Collimation
- Shapes the beam
- Not to exceed 2.75 inches or 7 cm at the patient's skin

Lead diaphragm
- PID
- Rectangular
- Cylindrical

Filtration
Types
- Aluminum filters remove low-energy x-rays
- Rare earth filters remove low- and high-energy x-rays

Methods of Filtration
Inherent
- Glass window
- Insulating oil
- Tube head seal

Added
- Aluminum disks
- 1.5 mm for 50 to 70 kVp
- 2.5 for >70 kVp

Total filtration
- Combination of inherent and added

Target–film distance
- Longer PID increases resolution of image
- Longer PID decreases scatter of radiation

Object–film distance
- Increased object–film distance achieves parallelism
- Decreased object–film distance decreases penumbra

Film speed
- Faster-speed film decreases definition; image is more grainy

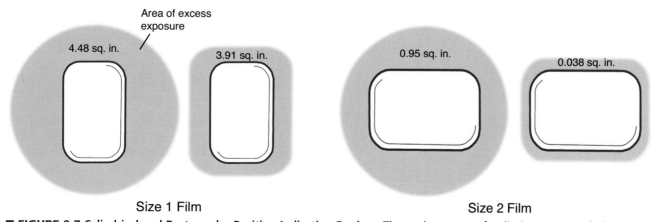

■ **FIGURE 9-7 Cylindrical and Rectangular Position-Indicating Devices.** The useless areas of radiation are greatly lessened when rectangular collimation is used. The patient can be spared exposure to excessive radiation. (Redrawn from Shannon, S.A.: Rectangular Versus Cylindrical Collimation, *Dent. Hyg., 61,* 173, April, 1987; copyright 1987 by the American Dental Hygienists' Association.)

2. *Rare earth filters* selectively remove both low- and high-energy photons from the x-ray beam. Examples of rare earth filters include samarium, erbium, yttrium, niobium, gadolinium, terbium-activated gadolinium oxysulfide, and thulium-activated lanthanum oxybromide.

B. Purpose

To minimize exposure of the patient's skin to unnecessary radiation.

C. Methods

1. *Inherent Filtration.* Includes the glass envelope encasing the x-ray tube and the glass window in the tube housing (Figure 9-1).
2. *Added Filtration.* Thin, pure, aluminum disks inserted between the lead diaphragm and the x-ray tube.
3. *Total Filtration.* The sum of inherent and added filtration.

The recommended total is the equivalent of 0.5 mm (below 50 kVp), 1.5 mm (50 to 70 kVp), and 2.5 mm (over 70 kVp) of aluminum.

III. KILOVOLTAGE

Kilovoltage is the potential difference of force that moves electrons between the negative anode and the positive cathode of an x-ray tube. When the kilovoltage is increased, the speed of electrons is increased and the resulting x-rays have a shorter wavelength and more penetrating power. The kilovoltage peak (kVp) refers to the crest value (in kilovolts) of the potential difference of a pulsating generator. When only one-half of the wave is used, the value refers to the useful half of the cycle.

A. How kVp Affects the Radiographic Image

1. Affects the **contrast**
   a. Low kilovoltage produces high contrast, with sharp black-white differences in densities between adjacent areas but a small range of distinction between subject thicknesses recorded.
   b. High kilovoltage produces low contrast, with a wide range of subject thicknesses recorded; greater range of densities from black to white (more gray tones), which provide more interpretive details.
2. Affects the **density**: increased kilovoltage results in increased density (other factors remaining constant).

3. To maintain the same film **density**: the milliampere seconds must be decreased as the kVp is increased.

B. Advantages of High kVp

1. Permits shorter exposure time.
2. Reduces exposure to tissues lying in front of the film packet.

C. Disadvantages of High kVp

1. Increased radiation to tissues outside the edges of the film.
2. More internal scattered radiation at 90 kVp than at 70 kVp.

IV. MILLIAMPERE SECONDS

A. Milliamperage

The measure of the electron current passing through the x-ray tube; it regulates the heat of the filament, which determines the number of electrons available to bombard the target. As the milliamperage is increased, the density of the image is increased.

B. Quantity of Radiation

Quantity of radiation is expressed in milliampere seconds (mAs).
1. Definition: mAs is the milliamperes multiplied by the exposure time in seconds; mAi is the milliamperes multiplied by the exposure time in impulses.
2. Example: At 10 milliamperes for ½ second, the exposure of the film would be 5 mAs. At 10 milliamperes for 15 impulses, the exposure of the film would be 150 mAi.

V. DISTANCE

Several distances are involved in x-ray film exposure. The object–film and the target–film distances must be considered for film placement.

A. Object–Film Distance

The object–film distance refers to the distance between the object (teeth of interest) and the film. With the paralleling technique and the use of a film holder, the object–film distance is greater than it is for the bisecting-angle technique. A collimated beam and increased source–film distance compensate to maximize definition and resolution.

B. Target–Film Distance

The PID on the x-ray machine is designed to indicate the direction of the x-ray beam and to serve as a guide in establishing desired target–surface and target–film distances. Techniques using 8-, 12-, and 16-inch target–film distances are common.

The *source* is the *tungsten target*. The target–film distance (sometimes called the source–film distance) is the sum total of the distance from the tungsten target to the film. The PID should lightly touch the face. Principles related to target–film distance are as follows:

1. The intensity of the x-ray beam varies inversely as the square of the target–film distance. For example, if two films of the same speed were used, one at a 16-inch target–film distance and one at an 8-inch distance, the film at 16 inches would require four times the exposure (time) to maintain the same density in the finished radiograph.
2. The exposure decreases as the distance increases; when the distance is doubled, the radiation exposure to the patient is reduced to one fourth.
3. To maintain film density when distance is increased, an increase in mAs, kVp, or time is required.

C. Advantages in the Use of a Long PID

1. Increased definition.
2. Decreased magnification.
3. Decreased skin exposure owing to decreased scatter.

VI. FILMS

With optimum filtration, collimation, and fast film, the skin dose to the face can be reduced significantly. In recent years, the manufacture of very-slow-speed films has been discontinued, the speed of films has been increased, and the use of higher-speed films has gained increased acceptance by the dental profession.

A. Film Composition

A film is a thin, transparent sheet of cellulose acetate coated on both sides with an emulsion of gelatin and silver halide crystals.

1. *Film Base.* A flexible piece of polyester plastic that is used to provide support for the emulsion.
2. *Halide Crystals.* Silver bromide and silver iodide crystals are used in dental x-ray film. They are sensitive to radiation and light.
3. *Emulsion.* A coating of gelatinous and nongelatinous materials attached to both sides of the film base that keeps the silver halide crystals evenly dispersed in a suspension.
4. *Adhesive Layer.* A thin layer of adhesive material that covers both sides of the film base and keeps the emulsion on the film base.

B. Film Packet

Sealed paper envelope that is small, light-proof, and moisture resistant, containing an x-ray film (or two) and a thin sheet of lead foil.

- Two-film packet: Useful for processing one film differently from the other to make diagnostic comparisons; for sending to specialist to whom patient may be referred; for legal evidence.
- Purposes of lead foil backing: To prevent exposure of the film by scattered radiation that could enter from back of packet and to protect the patient's tissues lying in the path of the x-ray.

C. Film Speed

Film speed or film emulsion speed refers to the sensitivity of the film to radiation exposure. The speed is the amount of exposure required to produce a certain image density. The smaller the grain size, the slower the film speed. The slower the film speed, the less grainy the resulting image.

1. *Classification.* Films have been classified by the American National Standards Institute (ANSI) in cooperation with the American Dental Association (ADA). The ANSI/ADA Specification No. 22 designates six groups, A through F. Speed groups A, B, and C, the slowest, are associated with excess radiation exposure and are no longer used.
2. *Choice.* F-speed film is recommended for use with rectangular collimation for marked reduction in radiation exposure.

■ EXPOSURE TO RADIATION

I. IONIZING RADIATION

Ionizing radiation is electromagnetic radiation (for example, x-rays or gamma rays) or particulate radiation (for example, electrons, neutrons, protons) capable of ionizing air directly or indirectly.

The phenomenon of separation of electrons from molecules to change their chemical activity is called ionization. The organic and inorganic compounds that make up the human body may be altered by exposure to ionizing radiation. The biologic effects following irradiation are secondary effects in that they result from physical, chemical, and biologic action set in motion by the absorption of energy from radiation.

Factors that would influence the biologic effects of radiation are outlined in Box 9-6. Radiation to *somatic* tissues will affect the irradiated individual only, whereas radiation to *genetic* tissues will affect offspring and possibly future generations.

BOX 9-6 Factors That Influence the Biologic Effects of Radiation

- Quality of the radiation
- Chemical composition of the absorbing medium
- Sensitivity of tissues
- Total dose and dose rate
- Blood supply to the tissues
- Size of the area exposed
- Somatic vs. genetic cells

II. EXPOSURE

A. Types of Exposure

Exposure is a measure of the x-radiation to which a person or object, or a part of either, is exposed at a certain place; this measure is based on its ability to produce ionization.

1. *Threshold Exposure.* The minimum exposure that produces a detectable degree of any given effect.
2. *Entrance or Surface Exposure.* Exposure measured at the surface of an irradiated body, part, or object. It includes primary radiation and backscatter from the irradiated underlying tissue. The term *skin exposure* is used with reference to the exposure measured at the center of an irradiated skin surface area.
3. *Erythema Exposure.* The radiation necessary to produce a temporary redness of the skin.

B. Exposure Units

The units of absorbed dose are expressed in joules/kilogram (1 rad = 0.01 J/kg). The units shown in Table 9-3 are the recommendations of the International Commission on Radiation Units and Measurements.[7]

The unit of measurement is the *gray* (Gy). An absorbed dose of 1 Gy is equal to 1 J/kg; therefore, an absorbed dose of 1 Gy is equal to 100 rad.

The unit of biologic equivalence is the *sievert* (Sv). 1 Sv = 100 rem.

C. Dose

The radiation dose is the amount of energy absorbed per unit mass of tissue at a site of interest. The kinds of doses are defined in Box 9-7.

D. Permissible Dose

The amount of radiation that may be received by an individual within a specified period without expectation of any significantly harmful result is called the *permissible dose.*

Assumptions on which permissible doses are calculated include the following:

1. No irradiation is beneficial.
2. There is a dose below which no somatic cellular changes can be produced.
3. Children are more susceptible than older people.
4. There is a dose below which, even though it is delivered before the end of the reproductive period, the probability of genetic effects is slight.

E. Radiation Hazard

A condition under which persons might receive radiation in excess of the maximum permissible dose. Exposure would be a risk in an area where x-ray equipment is being used or where radioactive materials are stored.

F. National Council on Radiation Protection and Measurements

1. *Limits for Dentists and Dental Personnel.* See Table 9-4.
2. *Limits for Patients.* Exposure to x radiation shall be kept to the minimum level consistent with clinical requirements.[8] This limitation is determined by the professional judgment of the dentist.

▪ TABLE 9-3 RADIATION UNITS

DEFINITION	TRADITIONAL UNIT	S.I. UNIT*	EQUIVALENT
Unit of radiation exposure	Roentgen (R)	Coulomb per kilogram (C/kg)	1 R = 2.58×10^{-4} C/kg
Unit of absorbed dose	Rad	Gray (Gy)	100 rad = 1 Gy
Unit of dose equivalent	Rem	Sievert (Sv)	100 rem = 1 Sv
Unit of radioactivity	Curie (Ci)	Becquerel (Bq)	1 Ci = 3.7×10^{10} Bq

*S.I. (System International) is from the French *Système International d'Unités.*

BOX 9-7 KEY WORDS AND ABBREVIATIONS: Types of Radiation Doses

Absorbed dose: the amount of energy imparted by ionizing radiation to a unit mass of irradiated material at a specific exposure point; the unit of absorbed dose is the gray (Gy).

Cumulative dose: the total dose resulting from repeated exposures to radiation of the same region or of the whole body.

Dose: the amount of energy absorbed per unit mass of tissue at a site of interest.

Dose equivalent: the product of absorbed dose and modifying factors, such as the quality factor, distribution factor, and any other necessary factors; different types of radiation cause differing biologic effects; the unit of dose equivalence is the sievert (Sv).

Dose rate: rate of exposure.

Erythema dose: the minimum quantity of x or gamma radiation that produces the appearance of redness (erythema).

Exit dose: the absorbed dose delivered by a beam of radiation to the surface through which the beam emerges from an object.

LD 50–30: the dose of radiation that is lethal for 50% of a large population in a specified period of time, usually 30 days.

Lethal dose: the amount of radiation that is, or could be, sufficient to cause the death of an organism.

Maximum permissible dose: the maximum dose equivalent that a person (or specified parts of that person) is allowed to receive in a stated period of time; the dose of radiation that would not be expected to produce any significant radiation effects in a lifetime.

Skin dose (surface absorbed dose): the absorbed dose delivered by a radiation beam and backscatter at the point where the central ray passes through the superficial layer of the object.

Threshold dose: the minimum dose that produces a detectable degree of any effect.

---

3. *ALARA Concept.* Radiation exposures must be kept As Low As Reasonably Achievable. This concept is accepted and enforced by all regulatory agencies.

III. SENSITIVITY OF CELLS

A. Factors Affecting Cell Sensitivity to Radiation

1. *Cell Differentiation.* Immature cells are most sensitive. Highly specialized cells are radioresistant.

2. *Mitotic Activity.* Rapidly reproducing cells are more sensitive; most sensitive when undergoing mitosis.
3. *Cell Metabolism.* Cells are more sensitive in periods of increased metabolism.

B. Radiosensitive and Radioresistant Tissues

1. Radiosensitive: a cell that is sensitive to radiation.
2. Radioresistant: a cell that is resistant to radiation.

■ TABLE 9-4 MAXIMUM PERMISSIBLE DOSE EQUIVALENT VALUES (MPD)* TO WHOLE BODY, GONADS, BLOOD-FORMING ORGANS, LENS OF EYE

AVERAGE WEEKLY EXPOSURE†	MAXIMUM 13-WEEK EXPOSURE	MAXIMUM YEARLY EXPOSURE	MAXIMUM ACCUMULATED EXPOSURE‡
0.1 R	3 R	5 R	5(N−18) R§
0.001 Sv	0.03 Sv	0.05 Sv	0.05(N−18) Sv

*Exposure of persons for dental or medical purposes is not counted against their maximum permissible exposure limits.

†Used only for the purpose of designating radiation barriers.

‡When the previous occupational history of an individual is not definitely known, it shall be assumed that the full dose permitted by the formula 5(N−18) has already been received.

§N = Age in years and is greater than 18. The unit for exposure is the roentgen (R) or sievert (Sv).

BOX 9-8 Radiation Sensitivity of Tissues and Organs

High

Bone marrow

Reproductive cells

Intestines

Lymphoid tissue

Moderately High

Oral mucosa

Skin

Moderate

Growing bone

Growing cartilage

Small vasculature

Connective tissue

Moderately Low

Salivary glands

Mature bone

Mature cartilage

Thyroid gland tissue

Low

Liver

Optic lens

Kidneys

Muscle

Nerve

3. Radiation sensitivity of tissues and organs: the relative sensitivities are shown in Box 9-8.

C. Tissue Reaction

1. *Latent Period.* Lapse between the time of exposure and the time when effects are observed. (May be as long as 25 years or relatively short, as in the case of the production of a skin erythema.)
2. *Cumulative Effect*
   a. Amount of reaction depends on dose; the reaction to radiation received in fractional doses is less than the reaction to one large dose.
   b. Partial or total repair occurs as long as destruction is not complete.
   c. Some irreparable damage may be cumulative as, little by little, more radiation is added (for example, hair loss, skin lesions, falling blood cell count).

▪ RISK OF INJURY FROM RADIATION

The risk of injury from dental diagnostic radiation is extremely low; however, the more radiation received, the higher the chance of cellular injuries. With each exposure to radiation, cellular damage is followed by repair. The effects of radiation exposure are cumulative, and any cellular changes that are not repaired result in damaged tissues. Most of the damage caused by dental diagnostic low-level radiation is repaired within the body cells.

▪ RULES FOR RADIATION PROTECTION

Dental X-Ray Protection, prepared by the National Council on Radiation Protection and Measurements,[8] provides specific information about radiation barriers, film speed group rating, film badge service sources, x-ray equipment data, and operating procedure regulations.

To protect the clinician and the patient from excessive radiation, attention should be paid to unnecessary radiation that may result from retakes due to inadequate clinical procedures. Perfecting techniques contributes to the accomplishment of minimum exposure for maximum safety.

▪ PROTECTION OF CLINICIAN

I. PROTECTION FROM PRIMARY RADIATION

A. Stand behind a protective barrier.
B. Avoid the useful beam of radiation.
C. Never hand-hold the film during exposure.

II. PROTECTION FROM LEAKAGE RADIATION

A. Do not hand-hold the tube housing or the PID of the machine during exposures.
B. Test machine for leakage radiation.
C. Wear monitoring device for testing exposure.

III. PROTECTION FROM SECONDARY RADIATION

The major sources of secondary radiation are the filter and the irradiated soft tissues of the patient. Other sources may be the leakage from the tube housing or scatter from furniture and walls contacted by the primary beam. Methods of protection are related to these sources.

A. Minimization of Total X-Radiation

1. Use high-speed films.
2. Have x-ray machines tested frequently for x-ray output and leakage.
3. Replace older x-ray machines with modern equipment.

B. Collimation of Useful Beam

Use diaphragms and long PIDs to collimate the useful beam to an area no larger than 2.75 inches or 7 cm in diameter at the patient's skin. Rectangular collimation has been shown to be more effective than round collimation (Figure 9-7).

C. Type of PID

Use a shielded cylinder that is rectangular, long, and open ended, or use some other form of rectangular collimation.

D. Position of Clinician While Making Exposures

The clinician shall stand behind the patient's head behind the major sources of secondary radiation to prevent direct exposure.
1. *Exposure of the Region of the Central Incisors.* Stand at a 45° angle to the path of the central ray. This position is approximately behind either the left or the right ear of the patient (Figure 9-8).
2. *Exposure of Other Regions.* Stand behind the patient's head and at an angle of 45° to the path of the central ray of the x-ray beam.

E. Distance

1. Safety increases with distance.
2. The correct position for the clinician is behind an appropriate radiation-resistant barrier wall, preferably with a leaded window to permit a view of the patient during exposures.
3. When protective barrier shielding is not available, the clinician shall stand as far as practical from the patient, at least 6 feet (2 meters)[9] in the zone between 90° and 135° to the primary central ray, as shown in Figure 9-8.

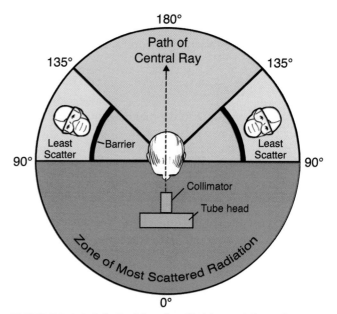

■ **FIGURE 9-8 Safe Position for Clinician.** While making an exposure, the clinician must stand behind the patient's head, between 90° and 135° from the primary beam.

IV. MONITORING

The amount of x-radiation that reaches the dental personnel can be measured economically with a film badge. Badges can be obtained from one of several laboratories. The film badge is:
- Worn at waist level for 1, 2, or 4 weeks.
- Returned on a routine basis to the laboratory by mail and processed; its exposure is evaluated.
- What is used to measure the exposure of the wearer. The wearer is notified by mail of the amount of exposure.
- Not to be shared with other clinicians.

■ PROTECTION OF PATIENT

I. FILMS

Use high-speed films. Use the largest intraoral film that can be placed skillfully in the mouth. Maximum coverage is provided in this manner with one exposure, whereas two exposures may be required if smaller films are used to examine the same area of the mouth. This factor is especially important when examining the mouths of children.

II. COLLIMATION

Use diaphragms and an open-ended, shielded (lead-lined), rectangular cylinder to collimate the useful beam.

III. FILTRATION

Use filtration of the useful beam to recommended levels (pages 146 and 148).

IV. PROCESSING

Process films according to the manufacturer's directions. When a choice of two periods of development is offered, the exposure of the patient can be reduced if the longer development time is employed.

V. TOTAL EXPOSURE

Do not expose the patient unnecessarily. There must be a good and valid reason for each exposure.

VI. PATIENT BODY SHIELDS

The use of leaded body shields for each patient is required by law in many states and countries. The purpose of the shield is to absorb scattered rays. Shields must contain a minimum of 0.25 mm of lead thickness.

A. Leaded Apron

1. *Types*
   a. General body coverage with extensions over the shoulders and down over the gonadal area.
   b. Body coverage, with cervical thyroid collar attached.
   c. Body coverage, with added coverage for the patient's upper back for wear during panoramic radiography.
2. *Care*
   a. Prevent cracks by hanging (Figure 9-9).
   b. Disinfect the apron before and after each use.

B. Thyroid Cervical Collar

Thyroid cancer can result from long-term exposure of the gland to x-rays.[10,11] The gland should be covered during exposure to x-rays. Figure 9-10 shows the position of a thyroid collar over the neckline of a body apron.

▪ CLINICAL APPLICATIONS

I. ASSESSMENT FOR NEED OF RADIOGRAPHS

A. Review health history.
B. Prepare or review radiation exposure history.
   1. Medical diagnostic or therapeutic radiation.
   2. Dates of dental surveys and availability of previous radiographs.
C. Review clinical examination.

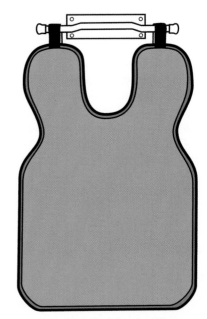

▪ **FIGURE 9-9 Care of Leaded Apron.** The apron can be kept on hooks or a hanging device near the x-ray machine to prevent cracks and prolong the usefulness of the apron.

D. Obtain dentist's prescription for number and type of radiographs. Refer to the *Guidelines for Prescribing Dental Radiographs* in Table 9-5.[2]

II. PREPARATION OF CLINIC FACILITY: INFECTION CONTROL ROUTINE (PAGES 76 TO 78)

A. Standard precautions should be followed for all radiographic equipment and materials.
B. Use barrier single-use plastic covers for all surfaces to be contacted, including x-ray machine controls.
C. Use disposable materials wherever possible.
D. Wear gloves or overgloves for handling of all radiographic materials.

III. PREPARATION OF CLINICIAN

A. Use full barrier protection that includes a mask, protective eyewear, and gloves.
B. Apply standard precautions throughout the radiographic procedure.

IV. PREPARATION OF PATIENT

A. Provide cup for holding removable dental prostheses.
B. For panoramic radiographs, request patient to remove all jewelry and other oral body piercing jewelry.
C. Provide antiseptic mouthrinse to lower bacterial contamination of radiographs and aerosols.

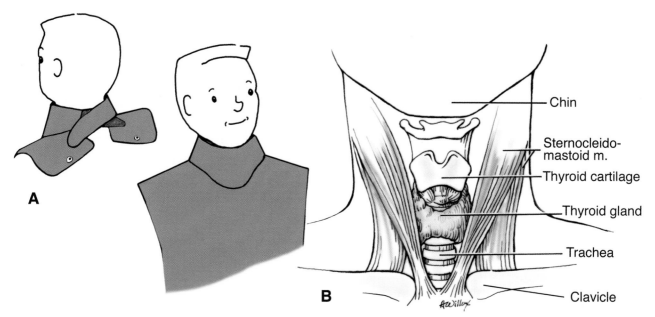

■ **FIGURE 9-10 Thyroid Cervical Collar. (A)** Thyroid collar in position, covering the neck and overlapping the leaded apron used for general body coverage. Velcro tabs facilitate overlap fastening at back of neck. Collars are available in child and adult sizes. **(B)** The thyroid gland is located over the trachea approximately halfway between the chin and the clavicles. Drawing shows anatomic relationship to the sternocleidomastoid muscle.

V. INTRAORAL EXAMINATION

A. Purpose

To determine necessary adaptations during film placement.

B. Factors of Particular Interest

1. Accessibility, determined by height and shape of palate, flexibility of muscles of orifice, floor of the mouth, possible gag reflex, and size of tongue.
2. Position of teeth and edentulous areas.
3. Apparent size of teeth.
4. Unusual features, such as tori, sensitive areas of the mucous membranes.

VI. PATIENT COOPERATION: PREVENTION OF GAGGING

Gagging may be the result of psychological or physiologic factors. It may present some problem in the placement of all films for molar radiographs and may be initiated in the patient who ordinarily does not gag when techniques are carried out efficiently.

A. Causes of Gagging

1. *Hypersensitive Oral Tissues.* Particularly common in posterior region of oral cavity.
2. *Anxiety and Apprehension*
    a. Fear of unknown, of the film touching a sensitive area.
    b. Previous unpleasant experiences with radiographic techniques.
    c. Failure to comprehend the clinician's instructions.
    d. Lack of confidence in the clinician.
3. *Techniques.* Film moved over the oral tissues or retained in the mouth longer than necessary.

B. Preventive Procedures

1. Inspire confidence in ability to perform the service.
2. Alleviate anxiety; explain procedures carefully. Smile and be cheerful.
3. Minimize tissue irritation.
    a. Request patient to swallow before film placement.
    b. Expose anterior films before posterior as placement is easier to tolerate.
    c. Place film firmly and positively without sliding the film over the tissue, especially the palate.
    d. Rub a finger over the tissues where the film placement is intended to desensitize the tissues.
    e. Instruct patient to breathe through nose with quick breaths; hold the breath during exposure.
    f. Use stick-on film cushions to make film placement more comfortable.
4. Use a premedicating agent prescribed by the dentist.
5. Use a topical anesthetic (page 605).

■ TABLE 9-5 GUIDELINES FOR PRESCRIBING DENTAL RADIOGRAPHS

The recommendations in this chart are subject to clinical judgment and may not apply to every patient. They are to be used by the dentist only after reviewing the patient's health history and completing a clinical examination. The recommendations do not need to be altered because of pregnancy.

Patient Category	Child Primary Dentition (before eruption of first permanent tooth)	Child Transitional Dentition (following eruption of first permanent tooth)	Adolescent Permanent Dentition (before eruption of third molars)	Adult Dentulous	Adult Edentulous
New Patient* All new patients to assess dental diseases and growth and development	Posterior bitewing examination if proximal surfaces of primary teeth cannot be visualized or probed	Individualized radiographic examination consisting of periapical/occlusal views and posterior bitewings or panoramic examination and posterior bitewings	Individualized radiographic consisting of posterior bitewings and selected periapicals. A full-mouth intraoral radiographic examination is appropriate when the patient presents with clinical evidence of generalized dental disease or a history of extensive dental treatment		Full-mouth intraoral radiographic examination or panoramic examination
Recall Patient* Clinical caries or high-risk factors for caries†	Posterior bitewing examination at 6-month intervals or until no carious lesions are evident		Posterior bitewing examination at 6- to 12-month intervals or until no carious lesions are evident	Posterior bitewing examination at 12- to 18-month intervals	Not applicable
No clinical caries and no high-risk factors for caries†	Posterior bitewing examination at 12- to 24-month intervals if proximal surfaces of primary teeth cannot be visualized or probed	Posterior bitewing examination at 12- to 24-month intervals	Posterior bitewing examination at 18- to 36-month intervals	Posterior bitewing examination at 24- to 36-month intervals	Not applicable
Periodontal disease or a history of periodontal treatment	Individualized radiographic examination consisting of selected periapical and/or bitewing radiographs for areas where periodontal disease (other than nonspecific gingivitis) can be demonstrated clinically		Individualized radiographic examination consisting of selected periapical and/or bitewing radiographs for areas where periodontal disease (other than nonspecific gingivitis) can be demonstrated clinically		Not applicable
Growth and development assessment	Usually not indicated	Individualized radiographic examination consisting of a periapical/occlusal or panoramic examination	Periapical or panoramic examination to assess developing third molars	Usually not indicated	Usually not indicated

*Clinical situations for which radiographs may be indicated include:

A. Positive historical findings
1. Previous periodontal or endodontic therapy
2. History of pain or trauma
3. Familial history of dental anomalies
4. Postoperative evaluation of healing
5. Presence of implants

B. Positive clinical signs/symptoms
1. Clinical evidence of periodontal disease
2. Large or deep restorations
3. Deep carious lesions
4. Malposed or clinically impacted teeth
5. Swelling

6. Evidence of facial trauma
7. Mobility of teeth
8. Fistula or sinus tract infection
9. Clinically suspected sinus pathology
10. Growth abnormalities
11. Oral involvement in known or suspected systemic disease
12. Positive neurologic findings in the head and neck
13. Evidence of foreign objects
14. Pain and/or dysfunction of the temporo-mandibular joint

15. Facial asymmetry
16. Abutment teeth or fixed or removable partial prosthesis
17. Unexplained bleeding
18. Unexplained sensitivity of teeth
19. Unusual eruption, spacing, or migration of teeth
20. Unusual tooth morphology, calcification, or color
21. Missing teeth with unknown reason

†Patients at high risk for caries may demonstrate any of the following:

1. High level of caries experience
2. History of recurrent caries
3. Existing restoration of poor quality
4. Poor oral hygiene
5. Inadequate fluoride exposure

6. Prolonged nursing (bottle or breast)
7. Diet with high sucrose frequency
8. Poor family dental health
9. Developmental enamel defects
10. Developmental disability

11. Xerostomia
12. Genetic abnormality of teeth
13. Many multisurface restorations
14. Chemo/radiation therapy

NOTE: **United States Food and Drug Administration,** Center for Devices and Radiological Health: *Selection of Patients for X-ray Examinations: Dental Radiographic Examinations.* Washington, D.C., Government Printing Office, No. 017-015-00236-5.

■ **TABLE 9-6 PRINCIPLES OF SHADOW CASTING**

1. Place the film as parallel as possible to the object.
2. Use as small an effective focal spot as practical.
3. Use as long a target–object distance as possible.
4. Use as short an object–film distance as possible.
5. Aim the x-ray beam perpendicular to the film.

■ PROCEDURES FOR FILM PLACEMENT AND ANGULATION OF RAY

The image projected onto the radiograph is a shadow of the teeth and the surrounding structures. The dental radiographer should follow as closely as possible the five principles of shadow casting, listed in Table 9-6, when exposing radiographs.

Basic intraoral procedures for periapical, bitewing, and occlusal radiographs are included in this chapter. The principles and uses of panoramic radiographs are also described.

Two fundamental periapical procedures are used in practice: the *paralleling* or right-angle and the *bisecting angle*. The principles for film/sensor placement are shown in Figure 9-11.

Clinicians vary in their application of the principles of the two techniques. Basic to both the paralleling technique and the bisecting-angle technique are:

- The primary beam should pass through the teeth of interest.
- The film/sensor should be placed in relation to the teeth so that all parts of the image are shown as close to their natural size and shape as possible.
- Dimensional distortion must be minimized.

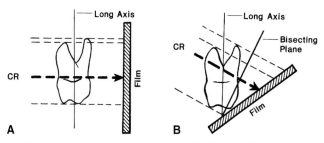

■ **FIGURE 9-11 Comparison of Paralleling and Bisecting-Angle Techniques. (A)** Paralleling technique. The film is parallel with the long axis of the tooth and the central ray (CR) is directed perpendicularly both to the film and to the long axis of the tooth. **(B)** Bisecting-angle technique. The central ray (CR) is directed perpendicularly to an imaginary line that bisects the angle formed by the film and the long axis of the tooth.

The development of a systematic, comfortable, smooth procedure saves time and energy for both patient and clinician. It increases the confidence of the patient, allows for consistency in technique, and leads to the production of good-quality radiographs. A basic objective during radiographic technique is to minimize the length of time the packet or sensor remains in the patient's mouth.

■ FILM SELECTION FOR INTRAORAL SURVEYS

I. PERIAPICAL SURVEYS

A. Area Covered

To obtain a view of the entire tooth and its periodontal supporting structures.

B. Film Sizes

1. *Child Size.*No. 0 (22 × 35 mm) for primary teeth and small mouths.
2. *Anterior.*No. 1 (24 × 40 mm) for anterior regions where width of arch makes positioning of standard film difficult or impossible.
3. *Standard.*No. 2 (31 × 41 mm) may be used for all positions.

C. Sensor Sizes

1. No. 0 for primary teeth and small mouths.
2. No. 1 for anterior teeth where the width of the arch makes positioning of the size 2 sensor difficult or impossible.
3. No. 2 may be used for all positions.

D. Number of Films or Sensors Used in a Complete Survey

14 to 16 projections plus bitewings depending on the clinician's preferences, the anatomy of the patient's mouth, and the size of the films used.

II. BITEWING (INTERPROXIMAL) SURVEYS

A. Area Covered

1. *Horizontal Bitewing Radiographic Images.* To show:
   - the crowns of the teeth and the alveolar crest in a dentition with normal to slight bone loss
   - proximal carious lesions
   - overhanging restorations
2. *Vertical Bitewing Radiographic Images.* To show:
   - the crowns of the teeth and the alveolar bone level with moderate to severe bone loss

▪ TABLE 9-7 BITEWING FILM SURVEYS

PATIENT	FILM PLACEMENT	FILM SIZE	NUMBER OF FILMS	REGION
Adult Posterior survey	Horizontal for dental caries Vertical for periodontal bone loss	2	4	Premolars and molars
Adult Anterior survey	Vertical	1 or 2	3	Centrals, laterals, canines
Child Survey: permanent dentition	Horizontal	2	2	Premolars and molars
Child Survey: mixed dentition	Horizontal	1 or 2	2	Premolars and/or primary molars and permanent molars
Child Survey: all primary teeth	Horizontal	0	2	Primary molars

Film size is determined by size of dental arch and patient tolerance. Use largest film the patient will tolerate.

- proximal root caries
- overhanging restorations

B. Films

Refer to Table 9-7 for film/sensor size and number guidelines.

The number and size of films/sensors used for bitewing surveys are determined by:
- the size of the dental arch
- the number of teeth present
- patient tolerance

III. OCCLUSAL SURVEYS

A. Purpose

To show large areas of the maxilla, mandible, or floor of the mouth.

B. Film

No. 4 (57 × 76 mm) for use in self packet or in intra-oral cassette.

C. Standard Film

No. 2 (31 × 41 mm) for child or individual areas of adult.

▪ DEFINITIONS AND PRINCIPLES

I. PLANES

A. Sagittal or Median

The plane that divides the body in the midline into right and left sides.

B. Occlusal

The mean occlusal plane represents the mean curvature from the incisal edges of the central incisors to the tips of the occluding surfaces of the third molars. The occlusal plane of the premolars and first molar may be considered as the mean occlusal plane.

II. ANGULATION

A. Horizontal

The angle at which the central ray of the useful beam is directed within a horizontal plane. Incorrect horizontal angulation results in *overlapping* or *superimposition* of parts of adjacent teeth in the radiograph.

B. Vertical

The plane at which the central ray of the useful beam is directed within a vertical plane. Variations:
- Elongation: inadequate vertical angulation
- Foreshortening: excessive vertical angulation

III. LONG AXIS OF A TOOTH

The long axis can be represented by an imaginary line passing longitudinally through the center of the tooth. Because of marked variations in tooth position and root curvature, estimation of the long axis of a tooth is difficult.

▪ PERIAPICAL SURVEY: PARALLELING TECHNIQUE

The paralleling technique is based on the principles that *the film/sensor is placed as parallel to the long axis of the tooth as the anatomy of the oral cavity permits, and the central ray is directed at right angles to the film or sensor.* In Figure 9-11A, the parallel relationship of the film or sensor with the long axis of the tooth and the right-angle direction of the central ray are shown.

- Maxillary Projections
  The film/sensor holder is placed toward the midline of the palate.
- Mandibular Projections
  The film/sensor is placed close to the teeth of interest as long as parallelism is maintained.

I. PATIENT POSITION

As long as the film/sensor is parallel to the long axis of the tooth and the central ray is directed at right angles to the film/sensor, the head may be in any position convenient to the clinician and comfortable for the patient. Slight modification of positioning may be needed for making radiographs in a supine position.

II. FILM/SENSOR PLACEMENT

A. Film/Sensor Position and Angulation of the Central Ray

Instructions for film/sensor placement and angulation are included in this section.

1. *Basic Principles.* Principles for film/sensor placement and angulation of the central ray are shown in Figures 9-12 and 9-13. The image objective in the completed radiograph is also illustrated.
2. *Horizontal Angulation.* The central ray is directed at the center of the film/sensor and through the interproximal area.
3. *Vertical Angulation.* The central ray is directed at a right angle to the film/sensor.

B. Film and Sensor-Positioning Holders

The use of a film/sensor holder (film-positioning device) facilitates obtaining the correct angulation of the central ray. Lining up the PID with coordinating parts of the film/sensor holder sets the correct vertical and horizontal angulation so that the central ray is perpendicular to the film/sensor. An example of a disposable film-positioning device is shown in Figure 9-14.

1. *Purposes.* The use of a beam-guiding, field size-limiting, film/sensor-holding instrument provides:
   - dose reduction
   - improved image quality
   - diagnostic radiographs without frequent retakes
   - improved infection control

2. *Characteristics.* An effective film/sensor-positioning device has such characteristics as the following:
   - Simple and adaptable to all positions.
   - Aids in reducing radiation exposure to patient.
   - Aids in alignment of x-ray beam.
   - Comfortable for the patient.
   - Minimal complexity for learning.
   - Disposable or conveniently sterilized.
3. *Types of Film Holders* Several types of film holders are listed in Box 9-9. Examples of widely used types include the following:
   - Styrofoam disposable film holder
     A disposable bite block used with the paralleling or bisecting-angle techniques (Figure 9-14).
   - Precision film holder
     A stainless steel film holder that offers rectangular collimation for the paralleling technique.
   - Rinn X-C-P film and sensor holders
     A plastic and stainless steel film holder with aiming devices that is used with the paralleling technique.
   - Rinn B-A-I film and sensor holders
     A plastic and stainless steel film/sensor holder with an aiming device that is used with the bisecting-angle technique.

III. PARALLELING TECHNIQUE: FEATURES

A. Accuracy

The paralleling technique gives a more accurate size and shape of dental structures with less distortion than when the bisecting-angle technique is used.

1. In Figures 9-12 and 9-13, an accurate crown:root ratio is shown with facial and lingual aspects in proper relation to each other.
2. Zygomatic bone can be shown in its normal position above the root apices of the molars and premolars.

B. Horizontal Ray Direction

No rays are directed toward the thyroid, whereas with the bisecting-angle technique, several maxillary radiographs require a relatively steep vertical angulation.

■ BITEWING SURVEY

I. PREPARATION

A. Patient Position

1. *Traditional.* Sagittal plane perpendicular to the floor and occlusal plane parallel with the floor.
2. *Patient in Supine Position.* The planes are reversed in their relation to the floor.

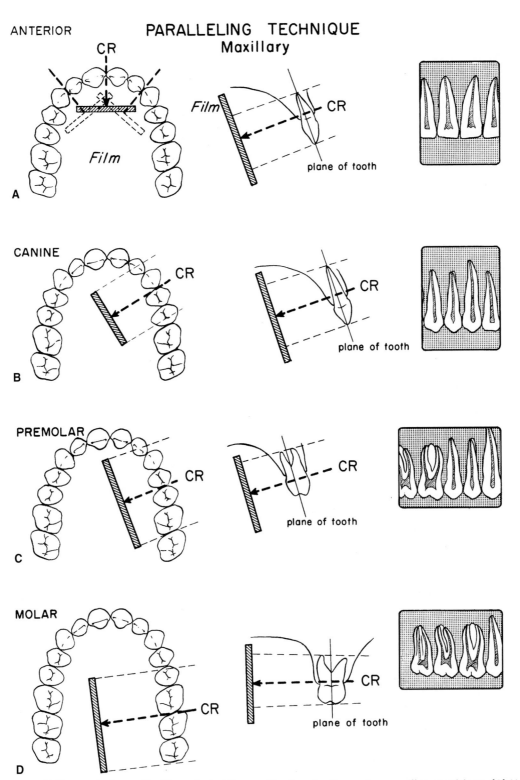

■ **FIGURE 9-12 Paralleling Technique, Maxillary Arch.** Film positioning for the major maxillary positions. **(A)** Horizontal angulation, with film placed parallel to the long axes of the teeth; central ray (CR) directed parallel with a line through the interproximal space. **(B)** Vertical angulation, with central ray (CR) directed at right angles to the film. **(C)** Image objective for the completed radiograph.

PARALLELING TECHNIQUE
Mandibular

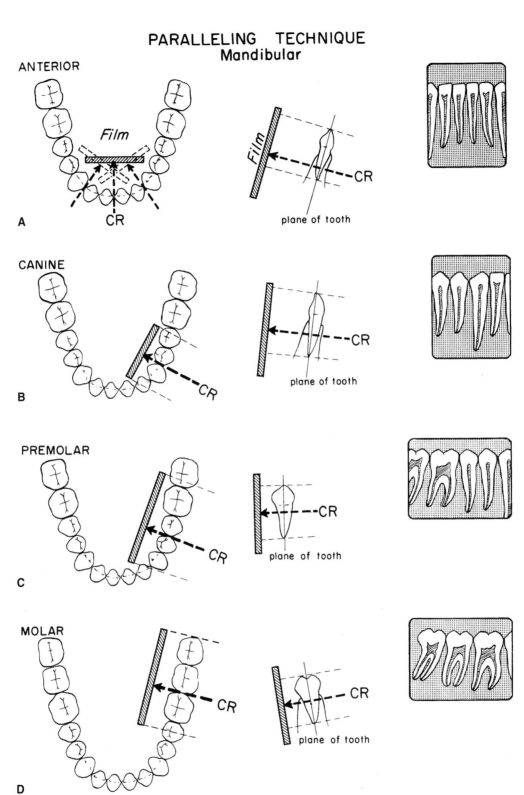

■ **FIGURE 9-13 Paralleling Technique, Mandibular Arch.** Film positioning for the major mandibular positions. **(A)** Horizontal angulation, with film placed parallel to the long axes of the teeth; central ray (CR) directed through the interproximal space. **(B)** Vertical angulation, with central ray (CR) directed at right angles to the film. **(C)** Image objective for the completed radiograph.

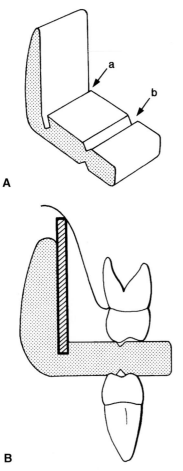

A

B

■ **FIGURE 9-14 Styrofoam Disposable Film Holder. (A)** Empty holder to show: **a,** slot for insertion of the film, and **b,** break-off point to shorten the bite surface for use in the mandibular posterior positions. **(B)** Film placement for maxillary molar radiograph for patient with a high palatal vault.

B. Vertical Angulation

Set at + 8° to + 10° for horizontal or vertical bitewings (Figure 9-15B).

C. Patient Instruction

Request patient to practice closing on posterior teeth prior to positioning film/sensor for posterior bitewing and to practice edge-to-edge closure for anterior bitewing (Figure 15-4).

II. FILM/SENSOR PLACEMENT: HORIZONTAL BITEWING SURVEY

Figure 9-15 shows in diagram form the position of the horizontal molar bitewing film/sensor in relation to the teeth, the horizontal and vertical angulation, and the

---

BOX 9-9 Film-Positioning Devices

Film Holders

Bite blocks, plastic or wooden

Stabe (Styrofoam disposable film holder)

Precision x-ray device

Snap-a-ray

X-C-P (Extension Cone Paralleling)

B-A-I (Bisecting-Angle Instrument)

V.I.P. (Versatile Intraoral Positioner)

Hemostat with rubber bite block

Supplements

Removable denture for stabilization of film holder

Cotton roll to achieve parallelism

---

image objective for both the premolar and the molar completed radiographs when standard film/sensor is used.

A. *Molar* (standard film/sensor in horizontal position). Center the film/sensor on the second molar with the mesial border of film/sensor placed to include the distal half of the mandibular second premolar. Distal surfaces of third molars can be examined clinically (see Figure 9-15A).

B. *Premolar* (standard film/sensor in horizontal position). Center the film/sensor over the second premolar with the mesial border of film/sensor at midline of the mandibular canine to include the distal surfaces of maxillary and mandibular canines and a clear view of both the first and second premolars.

III. FILM/SENSOR POSITION: VERTICAL BITEWING SURVEY

A. *Molar* (standard film/sensor in vertical position). Center of the film/sensor positioned over the middle of the second molar to include at least the distal portion of the first molar and the mesial portion of the third molar.

B. *Premolar* (standard film/sensor in vertical position). Position the mesial border of film/sensor at midline of the mandibular canine to include the distal portion of maxillary and mandibular canines and a clear view of the first and second premolars. Figure 9-16 shows in diagram form

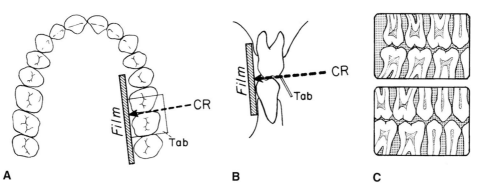

■ FIGURE 9-15 Horizontal Bitewing Radiograph. (A) Film position showing horizontal angulation for molar viewing, with central ray (CR) directed through the interproximal space to the center of the film. Film is centered over the second molar. **(B)** Vertical angulation set at +8° to +10°. **(C)** Image objective for molar (*above*) and premolar (*below*) regions.

the image objective for the vertical premolar bitewing, which includes the distal portion of the maxillary and mandibular canines, the first and second maxillary and mandibular premolars, and the mesial portion of the first maxillary and mandibular molars.

C. *Anterior.* Center of film/sensor at proximal space between the lateral and canine for the two canine/lateral bitewings; center of film/sensor at midline for central bitewing.

IV. HORIZONTAL ANGULATION (FOR HORIZONTAL AND VERTICAL BITEWINGS)

The horizontal angulation is adjusted to direct the central ray perpendicular to the center of the film/sensor. The central ray must pass through the interproximal space or parallel to a line through the interproximal spaces of the teeth of interest.

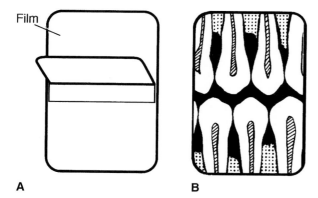

■ FIGURE 9-16 Vertical Bitewing Radiograph. (A) Vertical bitewing film with the tab positioned vertically over the center of the film. **(B)** Image objective of maxillary and mandibular premolar regions. Anterior edge of the film is placed behind the midline of the mandibular canine.

■ PERIAPICAL SURVEY: BISECTING-ANGLE TECHNIQUE

The bisecting-angle technique is based on the geometric principle that *the central ray is directed perpendicularly to an imaginary line that is the bisector of the angle formed by the long axis of the tooth and the plane of the film/sensor.* Figure 9-11B illustrates in diagram form the relationship of the long axis of the tooth, the film/sensor, and the bisector of the angle formed by these two.

■ OCCLUSAL SURVEY

The central midline films for maxillary and mandibular arches are described in this section. A variety of positions for the occlusal films is possible, depending on the area to be examined.

I. USES AND PURPOSES

A. To observe areas not shown on other image projections.

B. To position film when obtaining periapical image projections is impossible.

C. To supplement the angulation provided by other films for such conditions as fractures, impacted teeth, or salivary duct calculi.

II. MAXILLARY MIDLINE TOPOGRAPHIC PROJECTION

A. Position of Patient's Head

The line from the tragus of the ear to the ala of the nose is parallel with the floor.

B. Position of Film

- The stippled side of the film packet is toward the palate.
- Posterior border of film is brought back close to third molar region. Film is held between the teeth with edge-to-edge closure.

C. Angulation

The PID is directed toward the bridge of the nose at a +65° angle.

III. MANDIBULAR TOPOGRAPHIC PROJECTION

A. Position of Patient's Head

The head is tilted directly back.

B. Position of Film

The stippled side is toward the floor of the mouth, the posterior border of the film is in contact with the soft tissues of the retromolar area, and the film is held between the teeth in an edge-to-edge bite.

C. Angulation

- Incisal region: the PID is pointed at the tip of the chin at an angle of approximately −55°.
- Floor of the mouth: the PID is directed from under the chin, perpendicular to the film.

▪ PANORAMIC RADIOGRAPHIC IMAGES

Panoramic radiography, or pantomography, refers to methods that produce continuous radiographs showing the maxillary and mandibular arches with adjacent structures on a single radiograph.

The panoramic radiograph is an option to a periapical survey, but it is not a substitute because of the loss of sharpness and detail. The principal advantages of panoramic images are[12]:
- The broad coverage of facial bones and teeth.
- Low patient radiation dose.
- Convenience of the examination for the patient
- The short time required to make a panoramic image.

I. PANORAMIC RADIOGRAPHS AND TECHNIQUE

A panoramic radiograph is a radiographic projection that is positioned outside the mouth during x-ray exposure and is used to examine the maxillary and mandibular jaws in a single image receptor. The movement of the film and tube head produce an image through the process known as tomography. The prefix *tomo* means section; tomography is a radiographic technique that depicts one layer or section of the body in focus while surrounding structures in other planes are blurred. In a panoramic tomograph, the attempt is to radiograph the maxillary and mandibular dentitions in focus in one image receptor. The film/sensor and tube head rotate around the patient's head in opposite directions.

A. Patient Position

Patient positioning depends on the panoramic unit and the patient's height.
1. Seated or standing.
2. The head is stabilized with a chin support or one of several types of head holders characteristic of each machine.
3. Position the patient to ensure that the Frankfort plane (orbitale to tragus of the ear) is parallel to the floor.

B. Cassette

1. Curved or flat.
2. Rigid or flexible.
3. Must be marked for the left or right side of the patient.
4. Contains calcium tungstate or rare earth intensifying screens that provide for reduced radiation exposure to the patient.

II. USES

The numerous applications for panoramic radiographic images are outlined in Box 9-10. Routine use for patients seeking general oral care cannot be recommended as a substitute for a periapical survey as there is a loss of detail.

III. LIMITATIONS

- There is a loss of definition and detail compared with periapical radiographs.
- Distortion of structures and findings.
- Do not show proximal carious lesions except for large cavities, which can be seen by direct examination.
- Inadequate for examination of periodontal structures.

A. Inferiority of Definition and Detail

Causes of poor definition are:
1. Use of intensifying screens.

BOX 9-10 Uses for Panoramic Images

- Detection and diagnosis of oral pathologic lesions
- Evaluation of impacted teeth
- Examination of the extent of large lesions
- Survey for edentulous patients
- Detection of calcified carotid arteries: potential stroke victims
- Evaluation of growth and development for pedodontic patients
- Evaluation of teeth and jaw position for orthodontic patients
- Detection of fractured jaws and traumatic injuries
- When intraoral films are impossible

  Trismus

  Parkinson's disease

  Cerebral palsy

  Hyperactive gag reflex

2. Increased object–film/sensor distance.
3. Movement of x-ray tube and film/sensor.

B. Distortion

1. Magnified images are produced because of increased distance between the film/sensor and object.
2. Overlapping. In periapical techniques, each film/sensor is angulated with the central ray so that when a tooth is out of line, adjustment is made to prevent overlapping. With panoramic technique, the head and teeth remain fixed, and the ray and film/sensor are positioned for the average only.

IV. PROCEDURES

Learning to use panoramic equipment is not difficult. Each machine has its own characteristics that can be learned readily from the manufacturer's instructions.

A. Patient Preparation

A thyroid shield cannot be used because of superimposition on the image. A special shield for panoramic radiography is available with coverage over the shoulders and partway down the back.

B. Film/Sensor

Film and sensor sizes are usually either 5 × 12 or 6 × 12 inches. Fast-speed film should be used to minimize radiation.

C. Processing

Regular processing solutions are used for panoramic film. Special film holders for panoramic films are used during manual processing.

▪ PARACLINICAL PROCEDURES

Supplemental to the chairside clinical procedures are the processing of the films and the mounting of radiographs for diagnostic and clinical use. Standard procedures are outlined in the following sections.

▪ INFECTION CONTROL

I. PRACTICE POLICY

Personnel of each office or clinic must work out a specific protocol appropriate to their facility and the type of processing used. A written policy is necessary for infection control during film exposure, processing, and mounting and during management of the completed radiographs throughout clinical treatment appointments.[13,14]

II. BASIC PROCEDURES

Prevention of cross-infection during film exposure was addressed on page 154 with other clinical applications. Additional procedures must be followed to prevent cross-contamination during transport to the darkroom and during use of the processing equipment.[15,16]

A. Contamination of Films

Films become covered with contaminated saliva and should be confined to a disposable cup after exposure.

B. Gloves

Gloved hands fresh from contamination from the patient's mouth should not contact walls, doors, light switches, and other environmental surfaces when transporting a cup of contaminated exposed films to the darkroom.

C. During Processing

1. The darkroom work area is prepared by the disinfection of all touch surfaces, and the counter is covered with clean paper.

2. Research has shown that bacteria on radiographic film can survive the processing procedures. Processing procedures may reduce the bacterial counts, but the potential for cross-contamination still exists.[16,17]

D. Waste

Dispose of film wrappers, cups, and contaminated gloves with contaminated waste. Lead foil should be disposed of according to environmental waste guidelines.

III. NO-TOUCH METHOD

A. With gloved hands and under appropriate safelight, pull open packets by their tabs or from their barrier envelopes as shown in Figure 9-17.
B. Allow films to drop out into a cup or onto the clean barrier-covered surface.
C. Take care not to touch the film. Remove gloves, wash hands, and place films on hangers being careful to touch the films by the edges only.
D. Dispose of waste properly.
E. Alternative no-touch method.
   1. Wear overgloves over powder-free treatment gloves and remove them after dropping film into the cup.
   2. Films are then processed while wearing powder-free treatment gloves.

IV. DAYLIGHT LOADER METHOD

A. With powder-free regloved hands and exposed films in a paper cup, insert films in the daylight compartment.

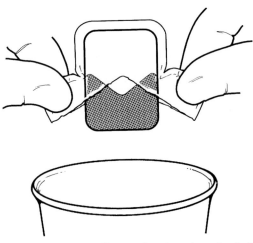

■ FIGURE 9-17 Plastic Film Barrier. Opening plastic film barrier using the no-touch method. Plastic film barriers placed over intraoral film are used to protect film from salivary contamination.

B. Remove films from packets with the no-touch method, dropping films into a clean cup.
C. Remove gloves. Process films with ungloved hands, being careful to touch film by the edges only.
D. Remove ungloved hands from daylight loader. Don new gloves.
E. Disinfect daylight loader.

■ FILM PROCESSING

Film processing is the chemical transformation of the latent image, produced in a film emulsion by exposure to radiation, into a stable image visible by transmitted light.

I. STANDARD PROCEDURES

Standardization of processing procedure goes hand in hand with standardized exposure techniques if consistently acceptable radiographs are to be prepared. Processing should be treated as an exacting chemical operation in which each step has specific objectives for the finished product.

II. FILM SENSITIVITY

Fast- and extra-fast-speed films are even more sensitive to variations in temperature, light, and processing chemicals than were the medium and slow films formerly in general use.

III. THE CHEMISTRY OF PROCESSING

A. Processing Chemicals

In Table 9-8, the developer and fixer ingredients are listed with the chemicals involved and their specific reactions.

B. Chemical Reactions

1. Development: selective reduction of affected silver halide salts to metallic silver grains.
2. Fixation: the selective removal of unaffected silver halide crystals.
3. Washing to remove the processing chemicals.

IV. HOW THE IMAGE IS PRODUCED

A. Film emulsion contains crystals of silver halides (bromide and iodide).
B. X-ray exposure changes the silver halides to silver and halide ions.
C. Developer reacts with the halide ions, leaving only the metallic silver in an arrangement

■ TABLE 9-8 PROCESSING CHEMICALS

DEVELOPER INGREDIENTS	CHEMICAL	ACTIVITY
Reducing agent	Hydroquinone Elon	Converts exposed silver halide crystals to black metallic silver Generates gray tones in the image
Accelerator	Sodium carbonate	Swells the emulsion and provides an alkaline medium
Restrainers	Potassium bromide	Blocks the action of the reducing agent on the unexposed crystals
Preservative	Sodium sulfite	Slows the oxidation and breakdown of the developer
Solvent	Water	Mixes the chemicals
FIXER INGREDIENTS		
Clearing agents	Ammonium thiosulfate or sodium thiosulfate	Removes all unexposed undeveloped silver halide crystals from emulsion
Acid or activator	Acetic acid Sulfuric acid	Stops development; neutralizes any remaining developer
Hardeners	Potassium alum	Toughens and shrinks the gelatin in the emulsion
Preservative	Sodium sulfite	Slows the oxidation of the fixer
Solvent	Water	Mixes the chemicals

corresponding with the radiolucency and radiopacity of the tissue being exposed.

D. Fixer removes only those crystals of silver halide that were not exposed to radiation.

E. End result is a *negative*, showing various degrees of lightness and darkness (microscopic grains of black metallic silver).

■ ESSENTIALS OF AN ADEQUATE DARKROOM

The work area must be free from chemicals, water, dust, and other substances that could contaminate the film either by splashing or by direct contact should a film touch the bench. The processing room should not be used as a storage room nor for other dental procedures in which dust or fumes may be produced.

■ LIGHTING

I. DARKROOM LIGHTING

A. Find and eliminate all possible light leaks.
B. Safelighting
   1. A 15-watt bulb or less is used.
   2. Placed a minimum of 4 feet above the working surface.
   3. A filter is selected for the light in accord with the type of film.
   4. GBX2 (red) filters are used for both intraoral and extraoral film.

II. SAFELIGHTING TEST

A. Unwrap film in the unlit darkroom.
B. Place film on work tabletop and place a coin on the film.
C. Turn on safelight and leave for 5 minutes.
D. Remove coin, process film.
E. Observe the radiograph; if any evidence exists of a light circle where the coin was placed, the darkroom safelight is excessive.

■ AUTOMATED PROCESSING

Automatic film processing refers to the use of equipment designed to transport film mechanically through a series of solutions under controlled conditions. Figure 9-18 illustrates the film being transported from the entry slot to the developer, the fixer, the water bath, the dryer, and the exit slot.

I. ADVANTAGES OF AUTOMATED PROCESSING

A. Consistency of results.
B. Conservation of time by dental personnel.
C. Finished radiographs in 4 to 6 minutes.
D. Radiographs available for immediate use.

II. PRINCIPLES OF OPERATION

Manufacturer's instructions must be followed and routine care and cleaning attended to for maintenance of equipment.

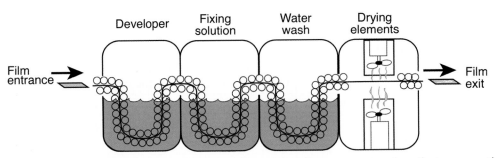

■ **FIGURE 9-18 Automatic Processor.** Diagram to show an automatic roller transport system that conveys the film over the rollers through the developer, fixer, water bath, and drying elements. (Adapted from Olson, S.S.: *Dental Radiography Laboratory Manual.* Philadelphia, W.B. Saunders, 1995, p. 86.)

A. Automated Film Transport

Rollers or tracks are used to carry the film through developing, fixing, washing, and drying. Some machines may process only standard intraoral films, whereas others may also accommodate extraoral sizes.

B. High Temperature

Increased temperature decreases processing time.

C. Care of Automatic Processor

The automatic processor requires meticulous routine maintenance. Manufacturer's instructions for each unit should be followed routinely.

D. Large films require more solution and would therefore necessitate more frequent change of the solutions.

■ MANUAL PROCESSING

The darkroom has three tanks of chemicals and water for processing by hand: the developing tank, fixing tank, and water bath. In most darkrooms, the developer is the left tank, the water bath is in the center tank, and the fixer is in the right tank. The fixer can be identified by a smell similar to vinegar.

I. MANUAL PROCESSING EQUIPMENT

A. Developer, water, fixer tanks, and stirring rods
B. Accurate, steel-based thermometer; timer
C. Safelights and white lights
D. Film hangers and drying rod for hangers, or electric dryer
E. Processing log

II. PROCESSING TEMPERATURE AND TIMES

The quality of the radiographic image depends greatly upon the processing time and temperature, with optimal developing conditions for manual processing being 68° F for 5 minutes.

Higher temperatures would produce films with excessive density; cooler temperatures, too little density. It is necessary to check the developer temperature and recommended time as outlined in Table 9-9.

III. STEPS FOR MANUAL PROCESSING

A. Check level and temperature of solutions; stir solutions.
B. Complete the processing log.

■ TABLE 9-9 PROCESSING TEMPERATURES AND TIMES*

SOLUTION TEMPERATURE	TIME IN DEVELOPER (MINUTES)	RINSE TIME (SECONDS)	TIME IN FIXER (MINUTES)	WASH TIME (MINUTES)
65°F	6	30	2–4	10
68°F	5	30	2–4	10
70°F	4.5	30	2–4	10
72°F	4	30	2–4	10
75°F	3	30	2–4	10
80°F	2.5	30	2–4	10

*These times and temperatures are for D-, E-, or F-speed film and Kodak GBX fixer and developer.

C. Turn on safelights and turn off the white lights.

D. Load films from the film packet or cassette onto hangers, making sure films are securely fastened.

E. Immerse film in the developer; activate timer.

F. When timer buzzes, rinse films in circulating water for 30 seconds.

G. Immerse the films in the fixer for 4 minutes.

H. Wash the films in circulating water for 10 minutes.

I. Dry films until they are no longer tacky.

IV. DISPOSAL OF LIQUID CHEMICALS

Fixer is considered an environmentally hazardous waste material and must be disposed of according to governmental regulations.

■ ANALYSIS OF COMPLETED RADIOGRAPHS

The completed radiographs are mounted and examined at a viewbox with an adequate light source. Interpretation of radiographs is difficult, and the determination of a pathologic condition requires keen evaluation. Attempting to base interpretation on inadequate, insufficient radiographs will result in guesswork rather than in an accurate, timely diagnosis.

I. MOUNTING

A. Legibly mark the mount with the name of patient, age, date, name of dentist; printing is preferred.

B. Handle radiographs only by the edges with clean, dry hands.

C. Keep films clean and free from dust, liquids, or other contaminants.

D. Arrange radiographs in front of the view box on clean, dry paper.

E. The embossed dot near the edge of the negative is the guide to mounting; the raised side of the dot is on the facial side.

F. Identify individual negatives by the teeth and other anatomic landmarks.

G. Approved mounting system is as follows: Looking at the teeth from outside the mouth, the teeth are viewed and mounted in the same manner as the approved numbering system.

II. ANATOMIC LANDMARKS

A. Definition

An anatomic landmark is an anatomic structure, the image of which may serve as an aid in the localization and identification of the regions portrayed by a radiograph. The teeth are the primary landmarks.

B. Landmarks that May Be Seen in Individual Radiographs

1. *Maxillary Molar.* Maxillary sinus, zygomatic process, zygomatic (malar) bone, hamular process, coronoid process of the mandible, maxillary tuberosity.

2. *Maxillary Premolar.* Maxillary sinus.

3. *Maxillary Canine.* Maxillary sinus, junction of the maxillary sinus and nasal fossa (Y-shaped, radiopaque).

4. *Maxillary Incisors.* Incisive foramen, nasal septum and fossae, anterior nasal spine (V-shaped), median palatine suture, symphysis of the maxillae.

5. *Mandibular Molar.* Mandibular canal, internal oblique line, external oblique ridge, mylohyoid ridge.

6. *Mandibular Premolar.* Mental foramen.

7. *Mandibular Incisors.* Lingual foramen, mental ridge, genial tubercles, symphysis of the mandible. Nutrient canals are seen most frequently in this radiograph.

III. IDENTIFICATION OF ERRORS IN RADIOGRAPHS

Table 9-10 outlines the more common errors, their causes, and the keys to correction.

A. Causes

Errors may be related to any step in the entire procedure, including film placement, angulation, exposure, processing, and care and handling of the film.

B. Types

Errors appear as problems of improper density or contrast, incomplete or distorted images, fogging, artifacts, or stains.

1. *Distortion:* an inaccuracy in the size or shape of an object in the radiograph. Distortion is brought about by misalignment of the PID relative to the object. Vertical distortion produces elongation or foreshortening of the object.

2. *Fog:* a darkening of the whole or part of a radiograph by sources other than the radiation of the primary beam to which the film was exposed. Types of fog include chemical, light, and radiation.

3. *Artifact:* a blemish or an unintended radiographic image that can result from faulty manufacture, manipulation, exposure, or processing of an x-ray film.

■ TABLE 9-10 ANALYSIS OF RADIOGRAPHS: CAUSES OF ERRORS

	ERROR	CAUSE: FACTORS IN CORRECTION
Image	Elongation Foreshortening	Insufficient vertical angulation Excessive vertical angulation
	Superimposition (overlapping)	Incorrect horizontal angulation (central ray not directed through interproximal space)
	Partial image	Cone-cut (incorrect direction of central ray or incorrect film placement) Incompletely immersed in processing tank Film touched other film or side of tank during processing
	Blurred or double image	Patient, tube, or packet movement during exposure Film exposed twice
	Stretched appearance of trabeculae or apices	Bent film
	No image	Machine malfunction from time-switch to wall-plug Failure to turn on the machine Film placed in fixer before developer
Density	Too dark	Excessive exposure Excessive developing Developer too warm Unsafe safelight Accidental exposure to white light (may be completely black)
	Too light	Insufficient exposure Insufficient development or excessive fixation Solutions too cool Use of old, contaminated, or poorly mixed solutions Film placement: leaded side toward teeth Film used beyond expiration date
Fog	Chemical fog	Imbalance or deterioration of processing solutions
	Light fog	Unintentional exposure to light to which the emulsion is sensitive, either before or during processing (1) Unsafe safelight (2) Darkroom leak (3) Holding unprocessed films too close to the safelight too long
	Radiation fog	Improper storage of unused film Film exposed prior to processing
Reticulation	(puckered or pebbly surface)	Sudden temperature changes during processing, particularly from warm solutions to very cold water
Artifacts	Dark lines	Bent or creased film Static electricity (1) Film removed from wrapper with excessive force (2) Wrapper sticking to film when opened with wet fingers, or if there was excessive moisture from patient's mouth Fingernail used to grasp film during placement on hanger
	Herringbone pattern (light film)	Packet placed in mouth backwards with foil next to teeth
Discoloration	Stains and spots	Unclean film hanger Spatterings of developer, fixer, dust Finger marks Insufficient rinsing after developing before fixing Splashing dry negatives with water or solutions Air bubbles adhering to surface during processing (insufficient agitation) Overlap of film on film in tanks or while drying Paper wrapper stuck to film (film not dried when removed from patient's mouth)
	At later date after storage of completed radiographs	Incomplete processing or rinsing Storage in too warm a place Storage near chemicals

IV. INTERPRETATION

Radiographs are used in conjunction with clinical assessment for a complete care program. Periodic radiographs permit continuing evaluation. As part of the permanent record, radiographs help to document the oral condition for comparison as well as for legal purposes.

The quality of the radiographs determines their usability for diagnostic interpretation. Procedures for the preparation of radiographs must be perfected so that the radiographs have maximum interpretability with minimum radiation exposure of the patient.

A. Prerequisites for Interpretation

1. *Mounting.* Mount radiographs in an opaque mount to prevent light between each radiograph from creating glare and producing a blinding effect.
2. *Viewbox.* Use an adequately lighted viewbox. Dimmed room light improves visibility for contrasting radiolucent and radiopaque areas. Holding the radiographs up to view by window, room, or unit light is inadequate, and only gross interpretation can be accomplished. When a viewbox is larger than the mount used, cover the edges to block out peripheral light.
3. *Hand Magnifying Glass.* Examine radiographs on a viewbox through a magnifying glass. A viewbox is available with a built-on magnifying glass.

B. Systematic Examination

1. Observe one radiographic feature at a time. Examine all of the radiographs in a survey for that feature, rather than taking each radiograph separately to find everything. It is important to note comparisons for each change over the entire survey.

2. When examining a particular tooth, compare the appearance of that tooth in each radiograph in which it appears, including bitewings. At different angulations, different findings may become apparent.

C. Correlation With Clinical Examination

A description of radiographic examination of the teeth may be found on page 272 and of the periodontal tissues on pages 241 to 244. Correlation of radiographic findings with the clinical examination, using probe and explorer, is basic to an understanding of the true oral condition of the patient.

■ RECORD KEEPING

I. RADIATION EXPOSURE HISTORY

Inquire whether the patient is receiving or has recently received radiation therapy. It may be necessary to minimize the number of exposures. A consultation with the patient's physician is recommended.

II. RADIATION EXPOSURE RECORD

A continuing record for each patient is kept to show the date, number of exposures, kVp, mA, time, and area exposed.

III. PATIENT SIGNATURE

After a careful explanation of the reasons why radiographs are essential to the diagnosis and treatment of a problem, the patient has the right to agree to or to refuse the recommended exposure(s). When a patient refuses to have radiographs made, record such in the patient's permanent record. Obtain patient's signature to a statement indicating such refusal in the event a legal issue should arise.

Everyday Ethics

A new patient to the practice, Mr. Glazier, brings a full series of radiographs (16 PAs and 4 BWs) from the previous dentist, prepared just 3 months ago. Following the oral examination, the dentist instructs the dental hygienist to make a panoramic radiograph and 4 BWs.

Mr. Glazier inquires why additional exposures are needed at this time.

Questions for Consideration

1. How will the dental hygienist question the prescriptive request by the dentist for additional radiographs? What would an appropriate response be? How can it be phrased?

2. What ethical standards of care and/or risks should be considered on behalf of the patient? Identify the moral duty of a dental hygienist in this situation.

✔ Factors To Teach The Patient

WHEN THE PATIENT ASKS ABOUT THE SAFETY OF RADIATION

- Patients ask questions about safety factors, and occasionally a patient may refuse to have any radiographs made. The patient must be reassured with confidence, instructed as to why radiographs are necessary at this time, and informed about how modern equipment and techniques are in accord with radiation standards.

- Adapt the answer to the patient. Certain patients have more fear; others have more knowledge about x-rays. The clinician who expresses confidence aids in allaying fears. Hesitation increases the patient's doubt.

- Radiographs are essential to diagnosis and treatment. Without the information provided, the clinician can only guess at conditions not visible clinically.

- The benefits resulting from the intelligent use of x-rays outweigh any possible negative effects.

- Modern x-ray machines are equipped for safety. Simple details about filtration, collimation, film speed, use of protective shields, and short exposure times can be explained.

EDUCATIONAL FEATURES IN DENTAL RADIOGRAPHS

- Position of unerupted permanent teeth in relation to primary teeth.

- Detection of early carious lesions not visible by clinical examination.

- Effects of loss of teeth and the importance of having replacements.

- Periodontal changes and other pathologic conditions appropriate to an individual patient.

IV. OWNERSHIP

Radiographs are the property of the dental practice even though they were paid for by the patient or the patient's insurance company. However, patients have a right to a copy of their records and radiographs.[17] When possible, a duplicate set can be made by using a two-film packet. If that is not possible, the original series must be duplicated so that the originals can be kept with the patient's complete record and the duplicated series given to the patient.

REFERENCES

1. Haring, J.I. and Jansen, L.: *Dental Radiography, Principles and Techniques,*2nd ed.Philadelphia, W.B. Saunders, 2000, p.4.
2. **United States Department of Health and Human Services,** Public Health Service, Food and Drug Administration, Center for Devices and Radiological Health: *Selection of Patients for X-ray Examinations: Dental Radiographic Examinations.*(HHS Publication FDA 88-8273). Washington, D.C., Government Printing Office, 1987.
3. **United States National Research Council:** *Health Effects of Exposure to Low Levels of Ionizing Radiation. BEIR-V,* Washington, D.C., National Academy Press, 1990.
4. **White, S.C. and Pharoah, M.J.:** *Oral Radiology, Principles and Interpretation,* 4th ed., St. Louis, Mosby, 2000, pp.11–12.
5. **Haring and Jansen,:** op.cit., pp. 384–394.
6. **Mauriello, S.M. and Platin, E.:** Dental Digital Radiographic Imaging, *J. Dent. Hyg.,* 75, 323, Fall, 2001.
7. **International Commission on Radiation Units and Measurements** (ICRU): *Radiation Quantities and Units.* Washington, D.C., ICRU Report No. 33, 1980.
8. **National Council on Radiation Protection and Measurements:** *Dental X-Ray Protection.* Washington, D.C., NCRP Report No. 35, 1970.
9. **Haring and Jansen:** op. cit., p.72.
10. **White, S.C.:** 1992 Assessment of Radiation Risk From Dental Radiography, *Dentomaxillofac. Radiol., 21,*118, August, 1992.
11. **Horner, K.:** Review Article: Radiation Protection in Dental Radiology, *Br. J. Radiol.,* 67,1041, November, 1994.
12. **White and Pharoah:** op.cit., p. 205.
13. **American Dental Association,** Council on Scientific Affairs: An Update on Radiographic Practices: Information and Recommendations, *J. Am. Dental. Assoc., 132,*234, February, 2001.
14. **Haring and Jansen:** op. cit., pp.194–207.
15. **Bachman,** C.E., White, J.M., Goodis, H.E., and Rosenquist, J.W.: Bacterial Adherence and Contamination During Radiographic Processing, *Oral Surg. Oral Med. Oral Pathol.,* 70, 669, November, 1990.
16. **Stanczyk,** D.A., Paunovich, E.D., Broome, J.C., and Fatone, M.A.: Microbiologic Contamination During Dental Radiographic Film Processing, *Oral Surg. Oral Med. Oral Pathol.,* 76, 112, July, 1993.
17. **Haring** and Jansen: op.cit, p. 190.

SUGGESTED READINGS

American Academy of Oral and Maxillofacial Radiology, Radiology Practice Committee, Goren, A.D., Lundeen, R.C., Deahl, S.T., Hashimoto, K., Kapa, S.F., Katz, J.O., Ludlow, J.B., Platin, E., Van Der Stelt, P.F., and Wolfgang, L.: Updated Quality Assurance Self-assessment Exercise in Intraoral and Panoramic Radiography, *Oral Surg.Oral Med. Oral Pathol. Oral Radiol. Endod.,* 89, 369, March, 2000.

Ludlow, J.B., Platin, E., and Mol, A.: Characteristics of Kodak Insight, an F-speed Intraoral Film, *Oral Surg. Oral Med., Oral Pathol. Oral Radiol. Endod.,* 91, 120, January, 2001.

Ludlow, J.B., Platin, E., Delano, E.O., and Clifton, L.: The Efficacy of Caries Detection Using Three Intraoral Films Under Different Processing Conditions, *J. Am. Dent. Assoc.,* 128, 1401, October, 1997.

Peterson, C.A., Mauriello, S.M., Overman, V.P., Platin, E., and Tangen, C.M.: Effects of Beam Collimation on Image Quality, *J. Dent. Hyg., 71*, 61, March–April, 1997.

Wyche, C.J.: Infection Control Protocols for Exposing and Processing Radiographs, *J. Dent Hyg., 70*, 122, May–June, 1996.

Technique

Bohay, R.N., Kogon, S.L., and Stephens, R.G.: A Survey of Radiographic Techniques and Equipment Used by a Sample of General Dental Practitioners, *Oral Surg. Oral Med. Oral Pathol., 78*, 806, December, 1994.

Dubrez, B., Jacot-Descombes, S., and Cimasoni, G.: Reliability of a Paralleling Instrument for Dental Radiographs, *Oral Surg. Oral Med. Oral Pathol. Oral Radiol. Endod., 80*, 358, September, 1995.

Stabulas, J.J.: Vertical Bitewings: The Other Option, *J. Pract. Hyg., 11*, 46, May/June, 2002.

Radiation Exposure Control

Atchison, K.A., White, S.C., Flack, V.F., and Hewlett, E.R.: Assessing the FDA Guidelines for Ordering Dental Radiographs, *J. Am. Dent. Assoc., 126*, 1372, October 1995.

Atchison, K.A., White., S.C., Flack, V.F., Hewlett, E.R., and Kinder, S.A.: Efficacy of the FDA Selection Criteria for Radiographic Assessment of the Periodontium, *J. Dent. Res., 74*, 1424, July, 1995.

Geist, J. and Katz, J.: Radiation Dose-reduction Techniques in North American Dental Schools, *Oral Surg. Oral Med. Oral Pathol. Oral Radiol. Endod., 93*, 496, April, 2002.

Rushton, V.E., Horner, K., and Worthington, H.V.: Factors Influencing the Frequency of Bitewing Radiography in General Dental Practice, *Community Dent. Oral Epidemiol., 24*, 272, August, 1996.

White, S.C., Atchison, K.A., Hewlett, E.R., and Flack V.F.: Efficacy of FDA Guidelines for Ordering Radiographs for Caries Detection, *Oral Surg. Oral Med. Oral Pathol., 77*, 531, May, 1994.

Digital Radiography

Alty, C.T.: Digital Exposure, *RDH, 20*, 20, July 2000.

Gakenheimer, D.C.: The Efficacy of a Computerized Caries Detector in Intraoral Digital Radiography, *J. Am. Dent. Assoc., 133*, 883, July, 2002.

Hausmann, E.: Radiographic and Digital Imaging in Periodontal Practice, *J. Periodontol., 71*, 497, March, 2000.

Hokett, S.D., Honey, J.R., Ruiz, F., Baisden, M.K., and Hoen, M.M.: Assessing the Effectiveness of Direct Digital Radiography Barrier Sheaths and Finger Cots, *J. Am. Dent. Assoc., 131*, 463, April, 2000.

Ludlow, J.B. and Mol, A.: Image-receptor Performance: A Comparison of Trophy RVG UI Sensor and Kodak Ektaspeed Plus Film, *Oral Surg. Oral Med. Oral Pathol. Oral Radiol. Endod., 91*, 109, January, 2001.

Paurazas, S.B., Geist, J.R., Pink F. E., Hoen, M.M., and Steiman, H.R.: Comparison of Diagnostic Accuracy of Digital Imaging by Using CCD and CMOS-APS Sensors With E-speed Film in the Detection of Periapical Bony Lesions, *Oral Surg. Oral Med. Oral Pathol. Oral Radiol. Endod., 89*, 356, March 2000.

Wenzel, A., Frandsen, E., and Hintze, H.: Patient Discomfort and Cross-infection Control in Bitewing Examination With a Storage Phosphor Plate and a CCD-based Sensor, *J. Dent., 27*, 243, March, 1999.

Panoramic

Almog, D.M., Illig, K.A., Khin, M., and Green, R.M.: Unrecognized Carotid Artery Stenosis Discovered by Calcification on a Panoramic Radiograph, *J. Am. Dent. Assoc., 131*, 1593, November, 2000.

Danforth, R.A. and Clark, D.E.: Effective Dose From Radiation Absorbed During a Panoramic Examination With a New Generation Machine, *Oral Surg. Oral Med. Oral Pathol. Oral Radiol. Endod., 89*, 236, February, 2000.

Flint, D. J., Paunovich, E., Moore, W.S., Wofford, D.T., and Hermesch, C.B.: A Diagnostic Comparison of Panoramic and Intraoral Radiographs, *Oral Surg. Oral Med.Oral Pathol. Oral Radiol. Endod., 85*, 731, June, 1998.

Legg, L.M.: Common Panoramic Positioning Practices and Errors, *J. Pract. Hyg., 8*, 15, March/April, 1999.

Extraoral and Intraoral Examination

A careful overall observation of each patient and a thorough examination of the oral cavity and adjacent structures are essential to total assessment prior to care planning. A variety of lesions may be observed for which the patient may or may not report subjective symptoms. Recognition, treatment, and follow-up of specific lesions may be of definite significance to the present and future general and oral health of the patient.

Despite the occurrence of many seemingly minor lesions, the danger of oral malignancies remains a definite possibility. Every effort must be made to detect potentially cancerous lesions early.

Each area of the mucous membrane must be examined, and minor deviations from normal must be given prompt attention. A life may depend on an oral examination. Routine examination for each new patient and at each maintenance appointment provides a realistic approach to the control of oral disease.

The oral tissues are sensitive indicators of the general health of the individual. Changes in these structures may be the first indication of subclinical disease processes in other parts of the body.

Prerequisite to the recognition of deviations from the normal appearance of the oral cavity is knowledge and understanding of the normal morphology, anatomy, and physiology of the oral cavity and the surrounding area. Box 10-1 defines terms used for extraoral and intraoral examination.

■ OBJECTIVES

A thorough examination is essential to the total care of the patient. The dental hygienist will:

- Observe the patient overall, as well as in all areas in and about the oral cavity, and record those areas that appear to deviate from normal and that may be evidence of disease.
- Screen each patient at each appointment to detect lesions that may be pathologic, particularly those that may be cancerous.

BOX 10-1 KEY WORDS: Extraoral/Intraoral Examination

Aphtha: a little white or reddish ulcer.

Crust: outer scablike layer of solid matter formed by drying of a body exudate or secretion.

Cyst: a closed, epithelia-lined sac, normal or pathologic, that contains fluid or other material.

Dorsal: back surface; opposite of ventral.

Epidermis: outermost and nonvascular layers of the skin composed of basal layer, spinous layer, granular layer, and horny layer.

   Corium: the dermis or true skin just beneath the epidermis; well supplied with nerves and blood vessels.

Erosion: soft tissue slightly depressed lesion in which the epithelium above the basal layer is denuded.

Erythema: red area of variable size and shape; reaction to irritation, radiation, or injury.

Exophytic: growing outward.

Exostosis: a benign bony growth projecting from the surface of bone.

Fissure: a narrow slit or cleft in the epidermis where infected ulceration, inflammation, and pain can result.

Forensic: pertaining to or used in legal proceedings.

Idiopathic: of unknown etiology.

Indurated: hardened; abnormally hard.

Lymphadenopathy: disease of the lymph nodes; regional lymph node enlargement.

Morphology: science that deals with form and structure.

Palpation: perceiving by sense of touch.

Papilla: small, nipple-shaped projection or elevation (papillary: adjective).

Patch: circumscribed flat lesion larger than a macule; differentiated from surrounding epidermis by color and/or texture.

Pedunculated: elevated lesion attached by a thin stalk.

Petechia: hemorrhagic spot of pinpoint to pinhead size.

Polyp: any growth or mass protruding from a mucous membrane.

Pseudomembrane: a loose membranous layer of exudate containing microorganisms, precipitated fibrin, necrotic cells, and inflammatory cells produced during an inflammatory reaction on the surface of a tissue.

Punctate: marked with points or punctures differentiated from the surrounding surface by color, elevation, or texture.

Purulent: containing, forming, or discharging pus.

Rubefacient: reddening of the skin.

Scar: cicatrix; mark remaining after healing of a wound or healing following a surgical intervention.

Sclerosis: induration or hardening.

Sessile: elevated lesion with a broad base.

Temporomandibular disorder (TMD): a collective term that includes a wide range of disorders of the masticatory system characterized by one or more of the following: pain in the preauricular area, temporomandibular joint (TMJ), and muscles of mastication, with limitation or deviation in mandibular motion and TMJ sounds during mandibular function.

Torus: bony elevation or prominence usually located on the midline of the hard palate (torus palatinus) and the lingual surface of the mandible in the premolar area (torus mandibularis).

Trismus: motor disturbance of the trigeminal nerve, especially spasm of the masticatory muscles with difficulty in opening the mouth.

Ventral: anterior or inferior surface; opposite of dorsal.

Verruca: a wartlike growth.

- Recognize a need for postponement of the current appointment because of evidence of communicable disease or in deference to the need for urgent medical consultation and/or treatment.
- Prevent the development of advanced, irreversible, or untreatable oral disease by early recognition of initial lesions.
- Identify suspected conditions that require additional testing and refer for medical evaluation.
- Identify extraoral and intraoral deviations from normal for which dental hygiene care and instruction may need special adaptations.
- Provide a means of comparison of individual oral examinations over a series of maintenance appointments, and thus determine the effects of dental and dental hygiene care and the success of patient instruction.
- Provide information for continuing records of the patient's diagnosis and treatment plan for legal purposes.

▪ COMPONENTS OF EXAMINATION

The current concept of patient care is that the total patient is being treated, not only the oral cavity, and particularly not only the teeth and their immediately surrounding tissues. The examination is, therefore, all-inclusive to detect any physical, mental, or psychological influences of the whole patient on the oral health.

Thorough examination becomes a routine part of each patient appointment so that treatment for the control and prevention of oral diseases will be effective.

I. PREPARATION FOR EXAMINATION

A. Review the patient's health histories and other parts of the records.
B. Examine radiographs on viewbox.
C. Explain the procedures to be performed.

II. METHODS OF EXAMINATION

The various examination methods are defined on page 96. The extraoral and intraoral examination is accomplished primarily by direct visual observation and palpation, but other methods may also be used.

A. Direct Observation

Patient position, optimum lighting, and effective retraction for accessibility and visibility contribute to the accuracy and completeness of the examination.

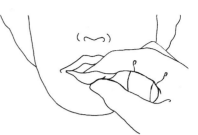

■ **FIGURE 10-1 Bidigital Palpation.** Palpation of the lip to illustrate the use of a finger and thumb of the same hand.

B. Palpation

Types of palpation include the following:
1. *Digital.* Use of a single finger. Example: index finger applied to inner border of the mandible beneath the canine–premolar area to determine the presence of a torus mandibularis.
2. *Bidigital.* Use of finger and thumb of the same hand. Example: palpation of the lips (Figure 10-1).
3. *Bimanual.* Use of finger or fingers and thumb from each hand applied simultaneously in coordination. Example: index finger of one hand palpates on the floor of the mouth inside, while a finger or fingers from the other hand press on the same area from under the chin externally (Figure 10-2).
4. *Bilateral.* The two hands are used at the same time to examine corresponding structures on opposite sides of the body. Comparisons may be made. Example: fingers placed beneath the chin to palpate the submandibular lymph nodes (Figure 10-3).

▪ SEQUENCE OF EXAMINATION

A recommended order for examination is outlined in Table 10-1, in which factors to consider during appointments are related to the actual observations made and recorded. The sequence presented in Table 10-1 is adapted from

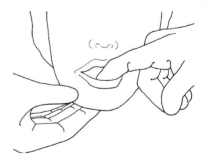

■ **FIGURE 10-2 Bimanual Palpation.** Examination of the floor of the mouth by simultaneous palpation with fingers of each hand in apposition.

▪ TABLE 10-1 EXTRAORAL AND INTRAORAL EXAMINATION

ORDER OF EXAMINATION	TO OBSERVE	INDICATION AND INFLUENCES ON APPOINTMENTS
1. Overall appraisal of patient	Posture, gait General health status; size Hair; scalp Breathing; state of fatigue Voice, cough, hoarseness	Response, cooperation, attitude toward treatment Length of appointment

2. Face	Expression: evidence of fear or
	    apprehension
	Shape: twitching; paralysis
	Jaw movements during speech
	Injuries; signs of abuse
		Need for alleviation of fears
		Evidence of upper respiratory or other
		    infections
		Enlarged masseter muscle (related to
		    bruxism)

3. Skin	Color, texture, blemishes Traumatic lesions Eruptions, swellings Growths	Relation to possible systemic conditions Need for supplementary history Biopsy or other treatment Influences on instruction in diet
4. Eyes	Size of pupil Color of sclera Eyeglasses (corrective) Protruding eyeballs	Dilated pupils or pinpoint may result from drugs, emergency state Eyeglasses essential during instruction Hyperthyroidism

5. Nodes (palpate) (Figure 10-4)
    a. Pre- and postauricular
    b. Occipital
    c. Submental; submandibular
    d. Cervical chain
    e. Supraclavicular
	Adenopathy; lymphadenopathy
	Induration
		Need for referral
		Medical consultation
		Coordinate with intraoral examination

6. Temporomandibular joint
    (palpate) (Figure 10-5)
	Limitations or deviations
	    of movement
	Tenderness; sensitivity
	Noises: clicking, popping, grating
		Disorder of joint; limitation of opening
		Discomfort during appointment and
		    during personal biofilm control

7. Lips
    a. Observe closed, then open
    b. Palpate (Figure 10-1)
	Color, texture, size
	Cracks, angular cheilosis
	Blisters, ulcers
	Traumatic lesions
	Irritation from lip-biting
	Limitation of opening; muscle
	    elasticity; muscle tone
	Evidences of mouthbreathing
	Induration
		Need for further examination: referral
		Immediate need for postponement of
		    appointment when a lesion may be
		    communicable or could interfere
		    with procedures
		Care during retraction
		Accessibility during intraoral
		    procedures
		Patient instruction: dietary, special
		    biofilm control for mouthbreather

8. Breath odor	Severity Relation to oral hygiene, gingival health	Possible relation to systemic condition Alcohol use history; special needs

9. Labial and buccal mucosa,
    left and right examined
    systematically
    a. Vestibule
    b. Mucobuccal folds
    c. Frena
    d. Opening of Stensen's duct
    e. Palpate cheeks
	Color, size, texture, contour
	Abrasions, traumatic lesions,
	    cheekbite
	Effects of tobacco use
	Ulcers, growths
	Moistness of surfaces
	Relation of frena to free gingiva
	Induration
		Need for referral, biopsy, cytology
		Frena and other anatomic parts that
		    need special adaptation for
		    radiography or impression tray
		Avoid sensitive areas during retraction

■ TABLE 10-1 EXTRAORAL AND INTRAORAL EXAMINATION (Continued)

ORDER OF EXAMINATION	TO OBSERVE	INDICATION AND INFLUENCES ON APPOINTMENTS
10. Tongue a. Vestibule b. Lateral borders c. Base of tongue (retract) (Figure 10-6) d. Deviation on extension	Shape: normal asymmetric Color, size, texture, consistency Fissures; papillae Coating Lesions: elevated, depressed, flat Induration	Need for referral, biopsy, cytology Need for instruction in tongue cleaning
11. Floor of mouth a. Ventral surface of tongue b. Palpate (Figure 10-2) c. Duct openings d. Mucosa, frena e. Tongue action	Varicosities Lesions: elevated, flat, depressed, traumatic Induration Limitation or freedom of movement of tongue Frena; tongue-tie	Large muscular tongue influences retraction, gag reflex, accessibility for instrumentation Film placement problems
12. Saliva	Quantity; quality (thick, ropy) Evidence of dry mouth; lip wetting Tongue coating	Reduced in certain diseases, by certain drugs Special dental caries control program Influence on instrumentation Need for saliva substitute
13. Hard palate	Height, contour, color Appearance of rugae Tori, growths, ulcers	Need for referral, biopsy, cytology Signs of tongue thrust, deviate swallow Influence on radiographic film placement
14. Soft palate, uvula	Color, size, shape Petechiae Ulcers, growths	Referral, biopsy, cytology Large uvula influences gag reflex
15. Tonsillar region, throat	Tonsils: size and shape Color, size, surface characteristics Lesions, trauma	Referral, biopsy, cytology Enlarged tonsils encourage gag reflex Throat infection, a sign for appointment postponement

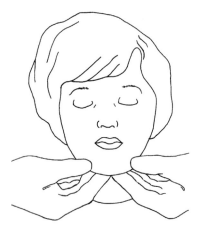

■ FIGURE 10-3 Bilateral Palpation. Bilateral palpation is used to examine corresponding structures on opposite sides of the body.

Detecting Oral Cancer, available from the National Institutes of Health.[1]

I. SYSTEMATIC SEQUENCE FOR EXAMINATION

The advantages of following a routine order for examination include the following:
  A. Minimal possibility of overlooking an area and missing details of importance.
  B. Increased efficiency and conservation of time.
  C. Maintenance of a professional atmosphere, which inspires the patient's confidence.

II. STEPS FOR THOROUGH EXAMINATION (TABLE 10-1)

A. Extraoral

1. Observe patient during reception and seating to note physical characteristics and abnormalities, and make an overall appraisal.

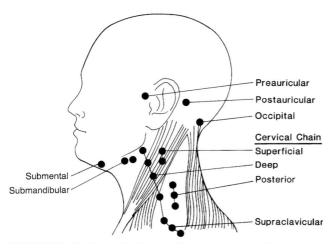

■ **FIGURE 10-4 Lymph Nodes.** The locations of the major lymph nodes into which the vessels of the facial and oral regions drain.

2. Observe head, face, eyes, and neck, and evaluate the skin of the face and neck.
3. Palpate the salivary glands and lymph nodes. Figure 10-4 shows the location of the major lymph nodes of the face, oral regions, and neck.
4. Observe mandibular movement and palpate the temporomandibular joint (Figure 10-5). Relate to items from questions in the medical/dental history.[2,3]

B. Intraoral

1. Make a preliminary examination of the lips and intraoral mucosa by using a mouth mirror or a tongue depressor.
2. View and palpate lips, labial and buccal mucosa, and mucobuccal folds.
3. Examine and palpate the tongue, including the dorsal and ventral surfaces, lateral borders, and base. Retract to observe posterior third, first to

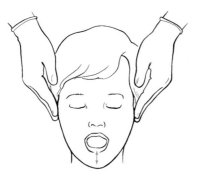

■ **FIGURE 10-5 Assessment of the Temporomandibular Joint.** The joint is palpated as the patient opens and closes the mouth.

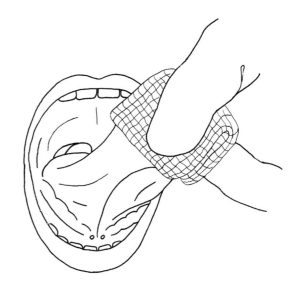

■ **FIGURE 10-6 Examination of the Tongue.** To observe the posterior third of the tongue and the attachment to the floor of the mouth, hold the tongue with a gauze sponge, retract the cheek, and move the tongue out, first to one side and then the other, as each section of the mucosa is carefully examined.

one side then the other (Figure 10-6). The papillae of the tongue are shown in Figure 12-2 (page 208).
4. Observe mucosa of the floor of the mouth. Palpate the floor of the mouth (Figure 10-2).
5. Examine the hard and soft palates, tonsillar areas, and pharynx. Use a mirror to observe the oropharynx, nasopharynx, and larynx.
6. Note amount and consistency of the saliva and evidence of dry mouth.

■ DOCUMENTATION OF FINDINGS

I. RECORDS

A. Record Form

1. Contains adequate space for complete descriptions of lesions observed; not merely a check sheet.
2. Contains spaces for successive examinations at follow-up and maintenance appointments.

B. Information to Record

A complete description of each finding includes the location, extent, size, color, surface texture or configurations, consistency, morphology, and history.

II. HISTORY

Questions directed to the patient provide necessary information in the management of an oral lesion. Because alarming the patient must be avoided, judgment is needed for selecting the appropriate time to obtain the history of a lesion.

A. Whether the lesion is known or not known to the patient; previous evaluation.

B. If known, when first noticed; if recurrence, previous date.

C. Duration; changes in size and appearance.

D. Symptoms.

III. LOCATION AND EXTENT

When a lesion is first seen, its location is noted in relation to adjacent structures. A printed diagram of parts of the oral cavity drawn into the record form can be a valuable aid for marking the location (Figure 10-7). Descriptive words to define the location and extent include the following:

A. *Localized.* Lesion limited to a small focal area.

B. *Generalized.* Involves most of an area or segment.

C. *Single Lesion.* One lesion of a particular type with a distinct margin.

D. *Multiple Lesions.* More than one lesion of a particular type. Lesions may be

1. Separate. Discrete, not running together; may be arranged in clusters.

2. Coalescing. Close to each other with margins that merge.

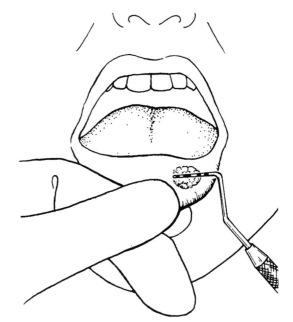

■ **FIGURE 10-8 Use of a Probe to Measure a Lesion.** In addition to the exact location, the width and length of a lesion should be recorded. Using the probe provides a convenient method.

IV. PHYSICAL CHARACTERISTICS

A. Size and Shape

Record length and width in millimeters. The height of an elevated lesion may be significant. Use a probe to measure, as shown in Figure 10-8.

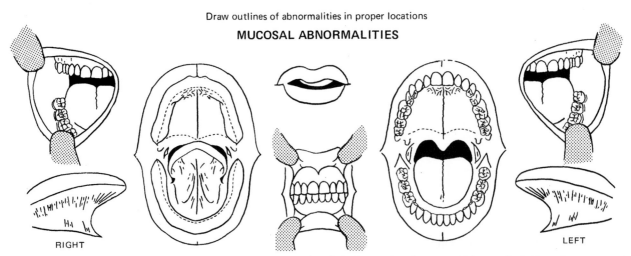

Draw outlines of abnormalities in proper locations
MUCOSAL ABNORMALITIES

RIGHT   LEFT

■ **FIGURE 10-7 Record Form for Clinical Findings.** As part of a clinical examination record form, deviations from normal can be drawn to show the location and relative size. (Courtesy, University of Southern California School of Dentistry.)

B. Color

Red, pink, white, and red and white are the most commonly seen. Other more rare lesions may be blue, purple, gray, yellow, black, or brown.

C. Surface Texture

A lesion may have a smooth or an irregular surface. The texture may be papillary, verrucous or wartlike, fissured, corrugated, or crusted. Other descriptive terms are defined in Box 10-1 with the key words.

D. Consistency

Lesions may be soft, spongy, resilient, hard, or indurated.

■ MORPHOLOGIC CATEGORIES[4]

Most lesions can be classified readily as *elevated, depressed,* or *flat* as they relate to the normal level of the skin or mucosa. Tables 10-2, 10-3, and 10-4 break down the terms used for describing lesions in each category.

I. ELEVATED LESIONS (TABLE 10-2)

An elevated lesion is above the plane of the skin or mucosa. Elevated lesions are considered *blisterform* or *nonblisterform*.

A. Blisterform

Blisterform lesions contain fluid and are usually soft and translucent. They may be vesicles, pustules, or bullae.

■ TABLE 10-2 DESCRIPTION OF ELEVATED SOFT TISSUE LESIONS

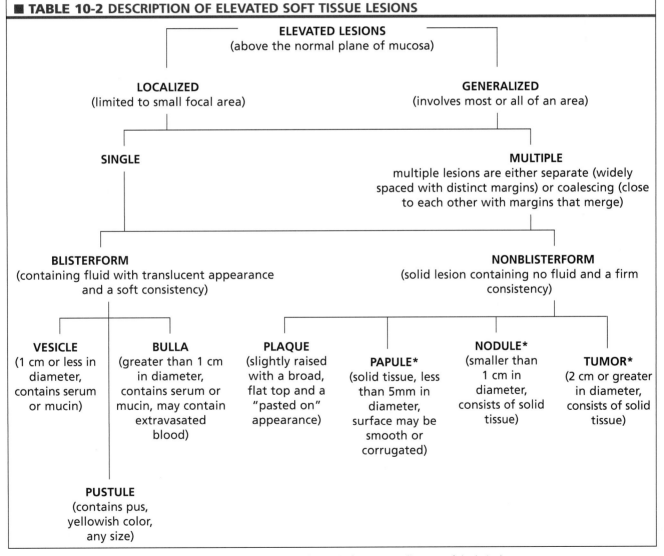

*May be pedunculated (on a stem or stalk) or sessile (base or attachment is the greatest diameter of the lesion)
(From McCann, A.: Describing Soft Tissue Lesions of the Oral Cavity, *DentalHygienistNews, 5,* 9, Spring, 1992. Used with permission.

■ **TABLE 10-3 DESCRIPTION OF DEPRESSED SOFT TISSUE LESIONS**

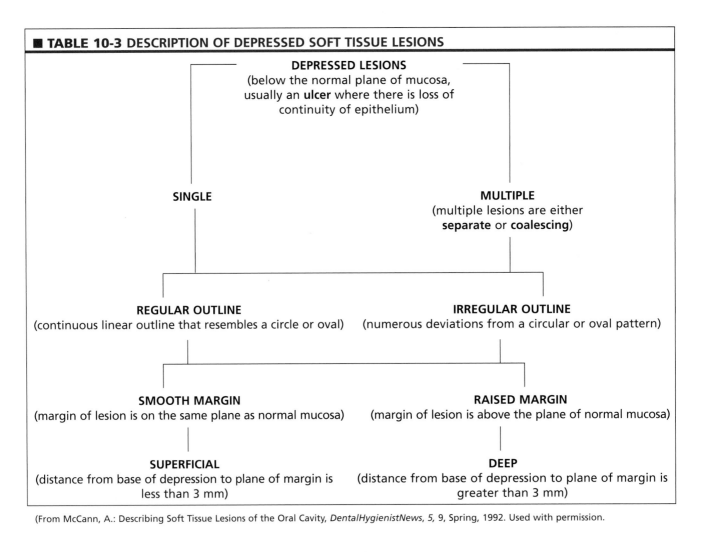

DEPRESSED LESIONS
(below the normal plane of mucosa,
usually an **ulcer** where there is loss of
continuity of epithelium)

SINGLE

MULTIPLE
(multiple lesions are either
separate or **coalescing**)

REGULAR OUTLINE
(continuous linear outline that resembles a circle or oval)

IRREGULAR OUTLINE
(numerous deviations from a circular or oval pattern)

SMOOTH MARGIN
(margin of lesion is on the same plane as normal mucosa)

RAISED MARGIN
(margin of lesion is above the plane of normal mucosa)

SUPERFICIAL
(distance from base of depression to plane of margin is
less than 3 mm)

DEEP
(distance from base of depression to plane of margin is
greater than 3 mm)

(From McCann, A.: Describing Soft Tissue Lesions of the Oral Cavity, *DentalHygienistNews*, *5*, 9, Spring, 1992. Used with permission.

■ **TABLE 10-4 DESCRIPTION OF FLAT SOFT TISSUE LESIONS**

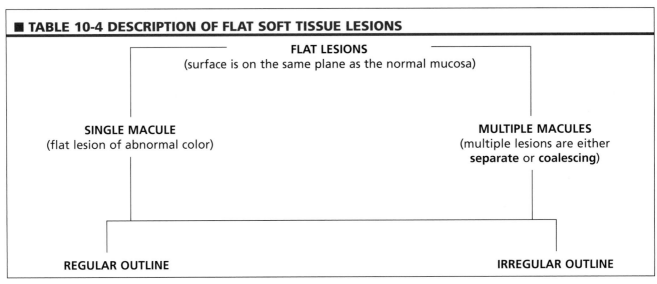

FLAT LESIONS
(surface is on the same plane as the normal mucosa)

SINGLE MACULE
(flat lesion of abnormal color)

MULTIPLE MACULES
(multiple lesions are either
separate or **coalescing**)

REGULAR OUTLINE

IRREGULAR OUTLINE

(From McCann, A.: Describing Soft Tissue Lesions of the Oral Cavity, *DentalHygienistNews*, *5*, 9, Spring, 1992. Used with permission.

1. *Vesicle.* A vesicle is a small (1 cm or less in diameter), circumscribed lesion with a thin surface covering. It may contain serum or mucin and appear white.
2. *Pustule.* A pustule may be more or less than 5 mm in diameter. It contains pus. Pus gives the pustule a yellowish color.
3. *Bulla.* A bulla is large (more than 1 cm). It is filled with fluid, usually mucin or serum, but may contain blood. The color depends on the fluid content.

B. Nonblisterform

Nonblisterform lesions are solid and do not contain fluid. They may be papules, nodules, tumors, or plaques. Papules, nodules, and tumors are also characterized by the base or attachment. As shown in Figure 10-9, the *pedunculated* lesion is attached by a narrow stalk or pedicle, whereas the *sessile* lesion has a base as wide as the lesion itself.

1. *Papule.* A papule is a small (pinhead to 5 mm in diameter), solid lesion that may be pointed, rounded, or flat-topped.
2. *Nodule.* A nodule is larger than a papule (greater than 5 mm but less than 1 cm).
3. *Tumor.* A tumor is 2 cm or greater in width. In this context, "tumor" means a general swelling or enlargement and does not refer to neoplasm, either benign or malignant.
4. *Plaque.* A plaque is a slightly raised lesion with a broad, flat top. It is usually larger than 5 mm in diameter, with a "pasted on" appearance.

II. DEPRESSED LESIONS (TABLE 10-3)

A depressed lesion is below the level of the skin or mucosa. The outline may be regular or irregular, and there may be a flat or raised border around the depression. The depth is usually described as superficial or deep. A deep lesion is greater than 3 mm deep.

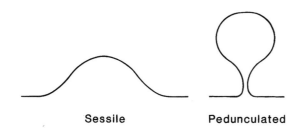

Sessile   **Pedunculated**

■ **FIGURE 10-9 Attachment of Nonblisterform Lesions.** The *sessile* lesion has a base as wide as the lesion itself; the *pedunculated* lesion is attached by a narrow stalk or pedicle.

A. Ulcer

Most depressed lesions are ulcers and represent a loss of continuity of the epithelium. The center is often gray to yellow, surrounded by a red border. An ulcer may result from the rupture of an elevated lesion (vesicle, pustule, or bulla).

B. Erosion

An erosion is a shallow, depressed lesion that does not extend through the epithelium to the underlying tissue.

III. FLAT LESIONS (TABLE 10-4)

A flat lesion is on the same level as the normal skin or oral mucosa. Flat lesions may occur as single or multiple lesions and have a regular or irregular form.

A *macule* is a circumscribed area not elevated above the surrounding skin or mucosa. It may be identified by its color, which contrasts with the surrounding normal tissues.

IV. OTHER DESCRIPTIVE TERMS

A. **Crust:** an outer layer, covering, or scab that may have formed from coagulation or drying of blood, serum, or pus, or a combination. A crust may form after a vesicle breaks; for example, the skin lesion of chicken pox is first a macule, then a papule, then a vesicle, and then a crust.
B. **Erythema:** red area of variable size and shape.
C. **Exophytic:** growing outward.
D. **Indurated:** hardened.
E. **Papillary:** resembling a small, nipple-shaped projection or elevation.
F. **Petechiae:** minute hemorrhagic spots of pinhead to pinpoint size.
G. **Pseudomembrane:** a loose membranous layer of exudate containing organisms, precipitated fibrin, necrotic cells, and inflammatory cells produced during an inflammatory reaction on the surface of a tissue.
H. **Polyp:** any mass of tissue that projects outward or upward from the normal surface level.
I. **Punctate:** marked with points or dots differentiated from the surrounding surface by color, elevation, or texture.
J. **Torus:** bony elevation or prominence usually found on the midline of the hard palate (torus palatinus) and the lingual surface of the mandible (torus mandibularis) in the premolar area.
K. **Verrucous** (verrucose): rough, wartlike.

■ ORAL CANCER

The objective is to detect cancer of the mouth at the earliest possible stage. Discovered later, when a cancer extends into adjacent structures and to the lymph nodes of the neck, the prognosis is less favorable.

Because the early lesions are generally symptomless, they may go unnoticed and unreported by the patient. Observation by the dentist or dental hygienist, therefore, is the principal method for the control of oral cancer. The first step in accomplishing this task is to examine the entire face, neck, and oral mucous membrane of each patient at the initial examination and at each maintenance appointment (Table 10-1).

It is necessary to know how to conduct the oral examination, where oral cancer occurs most frequently, what an early cancerous lesion may look like, and what to do when such a lesion is found. In addition to the early lesions of oral cancers, the oral manifestations of neoplasms elsewhere in the body as well as the oral manifestations of chemotherapy can be recognized (Chapter 52).

I. LOCATION

Neoplasms may arise at any site in the oral cavity. The most common sites are the floor of the mouth, the lateral parts of the tongue, the lower lip, and the soft palate complex.

Although patients may be instructed in self-examination to watch for changes in oral tissues, it is difficult for persons to see their own tissues, particularly the entire floor of the mouth and base of the tongue, by the usual mirror and lighting systems available in a private home. Self-examination should be routinely supplemented with professional examination.

II. APPEARANCE OF EARLY CANCER

Early oral cancer takes many forms and may resemble a variety of common oral lesions. All types should be looked at with suspicion. Five basic forms are listed here.

A. White Areas

These may vary from a filmy, barely visible change in the mucosa to heavy, thick, heaped-up areas of dry white keratinized tissue. Fissures, ulcers, or areas of induration in a white area are most indicative of malignancy.

Leukoplakia is a white patch or plaque that cannot be scraped off or characterized as any other disease. It may be associated with physical or chemical agents and the use of tobacco.

B. Red Areas

Lesions of red, velvety consistency, sometimes with small ulcers, should be identified.

The term *erythroplakia* is used to designate lesions of the oral mucosa that appear as bright red patches or plaques that cannot be characterized as any specific disease.

C. Ulcers

Ulcers may have flat or raised margins. Palpation may reveal induration.

D. Masses

Papillary masses, sometimes with ulcerated areas, occur as elevations above the surrounding tissues. Other masses may occur below the normal mucosa and may be found only by palpation.

E. Pigmentation

Brown or black pigmented areas may be located on mucosa where pigmentation does not normally occur.

III. DIAGNOSTIC AID: TOLUIDINE BLUE[5]

A. Uses

1. *Initial Examination.* To identify mucosal changes that may be malignant.[6]
2. *Maintenance.* For patients previously treated for oral cancer and at risk for recurrence, the test may be an aid in recognizing early tissue changes.[7]

B. Application and Results

The test solution is used as a mouthrinse or applied topically with a cotton-tipped applicator. Lesions that retain the dye after decolorization with a post-rinse solution containing 1% acetic acid are deemed highly suspicious and should be biopsied.

■ PROCEDURE FOR FOLLOW-UP OF A SUSPICIOUS LESION

As designated by the dentist, a lesion may be biopsied immediately, a cytologic smear may be obtained, or the patient may be referred to various specialists for additional diagnosis and biopsy.

I. BIOPSY

A. Definition

Biopsy is the removal and examination, usually by microscope, of a section of tissue or other material from the living body for the purposes of diagnosis. A biopsy is either *excisional,* when the entire lesion is removed, or *incisional,* when a representative section from the lesion is taken.

B. Indications for Biopsy[8,9]

1. Any unusual oral lesion that cannot be identified with clinical certainty must be biopsied.
2. Any lesion that has not shown evidence of healing in 2 weeks should be considered malignant until proven otherwise.
3. A persistent, thick, white, hyperkeratotic lesion and any mass (elevated or not) that does not break through the surface epithelium should be biopsied.
4. Any tissue surgically removed should be submitted for microscopic examination.

II. CYTOLOGIC SMEAR

A. Definition

The cytologic smear technique is a diagnostic aid in which surface cells of a suspicious lesion are removed for microscopic evaluation.

B. Indications for Smear Technique[8]

1. In general, a lesion for which a biopsy is not planned may be examined by smear. An exception is a keratotic lesion that is not suitable for exfoliative cytology.
2. A lesion that looks like potential cancer should be examined by smear if the patient refuses to have a biopsy specimen taken. A positive report from a smear should convince the patient of the need for treatment or biopsy.
3. The smear technique is used for follow-up examination of patients with oral cancer treated by radiation. The treated tissue may heal inadequately and cause persistent ulceration.
4. Cytology is useful for identifying *Candida albicans* organisms in patients with suspected candidiasis (moniliasis).
5. Cytology may be useful in identifying herpesvirus by taking a smear from an intact vesicle.
6. In mass screening programs for cancer detection, smears may be taken. However, all lesions of high suspicion should be referred for biopsy.

7. Research studies to show changes in surface cells, for example, the effects of topical agents, may use a smear technique.

C. Limitations of Smear Technique

1. When a clear-cut lesion, recognized as pathologic, is present, treatment must not be delayed by waiting for cytologic smear analysis.
2. The smear detects only surface lesions.
3. It is difficult or impossible to scrape deep enough to obtain representative cells from a heavily keratinized lesion.
4. Except for candidiasis, treatment cannot be determined by smear technique results only. After a positive smear, a biopsy is needed for definitive diagnosis.
5. Because research has shown that the smear technique is not diagnostically reliable (there can be "false negatives," which turn out to be positive biopsies), a negative report should not be considered conclusive.

■ EXFOLIATIVE CYTOLOGY

Stratified squamous epithelial cells are constantly growing toward the surface of the mucous membrane, where they are exfoliated. Exfoliated cells and cells beneath them are scraped off, and when these cells are prepared on a slide, changes in the cells can be detected by staining and studying them microscopically. The malignant cells stain differently from normal cells and take on unusual, abnormal forms.

I. PROCEDURE

A. Materials

Gauze sponges
Glass microscopic slides with frosted end
Plain lead pencil
Paper clips
Blade to scrape lesion (flexible metal spatula)
Fixative (70% alcohol)
Protective mailing container
History form or data sheet

B. Steps

1. *Prepare Materials.* Write the patient's name on the frosted ends of two glass slides (two for each lesion) in pencil, and place a paper clip on the end of one slide to prevent contact between the slides when packaged for mailing to the laboratory.

2. *Prepare the Lesion*. Irrigate the surface to remove debris. Wipe the surface gently with a wet gauze sponge as needed to remove debris or blood. Do not dry.

3. *Scrape the Lesion*. Use a flexible metal spatula. Scrape the entire surface of the lesion firmly several times (all strokes in the same direction) (Figure 10-10A). When a wooden tongue depressor is used, it must be wet before taking the sample so the material will not be absorbed into the wood. For intact vesicles, carefully rupture the vesicle so the fluid flows onto the glass slides.

4. *Smear the Glass Slide*. Spread the collected material on the glass slide. Start at the center of the clear end of the slide and smear evenly across the surface. Cover an area approximately 20 mm wide. Handle all glass slides by their edges to prevent fingerprints or other contamination (Figure 10-10B).

5. *Fix the Cells*. Immediately, to prevent drying of the cells, place the slide on a flat surface and flood with generous drops of 70% alcohol or use prepared commercial fixative spray.

6. *Obtain Second Smear*. Duplicate the previous smear technique. Apply fixing agent immediately.

7. *Complete the Fixation*. Leave slides for 30 minutes. After 20 minutes, tip the slide to let remaining alcohol run off. Air dry where dust or other foreign material cannot contaminate the smear.

8. *Prepare History or Data Sheet*. Basic information includes the following:

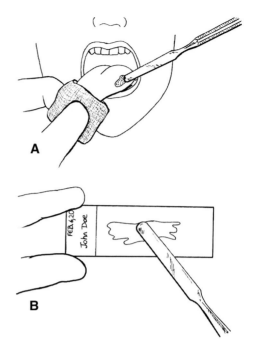

■ **FIGURE 10-10 Oral Cytology Technique. (A)** Tongue is held out with gauze sponge while a metal spatula is used to scrape a lesion. **(B)** Collected material is spread evenly on a glass slide. See text for details.

   a. Dentist. Name and address.
   b. Patient. Name and address.
   c. Lesion. Description (size, color, location, shape, consistency, and duration).
   d. Other. Additional related clinical findings or pertinent history.

Everyday Ethics

Abby and Sylvia are the two part-time dental hygienists in Dr. Anthony's practice. They work on different days at the office so rarely see each other except to attend local dental hygiene association meetings. Most patients know both hygienists and may be scheduled with either depending on available time.

Mr. Peters came in for his 3-month maintenance appointment carrying his unlit pipe as usual. This time his appointment was with Abby, and jokes were exchanged about the pipe. During the intraoral examination, Abby found a red lesion on the side of his tongue that was about 4 mm wide. She asked him if he had seen it and his answer was, "Oh yeah, Sylvia mentioned it when I was here last time." Abby glanced at the record and noted that his last date was over 4 months ago. Nothing could be found in the patient's dental record that mentioned any oral lesions.

Questions for Consideration

1. What ethical issues are involved here?

2. Since Dr. Anthony has never defined a policy for follow-up on such a finding, how should Abby proceed?

3. Privately, Abby is upset, and she is determined that this should be discussed with both Sylvia and Dr. Anthony. Where and how should she approach them and what recommendations does she need to propose for an office policy?

Factors To Teach The Patient

- Reasons for a careful extraoral and intraoral examination at each maintenance appointment.

- A method for self-examination. Examination should include the face, neck, lips, gingiva, cheeks, tongue, palate, and throat. Any changes should be reported to the dentist and the dental hygienist.

- General dietary and nutritional influences on the health of the oral tissues.

- How the oral cavity tends to reflect the general health.

- **The Warning Signs of Oral Cancer**

  - A swelling, lump, or growth anywhere, with or without pain.

  - White scaly patches, or red velvety areas.

  - Any sore that does not heal promptly (within 2 weeks).

  - Numbness or tingling.

  - Excessive dryness or wetness.

  - Prolonged hoarseness, sore throats, persistent coughing, or the feeling of a "lump in the throat."

  - Difficulty with swallowing.

  - Difficulty in opening the mouth.

9. *Prepare for Mailing.* Wrap slides to prevent breakage. Pack with the history or data sheet. Mailing containers provided by most laboratories list specific instructions.

II. LABORATORY REPORT

The pathologist makes the microscopic examination and classifies the specimen in one of the following categories:

Unsatisfactory: Slide is inadequate for diagnosis. The specimen may have been too thick or thin, or the cells may have dried before fixation. Another smear should be made promptly.

Class I: Normal.

Class II: Atypical, but not suggestive of malignant cells.

Class III: Uncertain (possible for cancer).

Class IV: Probable for cancer.

Class V: Positive for cancer.

III. FOLLOW-UP

A. Report of Class IV or V

Refer for biopsy.

B. Report of Class III

Reevaluate clinical findings; biopsy usually indicated.

C. Report of Class I or II

1. The patient must not be dismissed until the lesion has healed.
2. When lesion persists, the dentist either reevaluates the clinical findings and requests a repeat cytologic smear or performs a biopsy.

D. Negative Report

Either biopsy or smear requires careful follow-up when a negative report is obtained for an oral lesion that appears suspicious by clinical examination. False-negative reports are possible; that is, a malignancy may be present but the sample examined in the smear or biopsy may not have included cancerous cells.

REFERENCES

1. *Detecting Oral Cancer: A Guide for Health Care Professionals.* Available from National Oral Health Information Clearinghouse, 1 NOHIC Way, Bethesda, MD 20892-3500.
2. **Coakley,** M.C.: Temporomandibular Joint Dysfunction (TMJ): The Role of the Dental Hygienist, *J. Dent. Hyg., 62,* 521, November/December, 1988.
3. **McNeill,** C., Mohl, N.D., Rugh, J.D., and Tanaka, T.T.: Temporomandibular Disorders: Diagnosis, Management, Education, and Research, *J. Am. Dent. Assoc., 120,* 253, March, 1990.
4. **McCann,** A.L. and Wesley, R.K.: A Method for Describing Soft Tissue Lesions of the Oral Cavity, *Dent. Hyg., 61,* 219, May, 1987.
5. **OraScan,** Zila, Inc., 5227 North 7th Street, Phoenix, AZ 85014-2800.
6. **Warnakulasuriya,** K.A.A.S. and Johnson, N.W.: Sensitivity and Specificity of OraScan® Toluidine Blue Mouthrinse in the Detection of Oral Cancer, *J. Oral Pathol. Med., 25,* 97, March, 1996.
7. **Epstein,** J.B., Oakley, C., Millner, A., Emerton, S., van der Meij, E., and Le, N.: The Utility of Toluidine Blue Application as a Diagnostic Aid in Patients Previously Treated for Upper Oropharyngeal Carcinoma, *Oral Surg. Oral Med. Oral Pathol. Oral Radiol. Endod., 83,* 537, May, 1997.
8. **Sandler,** H.C. and Stahl, S.S.: Exfoliative Cytology as a Diagnostic Aid in the Detection of Oral Neoplasms, *J. Oral Surg., 16,* 414, September, 1958.
9. **Sabes,** W.R.: *The Dentist and Clinical Laboratory Procedures.* St. Louis, Mosby, 1979, pp. 109–113.

SUGGESTED READINGS

Abdel-Salam, M., Mayall, B.H., Chew, K., Silverman, S., and Greenspan, J.S.: Which Oral White Lesions Will Become Malignant? An Image Cytometric Study, *Oral Surg. Oral Med. Oral Pathol., 69,* 345, March, 1990.

Allen, C.M.: Diagnosing and Managing Oral Candidiasis, *J. Am. Dent. Assoc., 123,* 77, January, 1992.

Christian, D.C.: Computer-Assisted Analysis of Oral Brush Biopsies at an Oral Cancer Screening Program, *J. Am. Dent. Assoc., 133,* 357, March, 2002.

Cormier, L. and Lavelle, C.L.B.: The Dental Hygienist's Role in Screening for Oral Cancer, *Canad. Dent. Hyg. Assoc./Probe, 29,* 53, March/April, 1995.

DeMattei, R. and Aubertin, M.: Dental Hygiene Screening Reveals Childhood Neck Mass, *J. Dent. Hyg., 70,* 225, November–December, 1996.

Epstein, J.B. and Scully, C.: Assessing the Patient at Risk for Oral Squamous Cell Carcinoma, *Spec. Care Dentist., 17,* 120, July/August, 1997.

Flaitz, C.M. and Coleman, G.C.: Differential Diagnosis of Oral Enlargements in Children, *Pediatr. Dent., 17,* 294, July/August, 1995.

Hays, G.L., Lippman, S.M., Flaitz, C.M., Brown, R.S., Pang, A., Devoll, R., and Hong, W.K.: Co-carcinogenesis and Field Cancerization: Oral Lesions Offer First Signs, *J. Am. Dent. Assoc., 126,* 47, January, 1995.

Jones, A.C., Migliorati, C.A., and Stewart, C.M.: Oral Cytology: Indications, Contraindications, and Technique, *Gen. Dent., 43,* 74, January–February, 1995.

Layfield, L.L. Shopper, T.P., and Weir, J.C.: A Diagnostic Survey of Biopsied Gingival Lesions, *J. Dent. Hyg., 69,* 175, July–August, 1995.

Muzyka, B.C. and Glick, M.: A Review of Oral Fungal Infections and Appropriate Therapy, *J. Am. Dent. Assoc., 126,* 63, January, 1995.

Price, S.S. and Lewis, M.W.: Body Piercing Involving Oral Sites, *J. Am. Dent. Assoc., 128,* 1017, July, 1997.

Williamson, G.F. and Summerlin, D.-J.: Evaluating Oral Lesions: A Systematic Approach With Exercises, *J. Dent. Hyg., 66,* 264, July–August, 1992.

Zimmers, P.L. and Gobetti, J.P.: Head and Neck Lesions Commonly Found in Musicians, *J. Am. Dent. Assoc., 125,* 1487, November, 1994.

Temporomandibular Disorder

Dworkin, S.F.: Perspectives on the Interaction of Biological, Psychological and Social Factors in TMD, *J. Am. Dent. Assoc., 125,* 856, July, 1994.

Greene, C.S.: Managing TMD Patients: Initial Therapy is the Key, *J. Am. Dent. Assoc., 123,* 43, June, 1992.

Harriman, L.P., Snowdon, D.A., Messer, L.B., Rysavy, D.M., Ostwald, S.K., Lai, C.-H., and Soberay, A.H.: Temporomandibular Joint Dysfunction and Selected Health Parameters in the Elderly, *Oral Surg. Oral Med. Oral Pathol., 70,* 406, October, 1990.

Okeson, J.P.: Current Terminology and Diagnostic Classification Schemes, *Oral Surg. Oral Med. Oral Pathol., 83,* 61, January, 1997.

Pertes, R.A. and Cohen, H.V.: Guidelines for Clinical Management of Temporomandibular Disorders: Part 1, *Compend. Cont. Educ. Dent., 13,* 268, April, 1992.

Truelove, E.L., Sommers, E.E., LeResche, L., Dworkin, S.F., and von Korff, M.: Clinical Diagnostic Criteria for TMD: New Classification Permits Multiple Diagnoses, *J. Am. Dent. Assoc., 123,* 47, April, 1992.

Study Casts

As reproductions of the teeth, gingiva, and adjacent structures, study casts can be useful and frequently indispensable adjuncts in the assessment and care of a patient. Accurate and esthetically acceptable casts have a special use as visual aids for patient instruction.

The study casts, radiographs, and clinical examination with recordings and chartings, together with the medical and dental histories, are utilized in the diagnosis, total care planning, treatment, and subsequent maintenance.

I. PURPOSES AND USES OF STUDY CASTS

• To serve as a permanent record of the patient's present condition.
• To give sharper delineation to and corroboration of the observations made during the oral examination.
• To observe normal conditions and the variations of and departures from the normal at the outset

of treatment and, by comparison with subsequent periodic casts, to compare and evaluate certain aspects of treatment.

- During charting of the teeth, to note missing teeth; anomalies of size, shape, or number; partial eruption; tooth positions, such as drifting, tilting, rotation, and open or closed spacing.
- During examination of the occlusion, to observe the static relations (Angle's classification, malrelations of groups of teeth, and malpositions of individual teeth) and other features, such as wear patterns and the effects of premature loss of teeth.
- During periodontal charting, to record anatomic features, such as the position, size, and shape of the gingiva and interdental papillae and the position of frena.
- To be an effective visual aid to use when the oral conditions are explained and the dental and dental hygiene care plans are presented; to enable the patient to visualize and understand the need for the specific care outlined.
- To serve as a guide to clinical treatment procedures.
- To supplement clinical observations when the dental biofilm control program for the patient's daily self-care is explained.
- To provide assistance during forensic examination along with radiographs.

II. STEPS IN THE PREPARATION OF STUDY CASTS

Terms used to describe study casts and their preparation are defined in Box 11-1.

Procedures described in this chapter are as follows:

A. Clinical Procedures

1. Assemble materials and equipment.
2. Prepare the patient.

BOX 11-1 KEY WORDS: Study Casts*

Alginate: an aqueous impression material used for recording minimal detail such as for study casts.

Cast (model): a positive life-size reproduction of the teeth and adjacent tissues usually formed by pouring dental plaster or stone into a matrix or impression.

Diagnostic or study cast: used in the study of a patient's oral condition in preparation for treatment planning and patient instruction.

Master cast: used to fabricate a dental restoration or prosthesis.

Centric occlusion or habitual occlusion: the usual maximum intercuspation or contact of the teeth of the opposing arches.

Dental plaster: the beta form of calcium sulfate hemihydrate; a fibrous aggregate of fine crystals with capillary pores that are irregular in shape and porous in character; also referred to as plaster of Paris.

Dental stone: the alpha form of calcium sulfate hemihydrate with physical properties superior to those of the beta form (dental plaster); the alpha form consists of cleavage fragments and crystals in the form of rods and prisms and is therefore more dense than the beta form.

Impression: a negative imprint of an oral structure used to produce a positive replica of the structure; used to make casts for a permanent record or in the production of a dental restoration or prosthesis; usually identified by the type of material used, such as "hydrocolloid impression," "alginate impression," or "rubber base impression."

Interocclusal record: a registration of the positional relationship of the opposing teeth or dental arches made in a plastic material, such as a soft baseplate wax; also called the maxillomandibular relationship record or "wax-bite."

Occlusal plane: the average plane established by the incisal and occlusal surfaces of the teeth; generally not actually a plane, but the planar mean of the curvature of those surfaces.

Polish: to make smooth and glossy usually by friction; the act or process of making a cast smooth and glossy.

Prosthesis: an artificial replacement of an absent part of the human body; a therapeutic device to improve or alter function.

*Definitions in this chapter are taken or adapted from and in accord with *The Glossary of Prosthodontic Terms,* 7th ed. Academy of Prosthodontics Foundation, 1999.

3. Select and prepare the impression trays.
4. Make the interocclusal record for occluding the casts.
5. Make the mandibular impression.
6. Make the maxillary impression.

B. Paraclinical Procedures

1. Assemble materials and equipment.
2. Prepare the impression material for pouring.
3. Pour the casts.
4. Trim and finish the casts.
5. Polish the casts.

■ CLINICAL PREPARATION

I. ASSEMBLE MATERIALS AND EQUIPMENT

A. Coverall (plastic drape), towel, and mouthrinse.
B. Impression trays
   1. Perforated type generally used; small, medium, and large sizes are available.
   2. Trays for use in the patient's mouth must be disposable or clean, shiny, and sterilized metal.
C. Mixing bowl: clean, dry, flexible rubber or plastic with smooth, unscratched surface. Reserve separate bowls for each dental material: one always for impression material, another kept only for plaster or stone.
D. Spatula: clean, dry, stiff, with a smooth, rounded end that reaches every part of the bowl without scraping or cutting its surface.
E. Saliva ejector.
F. Dental materials
   1. Soft utility wax for preparation of tray rim.
   2. Alginate: irreversible hydrocolloid with manufacturer's measuring device.
   3. Soft baseplate wax for interocclusal record.
G. Water thermometer.

II. CLINICIAN PREPARATION

Standard precautions should be observed for all clinic procedures. A mask should always be worn when handling powder forms of dental materials to prevent inhalation.

III. PREPARE THE PATIENT

A. Antibiotic Premedication

- Review medical and dental histories for all possible precautionary needs.

- Plan for impressions when the patient who is at risk for bacteremia is protected and has received antibiotic coverage for other procedures.
- Check that the patient has taken the prescription one hour before.

B. Explain the Procedure to be Performed

The need for, and uses of, study casts are explained as with any procedure not familiar to the patient. The reactions of patients who have had an impression made previously may range from indifference to dread, and the conversation and approach can be directed accordingly.

C. Position the Patient

Position the patient upright for maximum visibility and accessibility and to minimize gagging. Stabilize the patient's head on the headrest.

D. Receive Removable Prostheses

Provide a container with water in which the patient can place removable oral prostheses.

E. Provide Preprocedural Mouthrinse

- To aid in the removal of saliva and debris and lessen the numbers of surface microorganisms.
- To lower the surface tension; aids in preventing bubbles in the impression.
- To provide a pleasant taste and feeling for the patient.
- To distract an anxious patient while the trays are being prepared.

F. Examine the Oral Cavity

Note facially displaced teeth, height of palate, undercut areas, mandibular tori, and other anatomic features that may influence the size or preparation of the impression tray and the procedures to be carried out during impression making.

G. Free the Mouth of Debris

When excess, tenacious debris is present, biofilm control instruction should be initiated or continued so that debris and biofilm can be removed during brushing by the patient.

H. Dry the Teeth

Use a cotton roll or compressed air stream to remove saliva from the teeth to prevent irregularities in the surface of the study cast.

I. Prevent Gagging

1. General approach
   - When the radiographic survey has been made for the new patient prior to the study casts, the clinician will have already determined whether precautions to prevent gagging are needed.
   - With all patients, a calm approach, an exhibition of confidence, a direct and efficient procedure, and a gentle handling of the patient's oral tissues increase rapport and contribute to a satisfactory result.
   - Suggestions are listed on page 155.
2. Technique considerations
   - Avoid excessive impression material in the tray.
   - Seat the maxillary tray from posterior to anterior, as described on page 193.
   - Instruct the patient to breathe deeply through the nose before the tray is inserted and to continue after insertion; bring head forward.

▪ THE INTEROCCLUSAL RECORD

I. PURPOSES

A. To relate the maxillary and mandibular casts correctly. Many, if not most, maxillary and mandibular casts orient to each other readily in only one position, but when such problems as open bite, crossbite, edentulous areas, and end-to-end or edge-to-edge relations interfere with direct occlusion of the casts, a bite registration is needed.

B. To place between the casts during trimming and storage to prevent breakage of teeth.

II. PROCEDURE

A. Numerous materials are available to obtain registration, such as wax and quick setting materials. Manufacturer's instructions for use are followed.

B. Request patient to practice opening and closing on the posterior teeth to ensure that the habitual position can be obtained.

C. Warm a shaped piece of soft baseplate wax or mix the bite registration material and place over the occlusal surfaces.

D. Guide patient to close in habitual occlusion.

E. Remove carefully to prevent distortion; chill wax in cold water. Disinfect.

▪ PREPARATION OF IMPRESSION TRAYS

I. SELECTION OF PROPER SIZE AND SHAPE

A. Width

1. Objective: to allow an adequate thickness of impression material on the facial and lingual surfaces of each tooth to provide strength and rigidity to the impression.
2. Tray flanges may be spread to accommodate for extra width in the molar regions, particularly lingual to the mandibular molars in the mylohyoid region.
3. When a tooth is in prominent labioversion, buccoversion, or linguoversion, a minimum thickness of 1/8 to 1/4 inch is suggested, but even then, the fragility of the impression material in that area is increased.
4. Tray: may appear in correct relation to the facial surfaces but may impinge on the lingual or palatal cusps of molars.

B. Length: Objectives

- To allow coverage of the retromolar area of the mandible and the tuberosity of the maxilla.
- Anterior: plan for at least 1/4-inch clearance labial to the most protruded incisor without impingement on lingual or palatal gingiva.

II. MAXILLARY TRAY TRY-IN

A. Position of Clinician

At side back of patient.

B. Retraction

1. With index finger of nondominant hand, retract the patient's lip and cheek.
2. At the same time, use the side of the tray to distend the other side of the patient's mouth to gain entry (Figure 11-1).

C. Insertion

1. With a rotary motion, insert the tray.
2. Orient the tray beneath the arch and center it by using the tray handle and the midline (usually between the central incisors and in line with the middle of the nose) as guides for positioning.
3. Bring the front of the tray to a position 1/4 inch labial to the most labially inclined incisor.

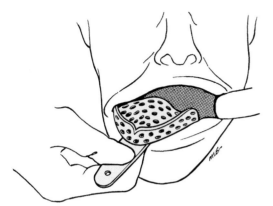

■ **FIGURE 11-1 Maxillary Tray Insertion.** The patient's lip and cheek are retracted with the fingers of the nondominant hand while the side of the tray is used to distend the other lip and cheek to gain entry. The tray is inserted with a rotary motion. The procedure for the mandibular tray is similar.

4. Seat the tray by bringing the posterior up before the anterior; retract the lip as the anterior is brought into place.

D. Evaluation of the Tray Size

1. Lower the front of the tray while holding the posterior border in place (Figure 11-2).
2. Examine the relationship of the posterior border to the most posterior molars and the tuberosity areas to determine whether the coverage will be ample.

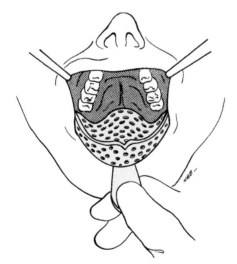

■ **FIGURE 11-2 Selection of Impression Tray.** Adequate coverage is determined as the posterior border of the tray is held in position while the front of the tray is lowered to observe the relationship of the posterior border to the maxillary tuberosity areas to be covered by the impression. The mandibular tray position is examined by lifting the tray to observe coverage of the retromolar areas.

3. Move the tray up and down to observe the relation to the facial surfaces of all teeth, malaligned teeth, protuberances, and other features and thus to assay the space allowed for the impression material.

III. MANDIBULAR TRAY TRY-IN

A. Position of Clinician

At side front of patient.

B. Retraction

1. With index and middle fingers of nondominant hand, retract the patient's lip and cheek.
2. At the same time, use the side of the tray to distend the side of the mouth to gain entry, similar to the procedure illustrated in Figure 11-1 for the maxillary tray.

C. Insertion

1. With a rotary motion, insert the tray.
2. Orient the tray over the dental arch and center it by using the tray handle and the midline (usually between the central incisors and in line with the center of the chin) as guides for positioning.
3. Bring the tray rim to about 1/4 inch anterior to the most labially positioned incisor; instruct the patient to raise the tongue to permit the lingual flange of the tray to pass by the lateral borders of the tongue without interference.
4. As the tray is lowered, retract the cheeks in the posterior regions to make certain the buccal mucosa is not caught beneath the edge of the tray; hold the lip out to ascertain that there is clearance to the base of the vestibule.

D. Evaluation of Tray Size

1. Lift the tray handle while keeping the posterior border of the tray in position, similar to the procedure illustrated in Figure 11-2 for the maxilla, to determine whether the coverage will be ample posteriorly to include the retromolar areas and laterally to allow for 1/4-inch thickness of impression material on the facial and lingual aspects of the teeth.
2. Reselect larger or smaller trays as indicated and repeat try-in. When in doubt, use the larger tray rather than the smaller.
3. Note tray sizes used in patient's permanent record for future reference.

IV. APPLICATION OF WAX RIM AROUND BORDERS OF TRAYS (BEADING)

A. Purposes

1. To prevent the metal tray rims from causing discomfort to the soft tissues.
2. To seat the vestibular periphery firmly into position with reduced pressure on the displaced tissues.
3. To prevent penetration of the incisal or occlusal surfaces through the impression material and thus to prevent a defective cast.
4. To provide a slight undercut at the rim as an aid in the retention of the alginate in the tray during placement and removal.
5. To create a posterior palatal seal to aid in preventing excess material from passing into the throat.

B. Procedure

1. *Application of Wax.* Attach a strip of soft utility wax firmly around the entire periphery of each tray (Figure 11-3).
2. *Mandibular Tray.* Add extra layers from canine to canine labially, and notch the wax to fit about the labial frenum.
3. *Maxillary Tray*
   a. Add extra layers as needed to extend the tray into the vestibule above the anterior teeth, and notch the wax to fit about the labial frenum (Figure 11-4A).
   b. Apply extra thickness across the posterior palatal seal area.
   c. When a patient has a high palatal vault, apply extra wax to support the impression material in that area.
4. *Try-in.* Try the rimmed trays in the mouth (Figure 11-4B); examine by retraction of the lips and cheeks and by use of a mouth mirror for lingual areas, hold the tray in position.

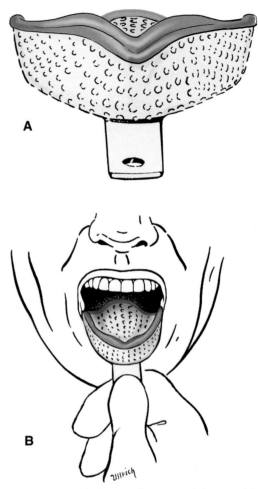

■ **FIGURE 11-4 Check the Beading Wax. (A)** Tray with double layer of beading wax about the labial frenum. The extra wax extends the tray, protects the soft tissue from the metal rim, and provides a more complete impression of the area. **(B)** Try-in after beading. The wax should contact all borders of the mucous membrane, displace the soft tissue outward, and prevent the teeth from contacting the tray.

5. *Characteristics of the Completed Molding.* When the tray is held firmly, all borders of the wax should contact the mucous membrane and displace the soft tissue outward and upward. The teeth do not touch the tray.

■ THE IMPRESSION MATERIAL

I. FACTORS RELATED TO THE IMPRESSION MATERIAL THAT CONTRIBUTE TO A SATISFACTORY IMPRESSION

Texts on dental materials should be reviewed for complete information about the irreversible hydrocolloids.[1,2] Properties related to the clinical procedures essential to

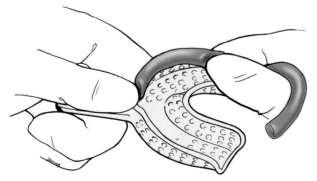

■ **FIGURE 11-3 Beading the Tray.** A strip of soft utility wax is applied around the periphery of each tray.

making an accurate impression are listed here. The manufacturer's directions are followed.

A. Powder

The alginate material deteriorates on standing, particularly at higher temperatures and humidity.
1. Keep metal container tightly closed; store in a cool place.
2. Use individually sealed packages to eliminate the problems of heat and moisture.
3. Individual package may be refrigerated in hot weather, provided the powder is used immediately on opening. If left exposed, water condenses on the powder. The bulk container cannot be refrigerated for that reason.
4. Do not agitate powders unnecessarily during mixing. Inhaled dust particles can cause serious irritation to the respiratory system.

B. Water

Temperature controls gelation time.
1. At room temperature, 20° to 21°C (68° to 70°F), an ideal gelation time between 3 to 4 minutes provides adequate working time.
2. Temperature of the water should be measured with a thermometer at the time of mixing.
3. For control in hot, humid weather, use cooler water and refrigerate the bowl and spatula.

C. Strength and Quality

The strength and quality of the finished impression depend on the following factors:
1. Powder/water ratio accurately weighed and measured.
2. Spatulation (1 minute) to homogenize, to remove bubbles, and to allow chemical reactions to proceed uniformly.
3. Holding the impression material in position for an optimum period in accord with manufacturer's specifications. The elasticity of most alginates improves with time; therefore, a superior reproduction can be obtained by waiting. Distortion can result when the impression is left in the mouth too long.

D. Surface Accuracy

The cast must be poured promptly to prevent loss of water from the impression. Permanent distortion can result.

II. MIXING THE IMPRESSION MATERIAL

Follow manufacturer's specifications precisely; total time lapse for mixing and insertion is approximately 2 minutes.
  A. Place measured water 20° to 21°C (68° to 70°F, measured with a thermometer) in a clean, dry mixing bowl.
  B. Sprinkle measured powder (from individually sealed package or premeasured from large container) into the water.
  C. Quickly incorporate the powder and water using a clean, dry, stiff spatula.
  D. Mix for 1 minute (clocked) vigorously, incorporating powder into the water, until a smooth, creamy mix is obtained.

III. TRAY PREPARATION

The mandibular impression is made first to introduce the patient to the procedure in an area where discomfort or gagging may be the least likely.

A. Working Time

The working time is 30 seconds.

B. Filling the Tray

1. Fill the tray from the posterior, being careful not to trap air bubbles.
2. Adapt the material to the tray thoroughly; press slightly through the perforations in the tray.
3. Do not overload; fill to a level just below the edge of the wax rim.
4. Wet index finger with cold water and pass lightly over the surface of the impression material; smooth the surface and make a slight indent where the teeth will insert.

C. Excess Material

Quickly gather the excess material from the bowl and bring the material on the spatula near to patient to use for precoating.

■ THE MANDIBULAR IMPRESSION

I. PRECOAT POTENTIAL AREAS OF AIR ENTRAPMENT

The precoat prevents air bubbles in the finished impression.
  A. Take a small amount of impression material from the spatula onto the index finger.

B. Apply quickly with a positive pressure to:
1. Undercut areas, such as distal surfaces of teeth adjacent to edentulous areas; cervical areas of erosion or abrasion; and gingival surfaces of fixed partial dentures.
2. Vestibular areas, particularly anterior areas about the frena.
3. Occlusal surfaces.

II. STEPS FOR INSERTION OF TRAY

A. Follow mandibular tray try-in. In summary, the procedure is as follows:
1. From 8 o'clock position (4 o'clock if left-handed), retract lip and cheek with fingers of nondominant hand.
2. Use side of tray to distend the other lip and cheek.
3. Rotate the tray into position, center it over the teeth, and introduce the tray 1/4 inch anterior to the facial surface of the most anterior incisor.
4. Instruct patient to raise the tongue while tray is lowered; retract cheeks and lip to clear the way for impression material to reach the base of the vestibule.
B. Seat the tray directly downward with a slight vibratory motion to aid in filling all crevices between the teeth.
C. Instruct the patient to extrude the tongue briefly to mold the lingual borders of the impression.
D. Apply equal bilateral pressure firmly, holding the middle fingers over the premolar regions and using the thumbs to support the mandible; or, if equal pressure can be maintained with one hand, place an index finger over the patient's premolar area on one side and the middle finger over the opposite side, with the thumb under the edge of the mandible for stabilization. Mold cheeks around the tray.
E. When the impression tray is held with one hand or when assistance is available, slip the saliva ejector in over the tray and then remove it before the tray is removed.
F. When the leftover material on the spatula has lost its surface stickiness (tackiness), hold the impression in position 2 more clocked minutes.

III. THE COMPLETED IMPRESSION

A. Removal of Impression

1. Hold tray with thumb and fingers.

2. Retract cheek and lip with fingers and release the edge of the impression by depressing the buccal mucosa.
3. Do not rock the impression back and forth to release it because these movements may cause permanent distortion of the final impression.
4. Remove the impression with a gentle jerk or snap.

B. Rinse

Rinse under cool running water to remove saliva, blood, and bacteria. Rinse carefully to prevent splashing contaminated saliva or blood over surroundings.

C. Examine and Evaluate the Impression

Observe surface detail, proper extension over retromolar area, and peripheral roll (rounded border of the impression) generally.

D. Repeat Procedure When Necessary

Correct mistakes rather than be satisfied with a substandard impression.

E. Storage

Disinfect then wrap mandibular impression in a wet towel while making the maxillary impression.

▪ THE MAXILLARY IMPRESSION

I. PREPARATION

A. Request Patient to Rinse

To clear particles left from the mandibular impression and to relax the oral muscles.

B. Examine the Maxillary Teeth

Examine for particles of mandibular impression material and remove. Request patient to use mouthrinse.

C. Prepare the Alginate

Fill the tray as described previously for the mandibular impression.

D. Precoat Undercut Areas

Precoat undercut areas, vestibular areas, and occlusal surfaces (see procedure for mandibular impression).

II. STEPS FOR INSERTION OF TRAY

A. Follow maxillary tray try-in. In summary, the procedure is as follows:
1. From 11 o'clock position (1 o'clock if left-handed), retract lip with fingers of nondominant hand.
2. Use side of tray to distend the lip and cheek.
3. Insert the tray with a rotary motion; center it over the teeth by using the small gap in the red wax border to relate to the labial frenum.
4. Introduce the material to the teeth so the wax rim is 1/4 inch facial to the most anterior incisor.

B. Seat the tray from posterior to anterior to direct the impression material forward and thus prevent irritation to the soft palate area.

C. Retract the lip and bring the tray to place with a slight vibratory motion to allow the material to flow into crevices and proximal areas.

D. The middle finger of each hand is placed over the premolar region to support and guide the tray; the index fingers and thumbs hold the lip out.

E. Request the patient to form a tight "O" with the lips to mold the impression material.

F. Maintain equal pressure on each side of the tray throughout the setting of the alginate. If assistance is available or if the pressure to hold the tray can be maintained with one hand, a saliva ejector can be inserted.

G. When the leftover material on the spatula has lost its surface stickiness, hold the impression in place for 2 more clocked minutes.

III. THE COMPLETED IMPRESSION

A. Remove Impression

Hold the tray handle with the thumb and fingers of the dominant hand, and retract the opposite lip and cheek with the fingers of the other hand. Elevate the cheek over the edge of the impression to break the seal, and remove the impression with a sudden jerk.

B. Rinse

Rinse under cool running water to remove saliva, blood, and bacteria. Rinse carefully to prevent dissemination of contaminated saliva and blood.

C. Examine

Examine surface detail and proper extension to include tuberosity areas and a complete reproduction of the height of the vestibule.

D. Repeat Procedure When Necessary

Repeat procedure rather than be satisfied with a substandard impression.

E. Disinfection

Proceed with disinfection for maxillary and mandibular casts.

■ DISINFECTION OF IMPRESSIONS[3,4]

To prevent cross-contamination during laboratory procedures, impressions should be disinfected in an approved disinfectant after rinsing. When impressions are to be sent to a laboratory, they should be isolated in a package. A sealable plastic bag can be used.

- Apply standard precautions; wear protective gloves, eyewear, and mask to handle contaminated impressions.
- Immerse to ensure maximum contact of the agent with all undercut areas. Impression then can be placed in the solution in a sealable plastic bag for 10 to 15 minutes.
- Discard disinfectant solution and rinse the impression under running water.

■ PARACLINICAL PROCEDURES

Supplemental to the chairside clinical procedures is the laboratory work involved in the production of the study casts from the impressions. These duties may be the responsibility of the dental laboratory technician or other dental team member.

The most frequent error in the use of the alginates for impressions is delay in pouring the cast. Undue dehydration or water loss from the alginate causes permanent distortion, an uneven surface, and hence an inaccurate cast. Regard for the sensitive properties of the dental materials, precision and practice in laboratory procedures, and pride in the production of neat, smooth, well-proportioned study casts determine the finished product's appearance, usefulness, and accuracy.

I. EQUIPMENT AND MATERIALS

A. Mixing bowl: clean, dry, flexible rubber or plastic, with smooth, unscratched surface. Separate bowls are reserved for each dental material.

B. Spatula: clean, dry, stiff, metal with a smooth, rounded end that can reach every part of the bowl without scraping or cutting its surface.

C. Plaster knife: sharp.
D. Vibrator with protective covering.
E. Mechanical mixer.
F. Model-base formers, glass or ceramic slab, waxed paper, or other nonabsorbent material.
G. Dental materials
1. Baseplate wax (and wax spatula).
2. White dental stone.
H. Water at room temperature, with measuring container.
I. Model trimmer.
J. Compass or dividers.
K. Plastic ruler.
L. Waterproof sandpaper.
M. Soap solution.

II. PREPARATION OF THE IMPRESSIONS

A. Rinse impressions under cool running water to remove residual disinfection that may affect the plaster or stone surface after pouring; shake out excess water gently and apply gentle blast of compressed air.
B. Create an artificial floor of the mouth in the mandibular impression to facilitate pouring and trimming of the cast.
1. Trim the lingual impression material all around so that the height is consistent from the occlusal and incisal surfaces to the base of the impression.
2. Using alginate:
a. Mix a small portion of alginate.
b. Hold the mandibular impression upright in the nondominant hand, with the middle and ring fingers extended from under the tray into the tongue area.
c. Apply alginate over the fingers to form a flat bridge slightly above the lingual flanges of the impression.
d. Smooth the surface with a finger moistened with cool water; hold until the alginate sets.
e. When assisted at the chair, the floor of the mandibular impression can be made while the maxillary impression is being held for setting. There is usually sufficient alginate mixed with that for the maxillary impression to use for this purpose.
3. Using baseplate wax:
a. Cut a piece of baseplate wax to the shape of the lingual periphery of the impression.
b. Seal into place with a warm spatula, taking care that no heat is applied to the anatomic portions of the impression.
c. Cool under running water.

■ MIXING THE STONE

I. FACTORS RELATED TO DENTAL STONE THAT CONTRIBUTE TO THE SUCCESSFUL CAST

Texts on dental materials should be reviewed for complete information about gypsum products.[5,6] Some pertinent properties are listed here as reference points.

A. Dental Stone

Sensitive to changes in the relative humidity of the atmosphere.
1. Store in airtight container; close soon after use; do not let water enter the container.
2. Keep the spoon or scoop (used to remove the powder) clean and dry.

B. Water

Controls the strength, rigidity, and hardness of the cast.
1. *Temperature.* Generally, cooler water decreases the setting time and warmer water increases it.
2. *Quantity.* Follow manufacturer's proportions exactly. Increasing the water over the specifications prolongs the setting time and reduces the strength.

C. Spatulation

Prolonged or very rapid mixing can hasten the chemical reaction and shorten the setting time.

II. THE MIX

A. Measure the water and powder by the manufacturer's specifications.
1. White stone is generally preferred for study casts. Plaster produces a cast more susceptible to breakage.
2. Ratio of 30 to 40 mL water to 100 g stone.
B. Place measured water (room temperature) in a clean, dry mixing bowl.
C. Sift in the powder gradually to prevent air trapping and to allow each particle to become wet.
D. Wait briefly until all powder is wet, then vibrate to release large bubbles.
E. Use vacuum mixer (follow manufacturer's directions).
F. The result is a smooth, homogeneous, creamy mix.

■ POURING THE CAST

The finished cast has two connected parts, the anatomic portion and the base or art portion (see Figure 11-5).

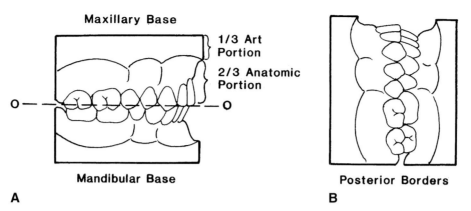

■ FIGURE 11-5 Finished Study Casts. (A) Proportions and planes. The *art* portion is one third and the *anatomic* portion two thirds of the total height of the cast. Note parallelism of the maxillary and mandibular bases with the mean occlusal plane (0—0). **(B)** Posterior borders are at right angles to the bases. When the maxillary and mandibular casts are placed on their posterior borders, the teeth intercuspate exactly.

I. POURING THE ANATOMIC PORTION

A. Shake water out of the impression.

B. Hold the impression tray by the handle and press handle against the vibrator.

C. With a small amount of stone mix on the end of the spatula, start at one posterior corner and allow the mix to flow through the impression. Use small amounts and vibrate continually.

1. Tip the impression so the material passes into the tooth indentations and flows slowly down the side, across the occlusal surface or the incisal edge, and up the other side of the impression of each tooth.

2. Air is trapped when the process is hurried or when too large a quantity of mix is poured in at one time without attentive control of the flow.

D. When all tooth indentations are covered, add larger amounts of mix to fill the impression slightly over the periphery. Vibrate.

II. ONE-STEP METHOD FOR FORMING THE BASE OF THE CAST

A. Fill rubber model-base former with the remainder of the mix, or form a mass of stone on a glass or ceramic slab or other nonabsorbent surface (waxed paper on a smooth surface). Add excess stone at the heel areas.

B. Invert the poured impression onto the base.

1. Use a slight back-and-forth motion to secure the two parts together.

2. Avoid the common error of inverting the impression before the stone is firm. The mix can flow out of the impression.

C. Adjust tray to proper position.

1. Occlusal plane (at premolars) should be parallel with the base of the model-base former or tabletop.

2. Midline (anterior as judged by handle of impression tray) centered at the midline of the model-base former.

3. Accommodate position so that a tooth in labioversion or buccoversion does not protrude over the trimming line of the art portion (see Figure 11-6).

D. Add stone on peripheral and heel areas to provide a smooth surface; remove excess so that wax periphery of the tray is visible. When excess stone above the edge of the tray rim is permitted to set, the tray is difficult to separate, and the use of a knife to carve the excess from the tray may damage the cast.

E. Final set occurs within 1 hour. Separate 1 hour after pouring to preserve the accuracy and prevent damage to the surface of the cast.

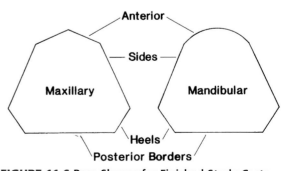
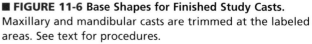

■ FIGURE 11-6 Base Shapes for Finished Study Casts. Maxillary and mandibular casts are trimmed at the labeled areas. See text for procedures.

III. OTHER METHODS FOR FORMING THE BASE OF THE CAST

A. Two-Step or Double-Pour

Both maxillary and mandibular impressions are poured and left upright (see "Pouring the Anatomic Portion," page 199). Stone is then prepared separately for the bases, and the model-base formers are filled or the mass is placed on the smooth nonabsorbent surface.

The impression is inverted and held on the surface of the new stone while the sides and periphery are shaped and smoothed. An advantage to this method is that there is no danger of inverting the poured impression too soon. If the cast is turned before it starts to set, the unset stone can fall away from the occlusal and incisal portions and leave bubbles in strategic places.

B. Boxing Technique

The object is to form a wall around the impression before pouring to provide a shape for the base as well as to prevent the need for inverting the poured impression. A strip of utility (beading) wax is attached slightly below the periphery of the impression and completely around the impression. Boxing wax or baseplate is applied around the strip of utility wax and attached to it by means of a warm spatula at a height that allows for proper thickness of the final cast, about 1/2 inch. Care must be taken not to displace the impression dimensionally or to touch the anatomic portions with the warm spatula. Pouring is carried out as described previously.

Work-model formers with side walls to provide the boxing effect are available. Such a mold has a slot through the rubber where the handle of the impression tray can be inserted.

IV. SEPARATION OF THE IMPRESSION AND THE CAST

A. Objective is to remove tray and impression material without breaking the teeth.
B. When model-based former is used, remove it first.
C. Cut away stone from the periphery to free the margin of the tray.
D. Remove the tray by itself.
E. Cut the impression material along the line of the occlusal surfaces and peel off the impression material (with care not to scratch the stone cast during cutting).
F. Direct removal is possible when the teeth are in reasonably normal alignment; remove the tray and the impression material with a straight pull after first releasing the anterior portion by a slight downward and forward movement. When this method is used, do not apply lateral pressures or

rock the tray back and forth, because the teeth are broken easily by such forces.
G. Trimming is started promptly, or if delayed, the cast must be thoroughly soaked in water before trimming.

▪ TRIMMING THE CASTS

The exact proportions of the study casts and the steps required to accomplish the trimming and finishing depend on several factors, including the measurements of the patient's dental arches, the positions of the teeth, and the preferences of the dentist. Development of a routine, systematic procedure for trimming can lead to the production of consistent, attractive, and useful diagnostic casts.

I. USE OF MODEL TRIMMER

- Precision-type model trimmer.
- Angulators that are available to fit on the table of the model trimmer to give average set angles for trimming the margins of the casts; when these are available, usually directions are supplied by the manufacturer.
- Use protective eyewear and mask while using a model trimmer. Goggles are indicated for laboratory procedures.

II. OBJECTIVES: CHARACTERISTICS OF THE FINISHED CASTS

Before the step-by-step description of the trimming procedure, an outline of the characteristics of the finished casts is provided as an overall guide. Table 11-1 lists the criteria for each cast feature.

III. PRELIMINARY STEPS TO TRIMMING THE CAST

A. Casts must be wet; soak at least 5 minutes.
B. Remove bubbles of stone on or about the teeth with a small sharp instrument; use care not to scar the cast.
C. Level down excess stone that is distal to the retromolar area and tuberosity so casts may be occluded. Do not shorten the cast anteriorly to posteriorly at this time.
D. Trim casts conservatively on the sides to make a smooth surface for marking.

IV. TRIMMING THE BASES

A. Objectives

1. To make bases parallel with the mean occlusal plane and to each other.

▪ TABLE 11-1 CRITERIA FOR AN ACCEPTABLE CAST		
CAST FEATURE	**CRITERIA**	**FIGURE NUMBER**
Overall base shape	See Figure 11-6 with labels	11-6
Proportions	1/3 art portion 2/3 anatomic portion	11-5A
Bases	Mean occlusal plane of the related casts = parallel with both bases Bases are parallel with each other	11-5A

Posterior borders	(1) At right angle with bases
	(2) Stand on the posterior borders: the casts rest
	  together in natural intercuspation
	(3) Posterior borders are perpendicular
	  (a) to median line from incisors through palate
	  (b) to middle of tongue
		11-5B
		11-5B
		
		11-7A
		11-7B

Sides	Symmetrical angulation with posterior border and heel cuts Parallel with line through the occlusal grooves of the premolars of each side	11-7 11-10A
Heels	1/2-inch cuts parallel with the mesiodistal plane of the opposite canine	11-10B
Anterior	Maxillary: pointed with the cuts extending from canine area Mandibular: arc shape	11-11A 11-11B

Borders	Posterior: includes retromolar area and tuberosity
	Sides: 1/4 to 5/16 inch from protuberance over premolars
	  and molars; anatomy of mucobuccal fold included
	Anterior: 1/4 to 5/16 inch from the most protruded tooth
	  or from the depth of the mucobuccal fold, whichever is most facial
		11-7
		
		11-11

Surfaces of the cast	Smooth and polished with air bubbles removed or filled	

2. To make correct proportions for the height of the casts; art portion one third and anatomic portion two thirds (Figure 11-7A).

B. Mandibular Cast Is Trimmed First

1. Measure the greatest height of the anatomic portion (usually this is from the tip of the canine to the depth of the vestibule) with a plastic ruler (Figure 11-8).

2. Divide by two to obtain the height of the art portion.

3. Add the measured height of the anatomic portion to the height of the art portion for the total height of the cast. Set compass or dividers at this measurement.

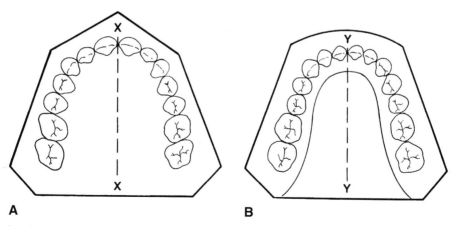

 A   B

▪ **FIGURE 11-7 Occlusal Views of Finished Casts. (A)** Maxillary. **(B)** Mandibular. The posterior border is perpendicular to the median line from the incisors through the palate (X—X) and the middle of the tongue (Y—Y). The tuberosity of the maxilla and the retromolar areas of the mandible are preserved.

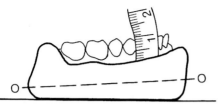

■ **FIGURE 11-8 Trimming the Base.** Measure the anatomic portion at its greatest height, which is usually from the tip of the canine to the depth of the vestibule. Note ruler in position. One half of the measurement is the height of the art portion. The trimming line (O—O) is parallel with the mean occlusal plane. See text for details.

4. Place the cast teeth down on a flat surface and mark a line around the art portion at the height calculated in step 3. This line should be parallel with the occlusal plane (line O—O in Figure 11-8). Trim the cast at the line.

C. Maxillary Cast Base

1. Measure the greatest depth of the anatomic portion (usually at the canine) and divide by two to obtain the height of the art portion.
2. Relate the two casts (use the wax bite if necessary) and place the mandibular base on the flat surface.
3. Measure from the base of the mandibular cast to the highest point of the maxillary anatomic portion (usually in the vestibule over the canine),

and add this figure to the height of the maxillary art portion calculated in step 1 above.

4. Set the compass at this measurement, and mark a line around the maxillary cast at the total height. The line must be parallel with the base of the mandibular cast and with the occlusal plane. Trim.

V. POSTERIOR BORDERS

A. *Select the longest cast to trim first* by measuring from the incisors to points distal to the retromolar and tuberosity areas.
B. On the longest cast, place the tip of the compass at the gingival border behind the midline anteriorly (usually this is between the central incisors) and mark an arc 1/4-inch distal to the tuberosity (if the maxillary cast) or retromolar area (if the mandibular cast) on each side.
C. Intersect the arc with a line through the central grooves of the molars (Figure 11-9A).
D. Connect the two points across the back of the cast (O—O in Figure 11-9A). Check that this line is perpendicular to the median line from the incisors through the palate or the tongue (X—Y in Figure 11-9B).
E. With the base of the cast flat on the model trimmer table, trim on the line marked for the posterior border.
F. For the shorter cast, relate the two casts with the wax bite and place flat on the base of the first

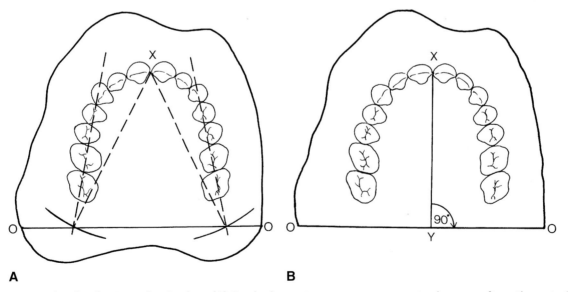

A   **B**

■ **FIGURE 11-9 Trim Line for Posterior Borders. (A)** On the longest cast, use a compass to draw arcs from the anterior midline point (X) to 1/4 inch distal to the tuberosity (maxilla) or retromolar area (mandible). Intersect the arc with a line through the central grooves of the molars and connect the two points across the cast (O—O). **(B)** Check that the O—O line is perpendicular to the median line from the incisors through the palate or tongue (X—Y) before trimming.

trimmed cast. Bring them carefully to the cutting surface of the model trimmer, and trim until the two posterior borders are even and parallel.

G. Check by placing the casts on their posterior borders and bringing them together. They should relate in their natural intercuspation (Figure 11-5B).

VI. SIDES AND HEELS

A. *Select the widest cast to trim first*; casts are usually widest at the molar region.

B. Mark with a ruler two symmetrical lines 1/4 inch buccal from the buccal bony prominence at the premolar regions and parallel with lines through the central grooves of the premolars (Figure 11-10A).
   1. Check that the lines form equal angles with the posterior border.
   2. Before trimming, make certain that the lines when cut would not remove any vestibular anatomy.
   3. Trim the sides with the base flat on the model trimmer table.

C. Mark trimming lines for the heels; cuts are 1/4-inch wide and parallel with a line through the mesiodistal plane of the opposite canine (Figure 11-10B). Trim with base flat on the model trimmer table.

D. Relate the opposite cast with the wax bite, and trim the sides and heels to match the previously trimmed cast.

VII. ANTERIOR

The maxillary cast is trimmed to a point, and the mandibular cast is rounded (Figure 11-6).

A. Maxillary

1. A ruler can be used to draw guidelines for trimming on each side of the midline to the canine areas. Note the broken lines in Figure 11-11A. The lines should be 1/4 inch labial to the depth of the mucobuccal fold (vestibule) or to the most labially inclined tooth.
2. Before trimming, check that both sides of the cast are the same length from the intersection of the front cut to the heels.

B. Mandibular

1. Sketch the shape of an arc from canine to canine to conform generally with the curvature of the anterior teeth and approximately 1/4 inch labial to the depth of the mucobuccal fold or the most labially inclined or positioned tooth (Figure 11-11B).
2. Before trimming, check that both sides of the cast are the same length from the intersection of the front cut to the heels.

VIII. FINISHING AND POLISHING

A. Trim rough edges and margins of both casts and the lingual portion of the mandibular cast to even

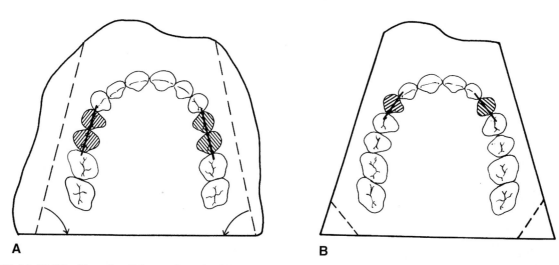

A   **B**

■ **FIGURE 11-10 Trim Lines for Sides and Heels. (A)** On the widest cast, trim lines for the sides are drawn parallel with lines through the central grooves of the premolars. The two symmetrical lines form equal angles with the posterior border of the cast. **(B)** Mark trim lines for heels 1/4 inch wide and parallel with lines through the mesiodistal plane of the opposite canine. The lines are symmetrical with each other and form equal angles with the posterior border.

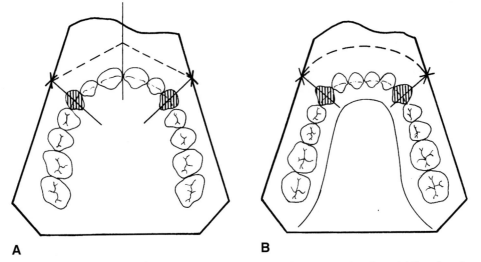

A   **B**

■ **FIGURE 11-11 Trim Lines for Anterior. (A)** Maxillary lines are drawn from opposite the middle of each canine to meet in a point at the midline and approximately 1/4 inch labial to the most labially positioned tooth. **(B)** Mandibular line forms an arc drawn from the middle of each canine approximately 1/4 inch labial to the most labially positioned tooth.

off irregularities and make the depth of the vestibule visible. Remaining bubbles are removed.

B. Use waterproof sandpaper and a plaster smoothing stone to remove marks left by the model trimmer on the art portion. Sandpaper is not used on the anatomic portion.

C. Fill any holes in the wet casts with stone applied with a spatula to the flat surfaces of the art portion or a camel's hair brush to the anatomic portion. Smooth off excess.

D. Finish and polish
1. Allow casts to dry thoroughly for 2 to 3 days.
2. Smooth the art portion with fine sandpaper.
3. Soak in heated soap solution for 30 to 60 minutes. Concentrated model gloss soap is available commercially.
4. Rub with chamois, cotton, or a soft cloth.

5. Talc or baby talcum powder with mineral oil may be used, followed by rubbing with a chamois or soft cloth.

IX. RECORDS AND STORAGE OF CASTS

- Label each cast with the patient's name and the date. These may be inscribed into the posterior border of the cast before soaping and polishing.
- Boxes of an appropriate size are available commercially for storage of one or more pairs of casts.
- Record in the patient's permanent record the size of impression tray used. When casts are made periodically for follow-up, time is saved both in the sterilization of all sizes for try-in and in the preparation of the wax rim in advance of the patient's appointment.

Everyday Ethics

? Everyone was rushing around the office trying to finish in time for lunch. Ylena was asked to take the impressions for whitening trays for Mrs. Lattoch. As Ylena places the maxillary tray, the patient begins to gag severely. Mrs. Lattoch pushes Ylena's arm out of the way and attempts to pull the tray out of her mouth. Ylena calls for assistance while forcefully restraining Mrs. Lattoch to keep the tray in until the impression material is set.

Questions for Consideration

1. Describe the ethical principle that best describes the actions of Ylena.

2. By restraining the patient, were the patient's rights violated? Why or why not? Explain the rationale.

3. Professionally, what choices could Ylena have exercised with Mrs. Lattoch to improve the outcome?

Factors To Teach The Patient

- Importance and purposes of study casts. Reasons for comparative casts following treatment or at a later date.

- Use the unidentified casts of other patients to show effects of treatment or what can happen if the prescribed treatment is not carried out.

- Areas that present difficulty in the dental biofilm control program:

    - Show anatomy of gingiva and teeth.

    - Demonstrate use of biofilm removal devices on the patient's own study casts.

- Make a duplicate cast for the permanent record when the dentist uses the original for the design of a prosthesis or fabrication of a secondary impression tray. The duplicate cast is made by taking an alginate impression of the original and pouring it in the same manner as the original.

REFERENCES

1. **Gladwin**, M. and Bagby, M.: *Clinical Aspects of Dental Materials.* Philadelphia, Lippincott Williams & Wilkins, 2000, pp. 99–100, 247–253.

2. **Ferracane**, J.L.: *Materials in Dentistry,* 2nd ed. Philadelphia, Lippincott Williams & Wilkins, 2001, pp. 179,184–188.

3. **American Dental Association**, Council on Scientific Affairs and Council on Dental Practice: Infection Control Recommendations for the Dental Office and the Dental Laboratory, *J. Am. Dent. Assoc., 127,* 672, May, 1996.

4. **Thouati**, A., Deveaux, E., Iost, A., and Behin, P.: Dimensional Stability of Seven Elastomeric Impression Materials Immersed in Disinfectants, *J. Prosthet. Dent., 76,* July 8, 1996.

5. **Gladwin** and Bagby: op. cit., pp. 107–113, 265–272.

6. **Ferracane**: op. cit., pp. 203–220.

SUGGESTED READINGS

Andrieu, S.C. and Springstead, M.C.: A Simplified Guide to Taking Accurate Alginate Impressions and Trimming Diagnostic Study Casts, *J. Pract. Hyg., 1,* 11, September, 1992.

Berry, T.G. and Berry, J.C.: Preparation of Study Models, in Woodall, I.R.: *Comprehensive Dental Hygiene Care,* 4th ed. St. Louis, Mosby, 1993, pp. 312–335.

Pratten, D.H. and Novetsky, M.: Detail Reproduction of Soft Tissue: a Comparison of Impression Materials, *J. Prosthet. Dent., 65,* 188, February, 1991.

Torres, H.O., Ehrlich, A., Bird, D., and Dietz, E.: *Modern Dental Assisting,* 5th ed. Philadelphia, W.B. Saunders, 1995, pp. 355–376.

Infection Control

Chia, W.K., Stevens, L., and Basford, K.E.: Dimensional Change of Impressions on Sterilization, *Aust. Dent. J., 35,* 23, February, 1990.

del Pilar Rios, M., Morgano, S.M., Stein, R.S., and Rose, L.: Effects of Chemical Disinfectant Solutions on the Stability and Accuracy of the Dental Impression Complex, *J. Prosthet. Dent., 76,* 356, October, 1996.

Gerhardt, D.E. and Williams, H.N.: Factors Affecting the Stability of Sodium Hypochlorite Solutions Used to Disinfect Dental Impressions, *Quintessence Int., 22,* 587, July, 1991.

King, B.B., Norling, B.K., and Seals, R.: Gypsum Compatibility of Antimicrobial Alginates After Spray Disinfection, *J. Prosthodont., 3,* 219, December 1994.

Mitchell, D.L., Hariri, N.M., Duncanson, M.G., Jacobsen, N.L., and McCallum, R.E.: Quantitative Study of Bacterial Colonization of Dental Casts, *J. Prosthet. Dent., 78,* 518, November, 1997.

Peutzfeldt, A. and Asmussen, E.: Effect of Disinfecting Solutions on Surface Texture of Alginate and Elastomeric Impressions, *Scand. J. Dent. Res., 98,* 74, February, 1990.

Samaranayake, L.P., Hunjan, M., and Jennings, K.J.: Carriage of Oral Flora on Irreversible Hydrocolloid and Elastomeric Impression Materials, *J. Prosthet. Dent., 65,* 244, February, 1991.

Touyz, L.Z.G. and Rosen, M.: Disinfection of Alginate Impression Material Using Disinfectants as Mixing and Soak Solutions, *J. Dent., 19,* 255, August, 1991.

Verran, J., Kossar, S., and McCord, J.F.: Microbial Study of Selected Risk Areas in Dental Technology Laboratories, *J. Dent., 24,* 77, January/March, 1996.

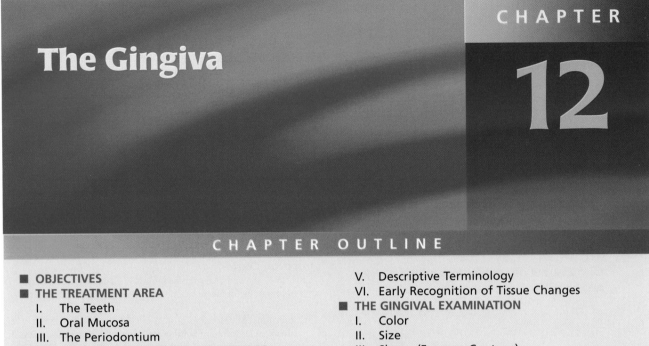

The Gingiva

CHAPTER OUTLINE

The true test of successful treatment, the real evaluation of the effects of scaling and related instrumentation, is the *health* of the gingival tissues. The objective of all treatment is to bring the diseased gingiva to a state of health that can be maintained by the patient. To do this, the first objective is to learn to recognize normal healthy tissue; to observe certain characteristics of color, texture, and form; to test for bleeding; and to apply this knowledge to the treatment and supervision of the patient's gingiva until health is attained.

An outline of the clinical features of the periodontal tissues in health and disease is included in this chapter. Key words are defined in Box 12-1.

■ OBJECTIVES

The ultimate objective is to apply knowledge and skill in examination and assessment of the periodontal tissues to patient care so that each patient attains and maintains optimum oral health. The dental hygienist must know when the treatment provided by dental hygiene services is definitive in restoring health and when additional treatment is needed. The patient can be properly informed so that complete treatment can be provided.

Specific objectives are to be able to

- Recognize normal periodontal tissues.
- Know the clinical features of the periodontal tissues that must be examined for a complete assessment.
- Recognize the markers that are the basic signs of periodontal infections and classify them by type and degree of severity.
- Identify the dental hygiene treatment and instruction needed.
- Outline the patient's preventive program.

BOX 12-1 KEY WORDS: Gingiva and Periodontium

Attachment apparatus: the cementum, periodontal ligament, and the alveolar bone.

Clinical attachment level: the probing depth measured from a fixed point, such as the cementoenamel junction.

Desmosome: cell junction; consists of a dense plate near the cell surface that relates to a similar structure on an adjacent cell, between which are thin layers of extracellular material.

Diastema: a space between two natural adjacent teeth. Plural, diastemata. See also Primate space, page 284.

Epithelium

    Oral: the tissue serving as a liner for the intraoral mucosal surfaces.

    Squamous: composed of a layer of flat, scalelike cells; or may be stratified.

Fibroblast: fiber-producing cell of the connective tissue; a flattened, irregularly branched cell with a large oval nucleus that is responsible in part for the production and remodeling of the extracellular matrix.

Fibrosis: a fibrous change of the mucous membrane, especially the gingiva, as a result of chronic inflammation; fibrotic gingiva may appear outwardly healthy, thus masking underlying disease.

Hemidesmosome: half of a desmosome that forms a site of attachment between junctional epithelial cells and the tooth surface.

Hyperkeratosis: abnormal thickening of the keratin layer (stratum corneum) of the epithelium.

Hyperplasia: abnormal increase in volume of a tissue or organ caused by formation and growth of new normal cells.

Hypertrophy: increase in size of tissue or organ caused by an increase in size of its constituent cells.

Keratinization: development of a horny layer of flattened epithelial cells containing keratin.

Marker: identifier; symptoms or signs by which a particular condition can be recognized; for example, clinical and microbiologic markers are used to identify gingival and periodontal infections.

Mastication: act of chewing.

Nonkeratinized mucosa: lining mucosa in which the stratified squamous epithelial cells retain their nuclei and cytoplasm.

Periodontium: tissues surrounding and supporting the teeth; in two sections are the **gingival unit,** composed of the free and attached gingiva and the alveolar mucosa, and the **attachment apparatus,** which includes the cementum, periodontal ligament, and alveolar process.

Probing depth: the distance from the gingival margin to the location of the periodontal probe tip inserted for gentle probing at the attachment.

Pus: a fluid product of inflammation that contains leukocytes, degenerated tissue elements, tissue fluids, and microorganisms.

Sharpey's fibers: penetrating connective tissue fibers by which the tooth is attached to the adjacent alveolar bone; the fiber bundles penetrate cementum on one side and alveolar bone on the other.

Stippling: the pitted, orange-peel appearance frequently seen on the surface of the attached gingiva.

Suppuration: formation of pus.

Taste bud: receptor of taste on tongue and oropharynx; goblet-shaped cells oriented at right angles to the surface of the epithelium.

■ THE TREATMENT AREA

The treatment procedures are applied directly to the teeth, the gingiva, and the gingival sulcus. Detailed knowledge and understanding of the anatomy and normal clinical appearance of the hard and soft oral tissues are prerequisite to meaningful examination and treatment.

I. THE TEETH

A. Clinical Crown

The part of the tooth above the attached periodontal tissues. It can be considered the part of the tooth where clinical treatment procedures are applied (Figure 12-1).

B. Clinical Root

The part of the tooth below the base of the gingival sulcus or periodontal pocket. It is the part of the root to which periodontal fibers are attached.

C. Anatomic Crown

The part of the tooth covered by enamel.

D. Anatomic Root

The part of the tooth covered by cementum.

II. ORAL MUCOSA

The lining of the oral cavity, the oral mucosa, is a mucous membrane composed of connective tissue covered with stratified squamous epithelium. There are three divisions or categories of oral mucosa.

A. Masticatory Mucosa

1. Covers the *gingiva* and the *hard palate,* the areas used most during the mastication of food.
2. Except for the free margin of the gingiva, the masticatory mucosa is firmly attached to underlying tissues.
3. The epithelial covering is generally keratinized.

B. Lining Mucosa

1. Covers the *inner surfaces of the lips and cheeks, the floor of the mouth, the under side of the tongue, the soft palate, and the alveolar mucosa.*
2. These tissues are not firmly attached to underlying tissue.
3. The epithelial covering is not generally keratinized.

C. Specialized Mucosa

1. Covers the *dorsum (upper surface) of the tongue.* It is composed of many papillae; some contain taste buds.
2. The distribution of the four types of papillae is shown in Figure 12-2.
   a. *Filiform.* Threadlike keratinized elevations that cover the dorsal surface of the tongue; they are the most numerous of the papillae.
   b. *Fungiform.* Mushroom-shaped papillae interspersed among the filiform papillae on the tip and sides of the tongue. They are redder than the filiform papillae and contain variable numbers of taste buds. The inset enlargement in Figure 12-2 shows the comparative shape and size of the filiform and fungiform papillae.

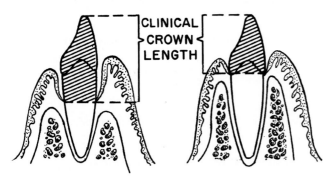

■ **FIGURE 12-1 Clinical Crown.** The clinical crown is the part of the tooth that is above the attached periodontal tissue. *Left,* When the periodontal pocket depth is increased, the clinical crown extends to a position at which the clinical crown length is greater than the clinical root length. The clinical root is that part of the tooth with attached periodontal tissues. *Right,* When the clinical attachment level is at the cementoenamel junction, the clinical crown and the anatomic crown are the same.

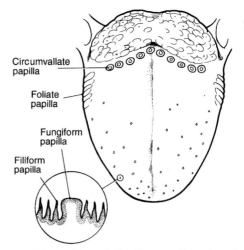

■ **FIGURE 12-2 Papillae of the Tongue.** Dorsal surface of a human tongue shows the four types of papillae. Inset enlargement shows the shape of filiform and fungiform papillae.

c. *Circumvallate (vallate)*. The 10 to 14 large round papillae arranged in a "V" between the body of the tongue and the base. Taste buds line the walls.

d. *Foliate*. Vertical grooves on the lateral posterior sides of the tongue; also contain taste buds.

III. THE PERIODONTIUM

The periodontium is the functional unit of tissues that surrounds and supports the tooth. The four parts are the gingiva, periodontal ligament, cementum, and bone; the last three make up the attachment apparatus.

A. Periodontal Ligament

The periodontal ligament is the fibrous connective tissue that surrounds and attaches the roots of teeth to the alveolar bone.

The ligament is located in the periodontal space between the cementum and the alveolar bone. It is composed of connective tissue cells and intracellular substance. The fibers that are inserted into the cementum on one side and the alveolar bone on the other are called *Sharpey's fibers*.

The two general groups of fibers are the *gingival groups* (around the cervical area within the gingival tissues) and the *principal fiber groups* (surrounding the root).[1]

1. *Gingival Fiber Groups* (Figure 12-3)

a. **Dentogingival fibers** (free gingival). From the cementum in the cervical region into the free gingiva to give support to the gingiva.

b. **Alveologingival fibers** (attached gingival). From the alveolar crest into the free and attached gingiva to provide support.

c. **Circumferential fibers** (circular). Continuous around the neck of the tooth to help to maintain the tooth in position.

d. **Dentoperiosteal fibers** (alveolar crest). From the cervical cementum over the alveolar crest to blend with fibers of the periosteum of the bone.

e. **Transseptal fibers**. From the cervical area of one tooth across to an adjacent tooth (on the mesial or distal only) to provide resistance to separation of teeth (Figure 12-4).

2. *Principal Fiber Groups* (Figure 12-4)

The five principal groups of collagen fibers are named for their location on the root and for their direction. They are also called the dentoalveolar fiber groups.

a. **Apical fibers**. From the root apex to adjacent surrounding bone to resist vertical forces.

b. **Oblique fibers**. From the root above the apical fibers obliquely toward the occlusal to resist vertical and unexpected strong forces.

c. **Horizontal fibers**. From the cementum in the middle of each root to adjacent alveolar bone to resist tipping of the tooth.

d. **Alveolar crest fibers**. From the alveolar crest to the cementum just below the cementoenamel junction to resist intrusive forces.

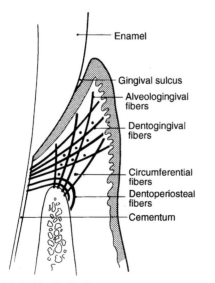

■ FIGURE 12-3 Gingival Fiber Groups. Cross section of the gingiva shows the relation of the gingival fiber groups to the gingival sulcus, the free gingiva, the cementum, and the alveolar bone.

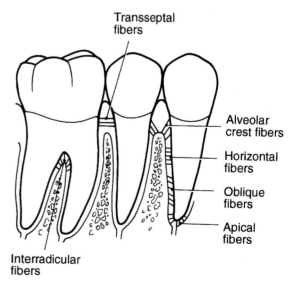

■ FIGURE 12-4 Principal Fiber Groups of the Periodontium. The five principal groups (apical, oblique, horizontal, alveolar crest, and interradicular) are shown. The transseptal fibers of the gingival fiber groups are also shown as they span across from the cervical area of one tooth to the neighboring tooth.

e. **Interradicular fibers.** From cementum between the roots of multirooted teeth to the adjacent bone to resist vertical and lateral forces.

B. Cementum

The cementum is a thin layer of calcified connective tissue that covers the tooth from the cementoenamel junction to, and around, the apical foramen.
1. *Functions*
   a. To seal the tubules of the root dentin.
   b. To provide attachment for the periodontal fiber groups.
2. *Characteristics*
   a. Thickness is 50 to 200 μm about the apex; 30 to 60 μm about the cervical area.
   b. Vascular and nerve connections are missing; therefore, cementum is insensitive.
   c. Relationship of enamel and cementum at the cervical area is shown elsewhere.

C. Alveolar Bone

The alveolar bone consists of the lamina dura, which surrounds the tooth socket, and the supporting bone. When teeth are lost, the alveolar bone is resorbed. The bone functions to support the teeth and provide attachment for the periodontal ligament fibers.

D. Gingiva

The part of the masticatory mucosa that surrounds the necks of the teeth and is attached to the teeth and the alveolar bone.

▪ THE GINGIVA AND RELATED STRUCTURES

The gingiva is made up of the free gingiva, the attached gingiva, and the interdental gingiva or interdental papilla.

I. FREE GINGIVA (MARGINAL GINGIVA)

In health, the free gingiva is closely adapted around each tooth. It connects with the attached gingiva at the free gingival groove and attaches to the tooth at the coronal portion of the junctional epithelium (Figure 12-5).

A. Free Gingival Groove

- The free gingival groove is a shallow linear groove that demarcates the free from the attached gingiva. Generally, about one-third of the teeth show a visible gingival groove when the gingiva is healthy.[2]

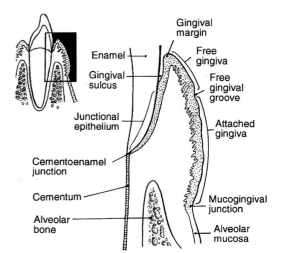

■ **FIGURE 12-5 Parts of the Gingiva.** Cross-sectional diagram shows the parts of the gingiva and adjacent tissues of a partially erupted tooth. Note that the junctional epithelium is on the enamel.

- In the absence of inflammation and pocket formation, the gingival groove runs somewhat parallel with and about 0.5 to 1.5 mm from the gingival margin,[3] and it is approximately at the level of the bottom of the gingival sulcus.

B. Oral Epithelium (outer gingival epithelium, Figure 12-6)

- Covers the free gingiva from the gingival groove over the gingival margin.
- Composed of keratinized stratified squamous epithelium.

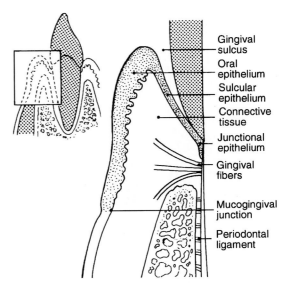

■ **FIGURE 12-6 The Gingival Tissues.** Cross-sectional diagram shows the histologic relationships of the oral, sulcular, and junctional epithelia and the connective tissue.

C. Gingival Margin (gingival crest, margin of the gingiva, or free margin, Figure 12-5)

- This is the edge of the gingiva nearest the incisal or occlusal surface.
- Marks the opening of the gingival sulcus.

II. GINGIVAL SULCUS (CREVICE)

A. Location

The crevice or groove between the free gingiva and the tooth.

B. Boundaries (Figure 12-6)

1. *Inner.* Tooth surface. May be the enamel, cementum, or part of each, depending on the position of the junctional epithelium.
2. *Outer.* Sulcular epithelium.
3. *Base.* Coronal margin of the attached tissues. The base of the sulcus or pocket is also called the "probing depth," the "depth of the sulcus," or the "bottom of the pocket."

C. Sulcular Epithelium

The continuation of the oral epithelium covering the free gingiva. Sulcular epithelium is not keratinized.

D. Depth of Sulcus

Healthy sulci are shallow and may be only 0.5 mm. The average depth of the healthy sulcus is about 1.8 mm.[4]

E. Gingival Sulcus Fluid (sulcular fluid, crevicular fluid)

1. A serumlike fluid that seeps from the connective tissue through the epithelial lining of the sulcus or pocket.

2. Occurrence is slight to none in a normal sulcus; increased with inflammation. It is part of the local defense mechanism and is able to transport many substances, including endotoxins, enzymes, antibodies, and certain systemically administered drugs.

III. JUNCTIONAL EPITHELIUM (ATTACHMENT EPITHELIUM)

A. Description

The junctional epithelium is a cufflike band of stratified squamous epithelium that is continuous with the sulcular epithelium and completely encircles the tooth. It is triangular in cross section, is widest at the junction with the sulcular epithelium, and narrows down to the width of a few cells at the apical end.

The junctional epithelium is not keratinized. It has two basement membranes: one adjacent to the connective tissue and one adjacent to the tooth surface.

B. Size

The junctional epithelium may be up to 15 or 20 cells in thickness where it joins the sulcular epithelium and tapers down to 1 or 2 cells in thickness at the apical end. The length ranges from 0.25 to 1.35 mm.

C. Position

1. As the tooth erupts, the attachment is on the enamel; during eruption, the epithelium migrates toward the cementoenamel junction (Figure 12-7).
2. At full eruption, the attachment is usually on the cementum, where it becomes firmly attached (Figure 12-7D).
3. With wear of the tooth on the incisal or occlusal surface and with periodontal infections, the attachment migrates along the root surface (Figure 12-7E).

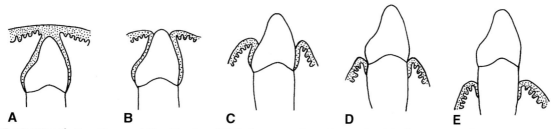

■ **FIGURE 12-7 Tooth Eruption and the Gingiva. (A)** Before eruption, the oral epithelium covers the tooth. **(B)** As the tooth emerges, the reduced epithelium joins the oral epithelium as the gingival sulcus is formed. **(C)** Partial eruption with the junctional epithelium along the enamel. **(D)** Eruption complete, with junctional epithelium at the cementoenamel junction. **(E)** From disease or other cause, the attachment migrates along the root surface, exposing the cementum.

D. Relation of Crest of Alveolar Bone to the Attached Gingival Tissue

The distance between the base of the attachment and the crest of the alveolar bone is approximately 1.0 to 1.5 mm. This distance is maintained in disease when the epithelium moves along the root surface and bone loss occurs.

E. Attachment of the Epithelium to the Tooth Surface

The junctional epithelium or attachment epithelium provides a seal at the base of the sulcus. The attachment, or connecting interface between the tooth and the tissue, is accomplished by hemidesmosomes and the basal lamina of the junctional epithelium.

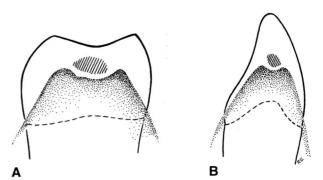

A   **B**

■ **FIGURE 12-8 Col.** A col is the depression between the lingual or palatal and the facial papillae under the contact area. The contact area is represented by the striped lines. **(A)** Mesial of mandibular molar to show wide col area. **(B)** Mesial of mandibular incisor to show a narrow col. The col deepens when gingival enlargement occurs.

IV. INTERDENTAL GINGIVA (INTERDENTAL PAPILLA)

A. Location

In health, the interdental gingiva occupies the interproximal area between two adjacent teeth. The tip and lateral borders are continuous with the free gingiva, whereas other parts are attached gingiva.

B. Shape

1. *Varies With Spacing or Overlapping of the Teeth.* The interdental gingiva may be flat or saddle-shaped when wide spaces are between the teeth, or it may be tapered and narrow when the teeth are crowded or overlapped.
2. *Between Anterior Teeth.* Pointed, pyramidal.
3. *Between Posterior Teeth*
   a. Flatter than anterior papillae because of wider teeth, wider contact areas, and flattened interdental bone.
   b. Two papillae, one facial and one lingual, connected by a col, are found when teeth are in contact.

C. Col

1. A col is the depression between the lingual or palatal and facial papillae that conforms to the proximal contact area (Figure 12-8).
2. The center of the col area is not usually keratinized and thus is more susceptible to infection. Most periodontal infection begins in the col area.

V. ATTACHED GINGIVA

A. Extent

1. The attached gingiva is continuous with the oral epithelium of the free gingiva and is covered with keratinized stratified squamous epithelium.
2. Maxillary palatal gingiva is continuous with the palatal mucosa.
3. The attached gingiva of the mandibular facial and lingual gingiva and maxillary facial gingiva is demarcated from the alveolar mucosa by the mucogingival junction.

B. Attachment

Firmly bound to the underlying cementum and alveolar bone.

C. Shape

Follows the depressions between the eminences of the roots of the teeth.

VI. MUCOGINGIVAL JUNCTION

A. Appearance

The mucogingival junction appears as a line that marks the connection between the attached gingiva and the alveolar mucosa. The anterior line is scalloped, but it is fairly straight posterior to the premolars.

A contrast can be seen between the pink of the keratinized, stippled, attached gingiva and the darker alveolar mucosa.

B. Location

A mucogingival line is found on the facial surface of all quadrants and on the lingual surface of the mandibular arch. There is no alveolar mucosa on the palate. The palatal tissue is firmly attached to the bone of the roof of the mouth.

The three mucogingival lines are facial mandibular, lingual mandibular, and facial maxillary. In Figure 12-9, the facial maxillary and mandibular mucogingival junctions are shown in relation to the attached gingiva and the alveolar mucosa.

VII. ALVEOLAR MUCOSA

A. Description

Movable tissue loosely attached to the underlying bone. It has a smooth, shiny surface with nonkeratinized, thin epithelium. Underlying vessels may be seen through the epithelium.

B. Frena (singular: frenum or frenulum)

1. *Description.* A frenum is a narrow fold of mucous membrane that passes from a more fixed to a movable part, for example, from the attached gingiva at the mucogingival junction to the lip, cheek, or undersurface of the tongue. A frenum serves to check undue movement.
2. *Locations*
   a. Maxillary and mandibular anterior frena. At midlines between central incisors. Figure 12-9 shows diagrammatically the location of the anterior frena.
   b. Lingual frenum. From undersurface of the tongue.
   c. Buccal frena. In the canine–premolar areas, both maxillary and mandibular.

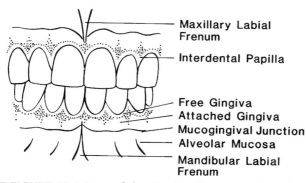

Maxillary Labial Frenum

Interdental Papilla

Free Gingiva
Attached Gingiva
Mucogingival Junction
Alveolar Mucosa

Mandibular Labial Frenum

■ **FIGURE 12-9 Parts of the Gingiva.** The mucogingival junction for each arch is shown in relation to the attached gingiva, alveolar mucosa, and labial anterior frena.

3. *Attachment of Frena in Relation to the Attached Gingiva*
   a. Closely associated with the mucogingival junction.
   b. When the attached gingiva is narrow or missing, the frena may pull on the free gingiva and displace it laterally. A "tension test" is used to locate frenal attachments and check the adequacy of the attached gingiva.

■ THE RECOGNITION OF GINGIVAL AND PERIODONTAL INFECTIONS

I. THE CLINICAL EXAMINATION

The recognition of normal gingiva, gingival infections, and deeper periodontal involvement depends on a disciplined, step-by-step examination. A basic examination performed to recognize the signs and effects of inflammation includes information about at least the following markers:
- Gingival tissue changes (color, size, shape, surface texture, position).
- Bleeding and exudates.
- Mucogingival involvement (adequate width of attached gingiva).
- Probing depths; pocket formation (attachment levels).
- Furcation involvement.
- Dental biofilm (and calculus) present.
- Mobility of teeth.
- Radiographic evidence.

It is also necessary to know the extent of the disease. *Gingival infections* are confined to the gingiva, whereas *periodontal infections* include all parts of the periodontium, namely, the gingiva, periodontal ligament, bone, and cementum.

II. SIGNS AND SYMPTOMS

Patients may or may not have specific symptoms to report because periodontal infections are insidious in development. Symptoms the patient notices or feels may include bleeding gingiva, sometimes only while brushing, sometimes with drooling at night, or sometimes spontaneously. Other possible symptoms are sensitivity to hot and cold, tenderness or discomfort while eating or some pain after eating, food retained between the teeth, unpleasant mouth odors, chronic bad taste, or a feeling that the teeth are loose. Most of these are symptoms of advanced disease.

III. CLINICALLY NORMAL

The terms "clinically normal" or "clinically healthy" may be used to designate gingival tissue that is characterized by the following: a shade of pale or coral pink varied by complexion and pigmentation; a knife-edged gingival margin that adapts closely around the tooth; stippling; firmness; and minimal sulcus depth with no bleeding when probed. Although "normal" varies with anatomic, physiologic, and other factors, general characteristics form a baseline for a contrast in the recognition of inflammation.

IV. CAUSES OF TISSUE CHANGES

Disease changes produce alterations in color, size, position, shape, consistency, surface texture, bleeding readiness, and exudate production.

To understand the changes that take place in the gingival tissues during the transition from health to disease, it is necessary to have a clear picture of what dental biofilm is, the role of biofilm microorganisms in the development of disease, and the inflammatory response by the body.

When the products of the biofilm microorganisms cause breakdown of the intercellular substances of the sulcular epithelium, injurious agents can pass into the connective tissue, where an inflammatory response is initiated. An inflammatory response means that there is increased blood flow, increased permeability of capillaries, and increased collection of defense cells and tissue fluid. The changes produce the tissue alterations, such as in color, size, shape, and consistency, that are described in the next section.

V. DESCRIPTIVE TERMINOLOGY

The degree of severity and distribution of a change should be noted when examining the gingiva. When a deviation from normal affects a single area, it can be designated by the number of the adjacent tooth and the surface of the tissue involved, namely, facial, lingual, mesial, or distal.

A. Severity

Severity is expressed as slight, moderate, or severe.

B. Distribution

Terms used for describing distribution are as follows:
1. *Localized*: The gingiva is involved only about a single tooth or a specific group of teeth.
2. *Generalized*: The gingiva is involved about all or nearly all of the teeth throughout the mouth. A condition may also be generalized throughout a single arch, the maxillary or mandibular.
3. *Marginal*: A change that is confined to the free or marginal gingiva. This is specified as either localized or generalized.
4. *Papillary*: A change that involves a papilla but not the rest of the free gingiva around a tooth. A papillary change may be localized or generalized.
5. *Diffuse*: Spread out, dispersed; affects gingival margin, attached gingiva, and interdental papillae; may extend into alveolar mucosa. A diffuse condition is more frequently localized, rarely generalized.

VI. EARLY RECOGNITION OF TISSUE CHANGES

Marked changes, such as moderate to severe generalized redness, enlargement, sponginess, deep pockets, and definite mobility, are relatively easy to detect even with limited experience, provided there is good light and accessibility for vision. In contrast, when changes are subtle, localized about one or a few teeth, and of a lesser degree of severity, more skillful application of knowledge is needed.

Early recognition and treatment of gingival and periodontal infections prevents neglect of conditions that can develop into severe disease. Treatment is less complicated, and the success of treatment and recovery to healthy tissue is predictable when early recognition makes early treatment possible.

▪ THE GINGIVAL EXAMINATION

The examination of the gingiva includes evaluation of color, size, shape, consistency, surface texture, position, mucogingival junctions, bleeding, and exudate. These are summarized in Table 12-1, which is a clinical reference chart.

I. COLOR

A. Signs of Health

1. *Pale Pink.* Darker in people with darker complexions.
2. *Factors Influencing Color*
   a. Vascular supply.
   b. Thickness of epithelium.
   c. Degree of keratinization.
   d. Physiologic pigmentation: melanin pigmentation occurs frequently in African Americans, Orientals, Indians, and Caucasians of Mediterranean countries.

B. Changes in Disease

1. *In Chronic Inflammation.* Dark red, bluish red, magenta, or deep blue.

■ TABLE 12-1 EXAMINATION OF THE GINGIVAL CLINICAL MARKERS

	APPEARANCE IN HEALTH	CHANGES IN DISEASE CLINICAL APPEARANCE	CAUSES FOR CHANGES
Color	Uniformly pale pink or coral pink	Acute: bright red	Inflammation Capillary dilation Increased blood flow
	Variations in pigmentation related to complexion, race	Chronic: bluish pink, bluish red	Vessels engorged Blood flow sluggish Venous return impaired Anoxemia Increased fibrosis
		Attached gingiva: color change may extend to the mucogingival line	Deepening of pocket, mucogingival involvement

Size	Not enlarged
	
	Fits snugly around the tooth
		Enlarged	Edematous:
			    inflammatory fluid
			    cellular exudate
			    vascular engorgement
			    hemorrhage
			Fibrotic: new collagen
			    fibers

Shape (contour)	Marginal gingiva:
	    knife-edged, flat, follows
	    a curved line about the
	    tooth
	Papillae:
	(1) normal contact: papilla
	    is pointed and
	    pyramidal; fills the
	    interproximal area
	(2) space (diastema)
	    between teeth; gingiva
	    is flat or saddle
	    shaped
		Marginal gingiva:
		    rounded
		    rolled
		
		Papillae:
		    bulbous
		    flattened
		    blunted
		    cratered
			Inflammatory changes:
			    edematous or fibrous
			
			Bulbous with gingival
			    enlargement
			    (see edematous and
			    fibrotic, above)
			
			Cratered in necrotizing
			    ulcerative gingivitis

Consistency	Firm
	
	Attached gingiva firmly
	    bound down
		Soft, spongy: dents readily
		    when pressed with probe
		Associated with red color,
		    smooth shiny surface, loss
		    of stippling, bleeding on
		    probing
			Edematous: fluid between
			    cells in connective tissue

		Firm, hard: resists probe
		    pressure
		Associated with pink color,
		    stippling, bleeding only
		    in depth of pocket
			Fibrotic: collagen fibers

Surface texture	Free gingiva: smooth
	
	Attached gingiva: stippled
		Acute condition: smooth,
		    shiny gingiva
		
		Chronic: hard, firm, with
		    stippling, sometimes
		    heavier than normal
			Inflammatory changes in the
			    connective tissue; edema,
			    cellular infiltration
			Fibrosis

▪ TABLE 12-1 EXAMINATION OF THE GINGIVAL CLINICAL MARKERS (Continued)

	APPEARANCE IN HEALTH	CHANGES IN DISEASE CLINICAL APPEARANCE	CAUSES FOR CHANGES
Position of Gingival Margin	Fully erupted tooth: margin is 1–2 mm above cementoenamel junction, at or slightly below the enamel contour	Enlarged gingiva: margin is higher on the tooth, above normal, pocket deepened Recession: margin is more apical; root surface is exposed	Edematous or fibrotic Junctional epithelium has migrated along the root; gingival margin follows
Position of Junctional Epithelium	During eruption along the enamel surface (Figure 12-7) Fully erupted tooth: the junctional epithelium is at the cemento-enamel junction	Position determined by use of probe, is on the root surface	Apical migration of the epithelium along the root
Mucogingival Junctions	Make clear demarcation between the pink, stippled, attached gingiva and the darker alveolar mucosa with smooth shiny surface	No attached gingiva: (1) Color changes may extend full height of the gingiva; mucogingival line obliterated (2) Probing reveals that the bottom of the pocket extends into the alveolar mucosa (3) Frenal pull may displace the gingival margin from the tooth	Apical migration of the junctional epithelium Attached gingiva decreases with pocket deepening Inflammation extends into alveolar mucosa
Bleeding	No spontaneous bleeding or upon probing	Spontaneous bleeding Bleeding on probing: bleeding near margin in acute condition; bleeding deep in pocket in chronic condition	Degeneration of the sulcular epithelium with the formation of pocket epithelium Blood vessels engorged Tissue edematous
Exudate	No exudate expressed on pressure	White fluid, pus, visible on digital pressure Amount not related to pocket depth	Inflammation in the connective tissue Excessive accumulation of white blood cells with serum and tissue makes up the exudate (pus)

2. *In Acute Inflammation.* Bright red.
3. *Extent.* Deep involvement can be expected when diffuse color changes extend into the attached gingiva, or from the marginal gingiva to the mucogingival junction, or through into alveolar mucosa.

II. SIZE

A. Signs of Health

1. *Free Gingiva.* Flat, not enlarged; fits snugly around the tooth.
2. *Attached Gingiva*

   a. Width of attached gingiva varies among patients and among teeth for an individual, from 1 to 9 mm.[5]

   b. Wider in maxilla than mandible; broadest zone related to incisors, narrowest at the canine and premolar regions.

B. Changes in Disease

1. *Free Gingiva and Papillae.* Become enlarged. May be localized or limited to specific areas or generalized throughout the gingiva. The col deepens as the papillae increase in size.

2. *Attached Gingiva.* Decreases in amount as the pocket deepens.

C. Enlargement From Drug Therapy

Certain drugs used for specific systemic therapy cause gingival enlargement as a side effect. Examples of such drugs are phenytoin, cyclosporine, and nifedipine.

III. SHAPE (FORM OR CONTOUR)

A. Signs of Health

1. *Free Gingiva*
    a. Follows a curved line around each tooth; may be straighter along wide molar surfaces.
    b. The margin is knife-edged or slightly rounded on facial and lingual gingiva; closely adapted to the tooth surface.
2. *Papillae*
    a. Teeth with contact area. Facial and lingual gingiva are pointed or slightly rounded papillae with a col area under the contact (Figure 12-8).
    b. Spaced teeth (with diastemata). Interdental gingiva is flat or saddle shaped.

B. Changes in Disease

1. *Free Gingiva.* Rounded or rolled.
2. *Papillae.* Blunted, flattened, bulbous, cratered (Figure 12-10).
3. *Festoon ("McCall's festoon").* An enlargement of the marginal gingiva with the formation of a lifesaver-like gingival prominence. Frequently, the total gingiva is very narrow, with associated apparent recession, as shown in Figure 12-10D.
4. *Clefts*
    a. "Stillman's cleft" (Figure 12-11). A localized recession may be V-shaped, apostrophe-shaped, or form a slitlike indentation. It may extend several millimeters toward the mucogingival junction or even to or through the junction.
    b. Floss cleft. A cleft created by incorrect floss positioning appears as a vertical linear or V-shaped fissure in the marginal gingiva.[6] It usually occurs at one side of an interdental papilla. The injury can develop when dental floss is curved repeatedly in an incomplete "C" around the line angle so the floss is pressed across the gingiva.

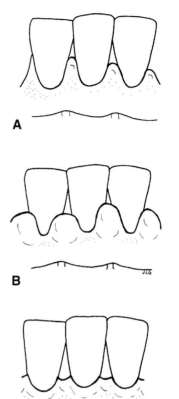

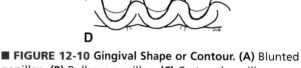

■ **FIGURE 12-10 Gingival Shape or Contour. (A)** Blunted papillae. **(B)** Bulbous papillae. **(C)** Cratered papillae. **(D)** Rolled, lifesaver-shaped "McCall's festoons."

IV. CONSISTENCY

A. Signs of Health

1. Firm when palpated with the side of a blunt instrument (probe).
2. Attached gingiva is bound down firmly to the underlying bone.

B. Changes in Disease

1. *To Determine Consistency.* Gently press side of probe on free gingiva. Soft, spongy gingiva dents readily; firm, hard tissue resists.
2. *Soft, Spongy Gingiva.* Related to acute stages of inflammation with increased infiltration of fluid

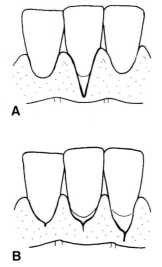

■ **FIGURE 12-11 Gingival Clefts. (A)** V-shaped Stillman's cleft. **(B)** Slit-like Stillman's clefts of varying degrees of severity in relation to the mucogingival junction.

and inflammatory elements. The tissue appears red, may be smooth and shiny with loss of stippling, has marginal enlargement, and bleeds readily on probing.

3. *Firm, Hard Gingiva.* Related to chronic inflammation with increased fibrosis. The tissue may appear pink and well stippled. Bleeding, when probed, usually occurs only in the deeper part of a pocket, not near the margin.

4. *Retraction of the Margin Away From the Tooth.* Normally, the free gingiva fits snugly about the tooth. When the margin tends to hang slightly away or is readily displaced with a light air blast, the gingival fibers that support the margin have been destroyed (Figure 12-3).

V. SURFACE TEXTURE

A. Signs of Health

1. *Free Gingiva.* Smooth.
2. *Attached Gingiva.* Stippled (minutely "pebbled" or "orange peel" surface).
3. *Interdental Gingiva.* The free gingiva is smooth; the center portion of each papilla is stippled.

B. Changes in Disease

1. *Inflammatory Changes.* May be loss of stippling, with smooth, shiny surface.
2. *Hyperkeratosis.* May result in a leathery, hard, or nodular surface.
3. *Chronic Disease.* Tissue may be hard and fibrotic, with a normal pink color and normal or deep stippling.

VI. POSITION

The *actual* position of the gingiva is the level of the attached periodontal tissue. It is not directly visible but can be determined by probing.

The *apparent* position of the gingiva is the level of the gingival margin or crest of the free gingiva that is seen by direct observation.

A. Signs of Health

For the fully erupted tooth in an adult, the apparent position of the gingival margin is normally at the level of, or slightly below, the enamel contour or prominence of the cervical third of a tooth.

B. Changes in Disease

1. *Effect of Gingival Enlargement.* When the gingiva enlarges, the gingival margin may be high on the enamel, partly or nearly covering the anatomic crown.
2. *Effect of Gingival Recession*
   a. Definition. Recession is the exposure of root surface that results from the apical migration of the junctional epithelium (Figure 12-12).
   b. Actual recession. The actual recession is shown by the position of the attachment level. The "receded area" is from the cementoenamel junction to the attachment.
   c. Visible recession. The visible recession is the exposed root surface that is visible on clinical

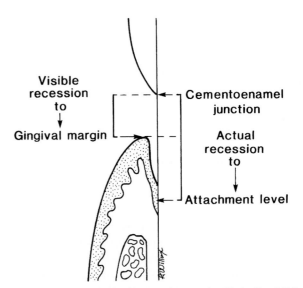

■ **FIGURE 12-12 Gingival Recession.** *Left,* Clinically visible recession of the gingival margin with root surface apparent to the eye. *Right,* The actual recession exposes the root surface as the periodontal attachment migrates along the root surface.

examination. It is seen from the gingival margin to the cementoenamel junction.

    d.   Localized recession (Figure 12-13). A localized recession may be narrow or wide, deep or shallow. The root surface is denuded, and the visible recession may extend to or through the mucogingival junction.

    e.   Measurement. Both actual and visible recession can be measured with a probe from the cementoenamel junction. Total recession is the actual and visible positions added together.

VII. BLEEDING

A. Signs of Health

1. No bleeding spontaneously or on probing.
2. Healthy tissue does not bleed.

B. Changes in Disease

1. Bleeding occurs spontaneously or when probed.
2. Sulcular epithelium becomes diseased *pocket epithelium*. The ulcerated pocket wall bleeds readily on gentle probing.

VIII. EXUDATE

A. Signs of Health

There is no exudate except slight gingival sulcus fluid. Gingival sulcus fluid cannot be seen by direct observation.

B. Changes in Disease

1. Increased gingival sulcus fluid.
2. Amount of exudate is not an indicator of the extent of disease or the depth of the periodontal pockets.

■ THE GINGIVA OF YOUNG CHILDREN[7,8]

I. SIGNS OF HEALTH

A. Primary Dentition

1. *Color.* Pink or slightly red.
2. *Shape.* Thick, rounded, or rolled.
3. *Consistency.* Less fibrous than adult gingiva; not tightly adapted to the teeth; may be easily displaced with a light air jet.
4. *Surface Texture.* May or may not have stippling; high percentage of patients has shiny gingiva.
5. *Attached Gingiva.* Width of attached gingiva in children aged 3 to 5 years: between 1 and 6 mm.[5]
6. *Interdental Gingiva*
   a. Anterior: diastemata are frequently present and the papillae are flat or saddle shaped.
   b. Posterior: col between facial and lingual papillae when teeth are in contact (Figure 12-8).

B. Mixed Dentition

- Constant state of change related to exfoliation and eruption.
- Free gingiva may appear rolled or rounded, slightly reddened, shiny, and with a lack of firmness.
- The gingiva covers a varying portion of the anatomic crown, depending on the stage of eruption (Figure 12-7).

II. CHANGES IN DISEASE

Examination of the periodontal tissues of a child is not different from that of an adult. A complete examination is necessary, including probing around each tooth.

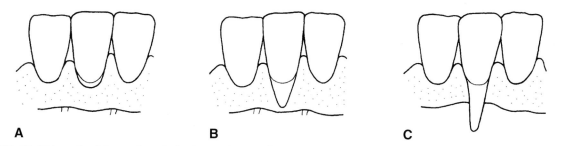

A   **B**   **C**

■ **FIGURE 12-13 Localized Recession.** A single tooth may show narrow or wide, deep or shallow recession. **(A)** Wide, shallow. **(B)** Wide, deep, with narrow attached gingiva. **(C)** Narrow, deep, with missing attached gingiva.

Everyday Ethics

? Britain and Nicholas were first-year dental hygiene students just beginning to practice on each other as student partners in the preclinic program. During the oral examination, Britain noticed that Nicholas had some areas of bleeding and changes in the contour of the marginal gingiva. In general, the soft tissue seemed more sponge-like and loose, but Britain was not sure she clearly understood what is considered "normal," remembering that the clinical instructor often referred to a "range" of normal.

Britain decided to focus on and document the areas that were pale pink, firm, and pointed in the interproximal areas. She carefully recorded this information with great detail and then signaled for her instructor to verify the findings. When the instructor sat down and reviewed the examination she was pleased with Britain's thoroughness. The instructor provided positive feedback and quickly moved on to the next pair of students. Britain began to feel uneasy that she should have pointed out the gingival tissues that she thought were possibly inflamed.

Questions for Consideration

1 Explain how the ethical principles of autonomy, beneficence, and veracity apply to this situation.

2 Indicate how Nicholas is the center of this dilemma both from the perspective of Britain, a student, and the clinical instructor who finds out from another faculty member that they think Nicholas has definite signs of periodontal disease.

3 Ethically, what alternatives or actions can Britain take at this time to address the "uneasy" feeling she has about Nicholas' gingival status?

Gingivitis occurs frequently in children but is usually reversible without leaving permanent damage.

Although relatively rare, periodontitis can occur in primary dentition.

Mucogingival problems occur in children.[9,10] The recognition of deficiencies of attached gingiva has particular significance for the child who will need orthodontic treatment.

▪ THE GINGIVA AFTER PERIODONTAL SURGERY

The characteristics of "normal healthy gingiva" take on different dimensions for the patient who has completed treatment for pockets, bone loss, and other signs of a periodontal infection. The junctional epithelium is apical to the cementoenamel junction. After healing, the sulcus depth may be within normal range and no bleeding should occur when probed.

Depending on the exact treatment performed, examination shows changes from the initial evaluation. For example, where the initial examination showed a deficiency of attached gingiva with frenal pull, mucogingival surgery may have been designed and treatment satisfactorily completed to create new attached gingiva. With each maintenance appointment, a thorough, careful examination is necessary to control factors that may permit recurrence of disease.

✓ Factors To Teach The Patient

- Characteristics of normal healthy gingiva.

- The significance of bleeding; healthy tissue does not bleed.

- Relationship of findings during a gingival examination to the personal daily care procedures for infection control.

- The special attention needed for an area of gingival recession to prevent abrasion, inflammation, and further involvement.

- How the method of brushing, stiffness of toothbrush filaments, abrasiveness of a dentifrice, and pressure applied during brushing can be factors in gingival recession.

REFERENCESS

1. **Avery**, J.K. and Steele, P.F.: *Essentials of Oral Histology and Embryology: A Clinical Approach*. St. Louis, Mosby, 1992, pp. 131–134.

2. **Ainamo**, J. and Löe, H.: Anatomical Characteristics of Gingiva: A Clinical and Microscopic Study of the Free and Attached Gingiva, *J. Periodontol.*, 37, 5, January–February, 1966.

3. **Orban**, B.: Clinical and Histologic Study of the Surface Characteristics of the Gingiva, *Oral Surg. Oral Med. Oral Pathol.*, 1, 827, September, 1948.

4. **Bhaskar**, S.N., ed.: *Orban's Oral Histology and Embryology,* 11th ed. St. Louis, Mosby, 1991, pp. 323–325.

5. **Bowers**, G.M.: A Study of the Width of Attached Gingiva, *J. Periodontol., 34,* 201, May, 1963.

6. **Hallman**, W.W., Waldrop, T.C., Houston, G.D., and Hawkins, B.F.: Flossing Clefts: Clinical and Histologic Observations, *J. Periodontol., 57,* 501, August, 1986.

7. **Carranza**, F.A. and Newman, M.G.: *Clinical Periodontics,* 8th ed. Philadelphia, W.B. Saunders Co., 1996, pp. 276–280.

8. **Casamassimo**, P.S.: Periodontal Conditions, in Pinkham, J.R., ed.: *Pediatric Dentistry: Infancy Through Adolescence,* 2nd ed. Philadelphia, W.B. Saunders Co., 1994, pp. 353–357, 607–615.

9. **Maynard**, J.G. and Ochsenbein, C.: Mucogingival Problems, Prevalence and Therapy in Children, *J. Periodontol., 46,* 543, September, 1975.

10. **Andlin-Sobocki**, A., Marcusson, A., and Persson, M.: 3-Year Observations on Gingival Recession in Mandibular Incisors in Children, *J. Clin. Periodontol., 18,* 155, March, 1991.

SUGGESTED READINGS

Ainamo, A., Ainamo, J., and Poikkeus, R.: Continuous Widening of the Band of Attached Gingiva From 23 to 65 Years of Age, *J. Periodont. Res., 16,* 595, November, 1981.

Carranza, F.A. and Newman, M.G.: *Clinical Periodontics,* 8th ed. Philadelphia, W.B. Saunders Co., 1996, pp. 12–29.

Fedi, P.F., and Vernino, A.R.: *The Periodontic Syllabus,* 3rd ed. Baltimore, Williams & Wilkins, 1995, pp. 1–12.

Grant, D.A., Stern, I.B., and Listgarten, M.A., eds.: *Periodontics,* 6th ed. St. Louis, Mosby, 1988, pp. 3–75.

Hassell, T.M.: Tissues and Cells of the Periodontium, *Periodontol. 2000, 3,* 9, 1993.

Hempton, T.J., Wilkins, E., and Lancaster, D.: Evaluation of Attached Tissue Aids in Treatment of Recession, *RDH, 16,* 34, June, 1996.

Hicks, M.J., Uldricks, J.M., Whitacre, H.L., Anderson, J., and Moeschberger, M.L.: A National Study of Periodontal Assessment by Dental Hygienists, *J. Dent. Hyg., 67,* 82, February, 1993.

Hoag, P.M. and Pawlak, E.A.: *Essentials of Periodontics,* 4th ed. St. Louis, Mosby, 1990, pp. 1–18.

Mariotti, A.: The Extracellular Matrix of the Periodontium: Dynamic and Interactive Tissues, *Periodontol. 2000, 3,* 39, 1993.

Melfi, R.C.: *Permar's Oral Embryology and Microscopic Anatomy,* 9th ed. Philadelphia, Lea & Febiger, 1994, pp. 227–242.

Serino, G., Wennström, J.L., Lindhe, J., and Eneroth, L.: The Prevalence and Distribution of Gingival Recession in Subjects With a High Standard of Oral Hygiene, *J. Clin. Periodontol., 21,* 57, January, 1994.

Vacek, J.S., Gher, M.E., Assad, D.A., Richardson, A.C., and Giambarresi, L.I.: The Dimensions of the Human Dentogingival Junction, *Int. J. Periodont. Restorative Dent., 14,* 155, Number 2, 1994.

Gingiva of Children

American Academy of Periodontology, Committee on Research, Science and Therapy: Position Paper: Periodontal Diseases of Children and Adolescents, *J. Periodontol., 67,* 57, January, 1996.

Andlin-Sobocki, A.: Changes of Facial Gingival Dimensions in Children: A 2-year Longitudinal Study, *J. Clin. Periodontol., 20,* 212, March, 1993.

Andlin-Sobocki, A. and Bodin, L.: Dimensional Alterations of the Gingiva Related to Changes of Facial/Lingual Tooth Position in Permanent Anterior Teeth of Children: A 2-year Longitudinal Study. *J. Clin. Periodontol., 20,* 218, March, 1993.

Bimstein, E. and Eidelman, E.: Longitudinal Changes in the Width of Attached Gingiva in Children, *Pediatr. Dent., 10,* 22, March, 1988.

Bimstein, E., Machtei, E., and Eidelman, E.: Dimensional Differences in the Attached and Keratinized Gingiva and Gingival Sulcus in the Early Permanent Dentition: A Longitudinal Study, *J. Pedod., 10,* 247, Spring, 1986.

Bimstein, E., Matsson, L., Soskolne, A.W., and Lustman, J.: Histologic Characteristics of the Gingiva Associated With the Primary and Permanent Teeth of Children, *Pediatr. Dent., 16,* 206, May/June, 1994.

Keszthelyi, G.: The Width of Plaque-Free Zones on Primary Molars With Attachment Loss, *J. Clin. Periodontol., 18,* 94, February, 1991.

Keszthelyi, G. and Szabo, I.: Attachment Loss in Primary Molars, *J. Clin. Periodontol., 14,* 48, January, 1987.

Saario, M., Ainamo, A., Mattila, K., and Ainamo, J.: The Width of Radiologically-defined Attached Gingiva Over Permanent Teeth in Children, *J. Clin. Periodontol., 21,* 666, November, 1994.

Saario, M., Ainamo, A., Mattila, K., Suomalainen, K., and Ainamo, J.: The Width of Radiologically-defined Attached Gingiva Over Deciduous Teeth, *J. Clin. Periodontol., 22,* 895, December, 1995.

Tenenbaum, H. and Tenenbaum, M.: A Clinical Study of the Width of the Attached Gingiva in the Deciduous, Transitional and Permanent Dentitions, *J. Clin. Periodontol., 13,* 270, April, 1986.

Parts of the gingival and dental examinations are made by direct *visual* observation, whereas other parts require *tactile* using a probe and an explorer. These two types of instruments, assisted by a mouth mirror, are key instruments in patient examination and assessment. Considerable skill is required for accurate and efficient probing and exploring.

General principles of instrumentation are described on pages 619 to 627. Box 13-1 contains definitions for key words used in or associated with this chapter.

I. PRECAUTION

A probe or an explorer should not be applied to the teeth and gingiva until an initial review of information from the patient history has been made. Of particular significance is knowledge of a patient's susceptibility to bacteremia. Patients at risk must receive prophylactic antibiotic premedication before instrumentation.

II. BASIC SET-UP

All tray arrangements need a basic set-up composed of a mouth mirror, probe, explorer, and cotton pliers. Wrapping these together for sterilizing increases efficiency. The packet should be labeled "basic set-up." Other packets can contain special instruments, such as a furcation probe, to use for supplemental examinations.

▪ THE MOUTH MIRROR

I. DESCRIPTION

A. Parts

The mirror has three parts: the handle, shank, and working end, which is the mounted mirror or mirror head.

BOX 13-1 KEY WORDS: Instruments of Examination

Calibration: determination of the accuracy of an instrument by measurment of its variation from a standard; (calibration between examiners).

Clinical attachment level: probing depth as measured from the cementoenamel junction (or other fixed point) to the location of the probe tip at the coronal level of attached periodontal tissues.

Explorer: a slender stainless steel instrument with a fine flexible, sharp point used for examination of the surfaces of the teeth to detect irregularities.

Fremitus: a vibration perceptible by palpation.

Periodontometer: instrument used to measure mobility.

Probe: smooth, slender instrument usually round in diameter with a rounded tip designed for examination of the teeth and soft tissues; except for a few probes made only for blunt examination, probes are calibrated in millimeter increments to facilitate recordings for comparison with periodic assessments.

Probing depth: the distance from the gingival margin to the location of the periodontal probe tip at the coronal border of attached periodontal tissues.

Tactile: pertaining to the touch.

> **Tactile discrimination:** the ability to distinguish relative degrees of roughness and smoothness, for example, on a tooth surface, using an explorer or a periodontal probe; also called tactile sensitivity.

Tension test: application of tension at the mucogingival junction by retracting cheek, lip, and tongue to tighten the alveolar mucosa and test for the presence of attached gingiva; area of missing attached gingiva is revealed when the alveolar mucosa and frena are connected directly to the free gingiva.

B. Mirror Surfaces

1. *Plane (Flat).* May produce a double image.
2. *Concave.* Magnifying.
3. *Front Surface.* The reflecting surface is on the front of the lens rather than on the back as with plane or magnifying mirrors. The front surface eliminates "ghost" images.

C. Diameters

Diameters vary from 5/8 to 1 1/4 inches. In addition, special examination mirrors are available in 1 1/2- to 2-inch diameters.

D. Attachments

Mirrors may be threaded plain stem or cone socket to be joined to a handle. Because mirrors tend to become scratched, replacement of the working end is possible without purchasing new handles.

E. Handles

1. Thicker handles contribute to a more comfortable grasp and greater control.
2. Wider mirror handles are especially useful for mobility determination.

F. Disposable Mirrors

1. May be plastic in one piece or may be a handle with replaceable head for professional use; may have front surface.
2. Take-home mirrors for patient instruction. Patient may observe lingual and posterior aspects. One type of mirror has a light attachment.

II. PURPOSES AND USES

The mouth mirror is used to provide:

A. Indirect Vision

This is particularly needed for distal surfaces of posterior teeth and lingual surfaces of anterior teeth.

B. Indirect Illumination

Reflection of light from the dental overhead light to any area of the oral cavity can be accomplished by adapting the mirror.

C. Transillumination

Reflection of light through the teeth.
1. Mirror is held to reflect light from the lingual aspect while facial surfaces of the teeth are examined.
2. Mirror is held for indirect vision on the lingual while light from the overhead dental light passes through the teeth. Translucency of enamel can be seen clearly, whereas dental caries or calculus deposits appear opaque.

D. Retraction

The mirror is used to protect or prevent interference by the cheeks, tongue, or lips.

III. PROCEDURE FOR USE

A. Grasp

Use modified pen grasp with finger rest on a tooth surface wherever possible to provide stability and control.

B. Retraction

1. Use a water-based lubricant on dry or cracked lips and corners of mouth.
2. Adjust the mirror position so that the angles of the mouth are protected from undue pressure of the shank of the mirror.
3. Insert and remove mirror carefully to avoid hitting the teeth because this can be very disturbing to the patient.

C. Maintain Clear Vision

1. Warm mirror with water, rub along buccal mucosa to coat mirror with thin transparent film of saliva, and request patient to breathe through the nose to prevent condensation of moisture on the mirror. Use a detergent or other means for keeping a clear surface.
2. Discard scratched mirrors.

IV. CARE OF MIRRORS

A. Dismantle mirror and handle for sterilization.
B. Examine carefully after ultrasonic cleaning or scrubbing with brush prior to sterilization to ensure removal of debris around back, shank, and rim of reflecting surface.
C. Handle carefully during sterilization procedures to prevent other instruments from scratching the reflecting surface.
D. Consult manufacturer's specifications for sterilizing or disinfecting procedures that may cloud the mirror, particularly the front surface type.

▪ INSTRUMENTS FOR APPLICATION OF AIR

I. PURPOSES AND USES

With appropriate, timely application of air to clear saliva and debris and/or dry the tooth surfaces, the following can be accomplished:

A. Improve and Facilitate Examination Procedures

- Make a thorough, more accurate examination.
- Dry supragingival calculus to facilitate exploring and scaling. Small deposits may be light in color and not visible until they are dried. Dried calculus appears chalky and presents a contrast to tooth color.
- Deflect the free gingival margin for observation into the subgingival area. Subgingival calculus usually appears darker than supragingival.
- Make identification of areas of demineralization and carious lesions easier.
- Recognize location and condition of restorations, particularly tooth-color restorations.

B. Improve Visibility of the Treatment Area During Instrumentation

- Dry area for finger rest to provide stability during instrumentation.
- Facilitate positive scaling techniques.
- Minimize appointment time.
- Evaluate complete removal of supragingival calculus after instrumentation.

C. Prepare Teeth and/or Gingiva for Certain Procedures

Examples are to dry surfaces for:
- Application of caries-preventive agents.
- Make impression for study cast.
- Apply topical anesthetic.

II. COMPRESSED AIR SYRINGE

A. Description

1. *Air Source.* Air compressor with tubing attachment to syringe.
2. *Air Tip.* Has angled working end that can be turned for maxillary or mandibular application. Tip may be disposable or removable for sterilization.

B. Procedure for Use

1. Use palm grasp about the handle of the syringe; place thumb on release lever or on button on handle.
2. Test the air flow so that the strength of flow can be controlled.
3. Make controlled, relatively short, gentle applications of air.
4. Supplement air drying with use of saliva ejector and folded gauze sponge placed in vestibule.

C. Precautions

- Avoid sharp blasts of air on sensitive cervical areas of teeth or open carious lesions. Such areas may be dried by blotting with a gauze sponge or cotton roll to avoid causing discomfort.
- Avoid applying air directly into a pocket. Subgingival biofilm may be forced into the tissues and may create a bacteremia.
- Avoid forceful application of air, which can direct saliva and debris out of the oral cavity, contaminate the working area and clinician, and create aerosols. Air directed toward the posterior region of the patient's mouth may cause coughing.
- Avoid startling the patient; forewarn when air is to be applied.

▪ PROBE

Early in the patient examination, the patient's periodontal disease status must be determined. Treatment planning varies depending on whether the condition is gingivitis, which may be reversible, or periodontitis with periodontal pockets, bone loss, and root surface involvement, which may require more extensive therapy.

Two general types of probes available are the traditional or standard manual probes and the controlled force or automated probes. Automated probes were developed and researched in an attempt to overcome the problems in obtaining consistent readings with traditional probes.

Factors that influence probe determinations are described later in this chapter. Included are variations in pressure (probing force) used, diameter, and other physical features, and the inconsistent depth or penetration during application.

A probe is used to make the initial assessment, followed by a detailed evaluation to determine the extent and degree of severity of disease and tissue destruction for specific treatment planning. During treatment, the probe is applied to assess progress. After treatment, use of the probe helps to determine completion of professional services as recognized by the health status of the tissues. At each maintenance appointment, a reevaluation with the probe is needed to ensure continued self-care by the patient and to identify early disease changes that require additional professional treatment.

I. PURPOSES AND USES

A probe is used to

A. Assess the Periodontal Status for Preparation of a Treatment Plan

1. Classify the disease as gingivitis or periodontitis by determining whether bone loss has occurred and whether the pockets are gingival or periodontal. A systematic screening method can be used (PSR).
2. Determine the extent of inflammation in conjunction with the overall gingival examination. Bleeding on probing is an early sign of inflammation in the gingiva.

B. Make a Sulcus and Pocket Survey

1. Examine the shape, topography, and dimensions of sulci and pockets.
2. Measure and record probing depths.
3. Evaluate tooth-surface pocket wall.
   a. Chart calculus location and severity.
   b. Record other root surface irregularities discerned by the probe.
4. Determine clinical attachment level.

C. Make a Mucogingival Examination

1. Determine relationship of gingival margin, attachment level, and mucogingival junction.
2. Measure the width of the attached gingiva (Figure 13-10).

D. Make Other Gingival Determinations

1. Evaluate gingival bleeding on probing and prepare a gingival bleeding index.
2. Measure the extent of visible gingival recession.
3. Determine the consistency of the gingival tissue.

E. Guide Treatment

1. Determine gingival characteristics, including probing depth, bleeding, and consistency (all determined using a probe), to provide a basis for patient instruction as part of the total treatment.
2. Define probing depth of sulcus or pocket for application of instruments for scaling, root planing and maintenance debridement, and define depth for use of an explorer for evaluation of these procedures.
3. Detect anatomic configuration of roots, subgingival deposits, and root irregularities that complicate instrumentation. For this, the probe is used in conjunction with the explorer.

F. Evaluate Success and Completeness of Treatment

1. Evaluate posttreatment tissue response to professional treatment on an immediate, short-term basis, as well as at periodic maintenance examinations.
2. Evaluate patient's self-treatment through therapeutic disease control procedures.
3. Signs of health revealed by probing
   a. No bleeding; healthy tissue does not bleed.
   b. Reduced probing depth; comparison of pretreatment and posttreatment probing depth.
   c. Tissue is firm, as shown by application of the probe to the surface of the free gingiva.

II. DESCRIPTION

A probe is a slender instrument with a smooth, rounded tip designed for examination of the depth and topography of an area. It has three parts: the handle, the angled shank, and the working end, which is the probe itself.

A. Materials

1. Stainless steel.
2. Plastic, for screenings and titanium implant probing.

B. Characteristics

1. *Straight Working End*
   a. Tapered, round, flat, or rectangular in cross section with a smooth rounded end.
   b. Calibrated in millimeters at intervals specific for each kind of probe; some have color coding. Figure 13-1 shows a comparison of a few typical markings; Table 13-1 lists probe markings with examples.
2. *Curved Working End.* Paired furcation probes have a smooth, rounded end for investigation of the topography and anatomy around roots in a furca. Examples are the Nabers 1N and 2N probes (Figure 13-8).

C. Selection

The probe chosen for use by a clinician is frequently the instrument first used when a particular technique

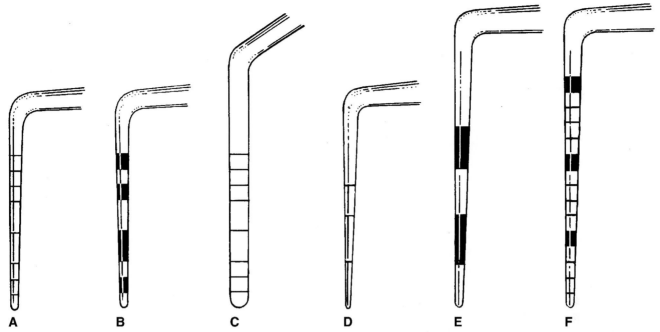

■ **FIGURE 13-1 Examples of Probes.** Names and calibrated markings shown are **(A)** Williams (1-1-1-2-2-1-1-1), **(B)** Williams, color-coded, **(C)** Goldman-Fox (1-1-1-2-2-1-1-1), **(D)** Michigan O (3-3-2), **(E)** Hu-Friedy or Marquis Color-coded (3-3-3-3 or 3-3-2-3), and **(F)** Hu-Friedy PCPUNC 15 (each millimeter to 15), color coded at 5-10-15. See Table 13-1 for additional data on probes.

was learned, or one that provides comfort and ease of manipulation. Another reason for selection is that consistency in reading can be accomplished.

Analysis of a probe and comparison with other probes are recommended. Important features to be considered in probe selection are

1. *Adaptability.* The probe should be adaptable around the complete circumference of each tooth, both posterior and anterior, so that no millimeter of probing depth can be neglected. Flat probes require more attention to adaptation and are useful primarily on facial and lingual surfaces.

TABLE 13-1 TYPES OF PROBES

PROBE MARKINGS (mm)	EXAMPLES	DESCRIPTION
Marks at 1-2-3-5-7-8-9-10	Williams	Round, tapered (available with color-code)
	University of Michigan with Williams marks	Round, narrow diameter, fine
	Glickman	Round, with longer lower shank
	Merritt A and B	Round, single bend to shank
Marks at 3-3-2	University of Michigan 0	Round, fine, tapered, narrow diameter
	Premier 0	
	Marquis M-1	
Marks at 3-6-9-12 3-6-8-11 (and other variations)	Hu-Friedy QULIX	Round, tapered, fine
	Marquis	Color-coded
	Nordent	
Marks at each mm to 15	Hu-Friedy PCPUNC 15	Round Color-coded at 5-10-15
Marks at 3.5-5.5-8.5-11.5	WHO Probe (World Health Organization)	Round, tapered, fine, with ball end Color-coded
No marks	Gilmore	Tapered, sharper than other probes
	Nabors 1N, 2N	Curved, with curved shank for furcation examination

2. *Markings.* Markings should be easy to read so that probing depth can be readily identified and measured, and no disease area is overlooked. Color coding contributes to readability.

▪ GUIDE TO PROBING

A pocket is a diseased gingival sulcus. The use of a probe is the only accurate, dependable method to locate, assess, and measure sulci and pockets.

I. POCKET CHARACTERISTICS

   A. A pocket is measured from the base of the pocket (top of attached periodontal tissue) to the gingival margin. Figure 13-2 shows two probing depths beneath gingival margins that are at the same level.
   B. The pocket (or sulcus) is continuous around the entire tooth, and the entire pocket or sulcus must be measured. "Spot" probing is inadequate.
   C. The depth varies around an individual tooth; probing depth rarely measures the same all around a tooth or even around one side of a tooth.
      1. The level of attached tissue assumes a varying position around the tooth.
      2. The gingival margin varies in its position on the tooth.
   D. Proximal surfaces must be approached by entering from both the facial and lingual aspects of the tooth.

1. Gingival and periodontal infections begin in the col area more frequently than in other areas.
2. Probing depth may be deepest directly under the contact area because of crater formation in the alveolar bone (Figure 13-3).
   E. Anatomic features of the tooth-surface wall of the pocket influence the direction of probing. Examples are concave surfaces, anomalies, shape of cervical third, and position of furcations.

II. EVALUATION OF TOOTH SURFACE

During the movement of the probe, calculus and tooth surface irregularities can be felt and evaluated. The information obtained is used to plan the scaling and root planing appointments.

III. FACTORS THAT AFFECT PROBE DETERMINATIONS

The general objectives of probing are accuracy and consistency so that recordings are dependable for comparison with future probings as well as with colleagues in

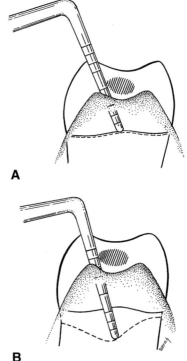

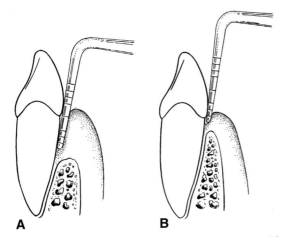

▪ **FIGURE 13-2 Probing Depth.** A pocket is measured from the gingival margin to the attached periodontal tissue. Shown is the contrast of probe measurements with gingival margins at the same level. **(A)** Deep periodontal pocket (7 mm) with apical migration of attachment. **(B)** Shallow pocket (2 mm) with the attachment near the cementoenamel junction.

▪ **FIGURE 13-3 Proximal Surface Probing. (A)** Probe must be applied more than half way across from facial to overlap with probing from the lingual. **(B)** Probe in area of crater formation. Probing is usually deeper on the proximal surface under the contact area than on the facial or lingual surfaces.

practice together. At the same time, patient discomfort and trauma to the tissues must be minimal. Probing is influenced by many factors, such as those that follow:

A. Severity and Extent of Periodontal Disease

With application of light pressure, the probe passes along the tooth surface to the attached tissue level. Diseased tissue offers less resistance, so that with increased severity of inflammation, the probe inserts to a deeper level.[1] Average levels show that the probe is stopped as follows:

1. *Normal Healthy Tissue.* The probe is at the base of the sulcus or crevice, at the coronal end of the junctional epithelium.
2. *Gingivitis and Early Periodontitis.* The probe tip is within the junctional epithelium.
3. *Advanced Periodontitis.* The probe tip penetrates through the junctional epithelium to reach attached connective tissue fibers.

B. The Probe Itself

1. *Calibration.* Must be accurately marked.
2. *Thickness.* A thinner probe slips through a narrow pocket more readily.
3. *Readability.* Aided by the markings and color-coding.

C. Technique

1. *Grasp.* Appropriate for maximum tactile sensitivity.
2. *Finger Rest.* Placed on nonmobile tooth with uniformity.

D. Placement Problems

1. *Anatomic Variations.* Tooth contours, furcations, contact areas, anomalies.
2. *Interferences.* Calculus, irregular margins of restorations, fixed dental prostheses.
3. *Accessibility, Visibility.* Obstructed by tissue bleeding, limited opening by patient, macroglossia.

E. Application of Pressure

Consistent pressure is accomplished by consistent grasp and finger rest in addition to keen tactile sensitivity.

▪ PROBING PROCEDURES

I. PROBE INSERTION

A. Grasp probe with modified pen grasp.
B. Establish finger rest on a neighboring tooth, preferably in the same dental arch.

C. Hold side of instrument tip flat against the tooth near the gingival margin. The cervical third of a primary tooth is more convex (Figure 13-4).
D. Gently slide the tip under the gingival margin.
1. *Healthy or Firm Fibrotic Tissue.* Insertion is more difficult because of the close adaptation of the tissue to the tooth surface; underlying gingival fibers are strong and tight.
2. *Spongy, Soft Tissue.* Gingival margin is loose and flabby because of the destruction of underlying gingival fibers. Probe inserts readily, and bleeding can be expected on gentle probing.

II. ADVANCE PROBE TO BASE OF POCKET

A. Hold side of probe tip flat against the tooth surface. Widespread roots of primary molars may make this probe position difficult unless the tissue is unduly distended by the probe (Figure 13-4).
B. Slide the probe along the tooth surface vertically down to the base of the sulcus or pocket.
1. Maintain contact of the side of the tip of the probe with the tooth.
   a. Gingival pocket. Side of probe is on enamel.
   b. Periodontal pocket. Side of probe is on the cemental or dentinal surface when inserted to a level below the cementoenamel junction.

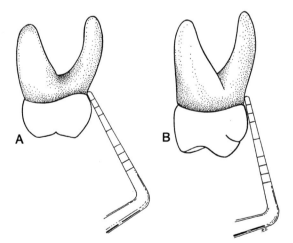

■ **FIGURE 13-4 Primary and Permanent Maxillary Molars. (A)** Accentuated convexity of the cervical third and widespread roots of the primary molar complicate probe placement. Probe may encounter the root. **(B)** Permanent tooth with less convexity of the cervical third and roots that are less widely spread.

2. As the probe is passed down the side of the tooth, roughness may be felt. Evaluation of the topography and nature of the tooth surface is important to instrumentation.

3. When obstruction by a hard bulky calculus deposit is encountered, lift the probe away from the tooth and follow over the edge of the calculus until the probe can move vertically into the pocket again.

4. The base of the sulcus or pocket feels soft and elastic (compared with the hard tooth surface and calculus deposits), and with slight pressure, the tension of the attached periodontal tissue at the base of the pocket can be felt.

C. Use only the pressure needed to detect by tactile means the level of the attached tissue, whether junctional epithelium or deep connective tissue fibers. A light pressure of 10 g, or of no more than 20 g, is ample.

D. Position the probe for reading.

1. Bring the probe to position as nearly parallel with the long axis of the tooth as possible for reading the depth.

2. Interference of the contact area does not permit placing the probe parallel for the measurement directly beneath the contact area. Hold the side of the shank of the probe against the contact to minimize the angle (Figure 13-3).

III. READ THE PROBE

A. Measurement for a probing depth is made from the gingival margin to the attached periodontal tissue.

B. Count the millimeters that show on the probe above the gingival margin and subtract the number from the total number of millimeters marked on the particular probe being used. A comparison of pocket measurement using probes with different calibrations is shown in Figure 13-5.

C. When the gingival margin appears at a level between probe marks, use the higher mark for the final reading.

D. Dry the area being probed to improve visibility for specific reading.

IV. CIRCUMFERENTIAL PROBING

A. Probe Stroke

Maintain the probe in the sulcus or pocket of each tooth as the probe is moved in a walking stroke.

- It is not necessary to remove the probe and reinsert it to make individual readings. Time would be wasted.
- Repeated withdrawal and reinsertion cause unnecessary trauma to the gingival margin and hence increase posttreatment discomfort.

B. Walking Stroke

1. Hold the side of the tip against the tooth at the base of the pocket.

2. Slide the probe up (coronally) about 1 to 2 mm and back to the attachment in a "touch . . . touch . . . touch . . ." rhythm (Figure 13-6).

3. Observe probe measurement at the gingival margin at each touch.

4. Advance millimeter by millimeter along the facial and lingual surfaces into the proximal areas.

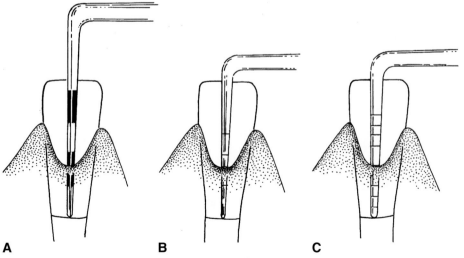

■ FIGURE 13-5 Comparison of Probe Readings. Measurement of same 5-mm pocket with three different probes. **(A)** Color-coded, **(B)** Michigan O, **(C)** Williams.

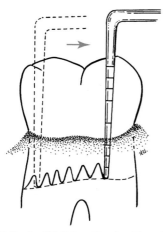

■ FIGURE 13-6 Probe Walking Stroke. The side of the tip of the probe is held in contact with the tooth. From the base of the pocket, the probe is moved up and down in 1- to 2-mm strokes as it is advanced in 1-mm steps. The attached periodontal tissue at the base of the pocket is contacted on each down stroke to identify probing depth in each area.

V. ADAPTATION OF PROBE FOR INDIVIDUAL TEETH

A. Molars and Premolars

1. Orient the probe at the distal line angle for both facial and lingual application.
2. Insert the probe at the distal line angle and probe in a distal direction; adapt the probe around the line angle; probe across the distal surface until the side of the probe contacts the contact area, then slant the probe to continue under the contact area.
3. Note the probing depth and slide the probe back to the distal line angle. Proceed in the mesial direction around the mesial line angle and across the mesial surface.

B. Anterior Teeth

1. Initial insertion may be at the distal line angle or from the midline of the facial or lingual surfaces.
2. Proceed around the distal line angle and across the distal surface; reinsert and probe the other half of the tooth.

C. Proximal Surfaces

1. Continue the walking stroke around each line angle and onto the proximal surface.
2. Roll the instrument handle between the fingers to keep the side of the probe tip adapted to the tooth surface at line angles and as the tooth contour varies.

3. Continue the strokes under the contact area. Overlap strokes from facial surface with strokes from lingual surface to ensure full coverage (Figure 13-3). Make sure that the col area under each contact has been thoroughly examined.

■ CLINICAL ATTACHMENT LEVEL

Attachment level refers to the position of the periodontal attached tissues at the base of a sulcus or pocket. It is measured from a fixed point to the attachment, whereas the probing depth is measured from a changeable point (the crest of the free gingiva) to the attachment (Figure 13-7A).

I. RATIONALE

A loss of attachment occurs in disease as the junctional epithelium migrates toward the apex. Stability of attachment is characteristic in health, and treatment procedures may be aimed to obtain a gain of attachment.

Evaluation can be made of the outcome of periodontal treatment and the stability of the attachment during maintenance examinations. When periodontal disease is active, pocket formation and migration of the attachment along the cemental surface continue.

II. PROCEDURE

A. Selecting a Fixed Point

1. Cementoenamel junction is usually used.
2. Margin of a permanent restoration.
3. For animal research, a notch may be made in the tooth; in human research studies, a template or splint may be made for each patient.

B. Measuring in the Presence of Visible Recession

1. Cementoenamel junction is visible directly.
2. Measure from the cementoenamel junction to the attachment (Figure 13-7B).
3. The clinical attachment level is greater than the probing depth when there is visible recession.

C. Measuring When the Cementoenamel Junction Is Covered by Gingiva

1. Slide the probe along the tooth surface, into the pocket, until the cementoenamel junction is felt (Figure 13-7C).
2. Remove the calculus when it covers the cementoenamel junction.

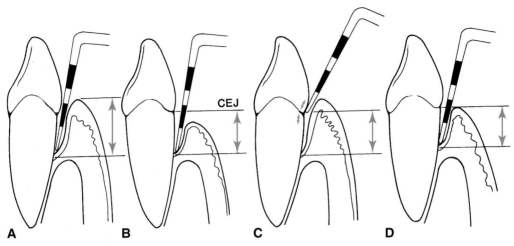

■ **FIGURE 13-7 Clinical Attachment Level. (A)** Probing depth: the pocket is measured from the gingival margin to the attached periodontal tissue. **(B)** Clinical attachment level in the presence of gingival recession is measured directly from the cementoenamel junction (CEJ) to the attached tissue. **(C)** Clinical attachment level when the gingival margin covers the cementoenamel junction: first the cementoenamel junction is located as shown, and then the distance to the cementoenamel junction is measured and subtracted from the probing depth. **(D)** The clinical attachment level is equal to the probing depth when the gingival margin is at the level of the cementoenamel junction.

3. Measure from the gingival crest to the cementoenamel junction.
4. Subtract the millimeters from cementoenamel junction to gingival crest from the total probing depth to the attachment.
5. Probing depth is greater than the clinical attachment level when the cementoenamel junction is covered by free gingiva.

D. Measuring When the Free Gingival Margin Is Level With the Cementoenamel Junction

1. Apply the probe as has been described.
2. The probing depth equals the clinical attachment level when the free gingival margin is level with the cementoenamel junction (Figure 13-7D).

■ FURCATIONS EXAMINATION

When a pocket extends into a furcation area, special adaptation of the probe must be made to determine the extent and topography of the furcation involvement.

I. ANATOMIC FEATURES

A. Bifurcation (teeth with two roots)

1. *Mandibular Molars.* The furcation area is accessible for probing from the facial and lingual surfaces (Figure 13-8).

2. *Maxillary First Premolars.* The furcation area is accessible from the mesial and distal aspects, under the contact area.
3. *Primary Mandibular Molar.* Widespread roots.

B. Trifurcation (teeth with three roots)

1. *Maxillary Molars.* A palatal root and two buccal roots, the mesiobuccal and the distobuccal roots. Access for probing is from the mesial, buccal, and distal surfaces.
2. *Maxillary Primary Molars.* Widespread roots (Figure 13-4).

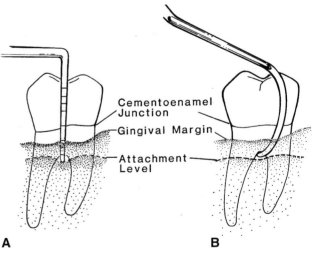

■ **FIGURE 13-8 Furcation Examination. (A)** Williams probe inserted into bifurcation in area of gingival recession shows probing depth of 3 mm. **(B)** Nabers furcation probe used to examine the topography of the furcation area.

II. EXAMINATION METHODS

A. Early Furcation

1. Measure probing depth.
2. Examine the area by adapting the probe closely to the tooth surface and moving the end of the probe over the anatomic curvatures of the roots.
3. Check radiograph for signs of furcation involvement (Figure 13-18).

B. Points of Access

Measure probing depths at points of access for each bifurcation or trifurcation area. Position of gingival margin will vary. Figure 13-8*A* shows apparent recession and 3-mm pocket in bifurcation.

C. Probe Adaptation

Use probe in diagonal or horizontal position to examine between roots when there is gingival recession or a flexible, short, soft pocket wall that permits access.

D. Use of Furcation Probe

Use a furcation probe, such as a Nabers 1N or 2N, to examine advanced furcation (Figure 13-8*B*).

E. Complications

Anatomic variations that complicate furcation examination are fused roots; anomalies, such as extra roots; or low or high furcations.

▪ MUCOGINGIVAL EXAMINATION

I. TENSION TEST[2]

A. Purposes

- To detect adequacy of the width of the attached gingiva.
- To locate frenal attachments and their proximity to the free gingiva.
- To identify promptly the mucogingival junction.

B. Procedures

1. *Facial*
    a. Retract cheeks and lips laterally by grasping the lips with the thumbs and index fingers. Watch at the mucogingival junction.
    b. Move the lips and cheeks up and down and across, creating tension at the mucogingival junction.
    c. Follow around from the molar areas on the right to molar areas on the left, both maxillary and mandibular.
2. *Lingual (Mandible)*
    a. Hold a mouth mirror to tense the mucosa of the floor of the mouth, gently retracting the side of the tongue, so that the mucogingival junction is clearly visible.
    b. Request patient to move the tongue to the left, to the right, and up to touch the palate.

C. Observations

1. Blanching at the mucogingival junction.
2. Frenal attachments.
3. Area(s) of apparent recession where there is very little keratinized gingiva and the base of the sulcus or pocket is near the mucogingival junction.
4. Area where color, size, loss of stippling, smooth shininess, or other characteristic indicates the need for careful probing to determine the amount of attached gingiva.
5. Area where tension pulls the free gingiva away from the tooth, thereby indicating no attached gingiva.

II. GINGIVAL TISSUE EXAMINATION

When inflammation is present and a pocket extends to or through the mucogingival junction, a streak of color (red, bluish-red) that shows the inflammatory changes from the gingival margin to the mucogingival junction may be apparent. When such an area does not pull away during a tension test or does not permit passage of a probe through to the alveolar mucosa, the area should be noted in the record for examination after elimination of inflammation.

III. PROBING

When a pocket extends to or beyond the mucogingival junction, the probe may pass through the pocket directly into the alveolar mucosa (Figure 13-9). Mucogingival involvement is present.

IV. MEASURE THE AMOUNT OF ATTACHED GINGIVA

A. Place the probe on the external surface of the gingiva and measure from the mucogingival junction to the gingival margin to determine the width of the total gingiva (Figure 13-10*A*).
B. Insert the probe and measure probing depth (Figure 13-10*B*).
C. Subtract the probing depth from the total gingival measurement to get the width of the attached gingiva.
D. Record findings.

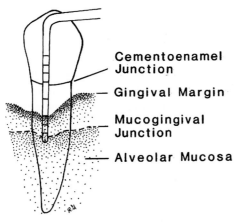

■ FIGURE 13-9 Mucogingival Examination. Probe in position for measuring probing depth where attached gingiva is missing. Absence of attached gingiva permits the probe to pass through the mucogingival junction into the alveolar mucosa.

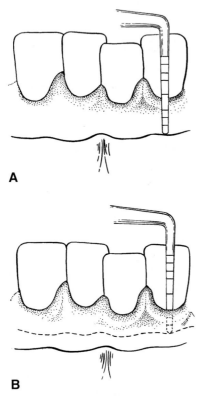

■ FIGURE 13-10 Measuring Attached Gingiva. (A) Measure the total gingiva by laying the probe over the surface of the gingiva and measuring from the free margin to the mucogingival junction. **(B)** Measure the probing depth. Dotted line represents the base of the pocket. Subtract the probing depth **(B)** from the total gingiva **(A)** to obtain the width of attached gingiva. The area illustrated shows 2 mm of attached gingiva.

■ PERIODONTAL CHARTING

Charting of findings while using the probe is a part of the complete periodontal record. The procedure described here assumes the use of a chart form with outline drawings of teeth with both facial and lingual root drawings. The exact procedure and format are entirely the choice of the individual dentist. A composite chart that includes dental as well as periodontal findings is frequently used.

In the preparation of the charting, contrasting colors should be used. For example, when red is used to chart dental caries on a composite charting, red would not be a good color selection for drawing the gingival margin because of possible interference with a drawing of a Class V carious lesion. One procedure for a relatively simple charting system is described here.

I. TEETH IDENTIFICATION

Mark missing, unerupted, or impacted teeth. When radiographs and study casts are available before the recording of clinical findings is scheduled, these markings can be made in advance of the patient's appointment.

II. DRAW GINGIVAL LINES

A. Gingival Margin

1. Draw the outline of the position and contour of the gingival margin on the chart form as it appears in relation to the teeth both facial and lingual.
2. Prepare in advance of the patient's appointment when new study casts are available.

B. Mucogingival Lines

1. *General Procedures*
   a. Use contrasting color to that used for drawing the gingival margin line.
   b. Draw on the facial aspect for all quadrants; draw the lingual line only on the mandibular chart.
2. *Three Methods.* For all, draw the gingival margin line first.
   a. Draw the lines directly, estimating distances between the gingival margin and the mucogingival junction.
   b. Measure with probe.
      i. Measure the total gingiva from gingival margin to mucogingival junction at the center of each tooth (facial and lingual). Write the millimeters on the tooth crown in light pencil to be erased later.
      ii. Place a dot on the tooth chart at the point of millimeters measured from the

margin; connect the dots in a relatively straight line representing the mucogingival junction for the molars and premolars and in a scalloped line for the anterior teeth, in keeping with the actual appearance.

   c. Study casts. When parts or all of the mucogingival lines show clearly on the casts, the drawing can be made in advance of the patient's appointment.

III. RECORD PROBING DEPTHS

  A. Record all diseased pockets of any depth.

  B. Record deepest millimeter measurement for each of the six areas around a tooth, as shown in Figure 13-11. Areas numbered 1, 3, 4, 6 extend from the line angle to under the contact area.

  C. Supplement the six recordings with additional readings to show particular areas of unusually deep pockets, furcation involvement, or mucogingival involvement.

  D. Record on the charting form. Figure 13-12 shows five possible methods for recording the millimeter depth.

IV. RECORD SPECIAL DISEASE PROBLEMS

Furcation involvement, mucogingival involvement, and frenal pull must be recorded either by a special symbol or by writing directly on the chart or in the record.

▪ EXPLORERS

I. GENERAL PURPOSES AND USES

An explorer is used to

  A. Detect, by tactile sense, the texture and character of the tooth surface.

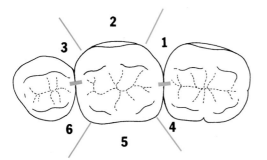

■ **FIGURE 13-11 Charting Probing Depths.** The pocket/sulcus is measured completely around each tooth. Record the deepest measurement for each of the six areas around the tooth. Areas 1, 3, 4, and 6 extend from the line angle to under the contact area.

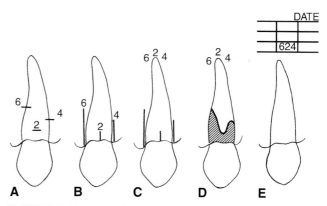

■ **FIGURE 13-12 Methods for Charting Probing Depths.** **(A), (B)** Chart forms with free-hand lines that designate relative depths. **(C)** Numeric notations written at the apex of each tooth. **(D)** A continuous line that defines the entire pocket and that can be shaded. **(E)** Multiple spaces over the apex of each tooth, used to record the probing depths. Each row can be dated, thus allowing comparisons of measurements at successive follow-up and maintenance examinations.

  B. Examine the supragingival tooth surfaces for calculus, demineralized and carious lesions, defects or irregularities in the surfaces and margins of restorations, and other irregularities that are not apparent to direct observation. An explorer is used to confirm direct observation.

  C. Examine the subgingival tooth surfaces for calculus, demineralized and carious lesions, diseased altered cementum, and other cemental changes that can result from periodontal pocket formation.

  D. Define the extent of instrumentation needed and guide techniques for

    1. Scaling and root planing.

    2. Finishing a restoration.

    3. Removing an overhanging filling.

  E. Evaluate the completeness of treatment as shown by the smooth tooth surface or the smooth restoration.

  F. Identify pits and fissures appropriate for sealant application.

II. DESCRIPTION

A. Working End

  1. Slender, wirelike, metal *tip* that is circular in cross section and tapers to a fine sharp *point*.

  2. Design

    a. Single. A single instrument may be universal and adaptable to any tooth surface, or it may be designed for specific groups of surfaces. In Figure 13-13, Nos. 2 through 7, 17, 18, 20, and 23 are single instruments.

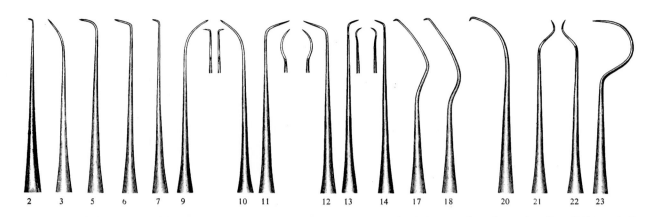

■ **FIGURE 13-13 Explorers.** This series from Nos. 2 through 23 shows standard shapes of explorer tips. Nos. 2 through 7, 17, 18, 20, and 23 are single instruments. Nos. 9 and 10, 11 and 12, 13 and 14, and 21 and 22 are paired instruments. (Courtesy of the S.S. White Company, Philadelphia, PA.)

   b.   Paired. Paired instruments are mirror images of each other, curved to provide access to contralateral tooth surfaces. In Figure 13-13, Nos. 9 and 10, 11 and 12, 13 and 14, and 21 and 22 are paired.

   c.   Design of a balanced instrument. Middle of working end should be centered over the long axis of the handle (Figure 13-14).

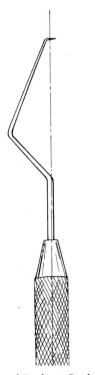

■ **FIGURE 13-14 Balanced Explorer Design.** With the middle of the tip centered over the long axis of the handle (shown by broken line from tip), the explorer can be positioned in a sulcus or pocket with ease and does not cause trauma to the gingival tissue. Shown is the balanced TU-17 explorer.

B. Shank

1. *Straight, Curved, or Angulated.* Whether a shank is straight, curved, or angulated depends on the use and adaptation for which the explorer was designed. In Figure 13-13, compare the straight shanks of Nos. 2, 5, 6, 7, 13, and 14 with the others in the series, which are not straight. A curved shank may facilitate application of the instrument to proximal surfaces, particularly of posterior teeth.

2. *Flexibility.* The slender, wirelike explorers have a degree of flexibility that contributes to increased sensitivity.

C. Handle

1. *Weight.* For increased acute tactile sensitivity, a lightweight handle is more effective.

2. *Diameter.* A wider diameter with serrations for friction while grasping can prevent finger cramping from too tight a grasp. With a lighter grasp, tactile sensitivity can be increased.

D. Construction

1. *Single-ended.* A single-ended instrument has one working end on a separate handle.

2. *Double-ended.* A double-ended instrument has two working ends, one on each end of a common handle. Most paired instruments are available double-ended. Other double-ended instruments combine two single instruments, for example, two unpaired explorers or an explorer with a probe.

III. PREPARATION OF EXPLORERS

Sharpen and retaper a dull explorer tip. With the explorer tip sharp and tapered, the following can be expected:

   A. Increased tactile sensitivity with less pressure required.

B. Prevention of unnecessary trauma to the gingival tissue, because less pressure allows greater control.

C. Decreased instrumentation time with increased patient comfort.

IV. SPECIFIC EXPLORERS AND THEIR USES

A variety of explorers is available, as shown by the examples in Figure 13-13. The function of each type is related to its adaptability to specific surfaces of teeth at particular angulations. Certain explorers can be used effectively for detection of dental caries in pits and fissures, and others are designed to be adapted to examine proximal surfaces for calculus or dental caries. By other criteria, some can be used subgingivally, whereas others cannot be adapted subgingivally without inflicting damage to the sulcular epithelium. Therefore, such explorers are limited to supragingival adaptation only.

A. Subgingival Explorer

1. *Names and Numbers.* Orban No. 20, TU-17, pocket explorer.

2. *Shape.* The pocket explorer has an angulated shank with a short tip (Figure 13-14). The tip should be measured to ensure that it is less than 2 mm. A longer tip cannot be adapted to the line angles of narrow roots.

3. *Features for Subgingival Root Examination*
   a. Back of tip can be applied directly to the attached periodontal tissue at the base of the pocket without lacerating. When a straight or sickle explorer is directed toward the base of the pocket, the sharp tip can pass into the epithelium without resistance.
   b. The short tip can be adapted to rounded tooth surfaces and line angles. Long tips of other explorers have a tangential relationship with the tooth and cause distention and trauma to sulcular or pocket epithelium.
   c. Narrow short tip can be adapted at the base where the pocket narrows without undue displacement of the pocket soft tissue wall.

4. *Supragingival Use of No. TU-17.* It may be adapted to all surfaces and is especially useful for proximal surface examination. It is not readily adaptable to pits and fissures.

B. Sickle or Shepherd's Hook (No. 23 in Figure 13-13)

1. *Use.* Examining pits and fissures and supragingival smooth surfaces; examining surfaces and margins of restorations and sealants.

2. *Adaptability*

a. Difficult to apply to proximal surfaces because the wide hook can contact an adjacent tooth and the straight long section of the tip can pass over a small proximal carious lesion.

b. Not adaptable for deep subgingival exploration. When the point is directed to the base of a pocket, trauma to the attachment area can result. In the attempt to prevent such damage, the clinician may not explore to the base of the pocket, thus providing incomplete service.

C. Pigtail or Cowhorn (Nos. 21 and 22 in Figure 13-13)

1. *Use.* Proximal surfaces for calculus, dental caries, or margins of restorations.

2. *Adaptability.* As paired, curved tips, they are applied to opposite tooth surfaces.

D. Straight (Nos. 2, 6, and 7 in Figure 13-13)

1. *Use.* Supragingival, for pits and fissures, tooth irregularities of smooth surfaces, and surfaces and margins of restorations and sealants.

2. *Adaptability*
   a. For pit and fissure caries, the explorer tip is held parallel with the long axis of the tooth and applied straight into a pit.
   b. Not adaptable deep in subgingival area. Straight shanked instruments or those with long tips cannot be adapted readily in the apical portion of the pocket near the attached tissue or on line angles.

■ BASIC PROCEDURES FOR USE OF EXPLORERS

Development of ability to use an explorer and a probe is achieved first by learning the anatomic features of each tooth surface and the types of irregularities that may be encountered on the surfaces. The second step is repeated practice of careful and deliberate techniques for application of the instruments.

The objective is to adapt the instruments in a routine manner that relays consistent comparative information about the nature of the tooth surface. Concentration, patience, attention to detail, and alertness to each irregularity, however small it may seem, are necessary.

I. USE OF SENSORY STIMULI

Both explorers and probes can transmit tactile stimuli from tooth surfaces to the fingers. A fine explorer usually gives a more acute sense of tactile discrimination to small irregularities than does a thicker explorer. Probes vary in diameter; the narrow types may provide greater sensitivity.

II. TOOTH SURFACE IRREGULARITIES

Three basic tactile sensations must be distinguished when probing or exploring. These may be grouped as normal tooth surface, irregularities created by excess or elevations in the surface, and irregularities caused by depressions in the tooth surface. Examples of these are listed here.

A. Normal

1. *Tooth Structure.* The smooth surface of enamel and root surface that has been planed; anatomic configurations, such as cingula, furcations.
2. *Restored Surfaces.* Smooth surfaces of metal (gold, amalgam) and the softer feeling of plastic; smooth margin of a restoration.

B. Irregularities: Increases or Elevations in Tooth Surface

1. *Deposits.* Calculus.
2. *Anomalies.* Enamel pearl; unusually pronounced cementoenamel junction.
3. *Restorations.* Overcontoured, irregular margins (overhangs).

C. Irregularities: Depressions, Grooves

1. *Tooth Surface.* Demineralized or carious lesion, abrasion, erosion, pits such as those caused by enamel hypoplasia, areas of cemental resorption on the root surface.
2. *Restorations.* Deficient margin, rough surface.

III. TYPES OF STIMULI

During exploring and probing, distinction of irregularities can be made through auditory and tactile means.

A. Tactile

Tactile sensations pass through the instrument to the fingers and hand and to the brain for registration and action. Tactile sensations, for example, may be the result of catching on an overcontoured restoration, dropping into a carious lesion, hooking the edge of a restoration or lesion, encountering an elevated deposit, or simply passing over a rough surface.

B. Auditory

As an explorer or probe moves over the surface of enamel, cementum, a metallic restoration, a plastic restoration, or any irregularity of tooth structure or restoration, a particular surface texture is apparent. With each contact, sound may be created. The clean smooth enamel is quiet; the rough cementum or calculus is scratchy or noisy. Sometimes a metallic restoration may "squeak" or have a metallic "ring." With experience, differentiations can be made.

■ SUPRAGINGIVAL PROCEDURES

I. USE OF VISION

Supragingival exploration for defects of the tooth surface differs from subgingival in that when a surface is dried, much of the actual exploration is performed to confirm visual observation. The exceptions are the proximal areas near and around contact areas that cannot be directly observed.

Unnecessary exploration should be avoided. With adequate light and a source of air, proper retraction, and use of a mouth mirror, dried supragingival calculus can generally be seen as either chalky white or brownish-yellow in contrast to tooth color. A minimum of exploration can confirm the finding.

II. FACIAL AND LINGUAL SURFACES

A. Adapt the side of tip with the point always on the tooth surface.
B. Move the instrument in short walking strokes over the surface being examined, or direct the side of the tip gently over a suspected carious lesion.
C. An intact surface where remineralization can be going on must not be vigorously explored. Careful noninvasive examination can be made using the side of the tip of an explorer gently to test whether the demineralized area has slight roughness. As described on pages 395 to 396 in Chapter 24, picking or scratching the surface can prevent further remineralization.

III. PROXIMAL SURFACES

A. Lead with the tip onto a proximal surface, rolling the handle between the fingers to ensure adaptation around the line angle. Keep the side of the point of the explorer in contact with the tooth surface at all times.
B. Explore under the proximal contact area when there is recession of the papilla and the area is exposed. Overlap strokes from facial and lingual surfaces to ensure full coverage.

▪ SUBGINGIVAL PROCEDURES

I. ESSENTIALS FOR DETECTION OF TOOTH SURFACE IRREGULARITIES

A. Definite but light grasp.

B. Consistent finger rest with light pressure.

C. Definite contact of the instrument with the tooth.

D. Light touch as the instrument is moved over the tooth surface.

II. STEPS

A. With the tip in contact with the tooth supragingivally, hold the lower shank (the part of the shank that is next to the tip) parallel with the long axis of the tooth. Gently slide the tip under the gingival margin into the sulcus or pocket.

B. Keep the point in contact with the tooth at all times to prevent unnecessary trauma to the pocket or sulcular epithelium. Adapt the tip closely to the tooth surface by applying the side of the point.

C. Slide the explorer tip over the tooth surface to the base of the pocket until, with the back of the tip, the resistance of the soft tissue of the attached periodontal tissue is felt (Figure 13-15A). Calculus deposits may obstruct direct passage of the instrument to the base of the pocket. Lift the tip slightly away from the tooth surface and follow over the deposit to proceed to the base of the pocket.

D. Use a "walking" stroke, vertical or diagonal (oblique).

  1. Lead with the tip. Move it ahead as the instrument progresses (Figure 13-15B).

  2. Length of stroke depends on the depth of a pocket.

    a. Shallow sulcus. The stroke may extend the entire depth, from the base of the pocket to just beneath the gingival margin.

    b. Deep pocket. Controlled strokes 2- to 3-mm long can provide more acute sensitivity to the surface and allow improved adaptation of the instrument. A deep pocket should be explored in sections. One should first explore the apical area next to the base of the pocket, then move up to a higher section, overlapping for full coverage.

  3. Do not remove the explorer from the pocket for each stroke on a particular surface because

    a. Trauma to the gingival margin caused by repeated withdrawal and reinsertion can cause the patient posttreatment discomfort.

    b. Concentration on the texture of the tooth surface is interrupted.

    c. More time is consumed.

E. Proximal surface

  1. Lead with tip of instrument; do not "back into" an area.

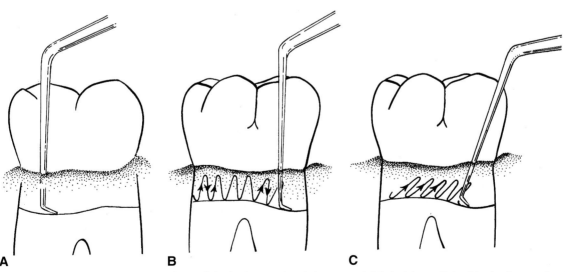

▪ **FIGURE 13-15 Use of Subgingival Explorer. (A)** The lower shank (next to tip) is held parallel with the long axis of the tooth. The explorer is passed into the pocket and lowered until the back of the working tip meets resistance from the attached periodontal tissue at the base of the pocket. **(B)** Vertical walking stroke. With the side of the tip in contact with the tooth surface at all times, the explorer is moved over the surface. **(C)** Diagonal walking stroke. Complete exploration of the surface is needed; therefore, groups of strokes are overlapped.

2. Continue the strokes around the line angle. Roll the instrument handle between the fingers to keep the tip closely adapted as the tooth contour changes.
3. Continue strokes under the contact area. Overlap strokes from facial and lingual aspects for full coverage.

■ RECORD FINDINGS

I. SUPRAGINGIVAL CALCULUS

A. Distribution

Supragingival calculus is generally localized. It is most commonly confined to the lingual surfaces of the mandibular anterior teeth and the facial surfaces of the maxillary first and second molars, opposite the openings to the salivary ducts.

B. Amount

Slight, moderate, heavy.

II. SUBGINGIVAL CALCULUS

A. Distribution

Subgingival calculus can be either localized or generalized.

B. Amount

Slight, moderate, heavy.

III. OTHER IRREGULARITIES OF TOOTH SURFACE

Note on the chart or in the record any other deviation from normal detected while using the explorer.

■ MOBILITY EXAMINATION

Because of the nature and function of the periodontal ligament, teeth have a slight normal mobility. Mobility can be considered abnormal or pathologic when it exceeds normal. Increased mobility can be an important clinical sign of disease.

I. CAUSES OF MOBILITY

A. Inflammation

Inflammation in the periodontal ligament leads to degeneration or destruction of the fibers.

B. Loss of Support

Loss of sufficient support by alveolar bone and periodontal ligament (destroyed by periodontal infection) can increase the mobility.

C. Trauma From Occlusion

Injury to the periodontal tissues can result from occlusal forces.

II. PROCEDURE FOR DETERMINATION OF MOBILITY

A. Position the patient for clear visibility with maximum light and ready accessibility through convenient retraction.
B. Stabilize the head. Motion of the head, lips, or cheek can interfere with a true evaluation of tooth movement.
C. Use two single-ended metal instruments with wide blunt ends, held with a modified pen grasp. Use of wooden tongue depressors or plastic mirror handles is not recommended because of their flexibility. Testing with the fingers without the metal instruments can be misleading because the soft tissue of the fingertips can move and give an illusion of tooth movement.
D. Apply specific, firm finger rests (fulcrums). A standardized finger rest pressure contributes increased consistency to the determinations. The teeth may be dried with air or sponge to prevent slipping of the instruments or the finger on the finger rest.
E. Apply the blunt ends of the instruments to opposite sides of a tooth, and rock the tooth to test horizontal mobility. Keep both instrument ends on the tooth as pressure is applied first from one side and then the other.
F. Test vertical mobility (depression of the tooth into its socket) by applying, on the occlusal or incisal surface, pressure with one of the mirror handles.
G. Test each primary abutment tooth of a fixed partial denture.
H. Move from tooth to tooth in a systematic order.

III. RECORD DEGREE OF MOVEMENT

A. Scale

N, 1, 2, 3 or I, II, III are frequently used, sometimes with a + to indicate mobility between numbers.

B. Recording

Although subjective, interpretation may be considered as follows.[3]

N = normal, physiologic

1 = slight mobility, greater than normal

2 = moderate mobility, greater than 1 mm displacement

3 = severe mobility, may move in all directions, vertical as well as horizontal.

C. The Letter N Means *Normal Mobility*

All teeth that have a periodontal ligament have normal mobility. No tooth has zero mobility except in a condition, such as ankylosis, in which there is no periodontal ligament.

D. Chart Form

A chart form should provide for a place to record mobility. Preferably more than one place should be reserved so that comparative readings may be recorded at successive maintenance appointments.

■ FREMITUS

I. DEFINITION

Fremitus means palpable vibration or movement. In dentistry it refers to the vibratory patterns of the teeth. A tooth with fremitus has excess contact, possibly related to a premature contact. Usually, the tooth also demonstrates some degree of mobility because the excess contact forces the tooth to move. The test is used in conjunction with occlusal analysis and adjustment.

Because fremitus depends on tooth contact, determination is made only on the maxillary teeth.

II. PROCEDURE FOR DETERMINATION OF FREMITUS

A. Seat the patient upright with the head stabilized against the headrest.

B. Press an index finger on each maxillary tooth at about the cervical third (Figure 13-16).

C. Request the patient to "click the back teeth" repeatedly.

D. Start with the most posterior maxillary tooth on one side, and move the index finger tooth by tooth around the arch.

E. Record by tooth number the teeth where vibration is felt and the teeth where actual movement is noted. The degree recorded may be subjective, but the following range has been suggested.

N = normal (without vibration or movement).

+ = One-degree fremitus; only slight vibration can be felt.

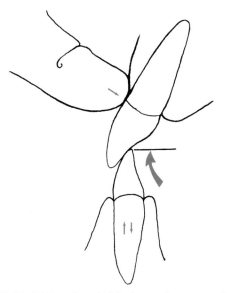

■ **FIGURE 13-16 Fremitus.** With the patient seated upright and the head stabilized against the headrest, an index finger is placed firmly over the cervical third of each maxillary tooth in succession starting with the most posterior tooth on one side and moving around the arch. The patient is requested to click the posterior teeth.

+ + = Two-degree fremitus; the tooth is clearly palpable but movement is barely visible.

+ + + = Three-degree fremitus; movement is clearly observed visually.

■ RADIOGRAPHIC EXAMINATION

Radiographs provide essential information to aid and supplement clinical findings. During other phases of the examination, and especially during probing, the mounted radiographs should be on a viewbox for viewing in conjunction with examination. When the radiographs have not been processed at the time of probing, areas of special confirmation can be marked on the record for review at the next appointment.

For observing evidence of periodontal involvement, periapical radiographs are needed. Horizontal bitewing radiographs do not show the complete periodontal tissues that extend around the roots. When bone loss is moderate to severe, the crest of the bone may be seen in a vertical bitewing survey.

Principles for use of radiographs are described elsewhere. The need for mounted radiographs free from errors of technique and viewed on an adequately lighted viewbox cannot be overemphasized. A magnifying reading glass is of special assistance when studying periodontal findings.

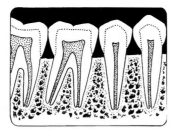

■ **FIGURE 13-17 Normal Bone Level.** Drawing of a radiograph to show normal bone level, 1 to 1.5 mm from the cementoenamel junction.

■ RADIOGRAPHIC CHANGES IN PERIODONTAL INFECTIONS

I. BONE LEVEL

A. Normal Bone Level

The crest of the interdental bone appears from 1.0 to 1.5 mm from the cementoenamel junction (Figure 13-17).

B. Bone Level in Periodontal Disease

The height of the bone is lowered progressively as the inflammation is extended and bone is resorbed.

II. SHAPE OF REMAINING BONE

A. Horizontal

1. When the crest of the bone is parallel with a line between the cementoenamel junctions of two adjacent teeth, the term "horizontal bone loss" is used (Figures 13-18 and 13-19).
2. When inflammation is the sole destructive factor, the bone loss usually appears horizontal.
3. When the amount of remaining bone is fairly evenly distributed throughout the dentition, the

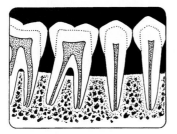

■ **FIGURE 13-18 Horizontal Bone Loss.** Bone level in periodontal disease is more than 1 to 1.5 mm from the cementoenamel junction. When bone loss is horizontal, the crest of the alveolar bone is parallel with a line between the cementoenamel junctions of adjacent teeth. Note early furcation involvement in the second molar and moderate furcation involvement in the first molar.

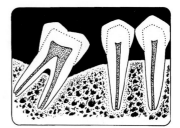

■ **FIGURE 13-19 Horizontal Bone Loss.** Second molar has drifted mesially into the space created when the first molar was removed. Note that the level of the crestal bone is parallel with a line between the cementoenamel junctions of the second premolar and the tipped second molar.

condition is described as *generalized* horizontal bone loss. It may be designated either by millimeters from the position of the normal bone level or by percentage. When making estimates, referral to the table of average root lengths can be helpful.

4. When bone loss is confined to specific areas, the condition is described as *localized* horizontal bone loss.

B. Angular or Vertical

1. Reduction in height of crestal bone that is irregular; the bone level is not parallel with a line joining the adjacent cementoenamel junctions (Figure 13-20); bone loss is greater on the proximal surface of one tooth than on the adjacent tooth.
2. Angular bone loss is more commonly localized; rarely generalized.
3. When inflammation and trauma from occlusion are combined in causing the destruction and irregular shape of the bone, the bone may appear with "angular defects" or with "vertical bone loss."

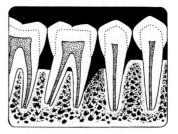

■ **FIGURE 13-20 Angular or Vertical Bone Loss; Mesial of the First Molar.** The level of the crestal bone between the second premolar and the first molar is not parallel with a line between the cementoenamel junctions of the same teeth.

III. CRESTAL LAMINA DURA

A. Normal

White, radiopaque; continuous with and connects the lamina dura about the roots of two adjacent teeth; covers the interdental bone (Figure 13-18).

B. Evidence of Disease

The crestal lamina dura is indistinct, irregular, radiolucent, fuzzy (Figure 13-20, mesial of first molar).

IV. FURCATION INVOLVEMENT

A. Normal

Bone fills the area between the roots (Figure 13-17).

B. Evidence of Disease

Radiolucent area in the furcation.
1. Early furcation involvement may appear as a small radiolucent black dot or as a slight thickening of the periodontal ligament space. It can be confirmed by probing. Early furcation involvement is shown in the second molar in Figure 13-18.
2. Furcation involvement of maxillary molars may become advanced before radiographic evidence can be seen. Superimposition of the palatal root may mask a small area of involvement. When the proximal bone level in the radiograph appears at the level where the furcation is normally located, furcation involvement should be suspected and probed for confirmation.
3. Maxillary first premolar furcation involvement cannot be seen in a radiograph except at an unusual angulation or unusual position of the tooth. With correct vertical and horizontal angulation, the roots are superimposed.
4. Furcations may show at one angulation but not at another; variations in technique can obscure a furcation involvement. All furcations must be carefully probed.

V. PERIODONTAL LIGAMENT SPACE

A. Normal

The periodontal ligament is connective tissue and, hence, appears radiolucent in a radiograph. It appears as a fine black radiolucent line next to the root surface. On its outer side is the lamina dura, the bone that lines the tooth socket and appears radiopaque (Figure 13-21).

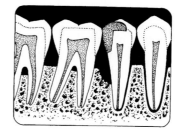

■ **FIGURE 13-21 Periodontal Ligament Space.** First and second molars have a normal periodontal ligament space, which appears as a fine black line about the roots. The first premolar shows thickening of the ligament space about the entire root, and the second premolar has thickening only about the mesial surface of the root.

B. Evidence of Disease

Widening or thickening.
1. *Angular Thickening or Triangulation.* The space is widened only near the coronal third, near the crest of the interdental bone.
2. *Complete Periodontal Ligament Thickened Along an Entire Side of a Root to the Apex, or Around the Root* (Figure 13-21). When viewed at different angulations (in the various radiographs of a complete survey), the ligament space may reveal varying thicknesses, thus showing that the disease involvement is not consistent around the entire root or that other structures are superimposed.

■ EARLY PERIODONTAL DISEASE

The real preventive service is to recognize *early signs* of periodontal involvement so that treatment can be initiated to arrest the disease and prevent more severe involvement, which could lead to tooth loss. The recognition of severe bone loss, advanced furcation involvement, and marked thickening of the periodontal ligament space is not difficult after a basic understanding has been gained. The difficult part is to watch carefully for incipient, often isolated indications of early periodontal disease. These changes can be seen in all age groups, from young children to elderly patients.

I. EARLIEST SIGNS

The earliest signs of periodontal involvement are not evident in a radiograph. Only after the inflammation has extended from the soft tissue (gingivitis) to the supporting periodontal tissues and bone resorption has become sufficient does radiographic evidence appear.

II. INITIAL BONE DESTRUCTION

A. The usual interproximal pathway of inflammation from gingivitis to periodontitis is directly from the inflamed gingival connective tissue into the crest of the interdental bone.

B. Initial bone destruction most frequently occurs at the crest of the interdental bone in the crestal lamina dura.

III. RADIOGRAPHIC EVIDENCE

A. Crestal lamina dura may appear slightly irregular, fuzzy, and radiolucent. At this stage it is best examined with a hand magnifying glass.

B. Angular thickening of the periodontal ligament space (triangulation) may also be apparent.

■ OTHER RADIOGRAPHIC FINDINGS

Any other radiographic findings that may be related directly or indirectly to periodontal involvement and its contributing factors should be noted in the record. Certain findings have a direct relation to dental hygiene care and instruction, particularly local factors that contribute to food impaction or biofilm retention.

I. CALCULUS

Gross deposits, primarily those on proximal surfaces, may be seen in radiographs. Observing these may be helpful, but the probe and explorer are needed to define the exact location and extent.

The density and contrast of the radiograph influence whether calculus is seen. Because all deposits are not visible, the use of radiographs has very limited value for specific calculus detection.

II. OVERHANGING RESTORATIONS

Some proximal overhanging margins may be seen on radiographs. The use of an explorer is necessary to detect irregular margins and to examine all proximal margins that do not reveal irregularities in the radiographs. Superimposition can mask an overhanging margin.

III. DENTAL CARIES

Clinical and radiographic identification of carious lesions is described elsewhere. Certain findings should be noted for their relationship to the periodontal tissues.

A. Large carious lesions may leave open contact areas that permit food impaction and hence damage the periodontal tissues.

B. Carious lesions, either enamel or root caries, hold biofilm and provide a rough surface for retention of food debris and dental biofilm.

C. Root caries and demineralization may interfere with techniques of root planing and require instruction in remineralization procedures.

IV. RELATIONSHIP TO POCKETS

Radiographs do not show pockets; soft tissue does not show in a radiograph. Because a pocket is measured from the gingival margin to the base of the pocket, both of which are soft tissue, pockets cannot be seen on a radiograph. Probing is necessary to identify pockets.

Everyday Ethics

Mrs. Claren, a neat-appearing lady in her 50s, was new to the practice. After a careful history recording, Doris, the dental hygienist, started the gingival examination and continued into the routine probing. Many of the probing depths were 3 and 4 mm, and some even 5 mm. Doris could feel subgingival calculus as she probed, and there was bleeding from her gentle probing.

Doris was nearly finished and was writing on the record when the patient raised her head and said, "You aren't cleaning my teeth. What is it you are doing?" Suddenly Doris realized that this lady may never have had a complete periodontal examination and was unaware of her moderate to severe chronic periodontitis with generalized subgingival calculus.

Questions for Consideration

1. What ethical responsibility does a dental hygienist have to first-time patients to explain all procedures and educate about observations made while gathering assessment information?

2. Should the hygienist have obtained informed consent in this scenario prior to developing the treatment plan for this patient? Why or why not?

3. After the appointment, what should the dental hygienist do as a follow-up for this patient to ensure a good outcome?

Factors To Teach The Patient

- The need for a careful, thorough examination if treatment is to be complete and effective.

- Information about the instruments and how their use makes the examination complete. Examples are the complete radiographic survey, probing 360° around each tooth, and exploring each subgingival tooth surface.

- Why bleeding can occur when probing. Healthy tissue does not bleed.

- Relation of probing depth measurements to normal sulci.

- Significance of mobility.

REFERENCES

1. Listgarten, M.A.: Periodontal Probing: What Does It Mean?, *J. Clin. Periodontol., 7,* 165, June, 1980.
2. Kopczyk, R.A. and Saxe, S.R.: Clinical Signs of Gingival Inadequacy: The Tension Test, *ASDC J. Dent. Child., 41,* 352, September–October, 1974.
3. Miller, S.C.: *Textbook of Periodontia,* 3rd ed. Philadelphia, The Blakiston Co., 1950, p. 125.

SUGGESTED READINGS

Armitage, G.C.: Clinical Evaluation of Periodontal Diseases, *Periodontol. 2000, 7,* 39, 1995.
Armitage, G.C.: Periodontal Diseases: Diagnosis, *Ann. Periodontol., 1,* 54-96, November, 1996.
Daly, C., Mitchell, D., Grossburg, D., Highfield, J., and Stewart, D.: Bacteraemia Caused by Periodontal Probing, *Austr. Dent. J., 42,* 77, April, 1997.
Eickholz, P.: Reproducibility and Validity of Furcation Measurements as Related to Class of Furcation Invasion, *J. Periodontol., 66,* 984, November, 1995.
Giargia, M. and Linde, J.: Tooth Mobility and Periodontal Disease, *J. Clin. Periodontol., 24,* 785, November, 1997.
McKechnie, L.B.: Root Morphology in Periodontal Therapy, *DentalHygienistNews, 6,* 3, Winter, 1993.
Nield-Gehrig, J.S. and Houseman, G.A.: *Fundamentals of Periodontal Instrumentation,* 3rd ed. Baltimore, Williams & Wilkins, 1996, pp. 215-245.
Papaioannou, W., Bollen, C.M.L., vanEldere, J., and Quirynen, M.: The Adherence of Periodontopathogens to Periodontal Probes: A Possible Factor in Intra-oral Transmission? *J. Periodontol., 67,* 1164, November, 1996.
Strassler, H.E.: Perio Charting Systems, *RDH, 12,* 23, January, 1992.
Svärdstrom, G. and Wennstrom, J.L.: Prevalence of Furcation Involvements in Patients Referred for Periodontal Treatment, *J. Clin. Periodontol., 23,* 1093, December, 1996.
Waerhaug, J.: The Furcation Problem: Etiology, Pathogenesis, Diagnosis, Therapy and Prognosis, *J. Clin. Periodontol., 7,* 73, April, 1980.

Probing

Aguero, A., Garnick, J.J., Keagle, J., Steflik, D.E., and Thompson, W.O.: Histological Location of a Standardized Periodontal Probe in Man, *J. Periodontol., 66,* 184, March, 1995.
Clerehugh, V., Abdeia, R., and Hull, P.S.: The Effect of Subgingival Calculus on the Validity of Clinical Probing Measurements, *J. Dent., 24,* 329, September, 1996.
Lang, N.P., Nyman, S., Senn, C., and Joss, A.: Bleeding on Probing as It Relates to Probing Pressure and Gingival Health, *J. Clin. Periodontol., 18,* 257, April, 1991.
Mayfield, L., Bratthall, G., and Attström, R.: Periodontal Probe Precision Using 4 Different Periodontal Probes, *J. Clin. Periodontol., 23,* 76, February, 1996.
Pattison, A.M. and Pattison, G.L.: *Periodontal Instrumentation,* 2nd ed. Norwalk, CT, Appleton & Lange, 1992, pp. 17–24.
Reddy, M.S., Palcanis, K.G., and Geurs, N.C.: A Comparison of Manual and Controlled-Force Attachment-Level Measurements, *J. Clin. Periodontol., 24,* 920, December, 1997.
Samuel, E.D., Griffiths, G.S., and Petrie, A.: In Vitro Accuracy and Reproducibility of Automated and Conventional Periodontal Probes, *J. Clin. Periodontol., 24,* 340, May, 1997.
Villata, L. and Baelum, V.: Reproducibility of Attachment Level Recordings Using an Electronic and a Conventional Probe, *J. Periodontol., 67,* 1292, December, 1996.
Zappa, U., Grosso, L., Simona, C., Graf, H., and Case, D.: Clinical Furcation Diagnoses and Interradicular Bone Defects, *J. Periodontol., 64,* 219, March, 1993.

Temperature Probe

Fedi, P.F. and Killoy, W.J.: Temperature Differences at Periodontal Sites in Health and Disease, *J. Periodontol., 63,* 24, January, 1992.
Haffajee, A.D., Socransky, S.S., and Goodson, J.M.: Subgingival Temperature (I). Relation to Baseline Clinical Parameters, *J. Clin. Periodontol., 19,* 401, July, 1992.
Haffajee, A.D., Socransky, S.S., and Goodson, J.M.: Subgingival Temperature (II). Relation to Future Periodontal Attachment Loss, *J. Clin. Periodontol., 19,* 409, July, 1992.
Haffajee, A.D., Socransky, S.S., Smith, C., Dibart, S., and Goodson, J.M.: Subgingival Temperature (III). Relation to Microbial Counts, *J. Clin. Periodontol., 19,* 417, July, 1992.
Kung, R.T.V., Ochs, B., and Goodson, J.M.: Temperature as a Periodontal Diagnostic, *J. Clin. Periodontol., 17,* 557, September, 1990.
Perdok, J.F., Lukacovic, M., Majeti, S., Arends, J., and Busscher, H.J.: Sulcus Temperature Distributions in the Absence and Presence of Oral Hygiene, *J. Periodont. Res., 27,* 97, March, 1992.

Radiographs

Åkesson, L., Håkansson, J., and Rohlin, M.: Comparison of Panoramic and Intraoral Radiography and Pocket Probing for the Measurement of the Marginal Bone Level, *J. Periodontol., 19,* 326, May, 1992.
Carranza, F.A. and Newman, M.G.: *Clinical Periodontology,* 8th ed. Philadelphia, W.B. Saunders Co., 1996, pp. 362-369.
Hausmann, E., Allen, K., and Clerehugh, V.: What Alveolar Crest Level on a Bite-wing Radiograph Represents Bone Loss?, *J. Periodontol., 62,* 570, September, 1991.
Hausmann, E., Allen, K., Norderyd, J., Ren, W., Shibly, O., and Machtei, E.: Studies on the Relationship Between Changes in Radiographic Bone Height and Probing Attachment, *J. Clin. Periodontol., 21,* 128, February, 1994.
Herzog, A. and Paarmann, C.: Enhancing Accurate Assessment of Periodontal Disease by Improving Radiographic Interpretation, *Can. Dent. Hyg. (Probe), 31,* 130, July/August, 1997.

Disease Development and Contributing Factors

CHAPTER OUTLINE

Early in the process of case assessment in preparation for care planning, the presence and severity of periodontal infection must be determined. Is the patient's disease limited to the gingival tissue without loss of periodontal attachment? Does the patient have bone loss, pocket formation, or other signs of periodontitis?

Table 14-1 shows the clinical case types. The case type designation for a patient is determined by first noting the gingival markers by direct observation, and then using the probe and studying the radiographs. The probe is utilized for many parts of the examination, one of which is assessment of the gingival and periodontal probing depths.

When the disease is limited to the gingiva, the possibility of reversal of the infection is considered first in the care planning objectives. Can the patient be guided to learn new habits of self-treatment through daily infection

control supplemented by periodic professional scaling? On the other hand, if there is apical positioning of the periodontal attachment with alveolar bone loss and other indications of periodontitis, can conservative procedures of *nonsurgical periodontal therapy* provide sufficient professional treatment? Is more complex periodontal therapy required?

Individual differences and the particular clinical features of each patient must be recognized. The oral tissues need treatment that can bring them to a state of maximum health that can be maintained by the patient.

Except in cases of advanced periodontitis, the need for additional treatment after initial nonsurgical periodontal therapy is rarely possible to predict. A reassessment of the treated tissues must be built into the care plan. The patient must be given a clear understanding of the purpose of such a reevaluation.

TABLE 14-1 PERIODONTAL CASE TYPES

CASE TYPE I—GINGIVAL DISEASE
Inflammation of the gingiva characterized clinically by changes in color, gingival form, position, surface appearance, and presence of bleeding and/or exudate.

CASE TYPE II—EARLY PERIODONTITIS
Progression of the gingival inflammation into the deeper periodontal structures and alveolar bone crest, with slight bone loss. There is usually a slight loss of connective tissue attachment and alveolar bone.

CASE TYPE III—MODERATE PERIODONTITIS
A more advanced stage of the preceding condition, with increased destruction of the periodontal structures and noticeable loss of bone support, possibly accompanied by an increase in tooth mobility. There may be furcation involvement in multirooted teeth.

CASE TYPE IV—ADVANCED PERIODONTITIS
Further progression of periodontitis with major loss of alveolar bone support usually accompanied by increased tooth mobility. Furcation involvement in multirooted teeth.

CASE TYPE V—REFRACTORY PERIODONTITIS
Includes those patients with multiple disease sites that continue to demonstrate attachment loss after appropriate therapy. These sites presumably continue to be infected by periodontal pathogens no matter how thorough or frequent the treatment provided. Also includes those patients with recurrent disease at single or multiple sites.

From American Academy of Periodontology: *Current Procedural Terminology for Periodontics and Insurance Reporting Manual,* 7th ed. Chicago, 1995, p. 15.

In this chapter, gingival and periodontal pockets and their development are described. Local and systemic risk factors for the initiation and progression of gingival and periodontal diseases are outlined. Key words are defined in Box 14-1.

▪ DEVELOPMENT OF GINGIVAL AND PERIODONTAL INFECTIONS

The stages of development of gingivitis are divided into the *initial lesion,* the *early lesion,* and the *established lesion.*[1] With an accumulation of dental biofilm on the cervical tooth surface adjacent to the gingival margin, an inflammatory reaction is set up, and the natural defense mechanisms respond.

I. THE INITIAL LESION

A. Inflammatory Response to Dental Biofilm

Occurs within 2 to 4 days.
1. Migration and infiltration of white blood cells into the junctional epithelium and gingival sulcus.
2. Increased flow of gingival sulcus fluid.
3. Early breakdown of collagen; fluid fills the spaces in the connective tissue.

B. Clinical Appearance

No clinical evidence of change appears in the earliest phases.

II. THE EARLY LESION

A. Increased Inflammatory Response

1. Dental biofilm becomes older and thicker (7 to 14 days; time reflects individual differences).
2. Infiltration of fluid, lymphocytes, and neutrophils with a few plasma cells into the connective tissue.
3. Breakdown of collagen fiber support to the gingival margin.
4. Epithelium proliferates and epithelial extensions and rete ridges are formed.

B. Clinical Appearance

1. Early signs of gingivitis become apparent with slight gingival enlargement; will become an established lesion if undisturbed.
2. Early gingivitis is reversible when biofilm is controlled and inflammation is reduced. Healthy tissue may be restored.
3. Susceptibility of individuals varies; time before lesion becomes established varies.

III. THE ESTABLISHED LESION

A. Progression From the Early Lesion

1. Fluid and leukocyte migration into tissues and sulcus increase; plasma cells are related to areas of chronic inflammation.
2. Formation of *pocket epithelium.*
   a. Proliferation of the junctional and sulcular epithelium continues in an attempt to wall out the inflammation.

BOX 14-1 KEY WORDS: Disease Development

Cicatrix: the fibrous tissue left after the healing of a wound; cicatricial: adj.

Collagen: white fibers of the connective tissue.

Collagenase: enzyme that catalyzes the degradation (hydrolysis) of collagen.

Desquamation: shedding of the outer epithelial layer of the stratified squamous epithelium of skin or mucosa.

Diastema: a space or abnormal opening; as a dental term, it is a space between two adjacent teeth in the same dental arch.

Edema: an accumulation of excessive fluid in cells, tissues, or a serous cavity.

Enzyme: a protein secreted by body cells that acts as a catalyst to induce chemical changes in other substances but remains unchanged itself.

Food impaction: forceful wedging of food into the periodontium by occlusal forces.

Gingivitis: inflammation of the gingival tissues.

Iatrogenic: resulting from treatment by a professional person.

Infiltration: the diffusion or accumulation in a tissue or cells of substances not normal to it or in amounts in excess of normal.

Lesion: any pathologic or traumatic discontinuity of tissue or loss of function of a part; broad term including wounds, sores, ulcers, tumors, and any other tissue damage.

Nonsurgical periodontal therapy: includes dental biofilm removal and biofilm control (by patient); supragingival and subgingival scaling; root planing; and the adjunctive use of chemotherapeutic agents for control of bacterial infection, desensitizing hypersensitive exposed root surfaces, and dental caries prevention as related to the health of the periodontium.

Periodontitis: inflammation in the periodontium affecting gingival tissues, periodontal ligament, cementum, and supporting bone.

Permeable: permitting passage of a fluid.

Refractory: not readily responsive to treatment.

Toxin: a poison; protein produced by certain animals, higher plants, and pathogenic bacteria.

  Bacterial toxin: poison produced by bacteria; includes exotoxins, endotoxins, and toxic enzymes.

Xerostomia: dryness of the mouth from a lack of normal secretions.

---

  b. Pocket epithelium is more permeable; areas of ulceration of the lining epithelium develop.
  c. Early pocket formation.
3. Collagen destruction continues; connective tissue fiber support lost.
4. Progression to early periodontal lesion may occur, or some established lesions may remain stable for extended periods of time.

B. Clinical Appearance

Clear evidence of inflammation is present with marginal redness, bleeding on probing, and spongy marginal gingiva. Later, chronic fibrosis develops.

IV. THE ADVANCED LESION

A. Extension of Inflammation

1. Bacteria from supragingival biofilm enter the sulcus and provide the source for subgingival biofilm.
2. Biofilm microorganisms produce irritants.
3. Alveolar bone destruction
  a. Inflammation spreads through the loose connective tissue along (beside) the blood vessels to the alveolar bone.[2]
  b. Most commonly, the inflammation enters the bone through small vessel channels in the alveolar crest.

c. Inflammation spreads through the bone marrow and out into the periodontal ligament.

B. Progressive Destruction of Connective Tissue

1. Connective tissue fibers below the junctional epithelium are destroyed; the epithelium migrates along the root surface.
2. Coronal portion of junctional epithelium becomes detached.
3. Exposed cementum where Sharpey's fibers were attached becomes altered by inflammatory products of bacteria and the sulcus fluid.
4. Diseased cementum contains a thin superficial layer of endotoxins from the bacterial breakdown.
5. Without treatment, the pocket becomes progressively deepened.

C. Characteristics of the Advanced Lesion

1. Pocket formation, mobility, bone loss; all signs of periodontitis.
2. Persistence of the chronic inflammatory process; plasma cells predominate.
3. Junctional epithelium continues to migrate; lesion extends through connective tissue.
4. Periods of inactivity alternating with periods of activity can be expected.

V. CLASSIFICATION

Periodontal disease is not a single pathologic entity. It is a term used to describe a variety of inflammatory and degenerative diseases that affect the supporting structures of the teeth. A widely used system for classifying the types and severity of periodontal disease has been prepared by the American Academy of Periodontology, as shown in Table 14-2.[3]

■ GINGIVAL AND PERIODONTAL POCKETS

A pocket is a diseased sulcus. The area of the sulcus and the pocket is the treatment area where calculus collects and instrumentation for nonsurgical periodontal therapy is applied.

It is the presence or absence of infection that distinguishes a pocket from a sulcus and the level of attachment on the tooth that distinguishes a gingival pocket from a periodontal pocket. A pocket has an *inner wall, the tooth surface,* and an *outer wall, the sulcular epithelium or pocket epithelium* of the free gingiva. The two walls meet at the base of the pocket (Figure 17-4, page 296).

The base of the pocket is the coronal margin of the attached periodontal tissues. Histologically, the base of a healthy sulcus is the coronal border of the junctional epithelium, whereas the base of a pocket (diseased sulcus) may be at the coronal border of the connective tissue attachment.

Pockets are divided into *gingival* and *periodontal* types to clarify the degree of anatomic involvement. They are then further categorized by their position in relation to the alveolar bone, that is, whether their pocket base is suprabony or intrabony (Figure 14-1).

I. GINGIVAL POCKET

A. Definition: A pocket formed by gingival enlargement without apical migration of the junctional epithelium (Figure 14-1B).
B. The margin of the gingiva has moved toward the incisal or occlusal without the deeper periodontal structures becoming involved.
C. The tooth wall is enamel.
D. During eruption, the base of the sulcus is at various levels along the enamel. The base of the sulcus of a fully erupted tooth is near the cementoenamel junction.
E. All gingival pockets are suprabony, that is, the base of the pocket is coronal to the crest of the alveolar bone.

II. PERIODONTAL POCKET

A. Definition: A pocket formed as a result of disease or degeneration that caused the junctional epithelium to migrate apically along the cementum.
B. The periodontal deeper structures (attachment apparatus) are involved, that is, the cementum, periodontal ligament, and bone.
C. The tooth wall is cementum or partly cementum and partly enamel.
D. The base of the pocket is on cementum at the level of attached periodontal tissue.
E. Periodontal pockets may be suprabony or intrabony.
   1. *Suprabony:* Pocket in which the base of the pocket is coronal to the crest of the alveolar bone (Figure 14-1C).
   2. *Intrabony:* Pocket in which the base of the pocket is below or apical to the crest of the alveolar bone (Figure 14-1D). "Intra" means located within the bone. The term "infrabony" is used in some texts. "Infra" means under or beneath.

TABLE 14-2A CLASSIFICATION OF GINGIVAL AND PERIODONTAL DISEASES AND CONDITIONS: GINGIVAL DISEASES

I. Gingival Diseases
  A. Dental plaque-induced gingival diseases*
    1. Gingivitis associated with dental plaque only
      a. Without other local contributing factors
      b. With local contributing factors
    2. Gingival diseases modified by systemic factors
      a. Associated with the endocrine system
        1) Puberty-associated gingivitis
        2) Menstrual cycle-associated gingivitis
        3) Pregnancy-associated
          a) Gingivitis
          b) Pyogenic granuloma
        4) Diabetes mellitus-associated gingivitis
      b. Associated with blood dyscrasias
        1) Leukemia-associated gingivitis
        2) Other
    3. Gingival diseases modified by medications
      a. Drug-influenced gingival diseases
        1) Drug-influenced gingival enlargements
        2) Drug-influenced gingivitis
          a) Oral contraceptive-associated gingivitis
          b) Other
    4. Gingival diseases modified by malnutrition
      a. Ascorbic acid-deficiency gingivitis
      b. Other
  B. Non-plaque-induced gingival lesions
    1. Gingival diseases of specific bacterial origin
      a. *Neisseria gonorrhea*-associated lesions
      b. *Treponema pallidum*-associated lesions
      c. Streptococcal species-associated lesions
      d. Other
    2. Gingival diseases of viral origin
      a. Herpesvirus infections
        1) Primary herpetic gingivostomatitis
        2) Recurrent oral herpes
        3) Varicella zoster infections
      b. Other

  3. Gingival diseases of fungal origin
    a. *Candida*-species infections
      1) Generalized gingival candidosis
    b. Linear gingival erythema
    c. Histoplasmosis
    d. Other
  4. Gingival lesions of genetic origin
    a. Hereditary gingival fibromatosis
    b. Other
  5. Gingival manifestations of systemic conditions
    a. Mucocutaneous disorders
      1) Lichen planus
      2) Pemphigoid
      3) Pemphigus vulgaris
      4) Erythema multiforme
      5) Lupus erythematosus
      6) Drug-induced
      7) Other
    b. Allergic reactions
      1) Dental restorative materials
        a) Mercury
        b) Nickel
        c) Acrylic
        d) Other
      2) Reactions attributable to
        a) Toothpastes/dentifrices
        b) Mouthrinses/mouthwashes
        c) Chewing gum additives
        d) Foods and additives
      3) Other
  6. Traumatic lesions (factitious, iatrogenic, accidental)
    a. Chemical injury
    b. Physical injury
    c. Thermal injury
  7. Foreign body reactions
  8. Not otherwise specified (NOS)

*Can occur on a periodontium with no attachment loss or on a periodontium with attachment loss that is not progressing.

(*continued*)

▪ TOOTH SURFACE POCKET WALL

I. TOOTH STRUCTURE INVOLVED

A sulcus or a pocket has a gingival side, which is the sulcular epithelium, and a tooth side. In gingival pockets, the tooth surface wall is enamel, whereas in periodontal pockets, the tooth surface wall is either cementum or a combination of cementum and enamel.

The positions of the periodontal attachment and the gingival margin determine whether the tooth surface wall is cementum or enamel. Pockets may be the same depth when measured with a probe, but because of the location of the attachment on the tooth surface, the tooth surface pocket wall varies.

II. CONTENTS OF A POCKET

A. Pocket Size

A pocket is narrow, and the pocket epithelial lining is adjacent to and follows the contour of the tooth. When calculus deposits are present, the pocket wall follows the contour of the calculus. The firmness of

TABLE 14-2B CLASSIFICATION OF GINGIVAL AND PERIODONTAL DISEASES AND CONDITIONS: PERIODONTAL DISEASES

II. Chronic Periodontitis†
  A. Localized
  B. Generalized
III. Aggressive Periodontitis†
  A. Localized
  B. Generalized
IV. Periodontitis as a Manifestation of Systemic Diseases
  A. Associated with hematological disorders
    1. Acquired neutropenia
    2. Leukemias
    3. Other
  B. Associated with genetic disorders
    1. Familial and cyclic neutropenia
    2. Down syndrome
    3. Leukocyte adhesion deficiency syndromes
    4. Papillon-Lefévre syndrome
    5. Chediak-Higashi syndrome
    6. Histiocytosis syndromes
    7. Glycogen storage disease
    8. Infantile genetic agranulocytosis
    9. Cohen syndrome
    10. Ehlers-Danlos syndrome (Types IV and VIII)
    11. Hypophosphatasia
    12. Other
  C. Not otherwise specified (NOS)
V. Necrotizing Periodontal Diseases
  A. Necrotizing ulcerative gingivitis (NUG)
  B. Necrotizing ulcerative periodontitis (NUP)
VI. Abscesses of the Periodontium
  A. Gingival abscess
  B. Periodontal abscess
  C. Pericoronal abscess
VII. Periodontitis Associated with Endodontic Lesions
  A. Combined periodontic-endodontic lesions
	VIII. Developmental or Acquired Deformities and Conditions
	  A. Localized tooth-related factors that modify or predispose to plaque-induced gingival diseases or periodontitis
	    1. Tooth anatomic factors
	    2. Dental restorations/appliances
	    3. Root fractures
	    4. Cervical root resorption and cemental tears
	  B. Mucogingival deformities and conditions around teeth
	    1. Gingival/soft tissue recession
	      a. Facial or lingual surfaces
	      b. Interproximal (papillary)
	    2. Lack of keratinized gingiva
	    3. Decreased vestibular depth
	    4. Aberrant frenum/muscle position
	    5. Gingival excess
	      a. Pseudopocket
	      b. Inconsistent gingival margin
	      c. Excessive gingival display
	      d. Gingival enlargement
	    6. Abnormal color
	  C. Mucogingival deformities and conditions on edentulous ridges
	    1. Vertical and/or horizontal ridge deficiency
	    2. Lack of gingiva/keratinized tissue
	    3. Gingival/soft tissue enlargement
	    4. Aberrant frenum/muscle position
	    5. Decreased vestibular depth
	    6. Abnormal color
	  D. Occlusal trauma
	    1. Primary occlusal trauma
	    2. Secondary occlusal trauma

†Can be further classified on the basis of extent and severity.
Used by permission from *1999 International Workshop for a Classification of Periodontal Diseases and Conditions. Papers. Oak Brook, Illinois, October 30-November 2, 1999. Ann Periodontol, 1999. 4(I): p. 2, 3.*

the free gingiva is influential in confining and shaping the subgingival calculus deposit.

Access of the opening of the pocket to the oral cavity provides an opportunity for dental biofilm to collect. The deeper the pocket, the less it can be cleaned by toothbrushing or other biofilm control devices.

B. Substances Found

Subgingival biofilm is described on page 296. The following may be inside a pocket in contact with the tooth surface on one side and with the surface of the pocket epithelium on the other side.
1. Microorganisms and their products: enzymes, endotoxins, and other metabolic products.
2. Gingival sulcus fluid.
3. Desquamated epithelial cells.
4. Leukocytes, the numbers of which increase with increased inflammation in the tissues.
5. Purulent exudate made up of living and broken down leukocytes, living and dead microorganisms, and serum.

III. NATURE OF THE TOOTH SURFACE

Knowledge of the characteristics and quality of the tooth surface pocket wall is of prime importance in instrumentation. During the examination of the tooth surface with probe and explorer, the various irregularities that can occur must be differentiated. The manner in which the

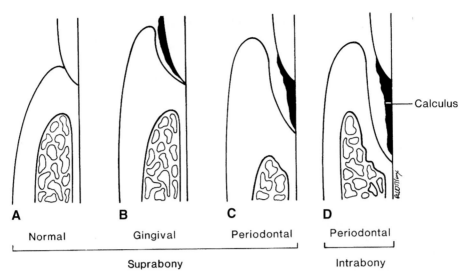

■ **FIGURE 14-1 Types of Pockets. (A)** Normal relationship of the gingival tissue and the cementoenamel junction in a fully erupted tooth. **(B)** Gingival pocket showing attachment at the cementoenamel junction and the pocket formed by enlarged gingival tissue. There is no bone loss. **(C)** Periodontal pocket showing attachment on cementum with root surface exposed. Gingival tissue has enlarged. **(D)** Periodontal intrabony pocket with the bottom of the pocket within the bone. See the text for further description of each type of pocket.

irregularities came into existence is important for interpretation and understanding.

A. Pocket Development Factors

1. The pocket deepens as a result of continuing action of the irritants and destructive agents from dental biofilm.
2. The periodontal ligament fibers become detached, and the junctional epithelium migrates apically.
3. The cementum becomes exposed to the open pocket and the oral fluids.
4. Physical, structural, and chemical changes alter the cementum.
5. Surface changes occur as a result of the exchange of minerals with oral fluids and exposure to biofilm bacteria and their products. On different surfaces of the same teeth or different teeth in the same mouth, any of the following can occur[4]:
   a. Hypermineralization of the surface cementum increases with time.
   b. Demineralization.
   c. Calculus formation.
   d. Dental biofilm and debris collection.

B. Tooth Surface Irregularities

Surface irregularities are detected supragingivally by drying the surface with air and observing under adequate direct or indirect light; an explorer is used as needed.

Subgingivally, examination is dependent, for the most part, on tactile and auditory sensitivity transmitted by a probe and an explorer. Causes of surface roughness include the following:

1. *Enamel Surface*
   a. Structural defects: cracks and grooves.
   b. Dental caries, demineralization.
   c. Calculus deposits and heavy stain deposits.
   d. Erosion, abrasion.
   e. Pits and irregularities from hypoplasia.
2. *Cementoenamel Junction.* Cementum overlaps enamel in 60% to 65% of teeth, cementum and enamel meet directly in 30%, and a small zone of dentin may be between the cementum and enamel in 5% to 10%.[5] The relationships of enamel and cementum at the cementoenamel junction are shown in Figure 14-2.

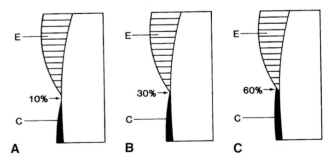

■ **FIGURE 14-2 Cementoenamel Junction.** The possible relationships of the enamel and the cementum of the cementoenamel junction. **(A)** The cementum and the enamel do not meet and there is a small zone of dentin exposed in 10% of teeth. **(B)** The cementum meets the enamel in approximately 30% of teeth. **(C)** The cementum overlaps the enamel in about 60% of teeth.

3. *Root Surface*
   a. Diseased altered cementum.
   b. Cemental resorption.
   c. Root caries.
   d. Abrasion.
   e. Calculus.
   f. Deficient or overhanging filling.
   g. Grooves from previous incomplete instrumentation.

▪ COMPLICATIONS OF POCKET FORMATION

I. FURCATION INVOLVEMENT

Furcation involvement means that the clinical attachment level and bone loss have extended into the furcation area, or furca, the area between the roots of a multirooted tooth.

A. Types of Furcations

Furcation involvement is usually classified by the amount of a furcation that has been exposed by periodontal bone destruction.

The four general classes, as shown in Figure 14-3, are as follows:
1. *Class I:* Early, beginning involvement. A probe can enter the furcation area, and the anatomy of the roots on either side can be felt by moving the probe from side to side.
2. *Class II:* Moderate involvement. Bone has been destroyed to an extent that permits a probe to enter the furcation area but not to pass through between the roots.
3. *Class III:* Severe involvement. A probe can be passed between the roots through the entire furcation.

4. *Class IV:* Same as Class III, with exposure resulting from gingival recession, especially after periodontal therapy.

B. Clinical Observations

1. When the gingiva over the furcation has not receded, the following may be seen:
   a. The furcation is covered by the gingival tissue pocket wall.
   b. No differences in color, size, or other tissue changes may exist to differentiate the area from adjacent gingiva, but when color changes do exist, they provide clues to supplement probe examination.
2. When the gingiva over a molar buccal furcation is receded, the root division may be seen directly (Figure 14-3, Class IV).

C. Detection

A suggested procedure for probing furcations is described on pages 232 to 233.

II. MUCOGINGIVAL INVOLVEMENT

A pocket that extends to or beyond the mucogingival junction and into the alveolar mucosa is described as *mucogingival involvement.* There is no attached gingiva in the area, and a probe can be passed through the pocket and beyond the mucogingival junction into the alveolar mucosa.

A. Significance of Attached Gingiva

1. *Functions of Attached Gingiva*
   a. Give support to the marginal gingiva.
   b. Withstand the frictional stresses of mastication and toothbrushing.

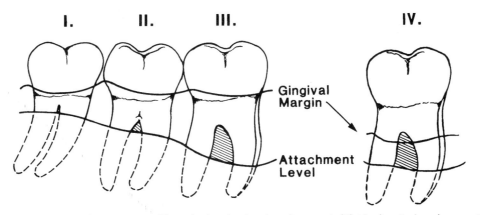

I.   **II.**   **III.**   **IV.**

Gingival Margin

Attachment Level

▪ **FIGURE 14-3 Classification of Furcations. (I)** Early, beginning involvement. **(II)** Moderate involvement, in which the furcation can be probed but not through and through. **(III)** Severe involvement, when the bone between the roots is destroyed and a probe can be passed through. **(IV)** Same as III, with clinical exposure resulting from gingival recession.

c. Provide attachment or a solid base for the movable alveolar mucosa for the action of the cheeks, lips, and tongue.

2. *Barrier to Passage of Inflammation.* Without attachment, inflammation from a pocket area can extend to the alveolar mucosa. The junctional epithelium (epithelial attachment) acts as a barrier to keep infection outside the body.

With destruction of the connective tissue and periodontal ligament fibers under the junctional epithelium, the epithelium migrates along the root. A pocket is created.

In mucogingival involvement, the bottom of the pocket extends into the alveolar mucosa. There, the unconfined inflammation can spread more rapidly in the loose connective tissue.

B. Clinical Observations

Color changes, tension test, and probe measurements are used during assessment of the mucogingival areas.

1. *Width of Attached Gingiva.* A narrow zone of gingiva from gingival margin to mucogingival junction, caused by recession or occurring naturally without recession, is more susceptible to developing mucogingival involvement because there is less attached gingiva at the start.

2. *Base of Pocket at Mucogingival Junction.* When the probe measures only 1 to 2 mm and there is no bleeding on probing, but the tip of the probe is at the mucogingival junction, the area should be charted and reevaluated at each successive maintenance review. A patient with such an area needs specific instruction in biofilm control procedures for preventive maintenance.

When an area of minimal attached gingiva (1 to 2 mm) is placed under stress by restorative, prosthetic, or orthodontic treatment procedures, an assessment should be made of the need for periodontal treatment to increase the zone of attached gingiva.

▪ LOCAL CONTRIBUTING FACTORS IN DISEASE DEVELOPMENT

Dental biofilm is the primary etiologic factor in the development of gingival and periodontal diseases. A variety of other factors predispose some patients to the retention of bacterial deposits and hence to the development of disease in the soft tissues.

Factors described in this section relate to dental biofilm retention. Although loose debris can be cleared away by self-cleansing, dental biofilm adheres firmly to the tooth surface and cannot be removed completely by self-cleansing. Retentive areas relate to rough surfaces of teeth and restorations, tooth contour and position, and gingival size, shape, and position.

Iatrogenic causes, that is, factors created by professionals during patient treatment or neglect of treatment, are significant. Other factors, such as mastication, saliva, the tongue, cheeks, lips, oral habits, and personal biofilm control procedures, contribute.

The patient's study casts can be especially useful for observing the physical factors. Irregularities, contour, position, malocclusion, and contact areas of the teeth, as well as features of the gingiva, may be partially or wholly noted. Problem areas can be explained to the patient by demonstration on the study casts. Changes in the patient's habits and daily personal care routine must be encouraged.

I. FACTORS INVOLVED

Complicating and risk factors to disease development may be etiologic, predisposing, or contributing. They are delineated as follows:

1. *Etiologic Factor:* A factor that is the actual cause of a disease or condition.

2. *Predisposing Factor:* A factor that renders a person susceptible to a disease or condition.

3. *Contributing Factor:* A factor that lends assistance to, supplements, or adds to a condition or disease.

4. *Risk Factor:* An exposure that increases the probability that disease will occur.

Etiologic, predisposing, and contributing factors may be local or systemic, defined as follows:

1. *Local Factor:* A factor in the immediate environment of the oral cavity or specifically in the environment of the teeth or periodontium.

2. *Systemic Factor:* A factor that results from or is influenced by a general physical or mental disease or condition.

II. DENTAL FACTORS

A. Tooth Surface Irregularities

Pellicle and biofilm microorganisms attach to defective or rough surfaces, including the following:

1. Pits, grooves, cracks.
2. Calculus.
3. Exposed altered cementum with irregularities.
4. Dental caries and demineralization.
5. Iatrogenic
   a. Rough or grooved surfaces left after scaling.
   b. Inadequately contoured and polished dental restorations (Figure 14-4B).

B. Tooth Contour

Altered shape may interfere with self-cleansing mechanisms and make personal care procedures difficult.

1. Congenital abnormalities

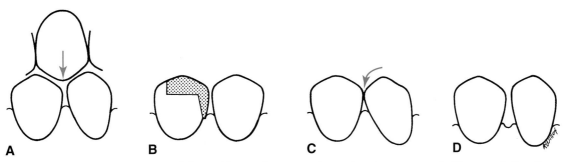

■ **FIGURE 14-4 Effect of Tooth Position. (A)** Food impaction area, shown by plunger cusp (with arrow) directing pressure between lower teeth with open contact area. **(B)** Inadequate restoration without proximal contact and with overhang. **(C)** Tipped tooth leaving irregular marginal ridge relation. **(D)** Natural open contact (diastema) with saddle-shaped gingival margin.

   a. Extra or missing cusps.
   b. Bell-shaped crown with prominent facial and lingual contours tends to provide deeper retentive area in cervical third.
2. Teeth with flattened proximal surfaces have faulty contact with adjacent teeth, thus permitting debris to wedge between.
3. Occlusal and incisal surfaces altered by attrition interrupt normal excursion of food during chewing. Marginal ridges have worn down.
4. Areas of erosion and abrasion.
5. Carious lesions.
6. Heavy calculus deposits; biofilm retained on rough surface.
7. Overcontoured and undercontoured restorations.

C. Tooth Position

1. Malocclusion: Irregular alignment of a single tooth or groups of teeth leaves areas conducive to collection of microorganisms for biofilm formation.
   a. Crowded or overlapped.
   b. Rotated.
   c. Deep anterior overbite
      i. Mandibular teeth force food particles against maxillary lingual surface.
      ii. Lingual inclination of mandibular teeth allows maxillary teeth to force food particles against mandibular facial gingiva.
2. Tooth adjacent to edentulous area may be inclined or migrated; contact missing.
3. Opposing tooth missing; tooth may extrude beyond the line of occlusion.
4. Related to eruption
   a. Incomplete eruption: below line of occlusion.
   b. Partially erupted impacted third molar.
5. Lack of function or use of teeth eliminates or decreases effectiveness of natural cleansing.
   a. Lack of opposing teeth.
   b. Open bite.

   c. Marked maxillary anterior protrusion.
   d. Crossbite with limited lateral excursion.
   e. Unilateral chewing.
6. Food impaction
   a. Created by the combined effect of tooth contour, missing proximal contact, proximal carious lesions, irregular marginal ridge relationship.
   b. Inclination related to loss of adjacent tooth, and a plunger cusp from the opposite arch (Figure 14-4A).
7. Defective contact area
   a. Restoration margin is faulty, and the contact area is missing, improperly located, or unnaturally wide (Figure 14-4B).
   b. Inclined tooth with irregular marginal ridge relation (Figure 14-4C).

D. Dental Prostheses

1. Orthodontic appliances provide retentive areas.
2. Fixed partial denture with deficient margin of an abutment tooth or an unusually shaped pontic.
3. Removable partial denture with inadequately adapted clasps.

III. GINGIVA

A. Position

Deviations from normal provide retentive areas.
1. Receded: depressed area is left at cementoenamel junction.
2. Enlarged: extended to or over the height of contour.
3. Reduced height of interdental papilla leaves open interdental area.
4. Tissue flap over occlusal surface of erupting tooth.
5. Periodontal pocket
   a. Free gingiva cannot adhere to tooth.

b. Shape of pocket conducive to dental biofilm collection.

c. Depth of pocket not available to toothbrush and cleaning aids.

d. Calculus provides rough retentive surface.

B. Size and Contour

1. Deviation of shape of enlarged gingiva: rolled, bulbous, cratered.

2. Combination with presence of irregular restorations or dental prosthesis can result in marked biofilm retention.

C. Effect of Mouth Breathing

Dehydration of oral tissues in anterior region leads to changes in size, shape, surface texture, and consistency.

IV. OTHER FACTORS

A variety of factors may predispose or contribute to the progression of periodontal infections. Some of the items listed here may have an indirect effect, whereas others have a direct effect on the oral tissues.

A. Personal Oral Care

1. *Neglect*: Neglect can lead to generalized dental biofilm accumulation and disease promotion.

2. *Faulty Biofilm Control Techniques*: Incorrect use of brush, abrasive dentifrice, and the effects of other harmful, detrimental procedures are described elsewhere.

3. *Awareness of Oral Cleanliness*: Cleansing habits, including both self-cleansing mechanisms and mechanical biofilm removal, depend in part on an individual's perception and feeling of debris through taste and tongue activity.

B. Diet and Eating Habits

1. Soft foods tend to adhere more than fibrous, firm foods.

2. Cariogenic food selection.

3. Masticatory deficiencies limit diet selection. Missing teeth, ill-fitting partial dentures, and various occlusal deficiencies alter diet selection and eating habits.

▪ SELF-CLEANSING MECHANISMS

The teeth, by their anatomy, alignment, and occlusion, function with the gingiva, tongue, cheeks, and saliva in a relationship called the self-cleansing mechanism of the oral cavity. A summary of the natural self-cleansing mechanisms during and following mastication is included here.

The following steps are described for food particles, but the same processes apply to any substances that enter the mouth and influence oral cleanliness and the formation of deposits on the teeth.

I. FOOD ENTERS THE MOUTH

Food is carried by the tongue, assisted by the lips and cheeks, to the occlusal surfaces for grinding.

A. Salivary flow increases as a result of sensory reflex stimulation.

B. Saliva begins lubrication of food and oral tissues.

II. THE TEETH ARE BROUGHT TOGETHER FOR CHEWING

The food moves over the occlusal surfaces.

A. Marginal ridges tend to force particles toward occlusal surfaces, away from the proximal region.

B. Contact areas prevent interdental entrance.

III. FOOD IS FORCED OUT BY PRESSURE OF BITE

Food passes over the smooth facial and lingual surfaces.

A. Embrasures provide spillways for the escape of particles.

B. Cervical enamel ridges deflect particles away from the free gingiva onto the attached gingiva.

C. Gingival crest prevents retention of particles by its position at a point below the height of contour of the cervical enamel ridge, by its knife-edge shape, and by its close adherence to the tooth surface.

D. Interdental papilla fills the interproximal area and prevents particles from entering.

IV. FOOD PARTICLES ARE BROUGHT BACK BY THE TONGUE TO THE OCCLUSAL SURFACES FOR ADDITIONAL CHEWING

The process is repeated until the food is ready for swallowing.

A. Salivary flow continues to be stimulated by repeated masticatory movements.

B. Saliva moistens food and oral mucosa and thus reduces the adhering capacity of the food.

V. FOOD PARTICLES REMAINING ON THE TEETH ARE REMOVED

A. Tip of tongue explores and attempts to dislodge remaining particles.

Everyday Ethics

Holly found it interesting that even after practicing dental hygiene for 5 years full-time, the "light bulb" of connecting certain conditions in the mouth with causative factors occurred. While listening to Mr. Zajek complain about food impaction, Holly noted the poor contours of crowns in the premolar area lacking proximal contact, as well as loss of both mandibular first molars.

Ideally, Mr. Zajek needed teeth to be repositioned and occlusal deviations to be corrected through orthodontic treatment. Holly hesitated to even mention it to Mr. Zajek since he was 55 years old. However, she found herself thinking that if this were Mr. Zajek's wife, she wouldn't hesitate to offer her a referral to address these contributing factors. Mr. Zajek was beginning to show signs of periodontal disease, including furcation involvement.

Questions for Consideration

1. Is age alone a factor in this scenario that precludes the hygienist from presenting an "optimal" dental hygiene diagnosis and care plan? Explain why or why not.

2. Using the step-approach decision model consider Mr. Zajek's existing oral findings and prioritize options for treatment that Holly can reference when developing a self-care plan for him.

3. Morally, is Holly obligated to spend extra appointment time convincing Mr. Zajek that he should seek referrals in another specialty dental office? Respond based on the duties and rights of both Holly and Mr. Zajek in the provider-patient relationship.

B. Lips and cheeks in conjunction with tongue aid in natural rinsing process by forcing saliva over and between the teeth.

C. Saliva continues to flow in increased amounts during rinsing and swallowing of particles, then gradually returns to its normal flow.

▪ RISK FACTORS FOR PERIODONTAL DISEASES

Identification of risk factors for periodontal disease can provide significant insight for the assessment and care planning for an individual patient. The various periodontal pathogenic microorganisms do not affect all people with the same degree of severity. It is clear that host factors play a significant role.

Certain risk factors are related to lifestyle, habits, treatable systemic diseases, and other controllable factors. On the other hand, factors derived from genetic predisposition, congenital immunodeficiencies, or other systemic conditions require a greater effort for the control of periodontal problems.

Many periodontal risk factors have been identified, and a few examples are described in this section. A list of outstanding articles from the literature is provided in the Suggested Readings at the close of this chapter.

I. EFFECT OF CERTAIN DRUGS

Medications for specific systemic conditions can lead to gingival enlargement.[6,7] The enlarged tissue encourages dental biofilm retention, thus increasing the potential for periodontal infections.

A. *Phenytoin-Induced Gingival Enlargement.* Phenytoin is a drug used to control seizures.

B. *Cyclosporine-Induced Gingival Enlargement.* Cyclosporine is an immunosuppressant drug used for patients with organ transplants to prevent rejection.

C. *Nifedipine-Induced Gingival Enlargement.* Nifedipine is used in the treatment of angina and ventricular arrhythmias.

II. TOBACCO

A. Smokers, especially cigarette users, have increased bone loss. An association between periodontal disease and all forms of tobacco use has been shown.[8,9]

B. Users of smokeless tobacco products experience oral effects, including predisposition to oral cancer. Periodontal lesions with severe recession and root exposure occur where the quid is held.[10]

III. DIABETES[11]

A. Increased susceptibility to periodontal infections.

B. Periodontal treatment improves the metabolic control of diabetes (page 1084).

C. Patient with well-controlled diabetes and healthy periodontal tissues is not at greater risk for susceptibility to infections, including periodontal.

✔ **Factors To Teach The Patient**

- What a pocket is and how it forms.

- How a pocket is measured with a probe and that, until the sulci and pockets are probed, it is not possible to tell whether disease is present and how far it has progressed. Probing depth must be checked regularly all around every tooth to be sure nothing is developing insidiously.

- Factors that contribute to disease development and progression.

- What a risk factor is and the importance of planning personal and professional care to include risk factor problems.

IV. OTHER SYSTEMIC CONDITIONS

A. Osteoporosis[12]

1. Many risk factors for osteoporosis are also risk factors for periodontitis, including cigarette smoking, nutritional deficiencies, corticosteroid use, and immune dysfunction.
2. Greater periodontal attachment loss in patients with osteoporosis.
3. Loss of alveolar bone results from osteopenia.

B. Psychosocial Factors

1. Higher levels of social strain are found in patients with periodontal infections.[13]
2. Stress is considered a factor in the etiology of necrotizing ulcerative gingivitis.

REFERENCES

1. **Page,** R.C. and Schroeder, H.E.: Structure and Pathogenesis, in Schluger, S., Yuodelis, R., Page, R.C., and Johnson, R.H.: *Periodontal Diseases,* 2nd ed. Philadelphia, Lea & Febiger, 1990, pp. 185–207.
2. **Weinmann,** J.P.: Progress of Gingival Inflammation Into the Supporting Structures of the Teeth, *J. Periodontol., 12,* 71, July, 1941.
3. **American Academy of Periodontology:** *Current Procedural Terminology for Periodontics and Insurance Reporting Manual,* 7th ed. Chicago, American Academy of Periodontology, 1995, pp. 1–2, 15.
4. **Selvig,** K.A.: Biological Changes at the Tooth-Saliva Interface in Periodontal Disease, *J. Dent. Res., 48,* 846, September–October, 1969.
5. **Bhaskar,** S.N., ed.: *Orban's Oral Histology and Embryology,* 11th ed. St. Louis, Mosby, 1991, p. 192.
6. **Fattore,** L., Stablein, M., Bredfeldt, G., Semla, T., Moran, M., and Doherty-Greenberg, J.M.: Gingival Hyperplasia: A Side Effect of Nifedipine and Diltiazem, *Spec. Care Dentist., 11,* 107, May/June, 1991.
7. **Payne,** J.B.: The Facts About Gingival Hyperplasia, *Dent. Teamwork, 5,* 22, September–October, 1992.

8. **Akef,** J., Weine, F.S., and Weissman, D.P.: The Role of Smoking in the Progression of Periodontal Disease: A Literature Review, *Compend. Cont. Educ. Dent., 13,* 526, June, 1992.
9. **Haber,** J., Wattles, J., Crowley, M., Mandell, R., Joshipura, K., and Kent, R.L.: Evidence for Cigarette Smoking as a Major Risk Factor for Periodontitis, *J. Periodontol., 64,* 16, January, 1993.
10. **Johnson,** R. and Herzog, A.: Oral Effects of Smokeless Tobacco Use, *Dent. Hyg., 61,* 354, August, 1987.
11. **American Academy of Periodontology,** Committee on Research, Science and Therapy: Position Paper: Diabetes and Periodontal Diseases, *J. Periodontol., 70,* 935, August, 1999.
12. **Wactawski-Wende,** J., Grossi, S.G., Trevisan, M., Genco, R.J., Tezal, M., Dunford, R.G., Ho, A.W., Hausman, E., Hreshchyshyn, M.M.: The Role of Osteopenia in Oral Bone Loss and Periodontal Disease, *J. Periodontol., 67,* 1076, October, Supplement, 1996.
13. **Moss,** M.E., Beck, J.D., Kaplan, B.H., Offenbacher, S., Weintraub, J.A., Koch, G.G., Genco, R.J., Machtei, E.E., and Tedesco, L.A.: Exploratory Case-control Analysis of Psychosocial Factors and Adult Periodontitis, *J. Periodontol., 67,* 1060, October, Supplement, 1996.

SUGGESTED READING

Atack, N.E., Sandy, J.R., and Addy, M.: Periodontal and Microbial Changes Associated With the Placement of Orthodontic Appliances: A Review, *J. Periodontol., 67,* 78, February, 1996.
Gagnon, F., Knoernschild, K.L., Payant, L., Tompkins, G.R., Litaker, M.S., and Schuster, G.S.: Endotoxin Affinity for Provisional Restorative Resins, *J. Prosthodont., 3,* 228, December, 1994.
Kornman, K.S. and Löe, H.: The Role of Local Factors in the Etiology of Periodontal Diseases, *Periodontol. 2000, 2,* 83, 1993.
Leknes, K.N., Lie, T., and Selvig, K.A.: Root Grooves: A Risk Factor in Periodontal Attachment Loss, *J. Periodontol., 65,* 859, September, 1994.
Tatakis, D.N.: The Inflammatory Response in Periodontitis, *DentalHygienistNews, 8,* 5, Special Issue, Spring, 1995.

Risk Factors

Alpagot, T., Wolff, L.F., Smith, Q.T., and Tran, S.D.: Risk Indicators for Periodontal Disease in a Racially Diverse Urban Population, *J. Clin. Periodontol., 23,* 982, November, 1996.
Clarke, N.G. and Hirsch, R.S.: Personal Risk Factors for Generalized Periodontitis, *J. Clin. Periodontol., 22,* 136, February, 1995.
Daniel, M.A. and Van Dyke, T.E.: Alterations in Phagocyte Function and Periodontal Infection, *J. Periodontol., 67,* 1070, October, Supplement, 1996.
Goulding, M.: Risk Assessment for Periodontal Disease, *Can. Dent. Hyg. Assoc./Probe, 30,* 100, May/June, 1996.
Michalowicz, B.S.: Genetic and Heritable Risk Factors in Periodontal Disease, *J. Periodontol., 65,* 479, Supplement, May, 1994.
Offenbacher, S., Katz, V., Fertik, G., Collins, J., Boyd, D., Maynor, G., McKaig, R., and Beck, J.: Periodontal Infection as a Possible Risk Factor for Preterm Low Birth Weight, *J. Periodontol., 67,* 1103, October, Supplement, 1996.
Page, R.C. and Beck, J.D.: Risk Assessment for Periodontal Diseases, *Internat. Dent. J., 47,* 61, April, 1997.
Schutte, D.W. and Donley, T.G.: Determining Periodontal Risk Factors in Patients Presenting for Dental Care, *J. Dent. Hyg., 70,* 230, November–December, 1996.

Drug-Induced Gingival Enlargement

Bredfeldt, G.W.: Phenytoin-Induced Hyperplasia Found in Edentulous Patients, *J. Am. Dent. Assoc., 123,* 61, June, 1992.
Daley, T.D., Wysocki, G.P., and Mamandras, A.H.: Orthodontic Therapy in the Patient Treated With Cyclosporine, *Am. J. Orthod. Dentofacial Orthop., 100,* 537, December, 1991.

Hefti, A.F., Eshenaur, A.E., Hassell, T.M., and Stone, C.: Gingival Overgrowth in Cyclosporine A Treated Multiple Sclerosis Patients, *J. Periodontol., 65,* 744, August, 1994.

Karpinia, K.A., Matt, M., Fennel, R.S., and Hefti, A.F.: Factors Affecting Cyclosporine-Induced Gingival Overgrowth in Pediatric Renal Transplant Recipients, *Pediatr. Dent., 18,* 450, November/December, 1996.

Montebugnoli, L., Bernardi, F., and Magelli, C.: Cyclosporine-A-induced Gingival Overgrowth in Heart Transplant Patients: A Cross-sectional Study, *J. Clin. Periodontol., 23,* 868, September, 1996.

Seymour, R.A., Thomason, J.M., and Ellis, J.S.: The Pathogenesis of Drug-Induced Gingival Overgrowth, *J. Clin. Periodontol., 23,* 165, March, 1996.

Somacarrera, M.L., Lucas, M., and Acero, J.: Reversion of Gingival Hyperplasia in a Heart Transplant Patient Upon Interruption of Cyclosporine Therapy, *Spec. Care Dentist., 16,* 18, January/February, 1996.

Thomason, J.M., Seymour, R.A., and Rice, N.: The Prevalence and Severity of Cyclosporin and Nifedipine-induced Gingival Overgrowth, *J. Clin. Periodontol., 20,* 36, January, 1993.

The Teeth

Clinical examination of the teeth is essential prior to treatment to provide guidelines for treatment planning, instrumentation, instruction, and follow-up evaluation. In general, patients may tend to be more concerned about their teeth than about their gingiva. The reasons may be related to personal appearance; degree of information, which may be greater about teeth than gingiva; and sensitivity and pain associated with ailments of the teeth.

Background study of histology, dental anatomy, and oral pathology is essential to this phase of clinical practice. Key words are defined in Box 15-1.

With information from the patient's personal and dental histories (see Tables 7-1 and 7-2) and a thorough clinical and radiographic examination, the objectives are to:

• Prepare a charting and provide a record of deviations from normal.

BOX 15-1 KEY WORDS AND ABBREVIATIONS: Teeth

Accessory root canal: a secondary canal extending from the pulp to the surface of the root; frequently found near the apex of a root but may occur higher and provide a connection to a periodontal pocket.

Amelogenesis: production and development of enamel.

Avulsion: the tearing away or forcible separation of a structure or part. Tooth avulsion is the traumatic separation of a tooth from the alveolus.

Bruxism: an oral habit of grinding, clenching, or clamping the teeth; involuntary, rhythmic, or spasmodic movements outside the chewing range; may damage teeth and attachment apparatus.

Cariogenic: adj. conducive to dental caries.

Carious: adj. used to define a carious lesion.

Cementicle: a calcified spherical body, composed of cementum, lying free within the periodontal ligament, attached to the cementum or imbedded within the cementum.

Dental caries: disease of the mineralized structures of the teeth characterized by demineralization of the hard components and dissolution of the organic matrix.

> **Arrested caries:** carious lesion that has become stationary and does not show a tendency to progress further; frequently has a hard surface and takes on a dark brown or reddish-brown color.

> **Primary caries:** occurs on a surface not previously affected; also called initial caries; early lesion may be referred to as incipient caries.

> **Rampant caries:** widespread formation of chalky white areas and incipient lesions that may increase in size over a comparatively short time.

> **Recurrent caries:** occurs on a surface adjacent to a restoration; may be a continuation of the original lesion; also called secondary caries.

Dentition: the natural teeth in the dental arch.

> **Primary (deciduous) dentition:** the first teeth; normally will be shed and replaced by permanent teeth.

> **Permanent dentition:** the natural 32 teeth that serve throughout life.

> **Mixed dentition:** combination of primary and permanent teeth between ages 6 and 12 when primary teeth are being replaced; starts with the eruption of the first permanent tooth.

> **Succedaneous:** the permanent teeth that erupt into the positions of exfoliated primary teeth.

Edentulous: without teeth; referred to as partially edentulous when some, but not all, teeth are missing.

Electrolyte: a conductor; a substance that, in solution, dissociates into electrically charged particles (ions) and thus is capable of conducting an electric current.

Etiology: the science or study of the cause of a disease or disorder.

Exfoliation: loss of primary teeth following physiologic resorption of root structure.

Facet: a small flattened surface on a hard body, such as a tooth; a wear facet can result from attrition or repeated parafunctional contact.

Hypoplasia: incomplete development or underdevelopment of a tissue or organ.

> **Enamel hypoplasia:** incomplete or defective formation of the enamel of either primary or permanent teeth. The result may be an irregularity of tooth form, color, or surface.

Idiopathic: denoting a condition of unknown cause.

KEY WORDS AND ABBREVIATIONS: Teeth, continued

Incipient: beginning; coming into existence.

pH: the symbol of hydrogen ion concentration expressed in numbers corresponding to the acidity or alkalinity of an aqueous solution; the range is from 14 (pure base) to 0 (pure acid); neutral is at 7.0.

Critical pH: the pH at which demineralization occurs; for enamel, pH 4.5 to 5.5; for cementum, pH 6.0 to 6.7.

Resorption: removal of bone or tooth structure; gradual dissolution of the mineralized tissue; may be internal or external; occurs during exfoliation of a primary tooth and from the pressure of orthodontic treatment.

- Identify the treatment and counseling needed in relation to the teeth for the particular patient.
- Outline the patient's preventive program (pages 362 and 375 to 377).
- Utilize the specific data during treatment for instrument selection and adaptation.

▪ THE DENTITIONS

Formation of the primary teeth begins *in utero*. Table 46-4 (page 790) shows the weeks *in utero* when each primary tooth begins to mineralize and the average months after birth when the enamel is completely formed before the date of eruption.

Mineralization of the permanent teeth starts at birth and continues into adolescence. The chronology of

development and eruption appears in Table 15-1. Roots normally are completed by 3 years after eruption.

The mixed dentition, when primary teeth are being exfoliated and permanent teeth move in to take their places, occurs between the ages of 6 and 12 years. Figure 15-1 illustrates the mixed dentition of a child approximately 6 years of age.

▪ DENTAL CARIES

The World Health Organization has defined dental caries as a "localized, post-eruptive, pathologic process of external origin involving softening of the hard tooth tissue and proceeding to the formation of a cavity."[1] Dental caries is a preventable disease.

▪ TABLE 15-1 TOOTH DEVELOPMENT AND ERUPTION: PERMANENT TEETH

		HARD TISSUE FORMATION BEGINS	ENAMEL COMPLETED (YEARS)	ERUPTION (YEARS)	ROOT COMPLETED (YEARS)
Maxillary	Central incisor	3–4 mo	4–5	7–8	10
	Lateral incisor	10 mo	4–5	8–9	11
	Canine	4–5 mo	6–7	11–12	13–15
	First premolar	1 1/2–1 3/4 yr	5–6	10–11	12–13
	Second premolar	2–2 1/4 yr	6–7	10–12	12–14
	First molar	at birth	2 1/2–3	6–7	9–10
	Second molar	2 1/2–3 yr	7–8	12–13	14–16
	Third molar	7–9 yr	12–16	17–21	18–25
Mandibular	Central incisor	3–4 mo	4–5	6–7	9
	Lateral incisor	3–4 mo	4–5	7–8	10
	Canine	4–5 mo	6–7	9–10	12–14
	First premolar	1 3/4–2 yr	5–6	10–12	12–13
	Second premolar	2 1/4–2 1/2 yr	6–7	11–12	13–14
	First molar	at birth	2 1/2–3	6–7	9–10
	Second molar	2 1/2–3 yr	7–8	11–13	14–15
	Third molar	8–10 yr	12–16	17–21	18–25

From Ash, M.M.: *Wheeler's Dental Anatomy, Physiology, and Occlusion,* 7th ed. Philadelphia, W.B. Saunders Co., 1993, p. 25.

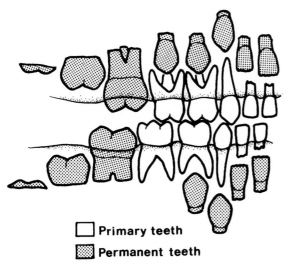

□ **Primary teeth**

▨ **Permanent teeth**

■ **FIGURE 15-1 Mixed Dentition at Approximately Age 6 Years.** The average child has 20 primary teeth in place, and root resorption of the incisors has started as the developing permanent incisors move into position. The first permanent molars are partially erupted.

I. DEVELOPMENT OF DENTAL CARIES

Requirements for the development of a carious lesion are microorganisms; carbohydrate, primarily sucrose; and a susceptible tooth surface. Figure 32-2 (page 528) is a diagram that shows four overlapping circles to illustrate the essential factors in the process of dental caries initiation.

Dental biofilm may contain numerous types of acid-forming bacteria. *Mutans streptococci* have been specifically implicated. The role of dental biofilm and the factors involved in dental caries initiation are described on pages 393 to 394.

II. CLASSIFICATION OF CAVITIES

A. G.V. Black's Classification[2]

The standard method for classifying dental caries was developed by Dr. G.V. Black, a noted dental educator who divided the categories into classes according to surfaces of the teeth; each class is represented by a Roman numeral. The categories customarily are used for carious lesions, cavity preparations, and finished restorations. Table 15-2 defines and illustrates the classifications.

B. Nomenclature by Surfaces

1. *Simple Cavity*: Involves one tooth surface. Example: occlusal cavity.
2. *Compound Cavity*: Involves two tooth surfaces. Example: mesio-occlusal cavity, referred to as an "M-O" cavity.

3. *Complex Cavity*: Involves more than two tooth surfaces. Example: mesio-occlusal-distal, referred to as an "M-O-D" cavity.

■ ENAMEL CARIES

I. STEPS IN THE FORMATION OF A CAVITY

A. Phase I: Incipient Lesion

1. *Subsurface Demineralization*: Acid products from cariogenic dental biofilm pass through microchannels (pores) of the enamel.
2. *Visualization*: Area of demineralization is not visible by clinical observation during initial changes; thin layer of enamel remains over the surface.
3. *First Clinical Evidence*: White spot appears with no breakthrough to enamel surface; with time, area may turn brown from food, beverages, or tobacco use.
4. *Remineralization*: Low concentrations of fluoride applied frequently during the early phase can provide sources for uptake by the demineralized zone. The porous demineralized area readily takes up fluoride from dentifrice, mouthrinse, fluoridated drinking water, and all possible sources. Figure 33-3 (page 547) shows examples of levels of concentration of fluoride in surface enamel and in a white spot area.

B. Phase II: Untreated Incipient Lesion

1. *Breakdown of Enamel Over the Demineralized Area (White Spot)*: Visible to observation and irregular to the gentle application of the side of an explorer tip.
2. *Progression of Carious Lesion*: Follows general direction of enamel rods.
3. *Spread of Carious Lesion*: Spreads at dentinoenamel junction; continues along the dentinal tubules (Figure 15-2).

II. TYPES OF DENTAL CARIES (DESCRIBED BY LOCATION)

A. Pit and Fissure

Caries begins in a minute fault in the enamel.
1. Pit or fissure irregularity occurs where three or more lobes of the developing tooth join; closure of the enamel plates is imperfect. Examples: occlusal pits of molars and premolars.

▪ TABLE 15-2 DENTAL CARIES CHARTING: CLASSIFICATION OF CAVITIES

CLASSIFICATION: LOCATION	APPEARANCE	METHOD OF EXAMINATION
Class I. Cavities in pits or fissures a. Occlusal surfaces of premolars and molars b. Facial and lingual surfaces of molars c. Lingual surfaces of maxillary incisors		Direct or indirect visual Exploration Radiographs not useful
Class II. Cavities in proximal surfaces of premolars and molars		Early caries: by radiographs only Moderate caries not broken through from proximal to occlusal: 1. Visual by color changes in tooth and loss of translucency 2. Exploration from proximal Extensive caries involving occlusal: direct visual
Class III. Cavities in proximal surfaces of incisors and canines that do not involve the incisal angle		Early caries: by radiographs or transillumination Moderate caries not broken through to lingual or facial: 1. Visual by tooth color change 2. Exploration 3. Radiograph Extensive caries; direct visual
Class IV. Cavities in proximal surfaces of incisors or canines that involve the incisal angle		Visual Transillumination
Class V. Cavities in the cervical 1/3 of facial or lingual surfaces (not pit or fissure)		Direct visual: dry surface for vision Exploration to distinguish demineralization: whether rough or hard and unbroken Areas may be sensitive to touch
Class VI. Cavities on incisal edges of anterior teeth and cusp tips of posterior teeth		Direct visual May be discolored

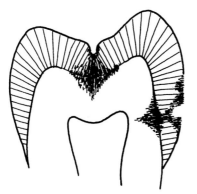

■ **FIGURE 15-2 Dental Caries.** Cones of dental caries in a pit and fissure and on a smooth tooth surface. Dental caries follows the general direction of the enamel rods, spreads at the dentinoenamel junction, and then continues along the dentinal tubules.

2. Occurs at the endings of grooves of the teeth. Example: the buccal groove of a mandibular molar.

B. Smooth Surface

Caries begins in smooth surfaces where there is no pit, groove, or other fault. It occurs in areas where dental biofilm collects, such as proximal tooth surfaces, cervical thirds of teeth, and other difficult-to-clean areas.

■ EARLY CHILDHOOD CARIES[3,4]

Baby bottle tooth decay is a form of rampant caries found in very young children who routinely have been given a nursing bottle when going to sleep or who have experienced prolonged at-will breast-feeding. Other names for the same condition are nursing bottle mouth, baby bottle syndrome, baby bottle caries, and prolonged nursing habit.

I. ETIOLOGY

A. Microbiology

High levels of *Mutans streptococci* have been cultured from the saliva and dental biofilm from the teeth of children with baby bottle tooth decay.[5,6] Lactobacilli also were found in large numbers in the biofilm.

B. Risk Factors

Additional information is included in Chapter 46, on pages 783 to 789. Teaching the parents about the cause and effects of baby bottle tooth decay must be a significant part of anticipatory guidance (see Table 46-2).

■ TABLE 15-3 RISK FACTORS: ROOT CARIES

- Periodontal infection: Root surfaces exposed
  All factors that contribute to bone loss and attachment loss
- Microorganisms: Caries-producing
  Potential transmission
- Local/Behavioral
  Inadequate personal hygiene
  Dental biofilm accumulations
  Poor compliance
- Diet: Frequent use of cariogenic foods
- Low fluoride exposure
  Outside fluoridated community water supply
  Insufficient daily self-application (dentifrice, mouthrinse, frequency)
- Xerostomia
  Medications with side effect
  Radiation to head/neck
  Salivary gland dysfunction
- History of dental caries
  Many restorations: coronal and root
  Overhanging margins, open contact areas, and other biofilm traps
  Poor compliance for dental care
- Prosthetic devices
  Inadequate biofilm removal daily
  Overdentures, clasps, provide biofilm-retentive areas
- Tobacco use: Sugar content of smokeless tobacco

C. Predisposing Factors

1. Nursing bottle that contains sweetened milk or other fluid sweetened with sucrose.
2. Pacifier dipped or filled with a sweet agent, such as honey.
3. Prolonged at-will breast-feeding.

II. EFFECTS

Maxillary anterior teeth and primary molars are the first to be affected (Figure 46-2). As the baby falls asleep, pools of sweet liquid can collect about the teeth. While the sucking is active, the liquid passes beyond the teeth. The nipple covers the mandibular anterior teeth; hence, they are rarely affected.

III. RECOGNITION

Children should be seen for an examination no later than 6 months after eruption of the first tooth.[7] Demineralization may be noted along the cervical third of the maxillary anterior teeth. The source of the problem may be detected and preventive procedures initiated through parental counseling.

At a later stage the lesions appear dark brown. Eventually, the crowns may be destroyed to the gum line, abscesses may develop, and the child may suffer severe pain and discomfort (Figure 46-4, page 790).

■ ROOT CARIES

Root caries is a soft, progressive lesion of cementum and dentin that involves bacterial infection and invasion. It is also called cemental caries, cervical caries, or radicular caries.

The incidence of root caries increases with age, but not because of age. Gingival recession is necessary for root caries, and gingival recession is related to periodontal conditions that lead to recession.

I. STEPS IN THE FORMATION OF A CAVITY

  A. Gingival recession exposes the cemental surface. Caries does not form in the root surface while periodontal fibers are still attached.

  B. Dental caries starts near the cementoenamel junction. Cementum is very thin and is soon destroyed; dentin is invaded.

  C. Enamel is not involved except by extension or when it is undermined. Root caries occurs in a mildly acidic environment. If the pH were lower, enamel would also become carious. The critical pH for enamel is 4.5 to 5.0; for cementum, 6.0 to 6.7.[8]

  D. Mutans streptococci and lactobacilli are primary organisms associated with root caries. Antibody levels to *Streptococcus mutans* are elevated.[9,10]

  E. Effects
    Root caries incidence has been shown to be directly related to the fluoride concentration in the drinking water.[11] Lifelong residence in a community with near-optimum levels of fluoride in the water was shown to be associated with at least an average 30% decrease in the incidence of root caries compared with that associated with lifelong residence in a nonfluoridated community.[12]

II. CLINICAL RECOGNITION

Root caries lesions are described as soft, leathery, or hard. Active lesions are soft or leathery, whereas inactive or arrested lesions are hard.

  A. Soft, shallow, ill-defined lesion.

  B. Increases laterally to coalesce with other small lesions and eventually may extend completely

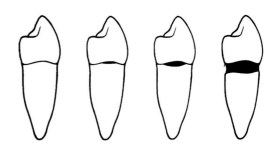

■ FIGURE 15-3 Root Caries. A root surface lesion starts near the cementoenamel junction after gingival recession has exposed the root surface. The lesion is progressive, undermines the enamel, and may eventually surround the cervical third of the cementum. (Modified from Banting, D.W. and Courtright, P.N.: Distribution and Natural History of Carious Lesions on the Roots of the Teeth, *Can Dent. Assoc. J., 41,* 45, January, 1975.)

around the tooth with undermining of the enamel (Figure 15-3).

  C. Yellowish, light brown, dark brown to black.

  D. Leathery in texture when explored (active lesion). Do not explore when remineralization is taking place.

  E. Arrested root caries displays cavitation and discoloration, but it is hard to the touch of the explorer.

III. RISK FACTORS FOR ROOT CARIES

The risk factors are shown in Table 15-3. Prevention and control of root caries depend on control of the risk factors.

■ NONCARIOUS DENTAL LESIONS

■ ENAMEL HYPOPLASIA

I. DEFINITION

Enamel hypoplasia is a defect that occurs as a result of a disturbance in the formation of the organic enamel matrix.

II. TYPES AND ETIOLOGY

A. Hereditary

Enamel is partly or wholly missing. An example is amelogenesis imperfecta, described on page 319.

B. Systemic (Environmental)

Factors that may contribute to enamel hypoplasia during tooth development include severe nutritional deficiency, particularly rickets; fever-producing diseases, such as measles, chickenpox, and scarlet fever; congenital syphilis; hypoparathyroidism; birth injury; prematurity; Rh hemolytic disease; fluorosis; or idiopathy.

C. Local

A single tooth can be affected; trauma or periapical inflammation about a primary tooth can injure the adjacent developing permanent tooth.

III. APPEARANCE

A. Hereditary

May appear brown (page 319).

B. Systemic

Called also "chronologic hypoplasia" because the lesions are found in areas of those teeth where the enamel was forming during the systemic disturbance.
1. *Single Narrow Zone* (smooth or pitted): Disturbance lasted a short period of time (Figure 15-4).
2. *Multiple*: Disturbance to the ameloblast occurred over a period of time, or several times.
3. *Teeth Most Frequently Affected*: First molars, incisors, canines, because the disturbances generally occur during the first year when those teeth are mineralizing.

C. Hypoplasia of Congenital Syphilis

Transmission of syphilis from mother to fetus after the 16th week of pregnancy may alter the development of the tooth germs. Figure 15-5 illustrates tooth forms that may result. The mesiodistal width may be reduced, and incisors are frequently narrowed at the incisal third.

Other conditions may also cause similar variations of tooth form.

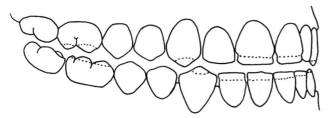

■ **FIGURE 15-4 Enamel Hypoplasia.** Chronologic hypoplasia, usually in the form of grooves or pits, appears in the enamel at a level corresponding with the stage of development of the teeth. For this patient, the disturbance in enamel development occurred at approximately 10 months of age.

D. Local Enamel Hypoplasia

A single tooth with a yellow or brown intrinsic stain.

■ ATTRITION

I. DEFINITION

Attrition is the wearing away of a tooth as a result of tooth-to-tooth contact (Figure 15-6).

II. OCCURRENCE

A. Location

May be found on occlusal, incisal, and proximal surfaces.

B. Age Factor

Increases with age, and more attrition is seen in men than in women of comparable age.

III. ETIOLOGY

A. Bruxism

Predisposing factors may be psychological, tension, or occlusal interferences.

B. Usage

Wear of surfaces on each other. Predisposing factors may be coarse foods, chewing tobacco, or abrasive dusts associated with certain occupations.

IV. APPEARANCE

A. Initial Lesion

Small polished facet on a cusp tip or ridge, or slight flattening of an incisal edge.

B. Advanced

Gradual reduction in cusp height, flattening of occlusal plane (Figure 15-6).

C. Staining of Exposed Dentin

May occur; stain usually is brown.

D. Radiographic

The pulp chamber and canals may be narrowed and sometimes obliterated as the result of formation of secondary dentin.

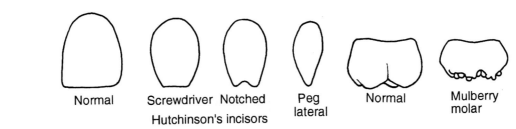

| Normal | Screwdriver | Notched | Peg lateral | Normal | Mulberry molar |

Hutchinson's incisors

▪ **FIGURE 15-5 Crown Forms of Enamel Hypoplasia.** Hutchinson's incisors and mulberry molars are typical crown forms that result from congenital syphilis. The central incisors are narrowed at the incisal third, and the lateral incisors may be conical or peg-shaped.

▪ EROSION

I. DEFINITION

Erosion is the loss of tooth substance by a chemical process that does not involve known bacterial action.

II. OCCURRENCE

A. Location

Facial or lingual surfaces, depending on cause.

B. Usually Involves Several Teeth

III. ETIOLOGY

The lesions are caused by some form of chemical dissolution.

A. May Be Idiopathic (Unknown)

B. Chronic Vomiting

Acid of chronic vomiting affects lingual surfaces, particularly anterior teeth.
1. Pregnancy.
2. Eating disorder, such as bulimia (page 1006).

C. Extrinsic

1. *Industrial.* Workers' teeth can be exposed to atmospheric acids.
2. *Dietary.* Facial surfaces are most frequently affected.
   a. Carbonated beverages or lemon juice used frequently.
   b. Lemons or other citrus fruit sucked frequently.

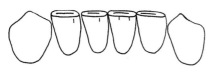

▪ **FIGURE 15-6 Attrition.** Attrition of the incisal surfaces of mandibular anterior teeth has extended to expose the dentin. Dentin usually appears as a brown line or ring.

IV. APPEARANCE

A. Smooth, shallow, hard, shiny (in contrast to dental caries, in which appearance is soft and discolored).
B. Shape varies from shallow saucer-like depressions to deep wedge-shaped grooves; margins are not sharply demarcated.
C. May progress to involve the dentin and stimulate secondary dentin.
D. May occur in combination with dental caries, calculus, or dental restorations.[13]

▪ ABRASION

I. DEFINITION

Abrasion is the mechanical wearing away of tooth substance by forces other than mastication.

II. OCCURRENCE

A. Location

Exposed root surfaces.

B. Other Types

At incisal edge.

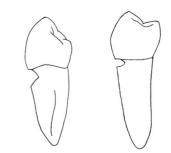

▪ **FIGURE 15-7 Abrasion.** Profile view of the facial surface of mandibular premolars shows shape of abrasion on the root. Note that the area of abrasion undermines the enamel.

III. ETIOLOGY

The lesion originates from a mechanical abrasive activity. The action of microorganisms is not essential for the development of abrasion. Dental caries may occur in the abraded area as a secondary lesion.

A. Abrasive Agent

The most common cause is an abrasive dentifrice applied with vigorous horizontal toothbrushing (Figure 15-7).

B. Other Types

Abrasion may occur at the incisal or occlusal surfaces.
1. Opening bobby pins may leave a small notch in one incisal edge. People with this habit usually utilize the same tooth each time.
2. Occupational causes include, for example, tacks held by carpenters, pins by dressmakers.
3. Pipe held between teeth; usually held in the same place over many years.

IV. APPEARANCE

A. V or wedge shaped with hard, smooth, shiny surface and clearly defined margins.
B. Except for incisal biting habits, the lesions occur initially on exposed cementum, then extend into the dentin.

■ FRACTURES OF TEETH

Trauma to the face may involve fractured bones and teeth in addition to soft tissue injuries. Fractured jaws and methods of treatment are described on pages 855 to 860.

I. CAUSES OF TOOTH FRACTURES

A. Automobile, bicycle, and diving accidents.
B. Contact sports when mouth protectors are not worn.
C. Blows incurred while fighting.
D. Falls.

II. DESCRIPTION

A. Line of Fracture

1. Horizontal.
2. Diagonal.
3. Vertical.

B. Radiographic Signs of Recent Trauma

1. Widened periodontal ligament space.
2. Radiolucent fracture line.
3. Radiopaque areas where fracture segments overlap.
4. Tooth displacement.

III. CLASSIFICATION: WORLD HEALTH ORGANIZATION[14]

Classification provided by the World Health Organization is numbered as a special section of the *International Classification of Diseases*. Both primary and permanent dentitions are included. Figure 15-8 illustrates fractures of a central incisor (page 273).

873.60 Fracture of enamel of tooth only. Includes chipping and incomplete fractures (cracks).

873.61 Fracture of crown of tooth without pulpal involvement.

873.62 Fracture of crown with pulpal involvement.

873.63 Fracture of root of tooth.

873.64 Fracture of crown and root of tooth with or without pulpal involvement.

873.65 Fracture of tooth, unspecified.

873.66 Luxation (dislocation) of tooth. This category may involve concussion, subluxation, and luxation. A tooth with concussion is sensitive to percussion but is not loosened or displaced. Loosening without displacement is subluxation, and loosening with displacement is luxation.

873.67 Intrusion or extrusion of tooth. Intrusion into the alveolar bone is usually accompanied by fracture of the alveolar socket. Extrusion from the socket is a partial displacement.

873.68 Avulsion of tooth. Avulsion is the complete displacement of the tooth out of its socket. Emergency care for a tooth forcibly displaced is found in Table 66-5.

■ CLINICAL EXAMINATION OF THE TEETH

Table 15-4 lists factors to observe during the examination of the teeth and suggests relationships to appointment procedures. Several of these are described in other chapters, for which page references are noted. Information about hypoplasia, attrition, erosion, abrasion, dental caries, and tooth vitality is included in this chapter.

■ RECOGNITION OF CARIOUS LESIONS

Both visual and exploratory means are used to identify dental caries.

I. PREPARATION

Dry each tooth or group of teeth with compressed air and carefully inspect each surface, first visually and then with an explorer as necessary to confirm visual findings.

▪ TABLE 15-4 EXAMINATION OF THE TEETH

FEATURE	TO OBSERVE	DENTAL HYGIENE IMPLICATION
Morphology	Number of teeth (missing teeth verified by radiographic examination) Size, shape Arch form Position of individual teeth Injuries: fractures of the crown (root fractures observed in radiographs)	Selection and adaptation of instruments Areas prone to dental caries initiation, particularly the difficult-to-reach areas during biofilm control Pulp test for vitality may be indicated
Development	Anomalies and developmental defects Pits and white spots	Distinguish hypoplasia and dental fluorosis from demineralization Identify pits for sealants
Eruption (Table 15-1)	Sequence of eruption: normal, irregular Unerupted teeth observed in radiographs	Care in using floss in the col area where the epithelium is usually less mature in young children Orthodontic needs Procedures for preservation of primary teeth
Deposits (Table 17-1, page 292) Food debris Biofilm Calculus Supragingival Subgingival	Overall evaluation of self-care and biofilm-control measures Relation of appearance of teeth to gingival health Extent and location of biofilm, debris, and calculus Calculus and the tooth surface pocket wall	Need for instruction and guidance Frequency of follow-up and maintenance appointments
Stains (pages 315 to 321) Extrinsic Intrinsic	Extrinsic: colors relate to causes Intrinsic: dark, grayish Tobacco stain	Need for test for pulp vitality Stain removal procedures; selection of polishing agent Dentifrice recommendation Biofilm-control emphasis for biofilm-related stains Provide information concerning the oral effects of tobacco use Tobacco cessation program (pages 513 to 515)
Regressive Changes	Attrition: primary and permanent Abrasion: physical agents that may be a cause Erosion	Evaluate causes and treat or counsel for prevention Dietary analysis: for finding foods that may be related Selection of nonabrasive dentifrice Habit evaluation
Exposed Cementum	Relation to gingival recession, pocket formation Areas of narrow attached gingiva Hypersensitivity	Special care areas where only slight attached gingiva remains Nonabrasive dentifrice advised Measures to prevent root-surface caries Care during instrumentation Indication for application of desensitizing agent
Dental Caries	Areas of demineralization Carious lesions (proximal lesions observed in radiographs) Arrested caries Root caries	Charting Treatment plan Preventive program for caries control, fluoride, dietary factors Follow-up and frequency of maintenance

(continued)

■ TABLE 15-4 EXAMINATION OF THE TEETH (Continued)

FEATURE	TO OBSERVE	DENTAL HYGIENE IMPLICATION
Restorations	Contour of restorations, overhangs Proximal contact (see separate heading later in this table) Surface smoothness Staining	Chart and correct inadequate margins Selection of instruments and polishing agents Dentifrice selection to prevent discoloration
Factors Related to Occlusion	Health of supporting structures; observation of radiographs for signs of trauma from occlusion	Need for study of bruxism and other parafunctional habits
Tooth wear	Facets; worn-down cusp tips	
Proximal contacts	Use of floss to find open contact areas Areas of food retention	Chart inadequate contacts for corrective measures Use of floss by patient
Mobility	Degree; comparison of chartings	Need for reduction of inflammatory factors that may be related
	Possible causes	Dentist will identify and treat factors related to trauma from occlusion
Classification	Position of teeth Angle's classification	Relationship to orthodontic treatment needs
Habits	Nail or object biting; lip or cheek biting Observe effects on lip, cheek, teeth Tongue thrust; reverse swallow	Guidance for habit correction when indicated
Edentulous Areas	Radiographic evaluation for impacted, unerupted teeth, retained root tips, other deviations from normal	Supplemental fulcrum selection during instrumentation Applied biofilm-control procedures for abutment teeth
Replacement for Missing Teeth Dentures Partial dentures Implants	Teeth and tissue that support a prosthesis Cleanliness of a prosthesis Factors that contribute to food and debris retention	Preventive measures for harm to supporting teeth and soft tissues Instruction in personal care of fixed and removable dentures; use of floss under fixed partial denture; other appropriate care
Saliva	Amount and consistency Dryness of mouth	Relation to instruction for prevention of dental caries: more caries can be expected in a dry mouth Use of saliva substitute; fluoride

II. VISUAL EXAMINATION: ENAMEL CARIES

Characteristic changes in the color and translucency of tooth structure may be observed. Such changes either are definite signs of dental caries progress or may lead the examiner to suspect dental caries, which can then be checked further with an explorer. Variations in color and translucency include the following:

A. Chalky white areas of demineralization.

B. Grayish-white discoloration of marginal ridges caused by dental caries of the proximal surface underneath.

C. Grayish-white color spreading from margins of restorations caused by lesions of secondary dental caries.

D. In relation to an amalgam restoration, dental caries appears translucent in outer portion and white and opaque adjacent to the amalgam.

E. Open carious lesions may vary in color from yellowish brown to dark brown.

F. Discoloration is generally less severe when dental caries progresses rapidly than when it progresses slowly.

G. Dull, flat white, opaque areas under direct light show loss of translucency, particularly of the enamel.

H. Dark shadow on a proximal surface may be shown by transillumination. This type of observation is especially useful for anterior teeth and unrestored posterior teeth.

III. EXPLORATORY EXAMINATION

A. Smooth Surface Caries

1. *Technique.* Adapt the side of the tip of the explorer closely to the tooth surface, as described on pages 238 to 240. Examine for roughness versus smoothness and continuity of tooth surface versus breaks in continuity. *Do not use pressure or break the surface when checking an area that may be remineralizing.*

2. *Restorations.* Follow the margins of all restorations around with an explorer. Overhanging margins may or may not appear in the radiographs, depending on superimposition. Types of overhangs are described on page 745. Chart all irregularities of existing restorations.

B. Pit and Fissure Caries

When a pit or fissure is discolored, one cannot determine visually whether dental caries is present except when a large obvious cavity can be seen. An obvious cavity should not be explored.

1. Direct the explorer tip so that it can pass straight into the pit or fissure. When the tip is not positioned correctly, caries in a small narrow pit can go undetected.

2. Explorer catches when dental caries is present and softening of tooth structure is evident.

IV. RADIOGRAPHIC EXAMINATION

During the clinical examination, information revealed by radiographs is utilized for supplementation and confirmation. Neither clinical nor radiographic examination is complete without the other. A few principal items to be seen in a radiographic examination of the teeth are:

Anomalies
Impactions
Fractures
Internal and root resorption
Dental caries
Periapical radiolucencies

A. Technique Principles

Periapical radiographs usually provide sufficient information concerning the teeth, but panoramic, extraoral, or occlusal radiographs may be needed for detecting or defining anomalies and pathologic lesions outside the scope of periapical radiographs. Bitewing radiographs or periapical radiographs made by a paralleling technique with no overlapping are most satisfactory for dental caries detection.

Mounted radiographs on an adequately lighted viewbox are a necessity during charting and treatment procedures. For the detection of early carious lesions, a hand-held magnifying glass can be of invaluable assistance.

B. Detection of Dental Caries

Radiographs are not needed for facial, lingual, or occlusal carious lesions because they are accessible and best observed by exploration and direct vision. Because of superimposition of other parts of the tooth, facial, lingual, and occlusal carious lesions need to be fairly well advanced before they are definitely discernible in a radiograph.

1. *Proximal Caries.* Proximal surface lesions may be missed if radiographs are not used. Clinical skills for caries discernment need to be perfected, however, to prevent excess exposure of a patient to unnecessary radiation.

   a. Proximal lesions. Properly angulated radiographs with no overlapping are required for the detection of small lesions that involve the enamel or extend slightly into the dentin.

   b. Proximal overhanging restorations. An overhanging filling or dental caries under that filling may be present, even if none can be seen in the radiograph because of superimposition. An explorer must be passed around the complete margin to confirm the condition.

2. *Root Caries*

   a. Location. Most root carious lesions occur in the vicinity of and just beneath the cementoenamel junction.

   b. Appearance. Root caries appears as a saucer-shaped lesion in a radiograph. It may appear to undermine the enamel, or it may be located beneath an overhanging filling.

■ TESTING FOR PULPAL VITALITY

Any tooth suspected of being nonvital must be tested for pulpal vitality or degree of vitality. The two basic types of pulp testing are thermal and electric.

Such testing is particularly significant prior to treatment involving periodontal surgery, any restorative procedures, and orthodontic appliance placement. Diagnosis of vitality is made not only on the basis of a pulp test but also on consideration of all data from the patient history and clinical and radiographic examinations.

A tooth may become nonvital from bacterial causes, particularly invasion of the pulp from dental caries or periodontal disease. Physical causes may be mechanical or thermal injuries. Examples of mechanical injuries are trauma, such as a blow, or iatrogenic dental procedures, such as cavity preparation or too-rapid orthodontic movement.

I. OBSERVATIONS THAT SUGGEST LOSS OF VITALITY

A. Clinical

1. Discoloration of a tooth crown (intrinsic stains, pages 318 to 320).
2. Fracture (part of the crown may be missing, Figure 15-8).
3. Large carious lesion or large restoration.
4. Fistula with opening into the oral cavity over the apical region of a tooth.

B. Radiographic

1. Apical radiolucency, which may indicate a granuloma, cyst, or abscess.
2. Bone loss with a widened periodontal ligament space extending to the apex.
3. Fractured root.

4. Large carious lesion or restoration that appears closely related to the pulp chamber.

II. RESPONSE TO PULP TESTING

A. Rationale

Pulp testing is based on the knowledge that a stimulus can create pain to which a patient can react. The pulp tester, therefore, determines the conduction of stimuli to the sensory receptors. The vitality of the pulp depends on its blood supply and not on its nerve supply. For that reason, a positive or negative pulp test may not always show the true condition of the pulp.

B. Factors That Influence a Patient's Response to a Pulp Test

1. *Degree of Pulpal Degeneration or Inflammation.* A necrotic pulp gives no response at all, whereas an acutely or chronically inflamed pulp responds at varying degrees between no response and full normal response.
2. *Pain Threshold.* The pain threshold is the lowest intensity of pain caused by a threshold stimulus. A threshold stimulus is the minimum stimulus necessary to induce patient response.
3. *Reaction to Pain.* May vary with a patient's attitude, age, sex, emotional security, fatigue, drugs used, as well as the size of the pulp and thickness of the dentin, particularly the amount of secondary dentin.
4. *Nerve Transmission Blocks.* Injuries or lesions of nerves, and anesthetics.
5. *Adjacent Metal.* Restorations or continuous bridgework.

C. Responses

An electric tester reveals only whether a pulp is vital or nonvital. Using thermal testing may show the following:
1. No response: necrotic pulp.

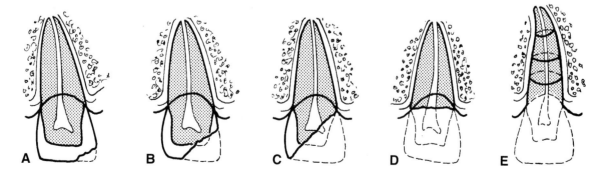

■ **FIGURE 15-8 Fractures of Teeth. (A)** Enamel fracture. **(B)** Crown fracture without pulpal involvement. **(C)** Crown fracture with pulpal involvement. **(D)** Fracture of crown and root near neck of tooth. **(E)** Root fractures involving cementum, dentin, and the pulp may occur in the apical, middle, or coronal third of the root.

2. Lingering pain after removal of stimulus: irreversible pulpitis.
3. Pain subsides promptly: reversible pulpitis.

III. THERMAL PULP TESTING

Cold or hot stimuli may be used. For all methods, a control test is performed on a healthy tooth on the opposite side of the arch. Inform the patient in advance about the procedure and what to expect.

A. Cold Test

1. *Materials.* Cold testing may be accomplished with an air blast, cold drink, ice stick, ethyl chloride in a spray or on a cotton swab, or a carbon dioxide dry-ice stick. Isolate the test teeth and dry with a gauze sponge.
2. *Preparation of ice stick.* Small icicles may be prepared by freezing water in anesthetic needle covers.
3. *Dry-ice stick.* Made from carbon dioxide and delivered using a special holder with a plunger.

B. Heat Test

1. *Temporary stopping.* Warm temporary stopping (gutta-percha). Apply to a tooth dried with cotton sponge.
2. *Water.* Warm to hot water. Isolate tooth and bathe in very warm water.

IV. ELECTRICAL PULP TESTER

A. Types

1. *Battery-operated*
   a. Advantages: Hand held so a clinician can work alone; portable.
   b. Disadvantage: Battery can run down. Some types have a light to indicate current in circuit.
2. *Plug-in*
   a. Advantage: More dependable than battery-operated.
   b. Disadvantage: Not self-contained; requires house-current plug.
   c. Newer models have grounding connection for patient to hold.

B. Precaution

The application of an electrical current to a patient with a cardiac pacemaker or any electronic life-support device by the use of a pulp tester, ultrasonic scaler, desensitizing equipment, or electrosurgical instrument may interfere with the function of the life-support device and may constitute a serious health hazard.[15] A review of the patient history and consultation with the patient's cardiologist are necessary prior to application of a pulp tester.

C. Preparation and Use of Equipment

Manufacturer's instructions are provided for each pulp tester and should be followed carefully. When the

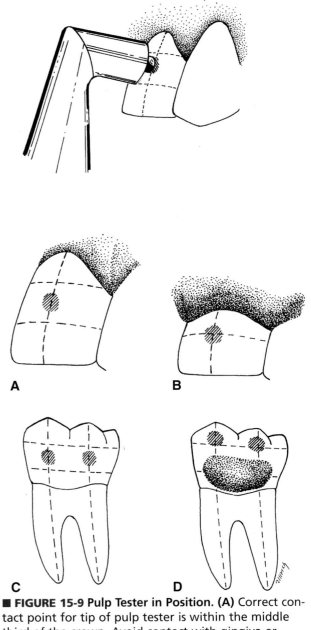

■ **FIGURE 15-9 Pulp Tester in Position. (A)** Correct contact point for tip of pulp tester is within the middle third of the crown. Avoid contact with gingiva or restorations. **(B)** Adjustment of position of contact point because of gingival enlargement. **(C)** Contact points on multirooted tooth. Place tip of pulp tester in the middle third over each root. **(D)** Adjustment of position of contact points because of large Class V restoration.

tester rheostat is separate from the applicator tip, an assistant is needed.

Consistency of procedures is essential to obtain consistent readings. The same pulp tester should be used for a particular patient at continuing comparative tests. Notes in a patient's record can indicate specific directions for that patient.

D. General Procedures

1. Assemble equipment.
2. Explain briefly to the patient what is to be done, but avoid detailed description, which could create anxiety or apprehension.
3. Dry the teeth to be tested to prevent the current from passing to the gingiva; isolate with cotton rolls and insert a saliva ejector, or use a rubber dam.
4. Moisten the end of the tip of the tester with a small amount of toothpaste. Another electrolyte (conductor) may be used if its consistency allows it to remain where placed and prevents it from flowing over the tooth surface.
5. Instruct the patient to signal when a sensation is felt; suggest raising a hand or making a sound.
6. Apply tester tip. The patient lightly holds the handle to complete the circuit.
   a. Apply first to at least one tooth other than the one in question, preferably an adjacent tooth and the same tooth on the contralateral side. Such a procedure determines a normal response for the patient.
   b. Place *without pressure* but with definite contact on sound tooth structure in a consistent location on the middle or gingival third. The middle third of the crown of a single-rooted tooth and the middle third of each cusp of a multirooted tooth are frequently used (Figure 15-9).

E. Readings

1. Avoid contact with gingival or other soft tissues. A low-resistance circuit can be formed, thus allowing the circuit to by-pass the tooth.
2. Avoid contact with metallic restorations. The metal forms a more rapid conductor than does tooth structure. When approximal restorations are in contact, the circuit can be transmitted across to the adjacent tooth. The reading obtained would not pertain to the tooth in question (Figure 15-10). A nonconductive clear plastic matrix strip may be inserted to separate the two metallic restorations.
3. Test each tooth at least twice. Average the readings.

Everyday Ethics

? Barbara, the dental hygienist, has just finished a thorough review of oral hygiene instruction with Mrs. Canavan when she is called out of the treatment room. In today's examination, Barbara had charted two possible carious lesions that will need to be restored. Barbara wanted her to realize all the things she could do to prevent dental caries. Her 12-year-old daughter, Millie, had several restorations today at her appointment with the dentist in another treatment room, had finished first, and was waiting for her mom.

When Barbara returned she could overhear Mrs. Canavan talking with her daughter and explaining how she got all the cavities. She described biofilm as green and painful and how "that's what happens when you eat a lot of candy and drink a lot of soft drinks instead of milk." Barbara stopped to watch quietly. Apparently Millie seemed to understand that it is the biofilm that causes all her cavities, but she was not getting accurate information on the mechanism of action. Mrs. Canavan seemed to be threatening her daughter.

Questions for Consideration

1. Would it be ethical for Barbara to join the conversation and attempt to clarify for both of them? Could she help them both understand the real prevention plan?

2. Describe the positive and negative effects that may occur if Barbara should correct the mother in front of the daughter, or instead, if she asks the daughter to go back to the reception room, and then tries to discuss daily biofilm removal again with Mrs. Canavan.

3. Which of the core values or principles of ethical behavior come into play in patient education efforts such as described in this scenario?

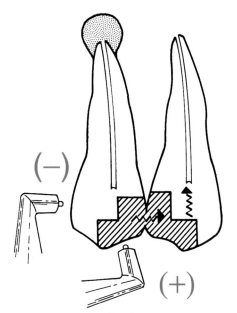

■ **FIGURE 15-10 Use of Pulp Tester.** False-positive response can result when the tester is placed on a metallic restoration. The current can be transmitted across a contact area to give a reading for the adjacent tooth rather than for the tooth in question. (Redrawn from Antel, J. and Christie, W.J.: Electrical Pulp Testing, *Can. Dent. Assoc. J. 45,* 597, November, 1979.)

4. Record on patient's record the average number at which a minimal stimulus induced a response. Record for all teeth tested, not only the tooth in question.

F. Reasons for False-Negative Responses[15]

1. Patient premedicated with analgesics, tranquilizers, narcotics, or alcohol.
2. Recently traumatized tooth.
3. Pulp canal narrow and calcified.
4. Newly erupted tooth with incomplete closure at the apex; immature tooth.

REFERENCES

1. **World Health Organization:** *The Etiology and Prevention of Dental Caries.* WHO Technical Report Series, No. 494, Geneva, World Health Organization, 1972, 19 pp.
2. **Blackwell,** R.E.: *G.V. Black's Operative Dentistry,* Volume II, 9th ed. Milwaukee, Medico-Dental Publishing Co., 1955, pp. 1–4.
3. **Ripa,** L.W.: Nursing Caries: A Comprehensive Review, *Pediatr. Dent., 10,* 268, December, 1988.
4. **Brice,** D.M., Blum, J.R., and Steinberg, B.J.: The Etiology, Treatment, and Prevention of Nursing Caries, *Compend. Cont. Educ. Dent., 17,* 92, January, 1996.
5. **Van Houte,** J., Gibbs, G., and Butera, C.: Oral Flora of Children With "Nursing Bottle Caries," *J. Dent. Res., 61,* 382, February, 1982.
6. **Berkowitz,** R.G., Turner, J., and Hughes, C.: Microbial Characteristics of the Human Dental Caries Associated With Prolonged Bottle-feeding, *Arch. Oral Biol., 29,* 949, Number 11, 1984.
7. **American Academy of Pediatric Dentistry:** Oral Health Policies, *Pediatr. Dent., 20,* 72, Special Issue, Number 6, November, 1998.
8. **Hoppenbrouwers,** P.M.M., Driessens, F.C.M., and Borggreven, J.M.P.M.: The Mineral Solubility of Human Tooth Roots, *Arch. Oral Biol., 32,* 319, Number 5, 1987.
9. **van Houte,** J., Lopman, J., and Kent, R.: The Predominant Cultivable Flora of Sound and Carious Human Root Surfaces, *J. Dent. Res., 73,* 1727, November, 1994.
10. **Zambon,** J.J. and Kasprzak, S.A.: The Microbiology and Histopathology of Human Root Caries, *Am. J. Dent., 8,* 323, December, 1995.
11. **Burt,** B.A., Ismail, A.I., and Eklund, S.A.: Root Caries in an Optimally Fluoridated and a High-Fluoride Community, *J. Dent. Res., 65,* 1154, September, 1986.

✔ **Factors To Teach The Patient**

- The cause and process of enamel or root caries formation and development for the patient at risk.

- A description of the hardness of the enamel and of why a cavity is sometimes larger in the dentin before there is evidence from the external surface.

- Why radiographs are needed to detect proximal incipient caries.

- Reasons for preservation of primary teeth.

- Frequency of complete oral examination in relation to a continuing preventive program.

- Preventive measures for control and prevention of tooth abrasion, such as dentifrice selection and correction of brush selection and use.

- Dietary factors related to erosion.

- Methods for prevention of dental caries, such as fluorides, biofilm prevention and control, and control of cariogenic foods in the diet.

- Methods for prevention of nursing caries. Nothing but plain water should be used in bedtime or naptime nursing bottles. Avoid the use of a sweetener on a pacifier. Use of a cup for milk or juice by the baby's first birthday.

- Medicines or vitamin preparations made with heavy syrup (sucrose) have been shown to cause dental caries. Parents must learn to clean (rinse, not brush) children's teeth after sugar exposures.[16]

- Discuss accident prevention procedures, such as always wearing a mouthguard for contact sports and wearing seat belts.

12. **Stamm**, J.W., Banting, D.W., and Imrey, P.B.: Adult Root Caries Survey of Two Similar Communities With Contrasting Natural Water Fluoride Levels, *J. Am. Dent. Assoc., 120,* 143, February, 1990.

13. **Sognnaes**, R.F., Wolcott, R.B., and Xhonga, F.A.: Dental Erosion. 1. Erosion-like Patterns Occurring in Association With Other Dental Conditions, *J. Am. Dent. Assoc., 84,* 571, March, 1972.

14. **World Health Organization:** *Application of the International Classification of Diseases to Dentistry and Stomatology,* ICD-DA, 2nd ed. Geneva, World Health Organization, 1978, pp. 88–89.

15. **Cohen**, S. and Burns, R.C., eds.: *Pathways of the Pulp,* 7th ed. St. Louis, Mosby, 1998, pp. 13–14.

16. **Rekola**, M.: *In vivo Acid Production From Medicines in Syrup Form, Caries Res., 23,* 412, November–December, 1989.

SUGGESTED READINGS

Anderson, M.H., Molvar, M.P., and Powell, L.V.: Treating Dental Caries as an Infectious Disease, *Oper. Dent., 16,* 21, January–February, 1991.

Choksi, S., Brady, J.M., Dang, D.H., and Rao, M.S.: Detecting Approximal Dental Caries With Transillumination: A Clinical Evaluation, *J. Am. Dent. Assoc., 125,* 1098, August, 1994.

Hirsch, J.M., Livian, G., Edward, S., and Noren, J.G.: Tobacco Habits Among Teenagers in the City of Göteborg, Sweden and Possible Association With Dental Caries, *Swed. Dent. J., 15,* 117, No. 3, 1991.

Ismail, A.I.: The Role of Early Dietary Habits in Dental Caries Development, *Spec. Care Dentist., 18,* 40, January/February, 1998.

Lagerlöf, F. and Oliveby, A.: Caries-Protective Factors in Saliva, *Adv. Dent. Res., 8,* 229, July, 1994.

Massler, M. and Schour, I.: *Atlas of the Mouth,* 2nd ed. Chicago, American Dental Association, Plates 7–16.

McCabe, R.P., Adamkiewicz, V.W., and Pekovic, D.D.: Invasion of Bacteria in Enamel Carious Lesions, *J. Can. Dent. Assoc., 57,* 403, May, 1991.

Newbrun, E.: Preventing Dental Caries: Current and Prospective Strategies, *J. Am. Dent. Assoc., 123,* 68, May, 1992.

Newbrun, E.: Preventing Dental Caries: Breaking the Chain of Transmission, *J. Am. Dent. Assoc., 123,* 55, June, 1992.

Öhrn, K., Crossner, C.-G., Borgesson, L., and Taube, A.: Accuracy of Dental Hygienists in Diagnosing Dental Decay, *Community Dent. Oral Epidemiol., 24,* 182, June, 1996.

Pitts, N.B. and Kidd, E.A.M.: Some of the Factors to Be Considered in the Prescription and Timing of Bitewing Radiography in the Diagnosis and Management of Dental Caries, *J. Dent., 20,* 74, April, 1992.

Tappuni, A.R. and Challacombe, S.J.: Distribution and Isolation Frequency of Eight Streptococcal Species in Saliva From Predentate and Dentate Children and Adults, *J. Dent. Res., 72,* 31, January, 1993.

Root Caries

Beighton, D., Lynch, E., and Heath, M.R.: A Microbiological Study of Primary Root-Caries Lesions With Different Treatment Needs, *J. Dent. Res., 72,* 623, March, 1993.

Faine, M.P., Allender, D., Baab, D., Persson, R., and Lamont, R.J.: Dietary and Salivary Factors Associated With Root Caries, *Spec. Care Dentist., 12,* 177, July/August, 1992.

Fejerskov, O.: Recent Advancements in the Treatment of Root Surface Caries, *Int. J. Dent., 44,* 139, April, 1994.

Galan, D. and Lynch, E.: Prevention of Root Caries in Older Adults, *J. Can. Dent. Assoc., 60,* 422, May, 1994.

Hicks, M.J., Flaitz, C.M., and Garcia-Godoy, F.: Root Surface Caries Formation: Effect of In Vitro APF Treatment, *J. Am. Dent. Assoc., 129,* 449, April, 1998.

Hunt, R.J., Eldredge, J.B., and Beck, J.D.: Effect of Residence in a Fluoridated Community on the Incidence of Coronal and Root Caries in an Older Adult Population, *J. Public Health Dent., 49,* 138, Summer, 1989.

Katz, R.V.: Clinical Signs of Root Caries: Measurement Issues From an Epidemiologic Perspective, *J. Dent. Res., 69,* 1211, May, 1990.

Keltjens, H., Schaeken, T., and van der Hoeven, H.: Preventive Aspects of Root Caries, *Int. Dent. J., 43,* 143, April, 1993.

Krasse, B. and Fure, S.: Root Surface Caries: A Problem for Periodontally Compromised Patients, *Periodontology 2000, 4,* 139, 1994.

Mitchell, T.L. and Forgay, M.G.E.: Root Surface Caries: Implications for Dental Hygienists, *Can. Dent. Hyg./Probe, 21,* 31, March, 1987.

Syed, S.A., Loesche, W.J., Pape, H.L., and Grenier, E.: Predominant Cultivable Flora Isolated From Human Root Surface Caries Plaque, *Infect. Immun., 11,* 727, April, 1975.

van der Veen, M.H., Tsuda, H., Arends, J., and ten Bosch, J.J.: Evaluation of Sodium Fluorescein for Quantitative Diagnosis of Root Caries, *J. Dent. Res., 75,* 588, January, 1996.

Vehkalahti, M. and Paunio, I.: Association Between Root Caries Occurrence and Periodontal State, *Caries Res., 28,* 301, July–August, 1994.

Noncarious Dental Lesions

Bishop, K., Kelleher, M., Briggs, P., and Joshi, R.: Wear Now? An Update on the Etiology of Tooth Wear, *Quintessence Int., 28,* 305, May, 1997.

Ellwood, R.P. and O'Mullane, D.: Enamel Opacities and Dental Esthetics, *J. Public Health Dent., 55,* 171, Summer, 1995.

Gabai, Y., Fattal, B., Rahamin, E., and Gedalia, I.: Effect of pH Levels in Swimming Pools on Enamel of Human Teeth, *Am. J. Dent., 1,* 241, December, 1988.

Gallien, G.S., Kaplan, I., and Owens, B.M.: A Review of Noncarious Dental Cervical Lesions, *Compend. Cont. Educ. Dent., 15,* 1366, November, 1994.

Grippo, J.O. and Simring, M.: Dental "Erosion" Revisited, *J. Am. Dent. Assoc., 126,* 619, May, 1995.

Harrison, J.L. and Roeder, L.B.: Dental Erosion Caused by Cola Beverages, *Gen. Dent., 39,* 23, January–February, 1991.

Järvinen, V.K., Rytömaa, I.I., and Heinonen, O.P.: Risk Factors in Dental Erosion, *J. Dent. Res., 70,* 942, June, 1991.

Krutchkoff, D.J., Eisenberg, E., O'Brien, J.E., and Ponzillo, J.J.: Cocaine-induced Dental Erosions (Correspondence), *N. Engl. J. Med., 322,* 408, February 8, 1990.

Lussi, A., Jaeggi, T., and Jaeggi-Schärer, S.: Prediction of the Erosive Potential of Some Beverages, *Caries Res., 29,* 349, September–October, 1995.

Owens, B.M. and Gallien, G.S.: Noncarious Dental "Abfraction" Lesions in an Aging Population, *Compend. Cont. Educ. Dent., 16,* 552, June, 1995.

Whittington, B.R. and Durward, C.S.: Survey of Anomalies in Primary Teeth and Their Correlation With the Permanent Dentition, *N. Z. Dent. J., 92,* 4, March, 1996.

Pulp Testing

Butel, E.M. and DiFiore, P.M.: Pulp Testing While Avoiding Dangers of Infection and Cross-contamination, *Gen. Dent., 39,* 42, January–February, 1991.

Certosimo, A.J. and Archer, R.D.: A Clinical Evaluation of the Electric Pulp Tester as an Indicator of Local Anesthesia, *Oper. Dent., 21,* 25, January–February, 1996.

Penna, K.J. and Sadoff, R.S.: Simplified Approach to Use of Electrical Pulp Tester, *NYSDJ, 61,* 30, January, 1995.

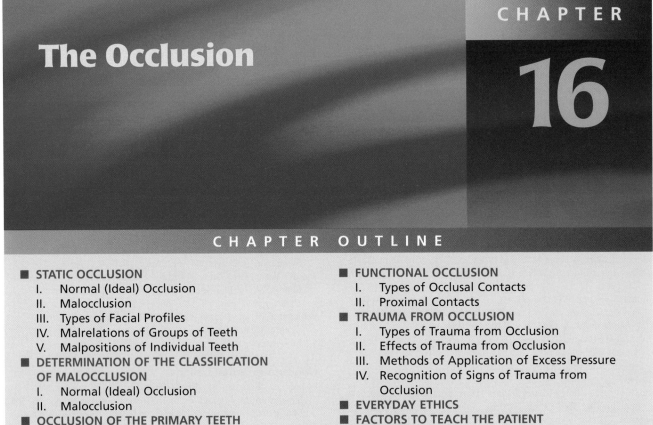

Occlusion is the relationship of the teeth in the mandibular arch to those in the maxillary arch as they are brought together. The occlusion is examined and recorded as part of the oral examination. Knowledge of the occlusion of each patient can contribute significantly to complete care and instruction. Recognition of malocclusion assists in the referral of patients to the orthodontist, gives many valuable points of reference for patient instruction, and determines necessary adaptations in techniques. Box 16-1 defines key words relating to occlusion and occlusal factors.

Recognizing a patient's occlusion and understanding the oral health problems of malocclusion can aid in accomplishing the following:

- Providing information for the comprehensive assessment and planning dental hygiene care.
- Planning personalized instruction in relation to such factors as oral habits, masticatory efficiency, personal oral care procedures, and predisposing factors to dental and periodontal infections.
- Adapting techniques of instrumentation to malpositioned teeth or groups of teeth.
- Planning the frequency of maintenance appointments for professional care on the basis of

deposit retention areas, particularly those that are difficult to reach in routine personal care.
- Providing the general features of malocclusion to consider when orthodontic referral is discussed with the patient.

STATIC OCCLUSION

Static occlusal relationships are seen when the jaws are closed in centric relation. The static occlusion can be efficiently observed in occluded study casts and seen directly in the oral cavity when the lips and cheeks are retracted. Classification of malocclusion and the variations that occur with each category are described here.

I. NORMAL (IDEAL) OCCLUSION

The ideal mechanical relationship between the teeth of the maxillary arch and the teeth of the mandibular arch is as follows:

A. All teeth in the maxillary arch are in maximum contact with all teeth in the mandibular arch in a definite pattern.

BOX 16-1 KEY WORDS: Occlusion

Ankylosis: union or consolidation of two similar or dissimilar hard tissues previously adjacent but not attached.

Dental ankylosis: rigid fixation of a tooth to the surrounding alveolus as a result of ossification of the periodontal ligament; prevents eruption and orthodontic movement.

Centric occlusion: the maximum intercuspation or contact of the teeth of the opposing arches; also called habitual occlusion.

Centric relation: the most unstrained, retruded physiologic relation of the mandible to the maxilla from which lateral movements can be made.

Cephalometer: an orienting device for positioning the head for radiographic examination and measurement.

Cephalometric analysis: the process of evaluating dental and skeletal relationships by way of measurements obtained directly from the head or from cephalometric radiographs and tracings made from the radiographs.

Cephalostat: a head-holding instrument used to obtain cephalometric radiographs; head is held in a precisely defined position relative to the film and to the central ray of the x-ray source.

Diastema: a space between two adjacent teeth in the same arch.

Occlusal guard: a removable dental appliance usually made of plastic that covers a dental arch and is designed to minimize the damaging effects of bruxism and other oral habits; also called bite guard, mouth guard, or night guard.

Occlusal prematurity: any contact of opposing teeth that occurs before the desirable intercuspation.

Orthodontic and dentofacial orthopedics: the specialty area of dentistry concerned with the diagnosis, supervision, guidance, and treatment of the growing and mature dentofacial structures; includes conditions that require movement of teeth and the treatment of malrelationships and malformations of the craniofacial complex.

Orthopedics: correction of abnormal form or relationship of bone structures; may be accomplished surgically (orthopedic surgery) or by the application of appliances to stimulate changes in the bone structure through natural physiologic response (orthopedic therapy); orthodontic therapy is orthopedic therapy.

Parafunctional: abnormal or deviated function, as in bruxism.

Pathologic migration: the movement of a tooth out of its natural position as a result of periodontal infection; contrasts with mesial migration, which is the physiologic process maintained by tooth proximal contacts in the normal dental arches.

Tongue thrust: the infantile pattern of suckle-swallow movement in which the tongue is placed between the incisor teeth or alveolar ridges; may result in an anterior open bite, deformation of the jaws, and abnormal function.

Trauma from occlusion: injury to the periodontium that results from occlusal forces in excess of the reparative capacity of the attachment apparatus; also called occlusal traumatism.

B. Maxillary teeth slightly overlap mandibular teeth on the facial surfaces.

II. MALOCCLUSION

Any deviation from the physiologically acceptable relationship of the maxillary arch and/or teeth to the mandibular arch and/or teeth.

III. TYPES OF FACIAL PROFILES (FIGURE 16-1)

A. Mesognathic

Having slightly protruded jaws, which give the facial outline a relatively flat appearance (straight profile).

B. Retrognathic

Having a prominent maxilla and a mandible posterior to its normal relationship (convex profile).

C. Prognathic

Having a prominent, protruded mandible and normal (usually) maxilla (concave profile).

IV. MALRELATIONS OF GROUPS OF TEETH

A. Crossbites

1. *Posterior.* Maxillary or mandibular posterior teeth are either facial or lingual to their normal position.

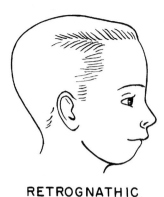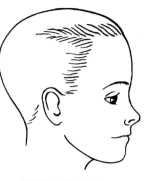

RETROGNATHIC   MESOGNATHIC   PROGNATHIC

▪ **FIGURE 16-1 Types of Facial Profiles.**

This condition may occur bilaterally or unilaterally (Figure 16-2).

2. *Anterior.* Maxillary incisors are lingual to the mandibular incisors (Figure 16-3).

B. Edge-to-Edge Bite

Incisal surfaces of maxillary teeth occlude with incisal surfaces of mandibular teeth instead of overlapping as in normal occlusion (Figure 16-4).

C. End-to-End Bite

Molars and premolars occlude cusp-to-cusp as viewed mesiodistally (Figure 16-5).

D. Open Bite

Lack of occlusal or incisal contact between certain maxillary and mandibular teeth because either or both have failed to reach the line of occlusion. The teeth cannot be brought together, and a space remains as a result of the arching of the line of occlusion (Figure 16-6).

E. Overjet

The horizontal distance between the labioincisal surfaces of the mandibular incisors and the linguoincisal surfaces of the maxillary incisors (Figure 16-7). One way to measure the amount of overjet is to place the tip of a probe on the labial surface of the mandibular incisor and, holding it horizontally against the incisal edge of the maxillary tooth, read the distance in millimeters.

F. Underjet

Maxillary teeth are lingual to mandibular teeth. The horizontal distance between the labioincisal surfaces of the maxillary incisors and the linguoincisal surfaces of the mandibular incisors (Figure 16-8).

G. Overbite

Overbite, or vertical overlap, is the vertical distance by which the maxillary incisors overlap the mandibular incisors.

1. *Normal Overbite.* An overbite is considered normal when the incisal edges of the maxillary teeth are within the incisal third of the mandibular teeth, as shown in Figure 16-9 in side view and in Figure 16-11A in anterior view.

2. *Moderate Overbite.* An overbite is considered moderate when the incisal edges of the maxillary teeth appear within the middle third of the mandibular teeth (Figure 16-11B).

3. *Deep (Severe) Overbite.*
   • Deep (severe): When the incisal edges of the maxillary teeth are within the cervical third of the mandibular teeth (Figure 16-11C).

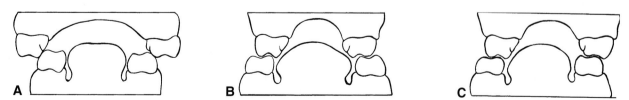

▪ **FIGURE 16-2 Posterior Crossbite. (A)** Mandibular teeth lingual to normal position. **(B)** Mandibular teeth facial to normal position. **(C)** Unilateral crossbite: right side, normal; left side, mandibular teeth facial to normal position.

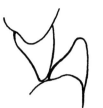

■ **FIGURE 16-3 Anterior Crossbite.** Maxillary anterior teeth are lingual to mandibular anterior teeth. Anterior crossbite occurs in Angle's Class III malocclusion.

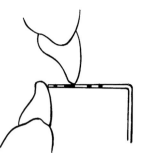

■ **FIGURE 16-7 Overjet.** Maxillary incisors are labial to the mandibular incisors. Measurable horizontal distance is evident between the incisal edge of the maxillary incisors and the incisal edge of the mandibular incisors. A periodontal probe can be used to measure for recording the distance.

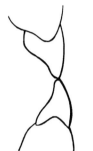

■ **FIGURE 16-4 Edge-to-Edge Bite.** Incisal surfaces occlude.

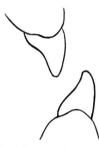

■ **FIGURE 16-8 Underjet.** Maxillary incisors are lingual to the mandibular incisors. Measurable horizontal distance is evident between the incisal edges of the maxillary incisors and the incisal edges of the mandibular incisors.

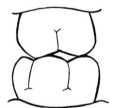

■ **FIGURE 16-5 End-to-End Bite.** Molars in cusp-to-cusp occlusion as viewed from the facial.

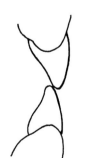

■ **FIGURE 16-9 Normal Overbite.** Profile view to show the position of the incisal edge of the maxillary tooth within the incisal third of the facial surface of the mandibular incisor.

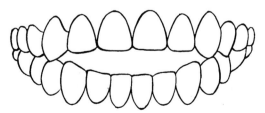

■ **FIGURE 16-6 Open Bite.** Lack of incisal contact. Posterior teeth in normal occlusion.

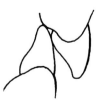

■ **FIGURE 16-10 Deep (Severe) Anterior Overbite.** Incisal edge of the maxillary tooth is at the level of the cervical third of the facial surface of the mandibular anterior tooth. See the facial view in Figure 16-11C.

- Very deep: When in addition the incisal edges of the mandibular teeth are in contact with the maxillary lingual gingival tissue. A side view of very deep overbite is shown in Figure 16-10.
4. *Clinical Examination of Overbite.*
   a. Direct observation: With the posterior teeth closed together, the lips can be retracted and the teeth observed, as in Figure 16-11. The degree of anterior overbite is judged by the position of the incisal edge of the maxillary teeth:
   - Normal (slight), within the incisal third of the mandibular incisors (Figure 16-11A).
   - Moderate overbite, within the middle third (Figure 16-11B).
   - Severe overbite, within the cervical third (Figure 16-11C).
   b. Mirror view: By placing a mouth mirror under the incisal edge of the maxillary teeth, one can sometimes see the mandibular teeth in contact with the maxillary palatal gingiva. When contact is not visible, an examination of the lingual gingiva may reveal teeth prints or at least enlargement and redness from the contact.

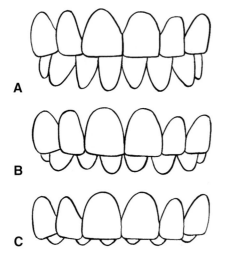

■ **FIGURE 16-11 Overbite, Anterior View. (A)** Normal overbite: incisal edges of the maxillary teeth are within the incisal third of the facial surfaces of the mandibular teeth. **(B)** Moderate overbite: incisal edges of maxillary teeth are within the middle third of the facial surfaces of the mandibular teeth. **(C)** Severe overbite: the incisal edges of the maxillary teeth are within the cervical third of the facial of the mandibular teeth. When the incisal edges of the mandibular teeth are in contact with the maxillary lingual gingival tissue, the overbite is considered very severe. See the profile view in Figure 16-10.

V. MALPOSITIONS OF INDIVIDUAL TEETH

A. Labioversion

A tooth that has assumed a position labial to normal.

B. Linguoversion

Position lingual to normal.

C. Buccoversion

Position buccal to normal.

D. Supraversion

Elongated above the line of occlusion.

E. Torsiversion

Turned or rotated.

F. Infraversion

Depressed below the line of occlusion, for example, primary tooth that is submerged or ankylosed.

■ DETERMINATION OF THE CLASSIFICATION OF MALOCCLUSION

The determination of the classification of occlusion is based upon the principles of Edward H. Angle, presented in the early 1900s. He defined normal occlusion as "the normal relations of the occlusal inclined planes of the teeth when the jaws are closed"[1] and based his system of classification upon the relationship of the first permanent molars.

Although authorities have since agreed that the maxillary first permanent molars do not occupy a fixed position in the dental arch, Angle's system serves to provide an acceptable basis for a useful classification. A more comprehensive picture of malocclusion is made by the orthodontist, who studies the relationships of the position of the teeth to the jaws, the face, and the skull.

Three general classes of malocclusion are described in the following sections. These classes are designated by Roman numerals. Because the mandible is movable and the maxilla is stationary, the classes describe the relationship of the mandible to the maxilla. For example, in distoclusion (Class II) the mandible is distal, whereas in mesioclusion (Class III) the mandible is mesial to the maxilla, as compared to the normal position.

I. NORMAL (IDEAL) OCCLUSION (FIGURE 16-12)

A. Facial Profile

Mesognathic (Figure 16-1).

B. Molar Relation

The mesiobuccal cusp of the maxillary first permanent molar occludes with the buccal groove of the mandibular first permanent molar.

C. Canine Relation

The maxillary permanent canine occludes with the distal half of the mandibular canine and the mesial half of the mandibular first premolar.

II. MALOCCLUSION

A. Class I or Neutroclusion (Figure 16-12)

1. *Facial Profile:* Same as normal occlusion.
2. *Molar Relation:* Same as normal occlusion.
3. *Canine Relation:* Same as normal occlusion.
4. *Malposition of Individual Teeth or Groups of Teeth*
5. *General Types of Conditions That Frequently Occur in Class I:*
    - Crowded maxillary or mandibular anterior teeth.
    - Protruded or retruded maxillary incisors.
    - Anterior crossbite.
    - Posterior crossbite.
    - Mesial drift of molars resulting from premature loss of teeth.

B. Class II or Distoclusion (Figure 16-12)

1. *Description:* Mandibular teeth posterior to normal position in their relation to the maxillary teeth.
2. *Facial Profile:* Retrognathic; maxilla protrudes; lower lip is full and often rests between the maxillary and mandibular incisors; the mandible appears retruded or weak (Figure 16-1, retrognathic).
3. *Molar Relation*
    a. The buccal groove of the mandibular first permanent molar is distal to the mesiobuccal cusp of the maxillary first permanent molar by at least the width of a premolar.
    b. When the distance is less than the width of a premolar, the relation should be classified as "tendency toward Class II."

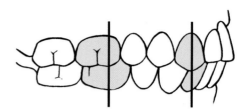

Normal (Ideal) Occlusion
Molar relationship: mesiobuccal cusp of maxillary first permanent molar occludes with the buccal groove of the mandibular first permanent molar.

Malocclusion
Class I: Neutroclusion.
Molar relationship: same as Normal, with malposition of individual teeth or groups of teeth.

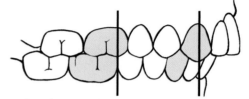

Class II: Distoclusion.
Molar relationship: buccal groove of the mandibular first permanent molar is distal to the mesiobuccal cusp of the maxillary first permanent molar by at least the width of a premolar.
  Division 1: mandible is retruded and all maxillary incisors are protruded.

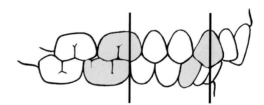

Class II: Distoclusion.
  Division 2: mandible is retruded and one or more maxillary incisors are retruded.

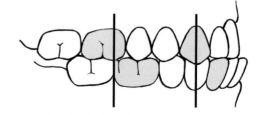

Class III: Mesioclusion.
Molar relationship: buccal groove of the mandibular first permanent molar is mesial to the mesiobuccal cusp of the maxillary first permanent molar by at least the width of a premolar.

■ **FIGURE 16-12 Normal Occlusion and Classification of Malocclusion.**

4. *Canine Relation*
   a. The distal surface of the mandibular canine is distal to the mesial surface of the maxillary canine by at least the width of a premolar.
   b. When the distance is less than the width of a premolar, the relation should be classified as "tendency toward Class II."
5. *Class II, Division 1*
   a. Description: The mandible is retruded and all maxillary incisors are protruded.
   b. General types of conditions that frequently occur in Class II, Division 1 malocclusion: Deep overbite, excessive overjet, abnormal muscle function (lips), short mandible, or short upper lip.
6. *Class II, Division 2*
   a. Description: The mandible is retruded, and one or more maxillary incisors are retruded.
   b. General types of conditions that frequently occur in Class II, Division 2 malocclusion: Maxillary lateral incisors protrude while both central incisors retrude, crowded maxillary anterior teeth, or deep overbite.
7. *Subdivision:* One side is Class I, the other side is Class II (may be Division 1 or 2).

C. Class III or Mesioclusion (Figure 16-12)

1. *Description:* Mandibular teeth are anterior to normal position in relation to maxillary teeth.
2. *Facial Profile:* Prognathic; lower lip and mandible are prominent (Figure 16-1).
3. *Molar Relation*
   a. The buccal groove of the mandibular first permanent molar is mesial to the mesiobuccal cusp of the maxillary first permanent molar by at least the width of a premolar.
   b. When the distance is less than the width of a premolar, the relation should be classified as "tendency toward Class III."
4. *Canine Relation*
   a. The distal surface of the mandibular canine is mesial to the mesial surface of the maxillary canine by at least the width of a premolar.
   b. When the distance is less than the width of a premolar, the relation should be classified as "tendency toward Class III."
5. *General Types of Conditions That Frequently Occur in Class III Malocclusion:*
   a. True Class III: Maxillary incisors are lingual to mandibular incisors in an anterior crossbite (Figure 16-3).

   b. Maxillary and mandibular incisors are in edge-to-edge occlusion.
   c. Mandibular incisors are very crowded but lingual to maxillary incisors.

■ OCCLUSION OF THE PRIMARY TEETH[2]

I. NORMAL (IDEAL)

A. Primary Canine Relation

Same as permanent dentition.
1. *With Primate Spaces**
   a. Mandibular: Between mandibular canine and first molar (Figure 16-13A).
   b. Maxillary: Between maxillary lateral incisor and canine (Figure 16-13B).
2. *Without Primate Spaces.* Closed arches.

B. Second Primary Molar Relation

The mesiobuccal cusp of the maxillary second primary molar occludes with the buccal groove of the mandibular second primary molar.
1. *Variations in Distal Surfaces Relationships.* Terminal step.
   a. The distal surface of the mandibular primary molar is mesial to that of the maxillary, thereby forming a mesial step (Figure 16-14A).
   b. Morphologic variation in molar size; maxillary and mandibular primary molars have approximately the same mesiodistal width.

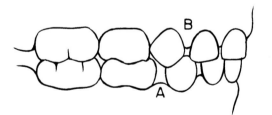

■ **FIGURE 16-13 Primary Teeth With Primate Spaces. (A)** Mandibular primate space between the canine and the first molar. **(B)** Maxillary primate space between the lateral incisor and the canine.

---

*Primate space: a diastema or gap in the tooth row occasionally observed in the human primary dentition. It is characteristic of nearly all species of primates except man. The maxillary primate spaces accommodate the mandibular canines, and the mandibular primate spaces accommodate the maxillary canines when the teeth are in occlusion. As a reduction in the length of canines accompanied man's evolution, the canines no longer protruded beyond the occlusal level. The diastema (primate space) was no longer functional.

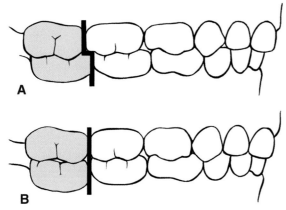

■ FIGURE 16-14 Eruption Patterns of the First Permanent Molars. (A) Terminal step. The distal surface of the mandibular second primary molar is mesial to the distal surface of the maxillary primary molar. **(B)** Terminal plane. The distal surfaces of the mandibular and maxillary second primary molars are on the same vertical plane; permanent molars erupt in end-to-end occlusion.

2. *Variation.* Terminal plane.
   a. The distal surfaces of the maxillary and mandibular primary molars are on the same vertical plane (Figure 16-14B).
   b. The maxillary molar is narrower mesiodistally than the mandibular molar (occurs in many patients).
3. *Effects on Occlusion of First Permanent Molars*
   a. Terminal step: First permanent molar erupts directly into proper occlusion (Figure 16-14A).
   b. Terminal plane: First permanent molars erupt end to end. With mandibular primate space, early mesial shift of primary molars into the primate space occurs, and the permanent mandibular molar shifts into proper occlusion. Without primate spaces, late mesial shift of permanent mandibular molar into proper occlusion occurs, following exfoliation of second primary molar (Figure 16-14B).

II. MALOCCLUSION OF THE PRIMARY TEETH

Same as permanent dentition.

■ FUNCTIONAL OCCLUSION

In contrast to static occlusion, which pertains to the relationship of the teeth when the jaws are closed, functional occlusion consists of all contacts during chewing, swallowing, or other normal action. Functional occlusion is associated with performance:

- Pressures or forces created by the muscles of mastication are transmitted from the teeth, after contact, to the periodontium.
- Such forces are necessary to maintain the occlusal relationship of the teeth and guide the teeth during eruption.
- The forces are also necessary to provide functional stimulation for the preservation of the health of the attachment apparatus, namely, the periodontal ligament, the cementum, and the alveolar bone.

I. TYPES OF OCCLUSAL CONTACTS

A. Functional Contacts

Functional contacts are the normal contacts that are made between the maxillary teeth and the mandibular teeth during chewing and swallowing. Each contact is momentary, so the total contact time is only a few minutes each day.

B. Parafunctional Contacts

Parafunctional contacts are those made outside the normal range of function.
1. They result from occlusal habits and neuroses.
2. They are potentially injurious to the periodontal supporting structures, but only in the presence of dental biofilm and inflammatory factors.
3. They create wear facets and attrition on the teeth. A facet is a shiny, flat, worn spot on the surface of a tooth, frequently on the side of a cusp.
4. They can be divided into the following:
   a. Tooth-to-tooth contacts: Bruxism, clenching, tapping.
   b. Tooth-to-hard-object contacts: Nail biting; occupational use of such objects as tacks or pins; use of smoking equipment, such as a pipe stem or hard cigarette holder.
   c. Tooth-to-oral-tissues contacts: Lip or cheek biting.

II. PROXIMAL CONTACTS

Proximal contacts serve to stabilize the position of teeth in the dental arches and to prevent food impaction between the teeth. Attrition or wear of the teeth occurs at the proximal contacts.

A. Drifting

- When proximal contact is lost, teeth can drift into spaces created by unreplaced missing teeth.

- There is also a natural tendency for mesial migration of teeth toward the midline.
- In the absence of disease, the surrounding periodontal tissues adapt to repositioned teeth.

B. Pathologic Migration

- With destruction of the supporting structures of a tooth as a result of periodontal infection, and with a force to move a tooth weakened by disease and bone loss, migration of the tooth can result.
- *Pathologic migration occurs when disease is present; in contrast, drifting is migration with a healthy periodontium.*

▪ TRAUMA FROM OCCLUSION

Periodontal tissue injury caused by repeated occlusal forces that exceed the physiologic limits of tissue tolerance is called *trauma from occlusion*. Other names are periodontal traumatism, occlusal traumatism, and periodontal trauma.

I. TYPES OF TRAUMA FROM OCCLUSION

A. *Primary trauma from occlusion results when:*
  - Excessive occlusal force is exerted on a tooth with normal bone support.
  - Example: the effect of a new restoration placed above the line of occlusion.
B. *Secondary trauma from occlusion occurs when:*
  - Excessive occlusal force is exerted on a tooth with bone loss and inadequate alveolar bone support.

- The ability of the tooth to withstand occlusal forces is impaired.
- A tooth has lost the support of the surrounding bone; even the pressures of what are usually considered normal occlusal forces may create lesions of trauma from occlusion.

II. EFFECTS OF TRAUMA FROM OCCLUSION

The attachment apparatus (periodontal ligament, cementum, and alveolar bone) has as its main purpose the maintenance of the tooth in the socket in a functional state. In a healthy situation, occlusal pressures and forces during chewing and swallowing are readily dispersed or absorbed and no unusual effects are produced.

A. Excess Forces

- When the forces of occlusion are greater than can be taken care of by the attachment apparatus, damage can result.
- Circulatory disturbances, tissue destruction from crushing under pressure, bone resorption, and other pathologic processes are initiated.

B. Relation to Inflammatory Factors

- *Trauma from occlusion does not cause gingivitis, periodontitis, or pocket formation.* The steps in the development of inflammatory disease and pockets are outlined on pages 247 to 249.
- In the presence of inflammatory disease, the existing periodontal destruction may be aggravated or promoted by trauma from occlusion.

Everyday Ethics

Many of the first-year dental hygiene students struggled to learn the specific classifications of malocclusion and how to recognize them in their patients.

The problem was often a locker room discussion item, and it was agreed that they noticed that the instructors didn't always look for the details of a patient's occlusion when the record was checked.

One clinic day Roxanne was confused, and she decided to just write anything down on the patient's chart. When the instructor came to check the oral examination, she questioned why Roxanne had the classification documented as a Class II

(distoclusion). The student just shrugged her shoulders and said, "I don't know."

Questions for Consideration

1. What are the issues with Roxanne's apparent lack of knowledge about occlusion and saying "I don't know" to her teacher?

2. What should Roxanne do to be more accurate with her clinical charting and documentation?

3. Can Roxanne "justify" her actions to the patient and to the instructor? Give a rationale.

III. METHODS OF APPLICATION OF EXCESS PRESSURE

To understand the nature of the occlusal forces that can cause periodontal trauma from occlusion, it is helpful to recognize types of tooth contacts that can overburden a tooth or a group of teeth.[3]

A. Individual Teeth That Touch Before Full Closure

The contact is premature and may put excessive force on an individual tooth.

B. Two or Only a Few Teeth in Contact During Movement of the Jaw

The teeth involved receive a disproportionate amount of force.

C. Initial Contacts on Inclined Planes of Cusps

Following the initial contact, when the teeth are brought together in a closed position, there may be excess pressure on the teeth where initial contact was made.

D. Heavy Forces Not in a Vertical or Axial Direction

Normal occlusal relationships imply a direct cusp-to-fossa position during closure, with the force of occlusion in a vertical direction toward the tooth apex and parallel with the long axis. When pressures are exerted laterally or horizontally, excess force is placed on the periodontal attachment apparatus.

E. Increased Frequency, Intensity, and Duration of Contacts

In the presence of parafunctional habits, such as bruxism, clenching, tapping, or biting objects, many more than the usual number of tooth contacts are made each day, and the intensity and duration are altered.

IV. RECOGNITION OF SIGNS OF TRAUMA FROM OCCLUSION

No one clinical or radiographic finding clearly defines the presence of trauma from occlusion. Diagnosis of the condition is complex. The possible observations listed as follows should be looked for specifically and recorded for evaluation and correlation with the patient history and all other clinical determinations.

✔ Factors To Teach The Patient

- Interpretation of the *general* purposes of orthodontic care (function and esthetics) to patients referred by the dentist to an orthodontist.

  - Dependence of masticatory efficiency on the occlusion of the teeth.

  - Influence of masticatory efficiency on food selection in the diet.

  - Influence of masticatory efficiency and diet on the nutritional status of the body and oral health.

- Interpretation of the dentist's suggestions for the correction of oral habits.

- The space-maintaining function of the primary teeth in prevention of malocclusion of permanent teeth.

- The role of malocclusion as a predisposing factor for dental biofilm retention in the formation of dental caries and periodontal infections.

- Dental biofilm removal methods for reducing dental calculus and soft deposit retention in areas where teeth are crowded, displaced, or otherwise not in normal occlusion.

- The relation of the occlusion and the position of the teeth to the patient's personal oral care procedures.

  - Selection of the proper type of toothbrush.

  - Application of thorough toothbrushing method or methods.

  - Use of dental floss.

- Specific reasons for frequency of maintenance examinations when related to malocclusion and while in the process of having orthodontic therapy.

A. Clinical Findings That May Occur in Trauma from Occlusion

1. Tooth mobility.
2. Fremitus.
3. Sensitivity of teeth to pressure and/or percussion.
4. Pathologic migration.

5. Wear facets or atypical incisal or occlusal wear.
6. Open contacts related to food impaction.
7. Neuromuscular disturbances in the muscles of mastication. In severe cases, muscle spasm can occur.
8. Temporomandibular joint symptoms.

B. Radiographic Findings

Characteristics that may occur in trauma from occlusion include:

1. Widened periodontal ligament spaces, particularly angular thickening (triangulation). This finding frequently occurs in conjunction with tooth mobility.
2. Angular (vertical) bone loss in localized areas (see Figure 13-20).
3. Root resorption.
4. Furcation involvement.
5. Thickened lamina dura. Although related to occlusal forces, thickened lamina dura should not be considered a detrimental or destructive effect of trauma from occlusion. It may be a defense reaction to strengthen tooth support against occlusal forces. Thickened lamina dura is frequently associated with teeth that have undergone orthodontic treatment.

C. Patient Management for Examination

1. Observe the facial profile as the patient enters and is seated in the dental chair to estimate the classification of occlusion before examination of the teeth.
2. Avoid mention of a dentofacial deformity that would make the patient feel self-conscious.
3. Avoid suggesting to the patient or a parent the possible procedures the orthodontist may use in treatment because complications become known only after the complete diagnosis.
4. Closing to centric relation can be performed most effectively by instructing the patient to curl the tongue and to try to hold the tip of the tongue as far back as possible while closing.
5. When a small child has difficulty in occluding, the clinician may firmly but gently press the cushions of the thumbs on the mucous membrane over the pterygomandibular raphe, holding the thumbs between the cheek and buccal surfaces of the teeth as the patient is requested to close.
6. Prepare mouth guards for patients in contact sports.
7. Study the occlusion of the patient with removable dentures with the dentures in and out of the mouth.

REFERENCES

1. **Angle**, E.H.: *Malocclusion of the Teeth,* 7th ed. Philadelphia, S.S. White, 1907.
2. **Baume**, L.J.: Physiological Tooth Migration and Its Significance for the Development of the Occlusion, I. The Biogenetic Course of the Deciduous Dentition, *J. Dent. Res., 29,* 123, April, 1950; II. The Biogenesis of the Accessional Dentition, *J. Dent. Res., 29,* 331, June, 1950; III. The Biogenesis of the Successional Dentition, *J. Dent. Res., 29,* 338, June, 1950; IV. The Biogenesis of Overbite, *J. Dent. Res., 29,* 440, August, 1950.
3. **Allen**, D.L., McFall, W.T., and Jenzano, J.W.: *Periodontics for the Dental Hygienist,* 4th ed. Philadelphia, Lea & Febiger, 1987, pp. 85–86.

SUGGESTED READINGS

Baker, I.M.: Record Taking in the Orthodontic Office, *Dent. Assist., 60,* 25, March/April, 1991.

Brezniak, N. and Wasserstein, A.: Root Resorption After Orthodontic Treatment: Part 1. Literature Review, *Am. J. Orthod. Dentofacial Orthop., 103,* 62, January, 1993.

Brezniak, N. and Wasserstein, A.: Root Resorption After Orthodontic Treatment: Part 2. Literature Review, *Am. J. Orthod. Dentofacial Orthop., 103,* 138, February, 1993.

Burden, D.J., Garvin, J.W., and Patterson, C.C.: Pilot Study of an Orthodontic Treatment Need Learning Package for General Dental Practitioners, *Br. Dent. J., 179,* 300, October 21, 1995.

Dyer, G.S., Harris, E.F., and Vaden, J.L.: Age Effects on Orthodontic Treatment: Adolescents Contrasted With Adults, *Am. J. Orthod. Dentofacial Orthop., 100,* 523, December, 1991.

Fink, D.F. and Smith, R.J.: The Duration of Orthodontic Treatment, *Am. J. Orthod. Dentofacial Orthop., 102,* 45, July, 1992.

Finkbeiner, R.L., Nelson, L.S., and Killebrew, J.: Case Reports. Accidental Orthodontic Elastic Band-Induced Periodontitis: Orthodontic and Laser Treatment, *J. Am. Dent. Assoc., 128,* 1565, November, 1997.

Khan, R.S. and Horrocks, E.N.: A Study of Adult Orthodontic Patients and Their Treatment, *Br. J. Orthod., 18,* 183, August, 1991.

Machen, D.E.: Legal Aspects of Orthodontic Practice: Risk Management Concepts. Oral Hygiene Assessment: Plaque Accumulation, Gingival Inflammation, Decalcification, and Caries, *Am. J. Orthod. Dentofacial Orthop., 100,* 93, July, 1991.

Martinez-Canut, P., Carrasquer, A., Magan, R., and Lorca, A.: A Study on Factors Associated with Pathologic Tooth Migration, *J. Clin. Periodontol., 24,* 492, July, 1997.

Massler, M.: Oral Habits: Development and Management, *J. Pedod., 7,* 109, Winter, 1983.

Newman, G.V.: Limited Orthodontics for the Older Population: Multidisciplinary Modalities, *Am. J. Orthod. Dentofacial Orthop., 101,* 281, March, 1992.

Ngan, P. and Fields, H.W.: Open Bite: A Review of Etiology and Management, *Pediatr. Dent., 19,* 91, March/April, 1997.

Robinson, H.B.G. and Miller, A.S.: *Color Atlas of Oral Pathology,* 5th ed. Philadelphia, J.B. Lippincott Co., 1990, pp. 52, 83–84, 93, 95.

Roe, S.: Treatment Recommendations for Nonnutritive Sucking Habits, *J. Pract. Hyg., 7,* 11, January/February, 1998.

Torres, H.O., Ehrlich, A., Bird, D., and Dietz, E.: *Modern Dental Assisting,* 5th ed. Philadelphia, W.B. Saunders Co., 1995, pp. 535–559.

Dental Biofilm and Other Soft Deposits

Dental caries and gingival and periodontal infections are caused by microorganisms in microbial or dental biofilms. Disease-producing microorganisms attach to the tooth surfaces and colonize. They bring about carious lesions of the enamel and root surfaces, in pits and fissures, and on smooth surfaces (pages 263 to 265). They also bring about inflammatory changes in the periodontium that can lead to destruction of tissues and loss of attachment. The morphologic forms of bacteria are shown in Figure 17-1.

During the clinical examination of the teeth and surrounding soft tissues, the soft and hard deposits that accumulate on the teeth and within the sulci or pockets must be recognized and assessed. From the findings, an initial care plan can be formulated based on the individual needs of the patient. Key words are defined in Box 17-1.

The soft deposits are acquired pellicle or cuticle, dental biofilm, materia alba, and food debris, each of which is an entity; the terms should not be interchanged. The hard, calcified deposit on teeth is dental calculus, which is described in Chapter 18. A classification with definitions of the dental deposits is presented in Table 17-1.[1]

■ ACQUIRED PELLICLE

The acquired pellicle is a tenacious membranous layer that is amorphous, acellular, and organic and that forms over exposed tooth surfaces, as well as over restorations and dental calculus. Its thickness, which varies from 0.1 to 0.8 µm, usually is greater near the gingival margin.

I. FORMATION

Within minutes after all external material has been removed from the tooth surfaces with an abrasive, the acquired pellicle begins to form. It is composed primarily of glycoproteins from the saliva that are selectively adsorbed by the hydroxyapatite of the tooth surface. The adsorbed material becomes a highly insoluble coating

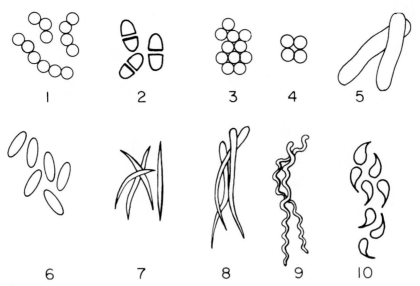

▪ **FIGURE 17-1 Morphologic Forms of Bacteria. (1)** Streptococci. **(2)** Diplococci. **(3)** Staphylococci. **(4)** Sarcina. **(5)** Bacilli. **(6)** Coccobacilli. **(7)** Fusiform bacilli. **(8)** Filamentous bacilli. **(9)** Spirochetes. **(10)** Vibrios. (From Hammond, B.: Bacterial Structure and Function, in Schuster, G.S., ed.: *Oral Microbiology and Infectious Disease,* 2nd student ed. Toronto, B.C. Decker, 1988, p. 23.)

over the teeth, calculus deposits, restorations, and complete and partial dentures.

II. TYPES OF PELLICLES[2]

A. Surface Pellicle, Unstained

The unstained pellicle is clear, translucent, insoluble, and not readily visible until a disclosing agent has been applied. When stained with a disclosing agent, it appears thin, with a pale staining that contrasts with the thicker, darker staining of dental biofilm.

B. Surface Pellicle, Stained

Unstained pellicle can take on extrinsic stain and become brown, grayish, or other colors, as described on pages 317 to 318.

C. Subsurface Pellicle

Surface pellicle is continuous with subsurface pellicle that is embedded in tooth structure, particularly where the tooth surface is partially demineralized.[3]

III. SIGNIFICANCE OF PELLICLE

A. Protective

Pellicle appears to provide a barrier against acids; thus, it may aid in reducing a dental caries attack.[3]

B. Lubrication

Keeps surfaces moist; prevents drying.

C. Nidus for Bacteria

Pellicle participates in biofilm formation by aiding the adherence of microorganisms.

D. Attachment of Calculus

One mode of calculus attachment is by the acquired pellicle (page 309).

▪ DENTAL BIOFILM

Dental biofilm is a dense, nonmineralized, complex mass of colonies in a gel-like intermicrobial matrix. It adheres firmly to the acquired pellicle and hence to the teeth, calculus, and fixed and removable restorations.

Dental biofilm may contain microorganisms other than bacteria. The organisms may include mycoplasmas, yeasts, protozoa, and viruses. Characteristics of supragingival and subgingival biofilms are shown in Table 17-2.

I. STAGES IN THE FORMATION OF BIOFILM

Biofilm is formed in three basic steps, namely, pellicle formation, bacterial colonization, and biofilm maturation (Figure 17-2). Biofilm formation does not occur randomly but involves a series of complex interactions.

A. Formation of a Pellicle

The pellicle forms on the tooth surface by selective adsorption of protein components from the saliva.

BOX 17-1 KEY WORDS: Dental Biofilm

Acellular: not made up of or containing cells.

Adsorption: attachment of one substance to the surface of another; the action of a substance in attracting and holding other materials or particles on its surface.

Aerobe: heterotrophic microorganism that can live and grow in the presence of free oxygen; some are obligate, others facultative; *adj.* aerobic.

Anaerobe: heterotrophic microorganism that lives and grows in complete (or almost complete) absence of oxygen; some are obligate, others facultative; *adj.* anaerobic.

Biofilm: matrix-enclosed bacterial populations adherent to each other and/or to surfaces or interfaces.

Calculogenesis: formation of calculus.

> **Calculogenic:** adjective applied to dental biofilm that is conducive to the formation of calculus.

Cariogenesis: development of dental caries.

> **Cariogenic:** adjective to indicate a conduciveness to the initiation of dental caries, such as a cariogenic biofilm or a cariogenic food.

Facultative: able to live under more than one specific set of environmental conditions; contrast with obligate.

Flora: the collective organisms of a given locale.

> **Oral flora:** the various bacteria and other microscopic organisms that inhabit the oral cavity. The mouth has an indigenous flora, meaning those organisms that are native to that area of the body. Certain organisms specifically reside in certain parts, for example, on the tongue, on the mucosa, or in the gingival sulcus.

Heterotrophic: not self-sustaining; feeding on others.

Intermicrobial matrix: material present between bacteria in dental biofilm; derived from saliva, gingival exudate, and microorganisms.

Infection: invasion and multiplication of a microorganism in body tissues.

Leukocyte: white blood corpuscle capable of ameboid movement; functions to protect the body against infection and disease. (For a description of the various white blood cells, see page 1061, and Figure 64-1.)

Materia alba: white or cream-colored cheesy mass that can collect over dental biofilm on unclean, neglected teeth; it is composed of food debris, mucin, bacteria.

Maturation: stage or process of attaining maximal development; become mature.

Microbiota: the microscopic living organisms of a region.

Microorganism: minute living organisms, usually microscopic; includes bacteria, rickettsiae, viruses, fungi, and protozoa.

Mycoplasma: pleomorphic, gram-negative bacteria that lack cell walls; many are regular oral cavity residents; some are pathogenic.

Obligate: ability to survive only in a particular environment; opposite of facultative.

Parasite: plant or animal that lives upon or within another living organism and draws its nourishment therefrom; may be obligate or facultative; *adj.* parasitic.

Pathogen: disease-producing agent or microorganism; *adj.* pathogenic.

Pleomorphism: assumption of various distinct forms by a single organism or within a species; *adj.* pleomorphic.

Saprophyte: any organism, such as bacteria, that lives upon dead or decaying organic matter.

▪ TABLE 17-1 TOOTH DEPOSITS

CATEGORY	TOOTH DEPOSIT	DESCRIPTION	DERIVATION
Nonmineralized	Acquired pellicle	Translucent, homogeneous, thin, unstructured film covering and adherent to the surfaces of the teeth, restorations, calculus, and other surfaces in the oral cavity	Supragingival: saliva Subgingival: gingival sulcus fluid
	Microbial (bacterial) biofilm	Dense, organized bacterial systems embedded in an intermicrobial matrix that adhere closely to the teeth, calculus, and other surfaces in the oral cavity Water irrigation removes only the outer layer of loose organisms	Colonization of oral microorganisms
	Materia alba	Loosely adherent, unstructured, white or grayish-white mass of oral debris and bacteria that lies over dental biofilm Vigorous rinsing and water irrigation can remove materia alba	Incidental accumulation
	Food debris	Unstructured, loosely attached particulate matter Self-cleansing activity of tongue and saliva and rinsing vigorously remove debris	Food retention following eating
Mineralized	Calculus	Calcified dental biofilm; hard, tenacious mass that forms on the clinical crowns of the natural teeth and on dentures and other appliances	Biofilm mineralization
	a. supragingival	Occurs coronal to the margin of the gingiva; is covered with dental biofilm	Supragingival: source of minerals is saliva
	b. subgingival	Occurs apical to the margin of the gingiva; is covered with dental biofilm	Subgingival: source of minerals is gingival sulcus fluid

Adapted from Schroeder, H.E.: *Formation and Inhibition of Dental Calculus.* Vienna, Hans Huber, 1969, pp. 14–15.

B. Bacteria Attach to the Pellicle

Initial attachment of bacteria to the pellicle is by selective adherence of specific bacteria from the oral environment. Innate characteristics of the bacteria and the pellicle determine the adhesive interactions that cause a particular organism to adhere to a particular pellicle.

C. Bacterial Multiplication and Colonization

1. Microcolonies form in layers as the bacteria multiply and grow.
2. With increased size, colonies meet and coalesce to form a continuous bacterial mass.
3. Organisms of the first few hours are gram-positive cocci and rods.

■ TABLE 17-2 CHARACTERISITICS OF SUPRAGINGIVAL AND SUBGINGIVAL BIOFILM

CHARACTERISTIC	SUPRAGINGIVAL BIOFILM	SUBGINGIVAL BIOFILM
Location	Coronal to the margin of the free gingiva	Apical to the margin of the free gingiva
Origin	Salivary glycoprotein forms pellicle Microorganisms from saliva are selectively attracted to pellicle	Downgrowth of bacteria from supragingival biofilm

Distribution	Starts on proximal surfaces and other protected areas
	Heaviest collection on
	  Areas not cleaned daily by patient
	  Cervical third, especially facial
	  Lingual mandibular molars
	  Proximal surfaces
	  Pit and fissure biofilm
		Shallow pocket: similar to supragingival biofilm
		Undisturbed; held by pocket wall
		Attached biofilm covers calculus
		Unattached biofilm extends to the periodontal attachment

Adhesion	Firmly attached to acquired pellicle, other bacteria, and tooth surfaces Surface bacteria (unattached): loose; washed away by saliva or swallowed	Adheres to tooth surface, subgingival pellicle, and calculus Subgingival flora: loose, floating, motile organisms in deep pocket do not adhere; they are between adherent biofilm on tooth and the pocket epithelium
Retention	Rough surfaces of teeth or restorations Malpositioned teeth Carious lesions	Pocket holds biofilm against tooth Overhanging margins of fillings that extend into pockets hold biofilm

Shape and size	Friction of tongue, cheeks, lips, limits shape and size
	Thickness: thicker at the cervical third and on proximal surfaces
	  Healthy gingiva: thin biofilm, 15 to 20 cells thick
	  Chronic gingivitis: thick biofilm, 100 to 300 cells thick
		Molded by pocket wall to shape of the tooth surface
		Follows form created by subgingival calculus
		May become thicker as the diseased pocket wall becomes less tight

Structure	Adherent, densely packed microbial layer over pellicle on tooth surface Intermicrobial matrix Onset: small isolated colonies 2 to 5 days; colonies merge to form a covering of biofilm	Three layers (see Figure 17–4) 1. Tooth-surface-attached biofilm: many gram-positive rods and cocci 2. Unattached biofilm in middle: many gram-negative, motile forms; spirochetes; leukocytes 3. Epithelium-attached biofilm: gram-negative, motile forms predominate; many leukocytes migrate through epithelium
Microorganisms	Early biofilm: primarily gram-positive cocci Older biofilm (3 to 4 days): increased numbers of filaments and fusiforms 4 to 9 days undisturbed: more complex flora with rods, filamentous forms 7 to 14 days: vibrios, spirochetes, more gram-negative organisms	Environment conducive to growth of anaerobic population Diseased pocket: primarily gram-negative, motile, spirochetes, rods See Table 17-3
Sources of nutrients for bacterial proliferation	Saliva Ingested food	Tissue fluid (gingival sulcus fluid) Exudate Leukocytes

Significance	Etiology of
	  Gingivitis
	  Supragingival calculus
	  Dental caries (Figure 17–6)
		Etiology of
		  Gingivitis
		  Periodontal infections
		  Subgingival calculus

Stage 1 Salivary glycoproteins are adsorbed onto dental enamel to form pellicle.

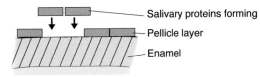

— Salivary proteins forming
— Pellicle layer
— Enamel

Stage 2 Selective colonization of the pellicle by microorganisms

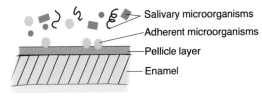

— Salivary microorganisms
— Adherent microorganisms
— Pellicle layer
— Enamel

Stage 3 Growth and maturation of biofilm

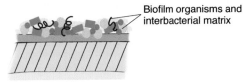

— Biofilm organisms and interbacterial matrix

■ **FIGURE 17-2 Stages of Biofilm Formation.**
Diagrammatic representation of the three stages of dental biofilm formation. (Redrawn from Katz, S., McDonald, J.L., and Stookey, G.K.: *Preventive Dentistry.* Upper Montclair, NJ, DCP Publishing, 1977.)

D. Biofilm Growth and Maturation

The increase in the mass and thickness of biofilm results from
1. Continued bacterial multiplication.
2. Continuous adherence of bacteria to the biofilm surface.

E. Matrix Formation

The intermicrobial substance is derived mainly from saliva for supragingival biofilm and from gingival sulcus fluid and exudate for subgingival biofilm. Other components of the intermicrobial substance are the polysaccharides, glucans, and fructans or levans produced by certain bacteria from dietary sucrose. The polysaccharides are sticky and contribute to the adhesion of the biofilm to the teeth.

II. CHANGES IN BIOFILM MICROORGANISMS

Dental biofilm consists of a complex mixture of microorganisms that occur primarily as microcolonies. The population density is very high and increases as biofilm ages.

The probability of the development of dental caries and/or gingivitis increases as the number of microorganisms increases.

Changes in the types of organisms occur within biofilm as the biofilm matures. When oral hygiene practices are discontinued, the numbers of bacteria increase rapidly. The changes in oral flora follow a pattern, such as that shown in Figure 17-3. The changes can be described as follows[4]:

A. Days 1 to 2

Early biofilm consists primarily of gram-positive cocci. Streptococci, which dominate the bacterial population, include *Streptococcus mutans* and *Streptococcus sanguis*.

B. Days 2 to 4

The cocci still dominate, and increasing numbers of gram-positive filamentous forms and slender rods may be seen on the surface of the cocci colonies. Gradually, the filamentous forms grow into the cocci layer and replace many of the cocci. Slow biofilm formers continue to form biofilm comprised primarily of cocci for a longer time than do fast biofilm formers.

C. Days 4 to 7

Filaments increase in numbers, and a more mixed flora begins to appear with rods, filamentous forms, and fusobacteria. Biofilm near the gingival margin thickens and develops a more mature flora, with gram-negative spirochetes and vibrios. As biofilm spreads coronally, the new biofilm has the characteristic coccal forms.

D. Days 7 to 14

Vibrios and spirochetes appear, and the number of white blood cells increases. As biofilm matures and thickens, more gram-negative and anaerobic organisms appear. During this period, signs of inflammation are beginning to be observable in the gingiva.

E. Days 14 to 21

Vibrios and spirochetes are prevalent in older biofilm, along with cocci and filamentous forms. The densely packed filamentous microorganisms arrange themselves perpendicular to the tooth surface in a palisade. Gingivitis is evident clinically.

III. EXPERIMENTAL GINGIVITIS[4]

Gingivitis develops in 2 to 3 weeks when biofilm is left undisturbed on the tooth surfaces. Most gingivitis is reversible, and when the gingiva is treated by biofilm

Accumulative Changes in Biofilm Bacteria at the Gingival Margin

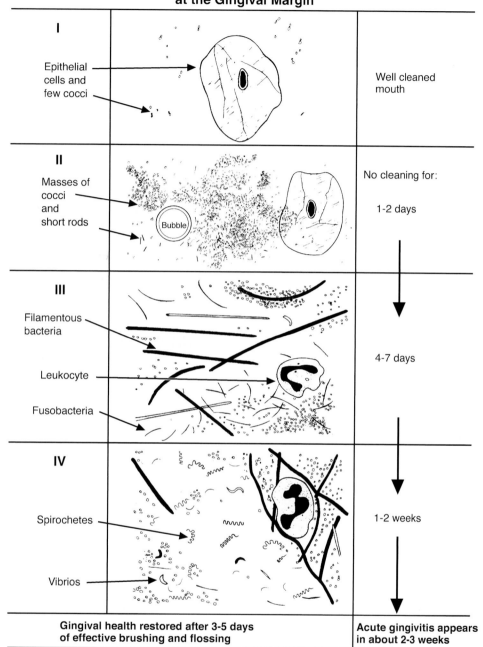

I Epithelial cells and few cocci		Well cleaned mouth
II Masses of cocci and short rods (Bubble)		No cleaning for: 1-2 days
III Filamentous bacteria / Leukocyte / Fusobacteria		4-7 days
IV Spirochetes / Vibrios		1-2 weeks
Gingival health restored after 3-5 days of effective brushing and flossing		**Acute gingivitis appears in about 2-3 weeks**

■ **FIGURE 17-3 Biofilm Microorganisms.** On the right are the time intervals from 1 day to 3 weeks. On the left are the changes in the biofilm content that take place as biofilm ages. As the numbers of microorganisms increase, the numbers of defense cells (leukocytes) also increase. (From Crawford, J.J.: Microbiology, in Barton, R.E., Matteson, S.R., and Richardson, R.E.: *The Dental Assistant,* 6th ed. Philadelphia, Lea & Febiger, 1988.)

removal procedures, the gingiva can return to health within a few days.

An experimental gingivitis program to demonstrate the effect of biofilm can be conducted as follows:

   A. Observe and record characteristics of the healthy gingiva at the outset. Record a gingival index (page 338), a biofilm index (pages 328 to 333), and a bleeding index (pages 336 to 338).

   B. Withhold all biofilm control procedures for a period of 3 weeks.

   C. Repeat clinical observations of tissues and record indices at least weekly during *the test period. Note initial evidence of gingivitis.*

D. Reinstate biofilm removal measures after 3 weeks. Make daily observations relative to gingival bleeding and indications that healing is taking place. In 1 week, repeat gingival and biofilm indices.

IV. SUBGINGIVAL DENTAL BIOFILM

A. Source

Subgingival biofilm results from the apical proliferation of microorganisms from supragingival biofilm. In the early stages of gingivitis and periodontitis, the supragingival biofilm is a strong influence on the accumulation and pathogenic features of the subgingival biofilm. As the periodontal pocket deepens, the supragingival biofilm only relates to the coronally situated pocket biofilm.

B. Microorganisms

The flora of the subgingival biofilm differs from that of the supragingival biofilm. The subgingival biofilm includes more anaerobic and motile organisms, and they are predominantly gram negative.

C. Organization of Subgingival Biofilm (Figure 17-4)

1. *Tooth-Surface-Attached Biofilm.* Over the pellicle, which covers the tooth surface, is a layer of densely packed microorganisms. Next to the tooth, on the innermost side of this layer, are many gram-positive rods and cocci. The biofilm of this area is associated with calculus formation, root caries, and root resorption.

2. *Unattached Biofilm.* Between the two layers of attached biofilm are many motile, gram-negative organisms. The "fluid" biofilm contains many white blood cells.

3. *Epithelium-Associated Biofilm.* Loosely attached to the pocket epithelium are many gram-negative microorganisms and numerous white blood cells. Many virulent pathogenic organisms in this layer may be considered a focus for the advancement of periodontal infection. From this layer, microorganisms invade the underlying connective tissue. Figure 17-4 shows bacteria within the connective tissue and on the bone surface.

D. Invasion of Microorganisms

Electron microscopy has made possible the detection of microorganisms within tissues.[5] Bacterial invasion

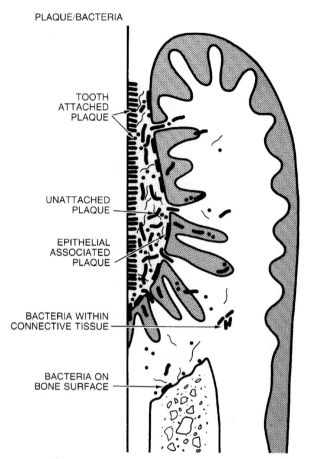

PLAQUE/BACTERIA

TOOTH ATTACHED PLAQUE

UNATTACHED PLAQUE

EPITHELIAL ASSOCIATED PLAQUE

BACTERIA WITHIN CONNECTIVE TISSUE

BACTERIA ON BONE SURFACE

■ **FIGURE 17-4 Bacterial Invasion.** Diagram of a periodontal pocket shows bacteria of attached and unattached biofilm bacteria within the pocket epithelium, in the connective tissue, and on the surface of the bone. (From Carranza, F.A.: *Glickman's Clinical Periodontology,* 6th ed. Philadelphia, W.B. Saunders Co., 1984, p. 368.)

provides a significant pathogenic mechanism for progress of periodontal infections. For example, bacteria that invade exposed dentinal tubules provide a source for recolonization within a pocket after treatment, which leads to the recurrence of the infection after a period of time.

V. COMPOSITION OF DENTAL BIOFILM

Biofilm is composed of microorganisms and intermicrobial matrix. Organic and inorganic solids constitute approximately 20%, and water accounts for 80%. Microorganisms make up at least 70% to 80% of the solid matter, which is higher in subgingival biofilm than in the supragingival form.

Composition differs among individuals and among different tooth surfaces of an individual. As biofilm ages, it changes.

A. Inorganic Elements[6,7]

1. *Calcium and Phosphorus.* The concentration of calcium, phosphorus, magnesium, and fluoride is higher in biofilm than in saliva, thus illustrating the ability of biofilm to concentrate inorganic elements.

   Biofilm on the lingual surfaces of the mandibular anterior teeth contains a higher concentration of calcium and phosphate than does biofilm on the other teeth, and the amount is even higher on those same surfaces in heavy calculus formers.

2. *Fluoride.* The concentration of fluoride in biofilm is higher when fluoridated water is used, and it increases following professional topical applications of fluoride and the use of fluoride-containing dentifrices and mouthrinses.

B. Organic Components

The organic intermicrobial substance surrounds the microorganisms of biofilm and contains primarily carbohydrates and proteins, with small amounts of lipids.

1. *Carbohydrates.* Carbohydrates, which are produced by several types of bacteria, include glucans and fructans or levans made from dietary sucrose. Dextran is a type of glucan. These carbohydrates contribute to the following:
   a. Adherence of the microorganisms to each other and the tooth. An example is *Streptococcus mutans,* which may be linked to glucans.
   b. Energy storage of carbohydrate for reserve use by biofilm bacteria.
2. *Proteins*
   a. Supragingival biofilm contains proteins derived from saliva.
   b. Subgingival biofilm contains proteins from gingival sulcus fluid.
3. *Lipids.* The lipid content may include lipopolysaccharide endotoxins from gram-negative bacteria.

■ CLINICAL ASPECTS

I. DISTRIBUTION

A. Location

1. *Supragingival Biofilm.* Biofilm is coronal to the gingival margin.
2. *Gingival Biofilm.* Biofilm forms on the external surfaces of the oral epithelium and attached gingiva.
3. *Subgingival Biofilm.* Biofilm is located between the periodontal attachment and the gingival margin, within the sulcus or pocket.

4. *Fissure Biofilm.* Biofilm also develops in pits and fissures and is referred to as *fissure* biofilm.

B. By Surfaces

1. *During Formation.* Supragingival biofilm formation begins at the gingival margin, particularly on proximal surfaces, and increases rapidly when left undisturbed. It spreads over the gingival third and on toward the middle third of the crown.
2. *Tooth Surfaces Involved*
   a. Biofilm occurs most frequently on proximal surfaces and around the gingival third, associated with protected areas (Figure 17-5).
   b. The least amounts occur on the palatal surfaces of maxillary teeth because of the activity of the tongue.

C. Factors Influencing Biofilm Accumulation

In Chapter 14, many factors that influence deposit accumulation and disease development are outlined. A review of those factors can be helpful in conjunction with the material in this section.

1. *Crowded Teeth.* Figure 17-5 illustrates the accumulation of dental biofilm around crowded mandibular anterior teeth. Research has shown that when personal biofilm removal efforts are made conscientiously, biofilm accumulation around crowded teeth is not greater than that around teeth in good alignment.[8]

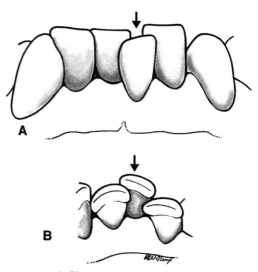

■ **FIGURE 17-5 Biofilm Accumulation in Protected Areas.** Crowded mandibular anterior teeth demonstrate dental biofilm after use of a disclosing agent. The thickest biofilm is on the proximal surfaces and at the cervical thirds of the teeth. Note the central incisors in facial view **(A)** and lingual view **(B)**, with thick extensive biofilm on the less accessible protected surfaces.

2. *Rough Surfaces.* More rapid collection occurs on rough surfaces of teeth, restorations, and calculus.

3. *Difficult to Clean.* Thick, dense deposits usually collect in difficult-to-clean areas, such as under overhanging margins of crowns or fillings, under ledges of calculus, and in areas associated with carious lesions.

4. *Out of Occlusion.* Deposits may extend over an entire crown of a tooth that is unopposed, out of occlusion, or not used during mastication.

5. *Bacterial Multiplication.* The thickness of biofilm results from constant cell division of the bacteria within the biofilm.

II. DETECTION

A. Direct Vision

1. *Thin Biofilm.* May be translucent and therefore not visible.

2. *Stained Biofilm.* May acquire extrinsic stains that make it visible, for example, yellow, green, tobacco, as described on pages 315 to 317.

3. *Thick Biofilm.* The tooth may appear dull, dingy, with a matted fur-like surface. Materia alba or food debris may collect over the biofilm.

B. Use of Explorer or Probe

1. *Tactile Examination.* When calcification has started, biofilm may feel slightly rough; otherwise the surface may feel only somewhat slippery because of the coating of soft, slimy biofilm.

2. *Removal of Biofilm.* When no biofilm is visible, it can be detected and removed by a probe passed over the tooth surface. When present, biofilm adheres to the probe tip.

C. Use of Disclosing Agent

When a disclosing agent is applied, biofilm takes on the color and becomes readily visible (Figure 17-5). Disclosing agent should not be applied until the evaluation of the oral mucosa and gingival color has been recorded.

D. Clinical Record

1. Record biofilm by location and extent (slight, moderate, or heavy). An index or biofilm score is recommended (pages 328 to 333).

2. Biofilm recordings and indices are kept for comparison in conjunction with the instructional plan for biofilm control by the patient, for both current and maintenance appointments.

3. Biofilm evaluation records are included with the complete charting and oral examination.

▪ SIGNIFICANCE OF DENTAL BIOFILM

Microbial biofilm plays a major role in the initiation and progression of both dental caries and periodontal diseases. Periodontal diseases and dental caries are infectious diseases caused by pathogenic microorganisms found in microbial biofilms. Particular groups of microorganisms are present in association with certain infections.

Biofilm is significant in the formation of dental calculus. Calculus is essentially mineralized dental biofilm.

General oral cleanliness depends on the daily removal of dental biofilm deposits. The accumulation of dental biofilm on the teeth and tongue contributes to an unpleasant personal esthetic appearance as well as to halitosis.

▪ DENTAL CARIES

Dental caries is a disease of the dental calcified structures (enamel, dentin, and cementum) that is characterized by demineralization of the mineral components and dissolution of the organic matrix. Clinical characteristics and types of cavities are described on pages 262 to 266.

I. ESSENTIALS FOR DENTAL CARIES

The sequence of events leading to demineralization and dental caries is shown in Figure 17-6. A diet high in cariogenic foods, along with specific microorganisms and a susceptible tooth surface, are essential (see Figure 32-2, page 528).

A. Susceptible Tooth Surface

A tooth with optimum fluoride content resists the process of dental caries.

B. Microorganisms[9]

Mutans streptococci (*Streptococcus mutans* and *Streptococcus sobrinus,* predominantly) play a major role in caries development and progression. They appear in large numbers in carious lesions.

Historically, acidogenic lactobacilli also have been implicated. The lactobacilli have a more important role in the progression of a carious lesion and may be less significant in its origin.

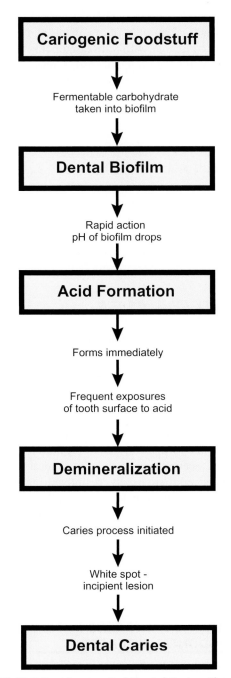

■ FIGURE 17-6 Development of Dental Caries. Flowchart shows the step-by-step action within the microbial biofilm on the tooth surface.

Dental biofilm contains many acidogenic microorganisms. In addition to mutans streptococci and lactobacilli, other predominant groups of microorganisms with acidogenic potential include nonmutans streptococci and actinomyces.

C. Cariogenic Foodstuff Source

1. Cariogenic foodstuff, particularly sucrose, enters the microbial biofilm.

2. Acid-forming bacteria break down the sugar to an acid.
3. Acid on the tooth surface causes subsurface demineralization.
4. Decreased salivary flow (xerostomia) and increased dietary carbohydrate promote the growth of mutans streptococci and lactobacilli in dental biofilm.

II. CONTRIBUTING FACTORS

A. Time

Acid formation begins *immediately* when the cariogenic substance is taken into the biofilm.

B. The pH of the Biofilm

The pH of the biofilm is lowered promptly, and 1 to 2 hours are required for the pH to return to a normal level, assuming the biofilm is left undisturbed.
1. Biofilm pH before eating ranges from 6.2 to 7.0; it is lower in the caries-susceptible person and higher in the caries-resistant person.
2. Immediately following sucrose intake into biofilm, a rapid drop in the pH of the biofilm occurs.[10,11]
3. Critical pH for enamel demineralization averages 4.5 to 5.5, below which the enamel demineralizes. The critical pH for root surface demineralization is approximately 6.0 to 6.7.[12]
4. The amount of demineralization depends on the length of time and the frequency with which the acid with a pH below the critical pH is in contact with the tooth surface.

C. Frequency of Carbohydrate Intake

With each meal or snack that contains sucrose, the pH of the biofilm is lowered (see Figure 32-6, page 537). Large amounts of sucrose eaten at mealtimes can be expected to be less cariogenic than small amounts eaten at frequent intervals during the day.[13] These and other related facts can be presented to the patient when the diet is discussed as a part of the basic instruction or as part of a total dental caries control program with dietary assessment.

III. THE CARIOUS LESION

The incipient carious lesion begins as subsurface demineralization. Acid from bacterial action on the tooth surface passes through microchannels in the enamel, demineralization occurs, and eventually a white spot can be seen clinically. Early and continuous use of fluoride for remineralization is necessary. Dental caries formation is described on pages 393 to 394, and the use of fluoride in remineralization is covered on page 395.

■ EFFECT OF DIET ON BIOFILM

I. CARIOGENIC FOODS

A. Dental Caries

The relationship of the cariogenic food content of the diet and its frequency of use to the development of dental caries is well defined in research and clinical application. Dental caries initiation is outlined in Figure 17-6.

B. Effect of Sucrose on Amount and pH of Biofilm

When a cariogenic diet is used, biofilm forms and grows more profusely.[14] Patients who were fed sucrose by stomach tube had a less acidogenic biofilm than did patients who were fed sucrose by mouth.[15]

II. FOOD INTAKE

Food particles are not needed in the mouth for biofilm to form. In one study, neither varying the number of meals nor feeding by stomach tube affected the development of biofilm.[16] In another study, less biofilm developed in a group of stomach-fed patients compared with those fed by mouth.[15]

III. TEXTURE OF DIET

The friction of mastication has been shown to affect only the occlusal and incisal thirds of the crowns of teeth. Biofilm on the gingival third collected in spite of a normal diet that included coarse bread and fresh fruit[4] or chewing raw carrots three times daily as the only methods for personal care.[17] Chewing apples did not affect moderate amounts of biofilm, but it did tend to remove food debris in a group of 12-year-olds.[18]

■ PERIODONTAL INFECTIONS

The microorganisms of dental biofilm cause the periodontal infections. The variations in clinical manifestations in different individuals can be accounted for by the differences in the bacterial activity within the biofilm, as well as by the tissue response and resistance to the microorganisms and their products.

More than 400 different species of bacteria have been known to colonize the human oral cavity. An individual may have as many as 150 at a given time.

I. BACTERIA OF HEALTHY GINGIVA

The microbiota of the healthy gingival sulcus differs from the bacteria of the diseased pocket. In health, there is a majority if aerobic, gram-positive streptococci and actinomyces. The total number of organisms and white blood cells is low compared with a diseased pocket.

Gram-negative, pathogenic forms may be found in apparently healthy gingiva. They may be an indication of change in the host response and future susceptibility to active disease.

II. PERIODONTAL BIOFILM PATHOGENS

Each of the various periodontal diseases (for example, aggressive, chronic, peri-implantitis) has its own microbial complex of subgingival pathogenic microorganisms. Not all have been specifically delineated, and research continues.[19,20]

Major microorganisms implicated in destructive periodontal infections are shown in Table 17-3.

■ MATERIA ALBA

Materia alba is a loosely adherent mass of bacteria and cellular debris that frequently occurs on top of dental biofilm where biofilm removal is neglected.

Materia alba ("white material") distinguishes itself clinically as a bulky, soft deposit that is clearly visible without application of a disclosing agent. It is white, or grayish-white, and characteristically may resemble cottage cheese.

Materia alba forms over dental biofilm. It is a product of informal accumulation of living and dead bacteria, desquamated epithelial cells, disintegrating leukocytes, salivary proteins, and particles of food debris.

Surface bacteria in contact with the gingiva contribute to gingival inflammation. Tooth surface demineralization and dental caries are seen frequently under materia alba.

Clinical distinction of materia alba, food debris, and dental biofilm is necessary, but patient instruction for the

---

■ TABLE 17-3 PATHOGENS IN DESTRUCTIVE PERIODONTAL DISEASES

STRONG EVIDENCE FOR ETIOLOGY
Actinobacillus actinomycetemcomitans
Porphyromonas gingivalis
Bacteroides forsythus
Treponema denticola

MODERATE EVIDENCE FOR ETIOLOGY
Campylobacter rectus
Eubacterium nodatum
Fusobacterium nucleatum
Prevotella intermedia
Peptostreptococcus micros
Streptococcus intermedius-complex

From: *Annals of Periodontology*, 1, 928, November, 1996.

Everyday Ethics

Daria was particularly excited to begin her patient schedule today because a student from the local community college was coming to observe her. Daria had graduated from the same dental hygiene program 4 years earlier and had volunteered to participate in the program for students to observe practitioners.

Roland, a second-year student, presented promptly at the receptionist's window 15 minutes prior to the first patient. Daria was already busily preparing her treatment room, and she quickly introduced herself to the student. She invited Roland to ask any questions and said she would introduce him to the patient at the beginning of each appointment. Daria said she would request verbal approval from the patient for his presence in the treatment room. Roland was impressed with Daria's professionalism.

After the first appointment was completed, Roland asked Daria why she was still using the term "plaque" during the homecare instruction instead of "biofilm" and why she didn't disclose the teeth before the selective polishing procedures? "Oh," Daria replied, "Is this something new you learned in school?"

Questions for Consideration

1. Explain the dialogue that might take place regarding use of the term "plaque" versus "biofilm," which was obviously a new concept for the dental hygienist.

2. Ethically, is Daria violating any ethical principles relative to beneficent care by not using disclosing agent to identify the biofilm?

3. What elements of the provider-patient relationship can Daria impress upon this student as a practicing hygienist in this scenario?

---

removal of all three involves the same basic biofilm control procedures. Materia alba can be removed with a water spray or oral irrigator, whereas dental biofilm cannot.

■ FOOD DEBRIS

Loose food particles collect about the cervical third and proximal embrasures of the teeth.

Factors To Teach The Patient

- Location, composition, and properties of dental biofilm, with emphasis on its role in dental caries and periodontal infections.

- The cause and prevention of dental caries.

- Effects of personal oral care procedures in the prevention of dental biofilm.

- Biofilm control procedures with special adaptations for individual needs.

- Sources of cariogenic foodstuff in the diet, with suggestions for control.

- Relationship of frequency of eating cariogenic foods to dental caries.

When there are open contact areas; mobility of teeth; or irregularities of occlusion, such as plunger cusps, food may be forced between the teeth during mastication, and vertical food impaction results. Horizontal or lateral food impaction occurs in facial and lingual embrasures, particularly when the interdental papillae are reduced or missing.

Food debris adds to a general unsanitary condition of the mouth. Cariogenic foods contribute to dental caries because liquefied carbohydrate diffuses rapidly into the biofilm and hence to the acid-forming bacteria.

Some self-cleansing through the action of the tongue, lips, saliva, and related factors takes place. Debris removal by toothbrushing, flossing, and other aids constitutes a total biofilm control program. Cleansing of debris from about fixed prostheses and orthodontic appliances is important to the plan for oral sanitation.

REFERENCES

1. Schroeder, H.E.: *Formation and Inhibition of Dental Calculus*, Vienna, Hans Huber Publishers, 1969, pp. 14–15.
2. Meckel, A.H.: Formation and Properties of Organic Films on Teeth, *Arch. Oral Biol.*, *10*, 585, July–August, 1965.
3. Meckel, A.H.: The Nature and Importance of Organic Deposits on Dental Enamel, *Caries Res.*, *2*, 104, No. 2, 1968.
4. Löe, H., Theilade, E., and Jensen, S.B.: Experimental Gingivitis in Man, *J. Periodontol.*, *36*, 177, May–June, 1965.
5. Saglie, R., Newman, M.G., Carranza, F.A., and Pattison, G.L.: Bacterial Invasion of Gingiva in Advanced Periodontitis in Humans, *J. Periodontol.*, *53*, 217, April, 1982.

6. **Mandel**, I.D.: Relation of Saliva and Plaque to Caries, *J. Dent. Res., 53,* 246, March–April, Supplement, 1974.

7. **Grøn**, P., Yao, K., and Spinelli, M.: A Study of Inorganic Constituents in Dental Plaque, *J. Dent. Res., 48,* 799, September–October, Supplement, 1969.

8. **Årtun**, J. and Osterberg, S.K.: Periodontal Status of Secondary Crowded Mandibular Incisors: Long-term Results After Orthodontic Treatment, *J. Clin. Periodontol., 14,* 261, May, 1987.

9. **Van Houte**, J., Sansone, C., Joshipura, K., and Kent, R.: Mutans Streptococci and Non-mutans Streptococci Acidogenic at Low pH, and *in vitro* Acidogenic Potential of Dental Plaque in Two Different Areas of the Human Dentition, *J. Dent. Res., 70,* 1503, December, 1991.

10. **Stephan**, R.M.: Intra-oral Hydrogen-Ion Concentrations Associated With Dental Caries Activity, *J. Dent. Res., 23,* 257, August, 1944.

11. **Rosen**, S. and Weisenstein, P.R.: The Effect of Sugar Solutions on pH of Dental Plaques From Caries-Susceptible and Caries-Free Individuals, *J. Dent. Res., 44,* 845, September–October, 1965.

12. **Hoppenbrouwers**, P.M.M., Driessens, F.C.M., and Borggreven, J.M.P.M.: The Mineral Solubility of Human Tooth Roots, *Arch. Oral Biol., 32,* 319, No. 5, 1987.

13. **Gustafsson**, B.E., Quensel, C.-E., Lanke, L.S., Lundquist, C., Grahnén, H., Bonow, B.E., and Krasse, B.: The Vipeholm Dental Caries Study: The Effect of Different Levels of Carbohydrate Intake on Caries Activity in 436 Individuals Observed for Five Years, *Acta Odontol. Scand., 11,* 232, Nos. 3–4, 1954.

14. **Carlsson**, J. and Egelberg, J.: Effect of Diet on Early Plaque Formation in Man, *Odont. Rev., 16,* 112, No. 1, 1965.

15. **Littleton**, N.W., Carter, C.H., and Kelley, R.T.: Studies of Oral Health in Persons Nourished by Stomach Tube. I. Changes in pH of Plaque Material After the Addition of Sucrose, *J. Am. Dent. Assoc., 74,* 119, January, 1967.

16. **Egelberg**, J.: Local Effect of Diet on Plaque Formation and Development of Gingivitis in Dogs. III. Effect of Frequency of Meals and Tube Feeding, *Odont. Rev., 16,* 50, No. 1, 1965.

17. **Lindhe**, J. and Wicén, P.-O.: The Effects on the Gingivae of Chewing Fibrous Foods, *J. Periodont. Res., 4,* 193, No. 3, 1969.

18. **Birkeland**, J.M. and Jorkjend, L.: The Effect of Chewing Apples on Dental Plaque and Food Debris, *Community Dent. Oral Epidemiol., 2,* 161, No. 4, 1974.

19. **Socransky**, S.S., Haffajee, A.D., Cugini, M.A., Smith, C., and Kent, R.L.: Microbial Complexes in Subgingival Plaque, *J. Clin. Periodontol., 25,* 134, February, 1998.

20. **Haffajee**, A.D. and Socransky, S.S.: Microbial Etiological Agents of Destructive Periodontal Diseases, *Periodontol. 2000, 5,* 78, 1994.

SUGGESTED READINGS

Alaluusua, S. and Maimivirta, R.: Early Plaque Accumulation: A Sign for Caries Risk in Young Children, *Community Dent. Oral Epidemiol., 22,* 273, October, 1994.

Corbet, E.F. and Davies, W.I.R.: The Role of Supragingival Plaque in the Control of Progressive Periodontal Disease: A Review, *J. Clin. Periodontol., 20,* 307, May, 1993.

Frisken, K.W.: The Incidence of Periodontopathic Microorganisms in Young Children, *Oral Microbiol. Immunol., 5,* 43, February, 1990.

Haffajee, A.D., Socransky, S.S., Smith, C., and Dibart, S.: Microbial Risk Indicators for Periodontal Attachment Loss, *J. Periodont. Res., 26,* 293, May, (Part 2), 1991.

Hellström, M.-K., Ramberg, P., Krok, L., and Lindhe, J.: The Effect of Supragingival Plaque Control on the Subgingival Microflora in Human Periodontitis, *J. Clin. Periodontol., 23,* 934, October, 1996.

Lang, N.P., Mombelli, A., and Attström, R.: Dental Plaque and Calculus, in Lindhe, J., Karring, T., and Lang, N.P., eds.: *Clinical Periodontology and Implant Dentistry,* 3rd ed. Copenhagen, Munksgaard, 1997, pp. 102–137.

Ramberg, P.W., Lindhe, J., and Gaffar, A.: Plaque and Gingivitis in the Deciduous and Permanent Dentition, *J. Clin. Periodontol., 21,* 490, August, 1994.

Sansone, C., Van Houte, J., Joshipura, K., Kent, R., and Margolis, H.C.: The Association of Mutans Streptococci and Non-mutans Streptococci Capable of Acidogenesis at a Low pH with Dental Caries on Enamel and Root Surfaces, *J. Dent. Res., 72,* 508, February, 1993.

Scannapieco, F.A., Stewart, E.M., and Mylotte, J.M.: Colonization of Dental Plaque by Respiratory Pathogens in Medical Intensive Care Patients, *Crit. Care Med., 20,* 740, June, 1992.

Socransky, S.S. and Haffajee, A.D.: Evidence of Bacterial Etiology: A Historical Perspective, *Periodontol. 2000, 5,* 7, 1994.

van Houte, J.: Role of Micro-organisms in Caries Etiology, *J. Dent. Res., 73,* 672, March, 1994.

Microbiology

Christersson, L.A., Fransson, C.L., Dunford, R.G., and Zambon, J.J.: Subgingival Distribution of Periodontal Pathogenic Microorganisms in Adult Periodontitis, *J. Periodontol., 63,* 418, May, 1992.

Columbo, A.P., Haffajee, A.D., Dewhirst, F.E., Paster, B.J., Smith, C.M., Cugini, M.A., and Socransky, S.S.: Clinical and Microbiological Features of Refractory Periodontitis Subjects, *J. Clin. Periodontol., 25,* 169, February, 1998.

Darveau, R.P., Tanner, A., and Page, R.C.: The Microbial Challenge in Periodontitis, *Periodontol. 2000, 14,* 12, 1997.

Liljenberg, B., Gualini, F., Berglundh, T., Tonetti, M., and Lindhe, J.: Composition of Plaque-Associated Lesions in the Gingiva and the Peri-implant Mucosa in Partially Edentulous Subjects, *J. Clin. Periodontol., 24,* 119, February, 1997.

Listgarten, M.A.: Electron Microscopic Observations on the Bacterial Flora of Acute Necrotizing Ulcerative Gingivitis, *J. Periodontol., 36,* 328, July–August, 1965.

Listgarten, M.A., Lai, C.-H., and Young, V.: Microbial Composition and Pattern of Antibiotic Resistance in Subgingival Microbial Samples From Patients With Refractory Periodontitis, *J. Periodontol., 64,* 155, March, 1993.

Mombelli, A., Marxer, M., Gaberthüel, T., Grunder, U., and Lang, N.P.: The Microbiota of Osseointegrated Implants in Patients With a History of Periodontal Disease, *J. Clin. Periodontol., 22,* 124, February, 1995.

Moore, W.E.C., Moore, L.H., Ranney, R.R., Smibert, R.M., Burmeister, J.A., and Schenkein, H.A.: The Microflora of Periodontal Sites Showing Active Destructive Progression, *J. Clin. Periodontol., 18,* 729, November, 1991.

Moore, W.E.C. and Moore, L.V.H.: The Bacteria of Periodontal Diseases, *Periodontol. 2000, 5,* 66, 1994.

Preber, H., Bergström, J., and Linder, L.E.: Occurrence of Peri-opathogens in Smoker and Non-smoker Patients, *J. Clin. Periodontol., 19,* 667, October, 1992.

Riviere, G.R., Smith, K.S., Carranza, N., Tzagaroulaki, E., Kay, S.L., and Dock, M.: Subgingival Distribution of *Treponema denticola, Treponema socranskii,* and Pathogen-related Oral Spirochetes: Prevalence and Relationship to Periodontal Status of Sampled Sites, *J. Periodontol., 66,* 829, October, 1995.

Russell, R.R.B.: Bacteriology of Periodontal Disease, *Curr. Opinion Dent., 2,* 66, September, 1992.

Shordone, L., Barone, A., Ramaglia, L., Ciaglia, R.N., and Iacono, V.J.: Antimicrobial Susceptibility of Periodontopathic Bacteria Associated With Failing Implants, *J. Periodontol., 66,* 69, January, 1995.

Socransky, S.S. and Haffajee, A.D.: The Bacterial Etiology of Destructive Periodontal Disease: Current Concepts, *J. Periodontol., 63,* 322, April, 1992 (Supplement).

Tanner, A., Maiden, M.F.J., Macuch, P.J., Murray, L.L., and Kent, R.L.: Microbiota of Health, Gingivitis, and Initial Periodontitis, *J. Clin. Periodontol., 25,* 85, February, 1998.

Zambon, J.J.: Periodontal Diseases: Microbial Factors, *Ann. Periodont., 1,* 879, November, 1996.

Dental Biofilm Structure and Formation

Dahlén, G., Lindhe, J., Sato, K., Hanamura, H., and Okamoto, H.: The Effect of Supragingival Plaque Control on the Subgingival Microbiota in Subjects With Periodontal Disease, *J. Clin. Periodontol., 19,* 802, November, 1992.

Gibbons, R.J. and van Houte, J.: On the Formation of Dental Plaques, *J. Periodontol., 44,* 347, June, 1973.

Katsanoulas, T., Reneé, I., and Allström, R.: The Effect of Supragingival Plaque Control on the Composition of the Subgingival Flora in Periodontal Pockets, *J. Clin. Periodontol., 19,* 760, November, 1992.

Listgarten, M.A.: The Structure of Dental Plaque, *Periodontol. 2000, 5,* 52, 1994.

Newman, H.N.: The Development of Dental Plaque: From Preeruptive Primary Cuticle to Acquired Pellicle to Dental Plaque to Calculus Formation, in Harris, N.O. and Christen, A.G.: *Primary Preventive Dentistry,* 4th ed. Norwalk, Conn., Appleton & Lange, 1995, pp. 19–38.

Quirynen, M., Dekeyser, C., and van Steenberghe, D.: The Influence of Gingival Inflammation, Tooth Type, and Timing on the Rate of Plaque Formation, *J. Periodontol., 62,* 219, March, 1991.

Ramberg, P., Axelsson, P., and Lindhe, J.: Plaque Formation at Healthy and Inflamed Gingival Sites in Young Individuals, *J. Clin. Periodontol., 22,* 85, January, 1995.

Ramberg, P., Lindhe, J., Dahlen, G., and Volpe, A.R.: The Influence of Gingival Inflammation on de novo Plaque Formation, *J. Clin. Periodontol., 21,* 51, January, 1994.

Scheie, A.A.: Mechanisms of Dental Plaque Formation, *Adv. Dent. Res., 8,* 246, July, 1994.

Transmission

Alaluusua, S., Asikainen, S., and Lai, C.-H.: Intrafamilial Transmission of *Actinobacillus actinomycetemcomitans, J. Periodontol., 62,* 207, March, 1991.

Greenstein, G. and Lamster, I.: Bacterial Transmission in Periodontal Diseases: A Critical Review, *J. Periodontol., 68,* 421, May, 1997.

Preus, H.R., Zambon, J.J., Dunford, R.G., and Genco, R.J.: The Distribution and Transmission of *Actinobacillus actinomycetemcomitans* in Families With Established Adult Periodontitis, *J. Periodontol., 65,* 2, January, 1994.

Van der Velden, U., Van Winkelhoff, A.J., Abbas, F., Arief, E.M., Timmerman, M.F., van der Weijden, G.A., and Winkel, E.G.: Longitudinal Evaluation of the Development of Periodontal Destruction in Spouses, *J. Clin. Periodontol., 23,* 1014, November, 1996.

Van Steenbergen, T.J.M., Petit, M.D.A., Scholte, L.H.M., van der Velden, U., and deGraaff, J.: Transmission of *Porphyromonas gingivalis* Between Spouses, *J. Clin. Periodontol., 20,* 340, May, 1993.

Von Troil-Linden, B., Torkko, H., Alaluusua, S., Wolf, J., Jousimies-Somer, H., and Asikainen, S.: Periodontal Findings in Spouses: A Clinical, Radiographic and Microbiological Study, *J. Clin. Periodontol., 22,* 93, February, 1995.

CHAPTER OUTLINE

Dental calculus, which is mineralized dental biofilm, is a hard, tenacious mass that forms on the clinical crowns of the natural teeth and on dentures and other dental prostheses. Terms and key words associated with calculus are defined in Box 18-1.

Calculus is significant in the progression of inflammatory periodontal disease. The rough surface of the subgingival calculus holds the disease-producing bacteria of the dental biofilm close to the gingival tissue and perpetuates the inflamed state.

The control of biofilm deposits by the patient, supplemented by complete professional calculus removal, can reduce or eliminate gingival inflammation. A major objective in nonsurgical periodontal therapy is to prepare the teeth, through calculus removal, to have biologically acceptable smooth surfaces.

Comprehensive understanding of the characteristics, origin, development, and methods of prevention of calculus is essential to patient examination, assessment, treatment, and instruction. For successful treatment and prevention, the patient needs to know the interrelationship between biofilm, calculus, and oral health; the need for complete removal of calculus; and the reasons for the painstaking manner in which scaling procedures must be carried out.

■ CLASSIFICATION AND DISTRIBUTION

Dental calculus is classified by its location on a tooth surface as related to the adjacent free gingival margin, that is, supragingival and subgingival (Figure 18-1).

BOX 18-1 KEY WORDS: Calculus

Amorphous: without definite shape or visible differentiation in structure.

Apatite: crystalline mineral component of bones and teeth that contains calcium and phosphate.

Calculus: abnormal concretion composed of mineral salts, usually occurring within the hollow organs or their passages; also called stones, such as gallstones or kidney stones.

Denture calculus: mineralized dental biofilm covered on the external surface with vital, tightly adherent, nonmineralized biofilm.

Ectopic: out of place; arising or produced at an abnormal site or in a tissue where it is not normally found.

   Ectopic oral calcification: examples are pulp stones, denticles, and salivary calculi.

Germ-free: free of microorganisms; a germ-free animal in research is reared under completely sterile conditions.

Matrix: intercellular or intermicrobial substance of a tissue, or the tissue from which a structure develops, gains support, and is held together.

Mineralization: addition of mineral elements, such as calcium and phosphorus, to the body or a part thereof with resulting hardening of the tissue.

Nidus: nucleus; focus; point of origin.

Pyrophosphate: inhibitor of calcification that occurs in parotid saliva of humans in variable amounts; anticalculus component of "tarter-control" dentifrices.

Saturated: holding all of a substance (solute) that can be dissolved in the solution.

Supersaturated: a solution containing more of an ingredient than can be held in solution permanently.

I. SUPRAGINGIVAL CALCULUS

A. Location

On the clinical crown coronal to the margin of the gingiva.

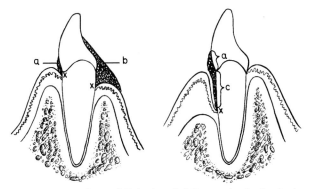

■ **FIGURE 18-1 Dental Calculus. (a)** Supragingival calculus on cervical third of a mandibular anterior tooth extends slightly subgingivally. **(b)** Supragingival calculus over crown, exposed root surface, and the margin of the gingiva. **(c)** Subgingival calculus along root to the bottom of a periodontal pocket. **(x)** Bottom of pocket.

B. Distribution

1. Most frequent sites are on the lingual surfaces of mandibular anterior teeth and the facial surfaces of maxillary first and second molars, opposite the openings of the ducts of the salivary glands.
2. Crowns of teeth out of occlusion; nonfunctioning teeth; or teeth that are neglected during daily biofilm removal (toothbrushing, flossing, or other personal care).
3. Surfaces of dentures, dental prostheses, and tongue piercings' barbells.

C. Other Names for Supragingival Calculus

1. Supramarginal.*
2. Extragingival.
3. Coronal, indicating that the calculus is on the anatomic crown.
4. Salivary, a term indicating that the source of the minerals is the saliva.

*The terms *supragingival* and *subgingival* are at present probably the most widely used. Supramarginal and submarginal are more specific in their definition because the margin of the free gingiva is the dividing line between the two categories. The gingiva includes free and attached.

II. SUBGINGIVAL CALCULUS

A. Location

On the clinical crown apical to the margin of the gingiva. It extends nearly to the bottom of the pocket. Calculus forms on the exposed root surfaces and on dental implants.

B. Distribution

1. May be generalized or localized on single teeth or a group of teeth.
2. Proximal surfaces have heaviest deposits.

C. Other Names for Subgingival Calculus

1. Submarginal.
2. Serumal, a term indicating that the source of the minerals is the blood serum.

III. OCCURRENCE

Calculus occurs at any age and on both permanent and primary teeth. Incidence increases with age, and in some populations nearly 100% of the people older than 30 years have calculus.

■ CLINICAL CHARACTERISTICS

I. APPEARANCE AND CONSISTENCY

Identification of calculus prior to removal depends on knowledge of its appearance, consistency, and distribution. Appointment planning, selection of instruments, and techniques depend on understanding the texture, morphology, and mode of attachment of calculus. Table 18-1 provides a summary of clinical characteristics.

II. SUPRAGINGIVAL EXAMINATION

A. Direct Examination

Supragingival deposits may be seen directly or indirectly, using a mouth mirror.

B. Use of Compressed Air

Small amounts of calculus may be invisible when they are wet with saliva. With light and drying with air, small deposits usually can be seen.

III. SUBGINGIVAL EXAMINATION

A. Visual Examination

1. Dark edge of calculus may be seen at or just beneath the gingival margin.

2. Gentle air blast can deflect the margin from the tooth for observation into the pocket.
3. Using transillumination, a dark, opaque, shadowlike area seen on a proximal tooth surface may be subgingival calculus. Without calculus, stain, or thick soft deposit, the enamel is translucent.

B. Gingival Tissue Color Change

Dark calculus may reflect through a thin margin and suggest the presence of subgingival calculus.

C. Tactile Examination

1. *Probe.* While probing for sulcus/pocket characteristics, a rough subgingival tooth surface can be felt when calculus is present.
2. *Explorer.* A fine subgingival explorer is needed that can be adapted close to the root surface all the way to the bottom of a pocket. Each subgingival area must be examined carefully to the bottom of the pocket, completely around each tooth.

D. Radiographic Examination

Thick, highly mineralized calculus may be detected on proximal tooth surfaces.

E. Perioscopy

Dental endoscope in deep pockets and furcations can show calculus otherwise undetectable, especially burnished calculus.

IV. CLINICAL RECORD

Calculus deposits are described in the examination record. The location of supragingival and subgingival deposits and their extent (slight, moderate, or heavy) must be designated.

■ CALCULUS FORMATION[1]

Subgingival calculus does not develop by direct extension from supragingival calculus. First, subgingival dental biofilm forms by extension of supragingival biofilm. Each biofilm mineralizes separately.

Calculus results from the deposition of minerals into a biofilm organic matrix. Calculus formation occurs in three basic steps: *pellicle formation, biofilm formation,* and *mineralization.* Mineralization of supragingival and subgingival calculus is essentially the same, although

■ TABLE 18-1 CLINICAL CHARACTERISTICS OF DENTAL CALCULUS

CHARACTERISTIC	SUPRAGINGIVAL CALCULUS	SUBGINGIVAL CALCULUS
Color	White, creamy yellow, or gray May be stained by tobacco, food, or other pigments Slight deposits may be invisible until dried with compressed air	Light to dark brown, dark green, or black Stains derived from blood pigments from diseased pocket
Shape	Amorphous, bulky Gross deposits may (1) Form interproximal bridge between adjacent teeth (2) Extend over the margin of the gingiva (Figure 18-1b) Shape of calculus mass is determined by the anatomy of the teeth, contour of gingival margin, and pressure of the tongue, lips, cheeks	Flattened to conform with pressure from the pocket wall Combination of the following calculus formations occur* (1) Crusty, spiny, or nodular (2) Ledge or ringlike (3) Thin, smooth veneers (4) Finger- and fernlike (5) Individual calculus islands
Consistency and Texture	Moderately hard Newer deposits less dense and hard Porous surface covered with nonmineralized biofilm	Brittle, flintlike Harder and more dense than supragingival calculus Newest deposits near bottom of pocket are less dense and hard Surface covered with dental biofilm
Size and Quantity	Quantity has direct relationship to (1) Personal oral care procedures and biofilm control measures (2) Physical character of diet (3) Individual tendencies (4) Function and use Increased amount in tobacco smokers	Related to pocket depth Increased amount with age because of accumulation Quantity is related to personal care, diet, and individual tendency as it is with supragingival. Subgingival is primarily related to the development and progression of periodontal disease
Distribution on Individual Tooth	Coronal to margin of gingiva May cover a large portion of the visible clinical crown, or may form fine thin line near gingival margin	Apical to margin of gingiva Extends to bottom of the pocket and follows contour of soft tissue attachment With gingival recession, subgingival calculus may become supragingival and become covered with typical supragingival calculus
Distribution on Teeth	Symmetrical arrangement on teeth except when influenced by (1) Malpositioned teeth (2) Unilateral hypofunction (3) Inconsistent personal care (4) Abrasion from food Occurs with or without associated subgingival deposits Location related to openings of the salivary gland ducts: (1) Facial surface of maxillary molars (2) Lingual surface of mandibular anterior teeth	Heaviest on proximal surfaces, lightest on facial surfaces Occurs with or without associated supragingival deposits

*Everett, F.G. and Potter, G.R.: Morphology of Submarginal Calculus, *J. Periodontol.*, 30, 27, January, 1959.

the source of the elements for mineralization is not the same.

I. PELLICLE FORMATION

The pellicle, or cuticle, is composed of mucoproteins from the saliva and is an acellular material. Its thickness and contour vary on the tooth surface. It begins to form within minutes after all deposits have been removed from the tooth surface.

II. BIOFILM MATURATION

A. Microorganisms settle in the pellicle layer.
B. Colonies are formed. Originally, the colonies consist primarily of cocci and rod-shaped organisms. By the fifth day, the biofilm is mostly made up of filamentous organisms.
C. The colonies grow together to form a cohesive biofilm layer.

III. MINERALIZATION

A. Mineralization Foci (Centers) Form

Within 24 to 72 hours, more and more mineralization centers develop close to the underlying tooth surface. Eventually, the centers grow large enough to touch and unite.

B. Organic Matrix

Mineralization first occurs within the intermicrobial matrix. The filamentous microorganisms provide the matrix for the deposition of minerals.

A calculus-like deposit has been observed on the teeth of germ-free animals that have no biofilm.[2-4] It may indicate that other organic substances, such as the pellicle, may mineralize. The pellicle is between the dental biofilm and the tooth surface. Since the attachment of calculus is very strong, it is expected that the pellicle must mineralize to create such a firm bond.

C. Sources of Minerals

1. *Supragingival Calculus.* The source of elements for supragingival calculus is the saliva.
2. *Subgingival Calculus.* The gingival sulcus fluid and the inflammatory exudate supply the minerals for the subgingival deposits. Because the amount of sulcus fluid and exudate increases with increases in inflammation, more minerals are available for mineralization of subgingival biofilm.

D. Crystal Formation

Mineralization consists of crystal formation, namely, hydroxyapatite, octocalcium phosphate, whitlockite, and brushite, each with a characteristic developmental pattern. The crystals form in the intercellular matrix and on the surface of bacteria, and finally within the bacteria.[5,6]

E. Mechanism of Mineralization[7]

The mineralization process is considered the same for both supragingival and subgingival calculus. Heavy calculus formers have higher salivary levels of calcium and phosphorus than do light calculus formers.[8] Light calculus formers have higher levels of parotid pyrophosphate.[9] Pyrophosphate is an inhibitor of calcification and is used in anticalculus dentifrices.

The process by which minerals, mainly calcium and phosphate, become incorporated from the saliva or gingival sulcus fluid into the biofilm matrix is still not completely understood.

Current research studies point to the probability that calcification of calculus may involve the same phenomena as those of other ectopic calcifications (such as urinary or renal calculi) and may be similar to normal calcification of bone, cartilage, enamel, or dentin.

IV. FORMATION TIME

Formation time means the average number of days required for the primary soft deposit to change to the mature mineralized stage. The average time is about 12 days, within a range from 10 days for rapid calculus formers to 20 days for slow calculus formers.[8] Mineralization can begin as early as 24 to 48 hours.

Formation time depends on individual tendency, but it is strongly influenced by the roughness of the tooth surface and the care and character of personal biofilm control measures. Determination of the approximate formation time for an individual is important to instruction and counseling as well as to treatment planning for professional care and frequency of maintenance appointments.

V. STRUCTURE OF CALCULUS

A. Layers

Calculus forms in layers that are more or less parallel with the tooth surface. The layers are separated by a line that appears to be a pellicle that was deposited over the previously formed calculus, and as mineralization progressed, the pellicle became imbedded.

The lines between the layers of calculus can be called incremental lines. They form around the tooth in supragingival calculus, but they form irregularly from crown to apex on the root surface in subgingival calculus. The lines are evidence that calculus grows or increases by apposition of new layers.

B. Surface

The surface of a calculus mass is rough and can be detected by use of an explorer. As observed by electron microscope, the surface roughness appears as peaks, valleys, and pits.

C. Outer Layer

The outer layer of subgingival calculus is partly calcified. On the surface is a thick, matlike, soft layer of dental biofilm. The outer surface of the biofilm on the subgingival calculus is in contact with the diseased pocket epithelium.

■ ATTACHMENT OF CALCULUS

Calculus is more readily removed from some tooth surfaces than from others. The ease or difficulty of removal can be related to the manner of attachment of the calculus to the tooth surface.

Several modes of attachment have been observed by conventional histologic techniques and by electron microscopy. On any one tooth and in any one area, more than one mode of attachment may be found.

When studying the attachment types, the character of the hard, smooth enamel surface and that of the rough, porous, cemental surface should be considered. Three general modes of attachment can be identified.[10]

I. ATTACHMENT BY MEANS OF AN ACQUIRED PELLICLE OR CUTICLE

A. The pellicle is a thin, acellular, homogeneous layer positioned between the calculus and the tooth surface.
B. Calculus attachment is superficial because no interlocking or penetration occurs.
C. Pellicle attachment occurs most frequently on enamel and newly scaled and planed root surfaces.
D. Calculus may be removed readily because of the smooth attachment.

II. ATTACHMENT TO MINUTE IRREGULARITIES IN THE TOOTH SURFACE BY MECHANICAL LOCKING INTO UNDERCUTS

A. Enamel irregularities include cracks, lamellae, and carious defects.

B. Cemental irregularities include tiny spaces left at previous locations of Sharpey's fibers, resorption lacunae, scaling grooves, and cemental tears.
C. Difficult to be certain all calculus is removed when it is attached by this method.

III. ATTACHMENT BY DIRECT CONTACT BETWEEN CALCIFIED INTERCELLULAR MATRIX AND THE TOOTH SURFACE

A. Interlocking of inorganic crystals of the tooth with the mineralizing dental biofilm.
B. Distinction between calculus and cementum is difficult during root debridement.

■ COMPOSITION

Calculus is made up of inorganic and organic components and water. Although the percentage varies depending on the age and hardness of a deposit and the location from which the sample for analysis is taken, mature calculus usually contains between 75% and 85% inorganic components; the rest is organic components and water. The chemical content of supragingival and subgingival calculus is similar.[11-13]

I. INORGANIC

A. Inorganic Components

The components are mainly calcium (Ca), phosphorus (P), carbonate (CO_3), sodium (Na), magnesium (Mg), and potassium (K).

B. Trace Elements

Various trace elements have been identified, including chlorine (Cl), zinc (Zn), strontium (Sr), bromine (Br), copper (Cu), manganese (Mn), tungsten (W), gold (Au), aluminum (Al), silicon (Si), iron (Fe), and fluorine (F).

C. Fluoride in Calculus

1. *Concentration.* The concentration of fluoride in calculus varies and is influenced by the amount of fluoride received from fluoride in the drinking water, topical application,[14] dentifrices,[15,16] or any form that is received by contact with the external surface of the calculus.
2. *Uptake.* The surface of the cementum, which is more permeable, has a content of fluoride higher than that of the enamel surface.

D. Crystals

At least two-thirds of the inorganic matter of calculus is crystalline, principally apatite. Predominating is hydroxyapatite, which is the same crystal present in enamel, dentin, cementum, and bone. Calculus also contains varying amounts of brushite, whitlockite, and octocalcium phosphate.[17]

E. Calculus Compared With Teeth and Bone

Dental enamel is the most highly mineralized tissue in the body and contains 96% inorganic salts; dentin contains 65%, and cementum and bone contain 45% to 50%.[18] Mature calculus has approximately 75% to 85% inorganic content. A comparison of calculus with the tooth parts provides insight into the effects of instrumentation, the difficulty of distinguishing calculus from cementum or dentin when scaling subgingivally, and the modes of attachment of calculus to the tooth surface.

II. ORGANIC

The organic proportion of calculus consists of various types of nonvital microorganisms, desquamated epithelial cells, leukocytes, and mucin from the saliva. Substances identified in the organic matrix include cholesterol, cholesterol esters, phospholipids, and fatty acids in the lipid fraction; reducing sugars and carbohydrate–protein complexes in the carbohydrate fraction; and keratins, nucleoproteins, and amino acids in the protein portion.[19,20]

The microorganisms are predominantly filamentous. In early calculus, during the first 5 days, cocci are found with some rods.[19,21] Most of the organisms within calculus are considered nonviable. The biofilm on the calculus surface contains viable organisms.

▪ SIGNIFICANCE OF DENTAL CALCULUS

Calculus has long been considered to have an important role in the development, promotion, and recurrence of gingival and periodontal infections.

Significant to the rationale for calculus removal and the production of a smooth tooth surface are the points summarized here concerning the relationship of calculus to periodontal and gingival diseases.

I. RELATION TO DENTAL BIOFILM

A. Subgingival biofilm develops as a result of downgrowth of supragingival biofilm bacteria.

B. Subgingival biofilm contains pathogenic bacteria that cause inflammation and destruction in the gingival tissue and lead to loss of attachment to the tooth surface and development and deepening of the pocket.

II. RELATION TO ATTACHMENT LOSS AND POCKET FORMATION

A. With increased pocket depth, greater amounts of biofilm can accumulate with increased numbers of pathogenic organisms. Irritation to the pocket lining stimulates greater flow of gingival sulcus fluid, which contains minerals for subgingival calculus formation.

B. Calculus is mineralized biofilm. The biofilm bacteria next to the tooth surface are mineralized first.

C. Subgingival calculus is always covered by masses of active biofilm bacteria. The bacterial mass is in contact with the diseased pocket epithelium and promotes gingivitis and periodontitis.

D. With its rough surface, permeable structure, and porosity, calculus can act as a reservoir for endotoxins and tissue breakdown products.

E. Calculus is a predisposing factor in pocket development in that it provides a haven for the collection of bacterial masses on the rough surface of the calculus deposit.

▪ PREVENTION OF CALCULUS

Dental calculus can be a cosmetic problem or a periodontal health problem (or both) for many patients. Patients at risk for calculus formation need individualized counseling. Risk factors related to calculus formation are the same as those for dental biofilm formation.

There are several methods for coping with the problem of calculus. The patient must understand the importance of individual daily biofilm removal and how professional maintenance appointments on a regular basis can supplement the personal care.

I. PROFESSIONAL REMOVAL OF CALCULUS

A. Removal of calculus provides a smooth tooth surface in an environment conducive to gingival healing.

B. The smooth surfaces can be easier for the patient to maintain.

C. With emphasis on good oral hygiene and routine professional removal, low levels of supragingival and subgingival calculus have been demonstrated on a long-term basis.[22]

Everyday Ethics

Coronal polishing legislation had just been passed at the state level. Certified dental assistants were now eligible to take a course and then begin polishing procedures on a patient after the dentist or the dental hygienist removes all calculus deposits. Mindy, the CDA in the office, completed the course and was ready to polish. As the hygienist in the office, Hilary was basically unaffected by the change in the dental practice act and continued to treat her patients in all aspects of the preventive protocol.

However, Dr. Bell found that additional services could be offered to his patients at the time of their restorative appointment by removing the calculus and then having Mindy finish with the polish. One day, as Hilary was on her way to find Dr. Bell to

check her patient, she saw Mindy using a curet to remove what she stated as, "slight subgingival deposits that didn't come off with the polishing cup."

Questions for Consideration

1. Would you consider what the hygienist observed the dental assistant doing as an ethical issue or dilemma? Explain your answer.

2. Is it necessary for the CDA to understand the attachment, maturation, and structure of calculus to provide 'beneficent' care to the patient? Why or why not?

3. If Dr. Bell dismisses the fact that Mindy was using instruments to remove calculus, what choices of action could Hilary pursue?

Factors To Teach The Patient

- Good oral hygiene and frequent professional care for complete scaling are consistent with low levels of supragingival and subgingival calculus.

- What calculus is and how it forms from dental biofilm.

- The effect of calculus on the health of the periodontal tissues and, therefore, on the general health of the oral cavity.

- Properties of calculus that explain the need for detailed, meticulous scaling procedures.

- Reasons for producing a calculus-free smooth tooth surface during scaling.

- Biofilm control measures that the patient may carry out to minimize calculus deposits.

- What to expect from use of an anticalculus dentifrice.

- Only selecting products with an ADA Seal of Acceptance.

II. PERSONAL DENTAL BIOFILM CONTROL

Removal of dental biofilm by appropriately selected brushing, flossing, and supplementary methods is a major factor in the control of dental calculus reformation.

III. ANTICALCULUS DENTIFRICE

Calculus-control dentifrices currently available contain either a pyrophosphate system or a zinc system. Their aim is to inhibit calculus crystal growth, which in turn should lessen the amount of calculus deposited on the teeth. The dentifrices do not have an effect on existing calculus deposits and are offered as a preventive measure against the formation of new calculus.

For a patient who cannot control supragingival calculus, and hence cannot achieve optimum gingival tissue health, an anticalculus dentifrice may provide motivation, as well as a supplement to mechanical biofilm removal efforts.[23]

REFERENCES

1. **Mandel**, I.D.: Calculus Update: Prevalence, Pathogenicity and Prevention, *J. Am. Dent. Assoc., 126*, 573, May, 1995.
2. **Fitzgerald**, R.J. and McDaniel, E.G.: Dental Calculus in the Germ-Free Rat, *Arch. Oral Biol., 2*, 239, August, 1960.
3. **Gustafsson**, B.E. and Krasse, B.: Dental Calculus in Germfree Rats, *Acta Odontol. Scand., 20*, 135, Number 2, 1962.
4. **Theilade**, J., Fitzgerald, R.J., Scott, D.B., and Nylen, M.U.: Electron Microscopic Observations of Dental Calculus in Germfree and Conventional Rats, *Arch. Oral Biol., 9*, 97, January–February, 1964.

5. **Gonzales**, F. and Sognnaes, R.F.: Electronmicroscopy of Dental Calculus, *Science, 131,* 156, January 15, 1960.
6. **Zander**, H.A., Hazen, S.P., and Scott, D.B.: Mineralization of Dental Calculus, *Proc. Soc. Exp. Biol. Med., 103,* 257, February, 1960.
7. **Ingram**, G.S. and Edgar, W.M.: Calcium Salt Precipitation and Mechanisms of Inhibition Under Oral Conditions, *Adv. Dent. Res., 9,* 427, December, 1995.
8. **Schroeder**, H.E.: *Formation and Inhibition of Dental Calculus.* Vienna, Hans Huber Publishers, 1969, pp. 73–74.
9. **Vogel**, J.J. and Amdur, B.H.: Inorganic Pyrophosphate in Parotid Saliva and Its Relation to Calculus Formation, *Arch. Oral Biol., 12,* 159, January, 1967.
10. **Canis**, M.F., Kramer, G.M., and Pameijer, C.M.: Calculus Attachment. Review of the Literature and New Findings, *J. Periodontol., 50,* 406, August, 1979.
11. **Mandel**, I.D.: Biochemical Aspects of Calculus Formation, *J. Periodont. Res., 9,* 10, No. 1, 1974.
12. **Glock**, G.E. and Murray, M.M.: Chemical Investigation of Salivary Calculus, *J. Dent. Res., 17,* 257, August, 1938.
13. **Mandel**, I.D. and Levy, B.M.: Studies on Salivary Calculus. I. Histochemical and Chemical Investigations of Supra- and Subgingival Calculus, *Oral Surg., 10,* 874, August, 1957.
14. **Schait**, A. and Mühlemann, H.R.: Fluoride Uptake by Calculus Following Topical Application of Fluorides, *Helv. Odont. Acta, 15,* 132, October, 1971.
15. **Kinoshita**, S., Schait, A., Schroeder, H.E., and Mühlemann, H.R.: Origin of Fluoride in Early Dental Calculus, *Helv. Odont. Acta, 9,* 141, October, 1965.
16. **Mühlemann**, H.R., Schait, A., and Schroeder, H.E.: Salivary Origin of Fluorine in Calcified Dental Plaques, *Helv. Odont. Acta, 8,* 128, October, 1964.
17. **Grøn**, P., van Campen, G.J., and Lindstrom, I.: Human Dental Calculus. Inorganic Chemical and Crystallographic Composition, *Arch. Oral Biol., 12,* 829, July, 1967.
18. **Melfi**, R.C.: *Permar's Oral Embryology and Microscopic Anatomy,* 9th ed. Philadelphia, Lea & Febiger, 1994, p. 85.
19. **Mandel**, I.D., Levy, B.M., and Wasserman, B.H.: Histochemistry of Calculus Formation, *J. Periodontol., 28,* 132, April, 1957.
20. **Mandel**, I.D.: Histochemical and Biochemical Aspects of Calculus Formation, *Periodontics, 1,* 43, March–April, 1963.
21. **Turesky**, S., Renstrup, G., and Glickman, I.: Histologic and Histochemical Observations Regarding Early Calculus Formation in Children and Adults, *J. Periodontol., 32,* 7, January, 1961.
22. **Anerud**, A., Löe, H., and Boysen, H.: The Natural History and Clinical Course of Calculus Formation in Man, *J. Clin. Periodontol., 18,* 160, March, 1991.
23. **Tilliss**, T.S.I.: A Closer Look at Tartar Control Dentifrices, *J. Dent. Hyg., 63,* 364, October, 1989.

SUGGESTED READINGS

Breuer, M.M., Mboya, S.A., Moroi, H., and Turesky, S.S.: Effect of Selected Beta-blockers on Supragingival Calculus Formation, *J. Periodontol., 67,* 428, April, 1996.

Brown, C.M., Hancock, E.B., O'Leary, T.J., Miller, C.H., and Sheldrake, M.A.: A Microbiological Comparison of Young Adults Based on Relative Amounts of Subgingival Calculus, *J. Periodontol., 62,* 591, October, 1991.

Carranza, F.A.: Dental Calculus, in Carranza, F.A. and Newman, M.G.: *Clinical Periodontology,* 8th ed. Philadelphia, W.B. Saunders Co., 1996, pp. 150–160.

Christersson, L.A., Grossi, S.G., Dunford, R.G., Machtei, E.E., and Genco, R.J.: Dental Plaque and Calculus: Risk Indicators for Their Formation, *J. Dent. Res., 71,* 1425, July, 1992.

Gaare, D., Rølla, G., Aryadi, F.J., and Van der Ouderaa, F.: Improvement of Gingival Health by Toothbrushing in Individuals With Large Amounts of Calculus, *J. Clin. Periodontol., 17,* 38, January, 1990.

Gaffar, A., LeGeros, R.Z., Gambogi, R.J., and Afflitto, J.: Recent Advances in Plaque, Gingivitis, Tartar and Caries Prevention Technology, *Int. Dent. J., 44,* 63, February, Supplement 1, 1994.

Galgut, P.N.: Supragingival Calculus Formation in a Group of Young Adults, *Quintessence Int., 27,* 817, December, 1996.

Hazen, S.P.: Supragingival Dental Calculus, *Periodontol. 2000, 8,* 125, 1995.

MacPherson, L.M.D., Girardin, D.C., Hughes, N.J., Stephen, K.W., and Dawes, C.: The Site-Specificity of Supragingival Calculus Deposition on the Lingual Surfaces of the Six Permanent Lower Anterior Teeth in Humans and the Effects of Age, Sex, Gum-Chewing Habits and the Time Since Last Prophylaxis on Calculus Scores, *J. Dent. Res., 74,* 1715, October, 1995.

Mandel, I.D.: Calculus Formation and Prevention: An Overview, *Compend. Cont. Educ. Dent.,* Special Issue No. 1, pp. S1–3, 1991.

Mandel, I.D. and Gaffar, A.: Calculus Revisited: A Review, *J. Clin. Periodontol., 13,* 249, April, 1986.

Nancollas, G.H. and Johnsson, M.A.S.: Calculus Formation and Inhibition, *Adv. Dent. Res., 8,* 307, July, 1994.

Okumura, H., Nakagaki, H., Kato, K., Ito, F., Weatherall, J.A., and Robinson, C.: Distribution of Fluoride in Human Dental Calculus, *Caries Res., 27,* 271, July–August, 1993.

Rolla, G., Rykke, M., and Gaare, D.: The Role of the Acquired Enamel Pellicle in Calculus Formation, *Adv. Dent. Sci., 9,* 403, December, 1995.

Turesky, S., Breuer, M., and Coffman, G.: The Effect of Certain Systemic Medications on Oral Calculus Formation, *J. Periodontol., 63,* 871, November, 1992.

Walsh, T.F., Figures, K.H., and Lamb, D.J.: *Clinical Dental Hygiene: A Handbook for the Dental Team.* Oxford, England, Wright, 1992, pp. 56–57, 88–89, 121–122.

Anticalculus Dentifrice

Adams, D.: Calculus-Inhibition Agents: A Review of Recent Clinical Trials, *Adv. Dent. Res., 9,* 410, December, 1995.

Beacham, B.E., Kurgansky, D., and Gould, W.M.: Circumoral Dermatitis and Cheilitis Caused by Tartar Control Dentifrices, *J. Am. Acad. Dermatol., 22,* 1029, June, 1990.

Chikte, U.M.E., Rudolph, M.J., and Reinach, S.G.: Anti-calculus Effects of Dentifrice Containing Pyrophosphate Compared With Control, *Clin. Prev. Dent., 14,* 29, July–August, 1992.

Disney, J.A., Graves, R.C., Cancro, L., Payonk, G., and Stewart, P.: An Evaluation of 6 Dentifrice Formulations for Supragingival Anticalculus and Antiplaque Activity, *J. Clin. Periodontol., 16,* 525, September, 1989.

Drake, D.R., Chung, J., Grigsby, W., and Wu-Yuan, C.: Synergistic Effect of Pyrophosphate and Sodium Dodecyl Sulfate on Periodontal Pathogens, *J. Periodontol., 63,* 696, August, 1992.

Gaengler, P., Kurbad, A., and Weinert, W.: Evaluation of Anti-calculus Efficacy: An SEM Method of Evaluating the Effectiveness of Pyrophosphate Dentifrice on Calculus Formation, *J. Clin. Periodontol., 20,* 144, February, 1993.

Hall, R.C., Embery, G., and Shellis, R.P.: Fluoride Modulates the Inhibition of *in vitro* Hydroxyapatite Crystal Growth by Small Dentin Proteoglycan: Relevance to Dental Calculus, *Adv. Dent. Res., 9,* 433, December, 1995.

Kazmierczak, M., Mather, M., Ciancio, S., Fischman, S., and Cancro, L.: A Clinical Evaluation of Anticalculus Dentifrices, *Clin. Prev. Dent., 12,* 13, April–May, 1990.

Kowitz, G., Jacobson, J., Meng, Z., and Lucatorto, F.: The Effects of Tartar-Control Toothpaste on the Oral Soft Tissues, *Oral Surg. Oral Med. Oral Pathol., 70,* 529, October, 1990.

Mellberg, J.R., Petrou, I.D., Fletcher, R., and Grote, N.: Evaluation of the Effects of a Pyrophosphate-Fluoride Anticalculus Dentifrice on Remineralization and Fluoride Uptake *in situ, Caries Res., 25,* 65, January–February, 1991.

Petrone, M., Lobene, R.R., Harrison, L.B., Volpe, A., and Petrone, D.M.: Clinical Comparison of the Anticalculus Efficacy of Three Commercially Available Dentifrices, *Clin. Prev. Dent., 13,* 18, July–August, 1991.

Scruggs, R.R., Stewart, P.W., Samuels, M.S., and Stamm, J.W.: Clinical Evaluation of Seven Anticalculus Dentifrice Formulations, *Clin. Prev. Dent., 13,* 23, January, 1991.

Segreto, V.A., Collins, E.M., D'Agostino, R., Cancro, L.P., Pfeifer, J., and Gilbert, R.J.: Anticalculus Effect of a Dentifrice Containing 0.5% Zinc Citrate Trihydrate, *Community Dent. Oral Epidemiol., 19,* 29, February, 1991.

Stephan, K.W., Saxton, C.A., Jones, C.L., Ritchie, J.A., and Morrison, T.: Control of Gingivitis and Calculus by a Dentifrice Containing a Zinc Salt and Triclosan, *J. Periodontol., 61,* 674, November, 1990.

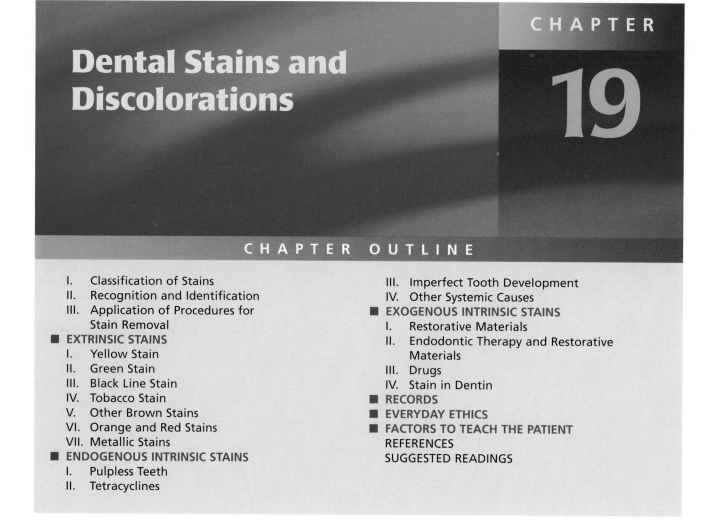

Discolorations of the teeth and restorations occur in three general ways: (1) stain adheres directly to the surfaces, (2) stain contained within calculus and soft deposits, and (3) stain incorporated within the tooth structure or the restorative material. Instructional and clinical procedures apply to all three. The first two types may be removed by scaling or polishing. Certain stains may be prevented by the patient's routine personal care.

The significance of stains is primarily the appearance or cosmetic effect. In general, any detrimental effect on the teeth or gingival tissues is related to the dental biofilm or calculus in which the stain occurs. Thick deposits of stain conceivably can provide a rough surface on which dental biofilm can collect and irritate the adjacent gingiva. Certain stains provide a means of evaluating oral cleanliness and the patient's habits of personal care. Key words that relate to dental stains and discolorations are defined in Box 19-1.

I. CLASSIFICATION OF STAINS

A. Classified by Location

1. *Extrinsic.* Extrinsic stains occur on the external surface of the tooth and may be removed by procedures of toothbrushing, scaling, and/or polishing.
2. *Intrinsic.* Intrinsic stains occur within the tooth substance and cannot be removed by techniques of scaling or polishing.

B. Classified by Source

1. *Exogenous.* Exogenous stains develop or originate from sources outside the tooth. Exogenous stains may be extrinsic and stay on the outer surface of the tooth or intrinsic and become incorporated within the tooth structure.
2. *Endogenous.* Endogenous stains develop or originate from within the tooth. Endogenous stains

BOX 19-1 KEY WORDS: Dental Stains and Discolorations

Amelogenesis imperfecta: imperfect formation of enamel; hereditary condition in which the ameloblasts fail to lay down the enamel matrix properly or at all.

Chlorophyll: green plant pigment essential to photosynthesis.

Chromogenic: producing color or pigment.

Chronologic: arranged in order of time.

Dentinogenesis imperfecta: hereditary disorder of dentin formation in which the odontoblasts lay down an abnormal matrix; can occur in both primary and permanent dentitions.

Endogenous: produced within or caused by factors within.

Exogenous: originating outside or caused by factors outside.

Extrinsic: derived from or situated on the outside; external.

Hypoplasia: incomplete development or underdevelopment of an organ or a tissue.

Intrinsic: situated entirely within.

are always intrinsic and usually are discolorations of the dentin reflected through the enamel.

II. RECOGNITION AND IDENTIFICATION

More than one type of stain may occur and more than one etiologic factor may cause the stains of an individual's dentition. A differential diagnosis may be needed.

A. Medical and Dental History

Developmental complications, medications, use of tobacco, and fluoride histories all contribute necessary information.

Accurately prepared medical and dental histories can provide information to supplement clinical observations.

B. Food Record

Assessment of a food record may aid in identifying certain contributing factors.

C. Oral Hygiene Habits

The history of personal biofilm removal with the type and frequency of use of toothbrush, floss, and other supplemental materials and devices may help explain the presence of certain stains. The state of oral hygiene and oral cleanliness is significant to the occurrence of dental stains.

III. APPLICATION OF PROCEDURES FOR STAIN REMOVAL

A. Stains Occurring Directly on the Tooth Surface

1. Stains that are directly associated with the biofilm or pellicle on the surface of the enamel or exposed cementum are removed as much as possible during toothbrushing by the patient. Certain stains can be removed by scaling, whereas others require polishing.
2. When stains are tenacious, excessive polishing should be avoided. As mild an abrasive agent as possible should be used. Precautions should be taken to prevent (1) abrasion of the tooth surface or gingival margin, (2) removal of a layer of fluoride-rich tooth surface, or (3) overheating with a power-driven polisher.

B. Stains Incorporated Within Tooth Deposits

When stain is included within the substance of a soft deposit or calculus, it is removed with the deposit.

▪ EXTRINSIC STAINS

The most frequently observed stains, yellow, green, black line, and tobacco, are described first; descriptions of the less common orange, red, and metallic stains follow.

I. YELLOW STAIN

A. Clinical Appearance

Dull, yellowish discoloration of dental biofilm.

B. Distribution on Tooth Surfaces

Yellow stain is associated with the presence of dental biofilm.

C. Occurrence

1. Common to all ages.
2. More evident when personal oral care procedures are neglected.

D. Etiology

Usually food pigments.

II. GREEN STAIN

A. Clinical Appearance

1. Light or yellowish green to very dark green.
2. Embedded in dental biofilm.
3. Occurs in three general forms:
    a. Small curved line following contour of facial gingival crest.
    b. Smeared irregularly, may even cover entire facial surface.
    c. Streaked, following grooves or lines in enamel.
4. The stain is frequently superimposed by soft yellow or gray debris (materia alba and food debris).
5. Dark green may become embedded in surface enamel and be observed as an exogenous intrinsic stain when superficial layers of deposit are removed.
6. Enamel under stain is sometimes demineralized as a result of cariogenic biofilm. The rough demineralized surface encourages biofilm retention, demineralization, and recurrence of green stain.

B. Distribution on Tooth Surfaces

1. Primarily facial; may extend to proximal.
2. Most frequently facial cervical third of maxillary anterior teeth.

C. Composition

1. Chromogenic bacteria and fungi.
2. Decomposed hemoglobin.

3. Inorganic elements include calcium, potassium, sodium, silicon, magnesium, phosphorus, and other elements in small amounts.[1]

D. Occurrence

1. May occur at any age; primarily found in childhood.
2. Collects on both permanent and primary teeth.

E. Recurrence

Recurrence depends on fastidiousness of personal care procedures.

F. Etiology

Green stain results from oral uncleanliness, chromogenic bacteria, and gingival hemorrhage.
1. Chromogenic bacteria or fungi are retained and nourished in dental biofilm where the green stain is produced.
2. Blood pigments from hemoglobin are decomposed by bacteria.
3. Predisposing factors are the presence of means for retention and proliferation of chromogenic bacteria, such as dental biofilm, and food debris.

G. Clinical Approach

1. Do not scale the area. Often, an area of demineralized tooth structure underlies the stain and soft deposits.
2. Ask the patient to remove the soft deposits during a dental biofilm control lesson. Initiate a daily fluoride remineralization program.

H. Other Green Stains

In addition to the clinical entity known as "green stain" that was just described, dental biofilm and acquired pellicle may become stained a green color by a variety of substances. Differential distinction may be determined by questioning the patient or from items in the medical or dental histories. Green discoloration may result from the following:
*   Chlorophyll preparations.
*   Metallic dusts of industry.
*   Certain drugs. The stain from smoking marijuana may appear grayish-green.

III. BLACK LINE STAIN

Black line stain is a highly retentive black or dark brown calculus-like stain that forms along the gingival third near the gingival margin. It may occur on primary or permanent teeth.

A. Other Names

Pigmented dental biofilm, brown stain, black stain.

B. Clinical Features

1. Continuous or interrupted fine line, 1 mm wide (average), no appreciable thickness.
2. May be a wider band or even occupy entire gingival third in severe cases (rare).
3. Follows contour of gingival crest about 1 mm above crest.
4. Usually demarcated from gingival crest by clear white line of unstained enamel.
5. Appears black at bases of pits and fissures.
6. Heavy deposits slightly elevated from the tooth surface may be detected with an explorer.
7. Gingiva is firm, with little or no tendency to bleed.
8. Teeth are frequently clean and shiny, with a tendency to lower incidence of dental caries.

C. Distribution on Tooth Surfaces

1. Facial and lingual surfaces; follows contour of gingival crest onto proximal surfaces.
2. Rarely on facial surface of maxillary anterior teeth.
3. Most frequently: lingual and proximal surfaces of maxillary posterior teeth.

D. Composition and Formation[2,3]

1. Black line stain, like calculus, is composed of microorganisms embedded in an intermicrobial substance.
2. The microorganisms are primarily gram-positive rods, with other bacteria, including cocci, in smaller percentages.

   The composition of black line stain is different from the composition of supragingival calculus, in which cocci predominate. Attachment to the tooth of black line stain is by a pellicle-like structure.[4]

   Oral disease does not result from the presence of black line stain. In contrast, gingivitis is related to the formation of supragingival biofilm, and in the presence of a cariogenic substrate, dental caries develops.
3. Mineralization in black line stain is similar to the formation of calculus.

E. Occurrence

1. All ages; more common in childhood.
2. More common in female patients.
3. Frequently found in clean mouths.

F. Recurrence

Black line stain tends to form again despite regular personal care, but quantity may be less when biofilm control procedures are meticulous.

G. Predisposing Factors

None apparent, except a natural tendency.

IV. TOBACCO STAIN

A. Clinical Appearance

1. Light brown to dark leathery brown or black.
2. Shape
   a. Diffuse staining of dental biofilm.
   b. Narrow band that follows contour of gingival crest, slightly above the crest.
   c. Wide, firm, tarlike band may cover cervical third and extend to central third of crown.
3. Incorporated in calculus deposit.
4. Heavy deposits (particularly from smokeless tobacco) may penetrate the enamel and become exogenous intrinsic.

B. Distribution on Tooth Surfaces

1. Cervical third, primarily.
2. Any surface, as well as pits and fissures.
3. Most frequently on lingual surfaces.

C. Composition

1. Tar and products of combustion.
2. Brown pigment from smokeless tobacco.

D. Predisposing Factors

1. Natural tendencies. The quantity of stain is not necessarily proportional to the amount of tobacco used.
2. Personal oral care procedures: increased deposits occur with neglect.
3. Extent of dental biofilm and calculus available for adherence.

V. OTHER BROWN STAINS

A. Brown Pellicle

The acquired pellicle is smooth and structureless and recurs readily after removal.[5] The pellicle can take on stains of various colors that result from chemical alteration of the pellicle.[6]

B. Stannous Fluoride[7-9]

Light brown, sometimes yellowish, stain forms on the teeth in the pellicle after repeated use of a stannous fluoride gel or other product, or after having a topical fluoride application. The brown stain results from the formation of stannous sulfide or brown tin oxide from the reaction of the tin ion in the fluoride compound.

C. Foodstuffs

Tea, coffee, and soy sauce are often implicated in the formation of a brownish-stained pellicle. As with other brown pellicle stains, less stain occurs when the personal oral hygiene and biofilm control are excellent.

D. Anti-Biofilm Agents[10,11]

Chlorhexidine and alexidine are used in mouthrinses and are effective against biofilm formation. A brownish stain of the tooth surfaces results, usually more pronounced on proximal and other surfaces less accessible to routine biofilm control procedures. The stain also tends to form more rapidly on exposed roots than on enamel. Tooth staining has been considered a significant side effect.

E. Betel Leaf[12]

Betel leaf chewing is common among people of all ages in eastern countries. Betel has a caries-inhibiting effect.

The discoloration imparted to the teeth is a dark mahogany brown, sometimes almost black. It may become thick and hard, with partly smooth and partly rough surfaces.

Microscopically, the black deposit consists of microorganisms and mineralized material with a laminated pattern characteristic of subgingival calculus. It should be removed by scaling.

VI. ORANGE AND RED STAINS

A. Clinical Appearance

Orange or red stains appear at the cervical third.

B. Distribution on Tooth Surfaces

1. More frequently on anterior than on posterior teeth.
2. Both facial and lingual surfaces of anterior teeth.

C. Occurrence

Rare (red more rare than orange).

D. Etiology

Chromogenic bacteria.

VII. METALLIC STAINS

A. Metals or Metallic Salts From Metal-Containing Dust of Industry

1. *Clinical Appearance.* Examples of colors on teeth:
   a. Copper or brass: green or bluish-green.
   b. Iron: brown to greenish-brown.
   c. Nickel: green.
   d. Cadmium: yellow or golden brown.
2. *Distribution on Tooth Surfaces*
   a. Primarily anterior; may occur on any teeth.
   b. Cervical third more commonly affected.
3. *Manner of Formation*
   a. Industrial worker inhales dust through mouth, bringing metallic substance in contact with teeth.
   b. Metal imparts color to biofilm.
   c. Occasionally, stain may penetrate tooth substance and become exogenous intrinsic stain.

B. Metallic Substances Contained in Drugs

1. *Clinical Appearance.* Examples of colors on teeth:
   a. Iron: black (iron sulfide) or brown.
   b. Manganese (from potassium permanganate): black.
2. *Distribution on Tooth Surfaces.* Generalized, may occur on all.
3. *Manner of Formation*
   a. Drug enters biofilm substance, imparts color to biofilm and calculus.
   b. Pigment from drug may attach directly to tooth substance.
4. *Prevention.* Use a medication through a straw or in tablet or capsule form to prevent direct contact with the teeth.

▪ ENDOGENOUS INTRINSIC STAINS

Stains incorporated within the tooth structure may be related to the period of tooth development.

I. PULPLESS TEETH

Not all pulpless teeth discolor. Improved endodontic procedures have contributed to the prevention of many discolorations formerly associated with that cause.

A. Clinical Appearance

A wide range of colors exists; stains may be light yellow-brown, slate gray, reddish-brown, dark brown, bluish-black, or black. Others have an orange or greenish tinge.

B. Manner of Formation

1. Blood and other pulp tissue elements may be made available for breakdown as a result of hemorrhages in the pulp chamber, root canal treatment, or necrosis and decomposition of the pulp tissue.
2. Pigments from the decomposed hemoglobin and pulp tissue penetrate the dentinal tubules.

II. TETRACYCLINES

A. Tetracycline antibiotics, used widely for combating many types of infections, have an affinity for mineralized tissues and are absorbed by the bones and teeth. They can be transferred through the placenta and enter fetal circulation.
B. Discoloration of the teeth of a child can result when the drug is administered to the mother during the third trimester of pregnancy or to the child in infancy and early childhood.
C. Color of teeth may be light green to dark yellow, or a gray-brown. The discoloration depends on the dosage, the length of time the drug was used, and the type of tetracycline. After eruption, the teeth may fluoresce under ultraviolet light, but that property is lost with age and exposure.[14]
D. Discoloration may be generalized or limited to specific parts of individual teeth that were developing at the time of administration of the antibiotic. Reference to the Table of Tooth Development (page 790) can assist in determining the patient's age at the time the drug was administered, and the patient's medical history at that age may reveal the illness for which the antibiotic was prescribed.

III. IMPERFECT TOOTH DEVELOPMENT

Defective tooth development may result from factors of genetic abnormality or environmental influences during tooth development.

A. Hereditary: Genetic[15]

1. *Amelogenesis Imperfecta*: The enamel is partially or completely missing because of a generalized disturbance of the ameloblasts. Teeth are yellowish-brown or gray-brown.

2. *Dentinogenesis Imperfecta ("Opalescent Dentin")*: The dentin is abnormal as a result of disturbances in the odontoblastic layer during development. The teeth appear translucent or opalescent and vary in color from gray to bluish-brown.

B. Enamel Hypoplasia

1. *Systemic Hypoplasia* (chronologic hypoplasia resulting from ameloblastic disturbance of short duration). Teeth erupt with white spots or with pits. Over a long period of time, the white spots may become discolored from food pigments or other substances taken into the mouth.
2. *Local Hypoplasia* (affects single tooth). White spots may become stained as in systemic hypoplasia.

C. Dental Fluorosis

Dental fluorosis was originally called "brown stain." Later, Dr. Frederick S. McKay, who studied the condition and described it in the dental literature, named it "mottled enamel."
1. *Manner of Formation*
    a. Enamel hypomineralization results from ingestion of excessive fluoride ion in drinking water (more than 2 parts per million) during the period of mineralization. The enamel alterations are a result of toxic damage to the ameloblasts.
    b. When the teeth erupt, they have white spots or areas that later become discolored from oral pigments and appear light or dark brown.
    c. Severe effects of excess fluoride during development may produce cracks or pitting; the discoloration concentrates in these. This condition and appearance led to the name mottled enamel.
2. *Classification*
    Dean provided the original definitions for five grades of fluorosis. They ranged from "questionable" (a few white flecks or spots) to "severe" (marked brown staining and pitting of the enamel surfaces).[16]
    More specific classifications have been developed for clinical and research purposes,[17,18] such as the Tooth Surface Index of Fluorosis (TSIF; page 549).

IV. OTHER SYSTEMIC CAUSES

Several types of tooth discolorations may result from blood-borne pigments.

Pigments circulating in the blood are transmitted to the dentin from the capillaries of the pulp. For example, prolonged jaundice early in life can impart a yellow or greenish discoloration to the teeth.

Erythroblastosis fetalis (Rh incompatibility) may leave a green, brown, or blue hue to the teeth.

▪ EXOGENOUS INTRINSIC STAINS

When intrinsic stains come from an outside source, not from within the tooth, the stain is called exogenous intrinsic. Extrinsic stains, such as tobacco and green stains, can provide stain that becomes intrinsic.

Restorative materials cause staining of teeth, as described in the section that follows. Tooth-color restorations may become stained from the various extrinsic staining substances mentioned in this chapter. A few references are included in "Suggested Readings" at the end of the chapter.

I. RESTORATIVE MATERIALS

A. Silver Amalgam

1. Silver amalgam can impart a gray to black discoloration to the tooth structure around a restoration.
2. Metallic ions migrate from the amalgam restoration into the enamel and dentin.
3. Silver, tin, and mercury ions eventually contact debris at the junction of the tooth and the restoration and form sulfides, which are products of corrosion.

B. Copper Amalgam

Copper amalgam used for filling primary teeth may impart a bluish-green color.

II. ENDODONTIC THERAPY AND RESTORATIVE MATERIALS

A. Silver nitrate: bluish-black.
B. Volatile oils: yellowish-brown.
C. Strong iodine: brown.
D. Aureomycin: yellow.
E. Silver-containing root canal sealer: black.

III. DRUGS

A. Stannous Fluoride Topical Application[7]

1. Light to dark brown staining from the formation of tin sulfide.
2. Located most frequently in occlusal pits and grooves of posterior teeth and cervical third facial surfaces of anterior teeth; in carious and precarious lesions; and in margins of tooth color and amalgam restorations.
3. Staining may accompany dental caries arrestment.

B. Ammoniacal Silver Nitrate

Used in treatment of such sensitive areas as exposed cementum or for inhibition of demineralization in dental caries prevention; imparts a dark brown to black discoloration.

Everyday Ethics

? Daniel returned to the dental office of Dr. Windum after 3 years of working on the East Coast at a large consulting firm. At the age of 32, Daniel was exhibiting signs of gingival inflammation and changes in the level of gingival attachment. Ruthie, the dental hygienist, immediately began talking to Daniel about biofilm and homecare techniques, including the use of chlorhexidine rinses.

Dr. Windum confirmed Ruthie's hygiene diagnosis and wrote a prescription for the agent. Daniel left the office only to call a few days later to complain about the "awful brown stain on his teeth and horrible taste of the mouthrinse." He further indicated that he had stopped using the product and wanted to come in and have the stain removed immediately.

Questions for Consideration

1. Was Ruthie unethical since it seems that she did not completely inform Daniel about the side effects of prescribed rinses? Use the ethical principles to support your answer.

2. Daniel seems to be more concerned about the staining that has occurred than the condition of his periodontium. How can Ruthie respect Daniel's feelings while helping him understand the potential outcomes of his daily homecare?

3. How could Ruthie and Dr. Windum "justify" the stain that results from the product while making Daniel "value" his gingival condition?

Factors To Teach The Patient

- Predisposing factors that contribute to stain accumulation.

- Personal care procedures that can aid in the prevention or reduction of stains.

- Advantages of starting a smoking cessation program.

- Reasons for not using an abrasive dentifrice with vigorous brushing strokes to lessen or remove stain accumulation.

- The need to avoid tobacco, coffee, tea, and other beverages or foodstuffs that can stain, to prevent discoloration of new restorations.

- Reasons for the difficulty of removing certain extrinsic stains during scaling and polishing.

- Effect of tetracyclines on developing teeth. Need to avoid use during pregnancy and by children to age 12.

IV. STAIN IN DENTIN

Discoloration resulting from a carious lesion is an example.

■ RECORDS

- Record color, type, extent, and location of stains with the patient's examination and assessment.
- Make additions to the dental history as information is gained concerning the origin of stains such as those related to tooth development, systemic disease, occupations, or medications.

REFERENCES

1. Shay, D.E., Haddox, J.H., and Richmond, J.L.: An Inorganic Qualitative and Quantitative Analysis of Green Stain, *J. Am. Dent. Assoc., 50,* 156, February, 1955.
2. Theilade, J., Slots, J., and Fejerskov, O.: The Ultrastructure of Black Stain on Human Primary Teeth, *Scand. J. Dent. Res., 81,* 528, No. 7, 1973.
3. Slots, J.: The Microflora of Black Stain on Human Primary Teeth, *Scand. J. Dent. Res., 82,* 484, No. 7, 1974.
4. Theilade, J.: Development of Bacterial Plaque in the Oral Cavity, *J. Clin. Periodontol., 4,* 1, December, 1977.
5. Meckel, A.H.: The Formation and Properties of Organic Films on Teeth, *Arch. Oral Biol., 10,* 585, July–August, 1965.
6. Eriksen, H.M. and Nordbø, H.: Extrinsic Discoloration of Teeth, *J. Clin. Periodontol., 5,* 229, November, 1978.
7. Horowitz, H.S. and Chamberlin, S.R.: Pigmentation of Teeth Following Topical Applications of Stannous Fluoride in a Nonfluoridated Area, *J. Public Health Dent., 31,* 32, Winter, 1971.
8. Shannon, I.L.: Stannous Fluoride: Does It Stain Teeth? How Does It React With Tooth Surfaces? A Review, *Gen. Dent., 26,* 64, September–October, 1978.
9. Leverett, D.H., McHugh, W.D., and Jensen, Ø.E.: Dental Caries and Staining After Twenty-eight Months of Rinsing With Stannous Fluoride or Sodium Fluoride, *J. Dent. Res., 65,* 424, March, 1986.
10. Flötra, L., Gjermo, P., Rölla, G., and Waerhaug, J.: Side Effects of Chlorhexidine Mouthwashes, *Scand. J. Dent. Res., 79,* 119, April, 1971.
11. Formicola, A.J., Deasy, M.J., Johnson, D.H., and Howe, E.E.: Tooth Staining Effects of an Alexidine Mouthwash, *J. Periodontol., 50,* 207, April, 1979.
12. Reichart, P.A., Lenz, H., König, H., Becker, J., and Mohr, U.: The Black Layer on the Teeth of Betel Chewers: A Light Microscopic, Microradiographic, and Electronmicroscopic Study, *J. Oral Pathol., 14,* 466, July, 1985.
13. Ehrlich, A. and Torres, H.O.: *Essentials of Dental Assisting.* Philadelphia, W.B. Saunders Co., 1992, pp. 389–393.
14. Robinson, H.B.G. and Miller, A.S.: *Color Atlas of Oral Pathology,* 5th ed. Philadelphia, J.B. Lippincott Co., 1990, p. 55.
15. Ibid., p. 41.
16. Dean, H.T.: Investigation of Physiological Effects by Epidemiological Method, in Moulton, F.R., ed.: *Fluorine and Dental Health.* Washington, D.C., American Association for the Advancement of Science, No. 19, 1942.
17. Thylstrup, A. and Fejerskov, O.: Clinical Appearance of Dental Fluorosis in Permanent Teeth in Relation to Histologic Changes, *Community Dent. Oral Epidemiol., 6,* 315, December, 1978.
18. Horowitz, H.S., Driscoll, W.S., Meyers, R.J., Heifetz, S.B., and Kingman, A.: A New Method for Assessing the Prevalence of Dental Fluorosis—The Tooth Surface Index of Fluorosis, *J. Am. Dent. Assoc., 109,* 37, July 1984.

SUGGESTED READINGS

Addy, M. and Moran, J.: Mechanisms of Stain Formation on Teeth, in Particular Associated With Metal Ions and Antiseptics, *Adv. Dent. Sci., 9,* 450, December, 1995.
Barta, J.E., King, D.L., and Jorgensen, R.L.: ABO Blood Group Incompatibility and Primary Tooth Discoloration, *Pediatr. Dent., 11,* 316, December, 1989.
Cuff, M.J.A., McQuade, M.J., Scheidt, M.J., Sutherland, D.E., and Van Dyke, T.E.: The Presence of Nicotine on Root Surfaces of Periodontally Diseased Teeth in Smokers, *J. Periodontol., 60,* 564, October, 1989.
Holan, G. and Fuks, A.B.: The Diagnostic Value of Coronal Dark-Gray Discoloration in Primary Teeth Following Traumatic Injuries, *Pediatr. Dent., 18,* 224, May–June, 1996.
Joiner, A., Jones, N.M., and Raven, S.J.: Investigation of Factors Influencing Stain Formation Utilizing an *in situ* Model, *Adv. Dent. Sci., 9,* 471, December, 1995.
Massler, M. and Schour, I.: *Atlas of the Mouth.* Chicago, American Dental Association, Plate 12.
Nathoo, S.A.: The Chemistry and Mechanisms of Extrinsic and Intrinsic Discoloration, *J. Am. Dent. Assoc., 128,* 6S, April, Supplement, 1997.
Nathoo, S.A. and Gaffar, A.: Studies on Dental Stains Induced by Antibacterial Agents and Rational Approaches for Bleaching Dental Stains, *Adv. Dent. Res., 9,* 462, December, 1995.
Tilliss, T.: Dental Stains and Chemotherapeutics: A Closer Look, *DentalHygienistNews, 2,* 12, January/February/March, 1989.

Chlorhexidine and Antibiotics

Addy, M., Moran, J., Griffiths, A.A., and Wills-Wood, N.J.: Extrinsic Tooth Discoloration by Metals and Chlorhexidine. I. Surface

Protein Denaturation or Dietary Precipitation?, *Br. Dent. J., 159,* 281, November 9, 1985.

Addy, M. and Moran, J.: Extrinsic Tooth Discoloration by Metals and Chlorhexidine. II. Clinical Staining Produced by Chlorhexidine, Iron and Tea, *Br. Dent. J., 159,* 331, November 23, 1985.

Addy, M., Al-Arrayed, F., and Moran, J.: The Use of an Oxidising Mouthwash to Reduce Staining Associated With Chlorhexidine: Studies *in vitro* and *in vivo, J. Clin. Periodontol., 18,* 267, April, 1991.

Addy, M., Mahdavi, S.A., and Loyn, T.: Dietary Staining *in vitro* by Mouthrinses as a Comparative Measure of Antiseptic Activity and Predictor of Staining *in vivo, J. Dent., 23,* 95, April, 1995.

Beiswanger, B.B., Mallatt, M.E., Mau, M.S., Jackson, R.D., and Hennon, D.K.: The Clinical Effects of a Mouthrinse Containing 0.1% Octenidine, *J. Dent. Res., 69,* 454, February, 1990.

Berger, R.S., Mandel, E.B., Hayes, T.J., and Grimwood, R.R.: Minocycline Staining of the Oral Cavity, *J. Am. Acad. Dermatol., 21,* 1300, December, 1989.

Leard, A. and Addy, M.: The Propensity of Different Brands of Tea and Coffee to Cause Staining Associated With Chlorhexidine, *J. Clin. Periodontol., 24,* 115, February, 1997.

Parkins, F.M., Furnish, G., and Bernstein, M.: Minocycline Use Discolors Teeth, *J. Am. Dent. Assoc., 123,* 87, October, 1992.

Sanz, M., Vallcorba, N., Fabreques, S., Müller, I., and Herkströter, F.: The Effect of a Dentifrice Containing Chlorhexidine and Zinc on Plaque, Gingivitis, Calculus and Tooth Staining, *J. Clin. Periodontol., 21,* 431, July, 1994.

Wade, W., Addy, M., Hughes, J., Milsom, S., and Doherty, F.: Studies on Stannous Fluoride Toothpaste and Gel (1). Antimicrobial Properties and Staining Potential in Vitro, *J. Clin Periodontol., 24,* 81, February, 1997.

Discoloration of Restorations

Chan, K.C., Fuller, J.L., and Hormati, A.A.: The Ability of Foods to Stain Two Composite Resins, *J. Prosthet. Dent., 43,* 542, May, 1980.

Kidd, E.A.M.: The Caries Status of Tooth-Coloured Restorations With Marginal Stain, *Br. Dent. J., 171,* 241, October 19, 1991.

Luce, M.S. and Campbell, C.E.: Stain Potential of Four Microfilled Composites, *J. Prosthet. Dent., 60,* 151, August, 1988.

Nordbö, H., Attramadal, A., and Eriksen, H.M.: Iron Discoloration of Acrylic Resin Exposed to Chlorhexidine or Tannic Acid: A Model Study, *J. Prosthet. Dent., 49,* 126, January, 1983.

Um, C.M. and Ruyter, I.E.: Staining of Resin-based Veneering Materials With Coffee and Tea, *Quintessence Int., 22,* 377, May, 1981.

Indices and Scoring Methods

Indices and scoring methods are used in clinical practice and community programs to determine and record the state of health of individuals and groups. Several well-known and widely used indices and scoring methods are described in this chapter. In addition, an index for scoring enamel fluorosis is included in the chapter on fluorides. "Suggested Readings" at the end of the chapter contains references to other indices. Box 20-1 defines related terminology.

Familiarity with the various types of indices may prove helpful when different evaluation criteria are needed. An individual oral health assessment score, a clinical trial, and a community health epidemiologic survey must be distinguished.

I. INDIVIDUAL ASSESSMENT SCORE

A. Purpose

In clinical practice, an index, biofilm record, or scoring system for an individual patient can be used for education, motivation, and evaluation. The effects of personal disease control efforts, the progress of healing between professional treatments, and the maintenance

---

BOX 20-1 KEY WORDS: Indices and Scoring Methods

Calibration: determination of accuracy and consistency between examiners to standardize procedures and gain reliability of recorded findings.

Epidemiology: the study of the relationships of various factors that determine the frequency and distribution of diseases in the human community; study of health and disease in populations.

Incidence: the rate at which a certain event occurs, as the number of new cases of a specific disease occurring during a certain period of time.

Index: a graduated, numeric scale with upper and lower limits; scores on the scale correspond to a specific criterion for individuals or populations; *pl.* indices or indexes.

Pilot study: a trial run of a planned study using a small sample to pretest an instrument, survey, or questionnaire.

Placebo: an inactive substance or preparation with no intrinsic therapeutic value given to satisfy a patient's symbolic need for drug therapy; used in controlled research studies in a form identical in appearance to the material being tested.

Prevalence: the total number of cases of a specific disease or condition in existence in a given population at a certain time.

Ramfjord Index Teeth: teeth used for epidemiologic studies of periodontal diseases: the maxillary right and mandibular left first molars, maxillary left and mandibular right first premolars, and maxillary left and mandibular right central incisors.

Reliability: ability of an index or test procedure to measure consistently at different times and under a variety of conditions; reproducibility; consistency.

Screening of a *population:* assessment of many individuals to disclose certain characteristics or a certain disease entity; *individual* screening: brief assessment for initial evaluation and classification of needs for additional examination and treatment planning.

Validity: ability of an index or test procedure to measure what it is intended to measure.

of health over time can be monitored. An example is the "plaque-free score," in which a patient is able to measure the effects of personal daily care efforts by the changes in the scores. This system may prove to be a valuable motivating device.

B. Uses

- Provides individual assessment to help a patient recognize an oral problem.
- Reveals the degree of effectiveness of present oral hygiene practices.
- Motivates the person in preventive and professional care for the elimination and control of oral disease.
- Evaluates the success of individual and professional treatment over a period of time by comparing index scores.

II. CLINICAL TRIAL

A. Purpose

A clinical trial is planned for the determination of the effect of an agent or procedure on the prevention, progression, or control of a disease. The trial is conducted by comparing an experimental group with a control group that is similar to the experimental group in every way except for the variable being studied.

Examples of indices used for clinical trials are the Plaque Index (Pl I) of Silness and Löe[1] and the Patient Hygiene Performance (PHP) of Podshadley and Haley.[2] These and other indices are described in this chapter.

B. Uses

- Determines baseline data before experimental factors are introduced.
- Measures the effectiveness of specific agents for the prevention, control, or treatment of oral conditions.
- Measures the effectiveness of mechanical devices for personal care, such as toothbrushes, interdental cleaning devices, or irrigators.

III. EPIDEMIOLOGIC SURVEY

A. Purpose

The word *epidemiology* denotes the study of disease characteristics of populations. An example of an index designed for a survey of population groups is the DMFT (Decayed, Missing, and Filled Teeth) Index.[3] It has been used with populations around the world to determine the extent of dental caries. Such a survey was not designed for evaluation of an individual patient.

B. Uses

- Shows the prevalence and incidence of a particular condition occurring within a given population.
- Provides baseline data to show existing dental health practices.
- Assesses the needs of a community.
- Compares the effects of a community program and evaluates the results.

IV. INDEX

An index is an expression of clinical observations in numeric values. It is used to describe the status of the individual or group with respect to a condition being measured. The use of a numeric scale and a standardized method for interpreting observations of a condition results in an index score that is more consistent and less subjective than a word description of that condition.

A. Descriptive Categories of Indices

1. *General Categories*
   a. Simple index: One that measures the presence or absence of a condition. An example is an index that measures the presence of dental biofilm without evaluating its effect on the gingiva.
   b. Cumulative index: One that measures all the evidence of a condition, past and present. An example is the DMFT Index for dental caries.
2. *Types of Simple and Cumulative Indices*
   a. Irreversible: One that measures conditions that will not change. An example is an index that measures dental caries.
   b. Reversible: One that measures conditions that can be changed. Examples are indices that measure dental biofilm.

B. Selection Criteria

A useful and effective index
- Is simple to use and calculate.
- Requires minimal equipment and expense.
- Uses a minimal amount of time to complete.
- Does not cause patient discomfort nor is otherwise unacceptable to a patient.
- Has clear-cut criteria that are readily understandable.
- Is as free as possible from subjective interpretation.
- Is reproducible by the same examiner or different examiners.
- Is amenable to statistical analysis; has validity and reliability.

V. SYSTEMS DESCRIBED IN THIS CHAPTER

A. Screening for Periodontal Health (PSR)

B. Dental Biofilm

- "Plaque Index" (Pl I).
- "Plaque Control Record."
- "Plaque-Free Score."

C. Biofilm, Debris, Calculus

- Patient Hygiene Performance (PHP).
- Simplified Oral Hygiene Index (OHI-S).

D. Gingival Bleeding

- Sulcus Bleeding Index (SBI).
- Gingival Bleeding Index (GBI).
- Eastman Interdental Bleeding Index (EIBI).

E. Gingival/Periodontal

- Gingival Index (GI).
- Community Periodontal Index of Treatment Needs (CPITN).

F. Dental Caries

- Decayed, Missing, and Filled Permanent Teeth (DMFT).
- Decayed, Missing, and Filled Permanent Tooth Surfaces (DMFS).
- Primary teeth indices.

▪ PERIODONTAL SCREENING AND RECORDING (PSR)

(American Academy of Periodontology and American Dental Association[4])

I. PURPOSE

To assess the state of periodontal health in a rapid and effective manner and to motivate the patient to seek necessary complete periodontal assessment and treatment.

II. SELECTION OF TEETH

The dentition is divided into sextants. Each tooth is examined. Posterior sextants begin distal to the canines.

III. PROCEDURE

A. Instrument

Specially designed probe used by the World Health Organization for the CPITN.
1. *Markings.* At intervals from tip: 3.5, 2.0, 3.0, and 3.0 mm (total 11.5 mm) (Figure 20-1).

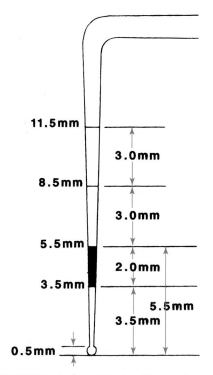

▪ **FIGURE 20-1 Periodontal Probe.** The probe, with markings as shown, is used to make determinations for the PSR and the Community Periodontal Index of Treatment Needs (CPITN). (From FDI: *A Simplified Periodontal Examination for Dental Practices.* Fédération Dentaire Internationale, 64 Wimpole Street, London W1M 8AL.)

2. *Working Tip.* A ball 0.5 mm in diameter. The functions of the ball are
    a. To aid in the detection of calculus, rough overhanging margins of restorations, and other tooth surface irregularities.
    b. To facilitate assessment at the probing depth and reduce risk of overmeasurement.
3. *Color Coding.* Color-coded between 3.5 and 5.5 mm.

B. Probe Application

1. Insert probe gently into a sulcus until resistance is felt.
2. Apply a circumferential walking step to probe systematically about each tooth through each sextant.
3. Observe color-coded area of the probe for prompt identification of probing depths.
4. Remember that each sextant receives one code number corresponding to the deepest position of the color-coded portion of the probe.

C. Criteria

1. Five codes and an asterisk are used. Table 20-1 shows the clinical findings, code significance, and patient management guidelines.

■ TABLE 20-1 PERIODONTAL SCREENING AND RECORDING (PSR)[†]

CLINICAL FINDINGS	CODE DESCRIPTION	MANAGEMENT GUIDELINES
Code 0	**Code 0** • Colored area of probe is completely visible in the deepest probing depth of the sextant • No calculus, no defective margins, no bleeding	**Code 0** • Dental biofilm control • Preventive care
Code 1	**Code 1** • Colored area of probe is completely visible in the deepest probing depth of the sextant • Smooth surfaces, no calculus, no defective margins • There is bleeding after gentle probing	**Code 1** • Dental biofilm control • Preventive care
Code 2	**Code 2** • Colored area of probe is completely visible in the deepest probing depth • Rough surface felt may be supragingival and/or subgingival calculus • Defective margins of restorations	**Code 2** • Dental biofilm control instruction • Complete preventive care • Calculus removal • Correction of irregular margins of restorations
Code 3	**Code 3** • Colored area of probe is only partly visible in the deepest probing depth • Requirements for Codes 1 and 2 may be present	**Code 3** • Comprehensive periodontal assessment is indicated[‡] • Patient is counseled concerning appropriate treatment plan
Code 4	**Code 4** • Colored area of probe completely disappears • Probing depth greater than 5.5 mm	**Code 4** • Comprehensive periodontal assessment is indicated[†] • Patient is counseled concerning appropriate treatment plan
✱ Clinical Abnormality	**Code✱** • Any notable feature such as furcation involvement • Mobility • Mucogingival problem • Marked recession area	**Code✱** • Abnormality in Codes 0, 1, or 2: specific treatment is planned • In Codes 3 or 4: included in comprehensive assessment and treatment plan

[†]American Dental Association and American Academy of Periodontology, 1992.
[‡]Comprehensive periodontal assessment includes but is not limited to radiographic and clinical examination (complete soft tissue record, identification of probing depths, mobility, gingival recession, mucogingival problems, and furcation involvements).

2. Each code may include conditions identified with the preceding codes; for example, Code 3 with probing depth from 3.5 to 5.5 mm also may include calculus, an overhanging restoration, and bleeding on probing.

3. One need not probe the remaining teeth in a sextant when a Code 4 is found. For Codes 0, 1, 2, and 3, the sextant is completely probed.

D. Recording

1. Use a simple six-box form to provide a space for each sextant. The form can be made into peel-off stickers or a rubber stamp to facilitate recording in the patient's permanent record.

2. One score is marked for each sextant; the highest code observed is recorded. When indicated, an asterisk is added to the score in the individual space with the sextant code number.

IV. SCORING

A. Follow-up Patient Management

Patients are classified into assessment and treatment planning needs by the highest coded score of their PSR (Table 20-1, right column).

B. Calculation Examples

Example 1.

PSR Sextant Score

Interpretation: With Codes 3 and 4, a comprehensive periodontal examination is indicated. Asterisks mean furcation involvement in two quadrants, and a possible mucogingival involvement in the mandibular anterior sextant. When the patient has not been aware of the presence of periodontal involvement, counseling is important if cooperation and compliance are to be obtained.

Example 2.

PSR Sextant Score

Interpretation: An overall Code 2 can indicate calculus and overhanging restorations that must be removed. All restorations must be checked for recurrent dental caries. Appointments for instruction in bacterial plaque control are of primary concern. The asterisks in two quadrants may indicate minimal attached gingiva.

▪ "PLAQUE INDEX" (PL I)

(Silness and Löe[1,5])

I. PURPOSE

To assess the thickness of biofilm at the gingival area.

II. SELECTION OF TEETH

The entire dentition or selected teeth can be evaluated.

A. Areas Examined

Examine four gingival areas (distal, facial, mesial, lingual) systematically for each tooth.

B. Modified Procedures

Examine only the facial, mesial, and lingual areas. Assign double score to the mesial reading, and divide the total by 4.

III. PROCEDURE

A. Dry the teeth and examine visually using adequate light, mouth mirror, and probe or explorer.

B. Evaluate dental biofilm on the cervical third; pay no attention to biofilm that has extended to the middle or incisal thirds.

C. Use probe to test the surface when no biofilm is visible. Pass the probe or explorer across the tooth surface in the cervical third and near the entrance to the sulcus. When no biofilm adheres to the probe tip, the area is scored 0. When biofilm adheres, a score of 1 is assigned.

D. Use a disclosing agent, if necessary, to assist evaluation for the 0 to 1 scores. When the Pl I is used in conjunction with the Gingival Index (GI), the GI must be completed first because the disclosing agent masks the gingival characteristics.

E. Include biofilm on the surface of calculus and on dental restorations in the cervical third in the evaluation.

F. Criteria
   0 = No biofilm.
   1 = a film of biofilm adhering to the free gingival margin and adjacent area of the tooth. The

biofilm may be recognized only after application of disclosing agent or by running the explorer across the tooth surface.

2 = Moderate accumulation of soft deposits within the gingival pocket that can be seen with the naked eye or on the tooth and gingival margin.

3 = Abundance of soft matter within the gingival pocket and/or on the tooth and gingival margin.

IV. SCORING

A. Pl I for Area

Each area (distal, facial, mesial, lingual, or palatal) is assigned a score from 0 to 3.

B. Pl I for a Tooth

Scores for each area are totaled and divided by 4.

C. Pl I for Groups of Teeth

Scores for individual teeth may be grouped and totaled and divided by the number of teeth. For instance, a Pl I may be determined for specific teeth or groups of teeth. The right side may be compared with the left.

D. Pl I for the Individual

Add the scores for each tooth and divide by the number of teeth examined. The Pl I ranges from 0 to 3.

E. Suggested Range of Scores for Patient Reference

Rating	Scores
Excellent	0
Good	0.1–0.9
Fair	1.0–1.9
Poor	2.0–3.0

F. Pl I for a Group

Add the scores for each member of a group and divide by the number of individuals.

■ "PLAQUE CONTROL RECORD"

(O'Leary, Drake, and Naylor[6])

I. PURPOSE

To record the presence of dental biofilm on individual tooth surfaces to permit the patient to visualize progress while learning biofilm control.

II. SELECTION OF TEETH AND SURFACES

A. All teeth are included. Missing teeth are identified on the record form by a single thick horizontal line.

B. Four surfaces are recorded: facial, lingual, mesial, and distal.

C. Six areas may be recorded. The mesial and distal segments of the diagram may be divided to provide space to record proximal surfaces from the facial separately from the lingual or palatal surfaces (Figure 20-2).[7]

III. PROCEDURE

A. Apply disclosing agent or give a chewable tablet. Instruct patient to swish and rub the solution over the tooth surfaces with the tongue before rinsing.

B. Examine each tooth surface for dental biofilm at the gingival margin. No attempt is made to differentiate quantity of biofilm.

C. Record by making a dash or coloring in the appropriate spaces on the diagram (Figure 20-2) to indicate biofilm on facial, lingual, palatal, mesial, and/or distal surfaces.

IV. SCORING

A. Total the number of teeth present; multiply by four (or six if modification is used) to obtain the number of available surfaces. Count the number of surfaces with biofilm.

B. Multiply the number of biofilm-stained surfaces by 100 and divide by the total number of available surfaces to derive the percentage of surfaces with biofilm.

C. Compare over subsequent appointments as the patient learns and practices biofilm control. Ten percent or fewer biofilm-stained surfaces can be considered a good goal, but if the biofilm is regularly left in the same areas, special instruction is indicated to prevent pocket formation.

D. Calculation example for biofilm control record:

Individual findings: 26 teeth scored 8 surfaces with biofilm

1. Multiply the number of teeth by 4:
   $26 \times 4 = 104$ surfaces

2. Percent with biofilm =

$$\frac{\text{Number of surfaces with biofilm} \times 100}{\text{Number of available tooth surfaces}}$$

$$= \frac{8 \times 100}{104} = \frac{800}{104} = 7.6$$

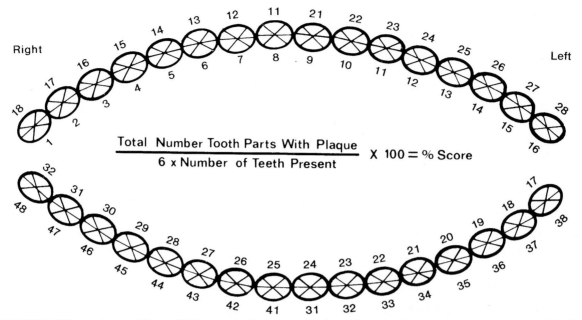

$$\frac{\text{Total Number Tooth Parts With Plaque}}{6 \times \text{Number of Teeth Present}} \times 100 = \% \text{ Score}$$

■ **FIGURE 20-2 "Plaque Control Record."** Diagrammatic representation of the teeth includes spaces to record biofilm on six areas of each tooth. The facial surfaces are on the outer portion and the lingual and palatal surfaces are on the inner portion of the arches. Teeth are numbered by the ADA System on the inside and by the FDI System on the outside. (Modified from Ramfjord, S.P. and Ash, M.M.: *Periodontology and Periodontics.* Philadelphia, W.B. Saunders Co., 1979, p. 273 and from O'Leary, T.J., Drake, R.B., and Naylor, J.E.: *J. Periodontol.,* 43, 38, 1972.)

Interpretation: Although 0% is ideal, fewer than 10% biofilm-stained surfaces has been suggested as a guideline in periodontal therapy. After initial therapy and when the patient has reached a 10% level of biofilm control or better, necessary additional periodontal and restorative procedures may be initiated.[6] In comparison, a similar evaluation using a biofilm-free score would mean that a goal of 90% or better biofilm-free surfaces would have to be reached before the surgical phase of treatment could be undertaken.

■ "PLAQUE-FREE SCORE"

(Grant, Stern, Everett[8])

I. PURPOSE

To determine the location, number, and percentage of biofilm-free surfaces for individual motivation and instruction. Interdental bleeding can also be documented.

II. SELECTION OF TEETH AND SURFACES

A. All erupted teeth are included. Missing teeth are identified on the record form by a single thick horizontal line through the box in the chart form.

B. Four surfaces are recorded for each tooth: facial, lingual or palatal, mesial, and distal.

III. PROCEDURE

A. "Plaque-Free Score"

1. Apply disclosing agent or give chewable tablet. Instruct patient to swish and rub the solution over the tooth surfaces with the tongue before rinsing.

2. Examine each tooth surface for evidence of biofilm. Use adequate light and a mouth mirror for visualizing all surfaces. The patient needs a hand mirror to see the location of the biofilm that has been missed during personal hygiene procedures.

3. Record in red the surfaces showing biofilm. Use an appropriate tooth chart form or a diagrammatic form, such as that shown in Figure 20-3. Red ink for recording the biofilm is suggested when a red disclosing agent is used to help the patient associate the location of the biofilm in the mouth with the recording.

B. Papillary Bleeding on Probing

1. The small circles between the diagrammatic tooth blocks in Figure 20-3 are used to record proximal bleeding on probing.

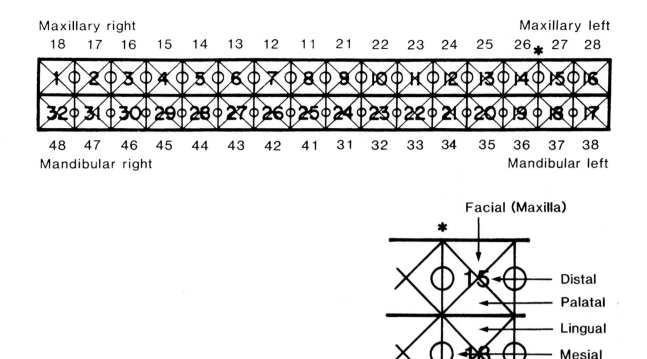

■ **FIGURE 20-3 "Plaque-Free Score."** Diagrammatic representation of the teeth used to record biofilm and papillary bleeding. Enlargement of teeth (*) shows tooth surfaces. Teeth are numbered by the ADA System inside each block and by the FDI System outside each block. (Adapted from Grant, D.A., Stern, I.B., and Listgarten, M.A.: *Periodontics,* 6th ed. St. Louis, Mosby, 1988, p. 613.)

2. Improvement in the gingival tissue health will be demonstrated over a period of time as fewer bleeding areas are noted.

IV. SCORING

A. "Plaque-Free Score"

1. Total the number of teeth present.
2. Total the number of surfaces with biofilm that appear in red on the tooth diagram.
3. Consult Table 20-2:
   a. Read across the top or bottom to locate the number of teeth and total surfaces.
   b. Read down the side to locate the number of surfaces with biofilm.
   c. Find the intersection of the top and side numbers; this number is the biofilm-free score, listed as a percentage.
4. To calculate without Table 20-2 for reference
   a. Multiply the number of teeth by four to determine the number of available surfaces.

   b. Subtract the number of surfaces with biofilm from the total available surfaces to find the number of biofilm-free surfaces.
   c. Biofilm-free score =

   $$\frac{\text{Number of biofilm-free surfaces} \times 100}{\text{Number of available surfaces}}$$

   = Percent biofilm-free surfaces

5. Evaluate biofilm-free score. Ideally, 100% is the goal. When a patient maintains a percentage under 85%, check individual surfaces to determine whether biofilm is usually left in the same areas. To prevent the development of specific areas of periodontal infection, remedial instruction in the areas usually missed is indicated.

B. Papillary Bleeding on Probing

1. Total the number of small circles marked for bleeding. A person with 32 teeth has 30 interdental areas. The mesial or distal surface of a

■ TABLE 20-2 "PLAQUE-FREE SCORE"

NUMBER OF TOOTH SURFACES

Number of Tooth Surfaces With Biofilm

	32–128	31–124	30–120	29–116	28–112	27–108	26–104	25–100	24–96	23–92	22–88	21–84	
1	99.2	99.2	99.2	99.2	99.2	99.1	99.1	99.0	99.0	99.0	98.9	98.9	
4	96.9	96.8	96.7	97.6	96.5	96.3	96.2	96.0	95.9	95.7	95.5	95.3	
7	94.6	95.4	94.2	94.0	93.8	93.6	93.3	93.0	92.8	92.4	92.1	91.7	
10	92.2	92.0	91.7	91.4	91.1	90.8	90.4	90.0	89.6	89.2	88.7	88.1	
13	89.9	89.6	89.2	88.8	88.4	88.0	87.5	87.0	86.5	85.9	85.3	84.5	
16	87.5	87.1	86.7	86.3	85.8	85.2	84.7	84.0	83.4	82.7	81.9	81.0	
19	85.2	84.7	84.2	83.7	83.1	82.5	81.8	81.0	80.3	79.4	78.5	77.4	
22	83.9	82.3	81.7	81.1	80.4	79.7	78.9	78.0	77.1	76.1	75.0	73.9	
25	80.4	79.9	79.2	78.5	77.7	76.9	76.0	75.0	74.0	72.9	71.6	70.3	
28	78.2	77.5	76.7	75.9	75.0	74.1	73.1	72.0	70.9	69.6	68.2	66.4	
31	75.8	75.0	74.2	73.3	72.4	71.3	70.2	69.0	67.8	66.4	64.8	63.1	
34	73.5	72.6	71.7	70.7	69.7	68.6	67.4	66.0	64.6	63.1	61.4	59.6	
37	71.1	70.2	69.2	68.2	67.0	65.8	64.5	63.0	61.5	59.8	58.0	56.0	
40	68.8	67.8	66.7	65.6	64.3	63.0	61.6	60.0	58.4	56.6	54.6	52.4	
43	66.5	65.4	64.2	63.0	61.7	60.2	58.7	57.0	55.3	53.3	51.2	48.9	
46	64.1	63.0	61.7	60.4	59.0	57.5	55.8	54.0	52.1	50.0	47.8	45.3	
49	61.8	60.5	59.2	57.8	56.3	54.7	52.9	51.0	49.0	46.8	44.4	41.7	
52	59.4	58.1	56.7	55.2	53.6	51.9	50.0	48.0	45.9	43.5	41.0	38.1	
55	57.1	55.7	54.2	52.6	50.9	49.1	47.2	45.0	42.8	40.3	37.5	34.6	
58	54.7	53.3	51.7	50.0	48.3	46.3	44.3	42.0	39.6	37.0	34.1	31.0	
61	52.4	50.9	49.2	47.5	45.6	43.6	41.4	39.0	36.4	33.7	30.7	27.4	
64	50.0	48.4	46.7	44.9	42.9	40.8	38.5	36.0	33.4	30.5	27.3	23.9	
67	47.7	46.0	44.2	42.3	40.2	38.0	35.6	33.0	30.3	27.2	23.9	20.3	
70	45.4	43.6	41.7	39.7	37.5	35.2	32.7	30.0	27.1	24.0	20.5	16.7	
73	43.0	41.2	39.2	37.1	34.9	32.5	29.9	27.0	24.0	20.7	17.1	13.1	
76	40.7	38.8	36.7	34.5	32.2	29.7	27.0	24.0	20.9	17.4	13.7	9.6	
79	38.3	36.3	34.2	31.9	29.5	26.9	24.1	21.0	17.8	14.2	10.3	6.0	
82	36.0	33.9	31.7	29.4	26.8	24.1	21.2	18.0	14.6	10.9	6.9	2.4	
85	33.6	31.5	29.2	26.8	24.2	21.3	18.3	15.0	11.5	7.7	3.3	—	
88	31.3	29.1	26.7	24.2	21.5	18.6	15.4	12.0	8.4	4.4	0.0	—	
91	29.0	26.7	24.2	21.6	18.8	15.8	12.5	9.0	5.3	1.1	—	1.3	79
94	27.6	24.2	21.7	19.0	16.1	13.0	9.7	6.0	2.1	—	0.0	5.0	78
97	24.3	21.8	19.2	16.4	13.4	10.2	6.8	3.0	—	—	4.0	8.8	73
100	21.9	19.4	16.7	13.8	10.8	7.5	3.9	0.0	—	2.8	7.9	12.5	70
103	19.9	17.0	14.2	11.3	8.1	4.7	1.0	—	1.5	7.0	11.9	16.3	67
106	17.2	14.6	11.7	8.7	5.4	1.9	—	0.0	5.9	11.2	15.8	20.0	64
109	14.9	12.1	9.2	6.1	2.7	—	—	4.7	10.3	15.3	19.8	23.8	61
112	12.5	9.7	6.7	3.5	0.0	—	3.4	9.4	14.8	19.5	23.7	27.5	58
115	11.2	7.3	4.2	.9	—	1.8	8.4	14.1	19.2	23.7	27.7	31.3	55
118	7.9	4.9	1.7	—	0.0	7.2	13.4	18.8	23.6	27.8	31.6	35.0	52
121	5.5	2.5	—	—	5.8	12.5	18.4	23.5	28.0	32.0	35.6	38.8	49
124	3.2	0.0	—	4.2	11.6	17.9	23.4	28.2	32.4	36.2	39.5	42.5	46
128	0.0	—	2.3	10.5	17.4	23.3	28.4	32.9	36.8	40.3	43.5	46.3	43
	—	0.0	9.1	16.7	23.1	28.6	33.4	37.5	41.2	44.5	47.4	50.0	40
	—	7.5	16.0	23.0	28.9	34.0	38.4	42.2	45.6	48.7	51.4	53.8	37
	5.6	15.0	22.8	29.2	34.7	39.3	43.4	46.9	50.0	52.8	55.3	57.5	34
	13.9	22.5	29.6	35.5	40.4	44.7	48.4	51.6	54.5	57.0	59.3	61.3	31
	22.3	30.0	36.4	41.7	46.2	50.0	53.4	56.3	58.9	61.2	63.2	65.0	28
	30.6	37.5	43.2	48.0	52.0	55.4	58.4	61.0	63.3	65.3	67.2	68.8	25
	38.9	45.0	50.0	54.2	57.7	60.8	63.4	65.7	67.7	69.5	71.1	72.5	22
	47.3	52.5	56.9	60.5	63.5	66.1	68.4	70.4	72.1	73.7	75.0	76.3	19
	55.6	60.0	63.7	66.7	69.3	71.5	73.4	75.0	76.5	78.8	79.0	80.0	16
	63.9	67.5	70.5	73.0	75.0	76.8	78.4	79.7	80.9	82.0	82.9	87.5	13
	72.3	75.0	77.3	79.2	80.8	82.2	83.4	84.4	85.3	86.2	86.9	87.5	10
	80.6	82.5	84.1	85.5	86.6	87.5	88.4	89.1	89.8	90.3	90.8	91.3	7
	88.9	90.0	91.0	91.7	92.4	92.9	93.4	93.8	94.2	94.5	94.8	95.0	4
	97.3	97.5	97.8	98.0	98.1	98.3	98.4	98.5	98.6	98.7	98.7	98.8	1
	9–36	10–40	11–44	12–48	13–52	14–56	15–60	16–64	17–68	18–72	19–76	20–80	

(From Grant, D.A., Stern, I.B., and Everett, F.G.: *Periodontics*, 5th ed. St. Louis, Mosby, 1979.)

tooth adjacent to an edentulous area is probed and counted.

2. Evaluate total interdental bleeding. In health, bleeding on probing does not occur.

C. Calculation Example for "Plaque-Free Score"

Individual findings: 24 teeth scored
                         37 surfaces with biofilm

1. With Table 20-2
    a. Locate the number of teeth across the top of Table 20-2 (24–96); the second number indicates the number of surfaces, which in this case total 96.
    b. Locate the number of surfaces with biofilm down the side (37); find the intersection.
    c. The percentage of biofilm-free surfaces is 61.5%.

2. Without reference to Table 20-2
    a. Multiply the number of teeth by 4:
        24 × 4 = 96 available surfaces
    b. Subtract the number of surfaces with biofilm from total available surfaces:
        96 − 37 = 59 biofilm-free surfaces
    c. Percentage of biofilm-free surfaces:

$$\frac{59 \times 100}{96} = 61.5\%$$

Interpretation: On the basis of the ideal 100%, 61.5% is poor. More instruction is indicated.

■ PATIENT HYGIENE PERFORMANCE (PHP)

(Podshadley and Haley[2])

I. PURPOSE

To assess the extent of biofilm and debris over a tooth surface. Debris is defined for the PHP as the soft foreign material consisting of dental biofilm, materia alba, and food debris that is loosely attached to tooth surfaces.

II. SELECTION OF TEETH AND SURFACES

A. Teeth Examined

(F.D.I. system tooth numbers are in parentheses.)

Maxillary	Mandibular
No. 3 (16) Right first molar	No. 19 (36) Left first molar
No. 8 (11) Right central incisor	No. 24 (31) Left central incisor
No. 14 (26) Left first molar	No. 30 (46) Right first molar

B. Substitutions

When a first molar is missing, is less than three-fourths erupted, has a full crown, or is broken down, the second molar is used. The third molar is used when the second is missing. The adjacent central incisor is used for a missing incisor.

C. Surfaces

The facial surfaces of incisors and maxillary molars and the lingual surfaces of mandibular molars are examined. These surfaces are the same as those used for the Simplified Oral Hygiene Index (see Figure 20-5).

III. PROCEDURE

A. Apply disclosing agent. Instruct the patient to swish for 30 seconds and expectorate, but not rinse.
B. Examination is made using a mouth mirror.
C. Each tooth surface to be evaluated is subdivided (mentally) into five sections (Figure 20-4A) as follows:
    1. *Vertically.* Three divisions—mesial, middle, and distal.
    2. *Horizontally.* The middle third is subdivided into gingival, middle, and occlusal or incisal thirds.
D. Each of the five subdivisions is scored for the presence of stained debris as follows:
    0 = No debris (or questionable).
    1 = Debris definitely present.

Identify by *M* when all three molars or both incisors are missing.

Identify by *S* when a substitute tooth is used.

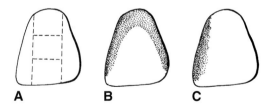

A   **B**   **C**

■ **FIGURE 20-4 Patient Hygiene Performance (PHP).**
(A) Oral debris is assessed by dividing a tooth into 5 subdivisions, each of which is scored 1 when debris is shown to be present after use of a disclosing agent. **(B)** Example of debris score of 3. Shaded portion represents debris stained by disclosing agent. **(C)** Example of debris score of 1. (From Podshadley, A.G. and Haley, J.V.: A Method for Evaluating Oral Hygiene Performance, *Public Health Rep., 83,* 259, 1968.)

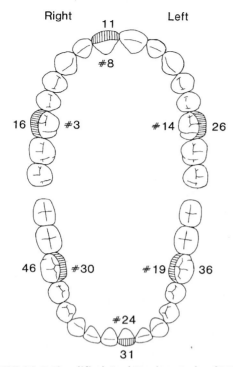

Right   Left

■ **FIGURE 20-5 Simplified Oral Hygiene Index (OHI-S).** Six tooth surfaces are scored as follows: facial surfaces of maxillary molars and of the maxillary right and mandibular left central incisors, and the lingual surfaces of mandibular molars. Teeth are numbered by the ADA System on the lingual surface and by the FDI System on the facial surface.

IV. SCORING

A. Debris Score for Individual Tooth

Add the scores for each of the five subdivisions. The scores range from 0 to 5.

B. PHP for the Individual

Total the scores for the individual teeth and divide by the number of teeth examined. The PHP ranges from 0 to 5.

C. Suggested Range of Scores for Evaluation

Rating	Scores
Excellent	0–(no debris)
Good	0.1–1.7
Fair	1.8–3.4
Poor	3.5–5.0

D. Calculation Example for an Individual

Tooth	Debris Score
No. 3 (16)	5
No. 8 (11)	3
No. 14 (26)	4
No. 19 (36)	5
No. 24 (31)	2
No. 30 (46)	3
Total	22

$$PHP = \frac{Total\ debris\ score}{Number\ of\ teeth\ scored} = \frac{22}{6} = 3.66$$

Interpretation: According to the suggested range of scores, this person with a PHP of 3.66 would be classified as exhibiting poor hygiene performance.

E. PHP for a Group

To obtain the average PHP score for a group or population, total the individual scores and divide by the number of people examined.

■ SIMPLIFIED ORAL HYGIENE INDEX (OHI-S)

(Greene and Vermillion[9] and Greene[10])

I. PURPOSE

To assess oral cleanliness by estimating the tooth surface covered with debris and/or calculus.

II. COMPONENTS

The OHI-S has two components, the Simplified Debris Index (DI-S) and the Simplified Calculus Index (CI-S). The two scores may be used separately or may be combined for the OHI-S.

III. SELECTION OF TEETH AND SURFACES

A. Identify the Six Specific Teeth (Figure 20-5)

1. *Posterior.* The first fully erupted tooth distal to each second premolar is examined. The facial surfaces of the maxillary molars and the lingual surfaces of the mandibular molars are used. Although usually the first molars are used, the second or third molars also may be used.
2. *Anterior.* The facial surfaces of the maxillary right and the mandibular left central incisors are used. When either is missing, the adjacent central incisor is scored.

B. Extent

A score represents half the circumference of the selected tooth; it includes proximal surfaces to the contact areas.

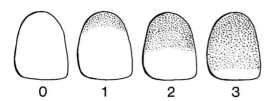

■ **FIGURE 20-6 Simplified Oral Hygiene Index.** For the Debris Index, 6 teeth (Figure 20-5) are scored. Scoring of 0 to 3 is based on tooth surfaces covered by debris as shown.

IV. PROCEDURE

A. Qualification

At least two of the six possible surfaces must have been examined for an individual score to be calculated.

B. Record Six Debris Scores

1. *Definition of Oral Debris.* Oral debris is the soft foreign matter on the surfaces of the teeth that consists of dental biofilm, materia alba, and food debris.
2. *Examination.* Run the side of the tip of a probe or explorer across the tooth surface to estimate the surface area covered by debris.
3. *Criteria* (Figure 20-6)
   0 = No debris or stain present.
   1 = Soft debris covering not more than one third of the tooth surface being examined, or the presence of extrinsic stains without debris, regardless of surface area covered.
   2 = Soft debris covering more than one third but not more than two thirds of the exposed tooth surface.
   3 = Soft debris covering more than two thirds of the exposed tooth surface.

C. Record Six Calculus Scores

1. *Definition of Calculus.* Dental calculus is a hard deposit of inorganic salts composed primarily of calcium carbonate and phosphate mixed with debris, microorganisms, and desquamated epithelial cells.
2. *Examination.* Use an explorer to estimate surface area covered by supragingival calculus deposits. Identify subgingival deposits by exploring and/or probing. Record only definite deposits of hard calculus.
3. *Criteria* (Figure 20-7)
   0 = No calculus present.
   1 = Supragingival calculus covering not more than one third of the exposed tooth surface being examined.

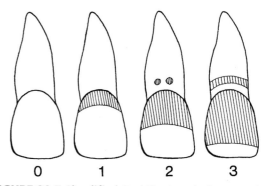

■ **FIGURE 20-7 Simplified Oral Hygiene Index.** For the Calculus Index, 6 teeth (Figure 20-5) are scored. Scoring of 0 to 3 is based on location and tooth surface area with calculus as shown. Note slight subgingival calculus recorded as 2 and more extensive subgingival calculus as 3.

   2 = Supragingival calculus covering more than one third but not more than two thirds of the exposed tooth surface, or the presence of individual flecks of subgingival calculus around the cervical portion of the tooth.
   3 = Supragingival calculus covering more than two thirds of the exposed tooth surface or a continuous heavy band of subgingival calculus around the cervical portion of the tooth.

V. SCORING

A. OHI-S for an Individual

1. *Determine Simplified Debris Index (DI-S) and Simplified Calculus Index (CI-S)*
   a. Divide total scores by number of sextants.
   b. DI-S and CI-S values range from 0 to 3.
2. *Simplified Oral Hygiene Index (OHI-S)*
   a. Combine the DI-S and CI-S.
   b. OHI-S value ranges from 0 to 6.

B. Suggested Range of Scores for Evaluation[10]

DI-S and CI-S

Rating	Scores
Excellent	0
Good	0.1–0.6
Fair	0.7–1.8
Poor	1.9–3.0

OHI-S

Rating	Scores
Excellent	0
Good	0.1–1.2
Fair	1.3–3.0
Poor	3.1–6.0

C. Calculation Example for an Individual

Tooth	DI-S	CI-S *Score*
No. 3 (16)	2	2
No. 8 (11)	1	0
No. 14 (26)	3	2
No. 19 (36)	3	2
No. 24 (31)	2	1
No. 30 (46)	2	2
Total	13	9

$$DI\text{-}S = \frac{\text{Total debris scores}}{\text{Number of teeth scored}} = \frac{13}{6} = 2.17$$

$$CI\text{-}S = \frac{\text{Total calculus scores}}{\text{Number of teeth scored}} = \frac{9}{6} = 1.50$$

$$OHI\text{-}S = DI\text{-}S + CI\text{-}S = 2.17 + 1.50 = 3.67$$

Interpretation: According to the suggested range of scores, the score for this individual (3.67) indicates a poor oral hygiene status.

D. OHI-S Group Score

Compute the average of the individual scores by totaling the scores and dividing by the number of individuals.

▪ BLEEDING INDICES

Bleeding on gentle probing or flossing is an early sign of gingival inflammation and precedes color changes and enlargement of the gingival tissues.[11,12] Based on the principle that healthy tissue does not bleed, testing for bleeding has become a significant procedure for evaluation prior to treatment planning, after therapy to show the effects of treatment, and at maintenance appointments to determine continued control of gingival inflammation.

For patient instruction and motivation, a variety of bleeding indices and scoring methods has been developed. The Gingival Index (GI) includes an estimate of bleeding on probing, along with other clinical observations to score the severity of gingivitis. The GI has been used extensively in research, as well as for patient instruction and motivation.

Another example is a "plaque-free score." The form illustrated in Figure 20-3 has small circles that can be colored to illustrate interproximal bleeding. A series of diagrams made over several weeks can show the patient's progress toward health, as less and less bleeding is charted.

Bleeding indices described here are the Sulcus Bleeding Index developed by Mühlemann, the Gingival Bleeding Index of Carter and Barnes, and the Eastman Interdental Bleeding Index.

▪ SULCUS BLEEDING INDEX (SBI)

(Mühlemann and Son[11])

I. PURPOSE

To locate areas of gingival sulcus bleeding upon gentle probing and thus recognize and record the presence of early (initial) inflammatory gingival disease.

II. AREAS EXAMINED

Four gingival units are scored systematically for each tooth: the labial and lingual marginal gingivae (M units), and the mesial and distal papillary gingivae (P units).

III. PROCEDURE

A. Use standardized lighting while probing each of the four areas.
B. Hold the probe parallel with the long axis of the tooth for M units, and direct the probe toward the col area for P units.
C. Wait 30 seconds after probing before scoring apparently healthy gingival units.
D. Dry the gingivae gently if necessary to observe color changes clearly.
E. Criteria
0 = Healthy appearance of P and M, no bleeding on sulcus probing.
1 = Apparently healthy P and M showing no change in color and no swelling, but bleeding from sulcus on probing.
2 = Bleeding on probing *and* change of color caused by inflammation. No swelling or macroscopic edema.
3 = Bleeding on probing *and* change in color and slight edematous swelling.
4 = (1) Bleeding on probing *and* change in color *and* obvious swelling.
(2) Bleeding on probing and obvious swelling.
5 = Bleeding on probing and spontaneous bleeding *and* change in color, marked swelling with or without ulceration.

IV. SCORING

A. SBI for Area

Each of the four gingival units (M and P) is scored 0 to 5.

B. SBI for Tooth

Scores for the four units are totaled and divided by four.

C. SBI for Individual

By totaling scores for individual teeth and dividing by the number of teeth, the SBI is determined. Indices range from 0 to 5.

▪ GINGIVAL BLEEDING INDEX (GBI)

(Carter and Barnes[13])

I. PURPOSE

To record the presence or absence of gingival inflammation as determined by bleeding from interproximal gingival sulci.

II. AREAS EXAMINED

Each interproximal area has two sulci, which are scored as one interdental unit or individually. Certain areas may be excluded from scoring because of accessibility, tooth position, diastemata, or other factors, and if exclusions are made, a consistent procedure should be followed for an individual and for a group if a study is to be made.

A full complement of teeth has 30 proximal areas. In the original studies, third molars were excluded, and 26 interdental units were recorded.[13]

III. PROCEDURE

A. Instrument

Unwaxed dental floss is used. Floss has the advantages of being readily available, disposable, and usable by the instructed patient.

B. Steps

1. Pass the floss interproximally first on one side of the papilla and then on the other.
2. Curve the floss around the adjacent tooth, and bring the floss below the gingival margin.
3. Move the floss up and down for one stroke, with care not to lacerate the gingiva. Adapt finger rests to provide controlled, consistent pressure.
4. Use a new length of clean floss for each area.
5. Retract for visibility of bleeding from both facial and lingual aspects.
6. Allow 30 seconds for reinspection of an area that does not show blood immediately either in the area or on the floss.

C. Criteria

Bleeding indicates the presence of disease. No attempt is made to quantify the severity of bleeding because no bleeding represents health.

IV. SCORING

The numbers of bleeding areas and scorable units are recorded. Patient participation in observing and recording over a series of appointments can increase motivation.

▪ EASTMAN INTERDENTAL BLEEDING INDEX (EIBI)

(Abrams, Caton, and Polson[14] and Caton and Polson[15])

I. PURPOSE

To assess the presence of inflammation in the interdental area by the presence or absence of bleeding.

II. AREAS EXAMINED

Each interdental area around the entire dentition.

III. PROCEDURE

A. Instrument

Triangular wooden interdental cleaner.

B. Steps

1. Insert gently, then immediately remove, a wooden cleaner into each interdental area in such a way as to depress the papilla 1 to 2 mm (Figure 20-8).
2. Make the path of insertion horizontal (parallel to the occlusal surface), taking care not to angle the point in an apical direction.
3. Insert and remove four times; move to next interproximal area.
4. Record the presence or absence of bleeding within 15 seconds for each area.

IV. SCORING

A. Number of Bleeding Sites

The number may be totaled for an individual score for comparison with scores over a series of appointments.

B. Percentage Scores

Index is expressed as a percentage of the total number of sites evaluated. Calculations can be made for total mouth, quadrants, or maxillary versus mandibular.

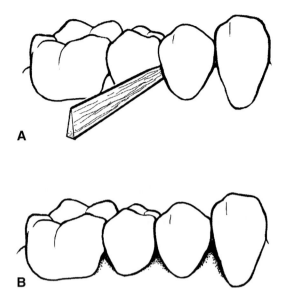

■ FIGURE 20-8 Eastman Interdental Bleeding Index. The test for interdental bleeding is made by inserting a wooden interdental cleaner into each interdental space. **(A)** Wooden interdental cleaner inserted in a horizontal path, parallel with the occlusal surfaces. **(B)** The presence or absence of bleeding is noted within a quadrant 15 seconds after final insertion. Bleeding indicates the presence of inflammation.

C. Calculation Example

An adult with a complete dentition has 15 maxillary and 15 mandibular interproximal areas. The EIBI revealed 13 areas of bleeding. To calculate percentage:

$$\frac{\text{Number of bleeding areas}}{\text{Total number of areas}} \times 100 = \text{Percent bleeding area}$$

$$\frac{13}{30} \times 100 = 43\% \text{ (EIBI expressed by \%)}$$

■ GINGIVAL/PERIODONTAL INDICES

Measurements for gingival and periodontal indices have varied over the years. Historically, the P-M-A (Papillary-Marginal-Attached) index is attributed to Schour and Massler,[16,17] two outstanding teacher-researchers. They developed the P-M-A to assess the extent of gingival changes in large groups for epidemiologic studies.

The Periodontal Index (PI) of Russell[18] was another acclaimed contribution to the study of disease incidence. As a complex index that accounted for both gingival and periodontal changes, its aim was to survey large populations.

For screening, the PSR is illustrated in Table 20-1. In this section, the Gingival Index (GI) of Löe and Silness[19] and the Community Periodontal Index of Treatment Needs (CPITN)[20,21] are described.

■ GINGIVAL INDEX (GI)

(Löe and Silness[5,19])

I. PURPOSE

To assess the severity of gingivitis based on color, consistency, and bleeding on probing.

II. SELECTION OF TEETH AND GINGIVAL AREAS

A gingival index may be determined for selected teeth or for the entire dentition.

A. Areas Examined

Four gingival areas (distal, facial, mesial, lingual) are examined systematically for each tooth.

B. Modified Procedure

The distal examination for each tooth can be omitted. The score for the mesial area is doubled, and the total score for each tooth is divided by four.

III. PROCEDURE

A. Dry the teeth and gingivae; under adequate light, use a mouth mirror and probe.
B. Use the probe to press on the gingivae to determine the degree of firmness.
C. Use the probe to run along the soft tissue wall near the entrance to the gingival sulcus to evaluate bleeding (Figure 20-9).

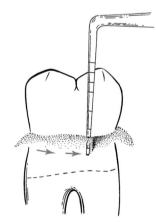

■ FIGURE 20-9 Gingival Index (GI). Probe stroke for bleeding evaluation. The broken line represents the level of attachment of the periodontal tissues. The probe is inserted a few millimeters and moved along the soft tissue pocket wall with light pressure in a circumferential direction. The stroke shown here is in contrast with the walking stroke used for probing depth evaluation and measurement.

D. Criteria

    0 = Normal gingivae.

    1 = Mild inflammation—slight change in color, slight edema. *No bleeding on probing.*

    2 = Moderate inflammation—redness, edema, and glazing. *Bleeding on probing.*

    3 = Severe inflammation—marked redness and edema. Ulceration. *Tendency to spontaneous bleeding.*

IV. SCORING

A. GI for Area

Each of the four gingival surfaces (distal, facial, mesial, lingual) is given a score of 0 to 3.

B. GI for a Tooth

Scores for each area are totaled and divided by four.

C. GI for Groups of Teeth

Scores for individual teeth may be grouped and totaled, and divided by the number of teeth. A GI may be determined for specific teeth, group of teeth, quadrant, or side of mouth.

D. GI for the Individual

By totaling scores and dividing by the number of teeth examined, the GI is determined. Indices range from 0 to 3.

E. Suggested Range of Scores for Patient Reference

Rating	Scores
Excellent (healthy tissue)	0
Good	0.1–1.0
Fair	1.1–2.0
Poor	2.1–3.0

F. Calculation Example for an Individual

(Using six teeth for an example of screening; teeth selected are known as the Ramfjord Index Teeth.[22])

	M	F	D	L
3 (16)	3	1	3	1
9 (21)	1	0	1	1
12 (24)	2	1	2	0
19 (36)	3	1	3	3
25 (41)	1	1	1	1
28 (44)	2	1	2	0
Total	12	5	12	6 = 35

$$\text{Gingival index} = \frac{\text{Total score}}{\text{Number of surfaces}}$$

$$= \frac{35}{24} = 1.45 \text{ GI}$$

Interpretation: According to the suggested range of scores, the score for this individual (1.45) indicates only fair gingival health (moderate inflammation). The ratings for each gingival area or surface can be used to help the patient compare gingival changes and improve oral hygiene procedures.

G. GI for a Group

Add the individual GI scores and divide by the number of individuals examined.

■ COMMUNITY PERIODONTAL INDEX OF TREATMENT NEEDS (CPITN)

(Fédération Dentaire Internationale[20] and Ainamo et al[21])

I. PURPOSE

To screen and monitor individual or group periodontal treatment needs.

II. SELECTION OF TEETH

A. Adults (20 years and older)

1. Divide the dentition into sextants. Evaluate all teeth.
   a. Posterior sextants begin distal to canines.
   b. A sextant must have two or more functional teeth. A functional tooth is not indicated for extraction. When only one functional tooth is present, it is assessed with the adjacent sextant. The sextant with no teeth or one tooth is recorded as missing and marked X on the record form.
2. Third molars are included only when they function in place of second molars.

B. Children and Adolescents (7 to 19 years of age)

1. Divide the dentition into sextants.
2. Evaluate one tooth per sextant: all first molars, maxillary right central incisor, and mandibular left central incisor.[20]
3. When a designated tooth is missing, the sextant is recorded as missing and marked with an X.

III. PROCEDURE

A. Instrument: Specially Designed Probe for CPITN and PSR (Figure 20-1)

1. *Markings.* At intervals from tip: 3.5, 2.0, 3.0, and 3.0 mm (total 11.5 mm).
2. *Working Tip.* A ball 0.5 mm in diameter. The functions of the ball tip are
   a. To aid in detection of calculus and other tooth surface roughness.
   b. To facilitate assessment of the base of the pocket and reduce the risk of overmeasurement.
3. *Color-Coding.* Color-coded between 3.5 and 5.5 mm.

B. Probe Application

1. Objectives are to determine probing depth, bleeding response, and presence of calculus.
2. Insert probe into sulcus/pocket gently. Keep light contact with tooth surface to detect calculus; use a pressure no greater than 15 to 25 grams to reveal disease without causing patient discomfort.
3. Observe color-coded area for prompt identification of probing depth below 3.5 mm, between 3.5 and 5.5 mm (within the color-coded zone), and above the 5.5-mm level to facilitate classification.

C. Criteria

Five codes are used. Each includes conditions identified with the preceding codes; for example, Code 3 with 4- or 5-mm pockets includes calculus and bleeding, typical of Codes 1 and 2.

Code 0 = Healthy periodontal tissues.
Code 1 = Bleeding after gentle probing.
Code 2 = Supragingival or subgingival calculus or defective margin of filling or crown.
Code 3 = 4- or 5-mm pocket.
Code 4 = 6-mm or deeper pathologic pocket.

D. Recording

1. Use a simple box chart for recording. The chart can be made into stick-on labels or a rubber stamp to facilitate the recording procedure on any examination form or individual patient record.
2. Place X for missing sextant.
3. Mark one score to represent each sextant. Record only the highest code that corresponds with the most severe condition.
4. Do not examine remaining teeth in a sextant after a Code 4 has been recorded.
5. The use of only Codes 0, 1, and 2 for patients aged 7 to 11 years may be advisable because of frequent occurrence of gingival ("false") pockets

without attachment loss. The possibility of periodontal disease with attachment loss, however, should not be overlooked in young patients, nor should the need to treat deep gingival pockets.

IV. SCORING

A. Periodontal Treatment Needs

Patients are classified (0, I, II, III) into treatment needs according to the highest coded score recorded during the examination.

0 = No need for treatment (Code 0).
I = Oral hygiene instruction (Code 1).
II = Oral hygiene instruction plus scaling and root planing, including elimination of plaque-retentive margins of fillings and crowns (Codes 2 and 3).
III = I + II + complex periodontal therapy that may include surgical intervention and/or deep scaling and root planing with local anesthesia (Code 4).

B. CPITN for an Individual

1. **Example 1.**

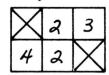

Interpretation: Two sextants are marked as missing (X). Codes 2, 3, and 4 indicate need for thorough periodontal examination, charting, and detailed treatment plan.

2. **Example 2.**

3	0	3
3	1	3

Interpretation: Code 1 indicates need for improved oral hygiene. Code 3 indicates need for scaling and root planing after a complete periodontal examination and charting.

C. CPITN for Groups

The recordings for a group may be presented in a variety of ways, such as the following[21]:

1. Treatment needs can be reported as the number or percentage of subjects in each treatment need category.
2. Mean number of sextants with bleeding, calculus, and moderate or deep pockets for each age group can be shown.

3. To identify high and low priorities for treatment in a community, calculations of the number and percentage of individuals with the following can be made:
   a. No sextant scoring each code.
   b. 1 to 2 sextants scoring Code 1, 2, 3, or 4.
   c. 3 to 4 sextants scoring Code 1, 2, 3, or 4.
   d. 5 to 6 sextants scoring Code 1, 2, 3, or 4.

■ DENTAL CARIES INDICES

The most widely used indices are DMFT (Decayed, Missing, Filled Teeth) and DMFS (Decayed, Missing, Filled Surfaces) for permanent teeth.[3] Their counterparts deft (decayed, extracted, filled teeth) and defs (decayed, extracted, filled surfaces) are used for the primary teeth.[23] For a mixed dentition, two separate indices are indicated, one for the permanent teeth and another for the primary teeth.

The indices show the number of persons affected by dental caries, the number of teeth that need treatment, and the proportion of teeth that have been treated.

■ DECAYED, MISSING, AND FILLED PERMANENT TEETH (DMFT)[24]

(Klein, Palmer, and Knutson[3])

I. PURPOSE

To determine total dental caries experience, past and present.

II. SELECTION OF TEETH

A. DMFT Is Based on 28 Teeth

B. Teeth Not Counted

1. Third molars.
2. Unerupted teeth. A tooth is considered erupted when any part projects through the gingiva. Certain types of research may require differentiation between clinical emergence, partial eruption, and full eruption.
3. Congenitally missing and supernumerary teeth.
4. Teeth removed for reasons other than dental caries, such as an impaction or during orthodontic treatment.
5. Teeth restored for reasons other than dental caries, such as trauma (fracture), cosmetic purposes, or use as a bridge abutment.
6. Primary tooth retained with the permanent successor erupted. The permanent tooth is evaluated because a primary tooth is never included in this index.

III. PROCEDURES

A. Instruments

Each tooth is examined in a systematic sequence, using a mouth mirror and adequate light. Explorers with standardized dimensions of the working ends are needed for consistency.

B. Examination

1. *Use of Explorer.* Teeth should be observed by visual means as much as possible. Unnecessary discomfort for the patient can be avoided by exploring only questionable small lesions.
2. *Criteria for Identification of Dental Caries.* In brief, for a dental caries index, a tooth can be considered carious when
   a. The lesion is clinically visible and obvious.
   b. The explorer tip can penetrate into soft, yielding material.
   c. Discoloration or loss of translucency typical of undermined or demineralized enamel is apparent.
   d. The explorer tip in a pit or fissure resists removal after moderate to firm pressure on insertion.

C. Criteria for Recording[24]

1. *Each Tooth Is Recorded Once.*
2. *"D" Recordings*
   a. When both dental caries and a restoration are present, the tooth is listed as D.
   b. When a crown is broken down as a result of dental caries, it may be recorded as D.
3. *"M" Recordings.* A tooth is considered missing
   a. When it has been extracted because of dental caries.
   b. When it is carious, nonrestorable, and indicated for extraction.
4. *"F" Recordings*
   a. Permanent and temporary fillings are recorded as F.
   b. A tooth with a defective filling but without evidence of dental caries is recorded as F.

IV. SCORING

A. Individual DMFT

1. Total each component separately.
2. Total D + M + F = DMF

Example:
a. $D = 3, M = 2, F = 5$
    $DMF = 3 + 2 + 5 = 10$
b. A DMF of 10 may have different derivations. An individual who had regular dental care may have a distribution: $D = 0, M = 0, F = 10$.

B. Group Average

1. Total the DMFs for each individual examined.
2. Divide the total DMFs by the number of individuals in the group.
    Example: 30 individuals with a total DMF of 210.

$$\frac{210}{30} = 7.0 = \text{average DMF for the group}$$

3. This DMF average represents accumulated dental caries experience. It can be presented by age groups.

C. Specific Treatment Needs of a Group

1. To calculate the percentage of DMF teeth needing restorations, divide the total D component by the total DMFT.
    Example: $D = 175, M = 55, F = 18$
    Total DMFT = 248

$$\frac{D}{DMF} = \frac{175}{248} = \begin{array}{l} 0.70 \text{ or } 70\% \text{ of the teeth} \\ \text{need restorations} \end{array}$$

2. To calculate the percent of *all* teeth lost by extraction because of dental caries: 20 individuals have $28 \times 20 = 560$ permanent teeth.

$$\frac{M}{\text{Total teeth}} = \frac{55}{560} = \begin{array}{l} 0.09 \text{ or } 9\% \text{ of all their teeth} \\ \text{lost because of dental caries} \end{array}$$

3. The same type of calculation can be used to determine the percentage of filled teeth.

▪ DECAYED, MISSING, AND FILLED PERMANENT TOOTH SURFACES (DMFS)[24]

(Klein, Palmer, and Knutson[3])

I. PURPOSE

To determine total dental caries experience, past and present, by recording tooth surfaces involved instead of teeth, as in the DMFT previously described.

II. SELECTION OF TEETH AND SURFACES

A. Teeth Not Counted

The same as listed for the DMFT.

B. Surfaces

1. *Posterior Teeth.* Each tooth has five surfaces examined and recorded: facial, lingual, mesial, distal, and occlusal.
2. *Anterior Teeth.* Each tooth has four surfaces for evaluation: facial, lingual, mesial, and distal.
3. *Total Surface Count for a DMFS.* 128 surfaces. Of 28 teeth, 16 are posterior ($16 \times 5 = 80$) and 12 are anterior ($12 \times 4 = 48$).
4. *Missing Posterior Teeth.* Recorded as five surfaces. The number of surfaces that were carious before extraction usually cannot be determined.

III. PROCEDURES

The same criteria for instruments and examination apply as listed previously for DMFT. In all surveys, specific criteria must be predetermined.

IV. SCORING

A. Individual DMFS

Teeth present = 24 (4 teeth have not yet erupted)
D (surfaces) = 3, M = 0, F (surfaces) = 8
DMFS = D + M + F = 3 + 0 + 8 = 11

B. Group DMFS

A group of 20 individuals 15 to 18 years old lives in a community with fluoridated water. All have lived there continuously except three who moved there from a nonfluoridated town after reaching 12 years of age. The following data show the distribution of DMFS:

10 individuals (each with 0 DMFS)	0
7 individuals (DMFS = 2,2,3,3,3,3,4)	20
3 individuals who had not lived continuously in the area (DMFS = 9,12,12)	33
Total DMFS	53

$$\text{Average DMFS for the group} = \frac{53}{20} = 2.65$$

Interpretation: The differences between those who had not lived with fluoridation are notable. The two groups should be presented separately because of the wide difference. The group average DMFS is 2.65, whereas the DMFS for those who lived in the fluoridated area all their lives is 1.18, and the DMFS for the other three is 11.0.

▪ DECAYED, INDICATED FOR EXTRACTION, AND FILLED PRIMARY TEETH OR SURFACES (dft AND dfs) (deft AND defs)[23]

(Gruebbel[23])

I. PURPOSE

To determine the dental caries experience as shown for the primary teeth present in the oral cavity by evaluating teeth or surfaces.

II. SELECTION OF TEETH OR SURFACES

A. deft or dft

20 teeth evaluated.

B. defs or dfs

88 surfaces evaluated.
1. *Posterior Teeth.* Each has five surfaces: facial, lingual or palatal, mesial, distal, and occlusal. (8 teeth × 5 surfaces = 40 surfaces.)
2. *Anterior Teeth.* Each has four surfaces: facial, lingual or palatal, mesial, and distal. (12 teeth × 4 surfaces = 48 surfaces.)

C. Teeth Not Counted

1. Missing teeth, including unerupted and congenitally missing.
2. Supernumerary teeth.
3. Teeth restored for reasons other than dental caries are not counted as f.

III. PROCEDURE

A. Instruments and Examination

Same as for DMFT.

B. Criteria for Identification of Dental Caries

Same as for DMFT.

C. Criteria for def

d = number of primary teeth or surfaces with dental caries but not restored.

e = number of teeth indicated for extraction because of dental caries.

f = number of filled primary teeth on surfaces that do not have dental caries (each surface is scored once only, "d" has first score).

D. Difference Between deft/defs and dft/dfs

In the deft and defs, both "d" and "e" are used to describe teeth with dental caries. Thus, d and e are sometimes combined, and the index becomes the "dft" or "dfs."

IV. SCORING

A. Individual dft

A 2 1/2-year-old child with nursing caries has 18 teeth. Teeth A (55) and J (65) are unerupted. There is no sign of dental caries in teeth M (73), N (72), O (71), P (81), Q (82), and R (83). All other teeth have two carious surfaces each, except B (54), which is broken down to the gum line.

Summary: Total teeth = 18
Caries-free = 6
"d" teeth = 12
"f" teeth = 0
dft = d + f = 12 + 0 = 12

Interpretation: 12 of 18 teeth with carious lesions indicates a serious need for dental treatment and a prevention program for the child.

B. Individual dfs

Using the same 2 1/2-year-old child to calculate dfs:
Total number of carious surfaces: 11 × 2 = 22
Tooth B: 1 × 5 = 5
Total dfs 27

Interpretation: The child has 48 anterior surfaces (12 teeth × 4 surfaces) and 30 posterior surfaces (6 teeth × 5 surfaces) to total 78 surfaces.

$$\frac{dfs}{\text{Number of surfaces}} = \frac{27}{78}$$

$$= \begin{array}{l} 0.34 \text{ or } 34\% \text{ of the surface} \\ \text{in need of dental treatment} \end{array}$$

C. Mixed Dentition

A DMFT or DMFS and a deft or defs are never added together. Each child is given a separate index for permanent teeth and another for primary teeth. The index for the permanent teeth is usually determined first, and then the index for the primary teeth is prepared separately.

Everyday Ethics

Susanna began practicing in the team clinic at the dental school and found the work to be very challenging. As a hygienist she was not only performing preventive treatment on maintenance patients but was also responsible for data collection for several research projects. Suddenly, the importance of understanding and calculating the various indices became critical. In particular, Susanna found herself reviewing the procedures for the OHI-S, bleeding indices, and the DMFT.

Susanna had always enjoyed her clinical interactions with patients, but now scoring and recording information on each and every tooth was beginning to cause her some stress. Generally Susanna worked without an assistant, and one day while recording the findings on a patient for Dr. Lowe's caries study she omitted several surfaces of the teeth. This was the patient's final visit to the dental school, so Susanna contemplated what to do when she realized the missing data at the end of day.

Questions for Consideration

1. According to the ADHA code, what role was the hygienist performing by collecting data on patients?

2. Can Susanna 'defend' her actions to Dr. Lowe by submitting the data she does have on the patient? Explain your rationale.

3. Which of the core values or principles of ethical behavior come into play in collecting research data such as described in this scenario?

▪ DECAYED, MISSING, AND FILLED PRIMARY TEETH (dmft OR dmfs)

(Gruebbel[23])

I. PURPOSE

To determine dental caries experience past and present for children older than 7 and up to 11 or 12 years of age.

II. SELECTION OF TEETH OR SURFACES

A. dmft: 12 teeth evaluated (8 primary molars; 4 primary canines).
B. dmfs: 56 surfaces evaluated.
   1. Primary molars: 8×5 surfaces each = 40.
   2. Primary canines: 4×4 surfaces each = 16.
C. A primary molar or canine is presumed missing because of dental caries when it has been lost before the normal exfoliation time.
D. Each tooth is counted only once. When both dental caries and a restoration are present, the tooth or surface is listed as *d*, dental caries.

III. PROCEDURE

A. Instruments and examination are the same as for DMFT or DMFS.
B. Criteria for dmft or dmfs
   d = number of primary molars and canines or number of surfaces that are carious (decayed).
   m = number of primary molars and canines missing.
   f = number of filled primary molars and canines without caries (teeth or surfaces).

IV. SCORING

A. Individual dmf

A 5-year-old boy has all primary molars and canines present.
   Examination reveals d = 2, m = 0, f = 1
   dmf = d + m + f = 2 + 0 + 1 = 3 dmf

B. Mixed Dentition

Permanent and primary teeth are evaluated separately. A DMFT or DMFS and a dmft and a dmfs are never added together.

✔ Factors To Teach The Patient

- How an index is used and calculated, and what the scores mean.

- Correlation of index scores with current oral health practices and procedures.

- Procedures to follow to improve index scores and bring the oral tissues to health.

REFERENCES

1. **Silness,** J. and Löe, H.: Periodontal Disease in Pregnancy. II. Correlation Between Oral Hygiene and Periodontal Condition, *Acta Odontol. Scand., 22,* 121, No. 1, 1964.

2. **Podshadley,** A.G. and Haley, J.V.: A Method for Evaluating Oral Hygiene Performance, *Public Health Rep., 83,* 259, March, 1968.

3. **Klein,** H., Palmer, C.E., and Knutson, J.W.: Studies on Dental Caries. I. Dental Status and Dental Needs of Elementary School Children, *Public Health Rep., 53,* 751, May 13, 1938.

4. **American Academy of Periodontology and American Dental Association:** *Periodontal Screening & Recording.* Sponsored by Procter & Gamble, June, 1992.

5. **Löe,** H.: The Gingival Index, the Plaque Index and the Retention Index Systems, *J. Periodontol., 38,* 610, November–December, 1967 (Part II).

6. **O'Leary,** T.J., Drake, R.B., and Naylor, J.E.: The Plaque Control Record, *J. Periodontol., 43,* 38, January, 1972.

7. **Ramfjord,** S.P. and Ash, M.M.: *Periodontology and Periodontics.* Philadelphia, W.B. Saunders Co., 1979, p. 273.

8. **Grant,** D.A., Stern, I.B., and Everett, F.G.: *Periodontics,* 5th ed. St. Louis, Mosby, 1979, pp. 529–531.

9. **Greene,** J.C. and Vermillion, J.R.: The Simplified Oral Hygiene Index, *J. Am. Dent. Assoc., 68,* 7, January, 1964.

10. **Greene,** J.C.: The Oral Hygiene Index—Development and Uses, *J. Periodontol., 38,* 625, November–December, 1967 (Part II).

11. **Mühlemann,** H.R. and Son, S.: Gingival Sulcus Bleeding—A Leading Symptom in Initial Gingivitis, *Helv. Odontol. Acta, 15,* 107, October, 1971.

12. **Meitner,** S.W., Zander, H.A., Iker, H.P., and Polson, A.M.: Identification of Inflamed Gingival Surfaces, *J. Clin. Periodontol., 6,* 93, April, 1979.

13. **Carter,** H.G. and Barnes, G.P.: The Gingival Bleeding Index, *J. Periodontol., 45,* 801, November, 1974.

14. **Abrams,** K., Caton, J., and Polson, A.: Histologic Comparisons of Interproximal Gingival Tissues Related to the Presence or Absence of Bleeding, *J. Periodontol., 55,* 629, November, 1984.

15. **Caton,** J.G. and Polson, A.M.: The Interdental Bleeding Index: A Simplified Procedure for Monitoring Gingival Health, *Compend. Cont. Educ. Dent., 6,* 88, February, 1985.

16. **Schour,** I. and Massler, M.: Prevalence of Gingivitis in Young Adults, *J. Dent. Res., 27,* 733, Abstract No. 33, December, 1948.

17. **Massler,** M.: The P-M-A Index for the Assessment of Gingivitis, *J. Periodontol., 38,* 592, November–December, 1967 (Part II).

18. **Russell,** A.L.: A System of Classification and Scoring for Prevalence Surveys of Periodontal Disease, *J. Dent. Res., 35,* 350, June, 1956.

19. **Löe,** H. and Silness, J.: Periodontal Disease in Pregnancy. I. Prevalence and Severity, *Acta Odontol. Scand., 21,* 533, No. 6, 1963.

20. **Fédération Dentaire Internationale:** A Simplified Periodontal Examination for Dental Practices, FDI WG6 and Joint FDI/WHO WG1, Fédération Dentaire Internationale, 64 Wimpole Street, London, WIM 8AL.

21. **Ainamo,** J., Barmes, D., Beagrie, G., Cutress, T., Martin, J., and Sardo-Infirri, J.: Development of the World Health Organization (WHO) Community Periodontal Index of Treatment Needs (CPITN), *Int. Dent. J., 32,* 281, September, 1982.

22. **Ramfjord,** S.P.: Indices for Prevalence and Incidence of Periodontal Disease, *J. Periodontol., 30,* 51, January, 1959.

23. **Gruebbel,** A.O.: A Measurement of Dental Caries Prevalence and Treatment Service for Deciduous Teeth, *J. Dent. Res., 23,* 163, June, 1944.

24. **United States Department of Health and Human Services, Public Health Service, National Institutes of Health:** Oral Health Surveys of the National Institute of Dental Research, Diagnostic Criteria and Procedures. NIH Publication No. 91–2870. Bethesda, MD, National Institute of Dental Research, 1991.

SUGGESTED READINGS

Ainamo, J., Etemadzadeh, H., and Kallio, P.: Comparability and Discriminating Power of 4 Plaque Quantifications, *J. Clin. Periodontol., 20,* 244, April, 1993.

Burt, B.A. and Eklund, S.A.: *Dentistry, Dental Practice, and the Community,* 4th ed. Philadelphia, W.B. Saunders Co., 1992, pp. 57–77.

Lobene, R.R., Mankodi, S.M., Ciancio, S.G., Lamm, R.A., Charles, C.H., and Ross, N.M.: Correlations Among Gingival Indices: A Methodology Study, *J. Periodontol., 60,* 159, March, 1989.

Marks, R.G., Magnusson, I., Taylor, M., Clouser, B., Maruniak, J., and Clark, W.B.: Evaluation of Reliability and Reproducibility of Dental Indices, *J. Clin. Periodontol., 20,* 54, January, 1993.

Palat, M., Gomez, C., Scherer, W., Hittelman, E., and LoPresti, J.: Indicators of Gingival Inflammation: The Gingival Index vs Sulcular Temperature Measurements, *J. Practical Hyg., 2,* 25, January/February, 1993.

Quirynen, M., Dekeyser, C., and van Steenberghe, D.: Discriminating Power of Five Plaque Indices, *J. Periodontol, 62,* 100, February, 1991.

Silness, J. and Røynstrand, T.: Partial Mouth Recording of Plaque, Gingivitis and Probing Depth in Adolescents, *J. Clin. Periodontol., 15,* 189, March, 1988.

Summers, C.J., Gooch, B.F., Marianos, D.W., Malvitz, D.M., and Bond, W.W.: Practical Infection Control in Oral Health Surveys and Screenings, *J. Am. Dent. Assoc., 125,* 1213, September, 1994.

Tal, H. and Rosenberg, M.: Estimation of Dental Plaque Levels and Gingival Inflammation Using a Simple Oral Rinse Technique, *J. Periodontol., 61,* 339, June, 1990.

Toevs, S.E. and Lukken, K.M.: Assessing Interproximal Gingival Health, *J. Dent. Hyg., 63,* 228, June, 1989.

Toevs, S.E. and Lukken, K.M.: Bleeding as an Indicator of Health or Disease: Clinical Application of this Parameter, *J. Dent. Hyg., 64,* 256, July–August, 1990.

Periodontal Disease Indices

Almas, K., Bulman, J.S., and Newman, H.N.: Assessment of Periodontal Status With CPITN and Conventional Periodontal Indices, *J. Clin. Periodontol., 18,* 654, October, 1991.

Barnett, M.L.: Suitability of Gingival Indices for Use in Therapeutic Trials: Is Bleeding a Sine Qua Non? *J. Clin. Periodontol., 23,* 582, June, 1996.

Bentley, C.D. and Disney, J.A.: A Comparison of Partial and Full Mouth Scoring of Plaque and Gingivitis in Oral Hygiene Studies, *J. Clin. Periodontol., 22,* 131, February, 1995.

Blieden, T.M., Caton, J.G., Proskin, H.M., Stein, S.H., and Wagener, C.J.: Examiner Reliability for an Invasive Gingival Bleeding Index, *J. Clin. Periodontol., 19,* 262, April, 1992.

Butler, B.L., Morejon, O., and Low, S.B.: An Accurate Time-Efficient Method to Assess Plaque Accumulation, *J. Am. Dent. Assoc., 127,* 1763, December, 1996.

Khocht, A., Zohn, H., Deasy, M., and Chang, K.-M.: Screening for Periodontal Disease: Radiographs vs. PSR, *J. Am. Dent. Assoc., 127,* 749, June, 1996.

Mojon, P., Chung, J.-P., Favre, P., and Budtz-Jorgensen, E.: Examiner Agreement on Periodontal Indices During Dental Surveys of Elders, *J. Clin. Periodontol., 23,* 56, January, 1996.

Newbrun, E.: Indices to Measure Gingival Bleeding, *J. Periodontol., 67,* 555, June, 1996.

Spolsky, V.W. and Gornbein, J.A.: Comparing Measures of Reliability for Indices of Gingivitis and Plaque, *J. Periodontol., 67,* 853, September, 1996.

Sterrett, J.D., Hawkins, C.H., Pelletier, L., and Murphy, H.J.: The Use of Accurate Gingival Indices in Current Periodontal Literature, *Can. Dent. Hyg./Probe, 24,* 85, Summer, 1990.

Other Indices

Addy, M., Renton-Harper, P., and Myatt, G.: A Plaque Index for Occlusal Surfaces and Fissures: Measurement of Repeatability and Plaque Removal, *J. Clin. Periodontol., 25,* 164, February, 1998.

Aherne, C.A., O'Mullane, D., and Barrett, B.E.: Indices of Root Surface Caries, *J. Dent. Res., 69,* 1222, May, 1990.

Donachie, M.A. and Walls, A.W.G.: Assessment of Tooth Wear in an Aging Population, *J. Dent., 23,* 157, June, 1995.

Katz, R.V.: Development of an Index for the Prevalence of Root Caries, *J. Dent. Res., 63,* 814, Special Issue, May, 1984.

Koch, A.L., Gershen, J.A., and Marcus, M.: A Children's Oral Health Status Index Based on Dentists' Judgment, *J. Am. Dent. Assoc., 110,* 36, January, 1985.

Lobene, R.R., Weatherford, T., Ross, N.M., Lamn, R.A., and Menaker, L.: A Modified Gingival Index for Use in Clinical Trials, *Clin. Prev. Dent., 8,* 3, January–February, 1986.

Massler, M. and Schour, I.: The P-M-A Index of Gingivitis, *J. Dent. Res., 28,* 634, Abstract Number 7, December, 1949.

Quigley, G.A. and Hein, J.W.: Comparative Cleansing Efficiency of Manual and Power Brushing, *J. Am. Dent. Assoc., 65,* 26, July, 1962.

Silberman, S.L., Trubman, A., Duncan, W.K., and Meydrech, E.F.: A Simplified Hypoplasia Index, *J. Public Health Dent., 50,* 282, Summer, 1990.

Care Planning

▪ INTRODUCTION

After the initial assessment is completed as described in Section III, the data are assembled, sequenced, and analyzed in preparation for planning strategies for helping the patient acquire and maintain oral health. Figure IV-1 shows the position of Care Planning in the total dental hygiene process of care.

The dental hygiene diagnosis will focus attention on the behavioral aspects as well as deviations from normal oral health. Chartings, radiographs, histories, and all recorded data are brought together with the clinical evaluation. A blueprint plan, such as that designed in Figure 22-1, clarifies thinking toward preparation of diagnostic statements. Examples of the diagnostic statements are shown in Table 22-2. Each diagnostic statement identifies with a significant oral hygiene problem of the patient.

The dental hygiene diagnosis and care plan identify those patient needs that the dental hygienist will treat in dental hygiene appointments. The care plan is selected to conform with and be integrated with the total treatment plan of the patient. *Dental* diagnoses are directed at those particular diseases and conditions for which the dentist will provide treatment.

The overall objectives of the dental health care team focus on the oral health of the patient. The ultimate goal will be the control of oral diseases.

▪ ETHICAL APPLICATIONS

Professional ethics is a part of each element in the provider-patient relationship between the dental hygienist and the patient. The potential for an ethical situation arises anytime a dental hygienist interacts with a patient, with members of the dental team, or with individuals involved in the special needs of the patient, such as family, caregivers, or members of specialty practices. It is necessary to maintain communication among all parties responsible for dental and dental hygiene treatment, cognizant of the respect each patient deserves.

A dental hygienist must maintain a level of knowledge through continuing education coursework and reading professional journal articles about new research. Additionally, a dental hygienist must be aware of such ethical issues as conflict of interest while treating patients, the legal scope of one's duties, dealing with impaired colleagues, and the ability to assess and justify the reporting of unacceptable practices.

The basic concepts in healthcare law apply to all dental hygiene professionals. The dental hygiene practice acts of each state or province govern the scope of duties and the criteria for licensure. Professional liability, standard of care, informed consent, privacy information, and malpractice are other concerns that affect the daily duties and rights of both the patient and the dental hygienist. Selected legal concepts and suggestions for application are described in Table IV-1.

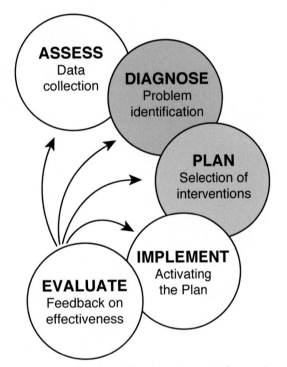

▪ **FIGURE IV-1** The dental hygiene process of care. Care planning.

▪ TABLE IV-1 LEGAL AND ETHICAL CONCEPTS

LEGAL CONCEPT	EXPLANATION	APPLICATION
Professional Liability	A licensed professional is legally accountable for all actions; bound by the law.	Scope and duties of the dental hygienist are defined in each state's Dental Practice Act.
Standard of Care	A professional must use the ordinary and reasonable skill that is commonly used by other reputable dental hygienists when caring for patients. Involves prudent judgment and use of all available resources.	Evaluating the patient's charting and examination data before determining what radiographs are needed according to individualized recall intervals.
Informed Consent	Affirmation by a patient to allow examination or treatment by authorized dental personnel.	Involves the ongoing process of communicating and educating a patient about oral health options, not only a printed form to sign.
Negligence/Malpractice	Failure to perform professional duties according to the accepted standard of care.	Patient must show that the dental hygienist owed a 'duty' to the patient, was 'derelict' and breached that duty, there was evidence of 'direct cause', and that 'damages' resulted.

Not performing circumferential probing and informing/referring a patient when periodontal concerns exist can be considered negligence. |

Planning for Dental Hygiene Care

Charlotte J. Wyche, RDH, MS

In the dental hygiene process of care described in Chapter 1 and illustrated in Figure IV-1, assessment data are used to formulate the dental hygiene diagnosis. Then, using an evidence-based approach, a dental hygiene care plan and appointment sequence can be formalized. Terms and key words used in conjunction with these steps are defined in Box 21-1.

ASSESSMENT FINDINGS

Assessment includes the gathering of details regarding the health status of the patient, followed by analysis and synthesis of that data. The application of clinical judgment and critical thinking skills are necessary to arrive at a dental hygiene diagnosis. Assessment procedures are described in detail in Chapters 6 through 20.

I. THE CHIEF COMPLAINT

The patient's statement regarding the reason for seeking dental and dental hygiene care is considered when plan-

ning. If a patient has a significant concern, such as pain, this need is addressed prior to initiating dental hygiene treatment.

II. RISK FACTORS

Whether or not the patient presents for dental hygiene care with current oral disease, several risk factors can be noted that increase the patient's potential for diminished oral health status. When a patient presents for dental hygiene care exhibiting one or more risk factors, it is essential to develop a care plan that addresses the need for preventive education and counseling.

A. Risk Factors for Periodontal Infections or Poor Response to Periodontal Therapy

- Behavioral factors (inadequate biofilm removal, diet, noncompliance with dental hygiene recommendations)

BOX 21-1 KEY WORDS AND ABBREVIATIONS: Planning for Dental Hygiene Care

ADLs (Activities of Daily Living): a measure of the ability to carry out the basic tasks needed for self-care.

IADLs (Instrumental Activities of Daily Living): a measure of the ability to perform more of the complex tasks necessary to function in our society; tasks that require a combination of physical and cognitive ability.

ASA: American Society of Anesthesiologists; originally developed the ASA Classifications to determine modifications necessary to provide general anesthetic to patients during surgical procedures.

Assessment: the critical analysis and valuation or judgment of a particular condition, situation, or other subject of appraisal.

Chief complaint: the patient's concern as stated during the initial health history preparation; may be the reason for seeking professional care; a complaint such as pain or discomfort may require emergency dental diagnosis.

Definitive care: complete care; end point at which all treatment required at the time has been completed.

Compromised therapy: initial therapy and continued periodontal maintenance provided as the therapeutic end point in cases where the severity and extent of the disease or the age and health of the patient preclude optimal results of periodontal therapy.

Diagnose: to identify or recognize a disease or problem.

Diagnosis: a concise technical description of the cause, nature, or manifestations of a condition, situation, or problem; identification of a disease or deviation from normal condition by recognition of characteristic signs and symptoms.

Dental hygiene diagnosis: identification of an existing or potential oral health problem that a dental hygienist is qualified and licensed to treat.

Differential diagnosis: determination of which one of several diseases or conditions may be producing the symptoms.

Evidence-based care: providing oral care based on relevant, scientifically sound research.

OSCAR: a mnemonic that stands for **O**ral, **S**ystemic, **C**apability, **A**utonomy, and **R**eality. Developed by the American Academy of Oral Medicine to provide a convenient, systematic approach to identifying dental, medical/pharmacologic, functional, ethical, and fiscal factors that need to be evaluated and weighed when planning treatment for geriatric or other disabled individuals.

Prognosis: prediction of outcome; a forecast of the probable course and outcome of an attack of disease and the prospects of recovery as expected by the nature of the specific condition and the symptoms of the case; usually expressed in general terms, such as "excellent," "good," "favorable," or "poor."

Dental hygiene prognosis: a judgment regarding the results (outcomes) expected to be achieved from oral treatment provided by the dental hygienist.

Risk factor: an attribute or exposure that increases the probability of disease, such as an aspect of personal behavior, environmental exposure, or an inherited characteristic associated with health-related conditions.

Modifiable risk factor: a determinant that can be modified by intervention, thereby reducing the probability of disease.

- Tobacco use
- Systemic conditions (diabetes, decreased immune factors, osteoporosis, osteopenia)
- Hormonal considerations (pregnancy, menopause)
- Nutritional status
- Iatrogenic factors (overhangs, open contacts, residual calculus)
- Genetic factors

B. Periodontal Disease as a Risk Factor for Systemic Conditions

Current research suggests that the presence of periodontal infection is a contributing factor to a variety of systemic conditions.

- Infective endocarditis
- Cardiovascular disease (CVD) and atherosclerosis
- Diabetes mellitus

- Respiratory disease
- Adverse pregnancy outcomes (pre-term, low-birth-weight infants)

C. Risk Factors for Dental Caries

- Behavioral factors (inadequate biofilm removal)
- Dietary factors (frequent use of cariogenic foods/beverages)
- Low fluoride
- Tooth morphology and position (deep occlusal pits and fissures, exposed root surfaces, rotated positioning)
- Xerostomia
- Personal and family history of dental caries/restorative dentistry
- Developmental factors (modifications of dental enamel)
- Genetic factors (immune response)

D. Risk Factors for Oral Cancer

- Tobacco use
- Alcohol use
- Sun exposure (lip and face)

III. PATIENT'S OVERALL HEALTH STATUS

A. Physical Status

The extent of the patient's medical, physical, and psychological risk determines modifications necessary during treatment. Patient positioning, sequence and timing of treatments, and prevention of medical complications need consideration.

The American Society of Anesthesiologists' (ASA) Classification System[1] (Table 21-1) and the OSCAR Planning Guide[2] (Table 21-2) are two examples of systematic approaches used to help determine modifications necessary when providing patient care.

B. Tobacco Use

The patient's use of tobacco will affect oral status and dental hygiene treatment outcomes. Information on planning dental hygiene interventions for the patient who uses tobacco is found on pages 513 to 515.

IV. ORAL HEALTHCARE KNOWLEDGE LEVEL OF THE PATIENT

Before planning individualized patient care, an attempt is made to assess the patient's oral health knowledge level. From that baseline, planned educational interventions can build on current knowledge rather than provide information too far above or below the patient's current understanding.

V. THE PATIENT'S ABILITY TO PERFORM ORAL CARE PROCEDURES

The patient's ability to manipulate a toothbrush and floss and to comply with suggested oral care regimens will determine the success of planned interventions. Patients with disabilities or physical limitations will require modifications to ensure adequate daily dental biofilm removal.

An Activities of Daily Living (ADL)[3] classification level, described in Table 21-3, will provide a guide to determine whether adaptive aids or caregiver training for home care procedures is necessary.

VI. DOCUMENTATION OF ASSESSMENT DATA

Complete and accurate records are essential. Data should be recorded in ink, and standardized abbreviations should be used to document all findings. Misunderstandings can lead to legal involvement.

■ THE PERIODONTAL DIAGNOSIS

Planning for the number and length of appointments in a treatment sequence will be determined by the patient's periodontal diagnosis.

I. CURRENT PERIODONTAL STATUS

A description of past and current periodontal conditions, as well as risk factors that affect the progress of disease, determine a patient's current periodontal status.

II. CASE TYPE

For purposes of determining the sequence and number of appointments required for initial nonsurgical periodontal therapy, it is useful to divide the periodontal diagnosis into case types as described in Table 14-1. However, this designation does not differentiate between patients with gingival tissue that is healthy at the present time or is in a currently active disease state.

III. CLASSIFICATION OF PERIODONTAL DISEASE

The classification of periodontal diseases is described on pages 250 to 251. The extent, severity, and chronic or aggressive nature of the patient's periodontal disease can be characterized.

▪ TABLE 21-1 ASA* PHYSICAL STATUS CLASSIFICATION SYSTEM

ASA CLASSIFICATION		EXAMPLES OF PHYSICAL OR PSYCHOSOCIAL MANIFESTATIONS	DENTAL TREATMENT CONSIDERATIONS
ASA I	Without systemic disease; a normal, healthy patient with little or no dental anxiety	Able to walk one flight of stairs with no distress	No modifications necessary
ASA II	Mild systemic disease or extreme dental anxiety	Must stop after walking one flight of stairs because of distress Well-controlled chronic conditions Upper respiratory infections Healthy pregnant woman Allergies	Minimal risk; minor modifications may be necessary
ASA III	Systemic disease that limits activity but is not incapacitating	Must stop en route walking one flight of stairs Chronic cardiovascular conditions Controlled insulin-dependent diabetes Chronic pulmonary diseases Elevated blood pressure	Elective treatment is not contraindicated, but serious consideration of treatment modifications may be necessary
ASA IV	Incapacitating disease that is a constant threat to life	Unable to walk up one flight of stairs Unstable cardiovascular conditions Extremely elevated blood pressure Uncontrolled epilepsy Uncontrolled insulin-dependent diabetes	Conservative, noninvasive management of emergency dental conditions; more complex dental intervention may require hospitalization during treatment
ASA V	Patient is moribund and not expected to survive	End-stage renal, hepatic, infectious disease, or terminal cancer	Only palliative treatment is delivered

*American Society of Anesthesiologists.

Adapted from: Malamed, S.F.: *Medical Emergencies in the Dental Office*, 5th ed. St.

Louis, Mosby, 2000, pp. 41–44.

▪ TABLE 21-2 TREATMENT PLANNING WITH OSCAR*

ISSUE	FACTORS OF CONCERN
Oral	Teeth, restorations, prostheses, periodontium, pulpal status, oral mucosa, occlusion, saliva, tongue, alveolar bone
Systemic	Normative age changes, medical diagnoses, pharmacologic agents, interdisciplinary communication
Capability	Functional ability, self-care, caregivers, oral hygiene, transportation to appointments, mobility within the dental office
Autonomy	Decision-making ability, dependence on alternative or supplemental decision makers
Reality	Prioritization of oral health, financial ability or limitations, significance of anticipated life span

*A systematic approach to identifying factors that need to be evaluated when planning dental hygiene care.

Used with permission from: The American Academy of Oral Medicine (Ship, J.A. and Mohammad, A.R., eds.): *The Clinician's Guide to Oral Health in Geriatric Patients* (Monograph). Baltimore, American Academy of Oral Medicine, 1999, p. 21.

■ TABLE 21-3 MEASURES OF PATIENT FUNCTIONING*

EXAMPLES OF ACTIVITIES OF DAILY LIVING (ADLs)	EXAMPLES OF INSTRUMENTAL ACTIVITIES OF DAILY LIVING (IADLs)	LEVELS
Brushing	*Maintaining self-care regimens*	**Level 0**
Flossing	*Ability to make and keep dental*	Ability to perform the task
Applying interdental aids	*appointments*	without assistance
Feeding	Writing	**Level 1**
Ambulation (walking)	Cooking	Ability to perform the task
Bathing	Shopping	with some human assistance;
Continence	Climbing stairs	may need a device or mechanical
Communication	Managing medication	aid but still independent
Dressing	Reading	**Level 2**
Toileting	Cleaning	Ability to perform the task
Transfer (from bed to toilet)	Using telephone	with partial assistance
Grooming		**Level 3**
		Requires full assistance to
		perform the task; totally
		dependent

*This scale provides a simple means of summarizing a person's ability to carry out the basic tasks needed for self-care.

Adapted from: Resnick, B.: Care of the Older Patient, in Nettina, S.M., ed.: *The Lippincott Manual of Nursing Practice,* 7th ed. Philadelphia, Lippincott Williams & Wilkins, 2001, pp. 167–168.

IV. PARAMETERS OF CARE

Clinical diagnosis, therapeutic goals, treatment considerations, and outcomes assessment for periodontal disease are outlined in the periodontal Parameters of Care.[4] Planning considerations are graded by the severity of infection. Examples are listed in Table 21-4.

■ THE DENTAL HYGIENE DIAGNOSIS

I. BASIS FOR DIAGNOSIS

A. Patient interview data (chief complaint, identification of oral problems, and comprehensive personal/social, medical, and dental health histories).

B. Physical assessment data (vital signs, extraoral and intraoral tissue examination, and dental and periodontal chartings).

C. Treatment or education needs that may be addressed by providing oral care services within the dental hygienist's legal scope of practice.

D. Treatment needs that may be addressed by consultation with another licensed healthcare professional.

II. DIAGNOSTIC STATEMENTS

A. Provide the basis for planning interventions that are within the scope of dental hygiene practice.

B. Reflect expected outcomes of dental hygiene interventions.

C. Identify patient responses that are changeable by dental hygiene interventions.

D. Exclude diagnoses requiring treatments that are legally defined as dental practice.

III. DIAGNOSTIC MODELS[5-9]

Medical and dental models of diagnosis evaluate assessment data and classify diagnostic statements according to disease processes. In contrast, dental hygiene models have been developed more like nursing models that encompass a broader focus. These models:

- address health functioning and behaviors.
- describe actual or potential health problems that dental hygienists are educated and licensed to treat.

The models, described in Table 21-5, give direction and a scientific basis from which to make diagnostic decisions and formulate patient care plans.

■ THE DENTAL HYGIENE PROGNOSIS

Prognosis means a look ahead to an anticipated outcome or end point. The dental hygiene prognosis is a statement of the possible outcomes that can be expected from the dental hygiene intervention selected for an individual patient.

▪ TABLE 21-4 PARAMETERS OF CARE

CLINICAL DIAGNOSIS	THERAPEUTIC GOALS	TREATMENT CONSIDERATIONS
Biofilm-induced gingivitis	To establish gingival health through elimination of etiologic factors	**Dental Hygiene Care Plan** • Customized patient education • Supragingival and subgingival debridement • Antimicrobial agents • Correction of biofilm-retentive factors **Dental Treatment Plan** • The dental treatment plan may indicate surgical correction of gingival deformities
Chronic periodontitis • With slight to moderate loss of periodontal support	To arrest progression of disease and prevent recurrence To preserve health, comfort, and function	**Dental Hygiene Care Plan** • Elimination and control of systemic risk factors • Biofilm control • Supragingival and subgingival scaling and root planing • Adjunctive antimicrobial agents • Elimination of contributing local factors **Dental Treatment Plan** • If resolution of the condition does not occur, periodontal surgery may be considered
• With advanced loss of periodontal support	To alter or eliminate microbial etiology and contributing risk factors To arrest the progression of disease	**Dental Hygiene Care Plan** • Initial therapy as described above **Dental Treatment Plan** • May include regeneration of periodontal attachment following the completion and evaluation of initial therapy **Compromised Therapy** • Severity/extent of disease or the age/health of the patient preclude optimal results • Initial therapy and continued periodontal maintenance become the end point
Periodontal maintenance	To minimize the recurrence and progression of the disease To reduce the incidence of tooth loss	**Dental Hygiene Care Plan** • Comparison of clinical data to previous baseline measurements • Assessment of personal oral hygiene status and compliance with maintenance intervals • Oral hygiene reinstruction or modification • Counseling on control of risk factors
Acute periodontal diseases Includes: • Gingival abscess • Periodontal abscess • Necrotizing diseases	To eliminate acute signs and symptoms of the condition as soon as possible	**Dental Hygiene Care Plan** • Collaborate with the attending dentist to prioritize treatment for the immediate need

■ TABLE 21-4 PARAMETERS OF CARE (Continued)

CLINICAL DIAGNOSIS	THERAPEUTIC GOALS	TREATMENT CONSIDERATIONS
• Herpetic gingivostomatitis • Pericoronitis • Periodontal-endodontic lesions		**Dental Treatment Plan** • Treatment considerations depend on the presenting condition
Aggressive periodontitis	To alter or eliminate microbial etiology and contributing risk factors To arrest or slow progression of the disease	**Dental Hygiene Care Plan** • Care parameters planned for chronic periodontitis **Dental Treatment Plan may include:** • General medical evaluation and consultation • Microbial identification • Antibiotic sensitivity testing • Alternative antimicrobial agents or delivery systems • Valuation/counseling of family members
Mucogingival conditions • Deviations from the normal anatomic relationship between the gingival margin and the mucogingival junction	To maintain and restore function and aesthetics	**Dental Hygiene Care Plan** • Careful comparison of baseline and follow-up findings • Control of inflammation through biofilm control, scaling, and root planing and/or antimicrobial agents **Dental Treatment Plan** • May include surgical treatment

From: American Academy of Periodontology: Parameters of Care, *J. Periodontol.*, 71, 849, May (Supplement), 2000.

I. FACTORS THAT DETERMINE OUTCOME

A. Assessment data regarding current disease status.
B. The patient's risk factors.
C. The patient's commitment to personal care and preventive regimens.
D. Interventions with the potential to reverse a patient's oral problem.
E. Treatment alternatives selected.
F. Evidence from the scientific literature.

II. EXPECTED OUTCOMES

Some examples of potential outcomes from dental hygiene interventions planned in a three-part care plan are listed below.

A. Gingival/Periodontal

• No bleeding on probing.
• Reduced probing depths.
• No further loss in attachment level.
• Decrease or no change in mobility.
• Resolution of erythematous tissue.
• Reduced swelling and edema.

B. Dental Caries

• No new demineralized areas.
• Demineralized areas resolved.
• No new carious lesions.
• Reduced intake of cariogenic foods/beverages.
• Dental sealants placed.

C. Prevention

• Elimination of iatrogenic factors (calculus, restoration overhangs).
• Increased percentage of biofilm-free areas.
• Demonstration of recommended oral care techniques
• Compliance with daily care recommendations.
• Compliance with recommended maintenance care interval.
• Tobacco-free status achieved.
• Modification/stabilization of systemic risk factors.

▪ **TABLE 21-5 DIAGNOSTIC MODELS USED IN PLANNING DENTAL HYGIENE CARE**	
MODEL NAME	**DIAGNOSTIC STATEMENTS**
Dental Hygiene Diagnostic Model[5-6]	• Developed by following six steps that form the process of diagnostic decision making: (1) Initial review (2) Hypothesis formation (3) Inquiry strategy (4) Problem synthesis (5) Diagnostic decision making (6) Learning from the process • Recorded in patient treatment records using the notation "DHDx" and accompanied by a treatment plan or treatment goal statement
The Human Needs Model[7]	• Based on whether specific criteria defining eight human needs are met or unmet by the patient's current oral health status • Written by outlining goals to be obtained for resolving each observed deficit
The Dental Hygiene Process Model[8]	• Identify patient's problem in terms of response rather than need and state the possible etiology • Classified into several categories, which include general systemic, soft tissue, periodontal, oral hygiene, and dental categories • Written by stating the problem and the etiologic factor joined by the phrase "related to"
The Oral Health–Related Quality of Life (OHRQL) Model[9]	• Diagnostic statements for individuals/populations are based on the assessment of domains related to health/preclinical disease; biological/physiological disease; and the broad-based sequelae to disease, such as symptom status, function status, health perceptions, and overall quality of life • Dental hygiene actions are formulated for each domain, incorporating a multidisciplinary approach to care

▪ CONSIDERATIONS FOR PROVIDING CARE

I. ROLE OF THE PATIENT

A. Purpose

The willingness and/or ability of the patient to participate in planned oral health behaviors will be the key to reaching goals set during planning.

B. Procedure

1. Determine the patient's level of understanding of dental diseases, risk factors, and oral health behaviors.
2. Determine the patient's physical ability to manipulate recommended oral care aids.
3. Determine lifestyle factors that impact the patient's ability to comply with oral health recommendations.
4. Educate patients regarding the importance of their role in setting oral health goals and complying with recommendations.

II. TISSUE CONDITIONING

Preparation or conditioning of the gingival tissue for scaling can be of particular significance when there is spongy, soft tissue that bleeds on slight provocation, and when the area is generally septic from dental biofilm and debris accumulation.

A. Purpose

Anticipated outcomes of a tissue conditioning program include:
1. Gingival healing
   • tissue becomes less edematous.
   • bleeding is minimized.
   • scaling procedures are facilitated.
2. Reduced bacterial accumulation
   • less likelihood that bacteremias will be produced during scaling.
   • reduced contamination in the aerosols produced.
3. Learning by the patient
   While conditioning the tissue for scaling, the patient can:
   • practice oral health behaviors.

- experience the benefits of a clean mouth.
- form lifetime habits for continued maintenance.

B. Procedure

- Initiate a pretreatment program of daily biofilm removal.
- Recommend daily use of an antibacterial rinse after thorough brushing and flossing before going to bed.
- Select affected quadrants for scaling only after patient cooperation has been demonstrated.

III. PREPROCEDURAL ANTIMICROBIAL RINSING

A. Purpose

Preprocedural removal of dental biofilm will lower the bacterial count in aerosols and decrease the potential for bacteremia.

B. Procedure

- The first choice is patient brushing and flossing.
- Vigorous rinsing with an antibacterial mouthwash is beneficial.[10]
- Forcing the fluid between the teeth, for 1 to 2 minutes can remove loose debris and surface bacteria approximately 1 mm below the gingival margin.[11]
- Even rinsing with water will have some effect on bacteria; however, chlorhexidine rinses have the most substantivity.[12]

IV. PAIN AND ANXIETY CONTROL

A. Purpose

Control of discomfort during treatment procedures will result in enhanced patient compliance with recommended interventions, including return for additional scheduled appointments.

B. Procedure

1. Quadrant selection
   Treat the patient's areas of discomfort first, unless tissue conditioning is required. Treat either the quadrant with the fewest teeth or the least severe periodontal infection first to:
   - make the first scaling less complicated.
   - help orient an anxious patient to clinical procedures.
2. Anesthesia
   The need for anesthesia is determined by:
   - severity of the periodontal infection.

- depth of pockets.
- consistency and distribution of calculus.
- potential patient discomfort during scaling.
- sensitivity of the patient's tissues.

When two quadrants are to be treated at the same appointment, it will minimize patient posttreatment discomfort to select a maxillary and mandibular quadrant on the same side.

V. MAINTENANCE DURING THERAPY

A. Purpose

When restorative, prosthetic, or orthodontic treatment extends over a period of time, periodic appointments with the dental hygienist are needed for monitoring the continued success of the patient's self-care.

B. Procedure

Dental hygiene care provided during extended dental therapy follows the dental hygiene process of care and includes:

1. gingival tissue assessment.
2. probing to determine bleeding.
3. biofilm check with disclosing agents.
4. reinforcement of daily oral care measures.
5. scaling and root planing to remove calculus.
6. additional instruction for care of new prostheses or implants.
7. motivational encouragement.

VI. FOUR-HANDED DENTAL HYGIENE

A. Purpose

Planning patient care while practicing with a dental assistant increases the dental hygienist's efficiency through the use of:

- flexible scheduling.[13]
- two treatment chairs in an overlapping time frame.

B. Procedure

A well-trained dental hygiene assistant can be delegated such duties as:

- patient reception and seating.
- medical history update prior to confirmation by the dental hygienist.
- radiographs (following individual state certification guidelines).
- reinforcement of oral hygiene instruction.
- assistance during sealant placement or ultrasonic scaling.
- cleanup/disinfection of the unit in preparation for the next patient.

Everyday Ethics

Victoria, a dental hygienist, is discussing the assessment findings for her patient, Mr. Rush, with the rest of the dental team. Mr. Rush has stated that he has already been told at his general dental office that he has extensive active periodontal disease. He was referred to this practice because he wants all of the most compromised teeth extracted and dental implants placed.

Mr. Rush has a number of risk factors, such as poorly controlled diabetes and smoking. Because his dental insurance is running out in 3 months, everyone is in a rush to get the treatment started, and the potential for a poor prognosis has not been discussed. In fact, Victoria's concerns about the patient's risk factors are being pushed aside.

Questions for Consideration

1. What is Victoria's obligation (duty) to make sure that Mr. Rush understands how his risk factors compromise the prognosis of his treatment plan?

2. What action can Victoria take if her concerns continue to be ignored and treatment progresses without interventions that address the risk factors involved in Mr. Rush's case?

3. How should Victoria proceed to obtain informed consent from Mr. Rush and ensure that his rights to optimal care are maintained?

■ EVIDENCE-BASED SELECTION OF DENTAL HYGIENE PROTOCOLS

Dental hygiene interventions are planned using scientific evidence of efficacy and efficiency. Scientific evidence from dental and medical literature can improve opportunities for achieving successful outcomes from dental hygiene treatment. The patient can benefit if the dental hygienist has developed skills in accessing and evaluating the scientific literature.

✔ Factors To Teach The Patient

- A clear explanation of how assessment data are used in planning dental hygiene care.

- The importance of using scientific evidence of success in the selection of patient-specific therapeutic and preventive interventions.

- Why disease control measures are learned before and in conjunction with scaling.

- Facts of oral disease prevention and oral health promotion relevant to the patient's current level of healthcare knowledge and individual risk factors.

- The long-term effects of comprehensive continuing care.

REFERENCES

1. **American Society of Anesthesiologists**: New Classification of Physical Status, *Anesthesiology, 24*, 111, January–February, 1963.
2. **The American Academy of Oral Medicine** (Ship, J.A. and Mohammad, A.R., eds.): *The Clinician's Guide to Oral Health in Geriatric Patients* (Monograph). Baltimore, MD, American Academy of Oral Medicine, 1999, p. 21.
3. **Resnick**, B.: Care of the Older Patient, in Nettina, S.M., ed.: *The Lippincott Manual of Nursing Practice*, 7th ed. Philadelphia, Lippincott Williams & Wilkins, 2001, pp. 167–168.
4. **American Academy of Periodontology**: Parameters of Care. *J. Periodontol., 71*, 847, May (Supplement), 2000.
5. **Gurenlian**, J.R.: Diagnostic Decision Making, in Woodall, I.R., ed.: *Comprehensive Dental Hygiene Care*, 4th ed. St Louis, Mosby, 1993, pp. 361–370.
6. **Gurenlian**, J.R.: Recording the Dental Hygiene Diagnosis, *Access, 8*, 16, November, 1994.
7. **Darby**, M.L. and Walsh, M.M.: Application of the Human Needs Conceptual Model to Dental Hygiene Practice. *J. Dent. Hyg., 74*, 230, Summer, 2000.
8. **Mueller-Joseph**, L. and Petersen, M.: *Dental Hygiene Process: Diagnosis and Care Planning*. Albany, Delmar, 1995, pp. 46–63.
9. **Williams**, K.B., Gadbury-Amyot, C.C., Krust Bray, K., Manne, D., and Collins, P.: Oral Health–Related Quality of Life: A Model for Dental Hygiene, *J. Dent. Hyg., 72*, 19, Spring, 1998.
10. **Fine**, D.H., Korik, I., Furgang, D., Myers, R., Olshan, A., Barnett, M.L., and Vincent, J.: Assessing Pre-procedural Subgingival Irrigation and Rinsing with an Antiseptic Mouthrinse to Reduce Bacteremia, *J. Am. Dent. Assoc., 127*, 641, May, 1996.
11. **Veksler**, A.E., Kayrouz, G.A., and Newman, M.G.: Reduction of Salivary Bacteria by Pre-procedural Rinses with Chlorhexidine 0.12%, *J. Periodontol., 62*, 649, November, 1991.

12. **Wunderlich**, R.C., Singleton, M., O'Brien, W.J., and Caffesse, R.G.: Subgingival Penetration of an Applied Solution, *Int. J. Periodontics Restorative Dent., 4*, 64, Number 5, 1984.

13. **Blitz**, P. and Wright, V.: It Takes Two, *RDH, 14,* 18, September, 1994.

SUGGESTED READINGS

Diagnosis and Care Planning

Calley, K.H.: Dental Hygiene Process of Care, in Darby M.L., ed.: *Mosby's Comprehensive Review of Dental Hygiene*, 5th ed. St. Louis, Mosby, 2002, pp. 577–578.

Doenges, M.E., Moorhouse, M.F., and Geissler, A.C.: *Nursing Care Plans: Guidelines for Individualizing Patient Care.* Philadelphia, F.A. Davis, 1997, pp. 6–10.

McCullough, C.: Diagnosis and Treatment Planning, *Access, 7,* 26, April, 1993.

Miller, S.S.: Dental Hygiene Diagnosis, *RDH, 2,* 46, July–August, 1982.

Pattison, A.M. and Pattison, G.L.: *Periodontal Instrumentation*, 2nd ed. Norwalk, CT, Appleton & Lange, 1992, pp. 329–335.

Stefanac, S.J.: Information Gathering and Diagnosis Development, in Stefanac, S.J. and Nesbit S.P., eds.: *Treatment Planning in Dentistry.* St. Louis, Mosby, 2001, pp. 20–25.

Risk Factors

American Academy of Periodontology, Research, Science and Therapy Committee: Position Paper: Periodontal Disease as a Potential Risk Factor for Systemic Diseases, *J. Periodontol.,69*, 841, July, 1998.

Caufield, P.W. and Griffen, A.L.: Dental Caries: An Infectious and Transmissible Disease, *Pediatr. Clin. North Am.,47*, 1001, October, 2000.

Dorsey, B. and Martin, B.S.: Implementation of a Caries Prevention Program Using Risk Assessment, *Contemp. Oral Hyg., 2,* 20, September/October, 2002.

Michalowicz, B.S., Diehl, S.R., Gunsolley, J.C., Sparks, B.S., Brooks, C.N., Koertge, T.E., Califano, J.V., Burmeister, J.A., and Schenkein, H.A.: Evidence of a Substantial Genetic Basis for Risk of Adult Periodontitis. *J. Periodontol., 71*, 1699, November, 2000.

Noack, B., Jachmann, I., Roscher, S., Sieber, L., Kopprasch, S., Luck, C., Hanefeld, M., and Hoffmann, T.: Metabolic Diseases and Their Possible Link to Risk Indicators of Periodontitis, *J. Periodontol., 71*, 898, June, 2000.

Page, R.C. and Beck, J.D.: Risk Assessment for Periodontal Diseases, *Int. Dent. J., 47,* 61, April, 1997.

Rethman, J.: Trends in Preventive Care: Caries Risk Assessment and Indications for Sealants, *J. Am. Dent. Assoc., 131,* 8S, June (Supplement), 2000.

Slots, J. and Kamma, J.J.: General Health Risk of Periodontal Disease, *Int. Dent. J., 51,* 417, December, 2001.

Wright, J.T. and Hart, T.C.: The Genome Projects: Implications for Dental Practice and Education, *J. Dent. Educ., 66,* 659, May, 2002.

Prognosis

Ghiai, S. and Bissada, N.F.: Prognosis and Actual Treatment Outcome of Periodontally Involved Teeth, *Periodontal Clin. Investig., 18,* 7, Spring, 1996.

Lloyd, P.M.: Users' Guide to the Dental Literature: How to Use an Article About Prognosis, *Dent. Clin. North Am., 46,* 127, January, 2002.

McGuire, M.K.: Prognosis vs Outcome: Predicting Tooth Survival, *Compend. Contin. Educ. Dent., 21,* 217, March, 2000.

Evidence-based Care

Anderson, J.D.: Applying Evidence Based Dentistry to Your Patients, *Dent. Clin. North Am., 46,* 157, January, 2002.

Carr, A.B. and McGivney, G.P.: Evidence-based Dentistry Series: Users' Guides to the Dental Literature: How to Get Started, *J. Prosthet. Dent., 83,* 13, January, 2000.

Chiappelli, F. and Prolo, P.: Evidence-based Dentistry for the 21st Century, *Gen. Dent., 50,* 270, May–June, 2002.

Forrest, J.L. and Miller, S.A.: Evidence-based Decision Making in Dental Hygiene Education, Practice, and Research, *J. Dent. Hyg., 75,* 50, Winter, 2001.

Laskin, D.M.: Finding the Evidence for Evidence-based Dentistry, *J. Am. Coll. Dent., 67,* 7, Spring, 2000.

Sutherland, S.E.: The Building Blocks of Evidence-based Dentistry, *J. Can. Dent. Assoc., 66,* 241, May, 2000.

Sutherland, S.E.: Evidence-based Dentistry: Part I. Getting Started, *J. Can. Dent. Assoc., 67,* 204, April, 2001.

Tavender, E.J. and Glenny, A.-M.: The Cochrane Collaboration: The Oral Health Group, *J. Dent. Educ., 66,* 612, May, 2002.

The Dental Hygiene Care Plan

Charlotte J. Wyche, RDH, MS

A written dental hygiene care plan is an essential part of the integrated components of the dental hygiene process of care illustrated in Figure 1-1. Terms and key words for this chapter are defined in Box 22-1.

■ PREPARATION OF A DENTAL HYGIENE CARE PLAN

Dental hygiene care is planned to address the needs of the entire oral cavity. The care plan is based on assessment of the oral mucosa, teeth, periodontal supporting structures, and health factors that influence the oral environment. A care plan that integrates a basic three-part plan to care for all of the patient's dental hygiene needs has a major influence on the future oral health of the patient.

I. PARTS OF A CARE PLAN

A. Periodontal/Gingival Health

The primary objective of the dental hygiene plan for periodontal therapy is to restore and maintain health of the gingival tissues.

B. Dental Caries Control

The plan for caries control includes a remineralization program, fluorides, dental sealants, and dietary control of fermentable carbohydrates.

C. Prevention

A plan for preventive care starts with the patient's personal daily bacterial control and includes interventions such as tobacco cessation, risk factor reduction, desensitizing exposed dentin, helping with halitosis, and much, much more.

II. DESCRIPTION

The written care plan is a prioritized sequence of evidence-based dental hygiene interventions that are:
A. Predicated on the dental hygiene diagnosis.
B. Composed of integrated plans for periodontal care, caries control, and other preventive interventions.
C. Integrated into a total treatment plan that encompasses the patient's restorative and surgical needs, as shown in Table 22-1.

BOX 22-1 KEY WORDS: Planning for Dental Hygiene Care

Consent: voluntary agreement to an action proposed by another.

Informed consent: a patient's voluntary agreement to a treatment plan after details of the proposed treatment have been presented and comprehended by the patient.

Informed refusal: a patient's decision to refuse recommended treatment after all options, potential risks, and potential benefits have been thoroughly explained.

Intervention: to happen or take place between other events; to intervene, as with a specific treatment.

Prioritize: to arrange in order of importance.

Sequence: a continuous or related series of things (such as dental hygiene interventions) following in a certain order or succession.

Total treatment plan: sequential outline of the essential services and procedures that must be carried out by the dentist, the dental hygienist, and the patient to eliminate disease and restore the oral cavity to health and normal function.

Dental hygiene care plan: the services within the framework of the total treatment plan to be carried out by the dental hygienist.

D. Contained within the scope of dental hygiene practice as defined by each practice act.

III. RATIONALE

A written dental hygiene care plan will help to:
- A. Focus on individualized patient needs when selecting dental hygiene interventions.
- B. Prioritize the sequence of planned treatment and education.
- C. Provide a checklist to ensure that all planned interventions are accomplished.

IV. OBJECTIVES

A well-prepared dental hygiene care plan:
- A. Is flexible and realistic.
- B. Plans care for patient needs based on assessment data collected.
- C. Contains treatment and education goals that address identified problems.
- D. Provides interventions and recommendations based on current scientific evidence.

■ COMPONENTS OF A WRITTEN CARE PLAN

A dental hygiene care plan may be written using a variety of formats. Components of a well-written care plan are described in this section. Figure 22-1 is a suggested template for a patient-specific care plan that follows

the dental hygiene process of care. The recommended components of a written care plan are described in this section.

I. DEMOGRAPHIC DATA

- A. Patient name, date of birth (age), and gender.
- B. A designation of initial or maintenance therapy.
- C. The name of the student or clinician who prepared the written plan.
- D. The date that the written plan was prepared.
- E. Notation of the patient's chief complaint or statement indicating the patient's reason for presenting for treatment.

II. ASSESSMENT FINDINGS AND RISK FACTORS

This section of the plan contains a thorough, summarized description of significant findings.

A. Medical History

- Systemic diseases and conditions
- Medications
- Overall health status
- Functional assessment

B. Dental History

- Treatment history
- Dental knowledge

▪ TABLE 22-1 COMPONENTS OF A MASTER TREATMENT PLAN

PHASE	PROCEDURES	INCLUDED IN THE DENTAL HYGIENE CARE PLAN
Preliminary phase	• Assessment data collection • Emergency care (pain, biopsy) • Removal of hopeless teeth • Provisional replacement to restore function	✓
Phase I therapy	• Dental biofilm control • Introduction of additional preventive measures (diet changes, fluorides, mouthguard) • Calculus removal • Correction of restorative and prosthetic irritants (biofilm traps, overhangs) • Restorative caries control (excavation and restoration) • Occlusal therapy • Minor orthodontic movement	✓ ✓ ✓
Outcomes evaluation of phase I	• Probing depths • Clinical signs of inflammation • Dental biofilm control • Patient's participation	✓ ✓ ✓ ✓
Phase II surgical	• Periodontal • Endodontic • Implant placement	
Phase III restorative	• Final restorations • Fixed/removable prostheses	
Evaluation of overall outcomes	• Final polish for restorations • Periodontal response to restorations/implants • Other response to restorations	✓ ✓
Phase IV maintenance	• Appointments for continuing care and supervision • Refining biofilm control techniques	✓ ✓

Adapted from: Carranza, F.A.: The Treatment Plan, in Carranza, F.A. and Newman, M.G.: *Clinical Periodontology*, 8th ed. Philadelphia, W.B. Saunders, 1996, p. 400.

C. Clinical Examination

- Extraoral and intraoral
- Soft and hard tissue

D. Link to Risk Factors

- Increased oral disease
- Increased risk of systemic disease due to oral infection
- Compromised treatment outcomes

III. PERIODONTAL DIAGNOSIS/CASE TYPE AND STATUS

The periodontal diagnosis formulated by the dentist is included in the dental hygiene care plan. Guidelines for noting the periodontal diagnosis and Parameters of Care, useful for planning dental hygiene interventions, are included in Chapter 21 on page 356.

IV. DIAGNOSTIC STATEMENTS

Table 22-2 contains examples of dental hygiene diagnostic statements that:
  A. Link observed or potential oral health problems identified during the patient assessment to probable etiology or risk factors.
  B. Relate to problems and solutions that can be addressed within the dental hygiene scope of practice.

V. PLANNED INTERVENTIONS

Dental hygiene interventions are measures applied to regenerate, restore, or maintain oral health. Selected interventions are specific to the individual patient's assessment findings and include:
  A. Clinical treatments, such as scaling, root planing, and debridement, selected for the purpose of arresting or controlling existing disease.

Patient-Specific Dental Hygiene Care Plan

Patient Name: _____   Age: _____   Gender: M   F   Initial Therapy
or
Student (Clinician) Name: _____   Date: _____   Maintenance

Chief Complaint:

ASSESSMENT FINDINGS

Medical History	Significant Findings	At Risk For:
• Systemic disease • Other conditions • Medications • ASA classification • ADL/IADL level		
Dental History • Treatment history • Dental knowledge		
Dental Examination • Extraoral examination • Intraoral examination • Teeth/restorations • Periodontal examination		

Periodontal Diagnosis / Case Type and Status:

DENTAL HYGIENE DIAGNOSIS

Problem		Cause (risk factors and etiology)
Extraoral:	Related to	
Intraoral:	Related to	
Restorative:	Related to	
Periodontal:	Related to	
Systemic health:	Related to	
Physical ability:	Related to	

■ **FIGURE 22-1 Patient-Specific Dental Hygiene Care Plan.** The written care plan includes a summary of assessment findings, the dental hygiene diagnosis, planned dental hygiene interventions, expected outcomes, and an appointment plan that sequences treatment procedures and education interventions for each appointment. (Adapted from a model by Dr. Laura Mueller-Joseph, State University of New York at Farmingdale, Farmingdale, New York.)

continued

PLANNED INTERVENTIONS

(to **arrest or control** disease and **regenerate, restore, or maintain** health)

Clinical	Education / Counseling	Oral Hygiene Instruction/Home Care

EXPECTED OUTCOMES

Goals	Evaluation methods	Time frame
1.		
2.		
3.		
4.		

APPOINTMENT PLAN

(**sequence** of planned interventions)

Appt #	Plan for Treatment and Services Quadrant		Plan for Education, Counseling, and Oral Hygiene Instruction
1.			
2.			
3.			
4.			

REEVALUATION FINDINGS

Re-treat   Refer   Maintain (interval _____)

Description of findings:

▪ **FIGURE 22-1 Patient-Specific Dental Hygiene Care Plan.** (continued).

■ TABLE 22-2 EXAMPLES OF DENTAL HYGIENE DIAGNOSTIC STATEMENTS

PROBLEM		CAUSE (RISK FACTORS AND ETIOLOGY)
Hypersensitivity	*Related to*	Exposed cementum/gingival recession
Gingival bleeding	*Related to*	Biofilm accumulation
Increased caries risk	*Related to*	Daily consumption of sugar-sweetened soft drinks
Probing depth and attachment loss increase (since last visit)	*Related to*	Uncontrolled diabetic condition
Risk for poor pregnancy outcomes	*Related to*	Periodontal infection
Biofilm Control Record fair to poor score	*Related to*	Physical disability (ADL level 3)

B. Preventive measures, such as dental sealants, that maintain tooth integrity.

C. Education and counseling in such topics as etiology and progression of oral disease and elimination of risk factors.

D. Individualized oral hygiene instructions and home care regimens based on patient needs and abilities.

VI. EXPECTED OUTCOMES

A plan for treatment or home care outcomes, created in consultation with the patient, contains:

A. At least one goal for each oral health problem identified in the dental hygiene diagnosis.

B. Evaluation methods that clearly identify how progress toward each goal will be measured.

C. A realistic time frame for measuring success.

VII. THE APPOINTMENT PLAN

A. An appointment plan for multiple appointments:
   • Outlines interventions sequenced in order of clinical performance.
   • Can be adapted at each appointment to respond to new information or immediate patient need.

B. Properly prioritized and sequenced treatment and education interventions will be:
   • More comfortable for the patient.
   • More effective in reaching planned oral health goals.

VIII. REEVALUATION

The reevaluation interval is identified during the initial planning and noted on the care plan. At the reevaluation appointment:

A. Interval is identified during the initial planning.

B. New assessment data are collected and analyzed.

C. A determination is made regarding whether expected outcomes of the care plan have been met.

■ SEQUENCING AND PRIORITIZING PATIENT CARE

I. OBJECTIVES

Reasons for preparing a well-sequenced dental hygiene care plan are:

A. To Provide Evidence-Based, Individualized Patient Care That Is:

• Determined by collection of assessment data.

• Based on documented evidence of success.

• Enhanced by the clinician's ability to assess the value of information available in product advertising and in the scientific literature.

B. To Eliminate or Control Etiologic and Predisposing Disease Factors

• The principal etiologic agents in both dental caries and periodontal and gingival diseases are the microorganisms of dental biofilm.

• Dental hygiene interventions can modify a variety of risk factors that predispose the patient to oral disease.

C. To Eliminate the Signs and Symptoms of Disease

Measures to eliminate signs of disease such as gingival bleeding and probing depths are included in the care plan.

D. To Promote Oral Health and Prevent Recurrence of Disease

Methods used to achieve optimum oral health are:
- Education on the etiology of oral disease.
- Counseling on prevention measures and elimination of risk factors.
- Instruction and supervision in daily self-care techniques.
- Encouragement of regularly scheduled maintenance follow-up for dental hygiene care.

II. FACTORS AFFECTING SEQUENCE OF CARE

Treatment sequence defines the order in which the parts of an individual appointment are to be carried out. Sequence planning involves:
- Identification of overall treatment and education patterns appropriate for an individual patient's needs.
- Outline of a series of appointments, with specific services, treatment procedures, and educational interventions included.

The sequence of care for an individual patient is determined by numerous factors.

A. Urgency

Discomfort or pain that requires first attention could apply to:
- An area of the gingiva that is particularly difficult to clean because of inaccessibility.
- An area with a periodontal abscess or with necrotizing ulcerative gingivitis (NUG).

B. Existing Etiologic Factors

In patients with gingival or periodontal infection or risk for dental caries, success of the treatment depends on thorough, daily biofilm removal. Biofilm control measures are introduced and success is evaluated before additional dental hygiene interventions will be effective.

C. Severity and Extent of the Condition

The number and length of appointments and the sequencing of procedures planned are affected by the severity of the condition. Findings that indicate the severity of gingival or periodontal infection include:
- Changes in color, size, shape, consistency, and bleeding of the gingiva.
- Probing depths.
- Mobility of the teeth.
- Clinical and radiographic signs of attachment loss.

D. Individual Patient Requirements

When writing the actual plan, each patient is considered individually. Items from the patient history that may require adaptation in appointment length, spacing, or sequencing when planning dental hygiene care include:
1. Antibiotic premedication.
   - Current recommended standard prophylactic regimens and a list of conditions that require antibiotic premedication appear on pages 122 to 125.
   - All instrumentation, including probing and exploring, as well as mobility determination, is done under antibiotic coverage.
   - Because bacteremias can occur, initial instruction and practice of biofilm-removing procedures are carried out while the patient is premedicated. Early introduction of biofilm control measures in the care plan is imperative.
   - Efficient use of appointment time and/or spacing of appointment dates will avoid unnecessary extra antibiotic coverage.
2. Systemic diseases.
   - Chronic disease will influence the content and length of appointments.
3. Physical disability.
   - Physical limitations will require adaptation of the appointment plan.
4. Other considerations.
   - An outline for maintenance appointments can be found on pages 759 to 760.
   - A treatment sequence for a patient with necrotizing ulcerative gingivitis is found on pages 693 to 695.
   - A suggested outline for conducting a biofilm control program using a series of lessons is found on pages 379 to 382.

▪ PRESENTING THE DENTAL HYGIENE CARE PLAN

Before treatment is begun, the care plan is discussed with the dentist and explained to the patient.

I. PRESENTING THE PLAN TO THE DENTIST

A. Purpose

- To integrate the dental hygiene care plan into the patient's total treatment plan.
- To provide a coordinated dental and dental hygiene statement to the patient regarding oral health needs.

B. Procedure

- Summarize major systemic and dental health assessment findings.
- Summarize risk factors.
- Indicate planned intervention strategies, goals, and expected outcomes.
- Outline planned appointment sequence and services to be provided.
- Be prepared to give greater detail and answer questions.

II. EXPLAINING THE PLAN TO THE PATIENT

A clinician with good verbal communication skills and the ability to build a trusting relationship can influence patient acceptance of treatment needs and compliance with recommendations.[1] Use of an intraoral camera during presentation of the plan for care provides visual documentation of need for oral health interventions.

A. Purpose

- To provide the patient with information needed to give informed consent for treatment.
- To reinforce the patient's role in setting and reaching oral health goals outlined in the plan.

B. Procedure

- Position the patient in an upright position, face to face with clinician.
- Use terminology that is appropriate to the patient's level of understanding.

- Educate the patient regarding systemic and dental health assessment findings and their link to oral disease.
- Educate the patient regarding planned interventions, appointment sequence, dental hygiene services, and expected outcomes.
- Present information using visual aids such as dental models, drawings or pictures, videotapes, brochures, or an intraoral camera.
- Engage the patient in planning and setting goals.
- Be prepared to give greater detail and answer questions.
- Obtained signed informed consent.

■ INFORMED CONSENT

It is every patient's right to possess knowledge that will allow shared decision making with the oral care provider while treatment is being planned.

- Informed consent is a legal concept that can exist even without a written document.
- Informed consent can be lacking even when a document has been signed if the patient has not had the opportunity to comprehend and evaluate the risks and benefits of the suggested treatment.
- "Expressed consent" is given either orally or in writing.
- "Implied consent," granted by the patient's presence in the dental chair, only applies to data collection procedures, data analysis, and treatment planning.[2]

Everyday Ethics

Ellen is responsible for explaining two alternative treatment plans to Mrs. Kwan, who is new to the practice. Mrs. Kwan must decide between several extractions, which would require expensive crown and bridge replacement, and treatment of periodontally involved teeth with poor prognosis. The decision must be made today if she is to begin treatment early next week, when there are several open appointments that must be filled.

English is not Mrs. Kwan's first language, and no one in the office speaks her language. Ellen has explained the information carefully, using pictures and patient-appropriate words, and she has gone over both treatment alternatives several times. When Ellen asks Mrs. Kwan to summarize her

understanding of the care plan she just nods her head, smiles, and says, "I'll sign whatever you say."

Questions for Consideration

1. Does it appear that Mrs. Kwan understands her treatment alternatives and is informed sufficiently to give consent? How can voluntary informed consent be ensured?

2. What is Ellen's responsibility, as the knowledgeable professional, in selecting the choice of treatments while ensuring Mrs. Kwan's autonomy?

3. In what ways does the pressure of making a timely decision reflect paternalistic treatment of Mrs. Kwan by the dental office?

BOX 22-2 Informed Consent

Information to Disclose

- *Diagnosis:* description of patient's problem(s)

- *Treatment:* nature and rationale for the proposed treatment(s)

- *Alternatives:* viable alternatives to the proposed treatment(s)

- *Consequences:* risks and benefits of all proposed treatment alternatives, including physical and psychological effects, costs, and potential resulting problems

- *Prognosis:* expected outcome with treatment(s), with alternative treatment(s), and without treatment

Principles of Informing

- Assess the patient's ability to give informed consent

- Simplify the terminology so that the patient can understand

- Encourage the patient and family to ask questions

- Continue to assess the patient's understanding and reeducate as often as necessary

- Document all relevant factors and include the signed form in patient record

I. INFORMED CONSENT PROCEDURES

Box 22-2 provides information for obtaining informed consent.

    A. The patient must be informed of all treatment options available and must consent to follow the recommendations in the agreed-upon care plan.

    B. When potential risks, complications, or failure are associated with therapy, consent must be obtained in writing prior to beginning treatment.[3]

    C. Informed consent includes recommendations for referral to other healthcare providers as necessary.[3]

✔ Factors To Teach The Patient

- Why a dental hygiene care plan is made.

- Why patient input into the final care plan is important.

- Which parts of the plan are to be carried out by the patient.

- How the roles of patient and members of the dental team are interrelated in eliminating the patient's oral problems.

- The patient's rights and responsibilities regarding informed consent.

    D. If necessary, use forms written in simpler terms, larger print, or the patient's primary language.[4]

    E. Create a duplicate copy for the patient to take home.[4]

II. INFORMED REFUSAL

The patient's right to autonomy in making decisions regarding oral treatment requires that practitioners respect a patient's decision to refuse treatment.[5] Refusal of care as well as any recommended treatment options are documented in the patient's permanent record.

REFERENCES

1. **Goldie,** G.: Enhance Verbal Skills to Get Patients to Accept What They Need, *Contemp. Oral Hyg., 2,* 14, May/June, 2002.

2. **Schoen,** D.H. and Dean, M.-C.: *Contemporary Periodontal Instrumentation.* Philadelphia, W.B. Saunders, 1996, p. 208.

3. **The American Academy of Periodontology:** Position Paper: Guidelines for Periodontal Therapy, *J. Periodontol.,72,* 1624, November, 2001.

4. **Pape,** T.: Legal and Ethical Considerations of Informed Consent, *AORN. J., 65,* 1122, June, 1997.

5. **Odom,** J.G. and Bowers, D.F.: Informed Consent and Refusal, in Weinstein, B.D.: *Dental Ethics.* Philadelphia, Lea & Febiger, 1993, pp. 65-80.

SUGGESTED READINGS

Doenges, M.E., Moorhouse, M.F., and Geissler, A.C.: *Nursing Care Plans: Guidelines for Individualizing Patient Care.* Philadelphia, F.A. Davis, 1997, pp. 6-10.

Mueller-Joseph, L. and Petersen, M.: *Dental Hygiene Process: Diagnosis and Care Planning.* Albany, Delmar, 1995, pp. 96–106.

Informed Consent

American Academy of Periodontology: *Informed Consent for Surgical Periodontics.* Chicago, American Academy of Periodontology, 1997, 28 pp.

Barsley, R.: Ethical and Legal Issues in Treatment Planning, in Stefanac, S.J. and Nesbit S.P.: *Treatment Planning in Dentistry.* St. Louis, Mosby, 2001, pp. 67–70.

Chiodo, G.T. and Tolle, S.W.: Informed Consent Across Cultures, *Gen. Dent., 45,* 421, September–October, 1997.

Christensen, G.J.: Informing Patients About Treatment Alternatives, *J. Am. Dent. Assoc., 130,* 730, May, 1999.

Graham, P.E. and Harel-Raviv, M.: The Future of Informed Consent and Patient-Dentist Communication, *J. Can. Dent. Assoc., 63,* 460, June, 1997.

Jerrold, L.: Litigation, Legislation, and Ethics: Informed Consent and the Fourth Dimension, *Am. J. Orthod. Dentofacial Orthop., 118,* 476, October, 2000.

Litch, C.S. and Liggett, M.L.: Consent for Dental Therapy in Severely Ill Patients, *J. Dent. Educ., 56,* 298, May, 1992.

Odom, J.G., Odom, S.S., and Jolly, D.E.: Informed Consent and the Geriatric Dental Patient, *Spec. Care Dentist., 12,* 202, September/October, 1992.

Robbins, K.S.: Medicolegal Considerations, in Malamed, S.F.: *Handbook of Medical Emergencies in the Dental Office,* 5th ed. St. Louis, Mosby, 2000, pp. 101–102.

Sfikas, P.M.: Informed Consent and the Law, *J. Am. Dent. Assoc., 129,* 1471, October, 1998.

Simonsen, R.J.: A Three-step Risk-protection Strategy (Editorial), *Quintessence Int., 25,* 297, May, 1994.

Van Dam, S. and Welie, J.V.M.: Requirement-driven Dental Education and the Patient's Right to Informed Consent, *J. Am. Coll. Dent., 68,* 40, Number 3, 2001.

Woodman, R.C. and Malz, V.L.: Informed Consent and the Elderly Dental Patient, *Spec. Care Dentist., 14,* 65, March/April, 1994.

PREVENTION

INTRODUCTION

Implementation of the prevention care plan is a specific part of the total care plan. The basic objectives are health promotion and disease prevention. The aim is to help each patient learn to accept the responsibility for daily self-care and how to prevent oral disease on a life-long basis. The influence of oral health on total body health may be a new concept for many patients to learn.

Teaching and learning, motivation, and adherence, are all part of the responsibilities of the dental hygienist with the patient. Section V provides detailed information on the personal care of the oral cavity, the teeth and their replacements, the influence of tobacco use, the basics of diet and nutrition for oral health, and the use of fluorides and sealants.

▪ ETHICAL APPLICATIONS

As ethical issues and dilemmas in the dental setting become more complex, other approaches to ethical decision making can be utilized. While a situation involving patient treatment may appear to be routine in nature, the competent dental hygienist is one who can view a concern from various perspectives. Understanding how the patient feels, or why the dentist-employer is responsible, proves critical when the dental hygienist must determine how to act within acceptable moral standards.

Using one's professional judgment, the dental hygienist reflects on the components of moral reasoning listed as topics in Table V-1 when making a decision. Solving an ethical dilemma often leads to the examination of other issues through the use of questions. Steps for solving an ethical dilemma are shown in Table V-1.

All individuals involved in the ethical situation can document their thoughts and communicate clearly with one another. It may be difficult at times, but sharing clear and concise evidence is extremely important when determining a morally acceptable decision.

▪ TABLE V-1 DECISION ALTERNATIVES THROUGH QUESTIONING

ETHICAL DECISION CONCEPT	QUESTIONING	DENTAL HYGIENE APPLICATION
Recognize Conflict	What are the specific details of the case? Are there issues of rights or moral character involved? At what level does the conflict exist?	Consider the role of the dental hygienist for each of the ethical principles outlined in the Code of Ethics.
Accumulate Possible Options	What alternative actions are available? Whose (or what) interests are at stake? What resources would other professionals use?	Review the dental practice act to determine the scope, duties and limitations of actions that can be taken by the dental hygienist, the dentist, and other practitioners for the patient.
Evaluate the Alternatives	Which decision would lead to the best consequences overall? Are all individuals involved being respected and treated in a fair manner? Which alternative would make a good general rule to follow?	Review the entries in a patient's record to determine if all points of view from the case have been included.
Reflect on the Decision	Can the action taken be justified as the best choice? What alternative actions also could be selected?	Discuss a similar situation at the next office/staff meeting to enhance responsiveness in ethical protocols.

Health Promotion and Disease Prevention

The dental hygienist is a primary care provider of preventive services. As a specialist in oral health care, the dental hygienist is involved at all levels of prevention, primary, secondary, and tertiary.

In Section V of this book, Prevention, for which this chapter is an introduction, objectives, information, and procedures for primary prevention are described. Box 23-1 defines key terms related to health promotion and disease prevention for the individual patient.

Within the process of dental hygiene care, the needs of a patient are assessed from the histories and clinical findings, a dental hygiene diagnosis is made, and the care plan is outlined. When planning the sequence of treatment for the patient, initiation of preventive measures precedes clinical services except in an emergency. One important reason is that the patient must learn and practice procedures of daily self-care if oral health is to be attained and maintained.

■ STEPS IN A PREVENTIVE PROGRAM

Each patient needs a preventive care plan. To plan and carry out a preventive program takes a cooperative effort by the patient and members of the dental team. Details of

BOX 23-1 KEY WORDS: Health Promotion and Disease Prevention

Behavior: manner in which an individual acts or performs.

Behavior modification: approach to correct undesirable behavior through systematic manipulation of environmental and behavioral variables; treatment procedure for certain mental and physical disorders.

Communication: verbal or nonverbal interaction or interchange; nonverbal, without spoken words, may be accomplished through pictures, gestures, facial expressions, or posture.

Compliance: extent to which a person's health behaviors coincide with dental/medical health advice; also called **adherence.**

Dental health education: the provision of oral health information to people in such a way that they can apply it in everyday living.

Dysphagia: difficulty in swallowing.

Evaluation: appraisal of changes in a patient's behavior or oral health status that have resulted from interventions by the professional health-care personnel.

Halitophobia: imaginary halitosis; constant fear of having bad breath; sometimes related to an underlying psychiatric condition.

Health education: combination of learning opportunities planned to facilitate and reinforce voluntary behavior conducive to the health of the individual or group.

Health promotion: planned combination of educational, economic, organizational, or environmental support for actions conducive to health of individuals or groups.

Learning: acquiring knowledge or skills through study, instruction, or experience; true learning means that knowledge acquired is applied in everyday living.

> **Affective domain:** the domain of learning concerned with attitudes, interests, and appreciations.
>
> **Cognitive domain:** the domain of learning concerned with knowledge outcomes and intellectual abilities.
>
> **Psychomotor domain:** the domain of learning concerned with levels of motor skills.

Marketing: the task of establishing, maintaining, and enhancing patient relationships so that the goals of the patient, the group, or the community can be achieved.

Motivation: inner driving force that prompts an individual to act to satisfy a need or desire or to accomplish a particular goal.

Noncompliance: failure to carry out a prescribed health-care plan, for example, failure to take medications as prescribed.

Organoleptic: stimulating any of the organs of sensation; susceptible to a sensory stimulus.

Preventive dental hygiene: sum total of the efforts to promote, restore, and maintain the oral health of the individual.

Putrefaction: enzymatic decomposition, especially of proteins with the production of foul-smelling compounds, such as hydrogen sulfide, ammonia, and mercaptans.

Volatile sulfur compounds (VSCs): hydrogen sulfide; methyl mercaptan; and, to a lesser extent, dimethyl sulfide and dimethyl disulfide produced by microbial metabolism and which create oral malodor.

Xerogenic: producing or causing dry mouth.

the basic steps listed below were described either in previous chapters or will be parts of the chapters to follow.

I. ASSESS THE PATIENT'S NEEDS

A. Review all information from the histories, radiographic and clinical examinations, and chartings.

B. Identify the presence and severity of infection and the risk factors for oral health.

C. Utilize indices to rate the extent of the needs and provide a baseline for continuing comparisons. For most patients, a dental biofilm score can be helpful for showing the patient the extent of the gingival problem, and a dietary record along with the charting of carious lesions help show the dental problem.

D. Does the patient show willingness and readiness to learn? How may cultural values and beliefs promote or block the patient's response and compliance?

II. PLAN FOR INTERVENTION

A. Apply information about the patient, such as educational level, occupation, socioeconomic background, and attitudes toward oral health and oral care.

B. Determine the current personal oral care procedures carried out by the patient and the frequency.

C. Note factors that may affect the patient's dexterity when using oral cleaning devices, such as an occupation that requires manual or digital skill.

D. Recognize the influence of age and physical and mental disabilities. Will another person (parent or other caregiver) be needed to carry out the necessary procedures?

E. Outline the procedures needed and work out goals with the patient.

F. Explain what can occur if the patient does not follow the care plan.

III. IMPLEMENTATION

A. How can the patient best be helped to be aware of personal oral health problems and to learn and practice more effective health behaviors?

B. Provide motivating demonstration and supervision for daily self-care, dental biofilm removal, self-applied fluoride, and other applicable preventive measures.

C. Introduce tobacco use cessation when indicated.

D. Show methods for self-evaluation.

E. Spread instruction over several appointments while clinical procedures are being completed. Learning takes time and reinforcement.

IV. PERFORM CLINICAL PREVENTIVE SERVICES

A. Complete scaling and bacterial debridement.

B. Apply caries-preventive agents: fluoride, sealants.

V. EVALUATE PROGRESSIVE CHANGES

A. Can the patient demonstrate the procedures for self-care? Do the teeth and gingiva show the benefits of learning?

B. Record a dental biofilm score at each appointment and compare previous recordings with the patient.

C. At appropriate intervals, probe to note improvement in tissue quality, bleeding on probing, and probing depths.

D. Provide preventive counseling for corrective action when goals are not met.

VI. PLAN SHORT- AND LONG-TERM MAINTENANCE

A. Determine appropriate maintenance intervals.

B. Reevaluate to monitor continuance of preventive practices.

C. Provide supplemental care for the patient who does not respond to basic therapy.

■ PATIENT COUNSELING

Personalized patient counseling contributes first to the knowledge, attitudes, and practices of the individual and then, through the individual, to the family and the community. Periodontal infections and dental caries can be prevented or controlled, and, therefore, teeth can be preserved throughout the lifetime of the individual.

For most patients, major attention must be placed on control of dental caries and/or periodontal infection, with emphasis on dental biofilm control and tobacco use cessation. Attention also should be paid to prevention of oral accidents such as those related to mouth protectors for contact sports, safety belts for automobiles, and children's accidents that lead to fractured anterior teeth.

Knowledge of and belief in health facts are not enough. Benefits result only when knowledge is put into action. Learning occurs when an individual changes behavior and when beneficial changes are incorporated into everyday living.

■ MOTIVATION

An individual is motivated to practice behavior that leads to achievement of goals that are valued. Instruction can be effective if the patient considers oral health a valuable asset.

Stimulation of behavior, or motivation, stems from basic physiologic or social needs. Peer group approval and the need to conform to group standards, as well as the fear of disapproval or rejection when, for example, appearance of the teeth or odor of the breath is unacceptable, are frequently much stronger motivating factors than is a health reason, such as freedom from infection or the ability to chew food.

■ THE LEARNING PROCESS

I. PRINCIPLES OF LEARNING

A. Learning is more effective when an individual is physiologically and psychologically ready to learn.

B. Individual differences must be considered if effective learning is to take place.

C. Motivation is essential for learning.

D. What an individual learns in a given situation depends on what is recognized and understood.

E. Transfer of learning is facilitated by recognition of similarities and dissimilarities between past experiences and the present situation.

F. An individual learns what is actually used.

G. Learning takes place more effectively in situations from which the individual derives feelings of satisfaction.

H. Evaluation of the results of instruction is essential to determine whether learning is taking place.

II. THE LEARNING LADDER[1]

Figure 23-1 illustrates the six steps from learner unawareness to habit formation. When beginning to help a patient learn about oral health and what the individual's needs are, one must determine where the patient stands on the ladder and start from there. Briefly, the ladder steps are as follows:

A. Unawareness

Many patients have little concept of the new information about dental and periodontal infections and how they are prevented or controlled.

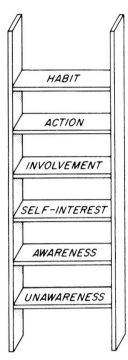

■ **FIGURE 23-1 The Learning Ladder.** Learning takes place in a series of steps from unawareness through interest and involvement to habit formation. See the text for the description of each step on the ladder. (From Harris, N.O. and Christen, A.G.: *Primary Preventive Dentistry*, 4th ed. Norwalk, CT, Appleton & Lange, 1995.)

B. Awareness

Patients may have a good knowledge of the scientific facts, but they do not apply the facts to personal action.

C. Self-interest

Realization of the application of facts/knowledge to the well-being of the individual is an initial motivation.

D. Involvement

With awareness and application to self, the response to action is forthcoming when attitude is influenced.

E. Action

Testing new knowledge and beginning of change in behavior may lead to an increased awareness that a real health goal is possible to attain.

F. Habit

Self-satisfaction in the comfort and value of sound teeth and healthy periodontal tissues helps to make certain practices become part of a daily routine. Ultimate motivation is finally reached.

■ INDIVIDUAL PATIENT PLANNING

Initial instruction for most new patients will be personal biofilm removal procedures. Each patient will have individual requirements.

All of the factors that apply to an individual patient are matched with the available dental biofilm removal procedures. These include the selection of a toothbrush, toothbrushing method, interdental care devices and methods, dentifrice, and applied techniques for implants and fixed and removable dental prostheses.

With a clear definition of the needs of a patient, a recommended regimen or program can be outlined. The patient is shown the oral condition, changes and benefits that can be expected are explained, and cooperation is solicited. In this framework, the patient helps to formulate the goals that must be accomplished.

I. WHEN TO TEACH

The initial instruction is best given *first,* before any clinical treatment. Reasons related to the educational aspects are as follows:

A. Emphasis on Importance of Self-care

Clinical professional services have only short-term effectiveness if the patient does not maintain tissue health through daily biofilm removal. If considered first, and first in succeeding appointments, the degree of importance placed on self-care procedures by the dental team will become apparent to the patient.

B. Teaching Is More Effective

If instruction is delayed until after the clinical procedures in an appointment,
1. Time may be limited.
2. The gingival margin may be sensitive from instrumentation.
3. Blood clots forming after scaling and root planing must not be disturbed so healing can progress favorably.
4. Patient may be tired, anxious to leave, and less receptive to instruction.

C. Biofilm on Patient's Teeth

1. *Biofilm Is the Lesson.* With removal of tooth deposits during scaling, the opportunity to utilize the patient's existing biofilm for demonstration is lost.
2. *Use a Disclosing Agent.* With the use of a disclosing agent, a method of instruction is available that clearly and dramatically can show the patient what is to be accomplished. Dental biofilm is not visible on most teeth without staining. Words fail to impress upon the patient that bacterial colonies exist on the teeth and that these multitudes of microorganisms are the responsible agents for dental and periodontal infections.

II. THE SETTING

A. Teaching Facility

A specific area may be set aside and furnished for biofilm control instruction in a dental office or clinic. Such an area should be planned with mirrors for the patient to use to observe the stained biofilm on posterior teeth and distal surfaces. The patient also should be able to see placement of the toothbrush and floss in all areas of the mouth.

B. At the Dental Unit

Because of the need for the light and rinsing facilities during the demonstration, instruction may be given best at the dental chair. Without an extensive display of instruments and other equipment to distract the patient, and with the clinician seated beside the dental chair at the patient's eye level, an atmosphere conducive to learning can be created.

■ PRESENTATION, DEMONSTRATION, PRACTICE

A suggested outline for conducting the dental biofilm control program follows. Various adaptations will be needed to tailor the plan to individual patients.

Each of the "lessons" described in the following outline is meant to represent the opening few minutes of each appointment before instrumentation for scaling. A biofilm index or score and/or a bleeding index is made at the start. The index or score is understood by the patient, and new and review instructions are provided as indicated.

I. FIRST LESSON

A. Objective

Orientation to dental biofilm removal.

B. Description

Describe the formation and composition of dental biofilm, its relationship to oral disease (dental caries and periodontal infection), and specifically the relationship to the patient's present condition. Present an overview of the biofilm control program, what it can accomplish, and its purposes in relation to professional treatment.

C. Illustration

Sketch on a pad of paper or use prepared materials. Show a tooth and gingiva and point out where the bacterial masses collect to form biofilm. Explain briefly how inflammation develops in the gingiva. Divide the material over more than one instruction period. Too long a "lecture" with too many facts and details at one time may mean the patient cannot absorb any of them.

1. *Patient With Gingivitis.* Show and explain the formation of dental calculus and how periodontal disease can develop if gingivitis is left untreated.
2. *Patient With Periodontitis.* Introduce pocket formation and the reasons for pocket elimination.
3. *Patient Whose Most Severe Problem Is Dental Caries.* When a food record for assessment is to be prepared, orientation to the preparation of the food record precludes discussion of biofilm, cariogenic foods, and dental caries until the dietary record is obtained.

D. Demonstration

1. While the patient observes in a mirror, a healthy area of gingiva and an inflamed area can be compared.
2. A probe is used to show a gingival sulcus and/or increased pocket depth related to periodontal involvement. Bleeding on probing is an important indicator of disease and should be recorded.
3. Remove a sample of biofilm with a curet to demonstrate the thickness and consistency of biofilm and to use for a phase microscope demonstration when available.

E. Application of a Disclosing Agent

1. *Explain Its Purpose.* Discoloration of biofilm shows where the masses of bacteria accumulate.
2. *Apply Disclosing Agent.* Use a topical application and provide diluted concentrate for a rinse; or request the patient to chew a tablet, swish for approximately 1 minute, and rinse.
3. *Examine the Teeth With the Patient.* Point out the stained biofilm and explain how the bacteria must be removed to control inflammation.
4. *Record Biofilm Score or Index.* Explain the score to the patient and use it to compare at future evaluations.

5. *Observe Location.* Observation of the location of disclosed biofilm guides the instruction for biofilm removal.

F. Instruction

1. *Keep Instruction Simple.* It may be better not to teach both flossing and brushing during the first control lesson, depending on the patient's background and experience.
2. *Floss First*
   a. Review objective.
   b. Show manner of holding the floss, inserting proximally, pressing around the tooth, and activating for biofilm removal.
   c. Examine in mirror to observe proximal areas where biofilm has been removed.
3. *Brush.* Select a soft brush and ask the patient to remove the stained biofilm. No specific brushing instructions should be given at this time so that the patient can concentrate on the single objective related to biofilm removal.
4. *After Brushing, Examine the Teeth With the Patient.* The patient will see where accessible biofilm was removed.
5. *Explain.* The use of a toothbrush is the most effective means of biofilm removal for facial and lingual surfaces. Dental floss and other interdental devices are needed for the proximal tooth surfaces.
6. *Additional Devices: Care of Fixed Prostheses and Implants.* Instruction for care of a new prosthesis must be provided at the same appointment as its placement. Dental implants need special attention.

G. Summary of Lesson I

1. Review the basic objectives of learning about biofilm composition, occurrence, and relationship to oral disease, and learning about the use of a disclosing agent to aid in biofilm detection and removal.
2. At the first lesson, a specific toothbrushing method is not necessarily presented. The basic objectives should not be obscured by inclusion of excess information or diversion of the patient's thinking by concentration on details of brush position. The exceptions are:
   a. The patient who demonstrates an acceptable brushing technique and whose mouth has been kept reasonably clean and shows no signs of detrimental brushing may only need to be shown a few special adaptations for the difficult-to-reach areas or other improvements.

b. The patient who demonstrates a brushing method that is detrimental, such as a vigorous horizontal stroke or a haphazard scrub-brush method, and whose teeth and/or gingiva show the effects of harmful brushing needs an introduction to a less destructive method.

H. Instruction at End of Appointment

1. Encourage use of disclosing agent at home; provide patient with tablets or instructions for purchasing. Suggest using a tablet for daily biofilm checks.

2. Emphasize the need for cleaning regularly for complete daily dental biofilm removal. Discuss carrying a toothbrush and dental floss for use when not at home.

3. When extra brushes cannot be supplied, explain that the toothbrush that has been used that day will be kept in the office for use during future appointments. Write down the specific name (number) of the brush for the patient to purchase for home use.

I. Patient Records

Methods, procedures, and patient progress and problems should be recorded following each appointment. The documented record can be reviewed before each appointment as a guide to continuing instruction.

II. SECOND LESSON

A. Objectives

To evaluate the patient's success to date and to review and expand the knowledge content of the previous lesson.

B. Evaluation

1. *Examine the Gingival Tissue With the Patient.* Evaluate and compare with notes recorded from previous examination. Changes in color, size, and bleeding on probing should be noted and recorded.

2. *Apply the Disclosing Agent.* Evaluate the biofilm as the patient self-evaluates, using a hand mirror. Chart biofilm index or other record and compare, with the patient, with previous scores or indices.

C. Review and Extension of Knowledge

1. Invite questions from patient concerning biofilm formation and gingival and periodontal infections to determine how clearly information from the previous lesson was understood and retained.

2. Always commend and compliment the patient for successes and improvements.

3. Discuss dentifrice recommendation when information from the dental history and the oral examination indicates the need for a change.

4. Explain why the patient needs a more scientific brushing method (or how a few alterations in the previous method can improve the oral condition).

5. Relate brushing to the treatment phase of oral care.

D. Demonstration

When not done previously, demonstrate the brushing technique of choice for this particular patient.

1. Show the basic stroke on the anterior teeth where the patient can observe brush position and activation. Explain each step. Demonstrate brush position for each quadrant.

2. Instruction is divided appropriately to permit the patient to learn at a comfortable pace. When a patient has a power-assisted brush, initial instruction is best given with the manual brush so that proficiency can be attained with both. The patient can be asked to bring the power-assisted brush to the next appointment for demonstration and instruction.

E. Practice

1. Each position around each arch must be practiced because of the variations in grasp of brush and hand positions; the difficulty of access; and the individual tooth positions, particularly malpositions.

2. A recommended sequence for biofilm removal that includes all areas and the tongue is discussed with the patient.

F. Instructions for Home Procedures

Use disclosing agent after flossing and brushing to test completeness of biofilm removal. A mouth mirror for the patient to use at home can be helpful. Inexpensive plastic mirrors are available specifically for this purpose.

III. CONTINUOUS INSTRUCTION

A. Number of Lessons

It is not possible to predict in advance the number of specific teaching sessions a patient will need to demonstrate mastery of the recommended procedures and to show by the appearance of the teeth and health of the gingiva that the practices have been carried out daily. When additional supervision is indicated after professional treatment has been completed, short appointments may be scheduled in conjunction with dental appointments.

One learning experience is rarely adequate. When a patient has been able to maintain relatively clean teeth and clinically healthy gingiva and can demonstrate an acceptable toothbrushing method, a review of difficult-to-reach areas can be made and reevaluated at a follow-up appointment.

B. Relationship to Gingival Health

When areas of gingival marginal redness and sponginess persist, tooth surfaces are checked carefully for residual calculus, and scaling and planing are completed as indicated. When the patient consistently fails to remove dental biofilm in certain areas, a reevaluation of the program is made. Perhaps the selected procedures are too difficult for the patient to accomplish, or perhaps supplementary measures are needed.

C. Maintenance

After the initial instruction series, a follow-up is scheduled after a short interval for the first maintenance appointment. One must evaluate the patient's ability to continue adequate self-care and determine whether true learning has resulted and new habits have been adopted. *Learning means that a change in behavior has occurred.*

At each maintenance appointment, a biofilm score or index is recorded, and the patient can evaluate the progress made.

IV. INSTRUCTION ADAPTABILITY

The methods for presentation, demonstration, practice, and evaluation described in the previous pages can be adapted readily to various age levels. Awareness of the changing motivation and interests of the young to the elderly, and adaptations of terminology with respect for the patient's level of understanding, ease the transition from patient to patient.

Others for whom instruction is provided are the caregivers who attend to patients who are unable to care for themselves. In Section VII, the various chapters that pertain to patients with disabilities include suggestions for patient care.

▪ THE PRESCHOOL CHILD

The establishment of positive health habits and attitudes in the adult has its beginnings in childhood. Even before birth and during the first year after birth, the parent's

education for prevention of dental caries and gingival infection should begin.

After birth, regular daily systemic fluoride in the absence of fluoridation, as well as attention to the control of cariogenic foods, can mean a great deal to the future oral health of the child.

Oral health during the preschool years is considered in detail in Chapter 46. Anticipatory Guidance for parents is described in Tables 46-2 and 46-3 on pages 786 to 788.

▪ THE TEACHING SYSTEM

A simple, direct approach, such as has been described, with specific content and unembellished material focuses the attention of the patient on the central theme: control of oral bacteria. The more practical, realistic, and goal centered the components of instruction can be, the more effective the outcomes will be in terms of treatment and prevention of recurrence of infection. An *informed,* knowledgeable patient will have reasons for *practicing* appropriate, scientifically based, self-care measures.

A teaching system must be reevaluated from time to time, particularly as new research reveals new aspects of prevention and treatment. New devices for biofilm removal and gingival care may become available, and these must be studied before recommendations to patients can be made.

The teaching system presented in this chapter has a built-in evaluation of patient learning. The outcomes of learning are shown by examination and demonstration: examination for the gingival characteristics consistent with health; demonstration of disclosable biofilm; and demonstration of the patient's ability to use floss and brush for biofilm removal without harm to the oral tissues.

Because the ultimate objective of biofilm control is to prevent dental caries and periodontal infections, the oral health history of the patient over several years can be used to document a true evaluation. The teaching system must involve development of the patient's attitudes relative to continuing professional supervision and regular appointments for examination and treatment.

▪ EVALUATION OF TEACHING AIDS

I. GENERAL CHARACTERISTICS

Evaluation of teaching aids involves consideration of the following:

A. Simplicity

Ease of management, ready obtainability, ease of understanding by the patient.

B. Content

Practical, scientifically sound, meaningful.

C. Level of Orientation

Appropriate for the individual patient.

D. Durability

If reusable, the teaching aids must maintain their cleanliness and freshness. Washable materials can be selected when available.

E. Cost

Reasonable. Cost relates to their essential value in reaching goals.

F. Objectives

1. Objective of a teaching aid must be clear and readily understood by the patient.
2. In teaching, activities should be reality centered, not fantasy centered. A well-intentioned visual aid may provide entertainment rather than education and have no transfer value, in terms of the actual oral health lesson, to the behavioral pattern of the patient.

II. READING MATERIAL FOR THE PATIENT

Effectively presented informational books and leaflets can supplement and reinforce individually presented instruction. Selected with a purpose, a booklet or other printed material may be presented to the patient to read while at the dental office, or it may be given for "homework." The booklet's contents must be reviewed with the patient; particular sections may be marked to personalize the instruction and encourage reading. Indiscriminate distribution of printed materials is pointless.

Obtaining copies of and reviewing newly available materials are essential parts of a dental hygienist's work, even as a teacher reviews new textbooks and materials for possible use in a classroom.

Instruction sheets and leaflets can be custom-made with the cooperation and recommendations of the dentist. It is especially helpful to have postcare instructions and biofilm control procedures outlined so that the patient can have a reference for home use. Materials can be personalized by writing on them the patient's name and special procedures or reminders.

III. USE OF MODELS

A. Patient's Study Cast

The cast can be useful to explain oral conditions or restorations, such as the need to replace missing teeth. With certain patients, aspects of dental biofilm control can be demonstrated, provided the patient is properly oriented to associate the cast with the teeth in the mouth.

B. Commercially Available Models

Although plastic models (dentoforms) have been used extensively for teaching toothbrushing methods, their meaningfulness to the patient has not been demonstrated. When a toothbrush is available for demonstration directly in the mouth and for a patient to use to practice brushing under supervision, the need for taking the time to demonstrate on a model first may be questioned.

When teaching is by means of the model and brush only, and particularly when the oversized model is used, the patient's learning should be carefully evaluated. All three of the patient evaluation methods described in this chapter (gingival status, disclosed biofilm, and ability of patient to brush) should be utilized.

The model and the large toothbrush probably do not represent a problem to the patient, and most patients can imitate the motions of the toothbrush on the model accurately when asked. The difficulty comes in transferring the motions to the mouth and relating such motions to the bacterial collections on the teeth. The more complex the technique, the greater the difficulty of transfer.

■ USE OF DISCLOSING AGENTS

A disclosing agent is a preparation in liquid, tablet, or lozenge form that contains a dye or other coloring agent. In dental hygiene, a disclosing agent is used to identify dental biofilm deposits for instruction, evaluation, and research. Key words related to disclosing agents are defined in Box 23-2.

Dental biofilm is nearly colorless unless stained by foods, beverages, or tobacco. After use of a disclosing agent, the soft deposits pick up and hold the color of the agent. On the other hand, the dye can be rinsed off readily from biofilm-free surfaces (Figure 23-2). After staining, the deposits that can be seen distinctly provide a valuable visual aid in patient instruction. Such a procedure can demonstrate dramatically to the patient the presence of deposits and the areas that need special attention during personal oral care.

BOX 23-2   KEY WORDS AND ABBREVIATIONS: Disclosing Agents

Diffusion: process of being widely spread.

　Diffusibility: refers to the ability of a disclosing agent to spread readily over a tooth surface and flow into the interproximal areas.

Disclosing agent: selective dye in solution, tablet, or lozenge form used to visualize and identify dental biofilm on the surfaces of the teeth.

Eosin: rose-colored dye used for preparing histologic specimens for microscopic study; companion dye with **hematoxylin** for the well-known "H & E" that stains nuclei blue and the cytoplasm pink.

Erythrosin: red-colored dye used in solution or tablet form for a disclosing agent in the identification of dental biofilm on teeth.

F.D.&C. (**F**ood **D**rug & **C**osmetic): United States Food, Drug, and Cosmetic Act regulates the packaging, labeling, importing, and exporting of such products as disclosing agents.

Fluorescein: bright yellow fluorescing dye effective for disclosing dental biofilm on teeth; used in ophthalmology to reveal corneal lesions of the eye.

I.   PURPOSES

A disclosing agent clearly demarcates soft deposits that might otherwise be invisible and therefore facilitates the following:

A. Personalized patient instruction in the location of soft deposits and the techniques for removal.

B. Self-assessment by the patient on a daily basis during initial instruction and periodic checks thereafter.

C. Continuing evaluation of the effectiveness of the instruction for the patient.
  1. Determining the need for revisions of the biofilm control procedures.
  2. Studying the long-term effects over successive maintenance appointments.

D. Preparation of biofilm indices.

E. Conducting research studies to gain new information about the incidence and formation of deposits on the teeth, the effectiveness of specific devices for dental biofilm control, and antibiofilm agents and to evaluate clinical and instructional group health programs.

II.   PROPERTIES OF AN ACCEPTABLE DISCLOSING AGENT

A.   Intensity of Color

A distinct staining of deposits should be evident. The color should contrast with normal colors of the oral cavity.

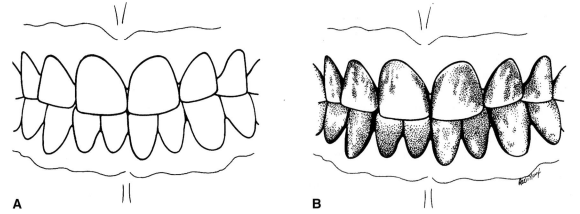

■ FIGURE 23-2 Use of Disclosing Agent. (A) Appearance of the teeth before application of a disclosing agent. Dental biofilm and pellicle are usually invisible. **(B)** After use of a disclosing agent on the same teeth as those shown in **A.** Dental biofilm and pellicle take on the color of the dye used in the disclosing agent. As noted, soft deposits are extensive, and are especially thick on the proximal surfaces.

B. Duration of Intensity

The color should not rinse off immediately with ordinary rinsing methods, and neither should it be removable by the saliva for the period of time required to complete the instruction or clinical service. The color should be removed from the gingival tissue and lips by the completion of the appointment, however, as the patient may have a personal reaction to color retained for a long period of time.

C. Taste

The patient should not be made uncomfortable by an unpleasant or highly flavored substance. The main reason for using the disclosant is to motivate the patient; therefore, the use of the agent should be pleasant and encourage cooperation.

D. Irritation to the Mucous Membrane

The patient should be questioned concerning the possibility of an idiosyncrasy to an ingredient. When this information is obtained, it should be entered on the patient's permanent history record. Because of the possibility of allergy, more than one type of disclosing agent should be available for use.

E. Diffusibility

A solution should be thin enough so it can be applied readily to the exposed surfaces of the teeth, yet thick enough to impart an intense color to dental biofilm.

F. Astringent and Antiseptic Properties

These properties may be highly desirable in that the disclosing agent may contribute other factors to the treatment procedures. The application of an antiseptic before scaling is frequently recommended, and if an antiseptic disclosing agent is used, one solution can serve a dual purpose.

A disclosant may inhibit the growth of microorganisms. In quantitative biofilm research studies, therefore, disclosing agents without antibacterial properties should be used.

III. FORMULAE

A variety of disclosing agents has been used. Skinner's iodine solution was formerly the most classic and widely used. In general, iodine solutions are less desirable because of their unpleasant flavor.

Aniline dyes have been shown to have carcinogenic potential. Therefore, the use of basic fuchsin and beta rose (flavored basic fuchsin) has been discouraged.

The formulae of a few disclosing agents are included in this chapter. Other well-known agents are Buckley's,

Berwick's, Talbot's iodo-glycerol, and Metaphen solutions.

A. Iodine Preparations

1. Skinner's Solution

Iodine crystals	3.3 g
Potassium iodide	1.0 g
Zinc iodide	1.0 g
Water (distilled)	16.0 mL
Glycerin	6.0 mL

2. Diluted Tincture of Iodine

Tincture of iodine	21.0 mL
Water (distilled)	15.0 mL

B. Mercurochrome Preparations

1. Mercurochrome Solution (5%)

Mercurochrome	1.5 g
Water (distilled) to make	30.0 mL

2. Flavored Mercurochrome Disclosing Solution

Mercurochrome	13.5 g
Water (distilled)	3.0 L
Oil of peppermint	3 drops

Artificial noncariogenic sweetener

C. Bismarck Brown (Easlick's Disclosing Solution)

Bismarck Brown	3.0 g
Ethyl alcohol	10.0 mL
Glycerin	120.0 mL
Anise (flavoring)	1 drop

D. Merbromin

Merbromin, N.F.	450.0 mg
Oil of peppermint	1 drop
Water (distilled) to make	100.0 mL

E. Erythrosin

1. Concentrate for Application by Rinsing

F.D.&C. Red No. 3 or No. 28	6.0 g
Water (distilled) to make	100.0 mL

2. For Direct Topical Application

Erythrosin	0.8 g
Water (distilled)	100.0 mL
Alcohol (95%)	10.0 mL
Oil of peppermint	2 drops

3. Tablet[3]

F.D.&C. Red No. 3	15.0 mg
Sodium chloride	0.747%
Sodium sucaryl	0.747%
Calcium stearate	0.995%
Soluble saccharin	0.186%

White oil   0.124%
Flavoring   2.239%
Sorbitol to make a 7-grain tablet

F. Fast Green

F.D.&C. Green No. 3.5% or 2.5%

G. Fluorescein[4]

F.D.&C. Yellow No. 8 (used with a special ultraviolet light source to make the agent visible)

H. Two-Tone[5]

F.D.&C. Green No. 3
F.D.&C. Red No. 3
Thicker (older) biofilm stains blue; thinner (newer) biofilm stains red.

IV. METHODS FOR APPLICATION

Make gingival tissue evaluation before application because disclosing agent masks tissue colors.

A. Solution for Direct Application (Painting)

1. Have patient rinse to remove food particles and heavy saliva.
2. Apply water-based lubricant generously to prevent staining of the lips.
3. Dry the teeth with compressed air, retracting cheek or tongue.
4. Use swab or small cotton pellet to carry the solution to the teeth.
5. Apply solution generously to the crowns of the teeth only.
6. Direct the patient to spread the agent over all surfaces of the teeth with the tongue.
7. Examine the distribution of agent and request the patient to rinse if indicated.

B. Rinsing

A few drops of a concentrated preparation are placed in a paper cup and water is added for the appropriate dilution. Instruct the patient to rinse and swish the solution over all tooth surfaces.

C. Tablet or Wafer

The patient chews the wafer (one half may be sufficient for some patients), swishes it around for 30 to 60 seconds, and rinses.

V. INTERPRETATION

A. Clean tooth surfaces do not absorb the coloring agent; when pellicle and dental biofilm are present, they absorb the agent and are disclosed (Figure 23-2).
B. Pellicle stains as a thin, relatively clear covering, whereas dental biofilm appears darker, thicker, and more opaque.
C. Two-Tone
   1. *Red Biofilm.* Newly formed, thin, usually supragingival.
   2. *Blue Biofilm.* Thicker, older, more tenacious; usually it is seen at and just below gingival margin, especially on proximal surfaces and where brush or floss is not easily applied; may be associated with calculus deposits.

VI. PATIENT INSTRUCTION

Because biofilm and pellicle are frequently invisible to a patient, a disclosing agent can provide a visual method for patient instruction.

A. Explain Dental Biofilm

The patient needs to be informed about the composition and effect of biofilm in the production of gingival and periodontal infections, with particular reference to the individual mouth.

B. Show Location and Distribution of Biofilm

With a mirror, the patient can observe the teeth and the disclosed dental biofilm. A small mouth mirror is needed to show the lingual surfaces and posterior facial areas.

Show the special areas of concern. Relate the tinted areas to the health of the gingiva.

C. Demonstrate Methods for Daily Biofilm Removal

A plan for instruction is outlined on pages 379 to 382. The techniques for toothbrushing and interdental care are described in Chapters 25 and 26.

■ TECHNICAL HINTS FOR DISCLOSING AGENTS

I. Avoid using disclosing or antiseptic solutions on teeth that have tooth-color restorations because these materials may be stained by coloring agents.

II.   Do not apply a disclosing agent before a sealant is to be placed.

III.   Purchase solutions in small quantities. Do not keep solutions containing alcohol longer than 2 or 3 months because the alcohol will evaporate and render the solution too highly concentrated.

IV.   Use small bottles with dropper caps for solutions. Transfer solution to a dappen dish for use. Do not contaminate the solution by dipping cotton pliers with pellet directly into the container bottle.

V.   Request local druggist to stock disclosing tablets for patients to purchase. Advise patients of the stores where the agents may be purchased.

VI.   Source for two-tone disclosing agent:
RHODES TO HEALTH
Marilyn Rhodes, R.D.H.
4335 Bermuda Avenue
Oakland, CA 94619-3020
Phone 510-531-0348
1-800-530-0348
www.rhodestohealth.com

■ XEROSTOMIA

Saliva has many functions in the oral cavity relating to the maintenance of health of the teeth and soft tissues. It is protective in its functions of lubrication and cleansing. It contains immunoglobulins, electrolytes, and other substances that aid in resistance to disease (Table 23-1).

Xerostomia means dryness of the mouth. It is caused by absence or diminished quantity of saliva. Lack of saliva and the resulting dry mouth are important contributing factors to oral discomfort and disease, particularly dental caries. Xerostomia is a symptom, not a disease entity.

I.   CAUSES OF XEROSTOMIA

Xerostomia may be permanent or temporary. Temporary dry mouth occurs in diseases accompanied by high fever with dehydration or fluid loss; with control of certain diseases, such as diabetes or hyperthyroidism, salivary flow returns to normal. Major causes of permanent xerostomia are as follows:

A.   Radiation to Head and Neck for Cancer Therapy

Permanent damage to the salivary glands can result.

B.   Surgical Removal of Glands

The glands may be removed because of neoplasm.

C.   Sjögren's Syndrome[6]

The syndrome is an autoimmune disorder of the salivary and lacrimal glands with symptoms of polyarthritis, enlarged parotid glands, marked xerostomia, and dryness of the eyes.

D.   Pharmacologically Induced Xerostomia

Many drugs that are common prescription items produce dry mouth as a side effect.[7] Table 23-2 shows a partial list of the classes of drugs that decrease salivary function.

II.   EFFECTS OF XEROSTOMIA

During patient examination and history preparation, questions and clinical observations can point to the existence of dry mouth even when a patient does not complain of the symptoms.

■ TABLE 23-1 FUNCTIONS OF SALIVA

Lubrication of membranes, gingiva, teeth
Cleansing in self-cleansing mechanism
Tasting
Digestion: Food breakdown: chewing
   Food bolus formation
   Swallowing
Protection against diseases
   Antibacterial
   Antifungal
   Antiviral
Buffering: pH control
Remineralization
   Protection against demineralization
Speech
Carrier of antibodies, hormones, enzymes
   Provide data for diagnostic testing

■ TABLE 23-2 PARTIAL LIST OF CLASSES OF DRUGS THAT DECREASE SALIVARY FUNCTION

Anticholinergics
Antihistamines
Antihypertensives
Antianxiety
Anticonvulsants
Diuretics
Narcotics
Antidepressants (tricyclic)

A. Clinical Symptoms

1. Feeling of oral dryness; tongue sticks to palate.
2. Difficulty with mastication, swallowing, or speech.
3. Impaired taste.
4. Thirst, with resultant increased use of fluids; licking of lips.
5. Smarting, burning, and soreness of mucosa and tongue.

B. Oral Effects

1. Heavy dental biofilm, materia alba, and debris accumulation can lead to increased severity of periodontal infection and dental caries.
2. Predisposition to dental caries, particularly root caries.
3. Problems of denture wearing.
4. Dietary changes because of discomfort during eating; may use large quantities of liquid to soften food for swallowing.

III. MANAGEMENT OF XEROSTOMIA[8,9]

A. Pilocarpine Therapy[9,10]

Pilocarpine acts to increase salivary output. Patients with Sjögren's syndrome or other causes of xerostomia can get relief.

B. Prevention of Dental Caries

Severe, rampant dental caries related to any cause needs prompt counseling and treatment. One example is radiation therapy. Even before the radiation treatments are started, oral hygiene and caries prevention instruction must start, and a fluoride program must be initiated.

C. Personal Care Program

1. Rigorous biofilm control effort by the patient for dental biofilm removal.
2. Multiple fluorides may be recommended; use of dentifrice, rinse, and brush-on gel (or tray).
3. Advise patient to avoid tobacco and alcohol and to use foods that are noncariogenic.

D. Environmental Factors

Patient may need to adjust air humidification in living quarters.

E. Use of a Saliva Substitute[10]

A saliva substitute is a preparation with physical and chemical properties similar to those of real saliva. The ideal substitute should be able to coat the mucosa and teeth to keep them moist, reduce enamel solubility, and remineralize the surface, as well as to help prevent accumulation of dental biofilm.

Saliva substitutes contain carboxymethylcellulose (CMC) and the minerals calcium and phosphorous, fluoride, and other ions typical of normal human saliva. A small amount is sprayed into the mouth and distributed over all surfaces with the tongue. Patients can use the preparation at will, as needed for comfort.

F. Early Recognition

Dental hygienists are often the first to observe dry mouth (during the intraoral examination) and the first to hear the complaints of the patient of the discomforts caused. Early diagnosis and early treatment of Sjögren's syndrome or other causes of xerostomia can provide a major contribution to the general and oral health of the patient.

▪ HALITOSIS

Halitosis, an unpleasant odor of exhaled air, is a symptom of importance in the complete consideration of health promotion and disease prevention. The sources or causes may be local or systemic. Bad breath can and should be a health concern.

The effects on the individual may be to create a sensitivity leading to a social handicap that can impair general daily living and personal relationships. When a patient asks about the breath, the request for help must be taken seriously.

Halitosis is also known as oral malodor, fetor ex ore, or just bad breath. It is sometimes called by names related to the cause such as "hunger breath," "menstrual breath," "tobacco breath," or "garlic breath."

I. ETIOLOGY

At least 90% of all malodor originates in the oral cavity, whereas the remaining 10% has systemic or nonoral causes.

A. Oral Causes and Contributing Factors

1. Periodontal Infections: odor from subgingival dental biofilm.
2. Tongue coating harbors microorganisms.
3. Xerostomia.
4. Faulty restorations retaining food and bacteria.
5. Unclean dentures.
6. Oral pathologic lesions: carcinomas.

Everyday Ethics

Jeremy was a favorite patient in the dental office. Jeremy had undergone extensive restorative work as a young child because he had collided on a swing set with an older sibling, which resulted in trauma to both maxillary and mandibular incisors and permanent tooth buds. Now 15 years old, Jeremy seemed to grow two or three inches each time he came for his maintenance appointments.

Tressa, the dental hygienist, always commented on what a handsome young man Jeremy was becoming. He received a "fair plus" on his oral homecare report card the last few visits, but this time something was different. Tressa noticed more biofilm on Jeremy's teeth, and a distinct unpleasant odor. "Jeremy," she teased, "have any of the girls refused to kiss you recently?" Turning very red, Jeremy pulled his cap over his eyes, crossed his arms, and mumbled,

"Nope." Tressa made a mental note to let him smell the dental floss she used in his mouth as part of her personal home care review.

Questions for Consideration

1. Professionally, was the dental hygienist approaching Jeremy according to his needs while developing a realistic dental hygiene treatment plan for educating him?

2. Was Tressa's assumption that Jeremy had halitosis as a result of poor oral hygiene correct? What other factors could have been considered or communicated to Jeremy?

3. Suggest which of the core values apply in this scenario. Is this something Tressa should keep confidential from Jeremy's parents? Why or why not?

---

7. Throat infection.
8. Cleft palate.

B. Systemic and Non-Oral Factors[11]

1. Renal or hepatic failure.
2. Carcinomas.
3. Diabetes.
4. Upper respiratory; nasal passages.
5. Cirrhosis of the liver.

II. ASSESSMENT

The normal breath of a healthy person with healthy oral tissues is nonodiferous or mildly sweet smelling. Suggestions for the assessment are included here. The list of predisposing and etiologic factors should provide a guide to specific areas of concern.

A. Medical, Dental, and Personal History[12]

1. Systemic influences: relate to list of causes.
2. Medications history: side effects of dry mouth.
3. Tobacco use.
4. Diet, eating habits.

B. Extraoral Examination

1. *Organoleptic.* Smelling of the exhaled air is the simplest and most common method for identification.

2. *Detection Oral Source.* When the odor is detected from the open mouth, but not from the nose when the mouth is closed, it can be assumed that the odor has an oral origin.

C. Intraoral Examination

1. Tongue coating.
2. Evidence of mouth breathing.
3. Xerostomia: dry mucosa.
4. Other: see "Oral Causes and Contributing Factors."

D. Complete Periodontal Examination

1. General personal care: state of oral hygiene.
2. Probing for attachment levels, probing depths; periodontal status.
3. Evidence of neglect; past history of dental hygiene care.

E. Measurement of Oral Malodor[13]

1. *Composition.* The majority of malodor arises in the mouth from microbial metabolism. Volatile sulphur compounds (VSCs) are produced consisting of hydrogen sulfide, methyl mercaptan, and lesser amounts of dimethyl sulfide and dimethyl disulfide. The VSCs are much higher in patients with periodontal diseases.[14]

2. *Instrumental Examination.* A VSC monitor has been developed especially for use in research to test the effects of mouthrinses and other

products on oral malodors. A portable sulfide monitor (halimeter) is available for obtaining either or both oral or nasal readings to differentiate the sources of malodor.[15]

III. INTERVENTIONS

A. Dental Hygiene Care Plan

Objectives are based on achieving optimum gingival and periodontal health. Daily dental biofilm control and cleaning of all fixed and removable prostheses and implants are mandatory. All potential sources of biofilm retention must be removed and carious lesions restored.

B. Plan for Instruction

For patients who want to use a mouthrinse to help produce pleasant oral odors, they should be advised that mouthrinses have only temporary effects on malodor. Rinses with alcohol, glycerin, or strong oxidizing agents that can have detrimental effects on the oral tissues when used extensively must be avoided.

C. Tongue Cleaning

Brushing and cleaning of the dorsal surface of the tongue is a daily requirement. The tongue is a major source of the organisms producing VSCs.[16]

Factors To Teach The Patient

- The relationship between preventive measures and clinical services.

- Why particular preventive measures were selected for the particular patient.

- Self-assessment and methods for determining health of gingiva; assessment of dental biofilm after use of a disclosing agent.

- Objectives for dental biofilm infection control.

- Treatment measures for xerostomia, such as diet, personal care, and where to obtain and how to use a saliva substitute.

- Purposes for use of disclosing agents; the appearance of stained dental biofilm and the methods of daily care necessary to keep biofilm controlled.

- For the parent, method of application of a disclosing agent to a small child's teeth to evaluate the presence of biofilm.

REFERENCES

1. **Christen**, A.G. and Katz, C.A.: Understanding Human Motivation, in Harris, N.O. and Christen, A.G.: *Primary Preventive Dentistry,* 4th ed. Norwalk, CT, Appleton & Lange, 1995, pp. 393–396.

2. **American Academy of Pediatric Dentistry:** A.A.P.D. Oral Health Policies, *Pediatr. Dent., 20,* 72, Special Issue, Number 6, November, 1998.

3. **Arnim**, S.S.: Use of Disclosing Agents for Measuring Tooth Cleanliness, *J. Periodontol., 34,* 227, May, 1963.

4. **Lang**, N.P., Ostergaard, E., and Löe, H.: A Fluorescent Plaque Disclosing Agent, *J. Periodont. Res., 7,* 59, Number 1, 1972.

5. **Block**, P.L., Lobene, R.R., and Derdivanis, J.P.: A Two-tone Dye Test for Dental Plaque, *J. Periodontol., 43,* 423, July, 1972.

6. **Fox**, P.C., Brennan, M., Pillemer, S., Radfar, L., Yamano, S., and Baum, B.J.: Sjögren's Syndrome: A Model for Dental Care in the 21st Century, *J. Am. Dent. Assoc., 129,* 719, June, 1998.

7. **Felder**, R.S., Millar, S.B., and Henry, R.H.: Oral Manifestations of Drug Therapy, *Spec. Care Dentist., 8,* 119, May–June, 1988.

8. **Fox**, P.C.: Management of Dry Mouth, *Dent. Clin. North Am., 41,* 863, October, 1997.

9. **Lockhart**, P.B., Fox, P.C., Gentry, A.C., Acharya, R., and Norton, J.: Pilot Study of Controlled-Release Pilocarpine in Normal Subjects, *Oral Surg. Oral Med. Oral Pathol. Oral Radiol. Endod., 82,* 517, November, 1996.

10. **Yagiela**, J.: Agents Affecting Salivation, in American Dental Association, Council on Scientific Affairs: *ADA Guide to Dental Therapeutics.* Chicago, ADA Publishing Co., 1998, pp. 186–198.

11. **Preti**, G., Clark, L., Cowart, B.J., Feldman, R.S., Lowry, L.D., Weber, E., and Young, I.M.: Non-oral Etiologies of Oral Malodor and Altered Chemosensation, *J. Periodontol., 63,* 790, September, 1992.

12. **Bosy**, A.: Oral Malodor: Philosophical and Practical Aspects, *J. Can. Dent. Assoc., 63,* 196, March, 1997.

13. **Rosenberg**, M. and McCulloch, C.A.G.: Measurement of Oral Malodor: Current Methods and Future Prospects, *J. Periodontol., 63,* 776, September, 1992.

14. **Yaegaki**, K. and Sanada, K.: Biochemical and Clinical Factors Influencing Oral Malodor in Periodontal Patients, *J. Periodontol., 63,* 783, September, 1992.

15. **Ratcliff**, R.: Current Concepts in the Causes and Treatment of Halitosis, *J. Pract. Hyg., 6,* 47, July/August, 1997.

16. **DeBoever**, E.H. and Loesche, W.J.: Assessing the Contribution of Anaerobic Microflora of the Tongue to Oral Malodor, *J. Am. Dent. Assoc., 126,* 1385, October, 1995.

SUGGESTED READINGS

Albandar, J.M., Buischi, Y.A.P., Mayer, M.P.A., and Axelsson, P.: Long-term Effect of Two Preventive Programs on the Incidence of Plaque and Gingivitis in Adolescents, *J. Periodontol., 65,* 605, June, 1994.

Al-Yahfoufi, Z., Mombelli, A., Wicki, A., and Lang, N.P.: The Effect of Plaque Control in Subjects With Shallow Pockets and High Prevalence of Periodontal Pathogens, *J. Clin Periodontol., 22,* 78, January, 1995.

Bader, J.D., Rozier, R.G., McFall, W.T., and Ramsey, D.L.: Association of Dental Health Knowledge With Periodontal Conditions Among Regular Patients, *Community Dent. Oral Epidemiol., 18,* 32, February, 1990.

Baker, K.A.: The Role of Dental Professionals and the Patient in Plaque Control, *Periodontol. 2000, 8,* 108, 1995.

Bruerd, B.: Focus Group: Evaluating Oral Health Education Materials, *DentalHygienistNews, 8,* 21, Spring, 1996.

Chopoorian, K.: How Adults Learn: The Dental Hygienist as an Educator, *DentalHygienistNews, 9,* 3, Number 2, 1996.

Christensen, G.J.: Educating Patients About Dental Procedures, *J. Am. Dent. Assoc., 126,* 371, March, 1995.

Chu, R. and Craig, B.: Understanding the Determinants of Preventive Oral Health Behaviours, *Can. Dent. Hyg. Assoc./Probe, 30,* 12, January/February, 1996.

Gluch-Scranton, J. and Tedesco, A.-M.: Individualizing Dental Hygiene Patient Management Throughout the Life Span, *Sem. Dent. Hyg., 4,* 1, January, 1994.

Ivanovic, M. and Lekic, P.: Transient Effect of a Short-term Educational Programme Without Prophylaxis on Control of Plaque and Gingival Inflammation in School Children, *J. Clin. Periodontol., 23,* 750, August, 1996.

Kiyak, H.A.: Behavioural Techniques in Oral Health Promotion, *Can. Dent. Hyg. Assoc./Probe, 26,* 112, Autumn, 1992.

Lachapelle, D., Desaulniers, G., and Bujold, N.: Dental Health Education for Adolescents: Assessing Attitude and Knowledge Following Two Educational Approaches, *Can. J. Public Health, 80,* 339, September–October, 1989.

Lang, W.P., Farghaly, M.M., and Ronis, D.L.: The Relation of Preventive Dental Behaviors to Periodontal Health Status, *J. Clin. Periodontol., 21,* 194, March, 1994.

Liebman, J.: Dental Hygienists as Adult Educators, *Access, 9,* 47, September–October, 1995.

Lim, L.P., Davies, W.I.R., Yuen, K.W., and Ma, M.H.: Comparison of Modes of Oral Hygiene Instruction in Improving Gingival Health, *J. Clin. Periodontol., 23,* 693, July, 1996.

McConaughy, F.L., Lukken, K.M., and Toevs, S.E.: Health Promotion Behaviors of Private Practice Dental Hygienists, *J. Dent. Hyg., 65,* 222, June, 1991.

McConaughy, F.L., Toevs, S.E., and Lukken, K.M.: Adult Clients' Recall of Oral Health Education Services Received in Private Practice, *J. Dent. Hyg., 69,* 202, September–October, 1995.

McCullough, C.: Personal Oral Hygiene: The Most Important Component in Managing Periodontal Health, *Access, 7,* 33, December, 1993.

Stabholz, A. and Mann, J.: Periodontal Health and the Role of the Dental Hygienist, *Int. Dent. J., 48,* 50, February, 1998.

Testa, M.A. and Simonson, D.C.: Assessment of Quality-of-Life Outcomes, *N. Engl. J. Med., 334,* 835, March 28, 1996.

Motivation, Compliance, Communication

Albrecht, G. and Hoogstraten, J.: Satisfaction as a Determinant of Compliance, *Community Dent. Oral Epidemiol., 26,* 139, April, 1998.

Bagley, J.G. and Low, K.G.: Enhancing Flossing Compliance in College Freshmen, *Clin. Prev. Dent., 14,* 25, November/December, 1992.

Brown, J.: Creating Agreement: Understanding the Resistant Patient, *DentalHygienistNews, 3,* 14, Summer, 1990.

DeVore, C.H., Beck, F.M., and Horton, J.E.: Plaque Score Changes Based Primarily on Patient Performance at Specific Time Intervals, *J. Periodontol., 61,* 343, June, 1990.

Feinstein, J.A.: Choosing Educational Materials Patients Understand, *DentalHygienistNews, 5,* 4, Winter, 1992.

Gluch-Scranton, J.: Motivational Strategies in Dental Hygiene Care, *Seminars in Dental Hygiene, 3,* 1, July, 1991.

Hellstadius, K., Åsman, B., and Gustafsson, A.: Improved Maintenance of Plaque Control by Electrical Toothbrushing in Periodontitis Patients With Low Compliance, *J. Clin. Periodontol., 20,* 235, April, 1993.

Levine, R.A. and Wilson, T.G.: Compliance as a Major Risk Factor in Periodontal Disease Progression, *Compend. Cont. Educ. Dent., 13,* 1072, December, 1992.

Stewart, J.E., Jacobs-Schoen, M., Padilla, M.R., Maeder, L.A., Wolfe, G.R., and Hartz, G.W.: The Effect of a Cognitive Behavioral Intervention on Oral Hygiene, *J. Clin. Periodontol., 18,* 219, April, 1991.

Tedesco, L.A., Keffer, M.A., Davis, E.L., and Christersson, L.A.: Effect of a Social Cognitive Intervention on Oral Health Status, Behavior Reports, and Cognitions, *J. Periodontol., 63,* 567, July, 1992.

Weinstein, P., Getz, T., and Milgrom, P.: Helping Patients Change Their Oral Self-care, *DentalHygienistNews, 6,* 11, Spring, 1993.

Weinstein, R., Tosolin, F., Ghilardi, L., and Zanardelli, E.: Psychological Intervention in Patients With Poor Compliance, *J. Clin. Periodontol., 23,* 283, March, 1996.

Weiss, B.D. and Coyne, C.: Communicating With Patients Who Cannot Read, *N. Engl. J. Med., 337,* 272, July 24, 1997.

Children

Hamilton, M.E. and Coulby, W.M.: Oral Health Knowledge and Habits of Senior Elementary School Students, *J. Public Health Dent., 51,* 212, Fall, 1991.

Macgregor, I.D.M. and Balding, J.W.: Self-esteem as a Predictor of Toothbrushing Behaviour in Young Adolescents, *J. Clin. Periodontol., 18,* 312, May, 1991.

Ogasawara, T., Watanabe, T., and Kasahara, H.: Readiness for Toothbrushing of Young Children, *ASDC J. Dent. Child., 59,* 353, September–October, 1992.

Raynor, J.A.: A Dental Health Education Programme, Including Home Visits, for Nursery School Children, *Br. Dent. J., 172,* 57, January 25, 1992.

Rise, J., Wold, B., and Aarö, L.E.: Determinants of Dental Health Behaviors in Nordic Schoolchildren, *Community Dent. Oral Epidemiol., 19,* 14, February, 1991.

Schneider, H.S.: Parental Education Leads to Preventive Dental Treatment for Patients Under the Age of Four, *ASDC J. Dent. Child., 60,* 33, January–February, 1993.

Schou, L., Currie, C., and McQueen, D.: Using a "Lifestyle" Perspective to Understand Toothbrushing Behavior in Scottish Schoolchildren, *Community Dent. Oral Epidemiol., 18,* 230, October, 1990.

Disclosing Agents

Baab, D.A., Broadwell, A.H., and Williams, B.L.: A Comparison of Antimicrobial Activity of Four Disclosant Dyes, *J. Dent. Res., 62,* 837, July, 1983.

Kipioti, A., Tsamis, A., and Mitsis, F.: Disclosing Agents in Plaque Control: Evaluation of Their Role During Periodontal Treatment, *Clin. Prev. Dent., 6,* 9, November–December, 1984.

Leknes, K.N. and Lie, T.: Erythrosin Staining in Clinical Disclosure of Plaque, *Quintessence Int., 19,* 199, March, 1988.

Lim, L.P., Tay, F.B.K., Waite, I.M., and Cornick, D.E.R.: A Comparison of 4 Techniques for Clinical Detection of Early Plaque Formed During Different Dietary Regimes, *J. Clin. Periodontol., 13,* 658, August, 1986.

Pitcher, G.R., Newman, H.N., and Strahan, J.D.: Access to Subgingival Plaque by Disclosing Agents Using Mouthrinsing and Direct Irrigation, *J. Clin. Periodontol., 7,* 300, August, 1980.

Rapley, J.W. and Brunsvold, M.A.: The Effects of Erythrosine on Alveolar Bone and Gingival Connective Tissue in Dogs, *J. Periodontol., 62,* 132, February, 1991.

Tan, A.E.S.: Disclosing Agents in Plaque Control: A Review, *J. West. Soc. Periodont. Periodont. Abstr., 29,* 81, Number 3, 1981.

Tan, A.E.S. and Wade, A.B.: The Role of Visual Feedback by a Disclosing Agent in Plaque Control, *J. Clin. Periodontol., 7,* 140, April, 1980.

Saliva

Edgar, W.M.: Saliva: Its Secretion, Composition and Functions, *Br. Dent. J., 172,* 305, April 25, 1992.

Epstein, J.B.: The Role of Saliva in Oral Health and the Causes and Effects of Xerostomia, *J. Can. Dent. Assoc., 58,* 217, March, 1992.

Hall, H.D.: Protective and Maintenance Functions of Human Saliva, *Quintessence Int., 24,* 813, November, 1993.

Mandel, I.D.: The Role of Saliva in Maintaining Oral Homeostasis, *J. Am. Dent. Assoc., 119,* 298, August, 1989.

Mandel, I.D.: The Diagnostic Uses of Saliva, *J. Oral Pathol. Med., 19,* 119, March, 1990.

NIDR, Public Information and Reports: Saliva: A Promising Diagnostic and Monitoring Tool, *J. Am. Dent. Assoc., 125*, 867, July, 1994.

Ship, J.A., Fox, P.C., and Baum, B.J.: How Much Saliva Is Enough? "Normal" Function Defined, *J. Am. Dent. Assoc., 122*, 63, March, 1991.

Shugars, D.C. and Wahl, S.M.: The Role of the Oral Environment in HIV-1 Transmission, *J. Am. Dent. Assoc., 129*, 851, July, 1998.

Xerostomia

Al-Hashimi, I.: Management of Xerostomia, *DentalHygienistNews, 7*, 17, Fall, 1994.

Butt, G.M.: Drug-Induced Xerostomia, *J. Can. Dent. Assoc., 57*, 391, May, 1991.

Ettinger, R.L.: Review: Xerostomia: A Symptom Which Acts Like a Disease, *Age Ageing, 25*, 409, September, 1996.

Garg, A.K. and Kirsch, E.R.: Xerostomia: Recognition and Management of Hypofunction of the Salivary Glands, *Compend. Cont. Educ. Dent., 16*, 574, June, 1995.

Kindelan, S.A., Yeoman, C.M., Douglas, C.W.I., and Franklin, C.: A Comparison of Intraoral *Candida* Carriage in Sjögren's Syndrome Patients With Healthy Xerostomic Controls, *Oral Surg. Oral Med. Oral Pathol. Oral Radiol. Endod., 85*, 162, February, 1998.

McDonald, E. and Marino, C.: Dry Mouth: Diagnosing and Treating Its Multiple Causes, *Geriatrics, 46*, 61, March, 1991.

Najera, M.P., Al-Hashimi, I., Plemons, J.M., Rivera-Hidalgo, F., Rees, T.D., Haghighat, N., and Wright, J.M.: Prevalence of Periodontal Disease in Patients With Sjögren's Syndrome, *Oral Surg. Oral Med. Oral Pathol. Oral Radiol. Endod., 83*, 453, April, 1997.

Sciubba, J.J.: Sjögren's Syndrome: Pathology, Oral Presentation, and Dental Management, *Compend. Cont. Educ. Dent., 15*, 1084, September, 1994.

Sreebny, L.M.: Dry Mouth and Salivary Gland Hypofunction, Part I: Diagnosis, *Compend. Cont. Educ. Dent., 9*, 569, July/August, 1988.

Sreebny, L.M.: Dry Mouth and Salivary Gland Hypofunction. Part II: Etiology and Patient Evaluation, *Compend. Cont. Educ. Dent., 9*, 630, September, 1988.

Sreebny, L.M.: Dry Mouth and Salivary Gland Hypofunction. Part III: Treatment, *Compend. Cont. Educ. Dent., 9*, 716, October, 1988.

Oral Lubricants

Furumoto, E.K., Barker, G.J., Carter-Hanson, C., and Barker, B.F.: Subjective and Clinical Evaluation of Oral Lubricants in Xerostomic Patients, *Spec. Care Dentist., 18*, 113, May/June, 1998.

Olsson, H. and Axéll, T.: Objective and Subjective Efficacy of Saliva Substitutes Containing Mucin and Carboxymethylcellulose, *Scand. J. Dent. Res., 99*, 316, August, 1991.

Olsson, H., Spak, C.-J., and Axéll, T.: The Effect of a Chewing Gum on Salivary Secretion, Oral Mucosal Friction, and the Feeling of Dry Mouth in Xerostomic Patients, *Acta Odontol. Scand., 49*, 273, October, 1991.

van der Reijden, W.A., Buijs, M.J., Damen, J.J.M., Veerman, E.C.I., ten Cate, J.M., and Amerongen, A.V.N.: Influence of Polymers for Use in Saliva Substitutes on De- and Remineralization of Enamel *in vitro, Caries Res., 31*, 216, May–June, 1997.

Halitosis

Bosy, A., Kulkarni, G.V., Rosenberg, M., and McCulloch, C.A.G.: Relationship of Oral Malodor to Periodontitis: Evidence of Independence in Discrete Subpopulations, *J. Periodontol., 65*, 37, January, 1994.

Carlson-Mann, L.: The Use of Tongue Cleaners in the Treatment of Halitosis, *Can. Dent. Hyg. Assoc./Probe, 32*, 114, May/June, 1998.

Kleinberg, I. and Westbay, G.: Salivary and Metabolic Factors Involved in Oral Malodor Formation, *J. Periodontol., 63*, 768, September, 1992.

Kozlovsky, A., Gordon, D., Gelernter, I., Loesche, W.J., and Rosenberg, M.: Correlation Between the BANA Test and Oral Malodor Parameters, *J. Dent. Res., 73*, 1036, May, 1994.

McDowell, J.D. and Kassebaum, D.K.: Diagnosing and Treating Halitosis, *J. Am. Dent. Assoc., 124*, 55, July, 1993.

Richter, J.L.: Diagnosis and Treatment of Halitosis, *Compend. Cont. Educ. Dent., 17*, 370, April, 1996.

Rosenberg, M.: Clinical Assessment of Bad Breath, *J. Am. Dent. Assoc., 127*, 475, April, 1996.

Rosenberg, M.: First International Workshop on Oral Malodor, *J. Dent. Res., 73*, 586, March, 1994.

Rosenberg, M., Kulkarni, G.V., Bosy, A., and McCulloch, C.A.G.: Reproducibility and Sensitivity of Oral Malodor Measurements With a Portable Sulphide Monitor, *J. Dent. Res., 70*, 1436, November, 1991.

Shimura, M., Watanabe, S., Iwakura, M., Oshikiri, Y., Kusumoto, M., Ikawa, K., and Sakamoto, S.: Correlation Between Measurements Using a New Halitosis Monitor and Organoleptic Assessment, *J. Periodontol., 68*, 1182, December, 1997.

Protocols for Prevention and Control of Dental Caries

Dental caries is an infectious, transmissible, communicable disease. As such, it is first, preventable, and when primary prevention has not been effective, the infection is controllable. Most patients have limited knowledge of the complex activity on the surfaces of their teeth that causes the teeth to develop cavities. Many patients take for granted the fact that they have a few cavities every year. Dental hygienists have new information from current research to impart to their patients.

- On the tooth surface, a constant process of demineralization and remineralization is going on.
- All ages are susceptible.
- Each step in the caries process has significance in the protocol for prevention and/or control that is planned with an individual patient.
- The basic caries process starts with certain acidogenic bacteria in dental biofilm acting to metabolize the fermentable carbohydrates ingested by the patient.[1]
- Acids are formed that in turn act to demineralize the enamel, cementum, and/or dentin and lead to cavity formation.
- Figure 32-2 (page 528) shows the interrelation of the essentials of the caries process.

- Terminology to describe dental caries is defined in Box 24-1.

I. ACIDOGENIC BACTERIA

- Specific bacteria in the biofilm on the tooth surfaces metabolize acid from the fermentable carbohydrates ingested by the individual.
- *Mutans streptococci* are infectious organisms that colonize the teeth and help to form the dental biofilm through their ability to create a sticky environment for survival and multiplication.
- Two groups of bacteria predominate in the caries process: the *Mutans streptococci* (including both *Streptococcus mutans* and *Streptococcus sobrinus*) and the *Lactobacillus* species.
- *Mutans streptococci* are most active during the initial stages of demineralization and cavity formation, whereas the lactobacilli are more active during the progression of the cavity.
- Permanent colonization of a child's teeth with *Mutans streptococci* can take place soon after tooth eruption. Transmission of the acid-forming organisms is usually from close family members, particularly the mother.[2]

BOX 24-1 KEY WORDS: Dental Caries

Acidogenic bacteria: bacteria in dental biofilm capable of metabolizing fermentable carbohydrates into acids.

Buffer: a substance that by its presence in solution increases the amount of acid or alkali necessary to produce a change in pH.

Caries risk assessment: procedure to predict future dental caries development before the clinical onset of the disease.

Cariology: science and study of dental caries.

Cavitation: process in the formation of cavities; final stage in the caries process.

Cavity: a hole; the final stage of demineralization and breakdown of tooth structure. The classification of cavities by tooth surfaces and anatomic location is defined on pages 263 to 265.

Demineralization: major stage in the dental caries process in which minerals, primarily calcium and phosphorous, are dissolved from tooth structure by acids formed by acidogenic bacteria, primarily *Mutans streptococci* and lactobacilli.

Dental caries: infectious disease of teeth caused by acidogenic bacteria with dissolution of enamel and dentin (coronal caries) and cementum and dentin (root caries).

> **Arrested caries:** after remineralization, the caries process is halted; the area usually becomes discolored with a brownish tinge, darker with age and in a tobacco user.
>
> **Rampant caries:** rapidly progressive caries occurring in many teeth simultaneously; also called acute caries in contrast to chronic caries (slow developing).
>
> **Secondary caries:** carious lesions at the margin of an existing restoration; also called recurrent caries.

Remineralization: healing process in which minerals are redeposited in the demineralized tooth structure; accomplished by the protective factors of the saliva and the action of fluoride to inhibit demineralization and interfere with the enzymatic requirements of bacteria.

II. FREQUENT FERMENTABLE CARBOHYDRATES

- Fermentable carbohydrates included are sucrose, glucose, fructose, and cooked starch.
- Acids produced during the metabolic processes include acetic, lactic, formic, and proprionic.
- Frequency of ingestion of sugary foods by the patient has a strong influence on the amount of acid produced and the extent of tooth destruction.

III. ACID PRODUCTION

- The acid formed passes rapidly into the tiny diffusion channels between the enamel rods or into the exposed root surfaces.
- The acid dissolves the calcium and phosphate mineral in the subsurface of the enamel or dentin structure.
- The subsurface initial carious lesion is formed as shown in Figure 33-3 (page 547). It is observed clinically as a white spot.

IV. DEMINERALIZATION

- Demineralization is the process by which the minerals of the tooth structure are dissolved by the organic acids produced from the fermentable carbohydrate by the acidogenic bacteria.
- With repeated bathing of the tooth surface with the acids produced in the course of a day, the tooth demineralization can progress in time to the final stage of dental caries, the dental cavity.
- Smooth surface caries as well as pits and fissures can result when cariogenic nutrients are available.

V. REMINERALIZATION

Remineralization can take over to halt or arrest the demineralization process. Saliva and fluoride provide protective factors in promoting remineralization. Fluoride therapy is an essential part of the protocol in dental caries control.[3]

A. Saliva

- Protective factors of the saliva can balance or reverse the destruction of the tooth structure.
- Saliva has many properties and functions, particularly to buffer the acids and to supply minerals to replace those calcium and phosphate ions dissolved from the tooth during demineralization.
- Saliva is a continuing source for fluoride transport to the tooth surfaces. Saliva derives fluoride from all its contacts, including fluoride from fluoridated water, fluoride products (toothpaste, mouthrinse used by the patient), and fluoride products for professional application (varnish, topical fluorides).

B. Fluoride Mechanisms of Action[3]

- *Inhibits demineralization*: When fluoride is present in the fluid of the biofilm around the enamel crystals (or dentin of the root), it will pass through the diffusion channels with the acid and increase the fluoride of the subsurface lesion to prevent the continued dissolution of the minerals.
- *Enhances remineralization*: As the saliva flows over the biofilm, its buffering properties neutralize the acid produced by the bacteria. The pH rises toward neutral and prevents further dissolution of the minerals. Minerals in the saliva can go back into the tooth for remineralization.
- *Inhibits bacteria in the biofilm*: Fluoride can change to HF when it is contacted by the acid produced by the bacteria from the carbohydrates in the patient's diet. In the HF form it can then diffuse over the cell membrane of the acidogenic bacteria. Inside it dissociates again and the fluoride ions interfere with essential enzyme activity within the bacterial cell.

■ DENTAL CARIES DIAGNOSIS AND DETECTION[4]

Formerly the term "dental caries" referred to the destructive lesion of the tooth structure that made a break in the tooth surface and created a cavity. Dental caries made its way through enamel and into dentin (coronal caries) or through the cementum and into the dentin (root caries). Diagnosis meant detection of decay with loss of tooth substance.

When unrestored, dental caries continued into the pulp, created a toothache, and required a root canal treatment or extraction. Patients went for their dental hygiene "recall" regularly to find out where their new cavities were.

Now that dental caries is treated as an infection, the *end-stage* of the infection is the hole or cavity that requires therapy for restoration. The diagnosis of dental caries as an infection has transformed what formerly was detection of *cavities-to-be-filled* to identification of each stage of the disease. The early stages of dental caries are usually eligible for remineralization of the natural tooth structure.

I. PREREQUISITES FOR CARIES DIAGNOSIS[5]

- Adequate lighting.
- Sharp eyes.
- Blunt probes: no sharp explorers used: remineralizing surfaces must not be scratched or altered in any way.
- Tri-syringe for viewing teeth wet and dry.
- Reproducible bitewing radiographs for showing coronal caries; *vertical bitewings* for root caries detection.

II. THE STAGES OF DENTAL CARIES

A. Initial Infection: Invisible lesion.

Mutans streptococci infect the tooth by:
- Clinging to the smooth tooth surface.
- Creating a biofilm.
- Producing acid from available fermentable carbohydrate.
- The acid produced diffuses through the microchannels between the enamel rods, dissolves the tooth minerals, and creates the subsurface lesion (Figure 33-3).

B. Early Subsurface Infection: Generally invisible.

C. White Spot Lesion

- Examination with air under bright light shows the white spot of subsurface demineralization.
- Surface smooth, with blunt probe run lightly over the surface.
- Careful examination: surface must not be broken or scratched.
- Picking or scratching a mineralizing surface can prevent further mineralization.[6,7]
- Remineralization process starts with saliva action and increased fluoride.

D. White Spot: Later Stage

- Examination: run blunt probe gently over the surface with no pressure.

- When there is slight surface roughness, beginning breakdown: **do not** scratch the surface.
- Remineralization may still be effective and should be continued.

E. Cavitation

1. *Visual Examination*
- Observation: open cavity can be observed directly.
- Open cavity with no intact tooth structure over the surface may be seen without exploration.
- Gentle airblast may be sufficient to clear loose biofilm and debris for direct vision.

2. *Instrumental*
- Avoid picking or scratching a surface undergoing remineralization.
- Probe or explorer not needed if visual examination of the occlusal, facial, palatal, or lingual identifies a cavity.
- Small proximal caries at the contact area needs radiograph for confirmation of depth.

3. *Radiographic Examination*
- Bitewing views: for cavities on proximal surfaces primarily; vertical bitewings for root caries detection.
- Early caries not extending into dentin: radiograph cannot reveal true depth because of tooth density.
- Large cavities do not need radiographic examination for detection, only for extension to pulpal involvement.
- Treatment plan for definite cavitation: appoint for restoration.

II. PREVIOUS MANAGEMENT OF DENTAL CARIES

- In the early half of the last century, the history of dental caries management shows many restorations placed, but also many diseased teeth removed and prosthetic replacements provided.
- Reductions in caries of 40% to 60% since 1945 in the United States were observed for those fortunate enough to live in the communities with fluoridation of the water supply.
- Recent history has shown reductions in dental caries prevalence generally related to the widespread home use of fluoride dentifrices and mouthrinses as well as professional topical applications of solutions, gels, and varnishes.
- Although the decline of dental caries in the general population has tapered off in more recent years, dental caries is still a major problem in the health and welfare of adults as well as children.

▪ SELECTIVE CARE PLANNING

The dental hygienist is challenged to select a management strategy for the individual patient to cover all needs. The care plan will need to provide for treatment of existing nonreversible carious lesions but also will open up a changed pattern of personal care previously unrealized by the patient so that new lesions can be prevented.

A variety of patients present for dental hygiene care. On the one side will be the patient with no current new dental caries, but a few simple questions may reveal that here is a patient with irregular habits of diet and personal oral care that could lead to serious problems later. At the opposite extreme is the need for as early recognition as possible of the lesions that have gone out of control and present as definite cavities in need of dental restorative care.

I. OBJECTIVES FOR CARIES MANAGEMENT

A. Determine Restorative Treatment Needs

- Chart existing restorations and sealants.
- Chart cavities (final stage of caries process in need of restoration).
- Chart secondary (recurrent) lesions.
- Chart sealants in need of repair.

B. Determine Areas That Require Remineralization

- Chart white spots and white cervical lines.
- Outline appropriate strategies for the patient.

C. Define Steps for Remineralization Program

- Explain needs and corrective methods for patient understanding.
- Prepare and explain risk assessment for the individual.
- Select and demonstrate procedures that must be followed.
- Plan for evaluation and reevaluation at continuing maintenance appointments.

II. RISK FACTORS

- Risk factors are habits, behaviors, lifestyles, or conditions that, when present, increase the probability of a disease occurring.
- The risk factors in Table 24-1 may apply to adult patients primarily. Table 46-1 (page 784) lists risk factors selected especially for the oral health of early childhood.

▪ TABLE 24-1 CARIES RISK ASSESSMENT DATA

FACTOR	HIGH RISK	LOW RISK
Social History	• Low knowledge of dental disease • Irregular dental visits • Family: generally poor oral care	• Dentally aware • Regularly scheduled appointments • Low caries in siblings
Medical History	• Medically compromised • Disabled/handicapped • Xerostomia (side effect of medications) • Radiation therapy	• No serious medical problems • No medications for chronic diseases • Normal salivary flow • No physical problems or handicaps
Use of Fluoride	• Does not live in a fluoridated community • Has fluoride toothpaste sometimes but brushing is irregular	• Lives in fluoridated community • Lived in fluoridated community as a small child • Fluoride toothpaste regularly • Uses fluoride mouthwash weekly
Dietary Habits	• Frequent sugar intake • Snacks frequently • Not familiar with Food Guide Pyramid • Uses chewing tobacco occasionally	• Infrequent sugar intake • Rarely snacks between meals • Uses xylitol gum when chews gum
Biofilm Control	• Irregular brushing and other oral care • Orthodontic appliance care • Poor manual dexterity or handicap • High biofilm scores	• Regular brushing at least 2 times daily • Uses dental floss daily • No prostheses, orthodontics, or other special care requirement • Good dexterity; no handicap • Low biofilm scores
Clinical/Oral	• Previous caries • New caries/white spots • Multiple restorations • Unsealed deep pits and fissures • Orthodontic appliances and/or prostheses to care for • Exposed root surfaces with previously restored root caries • Uses recreational drugs	• No new caries recently • Few restorations • Sealants in pits and fissures • No orthodontics or other prostheses to care for • Exposed root surfaces with special fluoride applications regularly

• Caries management begins with risk factor assessment so that specific needs of the individual patient can be identified.

III. RISK ASSESSMENT

A. Purposes and Uses of Individual Patient Risk Assessment

• The use of the patient's own list of risk factors can be a significant educational experience for the patient.
• Enlighten the patient of the existing individual oral problems.
• Provide factual information about the development and transmissibility of caries.

• Relate the patient's dental caries to behavioral and lifestyle habits that will need to change to arrest demineralization and initiate remineralization.
• Encourage the patient to apply caries preventive methods to family and other closely related individuals.
• Be a guide for the management of a caries preventive plan for reversing demineralizing lesions.

B. Sources and Selection of Risk Factors

1. *From the Patient's Medical, Dental, and Social Histories*[8]
• The regular history form can show answers to questions pertinent to a caries control program.

- The patient's *perception of needs* is guided by past dental experiences, family, and cultural influences.
- Immediate considerations of a patient that could show personal *value placed on oral health* often emphasize appearance, cost implications, and personal time involved.
- *Past dental experience* as shown by primary prevention, including sealants, secondary prevention by restorations, and tertiary prevention by extraction and replacement of teeth.
- *Fluoride history* showing residences and availability of community water supply fluoridation throughout life and currently. Other exposures to fluoride, including home dentifrice used over years and professional applications.
- *Success in changing habits*, such as the person who was a tobacco user but was able to cease use completely can be very indicative of the patient's ability to turn around caries-producing habits.

2. *Questioning the Patient Directly*
- Brief introductory checklist to show current daily care and fluoride.
- Example: Box 24-2 may introduce conversation and stimulate interest to encourage the patient to look at current habits as causes of oral problems.
3. *Food Diary*
- For analysis of sugar exposures Figure 32-4 (page 533).
- Food diary form is described on pages 528 to 531.

IV. APPLICATION

- The preparation and procedure for introducing a protocol for caries prevention or control with emphasis on remineralization of early, noncavitated lesions can lay the groundwork for a successful program.
- Most patients will learn very little about the seriousness of their problem if handed a checklist of things to be done every day.

BOX 24-2 Patient's Checklist

ORAL HEALTH CHECK SHEET

Name: _____

PLEASE CHECK "YES" OR "NO" OR FILL IN OTHER

	Yes	No	Other (please write)
1. Fluoride in your drinking water as a small child?			
2. Fluoride in your drinking water where you live now?			
3. Use toothpaste with fluoride in it now? Favorite kind? _____			
4. Brush at least twice each day?			
5. Use dental floss every day?			
6. Wear orthodontic appliances?			
7. Use sugar-free chewing gum when you chew gum?			
8. Have dry mouth most of the time?			
9. Sip on beverages other than water throughout the day? Mostly what?_____			
10. Snack frequently? Mostly what?_____			

Date: _____

- Participation in the process of selection can inform the patient (and parents) of the needs and ways of coping with change.
- Using the list in Table 24-1, help patients check off the topics that apply to their personal lifestyle and oral health habits.
- Beside each risk factor, the patients can identify possible changes to make to prevent future cavities.

V. THE PATIENT WITH NO DENTAL CARIES

- Primary prevention remains a top priority.
- The objective is to provide the patient with positive care and education so that dental health will be maintained indefinitely.
- A review is made with the patient of all the factors that classify the patient as "low risk." Such an understanding by the patient can encourage ideal personal daily biofilm removal.
- Supervision at routine maintenance appointments: necessary to prevent introduction of habit changes that can lead to caries infection.

■ A PROTOCOL FOR REMINERALIZATION[9,10]

A first approach to treating dental caries as an infectious disease is to eliminate as many of the causative factors as possible. That applies primarily to removal of the acid-forming bacteria and the fermentable carbohydrates that allow the harmful bacteria to survive and multiply.

At the same time that the infectious agents are being reduced in numbers, consideration for the contagious aspect of the microorganisms is needed. When possible, close personal contacts with the patient can be checked, advised relative to the potential communicability, have their own teeth checked, and dental caries eliminated.

I. REMOVE THE NIDUS OF INFECTION

A. Restoration of All Real Cavities

- Dental carious lesions contain large numbers of acidogenic bacteria, especially *Mutans streptococci* and lactobacilli.
- Well-placed restorations with marginal seal will help lower the bacterial counts in the oral cavity.
- Use of restorative materials containing fluoride should be used wherever possible.

B. Placement of Sealants

- Closing off the pits and fissures where microorganisms can live, multiply, and contribute to carious lesions.
- Live microorganisms cannot survive when sealed into a pit or fissure.

C. Family Members

- Encourage family members and other close contacts to have necessary restorative dentistry completed and to adopt measures for personal dental care that ensure optimum oral health.

II. SYSTEMIC DISEASE FACTORS

- Identify diseases and their medications with a side effect for dry mouth.
- Selected medically or nutritionally compromised patients may be at risk for dental caries and need additional preventive measures to be recommended.

III. INITIATE DAILY PREVENTIVE MEASURES

A. Personal Fluoride Use

- Use fluoridated water; fill personal drinking bottles.
- Dentifrice 2-3 times per day with brushing at least 3 minutes.
- Non–alcohol-containing fluoride mouthrinse daily; may recommend daily gel tray.
- Fluoride 1.1% dentifrice before bed with no further eating or drinking.

B. Dietary Modifications

- Fermentable carbohydrate exposures eliminated between meals and at the ends of meals; concentrated sweets eliminated.
- Select snacks from noncarbohydrate foods.

C. Chew Sugar-Free Gum at Ends of Meals

- Use sugar-free chewing gum, with xylitol.[11]
- Xylitol reduces levels of *Streptococcus mutans* and promotes remineralization.

IV. PROFESSIONAL APPLICATIONS

- Prescribe short-term chlorhexidine rinse: one 16-ounce bottle (0.12%); 30-second rinse just before going to bed; concentration remains high all night due to its substantivity.[12]
- Chlorhexidine is highly effective against *Mutans streptococcus* infections.

Everyday Ethics

? Sophie and Helen were two sisters who had been Dr. Newbury's patients for the past 30 years. Now in their 70s, they were experiencing new concerns with restorations and crowns that showed signs of occlusal wear and recurrent caries. Many margins of amalgam restorations had catches with the explorer upon examination.

Ken, the dental hygienist, continued to stress the importance of more frequent maintenance visits, but Sophie curtly reminded him that she "has been coming to the dentist since before he was born!" Ken suspected they did not want to hear about crowns that should be replaced or make decisions about the restorations that needed replacement.

A progress note in Helen's chart read, "the patient was not open to new homecare education techniques or interested in a proposed treatment plan to replace

amalgam restorations in tooth # 15, 18, 19, 30, and 31."

Questions for Consideration

1. What possible errors in judgment have Dr. Newbury and Ken made in discussing the current oral condition of Sophie's and Helen's restorative needs?

2. Is the entry in the patient's chart appropriate? Why or why not? Explain your rationale using ethical principles to defend your documentation.

3. What role can prevention play in the patient/provider relationship depicted in this scenario?

- Fluoride 1.1% dentifrice brush-on to start when the chlorhexidine short-term rinse is completed.
- Fluoride varnish applications at frequent dental hygiene appointments.[13]

▪ MAINTENANCE CARE PLANNING

Planning for maintenance is to monitor all of the special procedures for dental caries control. Frequent contact with the patient through telephone and e-mail messages during the first month can help to show the concern of the dental hygienist for the patient and the oral health problems.

✔ **Factors To Teach The Patient**

- What causes cavities and how they develop.

- Early dental caries is not a cavity: what demineralization means.

- How remineralization can be accomplished by using fluoride toothpaste and drinking fluoridated water daily

- Using fluorides is necessary throughout life.

- Biofilm control check: use disclosing agent and record the biofilm score.
- Check dental caries charting: sealants, margins of restorations.
- Radiographs are never routine; only use when specifically indicated by findings.
- Check details of the remineralization program.
- Patient compliance with fluoride details and all personal oral care.
- Need for repeat short-term chlorhexidine rinse schedule determined by other positive or negative results of the protocol thus far.
- Fluoride varnish application repeat.

REFERENCESS

1. **Featherstone**, J.D.B.: The Science and Practice of Caries Prevention, *J. Am. Dent. Assoc., 131*, 887, July, 2000.
2. **Caufield**, P.W., Cutter, G.R., and Dasanayake, A.P.: Initial Acquisition of *Mutans streptococci* by Infants: Evidence for a Discrete Window of Infectivity, *J. Dent. Res., 73*, 37, January, 1993.
3. **Featherstone**, J.D.B.: Prevention and Reversal of Dental Caries: Role of Low-Level Fluoride, *Community Dent. Oral Epidemiol., 27*, 31, February, 1999.
4. **Pitts**, N.B.: Clinical Diagnosis of Dental Caries: A European Perspective, *J. Dent. Educ., 65*, 972, October, 2001.
5. **Kidd**, E.A.M.: Caries Management, *Dent. Clin. North Am., 43*, 743, October, 1999.
6. **Van Dorp**, C.S.E., Exterkate, R.A.M., and ten Cate, J.M.: The Effect of Dental Probing on Subsequent Enamel Demineralization, *ASDC J. Dent. Child., 55*, 343, September–October 1988.
7. **Warren**, J.J., Levy, S.M., and Wefel, J.S.: Explorer Probing of Root Caries Lesions: An in vitro Study, *Spec. Care Dentist, 23*, 18, Number 1, 2003.

8. **Brown**, J.P: Indicators for Caries Management from the Patient History, *J. Dent. Educ., 61*, 855, November, l997.

9. **American Dental Association**, Council on Access, Prevention and Interprofessional Relations: Caries Diagnosis and Risk Assessment, *J. Am. Dent. Assoc., 126*, 1S, Special Supplement, June, 1995.

10. **Hildebrandt**, G.H.: Caries Risk Assessment and Prevention for Adults, *J. Dent. Educ., 59*, 972, October, 1995.

11. **Hayes**, C.: The Effect of Non-Cariogenic Sweeteners on the Prevention of Dental Caries: A Review of the Evidence, *J. Dent. Educ., 65*, 1106, October, 2001.

12. **Anderson**, M.H., Bales, D.J., and Omnell, K.-A.: Modern Management of Dental Caries: The Cutting Edge Is Not the Dental Bur, *J. Am. Dent. Assoc., 124*, 37, June, 1993.

13. **Anusavice**, K.J.: Chlorhexidine, Fluoride Varnish, and Xylitol Chewing Gum: Underutilized Preventive Therapies? *Gen. Dent., 46*, 34, January–February, 1998.

SUGGESTED READINGS

Barber, L.R., and Wilkins, E.M.: Evidence-based Prevention, Management, and Monitoring of Dental Caries, *J. Dent. Hyg., 76*, 270, Fall, 2002.

Caufield, P.W.: Dental Caries: A Transmissible and Infectious Disease Revisited: A Position Paper, *Pediatr. Dent., 19*, 491, November–December, 1997.

Clarkson, B.H.: Introduction to Cariology, *Dent. Clin. North Am., 43*, 569, October, 1999.

Dowd, F.J.: Saliva and Dental Caries, *Dent. Clin. North Am., 43*, 579, October, 1999.

Smith, D.J.: Caries Vaccines for the Twenty-first Century, *J. Dent. Educ., 67*, 1130, October, 2003.

Stookey, G.K., and González-Cabezas, C.: Emerging Methods of Caries Diagnosis, *J. Dent. Educ., 65*, 1001, October, 2001.

Trost, L.: Diagnodent, The Cornerstone for 21st Century Caries Management Protocol, *Woman Dent. J., 1*, 25, November/December, 2003.

Risk and Protocols

Anderson, M.: Risk Assessment and Epidemiology of Dental Caries: Review of the Literature, *Pediatr. Dent., 24*, 377, September/October, 2002.

Anusavice, K.J.: Treatment Regimes in Preventive and Restorative Dentistry, *J. Am. Dent. Assoc., 126*, 727, June, 1995.

Anusavice, K.J.: Efficacy of Nonsurgical Management of the Initial Caries Lesion, *J. Dent. Educ., 61*, 895, November, 1997.

Dorsey, B., and Martin, B.S.: Implementation of a Caries Prevention Program Using Risk Assessment, *Contemporary Oral Hyg., 2*, 20, September/October, 2002.

Habibian, M.: The Role of the Dental Hygienist in Prevention of Early Childhood Caries, *J. Pract. Hyg., 12*, 28, May/June, 2003.

Hausen, H., Kärkkäinen, S., and Seppa, L.: Application of the High-Risk Strategy to Control Dental Caries, *Community Dent. Oral Epidemiol., 28*, 26, February, 2000.

Mandel, I.D.: Caries Prevention, Current Strategies, New Directions, *J. Am. Dent. Assoc., 127*, 1477, October, 1996.

Newbrun, E.: Preventing Dental Caries: Current and Prospective Strategies, *J. Am. Dent. Assoc., 123*, 68, May, 1992.

Oral Infection Control: Toothbrushes and Toothbrushing

Tonya S. Ray, RDH, MA

INTRODUCTION

The toothbrush is the principal instrument in general use for accomplishing dental biofilm removal as a necessary part of oral disease control. Many different designs of both manual and power toothbrushes and supplementary devices have been manufactured and promoted.

Patients who have not previously received professional advice concerning the best brush for their particular oral conditions probably have used brushes selected on the basis of cost, availability, advertising claims, family tradition, or habit. Because of the variety of brushes currently available, and the constant development of new brushes, dental professionals must maintain a high level of knowledge on these products to advise patients appropriately.

Key words relating to toothbrushes are listed in Box 25-1 with their definitions.

■ DEVELOPMENT OF TOOTHBRUSHES

Crudely contrived toothpicks, presumably used for relief from food impaction, are believed to be the earliest implements devised for the care of the teeth. Excavations in Mesopotamia uncovered elaborate gold toothpicks used by the Sumerians about 3000 B.C.

The earliest record of the "chewstick," which has been considered the primitive toothbrush, dates back in the Chinese literature to about 1600 B.C. The care of the mouth was associated with religious training and ritual: the Buddhists had a "toothstick," and the Mohammedans used the "miswak" or "siwak." Chewsticks, made from various types of tasty woods by crushing an end and spreading the fibers in a brush-like manner, are still used in several regions of the world.

BOX 25-1 KEY WORDS: Toothbrushes

Abrasion (gingiva): lesion of the gingiva that results from mechanical removal of the surface epithelium.

Abrasion (tooth): loss of tooth structure produced by a mechanical cause (such as a hard-bristled toothbrush used with excessive pressure and an abrasive dentifrice); abrasion contrasts with erosion, which involves a chemical process.

Bristle: individual short, stiff, natural hair of an animal; historically, toothbrush bristles were taken from a hog or wild boar, but current toothbrush bristles are made of nylon and are called filaments.

End rounded: characteristic shape of each toothbrush filament; a special manufacturing process removes all sharp edges and provides smooth, rounded ends to prevent injury to gingiva or tooth structure during use.

Filament: individual synthetic fiber; a single element of a **tuft** fixed into a toothbrush head.

Angled filament: a nylon filament that is placed in the brush head at an angle.

Mechanical plaque control: oral hygiene methods for removal of dental biofilm from tooth surfaces using a toothbrush and selected devices for interdental cleaning; contrasts with chemotherapeutic biofilm control in which an antimicrobial agent is used.

Power toothbrush: a brush driven by electricity or battery; also called power-assisted, automatic, electric, or mechanical (in contrast with manual).

Stiffness: the reaction force exerted per unit area of the brush during deflection; the term stiffness is used interchangeably with **firmness** of toothbrush bristles or filaments; the stiffness depends primarily on the length and diameter of the filaments.

Sulcular brushing: a method in which the end-rounded filament tips are activated at the gingival margin for the purpose of loosening and removing dental biofilm from the gingival sulcus and tooth surface just below the gingival margin.

Toothbrush head: the part of the toothbrush composed of the tufts and the **stock** (extension of the handle where the tufts are attached).

Tuft: a cluster of bristles or filaments secured together in one hole in the head of a toothbrush.

The *Ebers Papyrus*, compiled about 1500 B.C. and dating probably at about 4000 B.C., contained reference to conditions similar to periodontal diseases and to preparations used as mouthwashes and dentifrices. The writings of Hippocrates (about 300 B.C.) include descriptions of diseased gums related to calculus and of complex preparations for the treatment of unhealthy mouths.[1-4]

I. EARLY TOOTHBRUSHES

It is believed that the first brush made of hog's bristles was mentioned in the early Chinese literature. Pierre Fauchard in 1728 in *Le Chirurgien Dentiste* described many aspects of oral health. He condemned the toothbrush made of horse's hair because it was rough and destructive to the teeth and advised the use of sponges or herb roots. Fauchard recommended scaling of teeth and developed instruments and splints for loose teeth, as well as dentifrices and mouthwashes.

One of the earlier toothbrushes made in England was produced by William Addis about 1780. By the early 19th century, craftsmen in various European countries constructed handles of gold, ivory, or ebony in which replaceable brush heads could be fitted. The first patent for a toothbrush in the United States was issued to H. N. Wadsworth in the middle of the 19th century.

Many new varieties of toothbrushes were developed around 1900, when celluloid was available for the manufacture of toothbrush handles. In 1919, the American Academy of Periodontology defined specifications for toothbrush design and brushing methods in an attempt to standardize professional recommendations.[5]

Nylon came into use in toothbrush construction in 1938. World War II complications prevented Chinese export of wild boar bristles, and synthetic materials were substituted for natural bristles. Since then, synthetic materials have been improved and manufacturer's specifications standardized. Most toothbrushes are made exclusively of synthetic materials. Power toothbrushes, although developed earlier, were not actively promoted until the 1960s.

II. EARLY BRUSHING METHODS

Historically, the purpose of brushing was to provide *massage* to increase the resistance of the gingival tissue. Massage or friction from a hard-bristled brush was believed to *increase keratinization*, which, in turn, resulted in the resistance to bacterial invasion.[6]

As quoted in Box 25-2, Koecker described, in 1842, a "new" method for daily care of teeth.[7] This early work proved to be the forerunner of contemporary oral care.

▪ MANUAL TOOTHBRUSHES

I. CHARACTERISTICS OF AN EFFECTIVE TOOTHBRUSH[8]

A. Conforms to individual patient requirements in size, shape, and texture.
B. Is easily and efficiently manipulated.
C. Is readily cleaned and aerated; impervious to moisture.
D. Is durable and inexpensive.
E. Has prime functional properties of flexibility, softness, and diameter of the bristles or filaments, and of strength, rigidity, and lightness of the handle.
F. Has end-rounded filaments.
G. Is designed for utility, efficiency, and cleanliness.

II. GENERAL DESCRIPTION

A. Parts (Figure 25-1)

1. *Handle*: The part grasped in the hand during toothbrushing.

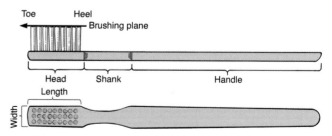

■ **FIGURE 25-1 Parts of a Toothbrush.**

2. *Head*: The working end; consists of tufts of bristles or filaments and the stock where the tufts are secured.

3. *Shank*: The section that connects the head and the handle.

B. Dimensions

1. *Total Brush Length*: About 15 to 19 cm (6 to 7.5 inches); junior and child sizes may be shorter.

2. *Head*: Should be only large enough to accommodate the tufts.
   a. Length of brushing plane, 25.4 to 31.8 mm (1 to 1¼ inches); width, 7.9 to 9.5 mm (⁵⁄₁₆ to ³⁄₈ inch).
   b. Bristle or filament height, 11 mm (⁷⁄₁₆ inch).

III. HANDLE

A. Composition

Most current brush handles are manufactured from a single type of plastic, or a combination of polymers that combine durability, imperviousness to moisture, pleasing appearance, low cost, and sufficient maneuverability.

B. Shape

1. **Preferred Characteristics**
   a. Easy to grasp.
   b. Does not slip or rotate during use.
   c. No sharp corners or projections.
   d. Light weight, consistent with strength.

2. **Variations**
   A twist, curve, offset, or angle in the shank with or without thumb rests may assist the patient in the adaptation of the brush to difficult-to-reach areas.

   A handle of larger diameter may be useful for patients with limited dexterity, such as children, aging patients, and those of any age with a disability (pages 898 to 899).

IV. BRUSH HEAD

A. Design

The brush head may be 5 to 12 tufts long and 3 to 4 rows wide. Tufts that are widely spaced allow for easy cleaning of the brush head. Those closely spaced provide a smooth brushing plane and allow the filaments to support each other. Tufts may be of a consistent shape on the brush head, or the shape of the tufts may be varied as shown in Figure 25-2.

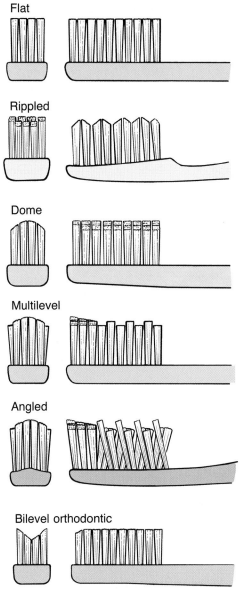

Flat

Rippled

Dome

Multilevel

Angled

Bilevel orthodontic

■ **FIGURE 25-2 Manual Brush Trim Profiles.** A variety of filament profiles are available. In addition to the classic flat planed brush, other trims include the rippled, dome, bilevel, multilevel, and angled. Brushes for use over orthodontic appliances are made with various bilevel shapes.

B. Brushing Plane (profile)

- *Trim.* Variously shaped filament profiles.
- *Length.* Range from filaments of equal lengths (flat planes) to those with variable lengths, such as dome-shaped, rippled, bilevel, multilevel, and angled (Figure 25-2).
- *Properties.* Soft and end-rounded for safety to oral soft tissues and tooth structure.
- *Efficiency in Biofilm Removal.* Efficiency for cleaning the hard-to-reach areas, such as extension

■ TABLE 25-1 COMPARISON OF NATURAL BRISTLES AND MAN-MADE FILAMENTS

	NATURAL BRISTLES	FILAMENTS
Source	Historically made from hair of hog or wild boar	Synthetic, plastic materials, primarily nylon
Uniformity	No uniformity of texture. Diameter or wearing properties depending upon the breed of animal, geographical location, and season in which the bristles were gathered	Uniformity controlled
Diameter	Varies depending on portion of bristle taken, age, and life of animal	Range from extra soft at 0.075 mm (0.003 inch) to hard at 0.3 mm (0.012 inch)
End shape	Deficient, irregular, frequently open-ended	End-rounded to ensure fewer traumas; research has shown a direct relation between gingival damage and the absence of end-rounding[10,11]; Figure 25-3 shows examples of nonrounded and end-rounded bristles[12]
Advantages and disadvantages[9]	• Cannot be standardized • Wear rapidly and irregularly • Hollow ends allow microorganisms and debris to collect inside	• Rinse clean, dry rapidly • Durable and maintain longer • End-rounded and closed, repel debris and water • More resistant to accumulation of microorganisms

onto proximal surfaces, malpositioned teeth, or exposed root surfaces, depends on individual patient abilities and understanding.

V.   BRISTLES AND FILAMENTS

Most current toothbrushes have nylon filaments. Natural bristles are relatively unsanitary, and their physical qualifications cannot be standardized. A comparison of natural bristles and man-made filaments is reviewed in Table 25-1.

The stiffness depends on the diameter and length of the filament. Brushes designated as soft, medium, or hard are not comparatively consistent between manufacturers.

A. Factors Influencing Stiffness

- *Diameter.* Thinner filaments are softer and more resilient.
- *Length.* Shorter filaments are stiffer and have less flexibility.
- *Number of Filaments in a Tuft.* Increased density of filaments and tufts give added support to adjacent filaments, thus increasing the feel of stiffness.
- *Angle of Filaments.* Angled filaments may be more flexible and less stiff than straight filaments of equal length and diameter; there is no straight end-line force applied as with the straight filament.

B. End-Rounding

- *Process of End-Rounding.* Each filament is sealed and rounded by heat treatment. The quality of

end-rounding varies depending on manufacturers.[10] Natural bristles cannot be end-rounded, but nylon filaments can be.

- *Effect.* Research has shown a direct relation between gingival damage and the absence of end-rounding.[11,12]
- *Examples.* Figure 25-3 shows examples of non-rounded and end-rounded filaments.

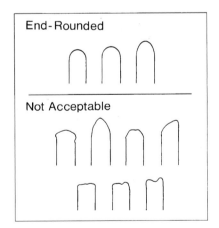

■ **FIGURE 25-3 End-Rounded Filaments.** Examples of the shape of acceptable end-rounding and of those that are not acceptable are shown. (From Silverstone, L.M. and Featherstone, M.J.: A Scanning Electron Microscope Study of the End Rounding of Bristles in Eight Toothbrush Types, *Quintessence Int.*, 19, 3, February, 1988.)

■ TOOTHBRUSH SELECTION FOR THE PATIENT

I. INFLUENCING FACTORS

Factors that influence the selection of the proper manual or power toothbrush for an individual patient include the following:

A. Patient

1. Ability of the patient to use the brush and remove dental biofilm from all tooth surfaces without damage to the soft tissue or tooth structure.
2. Manual dexterity of the patient.
3. Motivation, ability, and willingness to follow the prescribed procedures.
4. The age of the patient and the coinciding differences in the dentition and dexterity.

B. Gingiva

1. Status of gingival or periodontal health.
2. Anatomic configurations of the gingiva.

C. Position of Teeth

Displaced teeth require variations in brush placement.
1. Crowded teeth (Figure 17-5, page 297).
2. Open contacts (Figure 14-4D, page 255).

D. Shape of Teeth and Exposed Roots

E. Personal Preferences

1. Professional personnel may prefer to instruct patients in certain methods and with certain brushes.
2. Patient may have preferences and may resist change.

F. Method Selected

Method of brushing to be recommended and instructed.

II. TOOTHBRUSH SIZE AND SHAPE

The brush selected must be able to be adapted to all facial, lingual, palatal, and occlusal surfaces for dental biofilm removal.

III. SOFT NYLON BRUSH

The following are suggested as advantages for the use of a soft end-rounded brush that is applied appropriately.

- More effective in cleaning the cervical areas, both proximal and marginal.
- Less traumatic to the gingival tissue; therefore, patients can brush at the cervical areas without fear of discomfort or soft tissue laceration.
- Can be directed into the sulcus for sulcular brushing and into interproximal areas for cleaning the proximal surfaces.
- Applicable around fixed orthodontic appliances or fixation appliances used to treat a fractured jaw.
- Tooth abrasion and/or gingival recession can be prevented or may be less severe in an overvigorous brusher.
- More effective use for sensitive gingiva in such conditions as necrotizing ulcerative gingivitis or severe gingivitis, or during healing stages following scaling and debridement or periodontal surgery.
- Small size is ideal for a young child as a first brush on primary teeth.

■ GUIDELINES FOR MANUAL TOOTHBRUSHING

Complete toothbrushing instruction for a patient involves teaching what, when, where, and how. In addition to descriptions of specific toothbrushing methods, the succeeding sections consider the grasp of the brush, the sequence and amount of brushing, the areas of limited access, and supplementary brushing for the occlusal surfaces and the tongue. The possible detrimental effects from improper toothbrushing and variations for special conditions are described. The care of toothbrushes is outlined.

I. GRASP OF BRUSH

A. Objectives

Manipulation of the brush for successful removal of dental biofilm can be related to the manner in which the brush is held. Patients may need specific instruction in how to hold and place the brush. When they start to brush to remove the dental biofilm that has been colored with a disclosing agent, the tenaciousness of the biofilm and the need for controlled pressure can be realized. With a light, comfortable grasp, the following can be expected:
1. Control of the brush during all movements.
2. Effective positioning at the beginning of each brushing stroke, follow-through during the complete stroke, and repositioning for the next stroke.
3. Sensitivity to the amount of pressure applied.

B. Procedure

1. Grasp toothbrush handle in the palm of the hand with thumb against the shank.
   a. Near enough to the head of the brush so that it can be controlled effectively.
   b. Not so close to the head of the brush that manipulation of the brush is hindered or that fingers can touch the anterior teeth when reaching the brush head to molar regions.
2. Direct filaments in the direction needed for placement on the teeth; direction depends on the brushing method to be used.
3. Adapt grasp for the various positions of the brush head on the teeth throughout the procedure; adjust to permit unrestricted movement of the wrist and arm.
4. Apply appropriate pressure for removal of the dental biofilm. Too much pressure, however, bends the filaments and curves them away from the area where brushing is needed.

II. SEQUENCE

A. The procedure in brushing, for any method used, should ensure complete coverage for each tooth surface.
B. Start brushing from a molar region of one arch around to the opposite side, then back around the lingual or facial. Repeat in the opposing arch.
C. Each brush placement must overlap the previous one for thorough coverage (Figure 25-4).

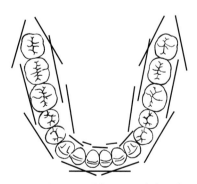

■ **FIGURE 25-4 Brushing Positions.** Each brush position, as represented by a black line, should overlap the previous position. Note placement at canines, where the distal aspect of the canine is brushed with the premolars and the mesial aspect is brushed with the incisors. Short lines on the lingual anterior aspect indicate brush placed vertically. The maxillary teeth require a similar number of brushing positions.

D. Encourage the patient to begin by brushing one of the areas of greatest individual need as shown by disclosing agent.
   1. Areas that are most frequently missed.
   2. Areas that are most difficult for brush placement and/or manipulation, such as the right side for the right-handed brusher or the left side for the left-handed brusher.
E. Suggest that the sequence be varied at least once each day so that the same areas are not always brushed last when time may be limited and biofilm removal may be less complete.

III. AMOUNT OF BRUSHING

The main consideration is the removal of the dental biofilm. All surfaces of all teeth need to be brushed clean. The number of strokes and length of time spent depends on the patient's ability and efficiency in accomplishing the task.

A. The Count System

To ensure thorough coverage with an even distribution of amount of brushing and to help the patient concentrate on the performance, a system of counting can be useful.

1. Count 6 strokes in each area (or 5 or 10, whichever is most appropriate for the particular patient) for modified Stillman or other method in which a stroke is used.
2. Count slowly to 10 for each brush position while brush is vibrated and filament ends are held in position for the Bass, Charters, or other vibratory method.

B. The Clock System

Some patients brush thoroughly while watching a clock or an egg timer for 3 or 4 minutes. Timed procedures cannot guarantee thorough coverage, because single areas that are most accessible may get more brushing time.

C. Combination

For many patients, use of the "count" system in combination with the "clock" system produces the most complete removal of dental biofilm.

D. Built-in Timers

Many power toothbrushes have built-in timers that signal the patient that a certain time period has elapsed. Some signal every 30 seconds, some every minute, and some every 2 minutes. These timers can be very effective methods of increasing the total time a patient spends on brushing.

IV. FREQUENCY OF BRUSHING

Because of individual variations, one set rule for frequency cannot be applied. The emphasis in patient education should be placed on complete biofilm removal daily rather than on the number of brushings.

For the control of dental biofilm, and for oral sanitation and halitosis prevention, at least two brushings, accompanied by appropriate interdental care, are recommended as a minimum for each day. The longer the bacteria remain undisturbed, the greater the pathogenic potential of the biofilm bacteria.

A clean mouth before going to sleep should be encouraged. Bacteria thrive in the dark, warm, moist climate of the oral environment. Patients who use a chewable fluoride tablet, mouthrinse, or gel application before going to bed should complete their biofilm removal before fluoride application.

■ METHODS FOR MANUAL TOOTHBRUSHING

Most toothbrushing methods can be classified based on the position and motion of the brush. Noted beside certain categories that follow are names of methods that utilize the designated motion as part or all of their particular procedure. Some of these methods are recorded for descriptive, comparative, or historic purposes only and are not currently recommended. A few may have been shown to be detrimental.

- A. Sulcular: Bass.
- B. Roll: Rolling stroke, modified Stillman.
- C. Vibratory: Stillman, Charters, Bass.
- D. Circular: Fones.
- E. Vertical: Leonard.
- F. Horizontal.
- G. Physiologic: Smith.
- H. Scrub-brush.

■ THE BASS METHOD: SULCULAR BRUSHING

The Bass method is widely accepted as an effective method for dental biofilm removal adjacent to and directly beneath the gingival margin. The area at the gingival margin is the most significant in the control of gingival and periodontal infections.

I. PURPOSES AND INDICATIONS

- A. For all patients for dental biofilm removal adjacent to and directly beneath the gingival margin.

- B. For open interproximal areas, cervical areas beneath the height of contour of the enamel, and exposed root surfaces.
- C. For the patient who has had periodontal surgery.
- D. For adaptation to abutment teeth, under the gingival border of a fixed partial denture, and orthodontic appliances (Figure 28-4, page 459).

II. PROCEDURE

A. Position the Brush

1. *Filaments.* Direct the filaments apically (up for maxillary, down for mandibular teeth). Even though the brush placement calls for directing the filaments at a 45° angle, it is usually easier and safer for the patient to first place the sides of the filaments parallel with the long axis of the tooth (Figure 25-6A). From that position the brush can be turned slightly and brought to the gingival margin to the 45° angle (Figure 25-6B).
2. *Gingival Sulcus.* Place the brush with the filament tips directed straight into the gingival sulcus. The filaments will be directed at approximately 45° to the long axis of the tooth, as shown in Figure 25-5A.

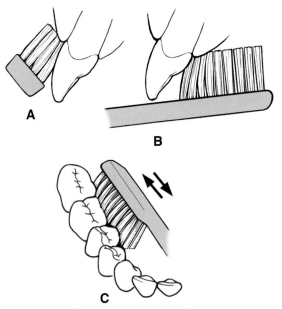

■ **FIGURE 25-5 Sulcular Brushing. (A)** Filament tips are directed into the gingival sulcus at approximately 45° to the long axis of the tooth. **(B)** Position for palatal surface of maxillary anterior teeth. **(C)** Brush in position for lingual surfaces of mandibular posterior teeth.

B. Strokes

1. *Press Lightly Without Flexing.* Press lightly so the filament tips enter the gingival sulci and embrasures and cover the gingival margin. Do not bend the filaments with excess pressure.
2. *Vibrate the Brush.* Vibrate the brush back and forth with very short strokes without disengaging the tips of the filaments from the sulci. Count at least 10 vibrations.

C. Reposition the Brush

Apply the brush to the next group of two or three teeth. Take care to overlap placement, as shown in Figure 25-4.

D. Repeat Stroke

The entire stroke (steps A through C) is repeated at each position around the maxillary and mandibular arches, both facially and lingually.

E. Position Brush for Lingual and Palatal Anterior Surfaces (Figure 25-5B)

Hold the brush the long narrow way for the anterior components. The filaments are kept straight and directed into the sulci.[13]

III. PROBLEMS

A. An overeager brusher may convert the previously mentioned "very short strokes" into a vigorous scrub that causes injury to the gingival margin.
B. Dexterity requirement may be too high for certain patients. Because a 45° angle can be difficult to visualize, emphasis should be on placing the tips of the filaments into the sulcus.
C. Rolling stroke procedure may precede the sulcular brushing when a patient believes it helps to clean the teeth. The two methods should be performed separately rather than trying to combine them in what has been referred to as a "modified Bass."

The procedure of rolling the brush down over the crown after the vibratory part of the sulcular brush stroke has several disadvantages: (1) too often the brush is hastily and carelessly replaced into the sulcus position, or the opposite is true, and considerable time is consumed in the attempt to replace the brush carefully; (2) gingival margin injury by the constant replacement of the brush can result; and (3) the patient may tend to roll the brush down over the crown prematurely, thereby accomplishing very little sulcular brushing.

■ THE ROLL OR ROLLING STROKE METHOD

I. PURPOSES AND INDICATIONS

A. Cleaning gingiva and removing biofilm, materia alba, and food debris from the teeth without emphasis on gingival sulcus.
   1. Meant for children with relatively healthy gingiva and normal tissue contour when a sulcular technique may seem difficult for the patient to master.
   2. Meant for general cleaning in conjunction with the use of a vibratory technique (Bass, Charters, Stillman).
B. Useful for preparatory instruction (first lesson) for modified Stillman method because the initial brush placement is the same. This can be particularly helpful when there is a question as to how complicated a technique the patient can master and practice.

II. PROCEDURE[5,14]

A. Position the Brush

1. *Filaments.* Direct filaments apically (up for maxillary, down for mandibular teeth).
2. *Place Side of Brush on the Attached Gingiva.* The filaments are directed apically. When the plastic portion of the brush head is level with the occlusal or incisal plane, generally the brush is at the proper height, as shown in Figure 25-6A.

B. Strokes

1. *Press to Flex the Filaments.* The sides of the filaments are pressed lightly against the gingiva. The gingiva will blanch.
2. *Roll the Brush Slowly Over the Teeth.* As the brush is rolled, the wrist is turned slightly. The filaments remain flexed and follow the contours of the teeth, thereby permitting cleaning of the cervical areas. Some filaments may reach interdentally.

C. Replace and Repeat Five Times or More

The entire stroke (steps A and B) is repeated at least five times for each tooth or group of teeth. When the brush is removed and repositioned, the wrist is rotated, the brush is moved away from the teeth, and the cheek is stretched facially with the back of the brush head. Care must be taken not to drag the filament tips over the gingival margin when the brush is returned to the initial position (Figure 25-6A).

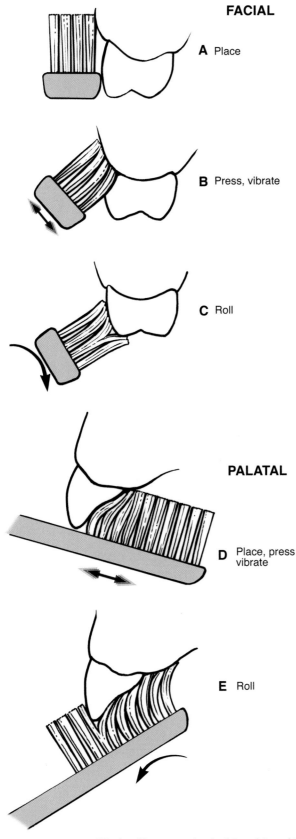

FIGURE 25-6 Modified Stillman Method of Brushing. (A) Initial brush placement with sides of bristles or filaments

D. Overlap Strokes

When moving the brush to an adjacent position, overlap the brush position, as shown in Figure 25-4.

E. Position Brush for Anterior Lingual or Palatal Surfaces

1. Use the brush the long, narrow way.
2. Hook the heel of the brush on the incisal edge (Figure 25-6D).
3. Press (down for maxillary, up for mandibular) until the filaments lie flat against the teeth and gingiva.
4. Press and roll (curve up for mandibular, down for maxillary teeth).
5. Replace and repeat five times for each brush width.

III. PROBLEMS

A. Brushing too high during initial placement can lacerate the alveolar mucosa.
B. Tendency to use quick, sweeping strokes results in no brushing for the cervical third of the tooth because the brush tips pass over rather than into the area; likewise for the interproximal areas.
C. Replacing brush with filament tips directed into the gingiva can produce punctate lesions.

■ THE STILLMAN METHOD

As originally described by Stillman,[15] the method was designed for massage and stimulation, as well as for cleaning the cervical areas. The brush ends were placed partly on the gingiva and partly on the cervical areas of the tooth and were directed slightly apically. Pressure was applied to effect a blanching. The handle was given a slight rotary motion, and the brush ends were maintained in position on the tooth surface. After several applications, the brush was moved to the adjacent tooth.

against the attached gingiva. **(B)** The brush is pressed and angled, then vibrated. **(C)** Vibrating is continued as the brush is rolled slowly over the crown. **(D)** Maxillary anterior lingual placement with the brush applied the long way. **(E)** Vibrating continues as the brush is rolled over the crown and interdental areas. Placement is similar for the lingual surfaces of the mandibular anterior teeth. The roll or rolling stroke brushing method has the same brush positions.

■ THE MODIFIED STILLMAN

A modified Stillman, which incorporates a rolling stroke after the vibratory (rotary) phase, frequently is used. The modifications minimize the possibility of gingival trauma and increase the biofilm removal effects.[16]

I. PURPOSES AND INDICATIONS

A. Dental biofilm removal from cervical areas below the height of contour of the crown and from exposed proximal surfaces.

B. General application for cleaning tooth surfaces and massage of the gingiva.

II. PROCEDURE (FIGURE 25-6)

A. Position the Brush

1. *Filaments.* Direct filaments apically (up for maxillary, down for mandibular teeth).
2. *Place Side of Brush on the Attached Gingiva.* The filaments are directed apically. When the plastic portion of the brush head is level with the occlusal or incisal plane, generally the brush is at the proper height, as shown in Figure 25-6A.

B. Strokes

1. *Press to Flex the Filaments.* The sides of the filaments are pressed lightly against the gingiva. The gingiva will blanch.
2. *Angle the Filaments.* Turn the handle by rotating the wrist so that the filaments are directed at an angle of approximately 45° with the long axis of the tooth.
3. *Activate the Brush.* Use a slight rotary motion. Maintain light pressure on the filaments, and keep the tips of the filaments in position with constant contact. Count to 10 slowly as the brush is vibrated by a rotary motion of the handle.
4. *Roll and Vibrate the Brush.* Turn the wrist and work the vibrating brush slowly down over the gingiva and tooth. Make some of the filaments reach interdentally.

C. Replace Brush for Repeat Stroke

Reposition the brush by rotating the wrist. Avoid dragging the filaments back over the free gingival margin by holding the brush out, slightly away from the tooth.

D. Repeat Stroke Five Times or More

The entire stroke (steps A through C) is repeated at least five times for each tooth or group of teeth. When moving the brush to an adjacent position, overlap the brush position, as shown in Figure 25-4.

E. Position Brush for Anterior Lingual and Palatal Surfaces

1. Position the brush the long, narrow way for the anterior components, as described for the rolling stroke technique and shown in Figure 25-6D and E.
2. Press and vibrate, roll, and repeat.

III. PROBLEMS

A. Without careful placement and using a brush with end-rounded filaments, tissue laceration can result. Light pressure is needed.

B. Patient may try to move the brush into the rolling stroke too quickly, and the vibratory aspect may be ineffective for biofilm removal at the gingival margin.

■ THE CHARTERS METHOD

During his long productive dental career, Dr. W. J. Charters emphasized the importance of prevention. The interproximal toothbrushing method that he taught had as its objectives cleanliness through removal of the "film and mucin" from the proximal surfaces and gingival massage through mechanical stimulation.

Among his many published papers, Charters described two brush positions, one at a right angle to the long axis of the tooth[17] and another at a 45° angle with the tips of the bristles toward the occlusal plane.[18] The right-angle position might have been intended primarily for patients with interdental periodontal tissue loss, where access permitted the bristles to enter the embrasure.

For either brush position, the instructions were to force the tips into the interproximal area. "With the bristles between the teeth, as much pressure as possible is exerted, giving the brush several slight rotary or vibratory movements. This causes the sides of the bristles to come in contact with the gum margin, producing an ideal massage."[18]

The classic periodontal textbooks[19] have described the Charters method with the bristles directed toward the occlusal plane at a 45° angle with the long axis. This method is described as follows.

I. PURPOSES AND INDICATIONS

A. Loosen debris and dental biofilm.

B. Massage and stimulate marginal and interdental gingiva.

C. Aid in biofilm removal from proximal tooth surfaces when interproximal tissue is missing, for example, following periodontal surgery.

D. Adapt to cervical areas below the height of contour of the crown and to exposed root surfaces.

E. Remove dental biofilm from abutment teeth and under the gingival border of a fixed partial denture (bridge) or from the undersurface of a sanitary bridge.

F. Cleansing orthodontic appliances (Figures 28-3 and 28-4).

II. PROCEDURE[17]

A. Apply Rolling Stroke Procedure

Instruct in a basic rolling stroke for general cleaning to be accomplished first.

B. Position the Brush

1. *Filaments.* Hold brush (outside the oral cavity) with filaments directed toward the occlusal or incisal plane of the teeth that will be brushed. The tips are pointed down for application to the maxillary and pointed up for application to the mandibular arch. Insert the brush held in the direction it will be used.

2. *Place the Brush.* Place the sides of the filaments against the enamel with the brush tips toward the occlusal or incisal plane.

3. *Angle the Filaments.* Angle at approximately 45° to the occlusal or incisal plane. Slide the brush to a position at the junction of the free gingival margin and the tooth surface (Figure 25-7B). Note contrast with position for the Stillman method (Figure 25-7A).

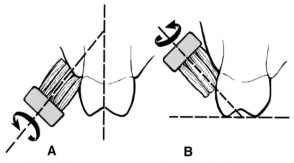

■ **FIGURE 25-7 Charters and Stillman Methods Compared. (A)** Stillman. The brush is angled at approximately 45° to the long axis of the tooth. **(B)** Charters. The brush is angled at approximately 45° to the occlusal plane, with brush tips directed toward the occlusal or incisal surfaces.

C. Strokes

1. *Press Lightly.* Press lightly to flex the filaments and force the tips between the teeth. The sides of the filaments are pressed against the gingival margin.

2. *Vibrate the Brush.* Vibrate gently but firmly, keeping the tips of the filaments in contact. Count to 10 slowly as the brush is vibrated by a rotary motion of the handle.

D. Reposition the Brush and Repeat

Repeat steps B and C, as described, several times in each position around the dental arches.

E. Overlap Strokes

When moving the brush to an adjacent position, overlap the brush position, as shown in Figure 25-4.

F. Position Brush for Anterior Lingual and Palatal Surfaces

Because the Charters brush position is difficult to accomplish on the lingual surfaces, a modified Stillman technique is frequently advised. When the Charters method is preferred, the positions are as follows:

1. *Posterior*
   a. With brush tips pointed toward the occlusal surfaces, extend the brush handle across the incisal edge of the canine of the side opposite that to be brushed.
   b. Place the sides of the toe-end filaments against the distal surface of the most posterior tooth and subsequently at each embrasure.
   c. Press and vibrate.

2. *Anterior*
   a. With brush handle parallel with the long axis of the tooth, place the sides of the toe-end filaments over the interproximal embrasure.
   b. Press and vibrate.

G. Application of Brush for Fixed Partial Denture

When placing the brush, check that the filament tips are directed under the gingival border of the pontic.

III. PROBLEMS

A. Brush ends do not engage the gingival sulcus to remove subgingival bacterial accumulations.

B. In some areas, the correct brush placement is limited or impossible; therefore, modifications become necessary, consequently adding to the complexity of the procedure.

C.   Requirements in digital dexterity are high.

■ OTHER TOOTHBRUSHING METHODS

The rolling stroke, modified Stillman, and Bass are probably the methods most used for patient instruction either directly or as guidelines with variations. Other methods that have been used are included here. The technique and intent of some of the methods overlap. Assessment prior to special instruction may reveal that a mixture of techniques may be in use by a patient.

I.   CIRCULAR: THE FONES METHOD

Alfred C. Fones, the founder of the first course for dental hygienists, advocated this method of brushing. He described the technique in the first dental hygiene text.

Although now considered possibly detrimental for adults, particularly when used by a vigorous brusher, this method may be recommended as an easy-to-learn first technique for young children. A soft brush with 0.006- to 0.008-inch filament diameter is selected. In abbreviated form, the technique described by Dr. Fones includes the following[20]:

A.   With the teeth closed, place the brush inside the cheek with the brush tips lightly contacting the gingiva over the last maxillary molar.

B.   Use a fast, wide, circular motion that sweeps from the maxillary gingiva to the mandibular gingiva with very little pressure, as shown in Figure 25-8.

C.   Bring anterior teeth in edge-to-edge contact, and hold lip out when necessary to make the continuous circular strokes.

D.   Lingual and palatal tooth surfaces require an in-and-out stroke. Brush sweeps across palate on the maxillary arch and back and forth to the molars on the mandibular arch.

II.   VERTICAL: LEONARD METHOD

As described by Hirschfeld,[21] the up-and-down stroke was employed when teeth were cleaned with a primitive crude twig toothbrush. The true vertical stroke passes from the gingiva over the maxillary teeth to the gingiva over the mandibular teeth, with a vigorous sweeping motion.

Leonard described and advocated a vertical stroke in which maxillary and mandibular teeth were brushed separately. Paraphrased, his method is described as follows[22]:

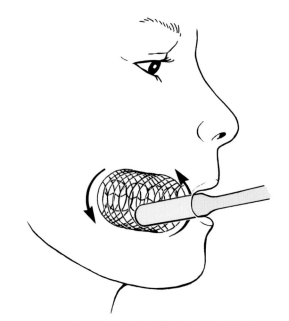

■ **FIGURE 25-8 Fones Method of Brushing.** With the teeth closed, a circular motion extends from the maxillary gingiva to the mandibular gingiva using a light pressure.

A.   With the teeth edge-to-edge, place the brush with the filaments against the teeth at right angles to the long axes of the teeth.

B.   Brush vigorously, without great pressure, with a stroke that is mostly up and down on the tooth surfaces, with just a slight rotation or circular movement after striking the gingival margin with force.

C.   Use enough pressure to force the filaments into the embrasures, but not enough to damage the brush.

D.   The upper and lower teeth are not brushed in the same series of strokes. The teeth are placed edge-to-edge to keep the brush from slipping over the occlusal or incisal surfaces.

III.   HORIZONTAL

Horizontal or crosswise brushing is generally recognized as detrimental. An unlimited sweep with a horizontal scrubbing motion bears pressure on teeth that are most facially inclined or prominent. With the use of an abrasive dentifrice, such brushing may produce tooth abrasion. Because the interdental areas are not touched by this method, dental biofilm can remain undisturbed on proximal surfaces.

IV.   PHYSIOLOGIC: SMITH'S METHOD

The physiologic method was described by Smith[23] and advocated later by Bell.[24] It was based on the principle that the toothbrush should follow the same physiologic pathway that food follows when it traverses over the tissues in a "natural" masticating act.

A soft brush with "small tufts of fine bristles arranged in four parallel rows and trimmed to an even length" was used in a brushing stroke directed down over the lower teeth onto the gingiva and upward over the teeth for the maxillary. Smith also suggested a few gentle horizontal strokes to clean the portion of the sulci directly over the bifurcations of the roots.

V. SCRUB-BRUSH

A scrub-brush procedure consists of vigorously combined horizontal, vertical, and circular strokes, with some vibratory motions for certain areas. Without caution, vigorous scrubbing can encourage gingival recession and, with a dentifrice of sufficient abrasiveness, can create areas of tooth abrasion.

■ POWER TOOTHBRUSHES

Power brushes are also known as power-assisted, automatic, mechanical, or electric brushes. The American Dental Association Council on Scientific Affairs evaluates and classifies power brushes for the reduction of dental biofilm and gingivitis (Figure 27-3, page 449).[25]

Power toothbrushes, like their manual counterparts, have evolved through time due to improved designs and features. The power toothbrushes of the 1960-1980 era mimicked the motions of manual brushing. During that time, research showed equivalence for power and manual brushes in biofilm removal and reduction of gingivitis.[26-29] However, current power brushes move in speeds and motions that cannot be duplicated by manual brushes, and research has shown consistently that power brushes are more effective than manual.[30-39] In addition, the safety of power brushes has been well-established.[33,39-44]

I. PURPOSES AND INDICATIONS

A. General Application

- To facilitate mechanical removal of dental biofilm and food debris from the teeth and the gingiva.
- Reduce calculus and stain buildup.[44]

B. Special Circumstances

Power brushes can be useful for many patients, including:
- Those undergoing orthodontic treatment (pages 456 to 459).
- Those undergoing complex restorative and prosthodontic treatment (pages 485 to 489).

- Those with dental implants (pages 491 to 495).
- Aggressive brushers—patients tend to use less pressure when using a power brush than with a manual brush.[45-47]
- Patients with disabilities or limited dexterity.
  - The large handles of power brushes can be of benefit.
  - Handle weight should be considered for these patients (pages 898 to 899).
- Patients unable to brush.
  - A power brush may be readily used by a parent or caregiver.

II. DESCRIPTION

A. Motion

There is great variety in the manner in which power brushes move, for example:
- The entire brush head moves as a unit in one type of motion.
- Groups of tufts on the same brush may move differently.
- The entire brush head moves as a unit, but in different, yet simultaneous motions.
- Different-shaped brush heads move separately, and in different, yet simultaneous motions.
- A synopsis of the types of motions of power brushes is seen in Table 25-2.

B. Brush Head Shape

- Adult. The variety of shapes is illustrated in Figure 25-9. They may be small and round, conical, or like traditional manual heads. Trim profiles include flat, bilevel, rippled, or angled.
- Child. A child's power brush should be smaller and specially designed to accommodate for the development of the dentition, as shown in Figure 25-10.
- Interdental. The interdental brushes pictured in Figure 25-11 are designed to fit a power brush handle and are similar in shape to manual interdental brushes, as shown in Figure 26-9.

C. Filaments

- Made of soft, end-rounded nylon.
- Diameters: from extra-soft, 0.075 mm (0.003 inch), to soft, 0.15 mm (0.006 inch).
- Some children's power brush heads feature specially manufactured filaments for extra softness.

D. Power Source

1. **Direct**
- Connects to electrical outlet

■ TABLE 25-2 POWER TOOTHBRUSH MOTION

MOTION	DESCRIPTION
Rotational	Moves in a 360° circular motion
Counter-rotational	Each tuft of filaments moves in a rotational motion; each tuft moves counter-directional to the tuft adjacent to it (if one tuft rotates to the left, the adjacent tuft rotates to the right)
Oscillating	Rotates from center to the left, and then to the right; degree of rotation from center varies from 25°–55°
Pulsating	When the brush head is on the tooth, the pulsations are in the direction toward the interproximal
Cradle or twist	Side to side with an arc
Side-to-side	Side-to-side in a direction that is perpendicular to the long axis of the brush handle
Translating	Up-and-down movements in a direction that is parallel to the long axis of the brush handle
Combination	Combination of simultaneous yet different types of movements

Rippled/teardrop

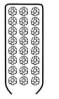

Bilevel/round

Bilevel, separated tufts/rectangle

Bilevel/round angled

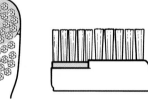

Multilevel/oval

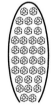

Bilevel/round

Orthodontic

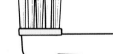

Multilevel/rectangle

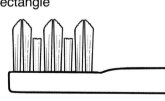
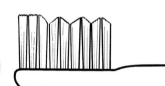
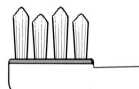
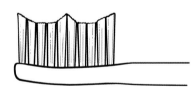
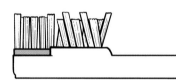

Regular

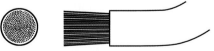

■ **FIGURE 25-9 Power Brush Trim Profiles.** Power brushes are made in a variety of brush head shapes, such as oval, teardrop, rectangular, and round. Some power brushes have two different-shaped heads on the same brush. In addition, there are a variety of brush head trims on power brushes, including, flat, bilevel, and multilevel.

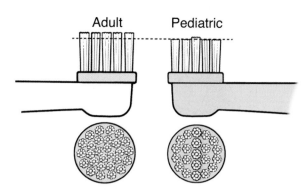

FIGURE 25-10 Child Power Brush Profile. Power brushes for children could necessitate smaller head sizes and shorter filaments to allow for distal reach in tight posterior areas.

2. **Replaceable Batteries**
   - Relatively inexpensive and convenient.
   - As the batteries lose their power, brush speed is reduced.
   - Advise patients to select a brush that has a water-tight handle to avoid corrosion of batteries.
3. **Rechargeable**
   - Rechargeable, nonreplaceable battery.
   - Recharges via a stand that is connected to the electrical outlet.
4. **Disposable**
   - Batteries can be neither replaced nor recharged.
5. **Switches**
   - Push-button switch that remains "on" until it is depressed once again.
   - Few models require that the push button be held down during operation, which may present difficulties for small children or persons with certain types of disabilities.

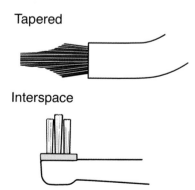

FIGURE 25-11 Interdental Power Brush Trim Profiles. Some power brushes offer brush heads especially for interdental and proximal surface dental biofilm removal and difficult-access areas such as around implants, orthodontic appliances, and exposed furcations.

E. Speeds
- Vary from low to high.
- Generally, power brushes with replaceable batteries move slower than those with rechargeable batteries.
- Movement varies from 3,800 to 40,000 movements per minute depending on the manufacturer and type.

III. INSTRUCTION

A. Basis for Brush Selection
- Quality of clinical research that supports the brush.
- Dental professional's experience with the product.
- Patient circumstances and preferences.
- Dexterity of the patient: hand motion by patient is not required as extensively as with manual brushes.

B. Preparation for Instructing Patient
- Review manufacturer's instructions as they can differ.
- If possible, use the product before teaching the patient.

C. Hands-on Instruction
- Teach patients that use of power brushes does require practice.
- Provide a demonstration model of the brush and a video of the brushing instructions, if available.
- Show and tell the patient how to turn the handle to reach all areas of the mouth.

IV. METHODS FOR USE
A. Select brush with soft end-rounded filaments.
B. Select dentifrice with minimum abrasivity.
C. Place a small amount of dentifrice on the brush and spread the dentifrice over the teeth to prevent splashing when the power is turned on.
D. Vary the brush position for each tooth surface. Brush each tooth and surrounding gingiva separately.
   - Apply the brush for sulcular brushing to the distal, facial, mesial, and lingual surfaces of each tooth as the brush is moved from the most posterior teeth toward the anterior, quadrant by quadrant.
   - Turn the brush to reach each proximal area.
   - Angulate for access to surfaces of rotated, crowded, or otherwise displaced teeth.

E.   Use slight steady pressure. Pressure should not be great enough at any time to bend the filaments.

SUPPLEMENTAL BRUSHING

I.   PROBLEM AREAS

A.   Adaptations

- Each surface of each tooth must be brushed.
- Initial instruction necessarily may be limited to a basic procedure, particularly when it varies from the patient's present procedures.
- At succeeding lessons, the special hard-to-get areas are shown.
- Suggestions are made and demonstrated for brush adaptation for areas that were missed.

B.   Areas for Special Attention

- Facially displaced teeth, especially canines and premolars, where the zone of attached gingiva on the facial may be minimal and where toothbrush abrasion frequently occurs.
- Inclined teeth, for example, lingual surfaces of mandibular molars that are inclined lingually.
- Exposed root surfaces; cemental and dentinal surfaces.
- Overlapped teeth or wide embrasures, which require use of vertical brush position (Figure 25-12).

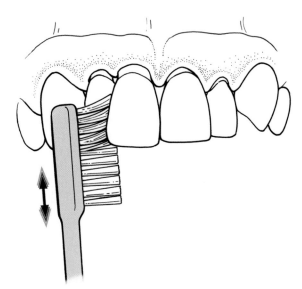

■ **FIGURE 25-12 Brush in Vertical Position.** For overlapped teeth, open interproximal areas, and selected areas of recession, the dental biofilm on proximal tooth surfaces can be conveniently removed with the brush held in a vertical position.

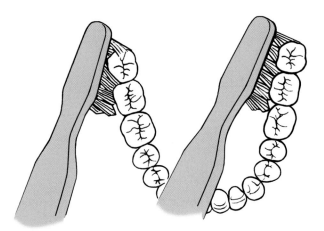

■ **FIGURE 25-13 Brushing Problems.** Brush placement to remove biofilm from the distal surfaces of the most posterior teeth. The distobuccal surface is approached by stretching the cheek; the distolingual surface is approached by directing the brush across from the canine of the opposite side.

- Surfaces of teeth next to edentulous areas.
- Exposed furcation areas.
- Right canine and lateral incisor, both maxillary and mandibular, which are commonly missed by right-handed brushers; the opposite is true for left-handed brushers.
- Distal surfaces of most posterior teeth (Figure 25-13). At best, the brush may reach only the distal line angles. Supplementation with dental floss or textured dental floss is needed for the distal surface (Figures 26-3G and 26-6C).

II.   OCCLUSAL BRUSHING

A.   Objectives

1.   Loosen biofilm microorganisms packed in pits and fissures.
2.   Remove biofilm deposits from occlusal surfaces of teeth out of occlusion or not used during mastication.
3.   Remove biofilm from the margins of restorations.
4.   Clean pits and fissures to prepare for sealants.

B.   Procedure

1.   Place brush on occlusal surfaces of molar teeth with filament tips pointed into the occlusal pits at a right angle. The handle should be parallel with the occlusal surface. The toe of the brush should cover the distal grooves of the most posterior tooth (Figure 25-14A).
2.   Two acceptable strokes are suggested.
     a.   Vibrate the brush in a slight circular movement while maintaining the filament tips on

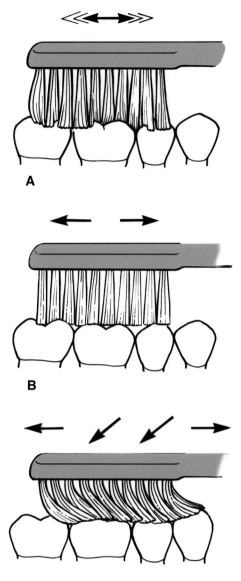

■ **FIGURE 25-14 Occlusal Brushing. (A)** Vibrating brush with light pressure while maintaining filament tips on the occlusal surface permits tips to work their way into pits and fissures. **(B)** Long horizontal strokes contact only the cusp tips. **(C)** Excess pressure curves the filaments so that tips cannot get into the pits and fissures.

> the occlusal surface throughout a count of 10. Press moderately so filaments do not bend but go straight into the pits and fissures (Figure 25-14B).
>
> b. Force the filaments against the occlusal surface with sharp, quick strokes; lift the brush off each time to dislodge debris; repeat about 10 times.

3. Move brush to premolar area, overlapping previous brush position.

C. Precaution

Long scrubbing strokes from anterior to posterior on an occlusal surface may contact only the prominent parts of the cusps (Figure 25-14B).

III. TONGUE CLEANING

Total mouth cleanliness includes tongue care.

A. Microorganisms of the Tongue

1. Main foci for oral microorganisms are:
   a. Dorsum of tongue.
   b. Gingival sulci and pockets.
   c. Dental biofilm on all teeth.
2. Microorganisms in saliva are principally from the tongue.
3. The microflora of the tongue is not constant, but changes frequently.[48]

B. Effects of Cleaning the Tongue

1. Retards dental biofilm formation and total biofilm accumulation.
2. Reduces number of microorganisms.
3. Reduces potential for halitosis (pages 388 to 390).
4. Contributes to overall cleanliness.

C. Anatomic Features of Tongue Conducive to Debris Retention

1. *Surface Papillae.* Numerous filiform papillae extend as minute projections, whereas fungiform papillae are not as high and create elevations and depressions that entrap debris and microorganisms (Figure 12-2, page 208).
2. *Fissured Tongue.* Fissures may be several millimeters deep and retain debris.

D. Brushing Procedure for Manual and Power Brushes

1. Hold the brush handle at a right angle to the midline of the tongue and direct the brush tips toward the throat.
2. With the tongue extruded, the sides of the filaments are placed on the posterior part of the tongue surface.
3. With light pressure, draw the brush forward and over the tip of the tongue. Repeat three or four times. Do not scrub the papillae.

E. Tongue Cleaner

Tongue cleaners may be made of plastic, stainless steel, or other flexible metal. They are curved and

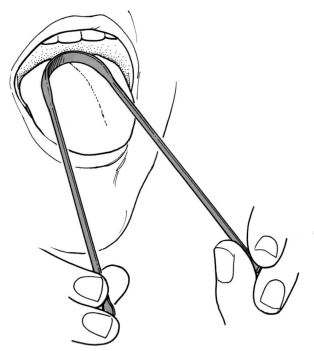

■ FIGURE 25-15 Tongue Cleaner. A variety of plastic or flexible metal cleaners are available to clean the dorsal surface of the tongue. The cleaner is pressed over the tongue with a light but firm stroke.

wide enough to fit over the tongue surface without hitting the teeth. Some are made with a single handle, whereas others have two ends to hold, as shown in Figure 25-15.

1. *Purpose.* By removing debris and microorganisms, the patient can expect tongue cleaning to contribute to overall mouth cleanliness, reduce the numbers of bacteria available for biofilm formation, and lessen mouth odors. The procedure can be especially helpful for the patient who has xerostomia, a coated tongue, deep fissures, or who smokes.

2. *Procedure.* Place the arch toward the posterior of the dorsal surface (Figure 25-15). Press with a light but firm stroke, and pull forward. Repeat several times, covering the entire surface of the tongue. Wash the tongue cleaner under running water.

■ TOOTHBRUSHING FOR SPECIAL CONDITIONS

Even when an unusual oral condition develops, a patient must be encouraged to brush wherever possible to reduce the possibility of infection and promote healing. Prolonged omission of techniques of biofilm

removal is never indicated. Examples of conditions that may require a temporary departure from personal care routines follow.

I. ACUTE ORAL INFLAMMATORY OR TRAUMATIC LESIONS

When an acute oral condition precludes normal brushing, the patient should be instructed to brush all areas of the mouth that are not affected and to resume regular biofilm control measures on the affected area as soon as possible. Rinsing with a warm, mild saline solution can encourage healing and debris removal.

II. FOLLOWING PERIODONTAL SURGERY

Patients must receive specific instructions concerning brushing while sutures and/or a dressing are in place. Because direct, vigorous brushing of a periodontal dressing could cause its displacement, brushing of the occlusal surfaces and light strokes over the dressing may be advised. Other teeth and gingiva should be brushed as usual. Additional instructions appear in Table 40-1 (page 708).

III. ACUTE STAGE OF NECROTIZING ULCERATIVE GINGIVITIS

A major contributing factor in the development of this disease is a lack of oral cleanliness. During the acute stage, the oral tissues are sensitive to any touch, and toothbrushing therefore is neglected. Instructions for these patients are on pages 694 to 695. A soft brush is indicated along with careful brush placement to avoid trauma.

IV. FOLLOWING DENTAL EXTRACTION

Instructions may be found on page 854 and include brushing all teeth and gingiva except the surgical wound area. Teeth adjacent to the extraction site need cleaning as soon as possible to reduce bacterial collections and to promote healing.

V. FOLLOWING DENTAL RESTORATIONS

Patients tend to avoid brushing a new crown, newly placed fixed partial denture, or other prosthesis. Specific instructions should be given at the time of insertion.

■ TOOTHBRUSH TRAUMA: THE GINGIVA

Trauma to the gingiva occurs most frequently on the facial surfaces over teeth prominent in the dental arch. The lesions frequently are found over canines and premolars.

Lesions are especially apt to occur after initial instruction in use of a new method of brushing. The patient may be overzealous or may have misunderstood correct brush placement. Examination of a patient's gingiva within a few days to a week after instruction can be important.

I. ACUTE ALTERATIONS

Acute lesions are usually lacerations or ulcerations. The severity of the lesion may depend on the frequency and extent of brushing, as well as on the stiffness of the filaments and the force applied.

A. Appearance

1. Scuffed epithelial surface with denuded underlying connective tissue.
2. Punctate lesions that appear as red pinpoint spots.
3. Diffuse redness and denuded attached gingiva.

B. Precipitating Factors

1. Horizontal or vertical scrub toothbrushing method.
2. Excess pressure applied using firm palm grasp of handle.[49]
3. Use of abrasive dentifrice.[50]
4. Overvigorous placement and application of the toothbrush.
5. Penetration of gingiva by filament ends.
6. Use of a toothbrush with frayed, broken bristles or filaments.
7. Application of filaments beyond attached gingiva.

II. CHRONIC ALTERATIONS

A. Changes in Gingival Contour

1. *Appearance*
   a. Rolled, bulbous, hard, firm marginal gingiva, in "piled up" or festoon shape ("McCall's festoon," Figure 12-10, page 217).
   b. Gingival cleft, which is a narrow groove or slit that extends from the crest of the gingiva to the attached gingiva ("Stillman's cleft," Figure 12-11, page 218).
2. *Location*
   a. Usually appear only on the facial gingiva, because of the vigor with which toothbrush is used.
   b. Frequently inversely related to the right- or left-handedness of the patient.
   c. Areas most often involved are around canines or teeth in labioversion or buccoversion.

B. Gingival Recession

1. *Appearance.* Margin has moved apically and root surface is exposed.
2. *Predisposing Factors*
   a. Anatomic: Narrow band of attached gingiva and thin facial bone over teeth malposed in labioversion.
   b. Toothbrushing habits: Vigorous pressured brushing with abrasive dentifrice and worn brush.

C. Suggested Corrective Measures

1. Recommend use of a soft toothbrush with end-rounded filaments.
2. Correct the patient's toothbrushing method; demonstrate a toothbrushing method better suited to the oral condition.
3. Temporary cessation of brushing the traumatized area may be needed. An antimicrobial rinse may assist in the healing process.

■ TOOTHBRUSHING TRAUMA: DENTAL ABRASION

I. APPEARANCE

Wedge-shaped indentations with smooth, shiny surfaces, as seen in Figure 15-7, page 268.

Abrasion is the loss of tooth substance produced by mechanical wear other than that caused by mastication. Abrasion also may be defined as the pathologic wearing away of tooth substance through some abnormal mechanical process, in contrast with erosion that generally involves a chemical process. It is understood that loss of tooth structure is a multifactorial issue. Classic controlled clinical trials are needed to establish a reliable base of information on the causative agents related to dental abrasion.[51]

II. LOCATION OF ABRADED AREAS

A. Primarily on facial surfaces, especially of canines, premolars, and sometimes first molars, or, on any tooth in buccoversion or labioversion, those most available to the pressure of the toothbrush. The canines are susceptible because of their prominence on the curvature of the dental arches.

B. Most abraded areas are on the cervical areas of exposed root surfaces, but occasionally they may occur on the enamel. When adjacent teeth are involved, the lesions appear in line with each other.

III. CONTRIBUTING FACTORS

A. Excessive brushing force with abrasive agent in the dentifrice.

B. Horizontal brushing with excessive pressure.

C. Form of filament ends: Abrasion is less frequent when filaments are end-rounded.

D. Prominence of the tooth surface labially or buccally.

IV. CORRECTIVE MEASURES

A. Explain the problem to the patient to ensure full cooperation.

B. Advise use of a specific brush with end-rounded filaments.

C. Change or correct the toothbrushing procedure.

D. Recommend a less abrasive dentifrice.

E. Use a smaller amount of dentifrice.

  1. Start brushing in the area of the dentition where the most biofilm and calculus are noted at a maintenance appointment.

  2. Avoid applying the dentifrice vigorously to the same tooth surfaces.

▪ CARE OF TOOTHBRUSHES

When discussing the type and features of the brush selected for an individual patient, the number of brushes needed and the frequency of replacement should be included. Perhaps an ideal time to teach cleaning and daily care of brushes would be after a practice session.

The condition of a brush depends on many factors, including the amount and manner of use, the type of care, and the quality of the brush at the start.

I. SUPPLY OF BRUSHES

A. Advise at least two brushes for home use and a third in a portable container for use at work, school, or travel.

B. Purchase of brushes should be staggered so that all brushes are not new at the same time and, more important, so that they are all not old at the same time, thereby resulting in less than optimum maintenance of the gingival condition.

II. BRUSH REPLACEMENT

A. Frequent replacement recommended; at least every 2 to 3 months.

B. Brushes should be replaced before filaments become splayed or frayed or lose resiliency. Duration of a brush is influenced by many factors, including frequency and method of use.

C. Brush contamination occurs with use.[52,53] Contamination has the potential for causing systemic or localized infection.

Everyday Ethics

Lucy is 19 years old and works in the sterilization center of a local hospital. In the past 6 months, her work schedule was changed from a day shift to a shift that requires her to work at night. At her maintenance appointment, Dorothy, the dental hygienist, reviewed the patient's history and noted that everything seemed the same except that Lucy had developed the habit of drinking many cups of coffee to help stay awake at work.

Lucy has noticed more staining on her teeth and tongue than ever before, and she complains of a bad taste in her mouth. Dorothy plans to recommend a power toothbrush and a tongue cleaner.

Questions for Consideration

1. Is it ethical for the dental hygienist to address Lucy's consumption of coffee before reviewing brushing techniques? From what role or perspective would this be appropriate?

2. Lucy interprets her change in oral health to be a result of working at night because she is not following her normal routine of brushing. What suggestions can Dorothy offer Lucy that would facilitate a regular routine of brushing?

3. The office in which Dorothy practices provides a specific brand of power brush to their patients as a part of the maintenance visit. Dorothy has never used the product, and neither has she read any research or literature about the product. She is basing her recommendation of the brush on the fact that she has seen some good results in other patients. Is there an ethical problem in recommending a product about which Dorothy knows very little? What types of questions might Dorothy's patients have that she would not be able to answer? Why is it the responsibility of a dental hygienist to know about a variety of over-the-counter products?

Factors To Teach The Patient

- How dental biofilm forms and its effects on the teeth and gingiva.

- Why it is necessary to remove dental biofilm from the teeth daily, especially before going to sleep.

- The type of brush—manual, power, or both—that is recommended to maintain optimal oral health for that patient.

- Individualized instruction on which type of manual brushing method is most appropriate.

- Individualized, hands-on instruction for the type of brush the patient is using.

- Proper care and maintenance of manual and power brushes.

- Indications for and use of a tongue cleaner.

D. Patients who are debilitated, immunosuppressed, have a known infection, or are about to undergo surgery for any reason can be advised to disinfect their brushes or use disposable brushes.[52]

III. CLEANING TOOTHBRUSHES

- Clean thoroughly after each use.
- Hold brush head under strong stream of warm water from faucet to force particles, dentifrice, and bacteria from between the filaments.
- Tap the handle on edge of sink to remove remaining particles.
- Use one toothbrush to clean another brush; filaments can be worked between those of the other brush to remove resistant debris.
- Rinse completely and tap out excess water.

IV. BRUSH STORAGE

- Brushes should be kept in open air with head in an upright position, apart from contact with other brushes, particularly those of another person.
- Portable brush container should have sufficient holes to give air temporarily until the brush can be completely exposed for drying. A closed container encourages bacterial growth.

REFERENCES

1. **Hirschfeld**, I.: *The Toothbrush: Its Use and Abuse.* Brooklyn, NY, Dental Items of Interest, 1939, pp. 1–27.

2. **Kimery**, M.J. and Stallard, R.E.: The Evolutionary Development and Contemporary Utilization of Various Oral Hygiene Procedures, *Periodont. Abstr., 16*, 90, September, 1968.

3. **McCauley**, H.B.: Toothbrushes, Toothbrush Materials and Design, *J. Am. Dent. Assoc., 33*, 283, March 1, 1946.

4. **Weinberger**, B.W.: *An Introduction to the History of Dentistry.* St. Louis, Mosby, 1948, pp. 43, 140–144.

5. **American Academy of Periodontology**, Committee Report: The Tooth Brush and Methods of Cleaning the Teeth, *Dent. Items Interest, 42*, 193, March, 1920.

6. **Alexander**, J.F.: Toothbrushes and Toothbrushing, in Menaker, L., ed.: *The Biologic Basis of Dental Caries.* Hagerstown, MD, Harper & Row, 1980, pp. 482–496.

7. **Koecker**, L.: *Principles of Dental Surgery, Exhibiting a New Method of Treating the Diseases of the Teeth and Gums.* Baltimore, MD, American Society of Dental Surgeons, 1842, Chapter III, pp. 155–156.

8. **American Dental Association**, Council on Dental Therapeutics: *Accepted Dental Therapeutics*, 40th ed. Chicago, American Dental Association, 1984, pp. 386–387.

9. **Massassati**, A. and Frank, R.M.: Scanning Electron Microscopy of Unused and Used Manual Toothbrushes, *J. Clin. Periodontol., 9*, 148, March, 1982.

10. **Checchi**, L., Minguzzi, S., Franchi, M., and Forteleoni, G.: Toothbrush Filaments End-Rounding: Stereomicroscope Analysis, *J. Clin. Periodontol., 28*, 360, April, 2001.

11. **Breitenmoser**, J., Mörmann, W., and Mühlemann, H.R.: Damaging Effects of Toothbrush Bristle End Form on Gingiva, *J. Periodontol., 50*, 212, April, 1979.

12. **Silverstone**, L.M. and Featherstone, M.J.: A Scanning Electron Microscope Study of the End Rounding of Bristles in Eight Toothbrush Types, *Quintessence Int., 19*, 3, February, 1988.

13. **Bass**, C.C.: An Effective Method of Personal Oral Hygiene, *J. Louisiana State Med. Soc., 106*, 100, March, 1954.

14. **Hard**, D.: Oral Prophylaxis, in Bunting, R.W.: *Oral Hygiene*, 3rd ed. Philadelphia, Lea & Febiger, 1957, pp. 280–283.

15. **Stillman**, P.R.: A Philosophy of the Treatment of Periodontal Disease, *Dent. Digest, 38*, 315, September, 1932.

16. **Hirschfeld**: op. cit., p. 380.

17. **Charters**, W.J.: Home Care of the Mouth. I. Proper Home Care of the Mouth, *J. Periodontol., 19*, 136, October, 1948.

18. **Charters**, W.J.: Eliminating Mouth Infections With the Toothbrush and Other Stimulating Instruments, *Dent. Digest, 38*, 130, April, 1932.

19. **Miller**, S.C.: *Textbook of Periodontia*, 3rd ed. Philadelphia, The Blakiston Co., 1950, pp. 327–328.

20. **Fones**, A.C., ed.: *Mouth Hygiene*, 4th ed. Philadelphia, Lea & Febiger, 1934, pp. 299–306.

21. **Hirschfeld**: op. cit., pp. 369–371.

22. **Leonard**, H.J.: Conservative Treatment of Periodontoclasia, *J. Am. Dent. Assoc., 26*, 1308, August, 1939.

23. **Smith**, T.S.: Anatomic and Physiologic Conditions Governing the Use of the Toothbrush, *J. Am. Dent. Assoc., 27*, 874, June, 1940.

24. **Bell**, D.G.: Home Care of the Mouth. III. Teaching Home Care to the Patient, *J. Periodontol., 19*, 140, October, 1948.

25. **American Dental Association**, Council on Scientific Affairs: *ADA Acceptance Program Guidelines for Toothbrushes.* Chicago, American Dental Association, May 1998.

26. **McKendrick**, A.J.W., Barbenel, L.M.H., and McHugh, W.D.: A Two-Year Comparison of Hand and Electric Toothbrushes, *J. Periodontal. Res., 3*, 224, Number 3, 1968.

27. **Powers**, G.K., Tussing, G.J., and Bradley, R.E.: A Comparison of Effectiveness in Interproximal Plaque Removal of an Electric Toothbrush and a Conventional Hand Toothbrush, *Periodontics, 5*, 37, January–February, 1967.

28. **Lobene**, R.R.: The Effect of an Automatic Toothbrush on Periodontitis , *J. Oral Ther. Pharmacol.*, 3, 284, April, 1967.

29. **Frandsen**, A.: Mechanical Oral Hygiene Practices: State of the Science Review, in Loe, H. and Kleinman, D.V., eds.: *Dental Plaque Control Measures and Oral Hygiene Practices*, Oxford, IRL Press, 1986, p. 94.

30. **Truhe**, T.F.: Powered Toothbrushes: Indications for Patient Use and Recommendations for Dental Professionals, *J. Esthetic Dent.*, 8, 20, January–February, 1996.

31. **Truhlar**, R.S., Morris, H.F., and Ochi, S.: The Efficacy of a Counter-Rotational Powered Toothbrush in the Maintenance of Endosseous Dental Implants, *J. Am. Dent. Assoc.*, 131, 101, January, 2000.

32. **McCracken**, G.I., Stacey F., Heasman, L., Sellers, P., Macgregor, I.D., Kelly, P.J., and Heasman, P.A.: A Comparative Study of Two Powered Toothbrushes and One Manual Toothbrush in Young Adults, *J. Clin. Dent.*, 12, 7, Special Issue, 2001.

33. **Warren**, P.R., Cugini, M., Marks, P., and King, D.W.: Safety, Efficacy and Acceptability of a New Power Toothbrush: A 3-Month Comparative Clinical Investigation, *Am. J. Dent.*, 14, 3, February, 2001.

34. **Barnes**, C.M., Russell, C.M., and Weatherford, T.W.: A Comparison of the Efficacy of 2 Powered Toothbrushes in Affecting Plaque Accumulation, Gingivitis, and Gingival Bleeding, *J. Periodontol.*, 70, 840, August, 1999.

35. **Cronin**, M., Dembling, W., Warren, P.R., and King, D.W.: A 3-month Clinical Investigation Comparing the Safety and Efficacy of a Novel Electric Toothbrush (Braun Oral-B® 3D Plaque Remover) With a Manual Toothbrush, *Am. J. Dent.*, 11, S17, Special Issue, 1998.

36. **Tritten**, C.B. and Armitage, G.C.: Comparison of a Sonic and a Manual Toothbrush for Efficacy in Supragingival Plaque Removal and Reduction of Gingivitis, *J. Clin. Periodontol.*, 23, 641, July, 1996.

37. **Killoy**, W.J., Love, J.W., Love, J., Fedi, P.F., and Tira, D.E.: The Effectiveness of a Counter-rotary Action Toothbrush and Conventional Toothbrush on Plaque Removal and Gingival Bleeding: A Short Term Study, *J. Periodontol.*, 60, 473, August, 1989.

38. **Boyd**, R.L., Murray, P., and Robertson, P.B.: Effect of Rotary Electric Toothbrush Versus Manual Toothbrush on Periodontal Status During Orthodontic Treatment, *Am. J. Orthod. Dentofac. Orthop.*, 96, 342, October, 1989.

39. **Ho**, H.P. and Niederman, R.: Effectiveness of the Sonicare® Sonic Toothbrush on Reduction of Plaque, Gingivitis, Probing Pocket Depth, and Subgingival Bacteria in Adolescent Orthodontic Clients, *J. Clin. Dent.*, 8, 15, Special Issue, 1997.

40. **Warren**, P.R., Ray, T.S., Cugini, M., and Chater, B.V.: A Practice-based Study of a Power Toothbrush: Assessment of Effectiveness and Acceptance, *J. Am. Dent. Assoc.*, 131, 389, March, 2000.

41. **Wilson**, S., Levine, D., Dequincey, G., and Killoy, W.J.: The Effect of Two Toothbrushes on Plaque, Gingivitis, Gingival Abrasion, and Recession: A 1-Year Longitudinal Study, *Compend. Contin. Educ. Dent.*, 14, S569, Supplement 16, 1993.

42. **Danser**, M.M., Timmerman, M.F., Ijzerman, Y., van der Velden, U., Warren, P.R., and van der Weijden, F.A.: A Comparison of Electric Toothbrushes in Their Potential to Cause Gingival Abrasion of Oral Soft Tissues, *Am. J. Dent.*, 11, S 35, September, 1998.

43. **Johnson**, B.D. and McInnes, C.: Clinical Evaluation of the Efficacy and Safety of a New Sonic Toothbrush, *J. Periodontol*, 65, 692, July, 1994.

44. **Sharma**, N.C., Galustians, H.J., Qaqish, J., Cugini, M.A., and Warren, P.R.: The Effect of Two Power Toothbrushes on Calculus and Stain, *Am. J. Dent.*, 15, 72, April, 2002.

45. **van der Weijden**, G.A., Timmerman, M.F., Reijerse, E., Snoek, C.M., and van der Velden, U.: Toothbrushing Force in Relation to Plaque Removal, *J. Clin. Periodontol.*, 23, 724, August, 1996.

46. **Heasman**, P., Wilson, Z., Macgregor, I., and Kelly, P.: Comparative Study of Electric and Manual Toothbrushes in Patients With Fixed Orthodontic Appliances, *Am. J. Orthod. Dentofacial Orthop.*, 114, 45, July, 1998.

47. **Boyd**, R.L., McLey, L., and Zahradnik, R.: Clinical and Laboratory Evaluation of Powered Electric Toothbrushes: *In vivo* Determination of Average Force for Use of Manual and Powered Toothbrushes, *J. Clin. Dent.*, 8, 72, Special Issue, 1997.

48. **Van der Weijden**, G.A. and Van der Velden, U.: Fluctuation of the Microbiota of the Tongue in Humans, *J. Clin. Periodontol.*, 18, 26, January, 1991.

49. **Niemi**, M.-L., Ainamo, J., and Etemadzadeh, H.: The Effect of Toothbrush Grip on Gingival Abrasion and Plaque Removal During Toothbrushing, *J. Clin. Periodontol.*, 14, 19, January, 1987.

50. **Niemi**, M.-L., Sandholm, L., and Ainamo, J.: Frequency of Gingival Lesions After Standardized Brushing as Related to Stiffness of Toothbrush and Abrasiveness of Dentifrice, *J. Clin. Periodontol.*, 11, 254, April, 1984.

51. **Dyer**, D., Addy, M., and Newcombe, R.G.: Studies in vitro of Abrasion by Different Manual Toothbrush Heads and a Standard Toothpaste, *J. Clin. Periodontol.*, 27, 99, February, 2000.

52. **Glass**, R.T.: The Infected Toothbrush, the Infected Denture, and Transmission of Disease: A Review, *Compend. Contin. Educ. Dent.*, 13, 592, July, 1992.

53. **Müller**, H.-P., Lange, D.E., and Müller, R.F.: *Actinobacillus actinomycetemcomitans* Contamination of Toothbrushes From Patients Harbouring the Organism, *J. Clin. Periodontol.*, 16, 388, July, 1989.

SUGGESTED READINGS

Clayton, N., Addy, M., Scratcher, C., Ley, F., and Newcombe, R.: Comparative Professional Plaque Removal Study Using 8 Branded Toothbrushes, *J. Clin. Periodontol.*, 29, 310, April, 2002.

Daly, C.G., Chapple, C.C., and Cameron, A.C.: Effect of Toothbrush Wear on Plaque Control, *J. Clin. Periodontol.*, 23, 45, January, 1996.

Dyer, D., Addy, M., and Newcombe, R.G.: Studies in vitro of Abrasion by Different Manual Toothbrush Heads and a Standard Toothpaste, *J. Clin. Periodontol.*, 27, 99, February, 2000.

Dyer, D., MacDonald, E., Newcombe, R.G., Scratcher, C., Ley, F., and Addy, M.: Abrasion and Stain Removal by Different Manual Toothbrushes and Brush Actions: Studies in vitro, *J. Clin. Periodontol*, 28, 121, February, 2001.

Mandel, I.D.: The Plaque Fighters: Choosing a Weapon, *J. Am. Dent. Assoc.*, 124, 71, April, 1993.

Sforza, N.M., Rimondini, L., di Menna, F., and Camorali, C.: Plaque Removal by Worn Toothbrush, *J. Clin. Periodontol*, 27, 212, March, 2000.

Waerhaug, J: Effect of Toothbrushing on Subgingival Plaque Formation, *J. Periodontol.*, 52, 30, January, 1981.

Power Brushes

Ainamo, J., Xie, Q., Ainamo, A., and Kallio, P.: Assessment of the Effect of an Oscillating/Rotating Electric Toothbrush on Oral Health: A 12-month Longitudinal Study, *J. Clin. Periodontol.*, 24, 28, January, 1997.

Barnes, C.M.: Powered Toothbrushes: Evidence Warrants Wider Recommendations, *Access*, 12, 56, May–June, 1998.

Bhanji, S., Williams, B., Sheller, B., Elwood, T., and Mancl, L.: Transient Bacteremia Induced by Toothbrushing: A Comparison of the Sonicare Toothbrush With a Conventional Toothbrush, *Pediatr. Dent.*, 24, 295, July/August, 2002.

Bowen, D.: An Evidenced-Based Review of Power Toothbrushes, *Compend. Cont. Educ. Oral Hyg.*, 9, 3, Number 1, 2002.

Boyd, R.L.: Clinical and Laboratory Evaluation of Powered Electric Toothbrushes: Review of the Literature, *J. Clin. Dent., 8*, 67, Number 3, 1997.

Dentino, A.R., Derderian, G., Wolf, M.A., Cugini, M.A., Johnson, R., Van Swol, R.L., King, D., Marks, P., and Warren, P: Six-month Comparison of Powered Versus Manual Toothbrushing for Safety and Efficacy in the Absence of Professional Instruction in Mechanical Plaque Control, *J. Periondontol., 73*, 770, July, 2002.

Haffajee, A.D., Smith, C., Torresyap, G., Thompson, M., Guerrero, D., and Socransky, S.S.: Efficacy of Manual and Powered Toothbrushes (II): Effect on Microbiological Parameters, *J. Clin. Periodontol., 28*, 947, October, 2001.

Haffajee, A.D., Thompson, M., Torresyap, G., Guerrero, D., and Socransky, S.S.: Efficacy of Manual and Powered Toothbrushes (1): Effect on Clinical Parameters, *J. Clin. Periodontol., 28*, 937, October, 2001.

O'Beirne, G., Johnson, R.H., Persson, G.R., and Spektor, M.D.: Efficacy of a Sonic Toothbrush on Inflammation and Probing Depth in Adult Periodontitis, *J. Periodontol., 67*, 900, September, 1996.

Perno Goldie, M.: Power Toothbrushing: An Easy, Effective Way to Improve Oral Health, *Contemp. Oral Hyg., 2*, 28, July/August, 2002.

Shultz, P.H., Killoy, W.J., Rapley, J.W., and Shultz, R.E.: A Clinical Comparison of Subgingival and Interproximal Plaque Removal Effectiveness: Electric vs. Manual Toothbrushing, *J. Pract. Hyg., 4*, 31, March/April, 1995.

Williams, K.B., Cobb, C.M., Taylor, H.J., Brown, A.R., and Bray, K.K.: Effect of Sonic and Mechanical Toothbrushes on Subgingival Microbial Flora: A Comparative in vivo Scanning Electron Microscopy Study of 8 Subjects, *Quintessence Internat., 32*, 147, February, 2001.

Chewing Sticks

Al-Mohaya, M.A., Darwazeh, A., and Al-Khudair, W.: Oral Fungal Colonization and Oral Candidiasis in Renal Transplant Patients: The Relationship to Miswak Use, *Oral Surg. Oral Med. Oral Pathol. Oral Radiol. Oral Endod., 93*, 455, April, 2002.

Darout, I.A., Albandar, J.M., and Skaug, N.: Periodontal Status of Adult Sudanese Habitual Users of Miswak Chewing Sticks or Toothbrushes, *Acta Odont. Scand., 58*, 25, February, 2000.

Darout, I.A., Albandar, J.M., Skaug, N, and Ali, R.W.: Salivary Microbiota Levels in Relation to Periodontal Status, Experience of Caries and Miswak Use in Sudanese Adults, *J. Clin. Periodontol, 29*, 411, May, 2002.

Eid, M.A. and Selim, H.A.: A Retrospective Study on the Relationship Between Miswak Chewing Stick and Periodontal Health, *Egyptian Dent. J., 40*, 589, January, 1994.

Toothbrush Contamination

Caudry, S.D., Klitorinos, A., and Chan, E.C.S.: Contaminated Toothbrushes and Their Disinfection, *J. Can. Dent. Assoc., 61*, 511, June, 1995.

Filho, P.N., Macari, S., Faria, G., Assed, S., and Ito, I.Y.: Microbial Contamination of Toothbrushes and Their Decontamination, *Pediatr. Dent., 22*, 381, September/October, 2000.

Meier, S., Collier, C., Scaletta, M.G., Stephens, J., Kimbrough, R., and Kettering, J.D.: An *in vitro* Investigation of the Efficacy of CPC for Use in Toothbrush Decontamination, *J. Dent. Hyg., 70*, 161, July–August, 1996.

Quirynen, M., de Soete, M., Pauwels, M., Goossens, K., Teughels, W., van Eldere, J., and van Steenberghe, D.: Bacterial Survival Rate on Tooth- and Interdental Brushes in Relation to the Use of Toothpaste, *J. Clin. Periodontol, 28*, 1106, December, 2001.

Warren, D.P., Goldschmidt, M.C., Thompson, M.B., Adler-Storthz, K., and Keene, H.J.: The Effects of Toothpastes on the Residual Microbial Contamination of Toothbrushes, *J. Am. Dent. Assoc., 132*, 1241, September, 2001.

Interdental Care

Carol A. Jahn, RDH, MS, and
Esther M. Wilkins, BS, RDH, DMD

CHAPTER OUTLINE

Traditionally, toothbrushing has been considered to be first in line as the method for cleaning the teeth and removing dental biofilm for the prevention of gingival and periodontal infections. Toothbrushing cannot accomplish biofilm removal for the proximal tooth surfaces and adjacent gingiva to the same degree that it does for the facial, lingual, and palatal aspects. Interdental biofilm control, therefore, is essential to complete the patient's self-care program.

Objectives and procedures for removal of dental biofilm from proximal tooth surfaces are included in this chapter. Key words are defined in Box 26-1. When the preventive treatment plan is outlined for an individual, assessment is made of the oral condition, the problem areas, and the

overall prognosis for improvement or maintenance of gingival health. Measures for interdental biofilm control are selected to complement biofilm control by toothbrushing.

THE INTERDENTAL AREA

In health, the interdental gingiva fills the interproximal area and under the contact of the adjacent teeth in a Type I embrasure. The three types of gingival embrasures are illustrated in Figure 26-1. When the interdental papilla is missing or reduced in height, which is common as a result of periodontal infection, the shape of the interdental gingiva

BOX 26-1 KEY WORDS: Interdental Care

Col: the depression in the gingival tissue under a contact area between the lingual (palatal) papilla and the facial papilla.

Embrasure: V-shaped spillway space next to the contact area of adjacent teeth, narrowest at the contact and widening toward the facial, lingual (palatal), and occlusal contacts.

Floss cleft: a cleft in the gingival margin usually at a mesial or distal line angle of a tooth where dental floss was repeatedly applied incorrectly. The lining of the cleft can be completely lined with epithelium.

Floss cut: unintentional incision at the gingival margin due to incorrect positioning and placement of dental floss.

Interproximal space: the triangular region bounded by the proximal surfaces of contacting teeth and the alveolar bone between the teeth, which forms the base of the triangle; the space is normally filled with the interdental papilla; also called the interdental area.

Keratinized epithelium: outer, protective surface of stratified squamous epithelium; covers the masticatory mucosa; interdental col area is not normally keratinized.

Proxabrush: another name for an interdental brush (Figure 26-9).

---

changes, and open Type II or Type III embrasures may be seen. Figure 26-2 shows a Type II embrasure from the proximal surface with the col and from the facial surface.

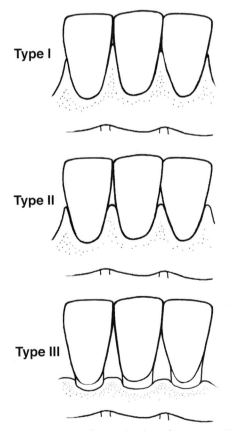

■ **FIGURE 26-1 Types of Gingival Embrasures.** Type I, interdental papilla fills the gingival embrasure. Type II, with slight to moderate recession of the interdental papilla. Type III, with extensive recession or complete loss of the interdental papilla.

I. ANATOMY OF THE INTERDENTAL AREA

A review of the gingival and dental anatomy of the interdental area can give meaning to and clarify the role and purpose of the various devices available for interdental care.

A. Posterior Teeth

- Between adjacent posterior teeth are two papillae, one facial and one lingual or palatal.
- The papillae are connected by a col, a depressed concave area that follows the shape of the apical border of the contact area (Figure 12-8, page 212).

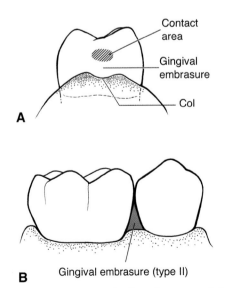

■ **FIGURE 26-2 Type II Gingival Embrasure. (A)** Embrasure shown from the proximal surface with the col. **(B)** Facial view, with gingival embrasure shown in blue.

B. Anterior Teeth

- Between anterior teeth in contact is a single papilla with a pyramidal shape.
- Tip of the papilla may form a small col under the contact area (Figure 12-8B).

C. Epithelium

- The epithelium covering a col is usually thin and not keratinized.
- Col epithelium is protected and is less resistant to infection than keratinized surfaces.
- Inflammation in the papilla leads to enlargement, with increased inflammatory cells and edema; the col becomes deeper.
- The col area is inaccessible for ordinary toothbrushing; microorganisms are harbored in the concave center.
- Most gingival disease starts in the col area.
- The incidence of gingivitis is greatest in the interdental tissues.[1]

II. PROXIMAL TOOTH SURFACES

- With bacterial infection and loss of gingival attachment, the interdental papillae are reduced in height.
- Proximal tooth surfaces become exposed.
- Dental biofilm can accumulate.
- Irregularities of tooth position, such as rotation or overlapping, and deviations related to malocclusion or tooth loss may be present.
- Easy access for removal of bacterial deposits by the individual is prevented.
- Root surface morphology of the proximal surfaces is typical for each tooth type.
- Concavities and grooves are predisposed to bacterial accumulations.[2,3]
- With advanced periodontitis, furcation areas of maxillary first premolars and molars open onto the proximal surfaces.

▪ PLANNING INTERDENTAL CARE

I. PATIENT ASSESSMENT

A. History of Personal Oral Care

- Type of toothbrush, dental floss, and other interdental devices currently used.
- Frequency and personal time spent.
- Estimate of the patient's apparent priorities on personal oral care.

B. Dental and Gingival Anatomy

- Position of teeth.
- Types and shapes of embrasures: variation throughout the dentition.
- Probing depths: classification of the periodontal condition.
- Prostheses present: special interdental care required for fixed and removable prostheses.
- Areas where toothbrush cannot reach.

C. Extent and Location of Dental Biofilm

- "Plaque score" to show patient the extent of biofilm needing removal on a daily basis.
- Use of a disclosing agent to show specific sites where biofilm accumulates.
- Evidence of the patient's ability to care for difficult access areas.

D. Personal Factors

- Handicap or disability that limits ability to carry out needed personal oral hygiene.
- Knowledge about and appreciation for interdental oral care.

II. DENTAL HYGIENE CARE PLAN

A. Objectives

- Select appropriate interdental aids to help the patient reach optimum oral cleanliness and health.
- Teach the patient correct system of oral care.
- Motivate the patient to accept responsibility for daily personal care.

B. Initial Care Plan

- At first, the simplest procedures are selected for the patient's convenience and ease of learning based on the patient's current knowledge and oral care habits.
- Minimum frequency: thoroughly once daily.
- Keep the daily oral care regimen at a realistic level with respect to the time the patient is able or willing to spend.
- As the values the patient places on oral health increase over time, and as the preventive maintenance program becomes a priority in the patient's lifelong self-care health goals, a more refined program can be introduced.

■ SELECTIVE INTERDENTAL BIOFILM REMOVAL

I. RELATION TO TOOTHBRUSHING

- Vibratory and sulcular toothbrushing, such as that performed with the Charters, Stillman, and Bass methods, can be successful to some degree in removing dental biofilm near the line angles of the facial and lingual or palatal embrasures.
- Brush in vertical position is effective for additional access around line angles onto the proximal surfaces (Figure 25-12, page 418).

II. SELECTION OF INTERDENTAL AIDS

- Dependent on oral health, disease status, and the risk for future recurrence.
- A patient working to control or arrest disease may need more frequent self-care than a patient practicing prevention.
- More than a toothbrush is needed for complete biofilm removal from exposed proximal tooth surfaces. With judicious selection and use of the various methods for interdental care, disease control can be accomplished by the motivated patient.
- Dental floss, interdental brushes, and other aids are described in this chapter.

■ DENTAL FLOSS AND TAPE

The effective use of dental floss contributes to gingival health by removing dental biofilm[4-7] and reducing interproximal bleeding.[8] Dental floss is most effective when interdental papillae are present and there has not been loss of attachment with root surface exposure.[9] As recession occurs, dental floss may still be used, but greater time, effort, and dexterity are required for complete removal of dental biofilm from the exposed proximal tooth surfaces.

I. TYPES OF FLOSS

Research has shown no difference in the effectiveness of waxed or unwaxed floss for biofilm removal.[4,6,10-12] Biofilm removal depends on how floss is applied. For optimal patient compliance, the patient may use a preferred type.[4,13]

A. Materials

1. *Silk.* Historically, floss was made of silk fibers loosely twisted together to form a strand and waxed for interproximal cleaning.

2. *Nylon.* Nylon multifilaments, waxed or unwaxed, have been widely used in circular (floss) or flat (tape) form for biofilm removal from proximal tooth surfaces.

3. *Expanded PTFE.* Plastic monofilament polytetrafluoroethylene with wax is used for proximal tooth surface biofilm removal.

B. Features of Waxed or Expanded PTFE

- Smooth surface provided by the wax covering helps to prevent trauma to soft tissue.
- Slides through contact area with ease.
- Monofilament type resists breakage or shredding when passed over irregular tooth surface, restoration, or calculus deposit.
- Wax gives strength and durability during application; shredding or breakage is rare.

C. Features of Unwaxed

- Thinner floss may be helpful when contact areas are tight; however, forcing the floss through may break the floss.
- Pressure against a tooth surface spreads the nylon fibers and gives a wider surface for biofilm removal.
- Sharper thin edge requires special attention to prevent injury to the gingival tissue when guiding floss through a tight contact area or when moving floss on the tooth surface in an apical direction.
- Squeaking sound effect when floss moves over a clean tooth surface may provide a motivation for patient thoroughness.
- Unwaxed floss, which frays when rubbed over an irregular tooth surface, rough surface of a restoration, or calculus deposit, might cause the patient to become aggravated and discouraged, thereby resulting in lost motivation to floss regularly.
- Floss that is tightly wound around fingers tends to cut, hurt, and cause discomfort. This problem is not usually as evident with wide dental tape or with waxed floss or tape.

D. Enhancements

Color and flavor have been added to dental floss. Therapeutic agents that have been added include fluoride and whitening agents. Limited research has been published relative to their effectiveness.

II. PROCEDURE

When dental floss is applied with firm pressure to a flat or convex proximal tooth surface, biofilm can be

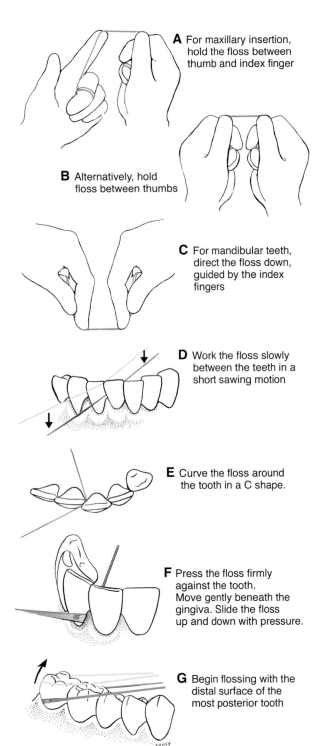

A For maxillary insertion, hold the floss between thumb and index finger

B Alternatively, hold floss between thumbs

C For mandibular teeth, direct the floss down, guided by the index fingers

D Work the floss slowly between the teeth in a short sawing motion

E Curve the floss around the tooth in a C shape.

F Press the floss firmly against the tooth. Move gently beneath the gingiva. Slide the floss up and down with pressure.

G Begin flossing with the distal surface of the most posterior tooth

■ **FIGURE 26-3 Use of Dental Floss.** For maxillary insertion, hold the floss between the thumb and index finger **(A)** or between thumbs **(B).** Grasp the floss firmly. Allow only 1/2-inch length between fingers. **(C)** For the mandibular teeth, direct the floss down, guided by the index fingers. **(D)** Work the floss slowly between the teeth in a short sawing motion. Avoid snapping through the contact area. **(E)** Curve the floss around the tooth in a C-shape. Hold the floss toward the mesial for cleaning the distal surfaces and toward the distal for cleaning the mesial surfaces. **(F)** Press the floss firmly against the tooth. Move gently beneath the gingiva until tissue resistance is felt. Slide the floss horizontally and vertically with pressure to remove biofilm. **(G)** Begin flossing with the distal surface of the most posterior tooth, and work systematically around the arch.

removed. Older biofilm is tenacious and may require several strokes for removal. When floss is placed over a concave surface, contact is not possible (Figure 26-10*A*), and supplementary devices are needed to remove a bacterial deposit completely.

A. When to Floss

For most patients, dental floss should be used before toothbrushing. The following reasons may apply:
1. When proximal tooth surfaces are flossed first and biofilm is removed, the fluoride from a dentifrice used while brushing reaches the proximal surfaces for prevention of dental caries.
2. When brushing is accomplished first, flossing may not be carried out.
    a. The mouth feels clean; the need for flossing may not be appreciated.
    b. Time may be short and flossing can be postponed.

B. Floss Preparation

1. Figure 26-3 outlines the flossing steps that are described in detail here in this section.
2. Hold a 12- to 15-inch length of floss with the thumb and index finger of each hand; grasp firmly with only 1/2 inch of floss between the finger tips. The ends of the floss may be tucked into the palm and held by the ring and little finger, or the floss may be wrapped around the middle fingers (Figure 26-3*A*, *B*, and *C*).
3. A circle of floss may be made by tying the ends together; the circle may be rotated as the floss is used (Figure 26-4).[14]

C. Application

1. *Maxillary Teeth.* Direct the floss up by holding the floss over two thumbs or a thumb and an index finger as shown in Figure 26-3*A* and *B*. Rest a side of a finger on teeth of the opposite side of the maxillary arch to provide balance and a fulcrum.
2. *Mandibular Teeth.* Direct the floss down by holding the two index fingers on top of the strand.

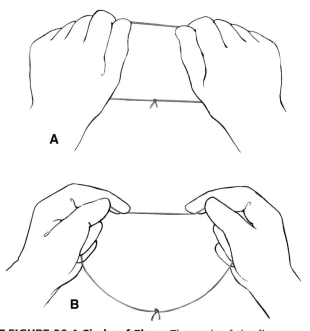

■ **FIGURE 26-4 Circle of Floss.** The ends of the floss are tied together for convenient holding. A child may be able to manage floss better with this technique. **(A)** Floss held for maxillary teeth. **(B)** Floss held for mandibular teeth.

One index finger holds the floss on the lingual aspect and the other on the facial aspect (Figure 26-3C). The side of the finger on the lingual side is held on the teeth of the opposite side of the mouth to serve as a fulcrum or rest.

D. Insertion

1. Hold floss firmly in a diagonal or oblique position (Figure 26-5).

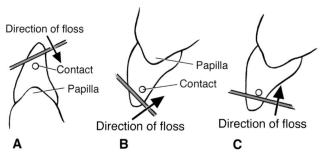

■ **FIGURE 26-5 Insertion of Floss.** Hold floss in a diagonal or oblique position over the teeth where the floss will be inserted. Arrows indicate the direction of movement of the floss. **(A)** Floss held for mandibular insertion. **(B)** Floss held for maxillary insertion. **(C)** Floss held incorrectly. When floss is held horizontally, the possibility for damage to the papilla is greater.

2. Guide the floss past each contact area with a gentle sawing motion (Figure 26-3D).
3. Control floss to prevent snapping through the contact area onto the gingival tissue.

E. Cleaning Stroke

1. Clean adjacent teeth separately; for the distal aspect, curve the floss mesially, and for the mesial aspect, curve the floss distally, around the tooth (Figure 26-3E and F).
2. Pass the floss below the gingival margin, curve to adapt the floss around the tooth, press, and slide up and down over the tooth surface. Repeat.
3. Loop the floss over the distal surfaces of the most posterior teeth in each quadrant and the teeth next to edentulous areas (Figure 26-3G). Hold firmly against the tooth and move the floss in both an up-and-down motion and a "shoe-shine" stroke.

F. Additional Suggestions

1. Slide the floss to a new, unused portion for succeeding proximal tooth surfaces.
2. Floss may be doubled to provide a wider rubbing surface.
3. When a dentifrice is used with the floss, dental tape may be better than floss in retaining the dentifrice against the tooth.

III. PRECAUTIONS

A. Pressure in Col Area

- The col area is not keratinized and is vulnerable to bacterial invasion.
- Biofilm control of the area is of great importance because most gingival and periodontal infection begins in the col area.
- Too great a pressure with floss one or more times daily, particularly very fine floss that tends to cut more easily than thicker floss, can be destructive to the attachment. Excess pressure of the floss against the attachment is particularly significant in children in whom teeth are in the process of eruption and the junctional epithelium is less firmly attached.

B. Prevention of Floss Cuts and Floss Clefts

1. *Location.* Floss cuts or clefts occur primarily on facial and lingual or palatal surfaces directly beside or in the middle of an interdental papilla. They appear as straight-line cuts from the gingival margin and may result in a floss cleft (page 217).

2. *Causes*
    a. Using too long a piece of floss between the fingers when held for insertion.
    b. Snapping the floss through the contact area.
    c. Not curving the floss about the teeth; holding floss straight across the papilla.
    d. Not using a rest to prevent undue pressure.

C. Aid for Flossing

A floss holder can be helpful for a person with a disability or for a parent or caregiver serving a child or patient. Floss holders are described on pages 900 and 901.

■ TUFTED DENTAL FLOSS

I. DESCRIPTION

Tufted dental floss is also called a floss/yarn combination. Regular dental floss is alternated with a thickened tufted portion. Two variations are available commercially.

A. Single, Precut Lengths

"Super Floss"[15] is available in a 2-foot length composed of a 5-inch tufted portion adjacent to a 3-inch stiffened end for inserting under a fixed appliance or orthodontic attachment (Figure 26-6A).

B. Roll

"NUFloss"[16] is available in a roll that is similar to that of regular floss and has a cutting device to allow selection of a preferred length. The tufted portions (about 1 inch long) alternate with the plain floss (about 1 1/2 inches long) (Figure 26-6B).

II. INDICATIONS FOR USE

A. Biofilm removal from tooth surfaces adjacent to wide embrasures where interdental papillae have been lost.
B. Biofilm removal from mesial and distal abutments and under pontic of a fixed partial denture or orthodontic appliance. The stiff end of "Super Floss" is inserted; "NUFloss" is threaded using a floss threader (see Figures 29-2 and 29-3, pages 472 and 473).

III. PROCEDURE

A. Individual Surface of Tooth or Implant

Curve floss and/or tufted portion around the tooth or implant in a "C" to remove dental biofilm. Move floss vertically and horizontally (Figure 26-6C).

B. Fixed Partial Denture

Thread tufted floss over pontic and apply to distal surface of the mesial abutment and mesial surface of the distal abutment (Figure 29-3).

■ KNITTING YARN

I. INDICATIONS FOR USE

A. For tooth surfaces adjacent to wide proximal spaces, dental floss is too narrow and does not remove biofilm efficiently.

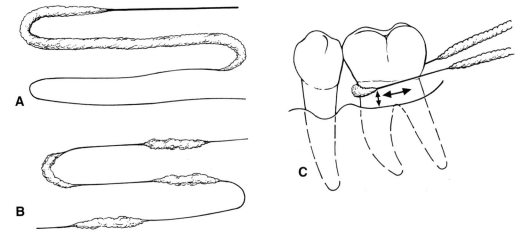

■ FIGURE 26-6 Tufted Dental Floss. The floss/yarn combination may be "Super Floss" **(A)** in a precut length with a tufted portion and a 3-inch stiffened end for insertion under a fixed prosthesis, or "NUFloss" **(B)** with tufted portions alternated with plain floss. A preferred length of "NUFloss" is obtained from the container. **(C)** "NUFloss" applied to the proximal surface of a molar. It may be used in an up-and-down and a shoe-shine stroke.

B. For mesial and distal abutments of fixed partial dentures and under pontics, use a floss threader.

C. For isolated teeth, teeth separated by a diastema, and distal surfaces of most posterior teeth.

II. PROCEDURE

A. Fold yarn double. Use about 8 inches of 3- or 4-ply smooth synthetic yarn. Loop through about 8 inches of dental floss; tie floss with one over-hand knot.

B. Insert floss through the contact area. Draw the yarn into the embrasure (Figure 26-7).

C. Clean adjacent teeth separately with a facial-lingual, back-and-forth stroke. Hold the ends of the yarn distally and then around mesially.

D. For specific areas where a papilla may be high or access is not otherwise sufficient for the wide

yarn, use the dental floss end of the combination.

E. Apply dentifrice.

F. For closed contacts, use a floss threader (see Figure 29-2, page 472).

■ GAUZE STRIP

I. INDICATIONS FOR USE

A. For proximal surfaces of widely spaced teeth. Gauze is too thick to pass through contact areas.

B. For surfaces of teeth next to edentulous areas.

C. For distal and mesial surfaces of abutment teeth.

D. For areas under posterior cantilevered section of a fixed appliance, such as the distal portion of a denture supported by implants.

II. PROCEDURE

A. Cut 1-inch gauze bandage into a 6- to 8-inch length, and fold in thirds or down the center.

B. Position the fold of the gauze on the cervical area next to the gingival crest and work back and forth several times; hold ends in a distal direction to clean a mesial surface, and in a mesial direction to clean a distal surface (Figure 26-8).

■ INTERDENTAL BRUSHES

I. TYPES

A. Small Insert Brushes With Reusable Handle

1. Soft nylon filaments are twisted into a fine stainless steel wire for insertion into a handle with an

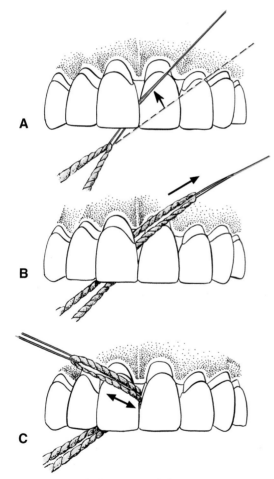

■ **FIGURE 26-7 Knitting Yarn. (A)** Yarn is looped through dental floss, and the floss is drawn through the contact area in the usual manner, shown by the arrow. **(B)** Yarn is drawn through the embrasure. **(C)** Yarn is positioned against the surface of the tooth for biofilm removal. When tooth contact is missing and space permits, the yarn is used without floss.

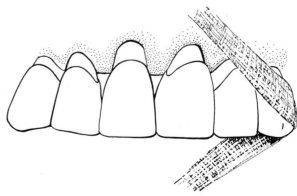

■ **FIGURE 26-8 Gauze Strip.** A 6- or 8-inch length of 1-inch bandage is folded in thirds and placed around a tooth adjacent to an edentulous area, a tooth with interdental spacing, or the distal surface of the most posterior tooth. A shoe-shine stroke is used to clean the dental biofilm from the surface.

angulated shank (Figure 26-9D). Select brush with plastic-coated wire.

2. The small tapered or cylindric brush heads are of varying sizes approximately 12 to 15 mm (1/2 inch) in length, with a diameter of 3 to 5 mm (1/8 to 1/4 inch).

B. Brush With Wire Handle

1. Soft nylon filaments are twisted into a fine stainless steel wire. The wire is continuous with the handle, which is approximately 35 to 45 mm (1 1/2 to 1 3/4 inches) in length (Figure 26-9C).

2. The filaments form a narrow brush approximately 30 to 35 mm (1 1/4 to 1 1/2 inches) in length and 5 to 8 mm (1/4 to 5/16 inches) in diameter.

II. INDICATIONS FOR USE

When sufficient space is available for the insertion of an interdental brush without excess force, the following applications are indicated:

A. For Removal of Dental Biofilm and Debris

1. Proximal tooth surfaces adjacent to open embrasures, orthodontic appliances, fixed prostheses, dental implants, periodontal splints, and space maintainers, and other areas that are hard to reach with a regular toothbrush.

2. Concave proximal surfaces where dental floss and other interdental aids cannot reach (Figure 26-10A). Floss bridges over a concave surface, whereas the interproximal brush can reach and cleanse (Figure 26-10B).[1,17]

3. Exposed Class IV furcations (Figure 14-3, page 253).

B. For Application of Chemotherapeutic Agents

1. Fluoride dentifrice, gel, and/or mouthrinse for prevention of dental caries, particularly root surface caries, and for surfaces adjacent to any prosthesis.

2. Antibacterial agents for control of dental biofilm and the prevention of gingivitis.

3. Desensitizing agents.

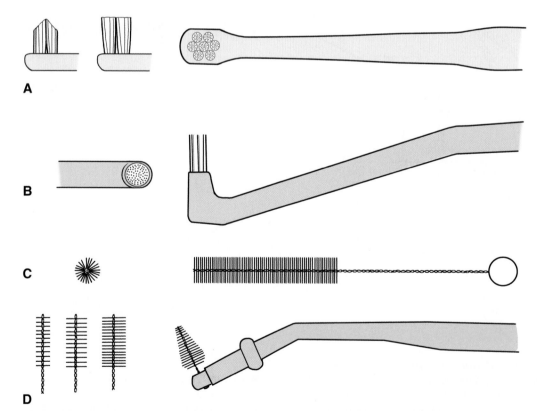

■ **FIGURE 26-9 Single-tuft and Interdental Brushes. (A)** Single-tuft brush with tapered and flat groups of filaments. **(B)** Single-tuft brush on handle with angulated shank. **(C)** Interdental brush with filaments twisted into a fine wire that ends in a handle. **(D)** Insert brushes for a reusable handle with an angulated shank.

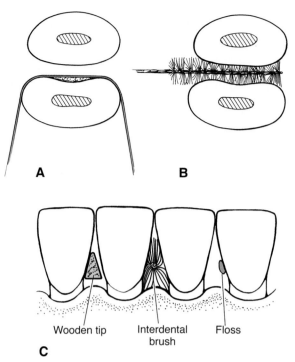

C

■ **FIGURE 26-10 Interdental Care. (A)** Floss positioned on the mesial surface of a maxillary first premolar shows the inability of the floss to remove dental biofilm on a concave proximal tooth surface. **(B)** Use of an interdental brush in the same interproximal area to show how the proximal surfaces can be cleaned free of dental biofilm. **(C)** Comparison of the access of a wooden tip, an interdental brush, and a piece of dental floss to an open interdental area.

Labels: Wooden tip · Interdental brush · Floss

III. PROCEDURE

A. Select brush of appropriate diameter.
B. Moisten the brush and insert at an angle in keeping with gingival form; brush in and out.

IV. CARE OF BRUSHES

A. Clean brush during use to remove debris and biofilm by holding under actively running water.
B. Clean thoroughly after use and dry in open air.
C. Discard when filaments become loose or deformed.

■ SINGLE-TUFT BRUSH (END-TUFT, UNITUFT)

I. DESCRIPTION

The single tuft, or group of small tufts, may be 3 to 6 mm in diameter and may be flat or tapered (Figure 26-9A and B). The handle may be straight or contra-angled.

II. INDICATIONS FOR USE

A. For Open Interproximal Areas

B. For Fixed Dental Prostheses

The single-tuft brush may be adaptable around and under a fixed partial denture, pontic, orthodontic appliance, precision attachment, or implant abutment.

C. For Difficult-to-Reach Areas

The lingual surfaces of the mandibular molars, abutment teeth, the distal surfaces of the most posterior teeth, and teeth that are crowded are examples of areas where an end-tuft brush may be of value. The shank may be bent for easy adaptation (Figure 26-11).

III. PROCEDURE

A. Direct the end of the tuft into the interproximal area and along the gingival margin.
B. Combine a rotating motion with intermittent pressure.
C. Use a sulcular brushing stroke.

■ INTERDENTAL TIP

I. COMPOSITION AND DESIGN

Conical or pyramidal flexible rubber or plastic tip is attached to the end of the handle of a toothbrush or is on a special plastic handle. The soft, pliable rubber tip is preferred because it can be adapted to the interdental area and below the gingival margin more easily than can the hard, more rigid plastic tip.

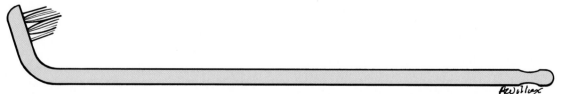

■ **FIGURE 26-11 Single-tuft Brush With Bent Shank.** Adaptation of brush with angulated handle permits easier access to lingual and palatal aspects of the natural teeth, as well as to orthodontic appliances, prostheses, and implant abutments.

II. INDICATIONS FOR USE

   A. For cleaning debris from the interdental area and for removal of biofilm by rubbing the exposed tooth surfaces.

   B. For biofilm removal at and just below the gingival margin.

III. PROCEDURE

   A. Trace along the gingival margin with the tip positioned just beneath the margin. The adaptation is similar to the toothpick in holder (see Figure 26-12).

   B. For additional cleaning of the proximal surfaces of the teeth, rub the tip against the teeth as it is moved in and out of an embrasure and under a contact area. Position tip with the gingival form; take care not to flatten the interdental tissue.

   C. Rinse the tip as indicated during use to remove debris, and wash thoroughly at the finish.

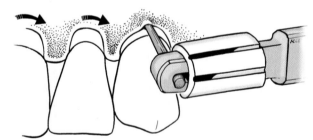

▪ **FIGURE 26-12 Toothpick in Holder for Dental Biofilm at Gingival Margin.** The tip is placed at or just below the gingival margin. Trace the margin around each tooth.

▪ TOOTHPICK IN HOLDER

I. DESCRIPTION

A round toothpick is inserted into a plastic handle with contra-angled ends for adaptation to the tooth surface at the gingival margin for biofilm removal. The device also is called a "Perio-Aid."

II. INDICATIONS FOR USE

A. Patient With Periodontitis

For biofilm removal at and just under the gingival margin, for interdental cleaning, particularly for concave proximal tooth surfaces, and for exposed furcation area.

B. Orthodontic Patient

For biofilm removal at gingival margin above appliances.

III. PROCEDURE

A. Prepare Instrument

1. Insert round tapered toothpick into the end of the holder. One type of holder has angulated ends for use in various positions.

2. Twist the toothpick firmly into place. Break off the long end cleanly so that sharp edges cannot scratch the inner cheek or the tongue during use.

B. Application

1. Apply toothpick at the gingival margin. At a right-angle application, with moderate pressure, trace the gingival margin around each tooth.

Everyday Ethics

A new patient, Jane, is excited about information she has just read on the internet about a powered flossing device. She begins to ask Glenna, the dental hygienist, detailed questions about the product such as whether it really works, where it can be purchased, and how much it costs. Glenna is unfamiliar with the flossing aid but doesn't want to be embarrassed in front of the patient so she tells Jane the product doesn't work and spends an extra 5 minutes at the end of the appointment going over manual flossing techniques.

Questions for Consideration

1. In ethical terms, how would Glenna's action be described?

2. From the patient's perspective, what is the role of the dental hygienist in this situation?

3. Is it unethical to mislead the patient about a product when the value is unknown or the dental hygienist prefers the benefits of another (perhaps rival) product? Why or why not?

2. To remove biofilm just below the gingival margin, apply the end at less than 45°, maintain the tip on the tooth surface, and follow around the sulcus or pocket (Figure 26-12).

3. Use a tip that has become frayed from use as a small cleaning "brush" to rub on tooth surfaces where biofilm has collected. Check for and remove loose bits of wood that could become deposited in the sulcus or gingiva.

4. For hypersensitive spots, usually at the cervical third of a tooth, the patient can use the tip daily to massage dentifrice for desensitization.

5. When a contact is inadequate and the patient indicates that floss or toothpicks are required to relieve pressure from impacted food, dental attention may be needed. The area should be charted or otherwise brought to the attention of the dentist.

■ WOODEN INTERDENTAL CLEANER

I. DESCRIPTION

The wooden cleaner is a 2-inch-long device made of bass wood or birchwood. It is triangular in cross section, as shown in Figure 26-13.

II. INDICATIONS FOR USE

A. Application

For cleaning proximal tooth surfaces where the tooth surfaces are exposed and interdental gingiva are missing. Space must be adequate otherwise the gingival tissue can be traumatized.

B. Limitation

- As with most interdental devices, the wooden cleaner is advised only for the patient who follows instructions carefully.
- A fresh cleaner may be advised for each arch or quadrant because the wood may become splayed.

III. PROCEDURE

A. Fulcrum (Rest)

First teach the patient to use a rest by placing the hand on the cheek or chin or by placing a finger on the gingiva convenient to the place where the tip will be applied. This precaution helps prevent insertion of the wedge with too much pressure.

B. Preparation

Soften the wood by placing the pointed end in the mouth and moistening with saliva.

C. Directions

1. Hold the base of the triangular wedge toward the gingival border of the interdental area and insert with the tip pointed slightly toward the occlusal or incisal surfaces to follow the contour of the embrasure (Figure 26-13*B* and *C*). When the wedge is held horizontally, the interdental tissue can be flattened.

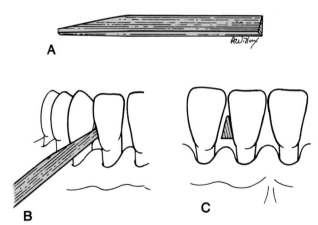

■ **FIGURE 26-13 Wooden Interdental Cleaner. (A)** The 2-inch wooden triangular cleaner. **(B)** Application on the proximal surface of a tooth with a Type III embrasure. The base of the triangle is on the gingival side. **(C)** The side of the triangle is rubbed in and out against the proximal surface to remove dental biofilm.

✔ Factors To Teach The Patient

- By demonstration with disclosing agent, how the toothbrush doesn't clean the interdental area thoroughly.

- About dental biofilm and how it collects on the proximal tooth surfaces when left undisturbed.

- How vulnerable the interdental area is to gingival infection.

- How to use each recommended interdental aid to clean the proximal tooth surfaces.

- To ask the dental hygienist and the dentist about new products they see advertised and whether the product should be tried.

2. Clean the tooth surfaces by moving the wedge in and out while applying a burnishing stroke with moderate pressure first to one side of the embrasure and then to the other, about four strokes each.

3. Discard the cleaner as soon as the first signs of splaying are evident.

REFERENCES

1. **Smukler**, H., Nager, M.C., and Tolmie, P.C.: Interproximal Tooth Morphology and Its Effect on Plaque Removal, *Quinessence Int.*, 20, 249, April, 1989.
2. **Gher**, M.E. and Vernino, A.R.: Root Morphology—Clinical Significance in Pathogenesis and Treatment of Periodontal Disease, *J. Am. Dent. Assoc.*, 101, 627, October, 1980.
3. **Fox**, S.C. and Bosworth, B.L.: A Morphological Survey of Proximal Root Concavities: A Consideration in Periodontal Therapy, *J. Am. Dent. Assoc.*, 114, 811, June, 1987.
4. **Ciancio**, S.G., Shibly, O., and Farber, G.A.: Clinical Evaluation of the Effect of Two Types of Dental Floss on Plaque and Gingival Health, *Clin. Prev. Dent.*, 14, 14, May/June, 1992.
5. **Abelson**, D.C., Barton, J.E., Maietti, G.M., and Cowherd, M.G.: Evaluation of Interproximal Cleaning by Two Types of Dental Floss, *Clin. Prev. Dent.*, 3, 19, July–August, 1981.
6. **Lobene**, R.R., Soparkar, P.M., and Newman, M.B.: Use of Dental Floss: Effect on Plaque and Gingivitis, *Clin. Prev. Dent.*, 4, 5, January–February, 1982.
7. **Hanes**, P.J., O'Dell, N.L., Baker, M.R., Keagle, J.G., and Davis, H.C.: The Effect of Tensile Strength on the Clinical Effectiveness and Patient Acceptance of Dental Floss, *J. Clin. Periodontol.*, 19, 30, January, 1992.
8. **Graves**, R.C., Disney, J.A., and Stamm, J.W.: Comparative Effectiveness of Flossing and Brushing in Reducing Interproximal Bleeding, *J. Periodontol.*, 60, 243, May, 1989.
9. **Killoy**, W.J., Chairman, Discussion Section II, Consensus Report: *Proceedings of the World Workshop in Clinical Periodontics.* American Academy of Periodontology, Princeton, NJ, 1989, pp. 11–15.
10. **Hill**, H.C., Levi, P.A., and Glickman, I.: The Effects of Waxed and Unwaxed Dental Floss on Interdental Plaque Accumulation and Interdental Gingival Health, *J. Periodontol.*, 44, 411, July, 1973.
11. **Lamberts**, D.M., Wunderlich, R.C., and Caffesse, R.G.: The Effect of Waxed and Unwaxed Dental Floss on Gingival Health. Part I. Plaque Removal and Gingival Response, *J. Periodontol.*, 53, 393, June, 1982.
12. **Wunderlich**, R.C., Lamberts, D.M., and Caffesse, R.G.: The Effect of Waxed and Unwaxed Dental Floss on Gingival Health. Part II. Crevicular Fluid Flow and Gingival Bleeding, *J. Periodontol.*, 53, 397, June, 1982.
13. **Beaumont**, R.H.: Patient Preference for Waxed or Unwaxed Dental Floss, *J. Periodontol.*, 61, 123, February, 1990.
14. **Masters**, D.H.: Oral Hygiene Procedure for the Periodontal Patient, *Dent. Clin. North Am.*, 13, 3, January, 1969.
15. **SUPER-FLOSS**, Oral-B Laboratories, Inc., 600 Clipper Dr., Belmont, CA 94002-4199.
16. **NU-FLOSS**, 1311 W. Webster Ave., Winter Park, FL 32789.
17. **Kiger**, R.D., Nylund, K., and Feller, R.P.: A Comparison of Proximal Plaque Removal Using Floss and Interdental Brushes, *J. Clin. Periodontol.*, 18, 681, October, 1991.

SUGGESTED READINGS

Bass, C.C.: The Optimum Characteristics of Dental Floss for Personal Oral Hygiene, *Dent. Items Int.*, 70, 921, September, 1948.

Beatty, C.F., Fallon, P.A., and Marshall, D.D.: A Comparison of the Effectiveness of Two Wooden Interdental Cleaners, *Contact Internat*, 12, 6, June, 1998.

Carter-Hanson, C., Gadbury-Amyot, C., and Killoy, W.: Comparison of the Plaque Removal Efficacy of a New Flossing Aid (Quik Floss®) to Finger Flossing, *J. Clin. Periodontol.*, 23, 873, September, 1996.

Caton, J.G., Blieden, T.M., Lowenguth, R.A., Frantz, B.J., Wagener, C.J., Doblin, J.M., Stein, S.H., and Proskin, H.M.: Comparison Between Mechanical Cleaning and an Antimicrobial Rinse for the Treatment and Prevention of Interdental Gingivitis, *J. Clin. Periodontol.*, 20, 172, March, 1993.

Checchi, L., Biagini, G., Zucchini, C., and DeLuca, M.: Clinical and Morphologic Response to Interdental Brushing Therapy, *Quinessence Int.*, 22, 483, June, 1991.

Dörfer, C.E., Wündrich, D., Staehle, J., and Pioch, T.: Gliding Capacity of Different Dental Flosses, *J. Periodontol.*, 72, 672, May, 2001.

Jahn, C.: Evidence-Based Self-care: Are You Informed? *Contemporary Oral Hyg.*, 2, 40, September/October, 2002.

Jahn, C.A.: Making Patient-Centered Self-care Recommendations: Interproximal Cleaning, *J. Pract. Hyg.*, 10, 45, November/December, 2001.

Kleisner, J. and Imfeld, T.: Evaluation of the Efficacy of Interdental Cleaning Devices: How to Design a Clinical Study, *J. Clin. Periodontol.*, 20, 707, November, 1993.

Kocher, T., Sawaf, H., Warncke, M., and Welk, A.: Resolution of Interdental Inflammation With 2 Different Modes of Plaque Control, *J. Clin. Periodontol.*, 27, 883, December, 2000.

Latcham, N.: The Effect of Overhang Removal on Increasing Patients' Flossing Frequency, *Clin. Prev. Dent.*, 12, 22, April–May, 1990.

Rodrigues, C.R., Ando, T., Singer, J.M., and Issáo, M.: The Effect of Training on the Ability of Children to Use Dental Floss, *ASDC J. Dent. Child.*, 63, 39, January–February, 1996.

Schmage, P., Platzer, U., and Nergiz, I.: Comparison Between Manual and Mechanical Methods of Interproximal Hygiene, *Quinessence Int.*, 30, 535, August, 1999.

Shibly, O., Ciancio, S.G., Shostad, S., Mather, M., and Boardman, T.J.: Clinical Evaluation of an Automatic Flossing Device vs. Manual Flossing, *J. Clin. Dent.*, 12, 63, Number 3, 2001.

Tillis, T.S.I. and Keating, J.G.: Interproximal Plaque Removal: The Case of the Missing Evidence, *Contemp. Oral Hyg.*, 1, 31, October, 2001.

Waerhaug, J.: Healing of the Dento-epithelial Junction Following the Use of Dental Floss, *J. Clin. Periodontol.*, 8, 144, April, 1981.

Chemotherapeutics and Topical Delivery Systems

Deborah M. Lyle, RDH, BS, MS

CHEMOTHERAPEUTICS

Recent advances in understanding the pathogenesis of periodontitis have led to alternative therapies that focus on disinfecting the oral cavity using both mechanical devices and chemotherapeutics. Either the clinician or the patient can administer chemotherapeutics. This chapter reviews the chemical agents and delivery methods available for patient self-care. Key words pertaining to chemotherapeutics are defined in Box 27-1.

The three general local self-care methods for delivering a chemical agent are (1) toothbrushing, (2) rinsing, and (3) irrigating. Dentifrices, delivered by a toothbrush, can provide both therapeutic and cosmetic benefits.

Mouthrinses can contain ingredients that are either cosmetic or therapeutic. Rinsing is a simple way to

BOX 27-1 KEY WORDS: Chemotherapeutics and Topical Delivery Systems

Antimicrobial agent: chemical that has a bacteriostatic or bactericidal effect on dental biofilm.

Astringent: a substance that causes contraction or shrinkage and arrests discharges.

Cannula: a tubular instrument placed into a cavity to introduce or drain fluid.

Chemotherapeutic agent: a chemical that is used for therapeutic reasons.

Chemotherapy: treatment of disease by means of chemical substances or pharmaceutical agents.

Humectant: substance contained in a product (such as in a dentifrice) to retain moisture and prevent hardening upon exposure to air.

Hydrokinetic activity: activity relating to motions of fluids or the forces that produce or affect such motions; opposite of hydrostatic.

Hydrostatic: relating to the equilibrium of a liquid and the pressure exerted by the liquid at rest.

Hydrotherapy: the use of forced intermittent or steady stream of water for cleansing or therapeutic purposes.

Irrigant: substance used for irrigation.

Irrigation: flushing of a specific site or area with a stream of fluid; application of a continuous or pulsated stream of fluid to a part of the body for a cleansing or therapeutic purpose.

> **Oral irrigation:** targeted delivery of water or solution to specific locations within the mouth.
>
> **Supragingival irrigation:** the point of delivery of the irrigation is at, or coronal to, the free gingival margin.
>
> **Marginal irrigation:** the point of delivery of the irrigation is angled at, or placed apically to, the gingival margin.
>
> **Subgingival irrigation:** the point of delivery of the irrigation is placed in the sulcus or pocket and may reach the apical border.

Irrigator: a device usually consisting of a reservoir with a flexible delivery tube that uses pressure to flush an area.

Isotonic: having a uniform tonicity or tension; denoting solutions with the same osmotic pressure.

Substantivity: the ability of an agent to be bound to the pellicle and tooth surface and to be released over an extended period of time with the retention of its potency.

Synergism: process whereby the joint action of separate agents is greater than the sum of their effects taken separately.

Synergistic effect: coordinated action; acting jointly; for example, one drug might enhance the effect of another drug.

Therapeutic rinse: a chemical with therapeutic properties that is delivered by rinsing.

deliver an antimicrobial, chemical, or cosmetic agent, but it has limited access subgingivally.

■ DENTIFRICES

A dentifrice is a substance used with a toothbrush or other applicator to remove the dental biofilm, materia alba, debris, and stain from the teeth, tongue, and gingiva for cosmetic, therapeutic, or preventive purposes. The recommendation of a specific dentifrice to a patient is dependent on patient need and desired treatment outcomes.

■ BASIC COMPONENTS[1,2]

Powder dentifrices contain abrasives, detergents, flavoring, and sweetener and are rarely used today. Paste and gel dentifrices contain the same ingredients plus binders, humectants, preservative, and water. Either may have a coloring agent. A therapeutic dentifrice has a chemical agent added for a specific preventive or treatment outcome.

The percentage of the ingredients in commercially available dentifrices is as follows:

Detergent   1% to 2%
Cleaning and polishing agents   20% to 40%
Binder (thickener)   1% to 2%
Humectants   20% to 40%
Flavoring   1% to 1.5%
Water   20% to 40%
Therapeutic agent   1% to 2%
Preservative, sweetener, and
    coloring agent   2% to 3%

A therapeutic dentifrice has a drug or chemical agent added for a specific preventive or therapeutic action. In manufacturing products, a challenge is to combine agents that are compatible with each other.

I. DETERGENTS (FOAMING AGENTS OR SURFACTANTS)

A. Purposes

To lower surface tension, penetrate and loosen surface deposits, emulsify debris for easy removal by the toothbrush, and contribute to the foaming action.

B. Characteristics

Nontoxic, neutral in reaction, active in acid or alkaline media, stable, compatible with other dentifrice ingredients, no distinctive flavor, and foaming characteristics.

C. Substances Used

Sodium lauryl sulfate USP
Sodium N-lauryl sarcosinate

II. CLEANING AND POLISHING AGENTS

A. Purposes

An abrasive is used to clean and a polishing agent is used to produce a smooth tooth surface.

B. Characteristics

The ideal abrasive cleans well with no damage to the tooth surface and provides a smooth surface that can prevent or delay the reaccumulation of stains and deposits.

C. Abrasives Used

Calcium carbonate
Calcium pyrophosphate
Dicalcium phosphate, dihydrate
Dicalcium phosphate, anhydrous
Insoluble sodium metaphosphate (IMP)
Hydrated aluminum oxide
Silica, silicates, and dehydrated silica gels

For gel dentifrices:
Synthetic amorphous silica zerogel
Synthetic amorphous complex aluminosilicate salt

III. BINDERS (THICKENERS)

A. Purpose

To prevent separation of the solid and liquid ingredients during storage.

B. Characteristics

Stable, nontoxic, compatible with other ingredients.

C. Types Used

Mineral colloids
Natural gums
Seaweed colloids
Synthetic celluloses
    Organic colloids require a preservative to prevent microbial growth.

IV. HUMECTANTS

A. Purposes

To retain moisture and prevent hardening on exposure to air; to stabilize the preparation.

B. Characteristics

Stable, nontoxic

C. Substances Used

Glycerol
Sorbitol
Propylene glycol
These agents require a preservative to prevent microbial growth.

V. PRESERVATIVES

A. Purposes

To prevent bacterial growth; to prolong shelf life.

B. Characteristics

Compatible with other ingredients

C. Substances Used

Alcohol
Benzoates
Formaldehyde
Dichlorinated phenols

VI. SWEETENING AGENTS

A. Purpose

To impart a pleasant flavor for patient acceptance.

B. Characteristics

Remain unchanged during manufacturing and storage; compatible with other ingredients.

C. Substances Used

Artificial noncariogenic sweetener
Sorbitol and glycerol, used as humectants, contribute to sweet flavor

VII. FLAVORING AGENTS

A. Purposes

To make the dentifrice desirable; to mask other ingredients that may have a less pleasant flavor.

B. Characteristics

Remain unchanged during manufacturing and storage; compatible with other ingredients

C. Substances Used

Essential oils (peppermint, cinnamon, wintergreen, clove)
Menthol
Artificial noncariogenic sweetener

VIII. COLORING AGENTS

A. Purpose

Attractiveness

B. Characteristics

Do not stain teeth or discolor other oral tissues or dental materials

C. Types

Vegetable dyes

▪ THERAPEUTIC AND COSMETIC BENEFITS

The therapeutic and cosmetic benefits of dentifrices fall into one or more of the following categories: dental caries prevention, reduction of sensitivity, reduction of calculus formation, reduction of gingivitis, or tooth-whitening effect.

I. DENTAL CARIES PREVENTION

The addition of an agent to help prevent dental caries was the focus of many manufacturers in the mid 1900s. Fluoride was recognized as an anticaries agent but the addition of fluoride to a dentifrice was problematic owing to lack of compatibility with abrasive agents.[3] The first caries-preventive dentifrice containing fluoride became available commercially in 1955.[4] Fluoride dentifrices are described in detail on page 560.

II. REDUCTION OF SENSITIVITY

The etiology of dentinal sensitivity may be multifactorial. Pain may be caused by mechanical, thermal, and/or chemical means. Antisensitivity therapy is designed either to occlude the dentinal tubules, coagulate or precipitate tubular fluids, stimulate secondary dentin formation, or block the pulpal neural response.[5] The most commonly used agent in a commercial dentifrice for the reduction of dentin sensitivity is potassium nitrate. Although there is evidence showing efficacy,[6,7] the sole use of a dentifrice may not be sufficient to reduce discomfort or pain. More information on reducing dentin hypersensitivity is on pages 718 to 722.

III. REDUCTION OF SUPRAGINGIVAL CALCULUS FORMATION

The reduction of supragingival calculus formation is a desired outcome of self-care. Some patients may benefit from the use of a dentifrice which contains ingredients that inhibit supragingival calculus formation. Tartar-control dentifrices that have been researched with significant results include those containing:
- Pyrophosphate salts, zinc salts (zinc chloride and zinc citrate).[8]
- Triclosan with a copolymer of polyvinyl methoxyethylene and maleic acid (PVM/MA) for increased substantivity.[9]
- Zinc citrate.[10]

IV. REDUCTION OF GINGIVITIS

The reduction or prevention of gingival inflammation is a primary outcome of brushing. The recommendation of an antigingivitis dentifrice can contribute to the prevention or improved health of gingival tissue. The primary agent available in the United States that has shown efficacy in reducing gingival inflammation when added to a dentifrice is triclosan. Studies using a commercially available dentifrice containing triclosan have shown significant reductions in supragingival biofilm formation and gingivitis.[11,12]

V. TOOTH-WHITENING AGENTS

Natural shades of teeth vary from white to gray and yellow to tan. Tooth color is affected by internal and external factors. Extrinsic staining is often promoted by tannin-rich foods, such as tea, coffee, and red wine; smoking; and certain cationic agents, such as chlorhexidine, tin, and iron. The pigment from foods, oral habits, or chemical agents are imbedded in the acquired pellicle and dental biofilm.[13,14] Dentifrices claiming to whiten teeth do so by either mechanical removal of the stained dental biofilm or the application of a chemical. Each commercially available product needs to be evaluated individually for its efficacy and patient acceptance.

■ ABRASIVITY OF DENTIFRICES

A dentifrice combined with toothbrushing needs to have sufficient abrasivity to clean the tooth surface and not damage the dental tissues.

- The ADA method of measuring toothpaste abrasiveness is called the Radioactive Dentin Abrasivity (RDA) Method.[15] It consists of comparing a special preparation of calcium pyrophosphate (set at 100) to a commercial dentifrice.
- The test measures quantitatively the amount of dentin removed by brushing the roots of extracted teeth that have been irradiated.
- Factors that affect abrasivity are hardness of abrasive; the particle size, shape, and pH of the dentifrice; and the amounts of glycerin and water.[16] Other variables to consider are stiffness of the bristles used, pressure used during brushing, and exposure of cementum and/or dentin.

■ CHEMOTHERAPEUTIC RINSES

Mechanical aids may not be sufficient to maintain optimum oral health for certain patients and may be supplemented with the use of a mouthrinse. Rinses are classified as cosmetic or therapeutic depending on the active ingredient included in the formula. Therapeutic rinses fall into one of five general categories listed in Box 27-2.

Chemotherapeutic rinses that have active ingredients to reduce inflammation or prevent oral disease help control the *supragingival* dental biofilm. A list of general functions of chemotherapeutic agents is provided in Box 27-3. Rinsing can deliver an agent less than 2 mm into the sulcus or pocket and therefore cannot be the delivery of choice for patients with moderate or deep pockets.[17]

BOX 27-2 Categories: Therapeutic Rinses

- Agents that can interfere with the attachment of all or some of the oral bacteria to the pellicle surface or to each other

- Antibiotics capable of inhibiting or killing a specific group of bacteria

- Antiseptics with a broad spectrum of antibacterial activity

- Nonenzymatic, dispersing, denaturing, or modifying agents that can alter the structure or metabolic activity of the biofilm

- Single or a combination of enzymes that can either break up or disperse the biofilm or modify bacterial activity

Adapted from Mandel, I.D.: Chemotherapeutic agents for controlling plaque and gingivitis, *J. Clin. Periodontol., 15*, 488, September, 1988.

■ COMMERCIAL MOUTHRINSE INGREDIENTS[1,2]

I. WATER

Makes up the largest percentage by volume.

II. ALCOHOL

Alcohol is used to increase the solubility of some active ingredients and to enhance flavor.

III. FLAVORING

Essential oils and their derivatives (eucalyptus oil, oil of wintergreen) or aromatic waters (peppermint, spearmint, wintergreen, or others) are used.

BOX 27-3 General Functions of Chemotherapeutic Agents

- Oxygenating: Cleansing

- Astringent: Shrink tissues

- Anodyne: Alleviate pain

- Buffering: Reduce oral acidity

- Deodorizing: Neutralize odor

- Antimicrobial: Bacteriocidal or bacteriostatic

IV. COLORING

Added for aesthetic purposes and must not discolor oral tissues.

V. SWEETENING AGENT

Artificial noncariogenic sweetener.

VI. ACTIVE INGREDIENTS

- Commercial mouthrinses generally contain more than one active ingredient and, therefore, may advertise multiple claims for use.
- Factors that influence how effective an agent may be, including the dilution by the saliva, the length of time the agent may be in contact with the tissue or bacteria, and the body of evidence supporting the particular product.
- General characteristics of an effective chemotherapeutic agent are shown in Box 27-4.

VII. PURPOSES AND USES

A. Prior to dental treatment to reduce intraoral microorganisms and reduce aerosol contamination during use of handpiece or ultrasonic scaler.[18,19]

B. As needed during treatment for patient comfort.

C. To promote shrinkage of soft tissue, facilitating an accurate impression.

D. As part of home self-care for specific needs, such as dental biofilm control, caries prevention, or reduction of infection.

E. As part of malodor control.

F. Posttreatment therapy.

BOX 27-4 General Characteristics of an Effective Chemotherapeutic Agent

- **Nontoxic:** The agent should not damage oral tissues or create systemic problems.

- **No or Limited Absorption:** The action should be confined to the oral cavity.

- **Substantivity:** The ability of an agent to be bound to the pellicle and tooth surface and be released over a period of time with retention of potency.

- **Bacterial Specificity:** May be broad spectrum, but with an affinity for the pathogenic organisms of the oral cavity.

- **Low Induced Drug Resistance:** Low or no development of resistant organisms to agent.

BOX 27-5 How to Rinse

1. Take a small amount of the fluid into the mouth.

2. Close lips; hold teeth slightly apart.

3. Force the fluid through the interdental areas with pressure.

4. Use the lips, cheeks, and tongue action to force the fluid back and forth between the teeth.

5. Balloon the cheeks, then suck them in, alternately several times.

6. Divide the mouth into three parts—front, right, and left.

7. Concentrate the rinsing first on the front, then on the right, and then on the left side.

8. Expectorate.

9. Follow manufacturer's directions on length and frequency of rinsing.

VIII.   PROCEDURE FOR RINSING

Many patients, particularly children, must be shown specifically how to rinse. The method can be practiced under supervision. Uninstructed patients may hold fluid in their mouths and bow the head from side to side, or perform some other action that cannot force the water about and between the teeth. Box 27-5 suggests steps for teaching a patient how to rinse.

IX. THERAPEUTIC AGENTS

A. Phenolic-Related Essential Oils

- *Action.* Phenolics disrupt cell walls and inhibit bacterial enzymes.[20]
- *Availability.* A combination of thymol, eucalyptol, menthol, and methylsalicylate is available as a brand and generic product.
- *Efficacy.* Long-term studies have reported significant reduction in the levels of biofilm and gingivitis.[21,22]
- *Considerations.* Research results are based on following the manufacturer's instructions and not casual use of the rinse.

B. Triclosan

- *Action.* A broad-spectrum antimicrobial effective against gram-negative and gram-positive bacteria. Triclosan acts on the microbial cytoplasmic membrane, causing leakage of the cell contents, or bacteriolysis.[20,23]

- *Availability.* Triclosan-containing mouthrinse is available in Europe and Canada.
- *Efficacy.* Reduction in plaque and bleeding has been recorded.[24]

C. Chlorhexidine

- *Action.* Chlorhexidine (CHX) is a cationic bis-biguanide with broad antibacterial activity. It can bind to oral tissue and alter the integrity of the bacterial cell membrane, thereby damaging the cytoplasm.[25] The ability to bind and remain in the oral cavity over a period of time is referred to as *substantivity.*
- *Availability.* Available by prescription in a 0.12% solution in the United States. Higher concentrations are available in Europe and Canada. Chlorhexidine is bacteriostatic at low concentrations and bactericidal at higher concentrations.[26]
- *Efficacy.* Studies have shown CHX to be safe and effective in preventing and controlling biofilm formation, reducing existing biofilm, and inhibiting and reducing the development of gingivitis.[27,28]
- *Consideration.* Reported adverse effects include staining of teeth and other soft tissues, increase in supragingival calculus formation, altered taste perception, minor irritation, and superficial desquamation of the oral mucosa.[29] Chlorhexidine interacts and is inactivated by sodium lauryl sulfate. The patient must be instructed to rinse well after brushing and to wait 30 minutes before rinsing with chlorhexidine.[30]

D. Quaternary Ammonium Compounds

- *Action.* Quaternary ammonium compounds are a group of cationic agents that bind to oral tissues. The mechanism of action is to rupture the cell wall and alter the cytoplasm. The initial attachment to oral tissue is very strong, but they are released rapidly and therefore have not shown the same efficacy as chlorhexidine.[31]
- *Availability.* The most commonly used agents are cetylpyridinium chloride (CPC), usually utilized at 0.05%, and domiphen bromide.
- *Efficacy.* The efficacy of current agents has not been thoroughly studied.
- *Considerations.* Adverse effects associated with this group of antiseptics are staining of teeth and increased supragingival calculus formation. A burning sensation and occasional desquamation have also been reported.[32,33]

E. Herbal Extracts

- *Action.* Some natural herbs, such as echinacea and goldenseal, are proposed to have antimicrobial and anti-inflammatory properties and are being marketed in over-the-counter mouthrinses and dentifrices.[34]
- *Availability.* Sanguinarine is an alkaloid extract from the bloodroot plant *Sanguinaria canadensis* and is currently available in both a mouthrinse and a dentifrice.
- *Efficacy.* Studies using only the mouthrinse have been inconclusive, but when the rinse and dentifrice were used together, a reduction in bleeding sites and inhibition of gingivitis were significantly better than the control.[35,36]
- *Considerations.* A reported adverse effect from using sanguinarine-containing products is a mild burning sensation.[35]

F. Oxygenating Agents

- *Action.* The efficacy of peroxide is limited with the antimicrobial effect based on the release of oxygen and the impact on anaerobic organisms.
- *Availability.* The use of peroxides is usually combined with other agents in commercial dentifrices and mouthrinses.
- *Efficacy.* Peroxides and perborates have been recommended for short-term use to reduce the symptoms of pericoronitis and necrotizing ulcerative gingivitis.[37]
- *Considerations.* Prolonged use of 3% hydrogen peroxide rinses has resulted in gingival irritation and delayed tissue healing.[38,39]

▪ ORAL IRRIGATION

Irrigation is the targeted application of a pulsated or steady stream of water or other irrigant for preventive or therapeutic purposes.

- The purpose of irrigation is to reduce the bacteria and chemical mediators that lead to the initiation or progression of periodontal diseases.
- For the patient, irrigation is a part of routine self-care for control of the supragingival and subgingival biofilm.

The control of gingival and periodontal infections requires the control of risk factors, including the microbial challenge.

- Oral irrigation helps keep the subgingival bacterial challenge at levels compatible with health.
- Endotoxins (lipopolysaccharides) are instrumental in initiating the inflammatory response, and

the subgingival area is a haven for pathogenic bacteria. Home irrigation with water can reduce subgingival pathogenic bacteria and inflammatory mediators.[40]

Mechanical devices, including toothbrushes and interdental aids, can accomplish dental biofilm removal supragingivally and slightly below the gingival margin for the motivated patient.

- Toothbrushes penetrate less than 1 mm into the gingival sulcus.[41]
- For selected patients in need of enhanced subgingival access, irrigation can supplement other efforts.
- Many patients can benefit from the addition of irrigation regardless of oral hygiene status.

▪ DESCRIPTION OF IRRIGATORS

I. POWER-DRIVEN DEVICE

A. Generates an intermittent or pulsating jet of fluid with an adjustable dial for regulation of pressure and flow.

B. Delivers irrigant through a hand-held interchangeable tip that rotates 360° for application at or below the gingival margin.

C. Maintains steady flow or pulsations of irrigant from a reservoir.

D. Provides reservoir container for convenient measurement of antimicrobial or other agent. Some reservoirs are calibrated for easy instruction and documentation.

II. NON–POWER-DRIVEN DEVICE

A. Attaches to a household water supply: faucet or shower.

B. Delivers water through a hand-held interchangeable tip that can be turned for application at the gingival margin.

C. Cannot definitively control water pressure.

D. Nonpulsating flow of irrigant.

E. Efficacy not tested in clinical studies.

▪ DELIVERY METHODS

When a standard delivery tip is directed perpendicularly to the long axis of the tooth, two zones of hydrokinetic activity are created. The first is the impact zone, where the irrigant makes initial contact, and the second is the flushing zone, where the irrigant is deflected from the tooth surface subgingivally.[42] A pulsating stream has been shown to be superior to a steady stream and should be considered when recommending products.[43]

Patient-applied irrigation is divided into three categories based on tip placement and design: supragingival, marginal, and subgingival. Regardless of tip placement, the reduction of clinical parameters is based on changes in the subgingival dental biofilm and gingival crevicular fluid.

I. STANDARD JET TIP

A. Delivery Tips

1. Monojet (single stream) (Figure 27-1A)
2. Fractionated microjet (Figure 27-1B)
3. Pulsating and nonpulsating

B. Procedure

1. Direct the jet tip toward the interdental area until almost touching the tooth surfaces; hold tip at a right angle (90°) to the long axis of the tooth. This is generally referred to as *supragingival irrigation* (Figure 27-1C).

2. Start on the lowest pressure setting; increase slightly over time depending on the condition of the gingiva and tissue comfort. Lean over the sink, allowing irrigant to flow from the oral cavity.

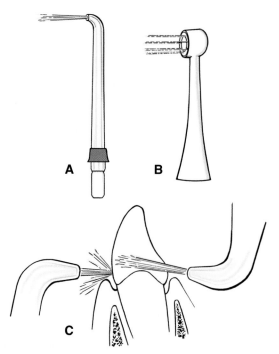

▪ **FIGURE 27-1 Supragingival Irrigation. (A)** Monojet tip (single stream). **(B)** Fractionated microjet tip (multiple streams). **(C)** Monojet delivery tip used in horizontal direction through interproximal area.

3. Follow a definite pattern around the mouth, maxillary arch first, then the mandibular; hold 5 to 6 seconds at each interdental area.

C. Special Instructions

1. Always read and follow manufacturer's instruction regarding use of an irrigator.
2. Irrigation imparts a clean feeling to the mouth; the patient must understand that irrigation is not a substitute for regular toothbrushing and interdental care.

II. SPECIALIZED TIPS

A. Delivery Tips

1. For application at or below the gingival margin for targeted delivery of water or antimicrobial agents.
2. Types
   a. Soft rubber tip designed to be placed 2 mm below the gingival margin (Figure 27-2A).

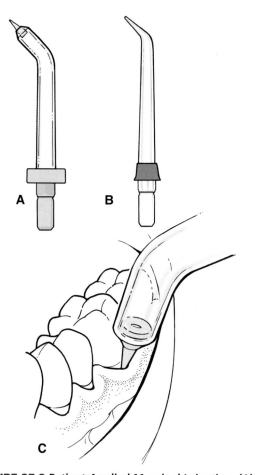

■ **FIGURE 27-2 Patient-Applied Marginal Irrigation. (A)** and **(B)** Special tips for use by the patient. **(C)** Soft rubber tip, designed to be placed 2 mm below gingival margin.

   b. Tapered plastic tip designed to be placed at the gingival margin (Figure 27-2B).
   c. Metal or plastic cannula tip for placement below the gingival margin, possibly to the base of pocket. May be difficult for patients to master.

B. Procedure

1. Identify appropriate areas for use (for example, specific pocket, furca, or implant).
2. Set unit pressure on lowest setting or follow the manufacturer's instructions.
3. Direct the tip at or below the gingival margin according to the manufacturer's directions. The use of a soft rubber tip or a tapered plastic tip is generally referred to as *marginal irrigation* (Figure 27-2C).
4. Activate flow of solution for 5 to 6 seconds into designated area; stop flow and move to next designated area.
5. When using a metal or plastic cannula, care must be given to ensure the patient can place the tip subgingivally and deliver the agent accurately and safely. Proper use of a cannula tip that reaches to the base of the pocket is considered *subgingival irrigation.*

■ BENEFICIAL EFFECTS FROM IRRIGATION

There are two bodies of evidence for oral irrigation: applied by the patient at home and professionally applied using a hand syringe, mechanized handpiece, or ultrasonic scaler. The evidence for home use is extensive and consistently shows positive benefits for multiple patient types.

Benefits that have been shown from the use of an oral irrigator include:

- Reduction of gingivitis and bleeding.[44]
- Reduction or alteration of dental biofilm and inflammatory mediators.[40,45]
- Subgingival access to pathogenic microorganisms.[46,47]
- Delivery of antimicrobial agents.
- Removal of bacteria and debris for oral disinfection and periodontal maintenance.[48]

I. REDUCTION OF GINGIVITIS AND BLEEDING

Supragingival and marginal irrigation are effective for removing loosely attached dental biofilm and reducing gingivitis. When an antimicrobial agent is used in the irrigator, reduction of the supragingival and subgingival biofilm and of gingivitis is enhanced.[44,49-51]

II. REDUCTION/ALTERATION OF DENTAL BIOFILM AND BY-PRODUCTS

Research has shown that irrigation with water can:
- Reduce the bacterial chemical mediators that promote or enhance the inflammatory process leading to bone loss.[40]
- Be effective with a pulsating device for both supragingival and marginal tip placement.[44,45,51,52]
- Alter or reduce the quality and quantity of the subgingival dental biofilm.[48]

III. PENETRATION INTO POCKET: SUBGINGIVAL ACCESS

- The standard jet tip placed supragingivally can penetrate below the gingival margin 44% to 71% of the pocket depth.[46]
- Specialized tips used for marginal or subgingival delivery have shown penetration between 41% and 90% depending on tip use, technique, and presence of calculus.[47,53,54]

IV. DELIVERY OF ANTIMICROBAL AGENTS

- The effectiveness of an antimicrobial agent is enhanced when delivered by an oral irrigator.
- Agents that have been researched for use in an irrigator include chlorhexidine gluconate, stannous fluoride, phenolic compounds (essential oils), hydrogen peroxide, and sanguinaria.

V. PERIODONTAL MAINTENANCE

The continuous absence of bleeding on probing is an important measurement for the success of therapy and the maintenance of periodontal health.[55] Oral irrigation has been shown to improve the following clinical parameters for periodontal maintenance patients:
- Gingival index.[40,44,49,51,52]
- Bleeding on probing.[40,44,45,49,52]
- Probing depths.[40,51]

▪ APPLICATIONS FOR PRACTICE

Regular use of daily home irrigation is beneficial. Even those with good oral hygiene can benefit from the use of daily irrigation. Use a patient-centered approach to evaluate each patient individually to determine which techniques, products, or devices are appropriate.

I. ADVANTAGES OF PATIENT-APPLIED DAILY IRRIGATION

A. Reduction of Bleeding

- The absence of bleeding is the best clinical measurement to predict minimal risk of periodontal breakdown.[55]
- Irrigation consistently has shown a significant reduction of bleeding even with water as the irrigant.

B. Removal of the Loosely Attached Biofilm From Subgingival and Problem Areas

Areas that are difficult to access with traditional mechanical methods, such as open interdental areas, malpositioned teeth, exposed furcas, periodontal pockets, and postperiodontal surgery problem areas, can benefit from daily irrigation.

C. Special Needs Areas

1. Prosthetic replacements and fixed partial dentures.
2. Orthodontic appliances.
3. Intermaxillary fixation appliances for orthognathic surgery and fractured jaw.
4. Complex restorations and other extensive rehabilitation.
5. Implant maintenance with soft rubber specialized tip.[56]
6. Individuals living with diabetes.[45]
7. Immunocompromised or physically challenged individuals.

II. CONTRAINDICATION

A. Premedication Requirement

A patient who requires antibiotic premedication for dental and dental hygiene treatment should be evaluated before introducing the use of an oral irrigator or other mechanical device.

B. Incidence of Bacteremia

- The incidence of bacteremia from irrigation ranges from a low of 6% in patients with gingivitis to a high of 50% in patients with periodontitis.[57,58] This is consistent with bacteremia observed following toothbrushing and flossing.[59-61]
- The incidence and magnitude of bacteremia of oral origin have been shown to be proportional to the degree of oral inflammation and

Everyday Ethics

Rachel worked in a dental office as a dental assistant prior to beginning her dental hygiene education. The office where she worked was opposed to recommending irrigation because "it does not remove biofilm," so she is adamant that it does not work and should not be recommended. She also expressed concern that if patients use irrigation they will not floss. Rachel has made a conscious decision that she will not recommend irrigation to any of her patients regardless of clinical findings.

Questions for Consideration

1. Using a framework for making choices, who might Rachel have to defend her decision to if she does not recommend irrigation for any of her patients? Include all individuals affected by this decision.

2. In this scenario, how does the principle of autonomy apply to the patients Rachel treats?

3. What suggestions would you offer this hygienist to make sure she continues to serve the needs of her patients as a licensed dental health professional?

---

infection.[61] Therefore, it is imperative that those at risk maintain optimal oral health. Detailed information on the incidence of bacteremia is on pages 1041 to 1042.

C. Consultation

The patient's physician should be contacted when a question arises about the use of adjunctive oral hygiene aids that can create a bacteremia, along with a review of the American Heart Association's most current recommendations for prevention of bacterial endocarditis (pages 122 to 125).

▪ AMERICAN DENTAL ASSOCIATION SEAL OF ACCEPTANCE PROGRAM

Approval of a product is shown by use of the ADA Seal of Acceptance (Figure 27-3). The depth and importance of the seal program is recognized internationally. Visit www.ada.org for a complete list of accepted products.

I. PURPOSE

A. To determine the safety and efficacy of a product.
B. To review advertising claims.
C. To inform members of the dental team and the public about the safety and efficacy of the product.

II. PRODUCTS CONSIDERED

A. Drugs and chemical agents used in the diagnosis, treatment, or prevention of oral diseases.

B. Chemicals that may affect the health of dental team, and the public.
C. Dental materials, instruments, and equipment.

III. REQUIREMENTS

A. Information to Be Provided

1. Composition: Properties and quantities of all ingredients and vehicles.
2. Objective data from clinical and laboratory studies.
   a. To support the product's safety and efficacy
   b. ADA guidelines and protocol to be followed
3. Advertising, promotional claims, and patient education materials.

B. Reapplication

1. Every 5 years for over-the-counter products; every 3 years for professional products.
2. Changes in the composition of any product require a new application at any time.

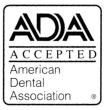

▪ **FIGURE 27-3 Seal of Acceptance, The American Dental Association,** Council on Scientific Affairs. The Seal is awarded to therapeutics, materials, instruments, and equipment that meet ADA guidelines for safety and effectiveness.

Factors To Teach The Patient

- Significance of American Dental Association product acceptance seal, especially that it is a voluntary program and no seal on a product does not signify it is unsafe or not effective.

- Ask dental hygienist and dentist about new mouthrinses, best way to use, and appropriateness for personal needs.

- Ask dental hygienist and dentist which oral irrigator and tip is appropriate since all products are not equivalent or clinically tested.

- Avoid impulse buying with regard to dentifrices, oral rinses, and other chemical agents. Seek professional advice to avoid contraindications with oral condition and restorations.

- Patient compliance to recommended use of chemical agent or mouthrinse and appropriate delivery vehicle are directly related to expected outcomes (results or improvements).

- The use of chemotherapeutics is not a substitute for proper and daily mechanical biofilm removal.

REFERENCES

1. **Volpe**, A.R.: Dentifrices and Mouth Rinses, in Stallard, R.E., ed.: *A Textbook of Preventive Dentistry*, 2nd ed. Philadelphia, W.B. Saunders Co., 1982, pp. 170–216.

2. **Forward**, G.C., James, A.H., Barnett, P., and Jackson R.J.: Gum Health Product Formulations: What Is in Them and Why? *Periodontol. 2000, 15*, 32, 1997.

3. **Melburg**, J.R.: Fluoride Dentifrices: Current Status and Prospectus, *Int. Dent. J., 41*, 9, February, 1991.

4. **Fischman**, S.L.: The History of Oral Hygiene Products: How Far Have We Come in 6000 Years? *Periodontol. 2000, 15*, 7, 1997.

5. **Muller**, H.P., Sicilia, A., Stoltze, K., and Zappa, U.: The Treatment of Dentinal Hypersensitivity, in Lang, N.P., Karring, T., and Lindhe, J.: *Proceedings of the 2nd European Workshop on Periodontology*, 1st ed. Berlin, Quintessence Verlag, 1997, p. 257.

6. **Shiff**,T., Zhang, Y.P., DeVizio, W., Stewart, B., Chaknis, P., Petrone, M.E., Volpe, A.R., and Proskin, H.M.: A Randomized Clinical Trial of the Desensitizing Efficacy of Three Dentifrices, *Compend. Contin. Educ. Dent., 27*, 4, Supplement, 2000.

7. **Orchardson**, R., and Gillam, D.G.: The Efficacy of Potassium Salts as Agents for Treating Dentin Hypersensitivity, *J. Orofac. Pain, 14*, 9, Winter, 2000.

8. **Lobene**, R.R., Soparkar, P. M. Newman, M.B., and Kohut, B.E.: Reduced Formation of Supragingival Calculus With Use of Fluoride-Zinc Chloride Dentifrice, *J. Am, Dent. Assoc., 114*, 350, March, 1987.

9. **Banoczy**, J., Sari, K., Schiff, T., Petrone, M., Davies, R., and Volpe, A.: Anticalculus Efficacy of Three Dentifrices, *Am. J. Dent., 8*, 205, August, 1995.

10. **Segreto**, V.A., Collins, E.M., D'Agostino, R., Cancro, L.P., Pfeifer, H.J., and Gilbert, R.J.: Anticalculus Effect of a Dentifrice Containing 0.5% Zinc Citrate Trihydrate, *Comm. Dent. Oral Epidemiol., 19*, 29, February, 1991.

11. **Bolden**, T.E., Zambon, J.J., Sowinski, J., Ayad, F., McCool, J.J., Volpe, A.R., and DeVizio, W.: The Clinical Effect of a Dentifrice Containing Triclosan and a Copolymer in a Sodium Fluoride/Silica Base on Plaque Formation and Gingivitis, *J. Clin. Dent., 3*, 125, 1992.

12. **Lindhe**, J., Rosling, B., Socransky, S.S., and Volpe, A.R.: The Effect of a Triclosan-Containing Dentifrice on Established Plaque and Gingivitis, *J. Clin. Periodontol., 20*, 327, May, 1993.

13. **Nordbo**, H., Eriksen, H.M., Rolla, G., Attramadal, A., and Solheim, H.: Iron Staining of the Acquired Enamel Pellicle After Exposure to Tannic Acid or Chlorhexidine: Preliminary Report, *Scand. J. Dent. Res., 90*, 117, Number 2, 1982.

14. **Addy**, M. and Moran, J.: Mechanisms of Stain Formation on Teeth in Particular Associated With Metal Ions and Antiseptics, *Adv. Dent. Res., 9*, 450, December, 1995.

15. **Grabenstetter**, R.J., Broge, R.W., Jackson, F.L., and Radike, A.W.: The Measurement of the Abrasion of Human Teeth by Dentifrice Abrasives: A Test Utilizing Radioactive Teeth. *J. Dent. Res., 37*, 1060, November–December, 1958.

16. **Barnes**, C.M.: An Evidenced-Based Review of Sodium Bicarbonate as a Dentifrice Agent. *Compend. Cont. Educ Oral Hyg., 6*, 3, Number 3, 1999.

17. **Wunderlich**, R.C., Singleton, M., O'Brien, W.J., and Caffesse, R.G.: Subgingival Penetration of an Applied Solution, *Int. J. Periodontics Restorative Dent., 4*, 64, Number 5, 1984.

18. **Veksler**, A.E., Kayrouz, G.A., and Newman, M.G.: Reduction of Salivary Bacteria by Pre-procedural Rinses with Chlorhexidine 0.12%, *J. Periodontol., 62*, 649, November, 1991.

19. **Fine**, D.H., Mendieta, C., Barnett, M.L., Furgang, D., Meyers, R., Olshan, A., and Vincent, J.: Efficacy of Preprocedural Rinsing With an Antiseptic in Reducing Viable Bacteria in Dental Aerosols, *J. Periodontol., 63*, 821, October, 1992.

20. **Scheie**, A.A.A.: Modes of Action of Currently Known Chemical Anti-Plaque Agents Other than Chlorhexidine, *J. Dent. Res., 68*, 1609, November, Special Issue, 1989.

21. **Overholser**, C.D., Meiller, T.F., DePaola, L.G., Minah, G.E., and Niehaus, C.: Comparative Effects of 2 Chemotherapeutic Mouthrinses on the Development of Supragingival Dental Plaque and Gingivitis, *J. Clin. Periodontol., 17*, 575, September, 1990.

22. **Lamster**, I.B.,., Alfano, M.C., Seiger, M.C., and Gordon, J.M.: The Effect of Listerine Antiseptic® on Reduction of Existing Plaque and Gingivitis, *Clin. Prev. Dent., 5*, 12, November–December, 1983.

23. **Volpe**, A.R., Petrone, M.E., DeVizio, W., and Davies, R.M.: A Review of Plaque, Gingivitis, Calculus and Caries Clinical Efficacy Studies With a Dentifrice Containing Triclosan and PVM/MA Copolymer, *J. Clin. Dent., 4*, Special Issue, 1993.

24. **Schaeken**, M.J.M., van der Hoeven, J.S., Saxton, C.A., and Cummins, D.: The Effect of Mouthrinses Containing Zinc and Triclosan on Plaque Accumulation, Development of Gingivitis and Formation of Calculus in a 28-Week Clinical Test, *J. Clin. Periodontol., 23*, 465, May, 1996.

25. **Davies**, A.: The Mode of Action of Chlorhexidine, *J. Periodontol. Res., 8* (Suppl.12), 68, 1973.

26. **Jones**, C.G.: Chlorhexidine: Is It Still the Gold Standard? *Periodontol. 2000, 15*, 55, 1997.

27. **Banting**, D., Bosma, M., and Bollmer, B.: Clinical Effectiveness of a 0.12% Chlorhexidine Mouthrinse Over Two Years, *J. Dent. Res., 68*, 1716, Special Issue, November, 1989.

28. **Grossman**, E., Reiter, G., Sturzenberger, O.P., De La Rosa, M., Dickinson, T.D., Ferretti, G.A., Ludlam, G.E., and Meckel, A.H.: Six-Month Study of the Effects of a Chlorhexidine Mouthrinse on Gingivitis in Adults, *J. Periodontal. Res., 21*(Suppl. 16.), 33, 1986.

29. **Mandel**, I.D.: Chemical Agents for Control of Plaque and Gingivitis, Committee on Research, Science and Therapy, American Academy of Periodontology, Chicago, April, Position Paper, *www.perio.org*, 1994.

30. **Barkvoll**, P., Rolla, G., and Svendsen, A.K.: Interaction Between Chlorhexidine Digluconate and Sodium Lauryl Sulfate In Vivo, *J. Clin. Periodontol., 16*, 593, October, 1989.

31. **Mandel**, I.D.: Chemotherapeutic Agents for Controlling Plaque and Gingivitis, *J. Clin. Periodontol, 15*, 488, September, 1988.

32. **Moran**, J. and Addy, M.: The Effect of Surface Adsorption and Staining Reactions on the Antimicrobial Properties of Some Cationic Antiseptic Mouthwashes, *J. Periodontol., 55*, 278, May, 1984.

33. **Roberts**, W.R. and Addy, M.: Comparison of In Vivo and In Vitro Antibacterial Properties of Antiseptic Mouthrinses Containing Chlorhexidine, Alexidine, Cetyl Pyridinium Chloride and Hexetidine: Relevance to Mode of Action, *J. Clin. Periodontol., 8*, 295, Number 4, 1981.

34. **Scherer**, W., Gultz, J., Lee, S.S., and Kaim, J.: The Ability of an Herbal Mouthrinse to Reduce Gingival Bleeding, *J. Clin. Dent., 9*, 97, Number 2, 1998.

35. **Kopczyk**, R.A., Abrams, H., Brown, A.T., Matheny, J.L., and Kaplan, A.L.: Clinical and Microbiological Effects of a Sanguinaria-containing Mouthrinse and Dentifrice With and Without Fluoride During 6 Months of Use, *J. Periodontol., 62*, 617, October, 1991.

36. **Harper**, D.S., Mueller, L.J., Fine, J.B., Gordon, J., and Laster, L.L.: Effect of 6 Months Use of a Dentifrice and Oral Rinse Containing Sanguinaria Extract and Zinc Chloride Upon the Microflora of the Dental Plaque and Oral Soft Tissues, *J. Periodontol., 61*, 359, June, 1990.

37. **Mandel**, I.D.: Antimicrobial Mouthrinses: Overview and Update, *J. Am. Dent. Assoc.,125*, 2S, August, Supplement,1994.

38. **Rees**, T.D. and Orth, C.F.: Oral Ulcerations With Use of Hydrogen Peroxide, *J. Periodontol., 57*, 689, November, 1986.

39. **Weitzman**, S.A., Weitberg, A.B., Niederman, R., and Stossel, T.P.: Chronic Treatment With Hydrogen Peroxide: Is It Safe? *J. Periodontol, 55*, 510, September, 1984.

40. **Cutler**, C.W., Stanford, T.W., Abraham, C., Cederberg, R.A., Boardman, T.J., and Ross, C.: Clinical Benefits of Oral Irrigation for Periodontitis Are Related to Reduction of Pro-Inflammatory Cytokine Levels and Plaque, *J. Clin. Periodontol., 27*, 134, February, 2000.

41. **Waerhaug**, J.: Effect of Toothbrushing on Subgingival Plaque Formation, *J. Periodontol., 52*, 30, January, 1981.

42. **Lugassy**,A.A., Lautenschlager, E.P., and Katrana, D.: Characterization of Water Spray Devices, *J. Dent. Res., 50*, 466, March–April, 1971.

43. **Bhaskar**, S.N., Cutright, D.E., Gross, A., Frisch, J., Beasley, J.D., and Perez, B.: Water Jet Devices in Dental Practice, *J. Periodontol., 42*, 658, October, 1971.

44. **Flemmig**, T.F., Newman, M.G., Doherty, F.M., Grossman, E., Meckel, A.H., and Bakdash, M.B.: Supragingival Irrigation with 0.06% Chlorhexidine in Naturally Occurring Gingivitis. I. 6 Month Clinical Observations, *J. Periodontol., 61*, 112, February, 1990.

45. **Al-Mubarak**, S., Ciancio, S., Aljada, A., Awa, H., Hamouda, W., Ghanim, H., Zambon, J., Boardman, T.J., Mohanty, P., Ross, C., and Dandona, P.: Comparative Evaluation of Adjunctive Oral Irrigation in Diabetics, *J. Clin. Periodontol., 29*, 295, April, 2002.

46. **Eakle**, W.S., Ford, C., and Boyd, R.L.: Depth of Penetration in Periodontal Pockets With Oral Irrigation, *J. Clin. Periodontol., 13*, 39, January, 1986.

47. **Braun**, R.E. and Ciancio, S.G.: Subgingival Delivery by an Oral Irrigation Device, *J. Periodontol., 63*, 469, May, 1992.

48. **Cobb**, C.M., Rodgers, R.L., and Killoy, W.J.: Ultrastructural Examination of Human Periodontal Pockets Following the Use of an Oral Irrigation Device In Vivo, *J. Periodontol., 59*, 155, March, 1988.

49. **Chaves**, E.S., Kornman, K.S., Manwell, M.A., Jones, A.A., Newbold, D.A., and Wood, R.C.: Mechanism of Irrigation Effects on Gingivitis, *J. Periodontol., 65*, 1016, November, 1994.

50. **Ciancio**, S.G., Mather, M.L., Zambon, J.J., and Reynolds, H.S.: Effect of a Chemotherapeutic Agent Delivered by an Oral Irrigation Device on Plaque, Gingivitis, and Subgingival Microflora, *J. Periodontol., 60*, 310, June, 1989.

51. **Jolkovsky**, D.L., Waki, M.Y., Newman, M.G., Otomo-Corgel, J., Madison, M., Flemmig, T.F., Nachnani, S., and Nowzari, H.: Clinical and Microbiological Effects of Subgingival and Gingival Marginal Irrigation With Chlorhexidine Gluconate, *J. Periodontol., 61*, 663, November, 1990.

52. **Newman**, M.G., Cattabriga, M. Etienne, D., Flemmig, T., Sanz, M., Kornman, K.S., Doherty, F., Moore, D.J., and Ross, C.: Effectiveness of Adjunctive Irrigation in Early Periodontitis: Multicenter Evaluation, *J. Periodontol., 65*, 224, March, 1994.

53. **Boyd**, R.L., Hollander, B.W., and Eakle, W.S.: Comparison of Subgingivally Placed Cannula Oral Irrigator Tip With a Supragingivally Placed Standard Irrigator Tip, *J. Clin. Periodontol, 19*, 340, May, 1992.

54. **Larner**, J.R. and Greenstein, G.: Effect of Calculus and Irrigator Tip Design on Depth of Subgingival Irrigation, *Int. J. Periodontics Restorative Dent.,13*, 289, Number 3, 1993.

55. **Lang**, N.P., Joss, A., and Tonetti, M.S.: Monitoring Disease During Supportive Periodontal Treatment by Bleeding on Probing, *Periodontol. 2000, 12*, 44, 1996.

56. **Felo**, A., Shibly, O., Ciancio, S.G., Lauciello, F.R., and Ho, A.: Effects of Subgingival Chlorhexidine Irrigation on Peri-implant Maintenance, *Am. J. Dent., 10*, 107, April, 1997.

57. **Romans**, A.R. and App, G. R.: Bacteremia: A Result From Oral Irrigation in Subjects With Gingivitis, *J. Periodontol., 42*, 757, December, 1971.

58. **Felix**, J.E., Rosen, S., and App., G.R.: Detection of Bacteremia After the Use of an Oral Irrigation Device in Subjects With Periodontitis, *J. Periodontol., 42*, 785, December, 1971.

59. **Donley**, T.G. and Donley, K.B.: Systemic Bacteremia Following Toothbrushing: A Protocol for the Management of Patients Susceptible to Infective Endocarditis, *Gen. Dent. 36*, 482, November–December, 1988.

60. **Berger**, S.A., Weitzman, S., Edberg, S.C., and Casey, J.I.: Bacteremia After the Use of an Oral Irrigation Device: A Controlled Study in Subjects With Normal-Appearing Gingiva: Comparisons With Use of Toothbrush, *Ann. Intern. Med., 80*, 510, April, 1974.

61. **Pallasch**, T.J. and Slots, J.: Antibiotic Prophylaxis and the Medically Compromised Patient, *Periodontol. 2000, 10*, 107, 1996.

SUGGESTED READINGS

Addy, M. and Moran, J.M.: Evaluation of Oral Hygiene Products: Science Is True; Don't Be Misled by the Facts, *Periodontol. 2000, 15*, 40, 1997.

Lyle, D.M.: The Role of Pharmacotherapeutics in the Reduction of Plaque and Gingivitis, *J. Pract. Hyg., 9*, 46, November/December, 2000.

Meyer, D.M.: Voluntary Programs: ADA Seal Program and International Implications, *Ann. Periodontol., 2*, 31, March, 1997.

Newman, M.G. and van Winkelhoff, A.J.: *Antibiotic and Antimicrobial Use in Dental Practice*, 2nd ed. Chicago, Quintessence Publishing Co., Inc., 2001.

Slots, J. and Jorgensen, M.G.: Effective, Safe, Practical and Affordable

Periodontal Antimicrobial Therapy: Where Are We Going, and Are We There Yet? *Periodontol. 2000, 28,* 298, 2002.

Dentifrices

Allen, D. R., Battista, G.W., Petrone, D.M., Petrone, M.E., Chaknis, P., DeVizio, W, and Volpe, A.R.: The Clinical Efficacy of Colgate Total Plus Whitening Toothpaste Containing a Special Grade of Silica and Colgate Total Fresh Stripe Toothpaste in the Control of Plaque and Gingivitis: A Six-Month Clinical Study, *J. Clin. Dent., 13,* 59, 2002.

Meredith, M.J.: Herbal Nutriceuticals: A Primer for Dentists and Dental Hygienists, *J. Contemp. Dent. Prac., 2,* 1, Spring, 2001.

Moran, J., Addy, M., Corry, D., Newcombe, R.G., and Haywood, J.: A Study to Assess the Plaque Inhibitory Action of a New Zinc Citrate Toothpaste Formulation, *J. Clin. Periodontol., 28,* 157, February, 2001.

Nogueira-Filho, G.R., Toledo, S., Cury, J.A.: Effect of 3 Dentifrices Containing Triclosan and Various Additives: An Experimental Gingivitis Study, *J. Clin. Periodontol., 27,* 494, July, 2000.

Sheen, S., Eisenburger, M., and Addy, M.: Effect of Toothpaste on the Plaque Inhibitory Properties of a Cetylpyridinium Chloride Mouth Rinse, *J. Clin. Periodontol., 30,* 255, March, 2003

Triratana, T., Rustogi, K.N., Volpe, A.R., DeVizio, W., Petrone, M., and Giniger, M.: Clinical Effect of a New Liquid Dentifrice Containing Triclosan/Copolymer on Existing Plaque and Gingivitis, *J. Am. Dent. Assoc., 133,* 219, February, 2002.

Mouthrinses

Charles, C.H., Sharma, N.C., Galustians, H.J., Qaqish, J., McGuire, J.A., and Vincent, J.W.: Comparative Efficacy of an Antiseptic Mouthrinse and an Antiplaque/Antigingivitis Dentifrice: A Six-Month Clinical Trial, *J. Am. Dent. Assoc., 132,* 670, May, 2001

Fine, D.H., Furgang, D., Barnett, M.L., Drew, C., Steinberg, L., Charles, C.H., and Vincent, J.W.: Effect of an Essential Oil-Containing Antiseptic Mouthrinse on Plaque and Salivary *Streptococcus mutans* Levels, *J. Clin. Periodontol., 27,* 157, March, 2000.

Keijser, J.A.M., Verkade, H., Timmerman, M.F., and Van der Weijden F.A.: Comparison of 2 Commercially Available Chlorhexidine Mouthrinses, *J. Periodontol., 74,* 214, February, 2003.

Leyes Borrajo, J.L., GarciaVarela, L., Lopez Castro, G., Rodriguez-Nunez, I., Garcia Figueroa, .M., and Gallas Torreira, M.: Efficacy of Chlorhexidine Mouthrinses With and Without Alcohol: A Clinical Study, *J. Periodontol., 73,* 317, March, 2002.

Owens, J., Addy, M., and Faulkner, J.: An 18-Week Home-Use Study Comparing the Oral Hygiene and Gingival Health Benefits of Triclosan and Fluoride Toothpastes, *J. Clin. Periodontol., 24,* 626, September, 1997.

Owens, J., Addy, M., Faulkner, J., Lockwood, C., and Adair, R.: A Short-term Clinical Study Design to Investigate the Chemical Plaque Inhibitory Properties of Mouthrinses When Used as Adjuncts to Toothpastes: Applied to Chlorhexidine, *J. Clin. Periodontol., 24,* 732, October, 1997.

Pilatti, G.L. and Sampaio, J.E.C.: The Influence of Chlorhexidine on the Severity of Cyclosporin A–induced Gingival Overgrowth, *J. Periodontol., 68,* 900, September, 1997.

Rosling, B., Dahlen, G., Volpe, A., Furuichi, Y., Ramberg, P., and Lindhe, J.: Effect of Triclosan on the Subgingival Microbiota of Periodontitis-Susceptible Subjects, *J. Clin. Periodontol., 24,* 881, December, 1997.

Irrigation

Drisko, C.H.: Non-Surgical Pocket Therapy: Pharmacotherapeutics, *Ann. Periodontol., 1,* 492, November, 1996.

Flemmig, T.F., Epp, B., Funkenhauser, Z., Newman, M.G., Kornman, K.S., Haubitz, I., and Klaiber, B.: Adjunctive Supragingival Irrigation With Acetylsalicylic Acid in Periodontal Supportive Therapy, *J. Clin. Periodontol., 22,* 427, June, 1995.

Jorgensen, M.G. and Slots, J.: Antimicrobials in Periodontal Maintenance, *J. Dent. Hyg., 75,* 233, Summer, 2001.

The Patient With Orthodontic Appliances

Marylou E. Gutmann, RDH, BS, MA
Su-yan Barrow, RDH, BS, MA

Without a strong and persistent preventive care program before, during, and following completion of orthodontic treatment, a high dental caries rate is probable due to the length of time appliances must be in place. Gingival and periodontal infections during and following treatment are not unusual. An individualized preventive program that includes a specific plan of instruction, motivation, and supervision is essential for the patient with orthodontic appliances. The patient must understand that much more effort is required while in treatment than was required before the appliances were placed. Terminology used in orthodontic therapy is defined in Box 28-1.

CEMENTED BANDS AND BONDED BRACKETS

Resin-bonded brackets and circumferential molar bands are used widely in orthodontic treatment. They aid in the application and control of applied forces necessary to accomplish tooth movement and bone remodeling for orthodontic therapy.

In contemporary orthodontic treatment, circumferential stainless steel bands are usually cemented to the permanent first molar teeth because of the strength needed to hold palatal bars, elastics, or other special devices. Stainless steel or ceramic brackets generally are bonded to facial surfaces of anterior and premolar teeth to retain the arch wire. Brackets are illustrated in Figure 28-1.

I. ADVANTAGES OF BONDED BRACKETS[1]

A. Improved aesthetics.
B. Improved gingival condition due to better access for control of dental biofilm at the cervical third of the teeth.
C. Proximal surface dental caries can be detected and treated without bracket removal.

453

BOX 28-1 KEY WORDS: Orthodontics*

Appliance: any device designed to influence the shape and/or function of the mouth/jaw system.

> **Fixed appliance:** a bonded or banded appliance affixed to individual teeth or groups of teeth.

> **Orthodontic appliance:** device used to influence growth and/or position of the teeth and jaws.

> **Orthopedic appliance:** device used to influence growth and/or position of bones.

Arch wire: curved wire positioned in the brackets around the dental arch and held in place by elastomers or ligatures.

Band: preformed stainless steel ring fitted around a tooth and cemented in place; available in shapes for each tooth form; each band has a bracket attached on the facial side, which is the mode of attachment for the arch wire.

Bonding: process by which orthodontic brackets are affixed to the tooth surface; a fluoride-releasing, light-activated resin is frequently used.

> **Direct bonding:** a single-step intraoral procedure in which orthodontic attachments are oriented and bonded individually.

> **Indirect bonding:** a two-step process by which orthodontic attachments are affixed temporarily to the teeth of a study cast from which they are transferred to the mouth at one time by means of a template or tray that preserves the predetermined orientation and permits them to be bonded simultaneously.

Bracket: attachment that is bonded to the enamel for the purpose of holding the arch wire.

Ceramic: alumina (Al_2O_3) used as a single-crystal material or as a polycrystalline material.

Debonding: removal of brackets and residual adhesive, after which the tooth surface is returned to its normal contour.

Elastomer: elastoplastic ring or latex elastic used to hold an arch wire in a bracket wing.

Fracture toughness: ability of bracket material to resist fracture.

Interceptive/preventive orthodontics: dental services intended to prevent the development of a malocclusion by maintaining the integrity of an otherwise normally developing dentition.

Ligature: cord, thread, elastic, or stainless steel wire used to secure the arch wire to the bracket.

Retainer: an orthodontic appliance, fixed or removable, used to maintain the position of the teeth following corrective treatment.

> **Hawley retainer:** a removable plastic and wire appliance used to stabilize teeth; may be modified for special applications during or after orthodontic therapy.

Space maintainer: prosthetic replacement for prematurely lost primary teeth to prevent closure of the space before eruption of the permanent successors.

Space regainer: appliance used for correction of tooth displacement resulting from premature loss of one or more teeth without timely space maintenance.

Tensile: susceptible to extension; capable of being stretched.

> **Tensile strength:** maximum stress that a material is capable of sustaining; usually expressed in pounds per square inch.

*Definitions in this chapter pertaining to orthodontics are taken from and are in accord with the *Glossary of Dentofacial Orthopedic Terms, Orthodontic Glossary*, 2002 Edition, American Association of Orthodontists, St. Louis, MO.

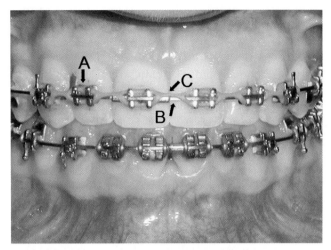

■ **FIGURE 28-1 Fixed Appliance System.** Bonded brackets **(A)** with arch wire **(B)** held in place by elastomers **(C)**.

D. Patient can be aware immediately when a bracket loosens, whereas an unsecured band may go undetected.
E. Placement factors
1. No need for tooth separation (as required for band placement); results in less patient discomfort and no band spaces to close at the end of treatment.
2. Bonded appliances can be placed on partially erupted teeth, so waiting for tooth eruption is unnecessary before treatment can be started.
3. Lingual brackets ("invisible braces") may be used for specially selected cases.
4. Placement of brackets is faster and easier than placement of bands.

II. DISADVANTAGES OF BONDED BRACKETS[1]

A. Attachment may be weaker because less surface area is in contact with tooth. Bracket may detach more readily than a band. Bond strength is technique sensitive and also dependent on the adhesive resin selected for the bonding procedure.[2,3]
B. Rebonding a loose bracket is more time consuming and requires more tooth preparation than does recementing a loose band.
C. Debonding at the end of treatment is more time consuming than debanding, with more potential for damage to the tooth surface because of the higher bond strength.
D. Lower fracture toughness; enamel is subject to cracks.[4]

III. FIXED APPLIANCE SYSTEM

Figure 28-1 shows the bonded brackets with arch wire held in place by elastomers.

A. Brackets

1. Materials
   a. Metal (stainless steel).
   b. Plastic (polycarbonate).
   c. Plastic with metal reinforcements.
   d. Ceramic.
2. Forms. Brackets are made in many styles, shapes, and sizes for different teeth, each designed to accomplish a specific objective of treatment. The basic forms are single or twin, as illustrated in Figure 28-2.
3. Base. The base of the bracket is prepared with a mesh backing to assist in retaining the resin bonding agent. The mesh backing, or bonding pad as it is also called, is made to the exact size of the bracket so that no area of tooth is left uncovered where demineralization can occur. Mesh backings retain less dental biofilm than do other types of backings.[5,6]

B. Arch Wire

The arch wire is used to generate and distribute forces that guide orthodontic tooth movement. Arch wires are made of stainless steel or an alloy of chromium or titanium, and they may be round, rectangular, or multistranded, as illustrated in Figure 28-1.

C. Elastomers

An elastomer is used to:
1. Hold wires in the brackets (Figure 28-1).
2. Apply force to close spaces between teeth.

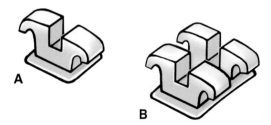

■ **FIGURE 28-2 Orthodontic Brackets. (A)** Single bracket with an incisal and a cervical wing. **(B)** Twin, or Siamese, bracket with two wings on each side of the central groove where the arch wire is held. The shape and style of each bracket vary with the tooth on which the bracket will be located.

▪ CLINICAL PROCEDURES FOR BONDING[1,7,8]

I. PREPARATION

Prior to bonding, it is important to document any irregularities of the patient's teeth, such as white spots or cracks, before orthodontic treatment begins and appliances are affixed, to prevent misunderstanding by the patient after debonding.[9]

II. PRINCIPLES

The principles described in Chapter 34, pages 573 to 575, for pit and fissure sealants apply for bonding orthodontic brackets. Details are not included here, except to point out that polishing the enamel surface prior to etching is unnecessary to achieve an acceptable bond.[10]

III. PROCEDURAL STEPS

A. Cleaning the Tooth Surface

Although polishing the enamel surface with pumice prior to etching is unnecessary to achieve an acceptable bond, cleaning of the tooth with pumice and a toothbrush or polishing with a rubber cup/brush pumice slurry may be done if desired, as this procedure will not affect the strength of the bond.

B. Conditioning the Enamel Surface

Follow procedures listed in Chapter 34, page 575, for sealant application.

C. Applying the Bonding Agent

Follow procedures listed in Chapter 34, page 575, for sealant application. After bonding, the area around the bracket must be cleaned of excess resin.

IV. CHARACTERISTICS OF BONDING RELATING TO DEBONDING

A. Nature of the Bond

The acid etch exposes the prism structure and creates microclefts, as illustrated in Figure 34-1. The average depth of the microclefts ranges from 50 to 80 μm.[11-13] Some fine tag extensions have been observed to depths of 100 to 170 μm.[13] On the bracket side, the resin becomes locked into the mesh base.

B. Effect of Filler Particles

- Physical property values increase from unfilled to heavily filled resins. Fillers increase bond strength, hardness, and wear resistance.

- Heavily filled resins (composites) perform better for the posterior teeth because posterior attachments are subject to high forces of mastication.
- Ease of debonding can be related to the type of resin and length of etching time. Heavily filled composites are thicker and less viscous; they may be more difficult to remove.[2] When etching time is decreased from 60 seconds to 15 seconds, less adhesive resin remains on the teeth.[3] This shorter etching time makes the enamel surface less retentive, but it is adequate for orthodontic bonding.[3]
- The bond is stronger when a smaller (thinner) layer of resin is placed between the tooth surface and the bracket.
- In summary, anterior brackets may be bonded with a lightly filled resin, whereas posterior teeth may need a heavily filled resin to prevent detachment.

V. USE OF FLUORIDE-RELEASING BONDING SYSTEM

Demineralization around brackets can result in a serious caries problem for even the most conscientious patient. Use of a fluoride-releasing bonding system has been shown to have positive preventive results.[14-16]

▪ DENTAL HYGIENE CARE

The patient may be under care with regular appointments for a long period, frequently over a few years. Periodic communication between the patient's referring dentist and dental hygienist is necessary to coordinate instruction along with other necessary dental and dental hygiene care.

I. COMPLICATING FACTORS: RISK FACTORS

A. Age Group

Many orthodontic patients are in the preteen and teenage years, periods when the incidence of gingivitis is high. The incidence of periodontal infection increases from early childhood to late teenage years.

B. Gingivitis

Dental biofilm retention by orthodontic appliances leads to gingivitis. The degree can vary from slight to severe with gingival enlargement, particularly of the interdental papillae. The tissue may greatly enlarge and cover the fixed appliance. The enlarged tissue with pockets provides additional biofilm-retentive areas.

C. Position of Teeth

Teeth that are irregularly positioned are naturally more susceptible to the retention of bacterial deposits and are more difficult to clean. With the severe malocclusions presented by orthodontic patients at the outset, this factor becomes even more significant.

D. Problems With Appliances

1. Orthodontic appliances retain biofilm and debris.
2. Accidents may cause a bracket to become detached.

E. Self-Care Is Difficult

Even the patient who tries to maintain oral cleanliness has difficulty because the appliances are in the way and interfere with the application of the toothbrush and other devices used for dental biofilm control.

II. DISEASE CONTROL

A rigid program for dental caries and periodontal disease control is needed. The selection of biofilm control procedures for an individual patient is determined by the anatomic features of the gingiva, the position of the teeth, and the type and position of the orthodontic appliance.

A. General Instructions

1. Give instructions before appliances are placed. Every attempt must be made to have the oral tissues in health and the patient motivated to perform thorough daily biofilm removal. Table 28-1 lists the advantages and disadvantages of various aids for the patient to use in the attempt to maintain optimal oral health.
2. Perform brushing before a mirror so that brush application is accurate and brushing is thorough.
3. Use a disclosing solution rinse to assist in self-evaluation. A patient wearing an orthodontic appliance may experience extreme difficulty in chewing disclosing wafers without discomfort or pain.
4. Recommend an approved fluoride dentifrice to aid in dental caries control.
5. Place emphasis in brushing on sulcular brushing and cleaning the area between the orthodontic bands and brackets and the gingiva.

B. Toothbrushing: Brush Selection

1. *Soft brush.* A soft brush with end-rounded filaments is recommended.

2. *Bilevel.* A special bilevel orthodontic brush designed with spaced rows of soft nylon filaments and a shorter middle row that can be applied directly over the appliance is shown in Figure 28-3. It is used with a short horizontal stroke.
3. *Power brush.* Used with soft filaments, a light stroke, and at a low speed, power brushes have been shown to be very effective for maintaining gingival health and cleaning around appliances. Figure 25-9 shows various designs of power brushes, including one designed especially for orthodontic use.

C. Brushing Procedure

1. *Sulcular brushing.* A sulcular method is needed by most patients for cleaning the appliances and maintaining the gingiva.
2. *Adapt for appliance.* Special adaptation is required for facial surfaces. Place the brush with filament ends directed toward the occlusal surface (Charters position, see Figure 28-4C) to clean over the wire and bracket (or under for mandibular arch); place in Stillman position for the opposite side (Figure 28-4D).
3. *Clean all surfaces.* To ensure cleanliness, one should brush the appliances in any way that the filaments can be manipulated. Insert the brush from below, over, and above the arch wire; rotate and vibrate to remove biofilm and debris.
4. *Lingual and palatal.* Approach to brushing is similar to the basic strokes used on the facial surfaces. When appliances are placed on the lingual or palatal surfaces, the approach to brushing is as shown in Figures 28-3 and 28-4).

D. Additional Measures

1. *Interdental aids.* Tables 28-1 and 28-2 list suggested interdental aids.

    A floss threader is needed for biofilm removal from proximal tooth surfaces when the appliance prevents passage of floss from the occlusal aspect. Tufted dental floss used in the floss threader can remove the biofilm more efficiently than can regular dental floss.

    An interdental brush and a single-tuft brush can be particularly beneficial around individual teeth. The entire system should be kept as simple as possible.

2. *Oral irrigation.* Most patients who wear orthodontic appliances can benefit from the regular use of water irrigation for removal of loose dental biofilm and food debris and prevention of gingival inflammation.

▪ TABLE 28-1 ADVANTAGES AND DISADVANTAGES OF VARIOUS DENTAL BIOFILM CONTROL AIDS

DENTAL BIOFILM CONTROL AIDS	INDICATION FOR USE	ADVANTAGES	DISADVANTAGES
Toothbrushes Manual Orthodontic End-tuft	• Sulcular (Bass) method for the areas adjacent to and beneath the gingival margin • Charters and Stillman brushing methods for cleaning the brackets and archwires on the facial and lingual surfaces • Applied to the surfaces of the tooth above and below brackets, short horizontal brushing stroke • Proximal surfaces adjacent to wide embrasures; used around orthodontic appliances	• Good for biofilm removal on the lingual and facial surfaces at the gingival area • Bilevel shape fits over fixed appliance brackets • Access to areas that are hard to reach with a regular toothbrush • Brush head is small, flat, or tapered in shape	• Improper angulations of the toothbrush can cause tissue trauma • Dexterity challenge • Improper horizontal stroke can cause tissue trauma; used only for orthodontic appliances • Time consuming, an additional aid
Power brushes Power toothbrush	• To facilitate the mechanical removal of dental biofilm; position filaments of the brush as with a manual toothbrush	• The action can be rotational, counter-rotational, or oscillating counter-rotational • Several small brush shapes to accommodate anatomical variations	• Need light, steady pressure to avoid abrasion
Interdental care Dental floss in floss threader Tufted dental floss Interdental brush (Single-tufted brush) Toothpick in holder	• Removal of biofilm from proximal tooth surfaces; indicated for wide embrasures where interdental papilla are missing • Removal of dental biofilm at the gingival margin	• A floss threader can be used for tight contact areas and inserting under the appliance • Cleaning around the appliance and subgingival area of the sulcus	• Requires good dexterity
Irrigators Oral irrigator	• An adjunctive method for the arrest and control of gingivitis • Can be used with antimicrobial agents	• Removal of loose dental biofilm and food debris	• Keep at a low pressure; keep tip at the gingival margin or tissue trauma can occur
Fluoride Self-applied fluoride	• Daily self-application of a rinse or brush-on gel, in addition to daily toothbrushing with fluoride toothpaste	• Prevents demineralization of the enamel and dental caries; acts as a desensitization agent • Surfaces of all teeth	

Adapted from Berglund, L.J. and Small, C.L.: Effective Oral Hygiene for Orthodontic Patients, *J. Clin. Orthod., 14,* 315, May, 1990.

▪ COMPLETION OF THERAPY

At the completion of therapy, patients are excited and are looking forward to the removal of the appliances. They may forget posttreatment instructions that are essential.

With this in mind, the dental hygienist provides written as well as verbal instructions on dental biofilm removal, the fluoride regimen, diet, care of the retainer, and follow-up appointments with the orthodontist and general practitioner. In addition, a description and careful

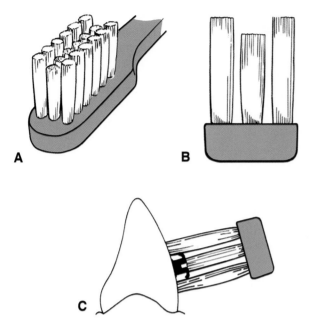

■ **FIGURE 28-3** Orthodontic Bilevel Toothbrush. **(A)** Middle row of filaments trimmed shorter to fit over a fixed appliance. **(B)** Cross section. **(C)** Brush held over a bracket.

explanation of each step in the procedure for debanding and debonding will alleviate patient apprehension about the process.

■ CLINICAL PROCEDURES FOR DEBANDING

I. BAND REMOVAL

Bands are generally removed with orthodontic band-removing pliers. Figure 28-5 shows the armamentarium used in debanding and debonding procedures.
   A. Open the pliers sufficiently to place tips on the apical and coronal portion of the band.
   B. Close the pliers by squeezing on the handle until the band slides off the tooth, as shown in Figure 28-6.

II. CEMENT REMOVAL

Cement remaining on the teeth following band removal is removed with an ultrasonic scaler.

■ CLINICAL PROCEDURES FOR DEBONDING

Mechanical, electrothermal, laser, and ultrasonic methods have been studied in an attempt to determine which method is the most efficient and effective, provides the least

discomfort for the patient, and causes the least damage to enamel.[17-21] Debonding with a CO_2 or YAG laser has shown promise but is still in the experimental stage.[18,22]

I. OBJECTIVES

An ideal debonding technique does not exist. The aim of debonding is to remove the bracket and residual resin with minimal damage to the enamel surface and minimal discomfort for the patient. Scratches and gouges of the enamel surface, as well as fractures of the enamel, have resulted from improperly applied techniques and materials.[1] An efficient and effective procedure is needed to minimize enamel damage.

II. EFFECTS ON ENAMEL

When debonding, each clinician must keep in mind that all the instruments and materials can lead to scratches,

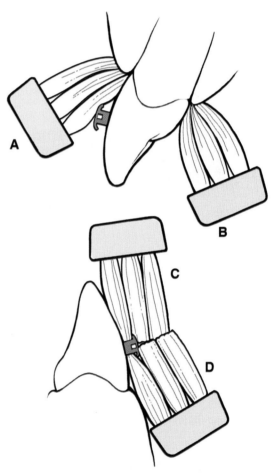

■ **FIGURE 28-4** Toothbrushing for Orthodontic Appliance. **(A)** Sulcular brushing for periodontal tissues. **(B)** Facial surface over bracket. **(C)** Cleaning the bracket using brush in Charters brushing position for the gingival side. **(D)** Brush in Stillman position for occlusal side of bracket and arch wire.

■ TABLE 28-2 RECOMMENDED DENTAL BIOFILM CONTROL AIDS	
I. Surfaces of all teeth	1. Fluoride treatments: daily application of a rinse, paste, or brush-on gel, in addition to professional topical applications 2. Professional fluoride applications
II. Toothbrushes	1. Manual, regular, and orthodontic 2. Power brushes
III. Interdental areas	1. Dental floss in floss threader 2. Tufted dental floss 3. Interdental drush (single-tufted brush) 4. Toothpick in holder
IV. Awkward areas to access Problematic maintenance areas	1. Single-tufted brush 2. Oral irrigation: water for debris removal 3. Oral irrigation with an antimicrobial agent
Adapted from Berglund, L.J. and Small, C.L.: Effective Oral Hygiene for Orthodontic Patients, *J. Clin. Orthod.*, *14*, 315, May, 1990.	

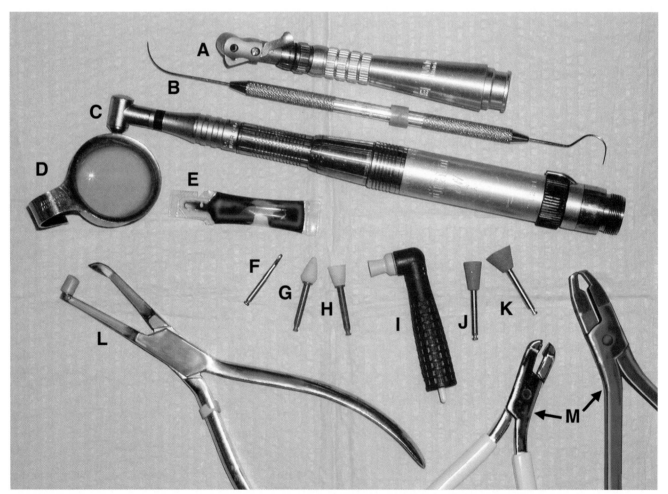

■ **FIGURE 28-5 Debanding and Debonding Armamentarium. (A)** Latch-type prophy angle. **(B)** Explorer. **(C)** Slow-speed handpiece with screw-type prophy angle. **(D)** Pumice slurry. **(E)** Disclosing solution. **(F)** Tapered tungsten-carbide finishing bur. **(G)** Aluminum finishing point. **(H)** Aluminum oxide finishing cup. **(I)** Disposable prophy angle and rubber cup. **(J)** Brown polishing cup. **(K)** Green polishing cup. **(L)** Debanding pliers. **(M)** Debonding pliers.

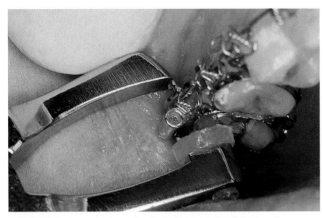

■ FIGURE 28-6 Removal of Molar Band With Band Removal Pliers.

grooves, or other irregularities of the tooth surface and that rotary instruments create heat that affects the pulp. Careful application of the instruments and frequent visual and tactile examination of the surface are necessary.

III. EXPOSURE CONTROL

Debonding procedures may expose the clinician to high levels of aerosol contamination.[23] In one study, use of a preprocedural chlorhexidine rinse was ineffective in reducing the level of microorganisms; therefore, use of standard barriers and high-speed evacuation is necessary.[23]

IV. BRACKET REMOVAL[1,19,24]

A. Technique Objectives

1. Create a fracture within the resin bonding material or between the bracket and the resin.
2. Leave the enamel surface intact.
3. Minimize patient discomfort.
4. Leave the arch wire in position with ligatures or elastomers.
   a. When all brackets have been released, it is safer to remove the entire assemblage together,[25] as shown in Figure 28-7.

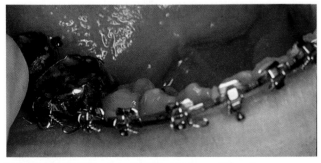

■ FIGURE 28-7 Removal of Brackets and Bands as a Single Unit.

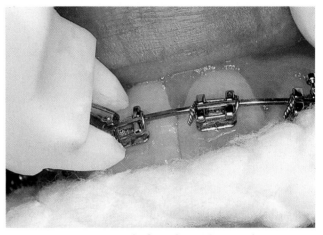

■ FIGURE 28-8 Removal of Bracket Using Bracket-Removal Pliers.

b. Having the brackets remain connected to the arch wire eliminates the threat of the patient swallowing or aspirating a loosened bracket.

B. The "Squeeze-Release" Technique[1,19,24]

1. Use a small pair of pliers with blunt beaks, as shown in Figure 28-8.
2. Apply the beaks to outside edges of the mesial and distal bracket wings (Figure 28-9A).
3. Squeeze the beaks together; do not twist.
   a. The wings bend together and cause the mesial and distal edges of the bracket base to pull away.

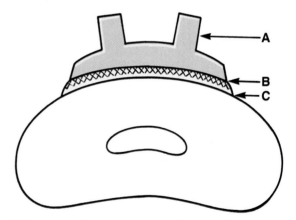

■ FIGURE 28-9 Cross Section of a Bracket. Viewed from the incisal aspect of a tooth. **(A)** Bracket wing. **(B)** Junction of bracket and mesh backing with resin at the adhesive–bracket interface. **(C)** Junction of resin and enamel. (Adapted from Bennett, C.G., Shen, C., and Waldron, J.M.: The Effects of Debonding on the Enamel Surface, *J. Clin. Orthod., 18,* 330, May, 1984.)

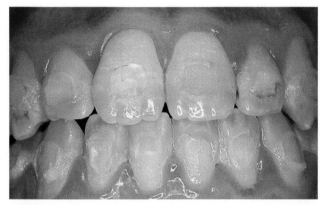

▪ **FIGURE 28-10 Facial View of Anterior Teeth With Adhesive Resin Remaining Following Removal of Orthodontic Brackets.** (Reprinted with permission from Journal of Practical Hygiene. Gutmann, M.E.: Composite Adhesive Resin Removal Following Active Orthodontic Treatment, *J. Pract. Hyg., 5*, 16, May–June, 1996.)

    b.   The break is at the adhesive–bracket interface, thereby leaving the enamel undisturbed.

    c.   Varying amounts of adhesive are left on the tooth surface, as seen in Figure 28-10; some may be attached to the mesh bracket base.

C. Precautions

1.   Mechanical Bracket Removal

Do not twist in a shearing stroke for the following reasons:

    a.   Potential fracture of enamel. The fragile projections of the etched enamel are susceptible to breaking.

    b.   Traumatic for patient. Teeth following orthodontic treatment are usually mobile, and twisting can be painful. Supporting the

tooth with the finger of the nondominant hand or asking the patient to close on a cotton roll to stabilize the tooth will decrease the discomfort.

    c.   Potential damage to periodontal ligament. Twisting stretches the fibers.

2.   Selection and Positioning of Pliers

    a.   Dull pliers are preferred to prevent scratching or gouging.

    b.   Pliers should be positioned for the A and B sites in Figure 28-9 at the adhesive–bracket interface. When cutting pliers are placed between the resin adhesive and the tooth, as shown in Figure 28-9C, and used in a cutting stroke, damage to the enamel can be severe.

V. REMOVAL OF RESIDUAL RESIN ADHESIVE

A. Procedure Objectives

1.   Remove resin bulk.
2.   Minimize damage to pulpal tissue.
3.   Avoid damage to enamel surface.
4.   Prevent excess enamel loss.

B. Examination

Varying amounts of resin remain after the bracket is removed, particularly in normal anatomic grooves, as shown in Figure 28-10. During debonding, frequent examination is necessary using visual and tactile methods. Box 28-2 contains a summary of the steps necessary to completely remove the orthodontic adhesive resin.

1.   Identification of Residual Resin

    a.   Patient reports feeling roughness with the tongue.

BOX 28-2 Steps for Orthodontic Adhesive Resin Removal Using Burs and Polishing Instruments

1. Identify the location and extent of the resin with an explorer, disclosing solution, and patient feedback.

2. Using a tapered, tungsten-carbide finishing bur in a low-speed handpiece, move the bur from the cervical to incisal/occlusal portion of the resin in a light, brushlike stroke.

3. Evaluate progress frequently by rinsing and drying the tooth surfaces.

4. Polish each surface with aluminum oxide polishing points followed by aluminum oxide polishing cups.

5. Use a rubber cup in a slow-speed handpiece to polish each surface with a fine pumice slurry. Use intermittent strokes.

6. Use a brown polishing cup in a slow-speed handpiece to polish the enamel surfaces.

7. Use a green polishing cup in a slow-speed handpiece to provide the final finish to the enamel surfaces.

b. Visual. When dry, the resin appears dull and opaque compared with clean, shiny enamel. Use of disclosing solution will also enhance the visibility of the adhesive resin remnant.[26]

c. Tactile. Application of an explorer reveals a rough surface, sometimes with catches along the margin of a resin tag. Filler particles from the resin may abrade the metal explorer tip, leaving a gray line on the resin surface.

2. *Use of Loupes for Magnification of the Tooth Surface.* A more accurate evaluation of the enamel surface can be made.

C. Removal of Resin From Tooth Surface[26,27]

1. *Bur selection.* Use a tapered, plain-cut, tungsten-carbide finishing bur with a low-speed handpiece, as illustrated in Figure 28-11.

2. *Speed.* Use low speed to control heat.

3. *Stroke.* Use a smooth, evenly applied, light brush stroke in one direction to prevent faceting.

4. *Direction.* Work systematically from cervical portion of the resin; move toward incisal or occlusal third. When removed, the resin resembles fine white shavings, as seen in Figure 28-12.

5. *Evaluate frequently* to prevent overinstrumentation, rinse frequently, dry, and evaluate the surface. The resin will appear opaque in contrast to the glossy enamel. Reapply disclosing solution as necessary to visualize small remaining resin particles. Patients may also be helpful in identifying resin remnants with their tongues.

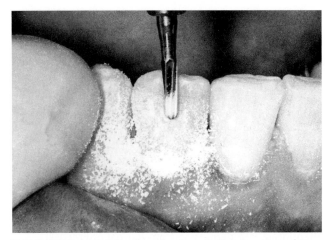

■ **FIGURE 28-12 Adhesive Shavings Following Use of Bur.** (Reprinted with permission from Journal of Dental Hygiene. Gutmann, M.: Debonding Orthodontic Adhesives, *J. Dent. Hyg., 59,* 369, August, 1985.)

D. Final Finish

1. Objective
   Restore pretreatment enamel surface finish.

2. Examination
   a. Perform visual and tactile examination to distinguish areas of normal enamel from irregularities.
   b. Request patients to examine their teeth by slowly sliding the tongue over the enamel surfaces.

3. Application of Aluminum Oxide Finishing Points and Cups[17,26,27]
   a. Use the finishing points first to remove any fine scarring resulting from the burs (Figure 28-13).

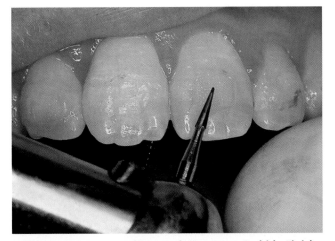

■ **FIGURE 28-11 Use of Tapered, Tungsten-Carbide Finishing Bur on Low-Speed Handpiece to Remove Bulk of Adhesive Resin.** (Reprinted with permission from Journal of Practical Hygiene. Gutmann, M.E.: Composite Adhesive Resin Removal Following Active Orthodontic Treatment, *J. Pract. Hyg., 5,* 16, May–June, 1996.)

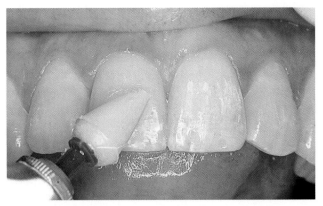

■ **FIGURE 28-13 Aluminum Oxide Finishing Point to Remove Any Enamel Scarring Resulting From Bur.** (Reprinted with permission from Journal of Practical Hygiene. Gutmann, M.E.: Composite Adhesive Resin Removal Following Active Orthodontic Treatment, *J. Pract. Hyg., 5,* 16, May–June, 1996.)

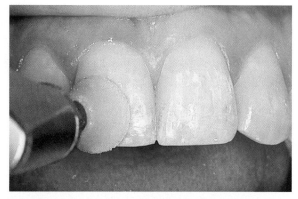

▪ FIGURE 28-14 Aluminum Oxide Finishing Cup to Remove Any Enamel Scarring Resulting From Bur. (Reprinted with permission from Journal of Practical Hygiene. Gutmann, M.E.: Composite Adhesive Resin Removal Following Active Orthodontic Treatment, *J. Pract. Hyg., 5,* 16, May–June, 1996.)

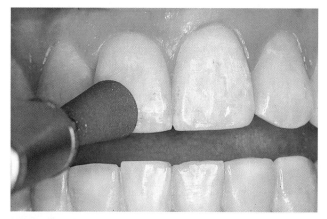

▪ FIGURE 28-16 Brown Polishing Cup Provides Maximum Gloss to Enamel Surface. (Reprinted with permission from Journal of Practical Hygiene. Gutmann, M.E.: Composite Adhesive Resin Removal Following Active Orthodontic Treatment, *J. Pract. Hyg., 5,* 16, May–June, 1996.)

    b.   Use a low-speed handpiece.
    c.   Follow with aluminum oxide cups and move from area to area in a cervical to incisal/occlusal direction (Figure 28-14).
  4. Application of the Rubber Cup
    a.   Use a fine pumice water slurry, as seen in Figure 28-15.
    b.   Polish in a wet field to prevent overheating.
    c.   Use intermittent strokes to avoid overheating and move from tooth to tooth.
  5. Final Polish
Use brown followed by green polishing cups to produce a natural-appearing, glossy enamel surface (Figures 28-16 and 28-17.[27]

▪ POST-DEBONDING EVALUATION

Each step of bonding and debonding has a deleterious effect on the enamel surface. Realization that the enamel surface can be damaged can help the clinician avoid unnecessary trauma during the various procedures.

I. ENAMEL LOSS

- Total enamel loss from etching, bracket removal, residual resin removal, surface finishing, and application of pumice averages approximately 30

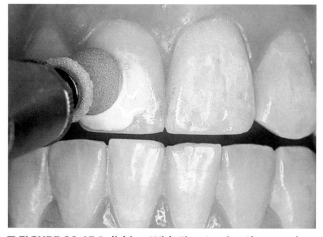

▪ FIGURE 28-15 Polishing With Fine Pumice Slurry and Rubber Cup. (Reprinted with permission from Journal of Practical Hygiene. Gutmann, M.E.: Composite Adhesive Resin Removal Following Active Orthodontic Treatment, *J. Pract. Hyg., 5,* 16, May–June, 1996.)

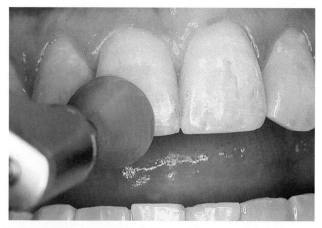

▪ FIGURE 28-17 Final Polishing With Green Polishing Cup. (Reprinted with permission from Journal of Practical Hygiene. Gutmann, M.E.: Composite Adhesive Resin Removal Following Active Orthodontic Treatment, *J. Pract. Hyg., 5,* 16, May–June, 1996.)

to 100 μm.[13,22,28,29] One laboratory study reported an average loss of enamel of only 7.4 μm with careful use of a tungsten-carbide finishing bur.[30]

- Enamel loss is greater when filled resins (composites) are used for bonding than when unfilled resins are used. The loss is also greater when a rotating bristle brush rather than a rubber cup is used with the abrasive for finishing.
- The outer layer of enamel is the most significant. The fluoride-rich surface enamel is approximately 50 μm deep. Therefore, the entire protective layer can be removed.
- When multiple bonding and debonding procedures are done, such as when a bracket becomes detached, the enamel loss is compounded. As much as 72 μm of enamel may be lost during a complete multiple procedure.[29]
- The need for careful selection of instruments and abrasives, along with minimal instrumentation, to prevent unnecessary enamel loss is apparent.

II. DEMINERALIZATION (WHITE SPOTS)

- White spots or dental caries have been relatively common findings after orthodontic treatment.
- Patients with teeth that have been banded or bonded tend to develop the spots significantly more often than do patients who have not had orthodontic therapy.
- Dental biofilm retention on the appliances and the resin, along with the difficulty of biofilm removal by the patient, contribute to demineralization and dental caries.

III. ETCHED ENAMEL NOT COVERED BY ADHESIVE

- Surface areas etched but not covered with adhesive resin become remineralized when the fluoride contact is high through personal and professional applications.
- Etched enamel has a high fluoride uptake.

■ RETENTION

After fixed appliances have been removed, a retainer is worn to give support to the teeth while the bone and other supporting tissues are stabilizing. One type of removable retainer is the Hawley appliance, shown in Figure 28-18. The use of a retainer provides another source for retention of dental biofilm. Special instruction for care and cleaning of a retainer is needed. General procedures are suggested here.

- Clean the appliance after each meal and before retiring. Instructions for cleaning procedures and

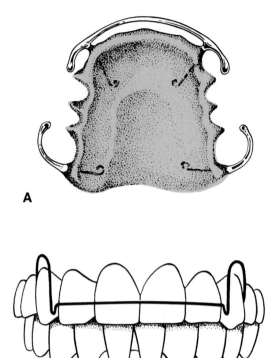

A

B

■ **FIGURE 28-18 Hawley Retainer. (A)** Removable acrylic retainer with facial retaining wire and clasps to be worn after removal of a fixed orthodontic appliance. **(B)** Anterior view shows a Hawley appliance in position. The method for cleaning the appliance is similar to that for cleaning a removable denture.

agents for removable appliances are described with the care of the removable denture (pages 474 to 475).

- Brush and rinse teeth and gingival tissue under the appliance each time the appliance is removed. Unless necessary as directed by the orthodontist, the health of the underlying tissues is best maintained when the appliance is not kept in the mouth continuously.
- Brush the mucosa under the appliance. Methods are described on pages 480 to 481.
- Keep appliance in a container with water when it is out of the mouth.

■ POST-DEBONDING PREVENTIVE CARE

I. PERIODONTAL EVALUATION

A complete examination with careful probing and charting is necessary because many changes take place during treatment. Calculus removal should be completed as

Everyday Ethics

? Dorothy, a patient who had recently completed orthodontic therapy, presents for a maintenance appointment with Caroline, the dental hygienist in her general dentist's practice. The facial surfaces of tooth numbers 4-13 and 20-29 appear to harbor remnants of composite adhesive resin.

Caroline, the dental hygienist, feels an obligation to remove these adhesive remnants but does not want to make any disparaging comments about the orthodontist, who should have removed the adhesive. There is not enough time to remove all of the resin and complete the exam, prophylaxis, and radiographs at the current appointment.

Questions for Consideration

1. Applying the principle of veracity, what obligation does Caroline have to tell Dorothy about the remaining adhesive resin on her teeth?

2. To maintain Dorothy's trust in her orthodontist, how can Caroline inform the patient of the accretions and explain the need for additional appointments?

3. Explain the treatment options that Caroline can consider, while keeping in mind the best interest of the patient.

needed. Clinical photographs assist the patient in comparing gingival tissue changes and teeth before and after disclosing agent application for documentation and patient instruction.

II. DENTAL CARIES

- Examination for demineralization (white spots) and dental caries is essential.
- Dental biofilm retention by orthodontic appliances can be extensive. The configurations of the appliances make biofilm control efforts by the patient extremely difficult. Biofilm collects on brackets and some resins even when the patient's oral hygiene is generally good.[5]
- Composite resin may be left on the tooth surface around the bracket. The surface of resins is difficult to make smooth; thus, biofilm collects.

✔ Factors To Teach The Patient

- The significance of dental biofilm around orthodontic appliances and the teeth.

- How to apply the toothbrush and adjunctive devices to remove dental biofilm from the bracket, the arch wire, and the teeth.

- How, when, and why to use fluoride rinses, toothpastes, and brush-on gels.

- The frequency for professional follow-up during and after orthodontic therapy.

- The bacteria of the biofilm, not the rough surface, cause the gingival inflammatory response and the white spots, or demineralization.

III. FLUORIDE THERAPY[31]

- A complete program of fluoride treatments, professionally applied at frequent maintenance appointments and used by the patient on a daily basis, is prerequisite both during and following orthodontic therapy.
- Application of a fluoride varnish immediately following bonding also can help to reduce demineralization by up to 50%.[32]
- With the loss of the fluoride-rich enamel surface during bonding and debonding procedures, the need for remineralization and replenishment of fluoride is clear.

REFERENCES

1. **Zachrisson**, B.U.: Bonding in Orthodontics, in Graber, T.M. and Vanarsdall, R.L.: *Orthodontics, Current Principles and Techniques,* 3rd ed. St. Louis, Mosby, 2000, pp. 557–639.

2. **David**, V.A., Staley, R.N., Bigelow, H.F., and Jakobsen, J.R.: Remnant Amount and Cleanup for 3 Adhesives after Debracketing, *Am J Orthod Dentofacial Orthop., 121,* 291, March, 2002.

3. **Osorio**, R., Toledano, M., and Garcia-Godoy, F.: Bracket Bonding With 15- or 60-Second Etching and Adhesive Remaining on Enamel After Debonding, *Angle Orthod., 69,* 45, February, 1999.

4. **American Dental Association**, Council on Dental Materials, Instruments, and Equipment: Ceramic Orthodontic Brackets: How and When to Use Them, *J. Am. Dent. Assoc., 123,* 243, July, 1992.

5. **Gwinnett**, A.J. and Ceen, R.F.: Plaque Distribution on Bonded Brackets: A Scanning Microscopic Study, *Am. J. Orthod., 75,* 667, June, 1979.

6. **Zachrisson**, B.U. and Brobakken, B.O.: Clinical Comparison of Direct Versus Indirect Bonding With Different Bracket Types and Adhesives, *Am. J. Orthod., 74*, 62, July, 1978.

7. **Gwinnett**, A.J., for the American Dental Association, Council on Dental Materials, Instruments, and Equipment: State of the Art and Science of Bonding in Orthodontic Treatment, *J. Am. Dent. Assoc., 105*, 844, November, 1982.

8. **Proffit**, W.R.: *Contemporary Orthodontics,* 2nd ed. St. Louis, Mosby, 1993, pp. 353–357.

9. **Zachrisson**, B.U., Skogan, Ö., and Höymyhr, S.: Enamel Cracks in Debonded, Debanded, and Orthodontically Untreated Teeth, *Am. J. Orthod., 77*, 307, March, 1980.

10. **Lindauer**, S.J., Browning, H., Shroff, B., Marshall, F., Anderson, R.H., and Moon, P.C.: Effect of Pumice Prophylaxis on the Bond Strength of Orthodontic Brackets, *Am. J. Orthod. Dentofacial Orthop., 111*, 599, June, 1997.

11. **Buonocore**, M.G., Matsui, A., and Gwinnett, A.J.: Penetration of Resin Dental Materials Into Enamel Surfaces With Reference to Bonding, *Arch. Oral Biol., 13*, 61, January, 1968.

12. **Retief**, D.H.: Effect of Conditioning the Enamel Surface With Phosphoric Acid, *J. Dent. Res., 52*, 333, March–April, 1973.

13. **Diedrich**, P.: Enamel Alterations From Bracket Bonding and Debonding: A Study With the Scanning Electron Microscope, *Am. J. Orthod., 79*, 500, May, 1981.

14. **Chan**, D.C.N., Swift, E.J., and Bishara, S.E.: *In Vitro* Evaluation of a Fluoride-releasing Orthodontic Resin, *J. Dent. Res., 69*, 1576, September, 1990.

15. **Bishara**, S.E., Swift, E.J., and Chan, D.C.N.: Evaluation of Fluoride Release From an Orthodontic Bonding System, *Am. J. Orthod. Dentofacial Orthop., 100*, 106, August, 1991.

16. **Basdra**, E.K., Huber, H., and Komposch, G.: Fluoride Released from Orthodontic Bonding Agents Alters the Enamel Surface and Inhibits Enamel Demineralization in Vitro, *Am. J. Orthod. Dentofacial Orthop., 109*, 466, May, 1996.

17. **Osorio**, R., Toledano, M., and Garcia-Godoy, F.: Enamel Surface Morphology after Bracket Debonding, *J. Dent. Child., 65*, 313, September–October, 1998.

18. **Smith**, S.C., Walsh, L.J., and Taverne, A.A.: Removal of Orthodontic Bonding Resin Residues by CO2 Laser Radiation: Surface Effects, *J. Clin. Laser Med. Surg., 17*, 13, February, 1999.

19. **Everett**, M.S.: Debonding Orthodontic Adhesives, *Dent. Hyg., 59*, 364, August, 1985.

20. **Bishara**, S.E. and Trulove, T.S.: Comparisons of Different Debonding Techniques for Ceramic Brackets: An In Vitro Study. Part I. Background and Methods, *Am. J. Orthod. Dentofacial Orthop., 98*, 145, August, 1990.

21. **Bishara**, S.E. and Trulove, T.S.: Comparisons of Different Debonding Techniques for Ceramic Brackets: An In Vitro Study. Part II. Findings and Clinical Implications, *Am. J. Orthod. Dentofacial Orthop., 98*, 263, September, 1990.

22. **Bishara**, S.E. and Fehr, D.E.: Ceramic Brackets: Something Old, Something New, a Review, *Semin. Orthod., 3*, 178, September, 1997.

23. **Toroglu**, M.S., Haytaç, M.C., and Köksal, F.: Evaluation of Aerosol Contamination During Debonding Procedures, *Angle Orthod., 71*, 299, August, 2001.

24. **Bennett**, C.G., Shen, C., and Waldron, J.M.: The Effects of Debonding on the Enamel Surface, *J. Clin. Orthod., 18*, 330, May, 1984.

25. **Koo**, B.C. and Chung, C.H.: A Safer Debonding/Debanding Technique, *J. Clin. Orthod., 32*, 374, June, 1998.

26. **Gutmann**, M.E.: Composite Adhesive Resin Removal Following Orthodontic Treatment, *J. Pract. Hyg., 5*, 16, May–June, 1996.

27. **Campbell**, P.M.: Enamel Surfaces After Orthodontic Bracket Debonding, *Angle Orthod., 65*, 103, Number 2, 1995.

28. **Pus**, M.D. and Way, D.C.: Enamel Loss Due to Orthodontic Bonding With Filled and Unfilled Resins Using Various Clean-up Techniques, *Am. J. Orthod., 77*, 269, March, 1980.

29. **Thompson**, R.E. and Way, D.C.: Enamel Loss Due to Prophylaxis and Multiple Bonding/Debonding of Orthodontic Attachments, *Am. J. Orthod., 79*, 282, March, 1981.

30. **van Waes**, H., Matter, T., and Krejci, I.: Three-Dimensional Measurement of Enamel Loss Caused by Bonding and Debonding of Orthodontic Brackets, *Am. J. Orthod. Dentofacial Orthop., 112*, 666, December, 1997.

31. **Boyd**, R.L.: Comparison of Three Self-applied Topical Fluoride Preparations for Control of Demineralization, *Angle Orthod., 63*, 25, Spring, 1993.

32. **Todd**, M.A., Staley, R.N., Kanellis, M.J., Donly, K.J., and Wefel, J.S.: Effect of a Fluoride Varnish on Demineralization Adjacent to Orthodontic Brackets, *Am. J. Orthod. Dentofacial Orthop., 116*, 159, August, 1999.

SUGGESTED READINGS

Bensch, L., Braem, M., Van Acker, K., and Willems, G.: Orthodontic Treatment Considerations in Patients With Diabetes Mellitus, *Am. J. Orthod. Dentofacial Orthop., 123*, 74, January, 2003.

Bowman, S.J.: Use of a Fluoride Varnish to Reduce Demineralization, *J. Clin. Orthodont., 34*, 377, June, 2000.

Boyd, R.L. and Baumrind, S.: Periodontal Considerations in the Use of Bonds or Bands on Molars in Adolescents and Adults, *Angle Orthod., 62*, 117, Summer, 1992.

Carstensen, W.: Direct Bonding With Reduced Acid Etchant Concentrations, *J. Clin. Orthod., 27*, 23, January, 1993.

Flores, D.A., Caruso, J.M., Scott, G.E., and Jeiroudi, M.T.: The Fracture Strength of Ceramic Brackets: A Comparative Study, *Angle Orthod., 60*, 269, Winter, 1990.

Frazier, M.C., Southard, T.E., and Doster, P.M.: Prevention of Enamel Demineralization During Orthodontic Treatment: An In Vitro Study Using Pit and Fissure Sealants, *Am. J. Orthod. Dentofacial Orthop., 110*, 459, November, 1996.

Gorton, J. and Featherstone, J.D.B.: In Vivo Inhibition of Demineralization Around Orthodontic Brackets, *Am. J. Orthod. Dentofacial Orthop., 123*, 10, January, 2003.

Gwinnett, A.J. and Gorelik, L.: Microscopic Evaluation of Enamel After Debonding: Clinical Application, *Am. J. Orthod., 71*, 651, June, 1977.

Howell, S. and Weekes, W.T.: An Electron Microscopic Evaluation of the Enamel Surface Subsequent to Various Debonding Procedures, *Aust. Dent. J., 35*, 245, June, 1990.

Øgaard, B., Rezk-Lega, F., Ruben, J., and Arends, J.: Cariostatic Effect and Fluoride Release From a Visible Light-Curing Adhesive for Bonding of Orthodontic Brackets, *Am. J. Orthod. Dentofacial Orthop., 101*, 303, April, 1992.

Staggers, J.A. and Margeson, D.: The Effects of Sterilization on the Tensile Strength of Orthodontic Wires, *Angle Orthod., 63*, 141, Summer, 1993.

Debonding Procedures

Bishara, S.E. and Fehr, D.E.: Comparisons of the Effectiveness of Pliers With Narrow and Wide Blades in Debonding Ceramic Brackets, *Am. J. Orthod. Dentofacial Orthop., 103*, 253, March, 1993.

Chate, R.A.C.: Safer Orthodontic Debonding With Rubber Dam, *Am. J. Orthod. Dentofacial Orthop., 103*, 171, February, 1993.

Gorbach, N.R.: Heat Removal of Ceramic Brackets, *J. Clin. Orthod., 25*, 247, April, 1991.

Herzberg, R.: A New Polishing System for Enhanced Esthetics after Debonding, *J. Clin. Orthod., 34*, 542, September, 2000.

Krell, K.V., Courey, J.M., and Bishara, S.E.: Orthodontic Bracket Removal Using Conventional and Ultrasonic Debonding Techniques, Enamel Loss, and Time Requirements, *Am. J. Orthod. Dentofacial Orthop., 103,* 258, March, 1993.

Oliver, R.G. and Griffiths, J.: Different Techniques of Residual Composite Removal Following Debonding: Time Taken and Surface Enamel Appearance, *Br. J. Orthod., 19,* 131, May, 1992.

Radlanski, R.J.: A New Carbide Finishing Bur for Bracket Debonding, *J. Orofac. Orthop., 62,* 296, July, 2001.

Rinchuse, D.J.: Pain-free Debonding With Occlusal Rim Wax, *J. Clin. Orthod., 28,* 587, October, 1994.

Sheets, C.G. and Paquette, J.M.: Postorthodontic Restoration of Enamel Surface Characteristics, *Signature, 4,* 1, Fall, 1997.

Strobl, K., Bahns, T.L., Willham, L., Bishara, S.E., and Stwalley, W.C.: Laser-Aided Debonding of Orthodontic Ceramic Brackets, *Am. J. Orthod. Dentofacial Orthop., 101,* 152, February, 1992.

Tocchio, R.M., Williams, P.T., Mayer, F.J., and Standing, K.G.: Laser Debonding of Ceramic Orthodontic Brackets, *Am. J. Orthod. Dentofacial Orthop., 103,* 155, February, 1993.

Turner, P.J.: Trouble-Free Debonding in Orthodontics: 2, *Dent. Update, 23,* 426, December, 1996.

Care of Dental Prostheses

Kathryn Ragalis, RDH, MS, DMD

Total cleanliness of the oral cavity for the health of the teeth and supporting structures involves specific procedures for the care of the natural teeth and all replacements, both fixed and removable. A *prosthesis* is an artificial replacement of a missing part of the body, and a dental prosthesis replaces one or more teeth. Other definitions may be studied in Box 29-1.

The fit and function of a dental prosthesis depend to a large degree on the cooperation of the patient in daily cleaning of the prosthesis and dental biofilm control for the remaining natural teeth. In turn, the patient's cooperation depends on the motivation, information, and sense of appreciation and concern imparted by the members of the dental team. For the natural teeth involved, instruction begins early, before construction of the prosthesis. When the appliance is inserted, instruction is supplemented to show specific techniques for daily care. Continuing supervision and review of procedures at succeeding appointments and during maintenance are needed.

BOX 29-1 KEY WORDS: Dental Prostheses*

Abutment: a tooth or implant used for the support or retention of a fixed or removable prosthesis.

Denture: artificial substitute for missing natural teeth and adjacent tissues.

> **Complete denture:** dental prosthesis that replaces the entire dentition and associated structures; may be a complete maxillary denture or a complete mandibular, or both.

> **Immediate denture:** a complete or removable partial denture fabricated in advance for placement immediately following the removal of natural teeth.

> **Fixed partial denture:** a replacement for one or more missing teeth that is securely retained to natural teeth and/or dental implant abutments that furnish the primary support for the prosthesis; also called a fixed prosthesis or bridge.

> **Removable partial denture:** a dental prosthesis that supplies teeth and/or associated structures in a partially edentulous jaw and can be removed and replaced at will.

Denture adhesive: a soft material used to adhere a denture to the underlying mucosa; also referred to as an adherent.

Obturator: a prosthesis used to close a congenital or acquired opening, such as for a cleft palate, an area lost because of trauma, or after surgery for removal of a diseased area.

Pontic: an artificial tooth on a partial denture that replaces a missing natural tooth, restores its function, and usually occupies the space previously filled by the natural crown.

Precision attachment: a type of connector that consists of a metal receptacle and a close-fitting part; the metal receptacle usually is included within the restoration of an abutment tooth, and the close-fitting part is attached to a pontic or removable partial denture framework.

Prosthesis: artificial replacement of an absent part of the body; may be a therapeutic device to improve or alter function; may be a device employed to aid in accomplishing a desired surgical result.

Rest: a rigid, stabilizing extension of a fixed or removable partial denture that contacts a remaining tooth or teeth; prevents movement toward the mucosa and transmits functional forces to the teeth.

*Definitions in this chapter that pertain to prosthodontics are taken or adapted from and are in accord with the *Glossary of Prosthodontic Terms,* 7th ed., 1999, of the Academy of Prosthodontics Foundation.

A patient may have more than one prosthesis. For example, a complete maxillary denture may be accompanied by both fixed and removable partial dentures in the mandibular arch. For this patient, the regimen for personal care involves the natural teeth as well as the fixed and removable dentures. A program of instruction must be worked out for each patient, depending on individual needs. Examples of fixed and removable prostheses and appliances are listed in Box 29-2.

▪ FIXED PARTIAL DENTURES

I. DESCRIPTION

Fixed partial dentures, commonly called dental *bridges,* are composed of abutments, connectors, and pontics, as shown in Figure 29-1.

II. CHARACTERISTICS

A. Types of Fixed Partial Dentures

1. *Natural Tooth Supported*
   - Bilateral: Supported by one or more natural teeth at each end (Figure 29-1A).
   - Cantilever: Pontic supported by one or more teeth at one end only (Figure 29-1B).
   - Resin-bonded cast metal bridge: Uses resin-bonded retainer attached to etched enamel; characterized by little or no removal of tooth structure. Also called a Maryland bridge.
2. *Implant Supported*
   - Shown in Figure 29-1C.
   - Blade, cylinder, and screw types of implants used for abutments are shown in Figure 30-5.

BOX 29-2 Types of Oral Prostheses and Appliances

FIXED

Fixed partial denture

Periodontal splint

Implant-supported complete denture

Orthodontic appliance

Space maintainer

REMOVABLE

Removable partial denture

    Natural tooth supported

    Implant supported

Complete denture

Overdenture

Obturator

Removable orthodontic appliance

Removable space maintainer

Hawley appliance

B. Criteria for Fixed Partial Denture[1]

- Biologically and aesthetically harmonious with the teeth and surrounding periodontium.
- All parts accessible for cleaning by the patient and the dental professional.
- Must not interfere with the cleaning regimen for the remaining natural dentition.
- Must not traumatize oral tissues.
- Restores function for missing tooth or teeth.

▪ CARE PROCEDURES FOR THE FIXED PROSTHESIS

I. DEBRIS REMOVAL

- When suggesting a procedure for the patient to follow for cleaning the oral cavity when a fixed partial denture is present, debris removal with an oral irrigator may be recommended as a first step.
- By removing food and debris, access of the toothbrush and other aids for biofilm removal is facilitated.
- Procedure for use of an oral irrigator is described on pages 445–447.

II. BIOFILM REMOVAL FROM ABUTMENT TEETH

- Nearly all the methods proposed for dental biofilm control in Chapters 25 and 26 may be applicable to abutment teeth.
- The proximal surface of an abutment tooth and the gingiva adjacent to a pontic require special attention.

A. Toothbrushing

- Sulcular brushing is generally indicated.

B. Dentifrice Selection

- A *nonabrasive* dentifrice is indicated to prevent the possibility of abrasion when pontic or crown facings are made of acrylic, when the gold of the partial denture is highly polished and could be scratched, and when areas of root are exposed on abutment teeth.

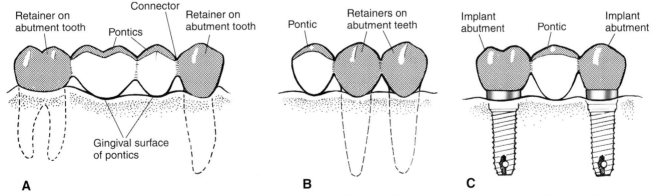

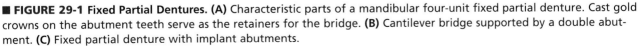

■ FIGURE 29-1 Fixed Partial Dentures. (A) Characteristic parts of a mandibular four-unit fixed partial denture. Cast gold crowns on the abutment teeth serve as the retainers for the bridge. **(B)** Cantilever bridge supported by a double abutment. **(C)** Fixed partial denture with implant abutments.

- *A fluoride-containing* dentifrice is important for protection of remaining tooth surfaces, particularly exposed cementum. Acidulated fluoride preparations are contraindicated for porcelain and composite restorations.[2]

C. Additional Interdental Care

- An interdental biofilm removal method is indicated.
- The method is selected on the basis of the individual patient and the prosthesis.
- The interdental cleaning device is adapted specifically to the distal surface of the mesial abutment and the mesial surface of the distal abutment, and from both facial and lingual aspects.
- The same interdental cleaning procedure usually can be applied to the gingival surface of the fixed partial denture.
- Interdental cleaning methods and devices are described on pages 429 to 436.

III. THE PROSTHESIS

A. Areas Requiring Emphasis

- Margins of the restorations may provide slight irregular areas for retaining biofilm and require the greatest attention.
- The gingival surfaces of the pontics and beneath the connectors are particularly prone to biofilm retention.

B. Toothbrushing

- A toothbrush in the Charters position may be helpful for cleaning the gingival surface of the pontic from the facial aspect.
- The filaments can be directed under the pontic to clean the gingival surface.
- Charters brush position is described on page 413.

C. Dental Floss in Threader

Tufted dental floss is most efficient for cleaning a fixed partial denture. As shown in Figure 26-6, two types are available.

1. *Floss threader*
   - Thread a 12- to 15-inch length into a floss threader. Several types are available and are shown in Figure 29-2.
   - Apply threader between abutment and pontic.
   - Draw the floss through, and using single or double thickness, remove loose debris, as in Figure 29-3.
   - Apply a new section of the floss with moderate pressure to the undersurface (gingival sur-

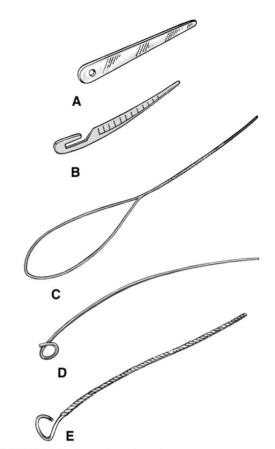

■ **FIGURE 29-2 Floss Threaders. (A)** Clear plastic with closed eye. **(B)** Tinted plastic with open eye. **(C)** Soft plastic loop. **(D)** Flexible wire. **(E)** Twisted wire.

face) of the pontic and then to the proximal surfaces of each abutment tooth to remove the biofilm.

2. *"Super floss"*
   - Available in 2-foot length with a tufted segment.
   - Has a stiffened end for threading.
   - Use in same manner as described above for floss threader.

D. Knitting Yarn

- Place length of synthetic yarn in floss threader.
- Apply under pontic and to abutment surfaces as described for floss and tufted floss.
- Figure 26-7 shows floss and yarn applied to proximal surfaces.

E. Other Interdental Devices

- An interdental brush shown in Figure 26-9 and a single-tuft brush shown in Figure 26-11 can be recommended and demonstrated as

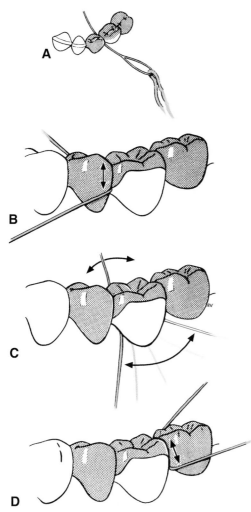

■ **FIGURE 29-3 Use of Floss Threader. (A)** Use floss threader to draw the floss (or yarn or tufted floss) between abutment and pontic. **(B)** Apply floss to the distal surface of the mesial abutment; pull through 1 or 2 inches. **(C)** Slide floss under pontic. Move back and forth several times, as shown by the arrows, to remove dental biofilm from the gingival surface of the pontic. **(D)** Apply new section of floss to the mesial surface of the distal abutment.

indicated by the requirements of the individual prosthesis.

- Interdental brushes may fit mesial and distal to the pontic and should not be forced to enter.

■ REMOVABLE PARTIAL DENTURES

I. DESCRIPTION

- A removable partial denture replaces one or more, but less than all, of the natural teeth and associated structures.

- It can be removed from the mouth and replaced at will.
- The denture base rests on the oral mucosa and carries the artificial teeth.

II. TYPES

- Depending on the location and number of remaining natural teeth, a partial denture may receive all its support from the teeth, or it may be partly tooth borne and partly tissue borne.
- The base is most frequently made of plastic acrylic resin, but alloys of gold or chrome have also been used.
- The teeth may be made of porcelain, plastic resin, or metal.
- The basic parts of a removable partial denture are shown in Figure 29-4 and defined in Box 29-1.

III. CHARACTERISTICS

- Self-care procedures for the patient with a removable prosthesis involve much more than cleaning the prosthesis.
- The abutment teeth, the gingival tissue, and the mucosa of edentulous areas require regular attention.
- Gingival health is unfavorably affected by a removable partial denture because biofilm tends to accumulate more readily and in greater quantities.
- Biofilm control is a major factor in maintaining the long-term effectiveness of abutment teeth for a removable partial denture.
- All removable appliances can be labeled for identification purposes. Methods of identification are described on pages 846 to 848.

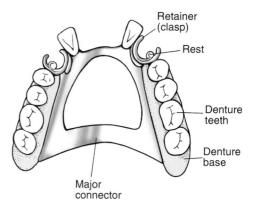

■ **FIGURE 29-4 Removable Partial Denture.** Components of a removable partial denture shown for a maxillary prosthesis.

IV. REMOVAL

It is usually most comfortable to ask the patient to remove the prosthesis because the patient is familiar with the path of insertion. When a patient is unable to remove the appliance, the dental hygienist proceeds as follows:

- Exert an even pressure on both sides of the denture simultaneously as the clasps are lifted over their abutment teeth.
- Usually, the line of insertion and removal of a partial denture is designed and constructed for an even, vertical movement.

V. RECEIVING A DENTURE

Prevent cross-contamination when receiving a removable prosthesis from a patient by:

- Wearing personal protective mask, eyewear, and gloves.
- Offering a container or disposable napkin in which the patient can place the prosthesis directly.
- Rinsing the prosthesis under slowing running water; taking care not to splash.
- Using ultrasonic cleaner.

■ CARE PROCEDURES FOR THE REMOVABLE PARTIAL PROSTHESIS

- The selection of cleansing agents and the procedures for cleaning are complicated by the intricacy of the metallic parts and their relation to the natural teeth, as well as by the dental materials used in construction.
- Rinsing, immersing, and brushing methods, as well as the cleansing agents described for the complete denture on pages 477 to 480, apply alike to various other removable prosthesis.
- Examples: removable space maintainers; appliances for orthodontic purposes, such as a Hawley biteplate or retainer; and obturators for closure of palatal openings, such as for cleft palate or for replacement of tissue removed in the treatment of oral cancer.
- After each meal, and at bedtime, the denture and the natural teeth should be cleaned.

I. OBJECTIVES FOR THE PATIENT

- Because natural teeth are adjacent to the prosthesis, objectives for cleaning the prosthesis take on added significance.

- The basic objectives are to remove irritants to the oral tissues (primarily biofilm), prevent mouth odors, and improve appearance.
- The objective for the natural teeth is to control biofilm for the prevention of dental caries and periodontal infection.

II. THE PROSTHESIS

A. Rinsing

- When regular cleaning facilities are not available, rinsing is important for both the natural teeth and the removable prosthesis.
- Partial denture is removed, the mouth is rinsed with water, and the denture is rinsed under running water. The method for rinsing the mouth is outlined in Box 27-5.
- Rinsing does not remove biofilm that is attached firmly, so it cannot be a substitute for complete care procedures.

B. Brushing

Precautions need to be taken during brushing a removable partial denture:

- Too tight a grasp of a partial prosthesis can result in bending or fracture of clasps or bars.
- Filaments of a brush can inadvertently catch the prosthesis and cause it to drop and break.
- Partial filling of the sink with water or lining of the sink with a face cloth or towel is necessary to prevent accidents that cause breakage should the prosthesis be dropped.

C. Types of Brushes

1. *Toothbrush*
   - The use of a regular toothbrush for care of a removable prosthesis is not recommended.
   - When a patient chooses to do so, however, a separate brush is definitely indicated.
   - Brushing the clasps and other metal parts can deform the filaments and make the brush ineffective for use on the natural teeth.
2. *Power Brush*
   - Should not be used on a removable prosthesis because of the danger of catching the brush and damaging the prosthesis.
   - May be appropriate for use on the natural teeth.
3. *Clasp Brush*
   - A specially designed narrow, tapered brush about 2 to 3 inches long that can be adapted to the inner surfaces of clasps is recommended (Figure 29-5).

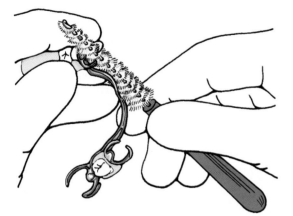

▪ FIGURE 29-5 Clasp Brush. A brush specially designed to remove dental biofilm from the inside surfaces of clasps is available. The denture must be held carefully to avoid accidents.

- Difficult-to-clean areas require special care because clasps and their connectors are closely adapted to the supporting teeth, and the protected internal surfaces are prone to biofilm accumulation.
4. *Denture Brush*
   - A denture brush is described on page 478.
   - It is an excellent brush for cleaning all the surfaces and the metal bars of the partial removable denture.

D. Immersion

- Before immersion, the denture must be cleaned by rinsing and brushing to remove all loose surface biofilm and debris.
- An agent known to corrode or discolor metal must be avoided.
- Procedures for immersion cleaning are described on pages 477 to 478.

III. THE NATURAL TEETH

A. Biofilm Control

- Toothbrushing and interdental cleaning methods selected for the particular needs of the patient must be followed meticulously.
- The longevity of the removable appliance depends on the health of the supporting teeth, and, in turn, the health of the natural teeth depends on the cleanliness of the prosthesis.

B. Dental Caries Control

- The topical application of fluoride, the use of a fluoride dentifrice and other self-applied fluoride

measures such as a daily mouthrinse or application of a gel, and the control of refined sugars in the diet, are definite parts of the complete program of oral care for the patient with a removable prosthesis.
- The patient's constant alertness to the control of biofilm retention by the prosthesis and to the need for rinsing immediately after eating when brushing is not possible is essential.
- For the patient who has been caries-susceptible and whose teeth are missing because of dental caries, a dietary assessment and specific dental caries control program can increase a patient's motivation for self-care.
- When an abutment tooth to a fixed or removable partial denture develops caries or periodontal disease, numerous complications can result, such as extraction with failure of the appliance and limited options for replacement.

▪ COMPLETE DENTURES

I. COMPONENTS OF A COMPLETE DENTURE (FIGURE 29-6)

In an effort to understand the effects of various cleansing agents and devices, information about the structure and material of the parts of a denture is pertinent.

A. Denture Base

- The part of a denture that rests on the oral mucosa and to which the teeth are attached.
- Most denture bases are made of plastic acrylic resin.
- Others may be metal, for example, chrome-cobalt or gold, in combination with a plastic resin.

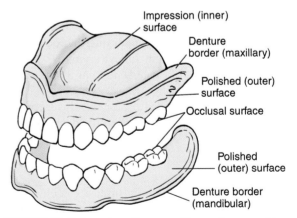

Impression (inner) surface
Denture border (maxillary)
Polished (outer) surface
Occlusal surface
Polished (outer) surface
Denture border (mandibular)

▪ FIGURE 29-6 Complete Denture. The surfaces and borders of maxillary and mandibular dentures.

B. Surfaces

1. *Impression Surface.* Also called the tissue or inner surface, the impression surface is the part that lies adjacent to the mucous membrane of the alveolar ridge and immediately associated parts; in the maxillary arch, the tissue surface is adjacent to the hard palate. This surface is occasionally lined with a:
   - Temporary soft liner.
   - Tissue conditioner.
   - Permanent silicone liner.
2. *Polished Surface.* The external or outer surface is highly polished. The occlusal and impression surfaces are not polished.
3. *Occlusal Surface.* The portion of the surface of a denture that makes contact or near contact with the corresponding surface of the opposing denture or natural teeth is the occlusal surface.

C. Teeth

- The denture teeth may be made of plastic acrylic resin, composite resin, or porcelain.
- Some have decorative or metal occlusal inserts.

II. DENTURE DEPOSITS

Accumulation of stains and deposits on dentures varies between individuals in a manner similar to that on natural teeth. The phases of deposit formation may be divided as follows:

A. Mucin and Food Debris on the Denture Surface

Readily removed by rinsing and brushing.

B. Denture Pellicle and Denture Biofilm

- Denture pellicle forms readily after a denture is cleaned. Denture biofilm is composed predominantly of gram-positive cocci, rods, and filamentous forms of bacteria in an intermicrobial substance. Biofilm also includes varying accumulations of *Candida albicans,* the yeast that causes candidiasis.
- Biofilm serves as a matrix for calculus formation and stain accumulation when the denture is not cleaned.

C. Calculus

Hard and fixed to the denture surface, calculus generally is located on the facial surfaces of the maxillary molars and the lingual surfaces of the mandibular anterior region.

III. REMOVAL OF DENTURE

- Usually, it is most comfortable for the patient to remove the denture.
- The clinician may have occasion to remove dentures for certain patients, particularly those who may be disabled, helpless, or in an emergency situation.
- Although denture removal may be complicated by anatomic features of an individual mouth, a general procedure is outlined here.
- The clinician follows standard procedures for infection control while removing and handling the denture from the patient's mouth.

A. Complete Maxillary Denture

1. Clinician is positioned at 11 to 12 o'clock; left-handed clinician is at 12 to 1 o'clock.
2. Grasp the denture firmly with the thumb on the facial surface at the height of the border of the denture under the lip and the index finger on the palatal surface.
3. With the other hand, elevate the lip to expose the border of the denture to break the seal.
4. Remove the denture gently in a downward and forward direction.
5. If the retention of the denture cannot be overcome by elevation of the lip, request the able patient to blow into the mouth with the lips closed to break the suction seal.

B. Complete Mandibular Denture

1. Clinician is positioned at 8 to 9 o'clock; left-handed clinician is at 3 to 4 o'clock.
2. Grasp the denture firmly on the facial surface with the thumb and on the lingual surface with the index finger.
3. With the other hand, retract the lower lip forward and remove the denture gently.

IV. CARE OF DENTURES DURING INTRAORAL PROCEDURES

- Provide a cleansing tissue for the patient's use when requesting the patient to remove or insert the denture.
- Rinse in water to remove any debris without splashing.
- Professionally clean denture with mechanical denture cleaner when indicated by the deposits on the appliance.
- Provide a cup or container with a fitted cover to hold the prosthesis after rinsing.

- Immerse in antimicrobial solution to disinfect and prevent drying.
- Place container in a safe place away from working area to prevent spilling or inadvertent discarding.
- At the end of the appointment, remember to return the denture before the patient rises from the dental chair.

V. MECHANICAL DENTURE CLEANSERS

- Commercially available devices include ultrasonic, sonic, magnetic, and agitating mechanisms that can be combined with an immersion agent.
- The action of the mechanical cleansing device seems to make the solution more efficient than a solution used alone.

■ CLEANING THE COMPLETE DENTURE

I. DESCRIPTION

- One should not assume that the patient who is wearing a denture knows the proper methods for caring for the prostheses and intraoral tissue.
- During questioning for the patient history, information about the method and frequency of oral care is recorded.
- Later, for a patient already wearing a denture, it is examined and the current method of care is reviewed.
- Alternate cleansing agents, devices, or procedures are recommended and demonstrated as needed.
- Instruction is individualized for each patient's need, for example, the patient receiving a maxillary and mandibular denture for the first time, for the patient whose dentures have been remade or relined, or for the patient with a single denture that opposes natural teeth.
- Types of dentures and characteristics of the edentulous mouth are described on pages 839 to 840.

II. PURPOSES FOR CLEANING

Inadequate oral tissue care and denture hygiene practices are major causes of oral lesions under dentures.

A. Prevent Irritation to the Oral Tissues

- *Mechanical Irritants.* Rough deposits of biofilm, calculus, thick stains.
- *Chemical Irritants.* Products of putrefaction of food debris and bacterial metabolic products.

B. Control Infection

Reactions to denture biofilm and/or secondary infections by way of traumatic lesions may occur.

C. Prevent Mouth Odors

D. Maintain Appearance

III. WHEN TO CLEAN

- Regularly after each meal, and at bedtime; the denture should be cleaned several times each day.
- Chemical immersion daily or twice weekly, depending on the rate of formation of calculus and stain and the type of solution used.
- Overnight if the denture is removed as instructed by the dentist.

IV. SELECTION OF PROCEDURE FOR CLEANING

Rinsing, immersion, followed by brushing, is recommended. When unable to clean, rinsing is advised.

V. PREPARATION FOR CLEANING

A. Rinse the denture thoroughly when it is taken from the mouth to remove saliva and loose debris.
B. Remove denture-adhesive material.
  1. *Definition.* A denture adhesive is a commercially available paste or powder preparation. A patient may use it under the direction of the dentist for temporary stabilization. An occasional patient may use an adhesive indefinitely in an attempt to get along with ill-fitting dentures that should be adjusted or remade.
  2. *Method.* Use a brush with light pressure to remove the adhesive.
C. Denture-bearing mucosa. Rinse and clean with a soft toothbrush twice or more times daily.

VI. CLEANING BY IMMERSION

The denture is soaked in a solvent or detergent in which chemical action removes or loosens stains and deposits that can then be rinsed or brushed away.

A. Advantages

- The solution reaches all areas of the denture for a complete cleaning.
- Minimizes the danger of dropping the appliance. Prevents need for handling, which is required during brushing.

- Offers safe storage when dentures are out of the mouth.
- Aids patients that have limited ability to manage a brush.
- When cleaning is distasteful, immersion involves the least handling and observation. This advantage is particularly attractive to a caregiver who must clean the denture of a patient.

B. Procedure

- Place denture in a plastic container with a fitted cover that is maintained specifically for this purpose.
- Use only warm water for rinsing and for mixing the solution.
- Warm water promotes the action of the cleanser.
- Hot water should never be used because it can distort plastic resin. Follow manufacturer's specifications to ensure correct dilution of cleanser.
- Check that the denture is completely submerged in the solution; cover the container.
- When the denture is removed, rinse under running water and remove loosened debris and chemicals before proceeding to clean by brushing.
- Empty and clean container daily. Mix fresh solution to prevent contamination and growth of microorganisms.[3]

C. Solutions

1. *Proprietary.* Available in powder or tablet form.
   a. *Preparation:* Add measured warm water as directed by the manufacturer.
   b. *Length of immersion:* Usually 10 to 15 minutes or as suggested by the manufacturer. Because the action depends on the mechanical bubbling effect of released oxygen, the solution has little value after the available oxygen has been released.
   c. *Effect:* The solutions are only effective against loose debris; denture cleanliness depends on regular daily immersion supplemented by brushing.
2. *Hypochlorite Solution:* Household bleach (5% sodium hypochlorite) and Calgone. Calgone acts to improve the penetrating and detaching power of the bleach.
   a. *Proportions:*
   - 1 tablespoon (15 ml) sodium hypochlorite (household bleach).
   - 2 teaspoons (8 ml) Calgone.
   - 4 ounces (114 ml) water.

   b. *Length of immersion:* Usually 10 to 15 minutes. When stains or calculus form, the patient should be instructed to soak the denture overnight provided there are no metal parts that can become corroded.

VII. CLEANING BY BRUSHING

Brush with water, soap, or other mild cleansing agent. Abrasive agents produce scratches, which promote biofilm accumulation.

A. Type of Brush

1. *Denture Brush*
   - A good-quality denture brush with end-rounded filaments is recommended. The styles of denture brushes vary.
   - One type shown in Figure 29-7 is designed with two arrangements of filaments: (1) round arrangement to access the inner, curved impression surface; (2) rectangular portion for convenient adaptation to the polished and occlusal denture surfaces.
   - Another brush design is shown in Figure 53-12.
2. *Other Brushes*
   - A few patients prefer not to have a denture brush for personal reasons.

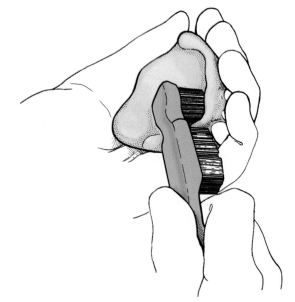

■ **FIGURE 29-7 Denture Brush.** The denture is held securely, but without squeezing, in the palm of the non-working hand. Place a face cloth in the bottom of the sink and partially fill with water. The specially designed brush is preferred because one group of tufts is arranged to provide access to the inner impression surface of the denture, as shown.

- A hand brush can be used, provided the filaments are long enough to reach into the deeper portions of the impression surfaces.
- Prerequisite is that each area of each surface of the denture be reached by the brush if denture biofilm formation is to be controlled.
- If a patient prefers to use an ordinary toothbrush, a multitufted soft nylon brush with end-rounded filaments should be acceptable if access to all the inner curvatures is possible without applying undue pressure on certain parts in the attempt to clean others.
- The patient who wears a single denture needs separate brushes for the natural teeth and the denture to maintain the brush for the natural teeth in the best condition possible.

B. Procedure

1. Grasp denture in palm of hand securely (Figure 29-7) but without a squeezing pressure because dentures can be broken.
2. Spread a towel, wash cloth, or rubber mat over the bottom of the sink to serve as a cushion should the denture be dropped; partially fill the sink with water.
3. Apply warm water, nonabrasive cleanser, and brush to all areas of the denture. Pay particular attention to the impression surfaces where configurations of the surface correspond with those of the oral topography. The anterior areas of the inner surfaces of both the maxillary and mandibular dentures require special adaptations of the brush.
4. Rinse denture and brush under running water. Use the brush to remove denture cleanser that may be retained in the grooves.
5. Visually check each area carefully for biofilm. Teach the patient to run a finger over the surfaces to find "slippery" biofilm areas.

C. Precautions Related to Brushing

1. Overzealous brushing with an abrasive cleansing agent on the impression surface could alter the fit of the denture.
2. Plastic resin can be abraded. Scratches make a rough surface; the denture may become more subject to the collection of debris and calculus.
3. Possibility of incomplete coverage during cleaning, particularly in the more inaccessible areas.
4. Possibility of cleaning with uneven pressure when the brush is applied more vigorously to accessible areas.

5. Danger of dropping and breaking the denture is increased when it is wet and, therefore, slippery.
6. Advise patient who wears eyeglasses to wear them when brushing to watch the procedure and to observe the cleanliness of the denture after brushing.

VIII. DENTURE CLEANSERS[4–7]

A. Requirements for a Denture Cleanser[4]

- Easy for a patient to use.
- Reasonably priced.
- Effective removal of denture deposits (organic and inorganic) without abrasion of the denture surface.
- Bactericidal and fungicidal action.
- Nontoxic.
- Harmless to the dental materials used for partial or complete dentures.

B. Chemical Solution Cleansers (Immersion)

1. *Alkaline Hypochlorite*
   a. Active ingredient: Dilute sodium hypochlorite with bleaching properties.
   b. Action: Loosens debris and light stains; bleaches; dissolves mucin; dissolves biofilm matrix.
   c. Example: Household bleach.
   d. Disadvantages: Odor; tarnish; surface pitting; bleaching effect on soft lining materials and denture materials containing fibers.
2. *Alkaline Peroxide*
   a. Active ingredient: Alkaline detergent with an oxygen-liberating agent (sodium perborate or percarbonate).
   b. Action: Loosens debris and light stains by an oxygen-liberating mechanism. A preventive cleanser should be used regularly from the day a denture has been cleaned professionally to prevent accumulation of heavy deposits.
   c. Examples: Most proprietary cleansers are in the form of a powder or tablet that is dropped into water to create the alkaline solution of hydrogen peroxide.
   d. Disadvantage: Does not remove heavy stains or calculus.
3. *Dilute Acids*
   a. Active ingredient: Inorganic acids.
   b. Action: Dissolves inorganic components of denture deposits.

c. Examples: 3% to 5% hydrochloric acid alone or with phosphoric acid; commercially prepared ultrasonic solutions. The strong acids (although in dilute forms) are not recommended for home use by the patient. Acetic acid (vinegar) has been used with some success when deposits were not old and hard.

d. Disadvantage: Corrosion of metal parts of a denture.

4. *Enzymes.* The enzymes act to break down biofilm proteins and polysaccharides. Enzyme agents have been incorporated into various immersion-type cleansers.

5. *Disinfectants*
   • A sanitary denture is necessary for the prevention of inflammation in the oral mucosa under the denture. Types of denture-induced lesions are described on pages 843 to 844.
   • Regular daily maintenance procedures must be carried out.
   • Patient instruction in disinfection of a denture is needed.
   • Full-strength, commercially available sodium hypochlorite (household bleach) has been shown to be an antimicrobial agent.
   • Before disinfection, preclean the denture under running water, taking care not to splash and thus contaminate the area.
   • To disinfect, immerse the denture for 5 minutes in full-strength bleach.[8] Because bleach can fade the color of a denture, immersion should be timed at 5 minutes, and the denture should be rinsed completely.

C. Abrasive Cleansers (Brushing)

1. *Denture Pastes and Powders, Toothpastes and Powders*
   a. Active ingredient: An abrasive, such as calcium carbonate.
   b. Action: Mechanical removal of biofilm and stains by brushing.
   c. Examples: Various commercial products.
   d. Disadvantages: Can abrade the plastic resin denture base and acrylic teeth. A paste with low abrasiveness should be selected.

2. *Household Agents*
   a. Active ingredient: Detergent and/or abrasive agent.
   b. Examples: Salt and bicarbonate of soda are mildly abrasive; hand soap is cleansing and not particularly abrasive. Scouring powders or other excessively abrasive cleansers should not be used.

IX. ADDITIONAL INSTRUCTIONS

A. Care of Plastic Resin

An appliance made with plastic resin should be immersed in water or cleansing solution when it is not in the mouth.

B. Prevention of Denture Deposits

When the denture is kept clean by regular procedures from the time of insertion, accumulation of heavy stains and calculus can be prevented.

C. Professional Maintenance

A denture should never be scraped by the patient with a sharp instrument in the attempt to remove calculus deposits. When the cleaning methods recommended in this chapter do not remove deposits, professional cleaning by the dental hygienist is needed. A regular maintenance plan is arranged.

D. Paste Cleansers

• Paste cleansers (dentifrices or denture pastes) may cling and be difficult to rinse from the denture.
• Residual chemical agents, such as essential oils, may cause inflammatory or allergic reactions of the oral mucosa, and phenolic agents can have deleterious effects on plastic resin.

E. Soft Lining Materials

• Temporary soft conditioning lining material may be sensitive to proprietary cleansers. Washing with cold water and a soft cloth, cotton, or soft brush (gently) can be suggested.
• Denture biofilm needs to be removed several times each day. Outer, polished surfaces should be thoroughly brushed in the usual manner.
• When the denture is placed in water overnight, the teeth should be placed down so that the soft material at the denture border cannot become deformed.
• Permanent silicone liners are softer and have a more porous surface to host biofilm accumulation, added diligence is required to remove biofilm and prevent build-up.

▪ THE UNDERLYING MUCOSA

I. RINSING

Each time the denture is removed, the mouth should be rinsed thoroughly with warm water or a mild salt solution. The patient can learn to clean the mucosa by rubbing over the edentulous areas with the tongue.

II. CLEANING

- At least once daily a soft toothbrush with end-rounded filaments is applied lightly over the ridges and in the vestibules using long, straight strokes from posterior to anterior.
- Concurrently, the tongue is cleaned. Use a tongue cleaner as described on pages 419 to 420.

III. MASSAGE

For stimulation of circulation and increased resistance to trauma, frequent massage is recommended. Methods for massage that may be suggested to the patient are the following:

A. Digital

Place thumb and index finger over the ridge and apply massage with a press-and-release stroke. The palate may be rubbed with the ball of the thumb.

B. Soft Toothbrush

Apply sides of filaments and vibratory motion to each area. Prevent trauma to the tissue by placing the brush carefully and avoiding scrubbing with undue pressure.

C. Power Brush

Apply to each area with smooth, even strokes.

IV. EXAMINATION

- Soft tissue examination and oral cancer screening are recommended at least yearly for all patients.
- Refer any concerns with appliance for evaluation.
- Record oral changes that may be indicative of systemic disease and refer for evaluation.
- Inform the patient to seek care when experiencing any oral changes or when concerns with a prosthesis arise.

■ COMPLETE OVERDENTURES

An overdenture is a complete denture supported by both retained natural teeth or implants and the soft tissue of the residual alveolar ridge. Overdentures also have been called overlay dentures, coping dentures, and tooth-mucosa–supported dentures.

I. PURPOSES

The advantages of an overdenture compared with a denture in a completely edentulous mouth are that the natural teeth

    A. Help preserve bone, which may improve retention of denture.

    B. Allow the remaining teeth to bear occlusal pressures, thereby reducing the pressures placed on edentulous areas.

    C. Improve stability and retention of the denture.

    D. Improve the patient's tactile and proprioceptive senses by having the periodontal ligament present.

    E. Increase the patient's psychologic acceptance of the denture. The patient does not feel that all natural teeth have been lost.

II. CRITERIA

The overdenture should be considered for any patient whose treatment plan calls for extraction of all teeth. Teeth to be preserved must meet certain standards of health.

A. Periodontal Condition

Because wearing the overdenture brings stress to the periodontium, the tissues must have, or be treatable to obtain, the following:

1. Healthy gingiva. There must be no bleeding or other signs of inflammation; minimal probing depth; and all requirements of health described in Table 12-1.
2. A band of attached gingiva, as described on page 233.

B. Bone Support

The bone level following tooth preparation must be adequate to withstand occlusal forces.

C. Teeth

Teeth must have minimal mobility. Teeth selected are frequently the mandibular canines and premolars and the maxillary canines.

III. PREPARATION OF THE TEETH

A. Endodontics

Most preserved teeth need endodontic therapy because the crowns will be reduced.

B. Periodontics

Treatment procedures depend on clinical findings but may include measures to eliminate inflammation and pockets, to increase the zone of attached gingiva, or to reshape the architecture of the bone or gingival tissue.

C. Restorative

1. Tooth crowns are reduced to short rounded preparations or, for some patients, to the level and contour of the gingival margin.

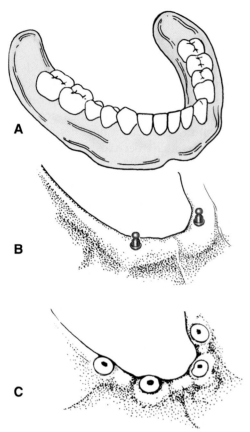

■ **FIGURE 29-8 Overdenture. (A)** Mandibular complete denture. **(B)** Support provided by implant copings. **(C)** Natural teeth with amalgam restoration in the coronal portion of the root canal opening.

2. An amalgam or composite restoration may cover the root canal fillings, as in Figure 29-8C.

IV. IMPLANT-RETAINED OVERDENTURE

Implants can be placed to help retain dentures, especially an implant placed in an area of each mandibular canine (Figure 29-8B). The advantages are similar to maintaining natural teeth and have the advantage regarding dental caries and periodontal health.

Peri-implant hygiene is described on page 494.

■ DENTAL HYGIENE CARE AND INSTRUCTION

I. GENERAL CARE

- The patient must be well informed concerning the care of the retained teeth, the periodontium, and all intraoral and extraoral tissues.
- A high degree of motivation to save the remaining teeth is a primary concern.

- Patient is provided with the individualized instructions that are appropriate for the type of prosthesis or prostheses present.

II. FLUORIDE PROGRAM

- A specific fluoride application plan is included for all natural tooth–retained overdentures and any patients with retained natural teeth.
- The requirements depend partly on the past history of dental caries.
- When the teeth have been extracted because of dental caries, caries control measures take on special significance, particularly if dietary habits remain the same.
- Current dietary habits must be checked by asking the patient to keep a daily food diary.
- Limitations on cariogenic food intake can be recommended accordingly.

A. Fluoride Self-application

- All patients need to use a fluoride dentifrice.
- In addition, a mouthrinse, prescription strength toothpaste, and/or a gel tray are recommended daily.
- After cleaning, the patient's denture can be used for a custom tray, and the gel drops can be placed inside at the locations of the natural teeth.
- Pressure of the denture as it is seated forces the gel about the teeth.
- Higher concentrations of sodium fluoride (5000 ppm) have been shown to be more protective for overdenture abutments.[9]

B. Professional Topical Applications

- Professional topical applications are made when daily fluoride is not carried out regularly by the patient or when additional fluoride is indicated.
- Because frequent maintenance appointments are needed to check the health of the gingival tissues, an application can be made at each such appointment.
- Benefit is derived from fluoride in direct proportion to the frequency of application: the more frequent the application of fluoride, the greater the benefit derived.
- Fluoride varnish may be used at every dental visit.

III. SEALANTS

Application of sealants to overdenture abutment teeth has been shown effective in the prevention of dental caries.[10]

Everyday Ethics

Mr. Samuel has a mandibular removable partial denture. It has never fit well, and he often goes days without wearing it. While he admits it affects his ability to chew, he says it is often painful. In the reception room he saw a pamphlet describing an overdenture and asked if this would be a good option for him. Mr. Samuel has been treated for periodontal disease due to generalized bone loss.

Questions for Consideration

1. What is the first suggestion that should be given to Mr. Samuel regarding his current complaints with his removable partial denture?

2. Given his periodontal condition, how much detail should the dental hygienist, Clara, share with this patient in reference to his request for an overdenture that he "might actually wear"?

3. Mr. Samuel is willing to pay anything for an appliance that works. He states that he'll find another dental practice that specializes in making overdentures if necessary. What action should be taken at this time?

4. What aspects of informed consent need to be addressed with Mr. Samuel?

IV. MAINTENANCE APPOINTMENTS

- Supervision by frequent maintenance appointments for scaling and biofilm debridement, topical fluoride applications, and motivation and instruction for biofilm control are essential.
- Check for integrity of each sealant and replace as necessary.
- More frequent maintenance appointment may be needed for patients at higher risk for periodontitis, dental caries, or other pathology.

✔ Factors To Teach The Patient

- How to make a self-examination of the oral tissues.

- Why all prostheses need cleaning more than once a day.

- How to handle a removable prosthesis while it is cleaned.

- The need to adapt toothbrushing, flossing, and use of other aids to the care of the abutment teeth.

- How tongue cleaning contributes to complete oral health.

- The significance of regular maintenance appointments to have the oral tissues checked and the prostheses professionally cleaned.

REFERENCES

1. Obreschkow, C.: Oral Hygiene and Periodontal Considerations in Restorative Treatment With Prefabricated Attachments and Precision-Milled Prosthetic Devices, *Int. J. Periodontics Restorative Dent., 4,* 73, No. 1, 1985.
2. American Dental Association, Council on Dental Materials, Instruments and Equipment and Council on Dental Therapeutics: Status Report: Effect of Acidulated Phosphate Fluoride on Porcelain and Composite Restorations, *J. Am. Dent. Assoc., 116,* 115, January, 1988.
3. DePaola, L.G. and Minah, G.E.: Isolation of Pathogenic Microorganisms from Dentures and Denture-Soaking Containers of Myelosuppressed Cancer Patients, *J. Prosthet. Dent., 49,* 20, January, 1983.
4. Abelson, D.C.: Denture Plaque and Denture Cleansers: Review of the Literature, *Gerodontics, 1,* 202, October, 1985.
5. Budtz-Jörgensen, E.: Materials and Methods for Cleaning Dentures, *J. Prosthet. Dent., 42,* 619, December, 1979.
6. Gallagher, J.B., Jr.: *Handbook for Complete Dentures.* Boston, Tufts University School of Dental Medicine, 1981.
7. American Dental Association, Council on Dental Materials, Instruments, and Equipment: Denture Cleansers, *J. Am. Dent. Assoc., 106,* 77, January, 1983.
8. Rudd, R.W., Senia, E.S., McCleskey, F.K., and Adams, E.D.: Sterilization of Complete Dentures With Sodium Hypochlorite, *J. Prosthet Dent., 51,* 318, March, 1984.
9. Ettinger, R.L., Olson, R.J., Wefel, J.S., and Asmussen, C.: In Vitro Evaluation of Topical Fluorides for Overdenture Abutments, *J. Prosthet. Dent., 78,* 309, September, 1997.
10. Kurtz, K.S.: Adjunctive Caries Control in Overdenture Abutment Teeth: A New Modality, *J. Am. Dent. Assoc., 126,* 213, February, 1995.

SUGGESTED READINGS

Asad, T., Watkinson, A.C., and Huggett, R.: The Effect of Disinfection Procedures on Flexural Properties of Denture Base Acrylic Resins, *J. Prosthet. Dent., 68,* 191, July, 1992.

Assery, M., Sugrue, P.C., Graser, G.N., and Eisenberg, A.D.: Control of Microbial Contamination With Commercially Available Cleaning Solutions, *J. Prosthet. Dent., 67,* 275, February, 1992.

Chan, E.C., Iugovaz, I., Siboo, R., Bilyk, M., Barolet, R., Amsel, R., Wooley, C., and Klitorimos, A.: Comparison of Two Popular Methods for Removal and Killing of Bacteria From Dentures, *J. Can. Dent. Assoc., 57,* 937, December, 1991.

Douglass, C.W. and Watson, A.S.: Future Needs for Fixed and Removable Partial Dentures in the United States, *J. Prosthet. Dent., 87,* 9, January, 2002.

Fernandes, A.: Denture Cleanliness?, *Br. Dent. J., 194,* 354, April 12, 2003.

Glass, R.T.: The Infected Toothbrush, the Infected Denture, and Transmission of Disease: A Review, *Compend. Cont. Educ. Dent., 13,* 592, July, 1992.

Keyf, F. and Gungor, T.: Comparison of Effects of Bleach and Cleansing Tablet on Reflectance and Surface Changes of a Dental Alloy Used for Removable Partial Dentures, *J. Biomater. Appl., 18,* 5, July, 2003.

Kulak-Ozan, Y., Kazazoglu, E. and Arikan, A.: Oral Hygiene Habits, Denture Cleanliness, Presence of Yeasts and Stomatitis in Elderly People, *J. Oral Rehabil., 29,* 300, March, 2002.

Ma, T., Johnson, G.H., and Gordon, G.E.: Effects of Chemical Disinfectants on the Surface Characteristics and Color of Denture Resins, *J. Prosthet. Dent., 77,* 197, February, 1997.

Merchant, V. and Molinari, J.A.: Infection Control in Prosthodontics: A Choice No Longer, *Gen. Dent., 37,* 29, January–February, 1989.

Nakamoto, K., Tamamoto, M., and Hamada, T.: Evaluation of Denture Cleansers With and Without Enzymes Against *Candida albicans, J. Prosthet. Dent., 66,* 792, December, 1991.

Nikawa, H., Jin, C., Makihira, S., Egusa, H., Hamada, T. and Kumagai, H.: Biofilm Formation of *Candida Albicans* on the Surfaces of Deteriorated Soft Denture Lining Materials Caused by Denture Cleaners in Vitro, *J. Oral Rehabil., 30,* 243, March, 2003.

Obatake, R.M., Collard, S.M., Martin, J., and Ladd, G.D.: The Effects of Sodium Fluoride and Stannous Fluoride on the Surface Roughness of Intraoral Magnet Systems, *J. Prosthet. Dent., 66,* 553, October, 1991.

Reeson, M.G.: A Modified Denture Cleaning Brush for Patients With Limited Manual Dexterity, *J. Prosthet. Dent., 90,* 205, August, 2003.

Shay, K.: Denture Hygiene: A Review and Update, *J. Contemp. Dent. Pract., 1,* 28, February, 15, 2000.

Overdentures

Ettinger, R.L. and Jakobsen, J.: Caries: A Problem in an Overdenture Population, *Community Dent. Oral Epidemiol., 18,* 42, February, 1990.

Gomes, B.C. and Renner, R.P.: Periodontal Considerations of the Removable Partial Overdenture, *Dent. Clin. North Am., 34,* 653, October, 1990.

Hong, L., Ettinger, R.L., Watkins, C.A., and Wefel, J.S.: In Vitro Evaluation of Fluoride Varnish on Overdenture Abutments, *J. Prosthet. Dent., 89,* 28, January, 2003.

Keltjens, H.M.A.M., Schaeken, M.J.M., van der Hoeven, J.S., and Hendriks, J.C.M.: Caries Control in Overdenture Patients: 18-Month Evaluation on Fluoride and Chlorhexidine Therapies, *Caries Res., 24,* 371, September–October, 1990.

The Patient With Oral Rehabilitation and Implants

Complete oral rehabilitation refers to the combined treatment of the teeth and periodontium to restore health, function, and physical form. As generally used, *oral rehabilitation* applies to involved extensive restorative procedures in a mouth that cannot be treated with routine dental care. It is also known as *mouth rehabilitation, occlusal rehabilitation, occluso-rehabilitation, complete reconstruction,* or *periodontal prosthesis.* Key words are defined in Box 30-1.

The term *periodontal prosthesis* is used to designate restorative and prosthodontic treatment that is neces-

sary for the treatment of advanced periodontal disease. The prosthesis used may be a splint for immobilization or stabilization of a group of teeth or an entire arch, maxillary or mandibular.

Periodontal, restorative, and prosthodontic treatments are interdependent. The function and duration of all restorative and prosthodontic treatments depend directly on the health of the periodontium, which provides the attachment and support necessary for the restored teeth. Periodontal health, in turn, is influenced by restorative and prosthodontic treatment.

BOX 30-1 KEY WORDS: Rehabilitation and Implants*

Crown: an artificial replacement that restores missing tooth structure by surrounding part or all of the remaining structure with a material, such as cast metal or porcelain, or a combination of materials, such as metal and porcelain fused (veneer crown).

Embrasure: the space defined by proximal surfaces of adjacent teeth where those surfaces diverge apically, facially, lingually, or occlusally from an area of contact.

Furcation invasion: pathologic resorption of bone within a furcation; a periodontal bony defect.

Hydroxyapatite ceramic: a composition of calcium and phosphate to provide a dense, nonresorbable, biocompatible ceramic used for dental implants; metal implants may be coated with tricalcium phosphate or hydroxyapatite.

Implant: an alloplastic (inert metal or plastic) material or device grafted or inserted surgically into intact tissues for diagnostic, prosthetic, therapeutic, or experimental purposes.

Inlay: a fixed restoration placed within tooth structure, prepared outside the mouth, and subsequently cemented into the tooth to restore intracoronal tooth structure; may be made of porcelain, composite resin, or cast gold.

Occlusal adjustment: treatment in which the occluding surfaces of teeth are reshaped by grinding to create harmonious contact relationships between maxillary and mandibular teeth; also known as occlusal equilibration or selective grinding.

Odontoplasty: the reshaping of a portion of a tooth; may be performed for therapeutic or esthetic purposes.

Onlay: a fixed restoration that is prepared outside the mouth and is subsequently cemented onto the tooth; it restores the occlusal surface, the mesial-distal or lingual-facial margins, and covers or replaces one or more cusps.

Osseous integration: the apparent direct attachment or connection of osseous tissue to an inert, alloplastic material without intervening connective tissue. Also called **osseointegration.**

Peri-implantitis: inflammation of the tissue around a dental implant.

Splint: an apparatus, appliance, or device used to prevent motion or displacement of fractured or movable parts.

   Dental splint: designed to immobilize and stabilize teeth in the same dental arch.

Supportive periodontal treatment: an extension of periodontal therapy; includes procedures performed at selected time intervals to review the general health history, reassess the status of periodontal health, and provide preventive oral hygiene care; also called **periodontal maintenance** or **preventive maintenance.**

Titanium: a uniquely biocompatible metal used for implants either in the commercially pure form or as an alloy.

Titanium alloy: the most common titanium alloy (Ti-6A1-4V) used for dental implants contains 6% aluminum to increase strength and decrease weight and 4% vanadium to prevent corrosion.

Tomography: a radiographic technique that provides a distinct image of a selected plane through the body; the images of structures that lie above and below that plane are blurred.

Veneer: a layer of tooth-color material (composite or porcelain) that is bonded or cemented to a prepared tooth surface.

*Definitions in this chapter that pertain to prosthodontics are taken or adapted from and are in accord with the *Glossary of Prosthodontic Terms,* 7th ed., 1999, of the Academy of Prosthodontics Foundation.
Definitions that relate to periodontics are taken or adapted from the *Glossary of Periodontal Terms,* 3rd ed., 1992, of the American Academy of Periodontology.

Many predisposing factors that contribute to the initiation, development, and progress of periodontal infections are a direct result of untreated dental caries, incomplete or inadequate restorations, unreplaced missing teeth, and inadequate occlusal relationships built into restorations or prostheses.

I. OBJECTIVES OF COMPLETE REHABILITATION

Objectives for complete rehabilitation involve the same principles as for all oral care and include the need to
   A. Restore optimal functional occlusion.
   B. Maintain the health of the periodontium.

C. Produce biologically contoured restorations in harmony with normal oral physiology.

D. Replace missing teeth.

E. Provide support to teeth with advanced bone loss and marked mobility.

F. Provide desirable esthetics.

G. Establish acceptable phonetics.

II. COMPONENTS OF TREATMENT

Complete oral reconstruction means total mouth involvement, which brings in many phases of dentistry, often accomplished by individual specialists. The overall treatment plan may include some or all of the following:

A. Extensive periodontal therapy involving various surgical procedures.

B. Occlusal adjustment.

C. Endodontic therapy.

D. Correction of oral habits.

E. Orthodontic tooth movement.

F. Splinting of teeth temporarily or permanently.

G. Dental implants.

H. Restorations involving individual teeth: crowns, inlays, onlays.

I. Replacement of teeth by fixed and/or removable prostheses.

III. ACCOMPLISHMENT OF TREATMENT

Treatment may be long and involved for the patient who undergoes complete oral rehabilitation. It requires patience, persistence, and dedication of the patient, the dental hygienist, and the dentist.

The dental hygiene treatment plan overlaps every phase of the total treatment, beginning with the initial preparation of the patient's mouth. Maintenance and supervision of the patient's self-care program are essential throughout restorative and prosthodontic therapy and continuing into the maintenance phase.

Specific measures for self-care in terms of biofilm removal and dental caries prevention must be selected and supervised. The patient is shown how to self-evaluate, so that minor deviations from normal can be recognized and called to the attention of the clinician.

▪ CHARACTERISTICS OF THE REHABILITATED MOUTH

To select the appropriate methods for dental biofilm control and dental caries prevention, one must assess existing conditions, such as contour and position of the gingiva, contour of restorations, and problem areas adjacent to fixed prostheses. When these are known, the variety of possible techniques and devices for biofilm removal can be reviewed and a plan for care outlined.

A patient who has undergone extensive periodontal therapy and restorative and prosthodontic rehabilitation may have some or all of the characteristics listed here. Each condition may require specially selected or adapted self-care measures for dental biofilm control. Fixed and removable appliances can provide many areas for dental biofilm and debris retention.

I. PERIODONTAL FINDINGS

A. Gingival recession.

B. Exposed root surfaces.

C. Exposed furcation areas.

D. Alterations of gingival contour; the gingival margins may be rolled or rounded.

E. Changes in size and shape of the gingival embrasures.

1. Missing interdental papillae; wide embrasures with gingival recession and increased root exposure (Figure 30-1).

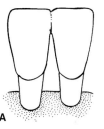

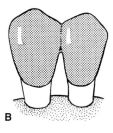

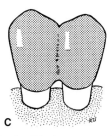

▪ **FIGURE 30-1 Gingival Embrasures. (A)** Wide embrasure between two central incisors with missing interdental papilla and gingival recession. **(B)** Double abutment with closed contact area with open embrasure provides access for biofilm removal. **(C)** Overcontoured crowns of a double abutment with a narrowed embrasure that provides limited access for dental biofilm and debris removal.

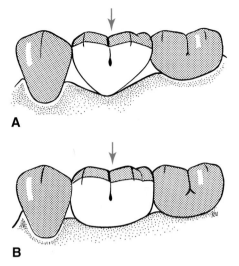

■ FIGURE 30-2 Shape of Pontics. Mandibular three-unit fixed partial denture. **(A)** "Bullet"-shaped pontic with wide embrasures for access for dental biofilm removal. **(B)** Improperly shaped pontic with closed embrasures and wide gingival surface for biofilm retention. Arrows indicate pontics.

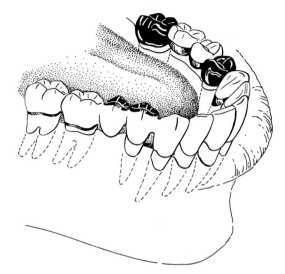

■ FIGURE 30-3 Complete-Arch Fixed Splint. A continuous therapeutic fixed appliance stabilizes periodontally involved teeth and replaces missing components to provide appropriate occlusal relationships. Numerous problem areas for dental biofilm removal exist.

2. Narrowed embrasures created by overcontoured restorations or variously shaped pontics (Figure 30-2).

II. SINGLE TOOTH RESTORATIONS

A. The gingival margin around a crown restoration may appear bluish or bluish-red when the crown margin is below the gingival margin.

B. Various restorations may require selective cleaning agents.

III. FIXED PROSTHESES

A patient may have
A. Fixed splinting around long segments of, or an entire, arch (Figure 30-3).
B. Natural abutment teeth with difficult access areas adjacent to a pontic.
C. Implant abutment surfaces.
D. Closed contacts between teeth involved in a multitooth prosthesis.
E. Gingival surfaces of pontics.
F. Wide and triangular embrasures created by pontics or narrow, unnatural, non–self-cleansing areas created by improperly shaped pontics (Figure 30-2B).

IV. REMOVABLE PROSTHESES

A. Complete denture may be used in one dental arch opposing natural teeth and partial dentures, fixed or removable.
B. Partial denture

1. Creation of potential areas of dental biofilm and debris retention.
   a. Alteration of tooth form by clasp, rest, or precision attachment.
   b. Improperly contoured edge of the partial denture at the junction of the partial denture and the abutment tooth.
2. Partial denture may impinge on the gingiva surrounding the abutment tooth.
3. Double abutment (two natural teeth with crowns that are soldered or cast together) has a closed contact requiring lateral (from facial or lingual aspects) access to the gingival embrasure (Figure 30-1B and C).
4. The mucosa under the partial denture needs special care.

■ SELF-CARE FOR THE REHABILITATED MOUTH

These special patients require greater than average attention, patience, and teaching skill to obtain a favorable result that will ensure continuing health of the patient's periodontal tissues. Total commitment on the part of the patient is necessary if the selected plan is to meet the requirements for daily care.

I. PLANNING THE DISEASE CONTROL PROGRAM

The control program should be planned as a concentrated effort to maintain the gingival tissue, the exposed tooth structure, and, hence, the underlying supporting periodontium, as well as the restorations and prostheses. The instructions have three parts: first, before the surgical, restorative, and prosthodontic treatment; second, during therapy; and third, after reconstruction.

A. Part 1

Basic biofilm control measures are learned and practiced by the patient during the preparatory phase. During these lessons, principles for self-evaluation can be presented.

B. Part 2

During therapy, adaptations are needed for applying techniques to temporary restorations. When the treatment extends over a long period, regular dental hygiene appointments for careful monitoring of the gingival health are essential.

C. Part 3

After therapy is completed, another set of self-care procedures is required to meet the needs of the rehabilitated mouth. Special devices and techniques are selected and tried until the most efficient and thorough procedures are determined.

II. BIOFILM CONTROL: SELECTION OF METHODS[1]

After assessment, methods selected must allow the patient to accomplish complete daily biofilm removal from each area around every tooth or replacement. A summary of devices and methods is provided in Table 30-1.

Most patients need a method for each of the following:
A. Debris removal, particularly from interproximal areas and around fixed implants and prostheses.
B. Sulcular brushing procedure adapted for complete coverage for anatomic variations.
C. Interdental biofilm removal
   1. Proximal surfaces of natural and restored teeth, including exposed roots where access exists from the incisal or occlusal surfaces.
   2. Proximal surfaces of abutment teeth under closed contact areas (Figure 30-4).
   3. Mesial and/or distal surfaces of teeth without proximal contact.
D. Removal of dental biofilm around a fixed partial denture must include the gingival and proximal surfaces of pontics.
E. Cleaning a removable prosthesis and care of the supporting tissues.

III. FLUORIDES

A. Selection of Fluorides

For the patient with porcelain or composite resin restorations, an acidulated fluoride preparation must be avoided. Porcelain and composite resin restorations become pitted and rough with repeated applications of a fluoride solution with an acidic pH.[2]

Neutral fluoride products with low viscosity and low fluoride concentration can be advised.

B. Personal Daily Program

Fluoride dentifrice, along with daily mouthrinse or brush-on gel, is recommended to prevent root caries. For certain patients in the root caries risk groups and those with multiple sensitive teeth, a custom-tray application should be used daily.

C. Professional Topical Applications

When the patient does not drink fluoridated water routinely or use self-treatment methods on a regular basis, additional topical fluoride may be deemed beneficial. Professional applications are recommended for each maintenance appointment.

IV. DIETARY ASSESSMENT

Whether the need for the rehabilitation was related to extensive dental caries or to a periodontal disease, dietary counseling is indicated. Every possible means must be taken to prevent carious lesions of the exposed root surfaces about the restorations. Overall dietary factors should be checked to ensure support from a nutritional standpoint.

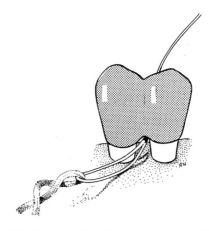

■ **FIGURE 30-4 Dental Biofilm Removal From Embrasure.** A floss threader is used with yarn or tufted floss to clean under a double abutment embrasure. Narrowed embrasure from overcontoured crown increases biofilm and debris retention and makes cleaning difficult.

■ TABLE 30-1 CARE OF THE REHABILITATED MOUTH

PROBLEM	DEVICE/METHOD	SPECIAL ADAPTATION
Debris removal	Water irrigation Toothbrush	Wide embrasures Under fixed partial dentures

Sulcular brushing	Toothbrush with soft,
	   end-rounded filaments
		Facial and lingual surfaces
		Distal surfaces of most-posterior teeth,
		   particularly terminal abutment

Proximal surfaces, biofilm removal	Floss Floss with threader Yarn with floss and/or threader Toothpick holder Pipe cleaner Interdental brush Single-tuft brush	Abutment teeth Proximal root surfaces Pontic surfaces Narrowed embrasures

Proximal surfaces,
   open contacts
	Gauze strip
	Yarn
		Terminal abutment of removable partial denture
		Distal surfaces of most-posterior teeth in the
		   dental arch

Exposed furcation, molars	Pipe cleaner Floss/yarn in threader Interdental brush Interdental rubber tip	Rotated tooth
Exposed furcation, maxillary first premolar	Interdental brush Interdental rubber tip	Fused root with groove
Exposed root surfaces	Fluoride dentifrice Dentifrice containing desensitizing agent	Desensitization Prevent abrasion of cementum or dentin
Fixed partial denture	Toothbrush (soft, end-rounded) Floss threader with floss/yarn Any other proximal surface procedures as applicable	Gingival surfaces of pontics Proximal surfaces of pontics and retainers

Edentulous gingiva
   under removable
   denture
	Toothbrush (soft nylon)
	   (manual or power-assisted)
	Digital massage
		Stimulation and biofilm removal

Tongue cleaning	Toothbrush (soft nylon) Tongue scraper	Deep fissures
Removable denture	Denture brush Clasp brush Chemical cleanser for immersion	Clasps

V. PROCEDURE

No fixed procedure applies to every patient. A personalized sequence must be worked out, often by trial and error.

  A. Outline a possible sequence
    1. Select methods and devices that can meet the requirements of the individual oral characteristics.
    2. Demonstrate the use of the methods and have the patient practice under supervision.

Avoid presenting too many procedures in one lesson, which can confuse and discourage the patient.

    3. Provide step-by-step written directions for home reference.
  B. Recheck successes within a few days and at least by 1 week.
    1. Assess gingival tissue.
    2. Assess biofilm. Use a disclosing agent to provide the patient with an evaluation of areas that need additional attention.

3. Assess performance
   a. Observe patient's dexterity in managing the self-care methods for biofilm removal.
   b. Note relationship of procedures used by the patient to areas where disclosing agent revealed biofilm retention.
4. Make necessary adjustments to simplify and clarify so that all areas are completely cleaned daily.

C. Reevaluate weekly or as frequently as needed to maintain the patient's motivation, to follow the health of the gingival tissues, and to recognize a need for changes in the procedures used.

VI. SAMPLE PROCEDURE

The patient described in this section has a complete maxillary fixed partial denture (splint), which has several natural teeth as abutments and four areas of double pontics; a mandibular removable partial denture with double abutments connecting mandibular canines and first premolars on each side; and wide embrasures between mandibular incisors caused by previous periodontal infection, which has since been treated with periodontal surgery.

The patient might use the following procedure:

A. Morning, After Eating

1. Completely brush with power toothbrush (containing softest filaments available); apply the brush to proximal surfaces.
2. Brush partial removable denture manually and rinse thoroughly.

B. Noon, After Eating (Away From Home)

1. Rinse partial denture under running water.
2. Use manual toothbrush, covering all surfaces as thoroughly as possible.
3. Rinse carefully, forcing the water under fixed partial denture areas.

C. Evening, After All Eating

1. Remove partial denture, rinse under running water, and place in cleansing solution.
2. Use water irrigator to remove debris from all parts of fixed splint and from all proximal surfaces of mandibular teeth.
3. Use toothbrush for facial and lingual sulcular brushing; apply the brush interdentally as much as possible. Use sodium fluoride dentifrice.
4. Brush tongue and edentulous gingiva under removable denture.
5. Use dental floss and/or yarn for accessible proximal surfaces.

6. Clean all gingival and proximal surfaces of fixed partial denture. Use floss and yarn with floss threader for all proximal and gingival surfaces not accessible from incisal or occlusal aspects. Interdental brush may be needed for certain wide embrasures.
7. Use yarn or gauze strip for distal surfaces of the abutment teeth for the mandibular removable denture (mandibular premolars).
8. Use toothpick holder with dentifrice containing a desensitizing agent to massage hypersensitive areas of exposed roots.
9. Rinse with fluoride mouthrinse; vigorously force the solution between the teeth and under fixed appliances.
10. Clean partial denture, using denture brush and clasp brush, and rinse the denture thoroughly.

VII. MAINTENANCE PLAN

Continuing supervision of the patient with oral rehabilitation is an absolute essential. The well-informed and conscientious patient who devotes up to an hour each day on personal care procedures expects a maintenance appointment that thoroughly evaluates the gingival tissue, the rehabilitation prostheses, and the completeness of biofilm control efforts.

What could seem like a minute area of gingival bleeding on probing, whether the pocket is shallow or has started to deepen, should be a warning signal that an area may not be covered by present self-care procedures and needs some form of treatment. *Each millimeter of gingival sulcus must be probed carefully to detect incipient changes.*

■ DENTAL IMPLANTS

A *dental implant* may be placed within or on mandibular or maxillary bone either to replace teeth or to provide a stable and retentive base for support of a fixed or removable prosthesis. The various plates and screws used in the treatment of fractured bones are also implants.

The success of an implant can depend on many factors, especially including patient understanding and skills for direct daily care of the prosthesis and the surrounding soft tissues. Frequent maintenance appointments for careful supervision and patient motivation are essential components for implant success.

■ TYPES OF DENTAL IMPLANTS

The three general categories of dental implants are described here. They are endosseous, subperiosteal, and transosteal. The endosseous implants are the most widely used.

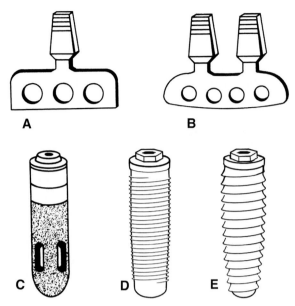

■ **FIGURE 30-5 Endosseous Implants. A** and **B.** Blade types. **C.** Cylinder types. **D** and **E.** Screw types.

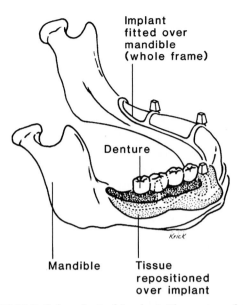

■ **FIGURE 30-6 Subperiosteal Implant.** The custom-fabricated framework is shown on the left side of the mandible; on the right side, the framework is shown by dotted lines under the denture.

I. ENDOSSEOUS (ENDOSTEAL)

A. Location

The implant is placed within the bone.

B. Examples

Blade, screw, and cylinder types are used (Figure 30-5).

C. Materials

The three basic types of biomaterials are metals and alloys, ceramics and carbon, and polymers.[3]

D. Description[4]

The support, body, or fixture is placed in bone during the first surgical step and left covered by mucosal tissue for several months while implant bonds with the bone. The abutment, post, or neck is then exposed through the soft tissue at a second-stage surgical procedure. Placement of the prosthesis follows.

II. SUBPERIOSTEAL

A. Location

The implant is placed over the bone, under the periosteum.

B. Example

A custom-fabricated framework of metal rests over the bone of the mandible or maxilla; it may be the complete arch or unilateral (Figure 30-6).

C. Material

Cobalt-chromium-molybdenum (Vitallium) or titanium are used.

D. Description[5,6]

1. *Two-step.* In the first step, a surgical flap is used to reflect mucosal tissues and to expose the underlying bone. An impression is made of the bony ridge. The metallic unit is cast and then placed in a second surgical step. Usually, four posts protrude into the oral cavity to hold the complete denture.
2. *One-step.* Computer-assisted tomography design and manufacturing have been applied, using a reformatted computed tomography scan from which approximate casts of the maxilla or mandible can be made. The implant is designed on this replica and is placed in one surgical procedure.

III. TRANSOSTEAL (TRANSOSSEOUS)

A. Location

The implant is placed through the bone.

B. Example

The mandibular staple bone plate (Figure 30-7).

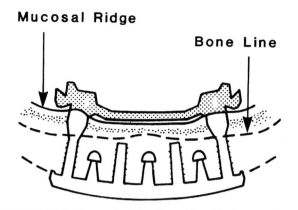

Mucosal Ridge

Bone Line

■ **FIGURE 30-7 Transosteal Implant.** Mandibular staple bone plate in the anterior region shows metal plate at the lower border of the mandible, with pins extending toward the occlusal surface. Terminal pins protrude into the oral cavity to hold the overdenture.

C. Materials

Stainless steel, ceramic-coated materials, and titanium alloy.

D. Description[7,8]

A metal plate, fitted to the inferior border of the mandible, has five to seven pins extending toward the occlusal surface. Usually, two terminal pins protrude into the oral cavity to hold the overdenture. The pins are connected by a crossbar. The transosteal implant can be used when the patient has an atrophic edentulous mandible or a congenital or traumatic deformity of the mandible.

■ PREPARATION AND PLACEMENT

I. PATIENT SELECTION

Careful screening is essential at the start. Generally acceptable physical health and a real desire to go through the required treatment are prerequisite. Diagnosis and treatment planning are based on a risk-benefit analysis and follow a detailed medical, dental, and behavioral history along with an oral and radiographic examination. Sometimes a psychologic examination is used.

A. Systemic Health

1. *Medical History.* The patient must be free of systemic conditions that can interfere with healing or acceptance of the implant. Biocompatibility of the implant with body tissues is essential.

2. *Contraindications.* Examples of conditions that may make a patient a poor risk include recent radiation therapy to the affected part, uncontrolled diabetes mellitus, alcoholism or heavy alcohol intake, substance abuse (including tobacco use), an immunosuppressive disease or medication, anticoagulant medication, psychosis, or paranoia.

B. Oral Examination

1. Radiographic evidence of adequate depth of alveolar bone is needed.
2. The presence of an active oral disease, such as periodontitis, contraindicates implant placement until the disease is treated and under control.

C. Oral Hygiene

The patient must demonstrate consistent and effective personal oral care.

II. INFORMATION FOR THE PATIENT

A. Explain procedures to be performed and the time schedule.
B. Explain possible complications.
C. Emphasize the role of personal oral care and the need for daily dental biofilm control.
D. Obtain an informed consent statement and agreement of understanding.

III. SURGICAL STEPS

Various systems are in use. Some are single-stage endosseous implants, and others use a two-stage procedure. The entire implant may not be inserted in one step because forces of occlusion (chewing, biting) may cause mobility and prevent bone healing. When the implant is first placed it must be stabilized. Movement of the implant may cause the formation of a fibrous tissue layer instead of osseointegration.

The surgical procedure requires atraumatic placement of the implant into the bone. Whenever microorganisms are introduced during a surgical procedure, healing can be impaired. Manufacturers prepare implants in sterile packages.

IV. PROSTHODONTIC STEPS

Attention to ideal requirements for acceptable prostheses is necessary. Margins, embrasure shapes, crown contours, contact areas, and occlusal harmony must be designed to prevent dental biofilm collection and permit thorough disease control procedures by the patient.

▪ IMPLANT INTERFACES

An implant has an inner interface with the *bone* and a *soft tissue* interface where the terminal pin, abutment, post, or other protruding portion of the implant is surrounded by the mucosal or gingival tissue.

I. IMPLANT/BONE INTERFACE

Osseointegration refers to direct structural and functional union between the implant and healthy living bone. No discernible connective tissue is between the bone and the implant.

II. IMPLANT/SOFT TISSUE INTERFACE

The external environment of an implant is the oral cavity, with saliva, dental biofilm, and debris.

A. Biologic Seal (Permucosal Seal)

Between the implant or post and the soft tissue, a biologic seal must exist to prevent microorganisms and inflammation-producing agents from entering the tissues.

B. Soft Tissue Connection

Sulcular epithelium is in contact with the implant surface. The attachment appears similar to the epithelial attachment of the junctional epithelium of a natural tooth. Hemidesmosomes and basal lamina have been identified. The epithelium resembles a long junctional epithelium.

▪ PERI-IMPLANT HYGIENE

A key requirement for implant success is the disease control program for the tissue surrounding the implant. Meticulous hygiene is a necessity for which repeated instruction may be needed.

I. CARE OF THE NATURAL TEETH

Transmission of microorganisms from the natural teeth and periodontal pockets to the peri-implant tissues can occur. The pockets around the teeth act as natural reservoirs, and periodontal pathogens from the pockets colonize in the tissue around the implants. It is therefore of utmost importance that, before placement of the implants, the periodontal condition be treated and brought to a healthy state. Then, after the placement of the implants, the maintenance program emphasizes care of the natural teeth and tissues as well as the peri-implant tissues.

II. DENTAL BIOFILM (IMPLANT BIOFILM)

Biofilm microorganisms around implants with healthy permucosal tissue have been shown to be like the flora around natural teeth. Gram-positive, nonmotile, coccoid, and other forms of bacteria predominate.[11-13]

The tissues around implant posts or abutments react to microorganisms and their toxic products in a manner similar to the gingiva surrounding natural teeth. When inflammation and pocket depths increase, the total number of microorganisms including spirochetes and motile rods increases also.[13]

III. PLANNING THE DISEASE CONTROL PROGRAM

A. Relation to Treatment

Supervision of a patient's oral hygiene must begin prior to the surgical phase for implant placement and carry on throughout the treatment phases.

B. Types of Prostheses

Implant-supported prostheses may be partial, complete, fixed, removable, or single-tooth replacements. Prostheses may be supported by natural teeth and/or implants. An individual may have a variety of areas and prostheses to care for.

IV. SELECTION OF BIOFILM-REMOVAL METHODS

Each patient needs an individually planned program so that each type of abutment and prosthesis can be maintained in a biofilm-free environment.

A. Conventional Prosthesis

Removable or fixed, partial or complete dentures made of conventional dental materials are to be cleaned by the usual methods described earlier. Suggestions provided here pertain primarily to the posts, abutments, or other protruding portions of implants.

B. Precautions

1. Prevent damage to implant materials. Care must be taken to use implements, dentifrices, or other cleaning agents that will not scratch or abrade the titanium or other material. Only smooth plastic or wooden implements should be used.
2. Each device should be checked before use. Toothbrush filaments must be smooth, soft, and end rounded to prevent damage to the peri-implant tissue. Soft, end-rounded, power toothbrushes can be applied effectively.

C. Subperiosteal Implant

The posts and surrounding tissue need to be cleaned completely around the circumference. Yarn or gauze strip can be used with a floss threader to position the material under the crossbar.

D. Endosseus Implant

1. *Abutments or Posts.* A floss threader can be used to position yarn or a gauze bandage strip around an abutment and under a fixed prosthesis. Tufted dental floss is also highly effective. Interdental brushes and single end-tuft brushes are adaptable. The end-tuft brush bent at the neck is particularly useful on lingual and palatal surfaces.

2. *Undersurface of Fixed Prosthesis With Cantilever.* Several endosseous implants may be placed anterior to the mental foramen, and the complete overdenture may have a cantilevered portion distal to the terminal implant. Cleaning biofilm from under the cantilever may be accomplished by using gauze strips.

V. RINSING AND IRRIGATION

A. General Cleaning

Use of an irrigator can remove debris before specific cleaning with toothbrush and auxiliary aids.

B. Chemotherapy

1. Rinsing or daily irrigation with an approved antimicrobial can be recommended to help minimize bacterial accumulation and inflammation. Specific directions for preparation of the solution and use of the irrigator must be demonstrated.

2. Chlorhexidine, 0.12%, has been shown to be effective. A cotton swab or interdental brush, dipped in the solution, can be applied directly to the gingival margins to help to prevent staining of oral tissues or tooth-color restorations.[14]

VI. FLUORIDE MEASURES FOR DENTAL CARIES CONTROL

For the patient with natural teeth, daily fluoride self-application should be incorporated into the regimen. Titanium implants may be corroded by acidic fluoride preparations or preparations with a high fluoride concentration.[15,16] Low-concentration neutral sodium fluoride is recommended.

■ MAINTENANCE

I. BASIC CRITERIA FOR IMPLANT SUCCESS

The long-term success of an implant is assessed by routine, frequent examinations. A healthy implant shows the following:
  A. No pain or discomfort reported by the patient.
  B. No mobility.
  C. No bleeding or increased probing depths on gentle probing.
  D. No bone loss or peri-implant radiolucency in a radiograph.
  E. No clinical signs of peri-implantitis.

II. FREQUENCY OF APPOINTMENTS

The patient's daily oral biofilm removal and regular supervision and monitoring through maintenance appointments directly influence the long-term success of an implant. When teeth were lost originally because of lack of daily biofilm control by the patient, a more intense program of education and practice may be needed. Neglect may have been caused by lack of knowledge about, or appreciation for, preventive measures.

Each patient must have a personalized appointment interval, depending on individual needs. The first series of appointments following placement of the implant(s) should start within a week and be scheduled weekly until healing is completed and the patient has demonstrated the ability to control the dental biofilm.

Maintenance appointments during the first year may be at 1- or 2-month intervals.

III. THE MAINTENANCE APPOINTMENT

Factors outlined for a maintenance appointment apply to a patient with an implant.

A. Health History Review; Vital Signs; Intraoral/Extraoral Examination

Basic review questions can reveal the present state of health, recent illnesses, changes in medications, and other current information. Comparisons with previous records permit assessment of vital signs and extraoral/intraoral observations.

B. Selective Radiographs

A standard procedure must be used so that comparisons can be made for bone level to determine status of implant stability. Special film placement devices have been developed.[17,18]

C. Periodontal Assessment

1. *Peri-Implant Tissue.* Visual examination should show no signs of inflammation as evidenced by the usual criteria of changes in color, size, shape, and consistency.
2. *Probing.* Probe gently to determine bleeding tendency. A plastic probe must be used.
3. *Mobility Determination.*
4. *Deposits.* Dental biofilm can be tested with a disclosing agent. The gingival surfaces of fixed prostheses should be checked carefully.

   Calculus is usually not extensive, hard, or firmly attached to implant abutments or other protruding parts, provided the patient has been faithful with daily procedures and professional maintenance appointments.

D. Review of Personal Dental Biofilm Control Procedures

The patient demonstrates self-care methods, and the clinician provides recommendations for improvements.

E. Instrumentation

Each type of implant requires attention to certain features. Manufacturer's instructions should be followed. Care must be taken not to scratch or alter in any way the surfaces of titanium and other materials making up the implant superstructures.

1. *Calculus Removal.* Plastic instruments are indicated for titanium. Figure 30-8 shows various

✔ Factors To Teach The Patient

I. IMPORTANCE OF DAILY CARE

The health of the periodontal tissues and the duration of the restorations and prostheses depend on daily self-care by the patient.

II. NEED FOR CONCENTRATION

More thought and concentration are required to maintain the mouth with advanced restorative dentistry, periodontal prostheses, or implants than are needed for an average mouth.

III. TIME REQUIREMENT

Cleaning a mouth with complex restorations takes longer. Time must be allotted in the daily schedule for complete cleaning and biofilm removal once each day, supplemented by cleaning at least three times each day, or after each meal.

IV. DILIGENCE AND THOROUGHNESS

Do not go easy with the brush and other devices in the attempt to protect the restorations from breakage. *Protection* is for the gingival tissues and the preservation of the periodontium and is accomplished only by thorough dental biofilm removal around every tooth.

V. IMPORTANCE OF MAINTENANCE

Frequent, regular appointments for professional supervision and cooperative care are necessary.

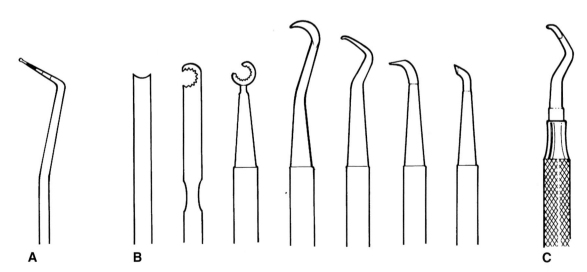

▪ **FIGURE 30-8 Plastic Instrument Designs for Implants. (A)** Plastic probe. **(B)** Scalers and curets. **(C)** Exchangeable plastic curet tip fitted to metal handle for convenient sterilization and replacement. (*Implacare,* HuFriedy, used with permission.)

Everyday Ethics

(?) Every time Larita treated Mrs. Talter she became frustrated because it was evident that significant rehabilitation had occurred in the past 5 years and yet the patient was recalcitrant to following prescribed guidelines for self-care. Dr. Langly had talked with Larita earlier in the week, showing her Mrs. Talter's most recent radiographs. He explained that he was going to suggest replacing tooth numbers 10 and 11 with implants.

Currently these anterior teeth had badly worn crowns and were not esthetically pleasing. Larita questioned the plan based on what she had observed about Mrs. Talter's interest in caring for the appliances she already had. "Wouldn't we be adding to her 'burden' with more specialized homecare procedures?" Larita questioned in a frustrated tone of voice.

Questions for Consideration

1. What "value" does Mrs. Talter appear to place on maintaining her oral cavity?

2. How is it, or is it not, ethically acceptable to change a treatment plan for a patient who has demonstrated such poor daily oral hygiene techniques?

3. With respect to the patient's autonomy, describe a dialogue that could ensue between Larita and Mrs. Talter at the next maintenance appointment.

---

plastic instruments that have been developed for use on implants.

2. *Prevention of Damage to the Implant Surface.* Severe abrasion can result from application of an ultrasonic scaler.

3. *Stain Removal.* Unless it is necessary for esthetics, stain removal is not included routinely. When selective stain removal with a rubber cup is indicated, only a nonabrasive agent should be used and applied gently. An airpowder polisher can be used with a light, sweeping, low-pressured application.[19-21]

4. *Professional Subgingival Irrigation.* The use of 0.12% chlorhexidine after professional instrumentation may be another treatment alternative when peri-implantitis has been present. Irrigation with chlorhexidine gluconate has been shown to be a safe procedure around implants.[22,23]

REFERENCES

1. **Bradbury**, E., Harvard University School of Dental Medicine, Boston, personal communication.

2. **American Dental Association**, Council on Dental Materials, Instruments, and Equipment and Council on Dental Therapeutics: Status Report: Effect of Acidulated Phosphate Fluoride on Porcelain and Composite Restorations, *J. Am. Dent. Assoc., 116,* 115, January, 1988.

3. **Lemons**, J.E.: Dental Implant Biomaterials, *J. Am. Dent. Assoc., 121,* 716, December, 1990.

4. **Albrektsson**, T., Zarb, G., Worthington, P., and Eriksson, A.R.: The Long-term Efficacy of Currently Used Dental Implants: A Review and Proposed Criteria of Success, *Int. J. Oral Maxillofac. Implants, 1,* 11, No. 1, 1986.

5. **Harris**, B.W.: A New Technique for the Subperiosteal Implant, *J. Am. Dent. Assoc., 121,* 422, September, 1990.

6. **Homoly**, P.A.: The Restorative and Surgical Technique for the Full Maxillary Subperiosteal Implant, *J. Am. Dent. Assoc., 121,* 404, September, 1990.

7. **Cranin**, A.N., Sher, J., and Schilb, T.P.: The Transosteal Implant: A 17-Year Review and Report, *J. Prosthet. Dent., 55,* 709, June, 1986.

8. **Small**, I.A.: The Fixed Mandibular Implant: Its Use in Reconstructive Prosthetics, *J. Am. Dent. Assoc., 121,* 369, September, 1990.

9. **Donley**, T.G. and Gillette, W.B.: Titanium Endosseous Implant-Soft Tissue Interface: A Literature Review, *J. Periodontol., 62,* 153, February, 1991.

10. **Cochran**, D.: Implant Therapy I, *Ann. Periodontol., 1,* 710, November, 1996.

11. **Mombelli**, A. and Lang, N.P.: Microbial Aspects of Implant Dentistry, *Periodontol. 2000, 4,* 74, 1994.

12. **Mombelli**, A., Marxer, M., Gaberthüel, T., Grunder, U., and Lang, N.P.: The Microbiota of Osseointegrated Implants in Patients With a History of Periodontal Disease, *J. Clin. Periodontol., 22,* 124, February, 1995.

13. **Schou**, S., Holmstrup, P., Hjorting-Hansen, E., and Lang, N.P.: Plaque-Induced Marginal Tissue Reactions of Osseointegrated Oral Implants: A Review of the Literature, *Clin. Oral Impl. Res., 3,* 149, December, 1992.

14. **Koutsonikos**, A., Federico, J., and Yukna, R.A.: Implant Maintenance, *J. Pract. Hyg., 5,* 11, March/April, 1996.

15. **Siirilä**, H.S. and Könönen, M.: The Effect of Oral Topical Fluorides on the Surface of Commercially Pure Titanium, *Int. J. Oral Maxillofac. Implants, 6,* 50, Number 1, 1991.

16. **Probster**, L., Lin, W., and Hüttemann, H.: Effect of Fluoride Prophylactic Agents on Titanium Surfaces, *Int. J. Oral Maxillofac. Implants, 7,* 390, Fall, 1992.

17. **Cox**, J.F. and Pharoah, M.: An Alternative Holder for Radiographic Evaluation of Tissue-Integrated Prostheses, *J. Prosthet. Dent., 56,* 338, September, 1986.

18. **Meijer**, H.J.A., Steen, W.H.A., and Bosman, F.: Standardized Radiographs of the Alveolar Crest Around Implants in the Mandible, *J. Prosthet. Dent., 68,* 318, August, 1992.

19. **Barnes**, C.M., Fleming, L.S., and Mueninghoff, L.A.: An SEM Evaluation of the In-vitro Effects of an Air-Abrasive System on

Various Implant Surfaces, *Int. J. Oral Maxillofac. Implants, 6,* 463, Number 4, 1991.

20. **Brookshire**, F.V.G., Nagy, W.W., Dhuru, V.B., Ziebert, G.J., and Chada, S.: The Qualitative Effects of Various Types of Hygiene Instrumentation on Commercially Pure Titanium and Titanium Alloy Implant Abutments: An in vitro and Scanning Electron Microscope Study, *J. Prosthet. Dent., 78,* 286, September, 1997.

21. **Chairay**, J.-P., Boulekbache, H., Jean, A., Soyer, A., and Bouchard, P.: Scanning Electron Microscopic Evaluation of the Effects of an Air-Abrasive System on Dental Implants: A Comparative in vitro Study Between Machined and Plasma-Sprayed Titanium Surfaces, *J. Periodontol., 68,* 1215, December, 1997.

22. **Lavigne**, S.E., Krust-Bray, K.S., Williams, K.B., Killoy, W.J., and Theisen, F.: Effects of Subgingival Irrigation With Chlorhexidine on the Periodontal Status of Patients With HA-coated Integral Dental Implants, *Int. J. Oral Maxillofac. Implants, 9,* 156, Number 2, 1994.

23. **Felo**, A., Shibly, O., Ciancio, S.G., Lauciello, F.R., and Ho, A.: Effects of Subgingival Chlorhexidine Irrigation on Peri-implant Maintenance, *Am. J. Dent., 10,* 107, April, 1997.

SUGGESTED READINGS

Bader, J.D., Rozier, R.G., McFall, W.T., and Ramsey, D.L.: Effect of Crown Margins on Periodontal Conditions in Regularly Attending Patients, *J. Prosthet. Dent., 65,* 75, January, 1991.

Brunsvold, M.A. and Lane, J.J.: The Prevalence of Overhanging Dental Restorations and Their Relationship to Periodontal Disease, *J. Clin. Periodontol., 17,* 67, February, 1990.

Cronin, R.J. and Cagna, D.R.: An Update on Fixed Prosthodontics, *J. Am. Dent. Assoc., 128,* 425, April, 1997.

Freilich, M.A., Breeding, L.C., Keagle, J.G., and Garnick, J.J.: Fixed Partial Dentures Supported by Periodontally Compromised Teeth, *J. Prosthet. Dent., 65,* 607, May, 1991.

Kois, J.C. and Spear, F.M.: Periodontal Prosthesis: Creating Successful Restorations, *J. Am. Dent. Assoc., 123,* 108, October, 1992.

Kourkouta, S., Walsh, T.F., and Davis, L.G.: The Effect of Porcelain Laminate Veneers on Gingival Health and Bacterial Plaque Characteristics, *J. Clin. Periodontol., 21,* 638, October, 1994.

Lundgren, D.: Prosthetic Reconstruction of Dentitions Seriously Compromised by Periodontal Disease, *J. Clin. Periodontol., 18,* 390, July, 1991.

Romberg, E., Wood, M., Thompson, V.P., Morrison, G.V., and Suzuki, J.B.: 10-Year Periodontal Response to Resin Bonded Bridges, *J. Periodontol., 66,* 973, November, 1995.

Van Dijken, J.W.V. and Sjöström, S.: The Effect of Glass Ionomer Cement and Composite Resin Fillings on Marginal Gingiva, *J. Clin. Periodontol., 18,* 200, March, 1991.

Wright, P.S. and Hellyer, P.H.: Gingival Recession Related to Removable Partial Dentures in Older Patients, *J. Prosthet. Dent., 74,* 602, December, 1995.

Dental Implants

Albrektsson, T. and Sennerby, L.: State of the Art in Oral Implants, *J. Clin. Periodontol., 18,* 474, July, 1991.

Balshi, T.J.: Candidates and Requirements for Single Tooth Implant Prostheses, *Int. J. Periodont. Restorative Dent., 14,* 317, August, 1994.

Berglundh, T. and Lindhe, J.: Dimension of the Periimplant Mucosa: Biological Width Revisited, *J. Clin. Periodontol., 23,* 971, October, 1996.

Eckert, S.E.: Food and Drug Administration Requirements for Dental Implants, *J. Prosthet. Dent., 74,* 162, August, 1995.

Meffert, R.M., Langer, B., and Fritz, M.E.: Dental Implants: A Review, *J. Periodontol., 63,* 859, November, 1992.

Meffert, R.M: Issues Related to Single-Tooth Implants, *J. Am. Dent. Assoc., 128,* 1383, October, 1997.

Nunn, P.J.: Peri-implant Disease: The New Kid in the Chair, *Access, 11,* 12, May–June, 1997.

Schnitman, P.A.: Implant Dentistry: Where Are We Now?, *J. Am. Dent. Assoc., 124,* 39, April, 1993.

Schulte, W.: Implants and the Periodontium, *Internat. Dent. J., 45,* 16, February, 1995.

Slavkin, H.C.: Biomimicry, Dental Implants and Clinical Trials, *J. Am. Dent. Assoc., 129,* 226, February, 1998.

Implant Applications

Bain, C.A.: Smoking and Implant Failure: Benefits of a Smoking Cessation Protocol, *Int. J. Oral Maxillofac. Implants, 11,* 756, November–December, 1996.

Bida, D.F.: The Use of Dental Implants in the Treatment of Athletic Injuries, *J. Oral Implantol., 17,* 172, Number 2, 1991.

Blanchaert, R.H.: Implants in the Medically Challenged Patient, *Dent. Clin. North Am., 42,* 35, January, 1998.

Block, M.S. and Kent, J.N.: Placement of Endosseous Implants Into Tooth Extraction Sites, *J. Oral Maxillofac. Surg., 49,* 1269, December, 1991.

Lemons, J.E., Laskin, D.M., Roberts, W.E., Tarnow, D.P., Shipman, C., Paczkowski, C., Lorey, R.E., and English, C.: Changes in Patient Screening for a Clinical Study of Dental Implants After Increased Awareness of Tobacco Use as a Risk Factor, *J. Oral Maxillofac. Surg., 55,* 72, Supplement 5, December, 1997.

Mengel, R., Stelzel, M., Hasse, C., and Flores-de-Jacoby, L.: Osseointegrated Implants in Patients Treated for Generalized Severe Adult Periodontitis: An Interim Report, *J. Periodontol., 67,* 782, August, 1996.

Silverstein, L.H., Koch, J.P., Lefkove, M.D., Garnick, J.J., Singh, B., and Steflik, D.E.: Nifedipine-Induced Gingival Enlargement Around Dental Implants: A Clinical Report, *J. Oral Implantol., 21,* 116, Number 2, 1995.

Smith, R.A., Berger, R., and Dodson, T.B.: Risk Factors Associated With Dental Implants in Healthy and Medically Compromised Patients, *Int. J. Oral Maxillofac. Implants, 7,* 367, Number 3, 1992.

Steiner, M., Windchy, A., Gould, A.R., Kushner, G.M., and Weber, R.: Effects of Chemotherapy in Patients With Dental Implants, *J. Oral Implantol., 21,* 142, Number 2, 1995.

Peri-Implant Microbiology

Bauman, G.R., Mills, M., Rapley, J.W., and Hallmon, W.W.: Plaque-Induced Inflammation Around Implants, *Int. J. Oral Maxillofac. Implants, 7,* 330, Number 3, 1992.

Ericsson, I., Persson, L.G., Berglundh, T., Marinello, C.P., Lindhe, J., and Klinge, B.: Different Types of Inflammatory Reactions in Peri-implant Soft Tissues, *J. Clin. Periodontol., 22,* 255, March, 1995.

George, K., Zafiropoulos, G.-G.K., Murat, Y., Hubertus, S., and Nisengard, R.J.: Clinical and Microbiological Status of Osseointegrated Implants, *J. Periodontol., 65,* 766, August, 1994.

Gouvoussis, J., Sindhusake, D., and Yeung, S.: Cross-Infection From Periodontitis Sites to Failing Implant Sites in the Same Mouth, *Int. J. Oral Maxillofac. Implants, 12,* 666, September/October, 1997.

Lambert, P.M., Morris, H.F., and Ochi, S.: The Influence of 0.12% Chlorhexidine Digluconate Rinses on the Incidence of Infectious Complications and Implant Success, *J. Oral Maxillofac. Surg., 55,* 25, Supplement 5, December, 1997.

Nelson, S.K., Knoernschild, K.L., Robinson, F.G., and Schuster, G.S.: Lipopolysaccharide Affinity for Titanium Implant Biomaterials, *J. Prosthet. Dent., 77,* 76, January, 1997.

Ong, E.S.-M., Newman, H.N., Wilson, M., and Bulman, J.S.: The Occurrence of Periodontitis-Related Microorganisms in Relation to Titanium Implants, *J. Periodontol., 63,* 200, March, 1992.

Quirynen, H.C., Van der mei, C.M.L., Bollen, A., Schotte, M., Marechal, G.I., Doornbusch, G.I., Naert, I., Busscher, H.J., and van Steenberghe, D.: An *in vivo* Study of the Influence of the Surface Roughness of Implants on the Microbiology of Supra- and Subgingival Plaque, *J. Dent. Res., 72,* 1304, September, 1993.

Quirynen, M., Papaioannou, W., and van Steenberghe, D.: Intraoral Transmission and the Colonization of Oral Hard Surfaces, *J. Periodontol., 67,* 986, October, 1996.

Rimondini, L., Fare, S., Brambilla, E., Felloni, A., Consonni, C., Brossa, F., and Carrassi, A.: The Effect of Surface Roughness on Early *in vivo* Plaque Colonization on Titanium, *J. Periodontol., 68,* 556, June, 1997.

Sbordone, L., Barone, A., Ramaglia, L., Ciaglia, R.N., and Iacono, V.J.: Antimicrobial Susceptibility of Periodontopathic Bacteria Associated With Failing Implants, *J. Periodontol., 66,* 69, January, 1995.

Instruments

Cross-Poline, G.N., Shaklee, R.L., and Stach, D.J.: Effect of Implant Curets on Titanium Implant Surfaces, *Am. J. Dent., 10,* 41, February, 1997.

Dmytryk, J.J., Fox, S.C., and Moriarty, J.D.: The Effects of Scaling Titanium Implant Surfaces With Metal and Plastic Instruments on Cell Attachment, *J. Periodontol., 61,* 491, August, 1990.

Fox, S.C., Moriarty, J.D., and Kusy, R.P.: The Effects of Scaling a Titanium Implant Surface With Metal and Plastic Instruments: An in vitro Study, *J. Periodontol., 61,* 485, August, 1990.

Hallmon, W.W., Waldrop, T.C., Meffert, R.M., and Wade, B.W.: A Comparative Study of the Effects of Metallic, Nonmetallic, and Sonic Instrumentation on Titanium Abutment Surfaces, *Int. J. Oral Maxillofac. Implants, 11,* 96, Number 1, 1996.

Kuempel, D.R., Johnson, G.K., Zaharias, R.S., and Keller, J.C.: The Effects of Scaling Procedures on Epithelial Cell Growth on Titanium Surfaces, *J. Periodontol., 66,* 228, March, 1995.

Kwan, J.Y., Zablotsky, M.H., and Meffert, R.M.: Implant Maintenance Using a Modified Ultrasonic Instrument, *J. Dent. Hyg., 64,* 422, November–December, 1990.

Parham, P.L., Cobb, C.M., French, A.A., Love, J.W., Drisko, C.L., and Killoy, W.J.: Effects of an Air-Powder Abrasive System on Plasma-Sprayed Titanium Implant Surfaces: An *in vitro* Evaluation, *J. Oral Implantol., 15,* 78, Number 2, 1989.

Implant Care and Maintenance

Ciancio, S.G., Lauciello, F., Shibly, O., Vitello, M., and Mather, M.: The Effect of an Antiseptic Mouthrinse on Implant Maintenance: Plaque and Peri-implant Gingival Tissues, *J. Periodontol., 66,* 962, November, 1995.

Daniels, A.H.: Home Care Parameters for the Implant Patient, *J. Pract. Hyg., 4,* 15, September/October, 1995.

DuCoin, F.J.: Dental Implant Hygiene and Maintenance: Home and Professional Care, *J. Oral Implantol., 22,* 72, Number 1, 1996.

Lang, N.P. and Nyman, S.R.: Supportive Maintenance Care for Patients With Implants and Advanced Restorative Therapy, *Periodontol. 2000, 4,* 119, 1994.

LeBeau, J.: Maintaining the Long-term Health of the Dental Implant and the Implant-borne Restoration, *Compend. Oral Hyg., 3,* 3, Number 3, 1997.

Lochhead, M.A.: Osseointegrated Implants. A Part of Our Future Here and Now, *Can. Dent. Hyg./Probe, 27,* 89, May/June, 1993.

McCollum, J., O'Neal, R.B., Brennan, W.A., Van Dyke, T.E., and Horner, J.A.: The Effect of Titanium Implant Abutment Surface Irregularities on Plaque Accumulation *in vivo, J. Periodontol., 63,* 802, October, 1992.

Speelman, J.A., Collaert, B., and Klinge, B.: Evaluation of Different Methods to Clean Titanium Abutments: A Scanning Electron Microscopic Study, *Clin. Oral Implants Res., 3,* 120, September, 1992.

Strong, S.S. and Strong, S.M.: The Dental Implant Maintenance Visit, *J. Pract. Hyg., 4,* 29, September/October, 1995.

Tomlinson, J.O.: Maintaining Implants at Home, *J. Pract. Hyg., 4,* 22, September/October, 1995.

Toumelin-Chemla, F., Rouelle, F., and Burdairon, G.: Corrosive Properties of Fluoride-Containing Odontologic Gels Against Titanium, *J. Dent., 24,* 109, January/March, 1996.

Yukna, R.A.: Optimizing Clinical Success With Implants: Maintenance and Care, *Compend. Cont. Educ. Dent., 14,* S5554, Supplement 15, 1993.

The Patient Who Uses Tobacco

Joan M. McGowan, RDH, MPH, PhD
Nancy L. J. Williams, RDH, MS, EdD

CHAPTER OUTLINE

Evidence began to accumulate many years ago that cigarette smoking poses an enormous threat to human health.[1] The Surgeon General's first report on tobacco made an unqualified announcement of tobacco's harm.[2] Subsequent reports

further documented the health hazards and discussed the social, economic, and cultural aspects of tobacco use.[3]

Advice from health professionals has been shown to be a powerful influence on patients' decisions to stop or not begin using tobacco. Oral effects of tobacco use are well documented and easily detected. Thus, dental and dental hygiene professionals are in an ideal position and have a responsibility to provide patients who use tobacco with the opportunity to enter a tobacco cessation program to try to prevent tobacco use.

Key words related to tobacco use and addiction are defined in Box 31-1. Box 31-2 defines the various forms of tobacco.

■ HEALTH HAZARDS

Tobacco is toxic to humans. Tobacco use is the single most preventable cause of disease and premature death in the world. Nearly 25% of adult Americans currently smoke, and thousands of children and adolescents become regular users of tobacco every day. Offspring of smokers are more likely to become smokers.[4]

As years of tobacco use accumulate, so do the systemic and oral health effects of all forms of tobacco. Life expectancy is shortened. The number of years lost depends on many factors. Those who quit prior to age 50 will have one-half the risk of dying within 15 years compared with smokers who continue.[5]

■ COMPONENTS OF TOBACCO PRODUCTS

The general public mistakenly believes that nicotine is the harmful substance in tobacco. While nicotine is the most addictive substance, other chemicals are more harmful. Pesticides, aldehydes, ketones, and amines are found in processed tobacco.

Once tobacco is ignited, carcinogenic nitrosamines, polonium 210, carbon monoxide, and other substances become part of mainstream smoke and are emitted in environmental tobacco smoke. Figure 31-1 illustrates the smoking process. The concentration of nicotine in tobacco ranges from 1 to 2 percent of the dry weight of the processed leaf in cigarette tobacco and between 1.45 and 8.00 percent in smokeless tobacco.[6]

■ METABOLISM OF NICOTINE

Absorption of nicotine occurs through the lungs, skin, and oral or nasal mucosa depending on the route of administration.[7,8] Several factors influence absorption of smoked tobacco (cigarettes, pipes, and cigars), as identified in Figure 31-1. Regardless of the type of tobacco used, nicotine is primarily eliminated by liver metabolism and excreted through the kidneys in acid urine.

I. NICOTINE FROM SMOKING

A. Absorption: Lungs

Nicotine enters the lungs and quickly passes into arterial circulation by way of blood vessels lining the sacs of the bronchi.

B. Distribution

1. *To the Brain.* Nicotine is delivered efficiently to the brain by the bloodstream in less than 20 seconds.
2. *Changes in the Liver.* Nicotine is metabolized in the liver into cotinine. Cotinine concentrations in the blood, urine, and saliva are used to assess (a) whether a person uses tobacco, (b) if so, to what extent, and (c) the level of exposure of nonsmokers to passive or environmental smoke.
3. *Peak Plasma Concentration.* Peak plasma concentration of nicotine occurs approximately 10 minutes after the onset of smoking and rapidly declines over the next 20 to 30 minutes.
4. *Dissemination.* Nicotine is spread to all body tissues.
5. *Duration.* The smallest amounts of nicotine from tobacco smoke (one puff) will remain in the body for 8 to 12 hours.

II. SMOKELESS TOBACCO

Smokeless tobacco is the term applied to snuff and chewing tobacco (defined in Box 31-2), which are not smoked but are placed in the mouth.[9]

A. Absorption: Oral Cavity

1. Nicotine is directly absorbed through the gingiva and oral mucous membranes.
2. Once the quid is placed in the mouth, the amount of nicotine absorbed is two to three times the amount delivered by a cigarette.
3. Nicotine concentration declines over 2 hours.
4. Smokeless tobacco users experience nicotine blood plasma levels similar to the nicotine blood levels of smokers.

B. Absorption: Intestinal

1. Most juice produced by smokeless tobacco is spit out.
2. Juice that is intentionally and/or accidentally swallowed by the user is absorbed through the blood vessels lining the small intestine.

BOX 31-1 KEY WORDS AND ABBREVIATIONS: Tobacco Use

Chemical dependency: generic term relating to psychological or physical dependency, or both, on an exogenous substance.

Cotinine: a by-product of nicotine found in body fluids; cotinine levels are used in behavioral research to determine recent use of nicotine-containing products and in clinical research to determine correlations between cotinine levels and oral disease.

Drug abuse: any use of a drug that causes physical, psychological, economic, legal, and/or social harm to the person who uses or other persons affected by the user's behavior.

Drug addiction: a chronic disorder leading to negative physical, psychological, or social consequences from compulsive use of substance; characterized by continued use despite negative effects encountered by use.

Dysphoria: generalized feeling of ill-being, malaise, restlessness, and discomfort.

Nicotine: a poisonous, addictive stimulant that is the chief psychoactive ingredient in tobacco.

Nicotine gum: polacrilex gum developed to aid in smoking cessation; available as an over-the-counter product.

Nicotine lozenge: lozenge developed to aid in smoking cessation; available as an over-the-counter product.

Nicotine nasal spray: a nicotine withdrawal product used nasally by the patient to aid in smoking cessation.

Nicotine patch: a transdermal form of nicotine withdrawal therapy; available as an over-the-counter product.

Nitrosamines: cancer-causing chemicals found in tobacco.

Oral cancer. in this chapter, the term "oral cancer" includes cancer of the lips, tongue, floor of the mouth, palate, gingiva, alveolar mucosa, buccal mucosa, and oropharynx.

Placenta abruptio: premature detachment of a normally situated placenta.

Placenta previa: placenta implanted in the lower segment of the uterus extending to the margin of the internal opening of the cervix; may obstruct opening partially or completely.

Psychoactive drug: possessing the ability to alter mood, behavior, cognitive processes, or mental tension.

Pyrolysis: chemical decomposition of a substance by heat.

Smoke: visible vapor and gases given off by a burning substance.

> **Environmental tobacco smoke (ETS) or passive smoke:** tobacco smoke present in room air resulting from ignited tobacco products burning in an ashtray or exhaled by a smoker (people who are currently smoking are also exposed to other smokers' sidestream smoke).

> **Mainstream smoke:** smoke that is inhaled directly into the user's lungs.

> **Sidestream smoke:** the aerosol emitted directly into the surrounding air from the lit end of a smoldering tobacco product; may be inhaled by the user; is a major component of environmental smoke.

Sudden infant death syndrome (SIDS): Sudden and unexpected death of an apparently healthy infant; typically occurring between the ages of 3 weeks and 5 months.

Thiocyanate: found in tobacco smoke, a byproduct of hydrogen cyanide used to determine recent use of smoked tobacco products.

Transdermal: method of drug delivery by patch on skin; a mode for slow release over extended time.

Transmucosal: type of drug delivery by infiltration of mucosal lining.

BOX 31-2 KEY WORDS: Tobacco Products

Smoking tobacco: any form of tobacco that is ignited and smoked by the user.

Cigar: a small, rolled form of tobacco leaf that is smoked by the user.

Cigarette: a cylindrical, paper-enclosed form of tobacco that is smoked by the user.

Pipe tobacco: ground leaf tobacco manufactured for smoking through a pipe.

Tobacco pipe: a tube with a bowl at one end used to smoke tobacco.

Smokeless (spit) tobacco: term used to define all forms of tobacco that are primarily used orally.

Chaw: a golf-ball-sized portion of chewing tobacco held in the user's mouth usually inside the cheek or between the lower lip, gingiva, and mucosa.

Chewing tobacco: tobacco available in loose-leaf, twist, and plug forms manufactured by air-drying tobacco leaves; held inside cheek and/or chewed (chaw).

Quid: a pinch of snuff held in the user's mouth for various periods of time.

Snuff: fire-cured, finely ground or powdered tobacco sold in both dry and moist forms; not chewed but a small amount ("pinch" or "quid") is placed and held between cheek and gingiva or lower lip, gingiva, and mucosa.

Spit tobacco: a synonymous term for smokeless tobacco products.

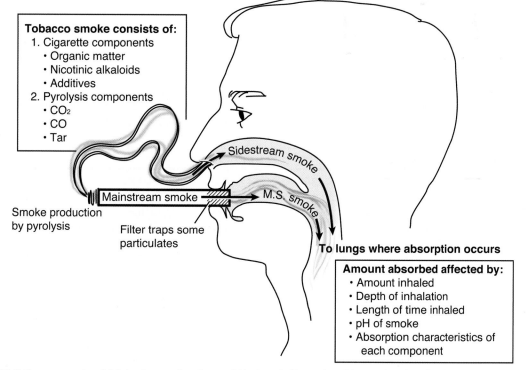

■ **FIGURE 31-1 Components of Mainstream Smoke and Factors Influencing Absorption by the Lungs.**

▪ SYSTEMIC EFFECTS

Use of tobacco products influences every system of the body. Table 31-1 shows smoking-related conditions. The diseases that affect each system have consequences ranging from mild to deadly. About half of today's smokers will die of a smoking-related disease.

I. CARDIOVASCULAR

Smoking aggravates and accelerates the development of atherosclerosis and is a major risk factor for coronary heart disease. Smokers who are over 50, who have used oral contraceptives, or who have a family history of coronary heart disease are at even greater risk.[10,11]

II. PULMONARY DISEASES

Smoking is the major cause of chronic obstructive pulmonary disease (COPD), which includes emphysema and chronic bronchitis. Emphysema slowly destroys a person's ability to breathe. Chronic bronchitis is a condition in which the airways produce excess mucous, which forces the smoker to cough frequently.[12]

III. CANCER

Smoking is responsible for 87% of lung cancers in the United States and is the chief neoplastic cause of death in the United Kingdom. Lung cancer is the leading cause of death for both black and white men and women. Approximately 75% of oral cancers are related to smoking and the use of smokeless tobacco.[13,14]

IV. TOBACCO AND USE OF OTHER DRUGS

Smokers are more likely to consume alcohol. The combined use of alcohol and tobacco places the patient at greater risk for neoplasms and other oral problems.

Heavy cigarette smoking is also highly correlated with cocaine and marijuana use.[15]

▪ ENVIRONMENTAL TOBACCO SMOKE (ETS)

ETS is a complex mixture of chemicals generated during the burning of tobacco products. The principal contributor to ETS is sidestream smoke, the material emitted from burning tobacco products between puffs. Other components of ETS include exhaled mainstream smoke and vaporized compounds diffused through a cigarette wrapper. ETS is also called passive, secondary, or second-hand smoke.[16]

In indoor areas, environmental smoke can last for many hours, depending on ventilation. Exposure for certain workers and family members can be extensive. Fortunately, many public areas, hospitals, and commercial work areas are now mandated smoke free.

Individuals exposed to environmental tobacco smoke are at risk for the same health problems as are active smokers. A nonsmoker may be more sensitive to the toxic effects than the habitual smoker because the system of the smoker adapts to compensate for the deleterious effects of continued smoking.

I. TOXICITY

Many chemicals are contained in passive smoke, including the same carcinogenic compounds as those in mainstream smoke. Some toxic components are actually in higher concentrations in sidestream smoke than in mainstream smoke. Chemicals present in ETS include irritants and systemic toxicants (hydrogen cyanide and sulfur dioxide), mutagens and carcinogens (benzo[a]pyrene and formaldehyde), and reproductive toxicants (nicotine, cadmium, and carbon monoxide).

▪ TABLE 31-1 DISEASE CONSEQUENCES OF TOBACCO USE*

CANCER	RESPIRATORY DISEASES	CARDIOVASCULAR DISEASES	PREGNANCY INFANT HEALTH	OTHER CONDITIONS
Oral cavity*	Chronic obstructive	Atherosclerosis	Abortion	Osteoporosis
Lung	pulmonary disease	Coronary artery disease	Fetal neonatal death	Alzheimer's
Larynx	(COPD)	Hypertension*	Placenta abruptio	disease
Pharynx	Emphysema	Aortic aneurysm	Placenta previa	Wrinkling
Esophagus	Bronchitis	Arterial thrombosis	Premature/prolonged	Concomitant
Stomach	Asthma	Stroke	membrane rupture	use of other
(peptic ulcer*)	Bacterial pneumonia		Preterm labor	drugs*
Bladder	Tuberculosis		Preeclampsia	Early
Uterine cervix			Growth retardation	menopause
Breast			Sudden infant death	
			syndrome	

*Associated with smoke and smokeless tobacco use.

II. LUNG AND RESPIRATORY EFFECTS

Smoking, whether active or passive, is the primary cause of lung cancer.[17] Eye and nasal irritation are the most commonly reported symptoms among adult nonsmokers.

III. CARDIOVASCULAR EFFECTS

Whether smoking is active or passive, its effects on the cardiovascular system are similar. Most deaths that occur annually from exposure to ETS are attributed to heart disease.[18-20]

■ PRENATAL AND CHILDREN

The involuntary ETS that reaches the fetus, the infant, and growing children comes from parents who smoke, the environment of day-care facilities, preschool, and other surroundings where ETS is present.[21,22] The nonsmoking mother who is exposed to passive smoke can also be a source. All exposure to smoke adversely affects the physical, behavioral, and mental health of children.

I. *IN UTERO*

1. Nicotine and carbon monoxide cross the placenta and enter the fetus.
2. Adverse pregnancy risks include miscarriage, placenta previa, low birth weight, and increased perinatal mortality.
3. Cleft lip, cleft palate, and delayed tooth formation have been associated with maternal smoking.[23,24]

II. INFANCY

1. Chemicals are passed to the baby in the breast milk of mothers who smoke.
2. Acute effects include increased incidence of lower respiratory tract illness.
3. Postnatal ETS exposure is an independent cause of sudden infant death syndrome.[25]

III. YOUNG CHILDREN

1. ETS affects lung development with symptoms of coughing, phlegm, and wheezing.
2. Children are at higher risk for asthma; asthma sufferers have additional episodes and a worsened condition.
3. Children have an increased incidence of middle ear infections.
4. Behavioral problems and lower academic achievement in school may be related to missing school during illnesses.

■ ORAL MANIFESTATIONS OF TOBACCO USE

The numerous oral conditions that are attributed to tobacco use vary with the type of tobacco used (smoking or smokeless) and the form in which it is used (cigarettes, pipes, cigars, chewing tobacco, moist snuff).[26] Frequency and duration of use also contribute to the pattern and severity of clinical presentation.

Table 31-2 lists examples of the wide variety of oral consequences of tobacco use; periodontal diseases and oral cancers provide the most serious destructive effects.[27, 28] A systematic extraoral/intraoral examination is the most efficient and effective method for detecting tobacco-related conditions in and around the mouth. The extraoral/intraoral examination gives visual examples for use in encouraging the patient to start a tobacco cessation program.

■ TOBACCO AND PERIODONTAL INFECTIONS

Tobacco use is a major risk factor for periodontal diseases. Users are at a high risk for developing more severe periodontitis at younger ages than nonusers.[29]

I. EFFECTS ON THE PERIODONTAL TISSUES

A. Gingivitis

The degree of inflammatory response to dental biofilm accumulation is reduced compared to nonsmokers.

B. Periodontitis in Tobacco Users

*   Increased rate and severity of periodontal destruction.
*   Increased bone loss, attachment loss, and pocket depths.
*   Pocketing is greater and gingival recession may be noted about anterior teeth.
*   Subgingival temperature lowered.[30]
*   Increased tooth loss from periodontal causes.
*   Increased prevalence with increased number of exposures to tobacco.
*   Prevalence and severity *lessen* with cessation.

II. MECHANISMS OF PERIODONTAL DESTRUCTION

*   No effect on the rate of dental biofilm accumulation.
*   Host response: lowered immune factors.

▪ TABLE 31-2 ORAL CONSEQUENCES OF TOBACCO USE

CANCER AND PRE-CANCER	PERIODONTAL PROBLEMS	SOFT TISSUE PROBLEMS	HARD TISSUE PROBLEMS	ESTHETIC FACTORS	EXACERBATION— ORAL SIGNS IN SYSTEMIC DISEASES
Squamous cell Leukoplakia (ST) Homogeneous Nonhomogeneous Verrucous	ANUG and ANUP Relapse during maintenance Increased risk for peri-implantitis and peri-implant bone loss Localized recession and clinical attachment loss	Nicotine stomatitis (P) Smoker's melanosis Black hairy tongue Median rhomboid glossitis Chronic hyperplastic candidiasis Leukodema (P) Hyperkeratosis (ST) Dry socket Delayed wound healing	Occlusal or incisal abrasion (P), (ST) Cervical abrasion (ST) Dehiscence of bone (ST) Tooth loss	Halitosis Dental stains Prosthesis stains Orthodontic appliance stains Discoloration of restorations Impaired taste and smell	HIV/AIDS Type 1 and Type 2 diabetes

Key: mainly associated with (ST) smokeless tobacco; (P) pipe; (C) cigars; no notation = smoked tobacco.

- Impaired neutrophils: decreased chemotaxis, phagocytosis, and adherence.[31,32]
- Altered antibody production; decreased serum IgG.[33]
- Impairment of revascularization: impact on healing.
- Negative effect on bone metabolism; after menopause, women smokers have a deficit in bone density; smoking can influence osteoporosis.

III. RESPONSE TO TREATMENT

- Resistance to conventional therapy.[34]
- Ideal personal dental biofilm control can minimize the effect.
- Implants have greater risk for failure due to implantitis.[35]
- Delayed healing after surgical and nonsurgical procedures

▪ NICOTINE ADDICTION

Nicotine is tobacco's psychoactive agent (one that produces feelings of pleasure and well-being), and its use leads to tolerance, dependence, and addiction.[36] No one starts using tobacco to become addicted to it. Users can seldom explain why they use tobacco but often say that it helps their physical performance, mood, or ability to think. In fact, physical performance does not improve, mood is not better, and intellectual stimulation is minor.

I. TOLERANCE

A. Physiologic Adaptation

Tolerance refers to the user's need for more smoking or chewing the same amount of the same product over time becomes less and less effective in creating the desired feeling of well-being.

B. Amount of Use

To sustain the positive feelings associated with tobacco use, more and more has to be taken as time goes by.

II. DEPENDENCE

A. Characteristics

As increased amounts are needed over time, the loss of control over the amount and frequency of tobacco use shows evidence of dependence. Facts about nicotine dependency are included in Box 31-3, and criteria for nicotine dependency are outlined in Box 31-4.

B. Reinforcing Effect

Nicotine intensifies the release of dopamine by the brain, thereby increasing a feeling of pleasure and the compulsion to use tobacco. Positive reinforcement is produced with tobacco use, and withdrawal symptoms are produced by abrupt stopping.

BOX 31-3 FACTS ABOUT NICOTINE DEPENDENCY

- Nicotine addiction is similar to that produced by other substances such as alcohol, cocaine, and heroin.

- Tolerance to nicotine is demonstrated as the user experiences less nausea and dizziness following initial use.

- Tobacco abuse: While moderate alcohol use is considered safe, any use of tobacco products is considered a health hazard. Therefore, use is not discussed since any amount is considered abuse.

- Nicotine addiction may be the most challenging of all addictions for complete recovery.

- 70% of smokers report that they would like to quit but only about 1/3 make a quit attempt each year; of these only about 2.5% are successful.

- Many tobacco users make many unsuccessful quit attempts before stopping use for indefinite or extended periods of time.

- Successfully quitting smokeless tobacco use may be equally or more difficult than stopping smoking and should not be considered a viable alternative for smokers who can quit.

Adapted from *American Psychiatric Association: Diagnostic and Statistical Manual of Mental Disorders* (DSM-IV), 4th ed. Washington, D.C., American Psychiatric Association, 1994, pp. 243–247; and Schmitz, J.M., Schneider, N.G., and Jarvik, M.E.: Nicotine, in Lowinson, J.H., Ruiz, P., Millman, R.B., and Langrod, J.G. eds.: *Substance Abuse: A Comprehensive Textbook,* 3rd ed. Baltimore, Williams & Wilkins, 1997, pp. 276–294.

BOX 31-4 Criteria for Nicotine Dependency

- Tolerance

- Withdrawal symptoms when use discontinued

- Used in greater amounts over longer period of time than intended

- A persistent desire or unsuccessful efforts to cut down or quit

- A great deal of time spent using the substance

- Giving up important social, occupational, or recreational activities because of use of the substance

- Continued use despite knowledge of medical problems related to use and/or social and legal problems resulting from use.

Adapted from *American Psychiatric Association: Diagnostic and Statistical Manual of Mental Disorders* (DSM-IV), 4th ed. Washington, D.C., Amerian Psychiatric Association, 1994, pp. 243–247, and Schmitz, J.M., Schneider, N.G., and Jarvik, M.E.: Nicotine, in Lowinson, J.H., Ruiz, P., Millman, R.B., and Langrod, J.G. eds.: *Substance Abuse: A Comprehensive Textbook,* 3rd ed. Baltimore, Williams & Wilkins, 1997, pp. 276–294.

III. ADDICTION

Addiction is a chronic, progressive, relapsing disease characterized by compulsive use of a substance. The effects result in physical, psychologic, and/or social harm to the user, but use continues despite that harm. Smoking is more addictive than alcohol and other drugs of abuse in terms of the proportion of those who are exposed and subsequently become dependent. The pattern of relapse is identical for tobacco, alcohol, and heroin. Factors affecting the development of addiction include:

- Properties of psychoactive drug (dose).
- Family, peer influences, and social acceptance.
- Existing psychiatric disorders.
- Cost and availability of the drug.
- Influence of advertising.

IV. WITHDRAWAL

Withdrawal refers to the effects of cessation of nicotine use by an individual in whom dependence is established. When users of nicotine products stop abruptly, within 24 hours they will likely experience maximal physical and/or psychological withdrawal symptoms. Box 31-5 identifies typical nicotine withdrawal symptoms.

A. Duration

Patients experience withdrawal symptoms almost immediately, and relapse within a week is not uncommon.

BOX 31-5 Criteria for Nicotine Withdrawal Syndrome

- Dysphoric or depressed mood

- Insomnia

- Irritability, frustration, and anger

- Anxiety

- Difficulty concentrating

- Restlessness

- Decreased heart rate

- Increased appetite or weight gain

- Cravings for tobacco

Adapted from *American Psychiatric Association: Diagnostic and Statistical Manual of Mental Disorders* (DSM-IV), 4th ed. Washington, D.C., American Psychiatric Association, 1994, pp. 243–247; and Schmitz, J.M., Schneider, N.G., and Jarvik, M.E.: Nicotine, in Lowinson, J.H., Ruiz, P. Millman, R.B., and Langrod, J.G. eds.: *Substance Abuse: A Comprehensive Textbook,* 3rd ed. Baltimore, Williams & Wilkins, 1997, pp. 276–294.

Most symptoms diminish over a few weeks when relapse does not occur. Cravings for tobacco, increased appetite, and weight gain may persist for months or years.

B. Alleviation of Symptoms

Table 31-3 lists activities that help to overcome withdrawal symptoms. The principle is to prevent relapse.

▪ TREATMENT

Tobacco cessation methods or treatment for nicotine addiction fall into two categories: **self-help** and **assisted strategies.**[7,37]

I. REASONS FOR QUITTING

Before any degree of success can be expected, the individual must make a concentrated effort and must believe in that effort's significance. Typical reasons include the following:
- General health awareness.
- Specific health problem directly or indirectly related to tobacco use.
- Effect on family.
  1. Need to act as a role model
  2. Awareness of effects of ETS
- Effect of smoking and/or ETS on fetus during pregnancy.
- Cost.

▪ TABLE 31-3 ALLEVIATING NICOTINE WITHDRAWAL SYMPTOMS

SYMPTOM	ACTIVITIES
Mood changes: anxiety, nervousness, stressed feelings	Breathe deeply; exhale through pursed lips Take a walk or other relaxation exercise Avoid caffeine Participate in self-reward activity such as purchasing new compact disk
Sleep disturbances	Avoid caffeine Avoid exercise immediately before bedtime Stay up later than usual Avoid resting or watching TV in bed; get in bed only at bedtime
Appetite increase	Eat only when you are hungry Eat low-fat, low-calorie snacks Chew sugarless gum or eat sugarless hard candy Drink additional glasses of water
Cravings	Delay smoking or dipping: Use tactics such as waiting 1 more minute; often cravings pass in 5 or 10 minutes Take deep breaths; exhale through pursed lips Exercise; take a walk Avoid places where you most commonly used tobacco

Taken from *Enough Snuff: A Guide to Quitting Smokeless Tobacco,* 1997, Applied Behavior Science, Point Richmond, CA, with permission from Dr. H.H. Severson.)

- Social pressure and restrictions on smoking in many settings.
- Personal recognition of the dangers of nicotine addiction and the desire to regain control of one's life.

II. SELF-HELP INTERVENTIONS

About one-third of adult smokers attempt to quit, but only 2 to 3 percent are able to achieve long-term abstinence on their own. The proportion of attempts and successes is similar among high school students.

- Go cold turkey. Consider changing lifestyle, including exercise and diet modifications.
- Reduce number of daily tobacco exposures and/or purchase a brand with lower nicotine content.
- Select over-the-counter nicotine replacement patches, gum, or lozenges.
- Join a family member or friend in the tobacco cessation effort.

III. ASSISTED STRATEGIES

A. Counseling

- Provision of practical counseling, including problem solving and skills training.
- Provision of intra-treatment social support: "Our office staff and I are willing to assist you."
- Help in securing extra-treatment social support: "Ask your spouse/partner, friends, and co-workers to support your attempt to quit."

B. Pharmacotherapies[38-40]

Table 31-4 provides an overview of FDA-approved first-line pharmacotherapies and second-line pharmacotherapies that may be considered if first-line pharmacotherapies are not effective.

C. Combination

Counseling combined with pharmacotherapy has been shown to be effective in helping patients to quit using tobacco.

■ PHARMACOTHERAPIES USED FOR TREATMENT OF NICOTINE ADDICTION

I. OBJECTIVES AND RATIONALE

A. Make it easier to abstain from tobacco by partial replacement of nicotine or by counteracting nicotine's action.
B. Reduce withdrawal symptoms.

C. Fulfill, in part, the craving for tobacco by sustaining tolerance.
D. Provide some effects (mood, cognitive changes) previously delivered from nicotine.

II. CONSIDERATIONS

A. Discourage casual use of pharmacotherapies. Failure as a result of improper use can discourage future quit attempts.
B. Inform patient of signs and symptoms of nicotine overdose: nausea, vomiting, dizziness, weakness, or rapid heartbeat.
C. Consult physician prior to use if under 18 years or contraindications are present.

III. CONTRAINDICATIONS

A. Self-medication without examination.
B. Pregnancy: nicotine in the bloodstream, even in small amounts, can still reach the fetus.
C. Nicotine gum: hypertension; using medication for asthma, depression, or diabetes; cardiovascular disease, stomach ulcers.
D. Nicotine patch: same as nicotine gum; in addition, some patients may be allergic to patch adhesives.

IV. NICOTINE REPLACEMENT THERAPY (NRT)

The nicotine gum is sweetened with xylitol and has either a mild mint or orange flavor, whereas the lozenge is sweetened with mannitol and aspartame and flavored with a mild mint.

A. Nicotine Gum

1. *Transmucosal delivery*: nicotine released in mouth during "chewing."
2. *Interference with absorption of nicotine*: avoid acidic foods and beverages while using gum.
3. *How to use*: chew, park, chew—take 3 or 4 chews until a "peppery" or "minty" taste emerges, then park between cheek and gingiva. Gum should be "chewed" and "parked" for about 30 minutes or until taste dissipates.

B. Nicotine Patch

1. *Transdermal delivery*: nicotine released through skin.
2. *Directions*: place a new patch on a hairless location upon rising; if sleep disruption occurs, remove 24-hour patch prior to bedtime or use 16-hour patch.

C. Nicotine Inhaler

1. *Transmucosal delivery*: nicotine released in mouth during inhalation or puffing.

■ TABLE 31-4 SUGGESTIONS FOR THE CLINICAL USE OF PHARMACOTHERAPIES FOR SMOKING CESSATION

PHARMACOTHERAPY	PRECAUTIONS/ CONTRAINDICATIONS	SIDE EFFECTS	DOSAGE	DURATION	AVAILABILITY
First-line pharmacotherapies	(approved for use for smoking cessation by the FDA)				
Bupropion SR	History of seizure History of eating disorder	Insomnia Dry mouth	150 mg every morning for 3 days then 150 mg twice daily (Begin treatment 1–2 weeks pre-quit)	7–12 weeks maintenance up to 6 months	Zyban (prescription only)
Nicotine gum	None	Mouth soreness Dyspepsia	1–24 cigs/day— 2-mg gum (up to 24 pcs/day) 25+ cigs/day— 4-mg gum (up to 24 pcs/day)	Up to 12 weeks	Nicorette, Nicorette Mint (OTC only)
Nicotine inhaler	None	Local irritation of mouth and throat	6–16 cartridges/ day	Up to 6 months	Nicotrol Inhaler (prescription only)
Nicotine nasal spray	None	Nasal irritation	8–40 doses/day	3–6 months	Nicotrol NS (prescription only)
Nicotine patch	None	Local skin reaction Insomnia	21 mg/24 hours 14 mg/24 hours 7 mg/24 hours	4 weeks then 2 weeks then 2 weeks	Nicoderm CQ, (OTC only), Generic patches (prescription and OTC) Nicotrol (OTC only)
Second-line pharmacotherapies	(not approved for use for smoking cessation by the FDA)				
Clonidine	Rebound hypertension	Dry mouth Drowsiness Dizziness Sedation	0.15–0.75 mg/day	3–10 weeks	Oral Clonidine-generic, Catapres (prescription only) Transdermal Catapres (prescription only)
Nortriptyline	Risk of arrythmias	Sedation Dry mouth	75–100 mg/day	12 weeks	Nortriptyline HCl-generic (prescription only)

Adapted from Fiore, M.C., Bailey, W.C., Cohen, S.J., et.al.: *Treating Tobacco Use and Dependence: Quick Reference Guide for Clinicians*. Rockville, MD; U.S. Department of Health and Human Services, Public Health Service, October 2000.

2. *Interference with absorption of nicotine*: avoid eating and/or drinking acidic beverages for 15 minutes before and during inhalation.
3. *Requirements*: store inhaler and cartridges in a warm place when temperatures drop below 40°F to prevent a decline in delivery of nicotine from the inhaler to the oral cavity.

D. Nicotine Nasal Spray

1. *Nasal mucous membrane delivery*: nicotine released through lining of nose.

2. *Dose delivery*: avoid sniffing, swallowing, or inhaling while administering doses, as these increase irritating effects.
3. *Directions*: tilt head slightly back while delivering spray.

E. Nicotine Lozenge

1. *Transmucosal delivery*: nicotine released in mouth as lozenge dissolves.
2. *Dose delivery*: is based on a new indicator "Time to First Cigarette" (TTFC):

- 4-mg lozenge for those who smoke the first cigarette within 30 minutes of waking.
- 2-mg lozenge for those who smoke the first cigarette after 30 minutes.

3. *Directions*: do not bite or chew lozenge as it dissolves in the mouth: this can cause more nicotine to be swallowed quickly and may result in indigestion and/or heartburn.

■ NICOTINE-FREE THERAPY

Bupropion SR is the first non-nicotine medication shown to be effective for smoking cessation and approved by the FDA for that use. Its mechanism of action is presumed to be mediated by its capacity to block neural uptake of dopamine and/or norepinephrine. Bupropion SR can be used in combination with nicotine replacement therapies. Table 31-4 provides an overview of non-nicotine pharmacotherapies.

Second-line medications are pharmacotherapies for which there is evidence of efficacy for treating tobacco dependence, but they have a more limited role because:

- The FDA has not approved them for a tobacco dependence treatment indication.
- There are more concerns about potential side effects than exist with first-line medications.
- Second-line treatments, clonidine and nortriptyline, should be considered for use on a case-by-case basis after first-line treatments have been used or considered.

■ DENTAL HYGIENE CARE FOR THE PATIENT WHO USES TOBACCO

The tobacco-using patient presents a unique challenge to the oral health team. Specific treatment modifications are indicated. Helping the patient to quit using tobacco becomes an integral part of the dental hygiene care plan.

■ ASSESSMENT

I. PATIENT HISTORY

Tobacco use status must be assessed at each appointment. The basic history form (pages 110–111) used by all patients should include one or two questions to determine whether the patient currently uses tobacco and, if so, the types of tobacco (smoking and/or smokeless). The National Cancer Institute's tobacco use assessment

form is shown as Figure 31-2. Concomitant use of alcohol, cocaine, or marijuana with tobacco may necessitate modifications of clinical procedures.

II. VITAL SIGNS[42]

Tobacco use status is considered a vital sign along with temperature, pulse, respiratory rate, and blood pressure (see Figure 8-1).

III. EXTRAORAL EXAMINATION

A. Breath and Body Odor

1. *Halitosis*
2. *Electropositive smoke*: smoke from cigars and other smoked tobacco products clings to skin, hair, and clothes and results in body odor.

B. Fingers

Smokers of nonfiltered cigarettes have a yellowish-brown discoloration of the fingers and fingernails.

C. Skin

Smokers experience premature and more extensive facial wrinkling.

D. Lips

Pipe and cigar smokers are at risk for development of precancerous and cancerous lip lesions.

IV. INTRAORAL EXAMINATION

An excellent outline for conducting the especially intensive intraoral examination the tobacco-using patient must receive is provided in Table 10-1 on pages 177 to 178. Oral consequences of tobacco use are listed in Table 31-2.

A. Detection of an Intraoral Lesion or Problem

Upon detecting a tobacco-related problem or lesion, the clinician will:

1. *Show the Patient.* Provide a simple but thorough explanation related to the nature of the condition.
2. *Explain.* Make certain that the patient understands the consequences of continuing tobacco use as it relates to the progress of the problem or lesion.
3. *Record.* Provide a detailed description of the problem or lesion and note the information given to the patient in the dental record for the dentist's review.

TOBACCO USE ASSESSMENT FORM

Name: _____   Date_____

1. Do you use tobacco in any form?   ☐ Yes   ☐ No

1A. If no, have you ever used tobacco in the past?   ☐ Yes   ☐ No

How long did you use tobacco?   Years____   Months____

How long ago did you stop?   Years____   Months____

If you are not currently a tobacco user, no other questions should be answered. Thank you for completing this form.

Question 2-10 are for current tobacco users only.

2. **If you smoke,** what type (check)   How many? (Number)
   ☐ Cigarettes   Cigarettes per day____
   ☐ Cigars   Cigars per day____
   ☐ Pipes   Bowls per day____

3. **If you chew/use snuff,** what type?   How much?
   ☐ Snuff   Days a can lasts____
   ☐ Chewing   Pouches per week____
   ☐ Other (describe)   Amount_____per_____

3A. **How long** do you keep a chew in your mouth? _____minutes

4. **How many days** of the week do you first use tobacco?   7   6   5   4   3   2   1

5. **How soon** after you wake do you first use tobacco?
   Within 30 minutes?____   More than 30 minutes?____

6. Does the person **closest to you** use tobacco?   ☐ Yes   ☐ No

7. **How interested are you** in stopping your use of tobacco?
   ☐ not at all   ☐ a little   ☐ somewhat   ☐ Yes   ☐ very much

8. Have you ever **tried to stop** using tobacco before?   ☐ Yes   ☐ No

9. Have you **discussed stopping** with your physician?   ☐ Yes   ☐ No

10. If you decided to stop using tobacco completely during the next two weeks, **how confident are you** that you would succeed?
    ☐ not at all   ☐ a little   ☐ somewhat   ☐ very confident

---

▪ **FIGURE 31-2 Tobacco Use Assessment Form.**

B. Referral Indications

Should a lesion persist for more than 2 weeks, a biopsy is indicated (Chapter 10, pages 184 to 185).

1. *Refer* the patient for biopsy.
2. *Ascertain*. Check to be certain that the patient undergoes the biopsy and receives results.
3. *Consult*. Pathologist that reviews the biopsy provides the pertinent information.
4. *Document*. Results are entered into the patient's treatment record.

C. Oral Self-examination

Oral self-examination must be taught to all patients who use tobacco. The significance of oral self-examination in this high-risk group cannot be overstated. Teach patients to perform an oral self-examination by using the same techniques and components of the professional extraoral and intra-oral examinations, as illustrated and explained in Chapter 10 (pages 176 to 179).

D. Detect, Relate, Motivate

Lesions that are a direct consequence of use are pointed out to the patient. The presence of tobacco-related problems/lesions can serve as a powerful motivational tool to encourage a quit attempt. The demonstration of the arrest or elimination of tobacco-related problems/lesions as the patient continues a nonuse status will aid in achieving permanent cessation.

V. CONSULTATION

Patients who do not seek routine medical care need referral to a physician for evaluation. Detection of underlying medical problems is essential so that necessary dental treatment modifications may be utilized.

▪ CLINICAL TREATMENT PROCEDURES

Patients who use tobacco have more dental stain, calculus, and periodontal problems, and therefore require longer and more frequent appointments, than nonusers.

I. DENTAL BIOFILM CONTROL

Self-care for daily dental biofilm control is the first priority in the care plan. Immaculate oral hygiene is required by this group of high-risk patients owing to their susceptibility to dental caries, periodontal infections, and other soft-tissue alterations.

II. SCALING AND ROOT PLANING

A. Inform the patient that healing will be jeopardized by continued tobacco use and that users cannot expect the same treatment results as nonusers.[34]

B. When using power-driven instruments:
   - Take precautions to prevent the patient from ingesting bacteria, water, and debris (smokers often have pulmonary and cardiovascular complications).
   - Take precautions (as described on pages 1051 to 1053) with smokers who have a cardiac pacemaker.

III. OTHER PATIENT INSTRUCTION

A. Diet and Nutrition

- Tobacco users may be poorly nourished because use decreases appetite. Conversely, the desire to control body weight through tobacco use may impede a patient's willingness to quit.
- Suggestions about diet and exercise can be provided.
- Most smokeless tobacco products are sweetened with sugar or molasses, which increases their cariogenic potential. Appropriate instruction can be provided.

B. Nonalcoholic Rinses

Tobacco users may be aware of halitosis and frequently use alcohol-containing mouth rinses to mask unpleasant odors. Long-term use of alcohol-containing antibacterial agents, mouthrinses, and other oral hygiene products cannot be recommended owing to the synergistic effect of alcohol and tobacco in the initiation of head and neck cancers.

▪ TOBACCO CESSATION PROGRAM

A program for tobacco cessation is an essential component of the dental hygiene care plan for all tobacco-using patients.[41,43] The majority of users admit that they would like to quit or "know" that they should, and about one-third of them are willing to try.

Interventions and their outcomes will vary depending on the motivation and experience of the clinician and the patient's acceptance of and adherence to the regimen. Even a minimal intervention conducted by a clinician may help a patient become tobacco free.

▪ THE "5 A's"

The "5 A's"—Ask, Advise, Assess, Assist, Arrange—provide the basis for a brief, simple, but effective tobacco dependence intervention. A cessation program flow chart is presented in Figure 31-3.

I. ASK

A. Health History

Ask all patients about tobacco use. Include questions about tobacco use on the health history. (See the ADA Health History Form on page 110.)

B. Present Questions Carefully

When reviewing the health history with the patient, present questions related to tobacco nonjudgmentally. Address tobacco use as a health issue, not as a moral and/or social issue. Obtain facts without placing the patient on the defensive.

C. Obtain Patient's Confidence

Many minors use tobacco without their parents' knowledge or consent. Social disapproval of tobacco use is increasing, and patients may hesitate to disclose their habit.

D. Children

1. By age 5, children are taking responsibility for themselves in many ways; therefore, it is recommended that this is the appropriate age to begin asking about tobacco use.

2. Children ages 3 to 6 can identify cartoon figures and relate them to a tobacco product. Children should hear messages that counter those produced by the tobacco industry.

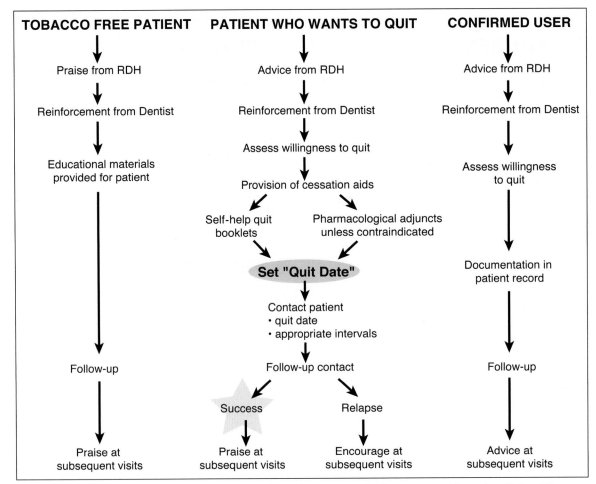

FIGURE 31-3 Tobacco Cessation. Flow chart to show how the **5 A's** can be incorporated into the clinic setting.

3. Ask parents about tobacco use in the home.
4. Discuss effects of ETS on health, developmental risks, the example that use of tobacco sets for children with the parents.

II. ADVISE

A. Never Users/Former Users

Advise every patient about tobacco use. Praise never-users and former users for their tobacco-free behavior. Reinforcement counters the tobacco industry's message and other enticements to begin.

B. Stop-Look-Listen Approach

1. **Stop Now.** Clearly advise the patient about the importance of *stopping* now. Present the advice in a caring, compassionate manner so that patients realize that clinicians are interested in their health and well-being.
2. **Show.** Have patients *look* in their mouths and observe the clinical effects of tobacco use.

Existing conditions such as stains, calculus, halitosis, periodontal disease, and abnormal lesions may serve as strong motivators in getting a patient to quit. Generally, patients are not impressed by a discussion of possible future health problems or of the effect of tobacco use on others. Advice should be relevant to existing conditions.

3. **Listen.** Ask patients their reasons for wanting to quit. Most users want to quit. Their reasons may have little to do with health, but speaking out forces patients to focus and strengthen their reasons. *Listening* to the patient allows the clinician to support the patient's thoughts and provide appropriate reinforcement.

C. Brief Advice to Patients

1. Significantly increases long-term abstinence rates.
2. Dentists and dental hygienists can and should offer brief advice.

III. ASSESS

A. Ask the patient: "Are you ready to quit?"
B. If the patient is ready:
1. Determine if the patient should be treated in your office. (Patients may have multiple problems that might necessitate a referral, e.g., alcoholic, psychotic.)
2. If treatment is to be provided in your office, go to the **ASSIST** step.
C. If the patient is not ready to quit, use the "5 R's":
1. **Relevance:** tailor advice and discussion to each patient.
2. **Risks:** discuss risks of continued tobacco use.
3. **Rewards:** discuss benefits of quitting.
4. **Roadblocks:** identify barriers to quitting.
5. **Repetition:** reinforce the motivational message at every visit.

IV. ASSIST

A. Establish a Quit Plan

1. Set a quit date, preferably within 2 weeks.
2. Have the patient tell family, friends, and coworkers about quitting and request their understanding and support.
3. Warn the patient to anticipate challenges to the planned quit attempt, particularly during the first few weeks. This includes nicotine withdrawal symptoms.
4. Ask the patient to remove all tobacco-related products from home and work sites.

B. Provide Practical Counseling

1. Total abstinence is essential: "not even a single puff or dip after the quit date."
2. Review past quit attempts and identify what helped and what factors contributed to relapse.
3. Discuss challenges/triggers and how the patient will overcome them successfully.
4. Because alcohol can cause relapse, limit/abstain from alcohol use.
5. Quitting is more difficult when there is another smoker in the household. Encourage housemates to quit or not to smoke in their presence.

C. Pharmacotherapy

Recommend the use of approved pharmacotherapy. See Table 31-4.

D. Provide Educational Materials

Many agencies publish motivational materials appropriate for various cultures and ethnic groups and are sensitive, as well, to different levels of education and differences in age of their readers. Keep a supply of these materials in the office for distribution to patients.

V. ARRANGE

Follow-up is essential to achieving a significant patient quit rate. Prepare a note, prescription, or other reminder showing the quit date for the patient. Suggest posting it in a suitable place in the patient's home.

A. Contact the Patient Before the Quit Date

1. A telephone call assures the patient that the interest is sincere.
2. Ask if the booklet provided has been read, if there are any questions, and if others have been asked to help.

B. Follow-up Contact

1. Follow-up, either in person or via telephone, is essential.
2. Timely intervals would be once within the first week after the quit date when the patient's physical withdrawal symptoms are most intense, and again at the end of the first, second, and third months.
3. More than four contacts help to increase long-term abstinence.

C. Actions During Follow-up Contact

1. Congratulate and praise patients who have remained tobacco free.
2. Provide the opportunity for patients to ask questions. If they have none, encourage the patient to contact you if questions should arise.
3. If relapse has occurred, ask the patient to recall and record the circumstances that led to reuse.
4. Encourage the patient to set another quit date, reminding the patient that a lapse can be a learning experience.
5. Review the use of pharmacotherapy.
6. Provide agencies and contact numbers for the patient who requests a more intensive cessation program.

▪ THE TEAM APPROACH

I. ORGANIZE THE CLINIC TEAM

A. Select a Team Coordinator

The coordinator does not do everything, but sees that everything is done.

Everyday Ethics

(?) Fifteen-year-old Jason comes with his mom for a regular maintenance appointment with the dental hygienist. During the oral examination the hygienist notices small red and white patches in the vestibular areas of the mandible adjacent to the molar teeth. She also records moderate brownish staining on the teeth and plans to use the air-powder polisher after scaling. She questions Jason about smoking and the use of smokeless tobacco, but he states that he has only tried cigarettes once or twice.

Questions to Consider

1. What beneficial approach can the dental hygienist use with Jason if she suspects he is not telling the truth about his smoking habits?

2. How can the dental hygienist maintain Jason's right to confidentiality but inform his mom of potentially serious changes in the gingival tissues?

3. Which of the ethical principles apply to this situation? Explain your response from both the dental hygienist's perspective and the patient's perspective.

B. Responsibilities

1. Identify tobacco use status at patient's first visit.
2. Record appropriate documentation in patient's records.

✔ Factors To Teach The Patient

- The most effective method to stop using tobacco is never to start.

- How to perform a regular self-examination of the oral cavity.

- Pregnant women who use tobacco products may harm the developing fetus and the newborn infant.

- Young children may experiment with or use tobacco products. Parents must be prepared to provide guidance.

- All forms of social tobacco use can lead to addiction.

- Nonsmokers who breathe ETS can incur the same serious health problems as smokers. Children are especially susceptible.

- Smokeless tobacco use is *not* a safe alternative to smoking.

- Oral health team members can help patients become tobacco free.

- Learn about local or state tobacco legislation and public health policy to make informed choices related to a tobacco smoke–free society.

3. Ensure that all tobacco-using patients are offered the opportunity to enter a cessation program.
4. Contact patients for follow-up.
5. Act as a coach for patients who relapse.
6. Maintain a supply of literature for patients.

C. Team Members

Tobacco users should be encouraged to quit and/or enter a cessation program.

II. ORGANIZE A TOBACCO-FREE ENVIRONMENT

A. Remove ashtrays and post positive "no smoking" signs.
B. Display tobacco use prevention and cessation materials prominently.
C. Eliminate magazines that contain tobacco advertising from reception area.

III. ORGANIZE A TOBACCO USER TRACKING SYSTEM

A. **Tobacco Use Assessment Form:** see Figure 31-2.
B. **Patient Permanent Progress Report:** records include dated case notes for all advice to quit, responses and interest in quitting, and progress.
C. **Tobacco Status on Charts:** clearly mark charts so that status can be immediately seen by any clinic staff.

■ ADVOCACY

I. PUBLIC HEALTH POLICY

The first-ever Surgeon General's Report on Oral Health[2] specifically identified tobacco use as a risk factor for oral cavity and pharyngeal cancer. Healthcare providers can help users quit and can become partners with one another and with community programs to prevent diseases and promote good health habits.

The Centers for Disease Control and Prevention has been supporting state-based tobacco control coalitions in all 50 states. Many local communities and municipalities are considering the adoption of a smoke-free workplace ordinance, or may be in the process of enacting such an ordinance. Oral health professionals can be valuable and welcome partners in these programs.

II. COMMUNITY ORAL HEALTH EDUCATIONAL PROGRAMS

Early signs of tobacco use may be seen in the oral cavity. No community oral health program can be considered complete without inclusion of tobacco prevention, control, and cessation education. Excellent materials are available from many nonprofit and professional organizations.

REFERENCES

1. **Pearl**, R.: Tobacco Smoking and Longevity, *Science, 87,* 216, March 4, 1938.

2. **Advisory Committee on Smoking and Health to the U.S. Surgeon General**: *Report*. Washington, D.C., U.S. Department of Health, Education, and Welfare, 1965, pp. 31–40.

3. **United States Department of Health and Human Services**: *Reducing Tobacco Use: A Report of the Surgeon General*. Atlanta, Centers for Disease Control and Prevention, National Center for Chronic Disease Prevention and Health Promotion, Office on Smoking and Health, 2000, p. I.

4. **Stein**, Z.: Smoking and Reproductive Health, *J. Am. Med. Women's Assoc., 51,* 29, January/April, 1996.

5. **United States Department of Health and Human Services**: *The Health Benefits of Smoking Cessation: A Report of the Surgeon General, Executive Summary*, Public Health Service, Centers for Disease Control, Center for Chronic Disease Prevention and Health Promotion, DHHS Pub. No. (CDC) 90-8416, 1990, in *MWWR, 39,* RR-12, October 5, 1990, p. vi.

6. **National Cancer Institute**: *Smokeless Tobacco or Health, An International Perspective. Smoking and Tobacco Control Monograph No. 2,* Bethesda, MD, U. S. Department of Health and Human Services, National Institutes of Health, National Cancer Institute, NIH Pub. No. 93-3461, 1992, p. 153.

7. **Schmitz**, J.M., Schneider, N.G., and Jarvik, M.E.: Nicotine, in Lowinson, J.H., Ruiz, P., Millman, R.B., and Langrod, J.G., eds.: *Substance Abuse: A Comprehensive Textbook*, 3rd ed. Baltimore, Williams & Wilkins, 1997, pp. 276–294.

8. **Benowitz**, N.L., Porchet, H., Scheiner, L., and Jacob, P.: Nicotine Absorption and Cardiovascular Effects With Smokeless Tobacco Use: Comparison With Cigarettes and Nicotine Gum, *Clin. Pharmacol. Ther., 44,* 23, July, 1988.

9. **Hatsukami**, D., Nelson, R., and Jensen, J.: Smokeless Tobacco: Current Status and Future Directions, *Brit. J. Addict., 86,* 559, May, 1991.

10. **Holbrook**, J.H., Grundy, S.M., Hennekens, C.H., Kannel, W.B., and Strong, J.P.: Cigarette Smoking and Cardiovascular Diseases: A Statement for Health Professionals by a Task Force Appointed by the Steering Committee of the American Heart Association, *Circulation, 70,* 1114A, December, 1984.

11. **Howard**, G., Wagenknecht, L.E., Burke, G.L., Diez-Roux, A., Evans, G.W., McGovern, P., Nieto, F. J., and Tell, G.S.: Cigarette Smoking and Progression of Atherosclerosis: The Atherosclerosis Risk in Communities (ARIC) Study, *JAMA, 279,* 119, January 14, 1998.

12. **Zielinski**, J. and Bednarck, M.: Early Detection of COPD in a High-Risk Population Using Spirometric Screening, *Cardiopulmonary and Critical Care J, 119,* 731, March, 2001.

13. **American Cancer Society**, *Cancer Facts and Figures 2002*, Atlanta, American Cancer Society, 2002, pp. 29–31.

14. **Peto**, R., Darby, S., Deo, H., Silcocks, P., Whitley, E., and Doll, R.: Smoking, Smoking Cessation, and Lung Cancer in the UK Since 1950: Combination of National Statistics With Two Case-Control Studies, *Brit. Med. J., 7257,* 323, August, 2000.

15. **Ford**, D.E., Vu, H.T., and Anthony, J.C.: Marijuana Use and Cessation of Tobacco Smoking in Adults From a Community Sample, *Drug and Alcohol Dependence, 67,* 243, August 1, 2002.

16. **National Cancer Institute**: *Health Effects of Exposure to Environmental Tobacco Smoke: The Report of the California Environmental Protection Agency. Smoking and Tobacco Control Monograph No. 10,* Bethesda, MD, U.S. Department of Health and Human Services, National Institutes of Health, National Cancer Institute, NIH Pub. No. 99-4645, 1999, pp. ES-3–10.

17. **Fontham**, E.T.H., Correa, P., Reynolds, P., Wu-Williams, A., Buffler, P.A., Greenberg, R.S., Chen, V. W., Alterman, T., Boyd, P., Austin, D.F., and Liff, J.: Environmental Tobacco Smoke and Lung Cancer in Nonsmoking Women: A Multicenter Study, *JAMA, 271,* 1752, June 8, 1994.

18. **Taylor**, A.E., Johnson, D.C., and Kazemi, H.: Environmental Tobacco Smoke and Cardiovascular Disease: A Position Paper From the Council on Cardiopulmonary and Critical Care, American Heart Association, *Circulation, 86,* 700, August, 1992.

19. **Glantz**, S.A. and Parmley, W.W.: Passive Smoking and Heart Disease. Mechanisms and Risk, *JAMA, 273,* 1047, April 5, 1995.

20. **Wells**, A. J.: Passive Smoking as a Cause of Heart Disease, *J. Am. Coll. Cardiol., 24,* 546, August, 1994.

21. **Charlton**, A.: Children and Passive Smoking: A Review, *J. Fam. Pract., 38,* 267, March, 1994.

22. **American Heart Association**, Committee on Atherosclerosis and Hypertension in Children, Council on Cardiovascular Disease in the Young: Active and Passive Tobacco Exposure: A Serious Pediatric Health Problem, *Circulation, 90,* 2581, November, 1994.

23. **Khoury**, M. J., Gomez-Farias, M., and Mulinare, J.: Does Maternal Cigarette Smoking During Pregnancy Cause Cleft Lip and Palate in the Offspring? *Am. J. Dis. Child., 143,* 333, March, 1989.

24. **Kieser**, J.A., Groeneveld, H.T., and da Silva, P.: Delayed Tooth Formation in Children Exposed to Tobacco Smoke, *J. Clin. Pediatr. Dent., 20,* 97, Winter, 1996.

25. **Klonoff-Cohen**, H.S., Edelstein, S.L., Lefkowitz, E.S., Srinivasan, I.P., Kaegi, D., Chang, J.C., and Wiley, K. J.: The Effect of Passive Smoking and Tobacco Exposure Through Breast Milk on Sudden Infant Death Syndrome, *JAMA, 273,* 795, March 8, 1995.

26. **Mecklenburg**, R.E., Greenspan, D., Kleinman, D.V., Manley, M. W., Niessen, L.C., Robertson, P.B., and Winn, D.E.: *Tobacco Effects in the Mouth: A National Cancer Institute and National Institute of Dental Research Guide for Health Professionals*, U.S. Department of Health and Human Services, Public Health Service, NIH Publication No. 00-3330, September, 2000.

27. **Tomar**, S.L. and Asma, S.: Smoking-Attributable Periodontitis in the United States: Findings From NHANES III, *J. Periodontol., 71,* 743, May, 2000.

28. **American Academy of Periodontology**, Research, Science, and Therapy Committee: Tobacco Use and the Periodontal Patient, *J. Periodontol., 70,* 1419, November, 1999.

29. **Haber**, J., Wattles, J. Crowley, M., Mandell, R., Joshipura, K., and Kent, R.L.: Evidence for Cigarette Smoking as a Major Risk Factor for Periodontitis, *J. Periodontol., 64*, 16, January, 1993.

30. **Trikilis**, N., Rawlinson, A., and Walsh, T.F.: Periodontal Probing Depth and Subgingival Temperature in Smokers and Non-Smokers, *J. Clin. Periodontol., 26*, 38, January, 1999.

31. **MacFarlane**, G.D., Herzberg, M.C., Wolff, L.F., and Hardie, N.A.: Refractory Periodontitis Associated With Abnormal Polymorphonuclear Leukocyte Phagocytosis and Cigarette Smoking, *J. Periodontol., 63*, 908, November, 1992.

32. **Pabst**, M.J., Pabst, K.M., Collier, J.A., Coleman, T.C., Lemons-Prince, M.L., Godat, M.S., Waring, M.B., and Babu, J.P.: Inhibition of Neutrophil and Monocyte Defensive Functions by Nicotine, *J. Periodontol., 66*, 1047, December, 1995.

33. **Tew**, J.G., Zhang, J.-B., Quinn, S., Tangada, S., Nakashima, K., Gunsolley, J.C., Schenkein, H.A., and Califano, J.V.: Antibody of the IgG2 Subclass, *Actinobacillus actinomycetemcomitans*, and Early-Onset Periodontitis, *J. Periodontol., 67*, 317, March, Supplement, 1996.

34. **Grossi**, S.G., Zambon, J., Machtei, E.E., Schifferle, R., Andreana, S., Genco, R.J., Cummins, D., and Harrap, G.: Effects of Smoking and Smoking Cessation on Healing After Mechanical Periodontal Therapy, *J. Am. Dent. Assoc., 128*, 599, May, 1997.

35. **Haas**, R., Haimböck, W., Mailath, G., and Watzek, G.: The Relationship of Smoking on Peri-Implant Tissue: A Retrospective Study, *J. Prosthet. Dent., 76*, 592, December, 1996.

36. **Leshner**, A.I.: Understanding Drug Addiction: Implications for Treatment, *Hospital Practice, 37*, 47, October 15, 1996.

37. **Mecklenburg**, R.E., Christen, A.G., Gerbert, B., Gift, H.C., Glynn, T. J., Jones, R.B., Lindsay, E., Manley, M.W., and Severson, H.: *How to Help Your Patients Stop Using Tobacco: A National Cancer Institute Manual for the Oral Health Team*, Smoking and Tobacco Control Program, National Cancer Institute, U.S. Department of Health and Human Services, Public Health Service, NIH Publication 91-3191, December, 1990.

38. **Henningfield**, J.E.: Nicotine Medications for Smoking Cessation, *N. Engl. J. Med., 333*, 1196, November 2, 1995.

39. **Hurt**, R.D., Sachs, D.P.L., Glover, E.D., Offord, K.P., Johnston, J.A., Dale, L.C., Khayrallah, M.A., Schroeder, D.R., Glover, P.N., Sullivan, C.R., Croghan, I.T., and Sullivan, P.M.:A Comparison of Sustained-Release Bupropion and Placebo for Smoking Cessation, *N. Engl. J. Med., 337*, 1195, October 23, 1997.

40. **Benowitz**, N.L.: Treating Tobacco Addiction: Nicotine or No Nicotine? (Editorial), *N. Engl. J. Med., 337*, 1230, October 23, 1997.

41. **Fiore**, M.C., Panel Chairman: *Treating Tobacco Use and Dependence: Clinical Practice Guideline.* Rockville, MD, U.S. Department of Health and Human Services, Public Health Service, June 2000, pp. 24–39.

42. **Fiore**, M.C.: The New Vital Sign: Assessing and Documenting Smoking Status, *JAMA, 266*, 3183, December 11, 1991.

43. **Mecklenburg**, R.E.: *How to Help Your Patient be Tobacco-Free.* National Cancer Institute, U.S. Department of Health and Human Services, Public Health Service, June, 2000, pp.1–14.

SUGGESTED READINGS

Bánócyz, J., Gintner, Z., and Dombi, C.: Tobacco Use and Oral Leukoplakia, *J. Dent. Educ., 65*, 322, April, 2001.

Brandt, A.M.: Recruiting Women Smokers: The Engineering of Consent, *J. Am. Med. Wom. Assoc., 51*, 63, January/April, 1996.

Christen, A.G. and Klein, J.A.: *Tobacco and Your Oral Health.* Carol Stream, IL, Quintessence, 1997, 35 pp.

Damiano, P.C.: The Question of Lost Reimbursement and Remuneration, *J. Dent. Educ., 65*, 364, April, 2001.

Elliot, J. Vullermin, P., and Robinson, P.: Maternal Cigarette Smoking Is Associated With Increased Inner Airway Wall Thickness in Children Who Die From Sudden Infant Death Syndrome, *Am. J. Respir. Critical Care Medicine, 158*, 802, September, 1998.

Fichtenberg, C.M. and Glantz, S.A.: Effect of Smoke-Free Workplaces on Smoking Behaviour: Systematic Review, *Brit. Med. J., 325*, 188, July 27, 2002.

Fried, J. L.: Women and Tobacco: Oral Health Issues, *J. Dent. Hyg., 74*, 49, Winter, 2000.

Kotlyar, M. and Hatsukami, D.K.: Managing Nicotine Addiction, *J. Dent. Educ., 66*, 1061, September, 2002.

Mecklenburg, R.E.: Tobacco Prevention and Control in Dental Practice: The Future, *J. Dent. Educ., 65*, 375, April, 2001.

Warner, K. E.: The Economics of Tobacco: Myths and Realities, *Tobacco Control, 9*, 78, March, 2000.

Periodontal Diseases and Implants

Albandar, J.M., Streckfus, C.F., Adesanya, M.R., and Winn, D.M.: Cigar, Pipe, and Cigarette Smoking as Risk Factors for Periodontal Disease and Tooth Loss, *J. Periodontal., 71*, 1874, December, 2000.

Bergstrom, J., Eliasson, S., and Dock, J.A.: A 10-Year Prospective Study of Tobacco Smoking and Periodontal Health, *J. Periodontol, 71*, 1338, August, 2000.

Haber, J., Cigarette Smoking: A Major Risk Factor for Periodontitis, *Compend. Cont. Educ. Dent., 15*, 1002, August, 1994.

Haffajee, A.D. and Socransky, S.S.: Relationship of Cigarette Smoking to the Subgingival Microbiota, *J. Clin. Periodontol., 28*, 377, May, 2001.

Hyman, J.J., Winn, D.M., and Reid, B.C.: The Role of Cigarette Smoking in the Association Between Periodontal Disease and Coronary Heart Disease, *J. Periodontol., 73*, 988, September, 2002.

Johnson, G. K. and Slach, N.A.: Impact of Tobacco Use on Periodontal Status, *J. Dent. Educ., 65*, 313, April, 2001.

Mecklenburg, R.E. and Grossi, S.G.: Tobacco Use and Intervention, in Rose, L.F., Genco, R.J., Cohen, D.W., and Mealey, B.L., eds.: *Periodontal Medicine.* Hamilton, Ont., B. C. Decker, Inc., 2000, pp. 99–120.

Shiloah, J., Patters, M.R., and Waring, M.B.: The Prevalence of Pathogenic Periodontal Microflora in Healthy Young Adult Smokers, *J. Periodontal., 71*, 562, April, 2000.

Smokeless Tobacco

Ayo-Yusuf, O.A., Swart, T.J.P., and Ayo-Yusuf, I. J.: Prevalence and Pattern of Snuff Dipping in a Rural South African Population, *S. Afr. Dent. J., 55*, 610, November, 2000.

Gansky, S.A., Ellison, J.A., Kavanagh, C., Hilton, J.F., and Walsh, M.M.: Oral Screening and Brief Spit Tobacco Cessation Counseling: A Review and Findings, *J. Dent. Educ., 66*, 1088, September, 2002.

Goebel, L. J., Crespo, R.D., Abraham, R.T., Masho, S.W., and Glover, E.D.: Correlates of Youth Smokeless Tobacco Use, *Nicotine and Tobacco Research, 2*, 319, May, 2000.

Martin, G.C., Brown, J.P., Eifler, C.W., and Houston, G.D.: Oral Leukoplakia Status Six Weeks After Cessation of Smokeless Tobacco Use, *J. Am. Dent. Assoc., 130*, 945, July, 1999.

McGowan, J.M. and Ship, J.A.: Fighting the Use of Smokeless Tobacco, *J. Pract. Hyg., 6*, 29, November/December, 1996.

Robertson, P.B., Walsh, M.M., and Greene, J.C.: Oral Effects of Smokeless Tobacco Use by Professional Baseball Players, *Adv. Dent. Res., 11*, 307, September, 1997.

Tomar, S.I. and Henningfield, J.E.: Review of the Evidence That pH Is a Determinant of Nicotine Dosage From Oral Use of Smokeless Tobacco, *Tobacco Control, 6*, 219, Autumn, 1997.

Wetter, D.W., McClure, J.B., deMoor, C., Cofta-Gunn, L., Cummings, S., Cinciripini, P.M., and Gritz, E.R.: Concomitant Use of

Cigarettes and Smokeless Tobacco: Prevalence, Correlates, and Predictors of Tobacco Cessation, *Preventive Med., 34,* 638, June, 2002.

TOBACCO CESSATION

Barker, G. J., Williams, K.B., Taylor, T. S., and Barker, B.F.: Practice Behaviors of Alumni Trained as Students in Tobacco Use Cessation Interventions, *J. Dent. Hyg.., 75,* 165, Spring, 2001.

Christen, A.G.: Tobacco Cessation, the Dental Profession, and the Role of Dental Education, *J. Dent. Educ., 65,* 368, April, 2001.

Covino, N.A. and Bottari, M.: Hypnosis, Behavioral Theory, and Smoking Cessation, *J. Dent. Educ., 65,* 340, April, 2001.

Doescher, M.P., Whinston, M.A., Goo, A., Cummings, D., Huntington, J., and Saver, B.G.: Pilot Study of Enhanced Tobacco-Cessation Services Coverage for Low-Income Smokers, *Nicotine and Tobacco Research, 4,* S19, Spring, 2002.

Gelskey, S.C.: Impact of a Dental/Dental Hygiene Tobacco-Use Cessation Curriculum on Practice, *J. Dent. Educ., 66,* 1074, September, 2002.

Gordon, J.S. and Severson, H.H.: Tobacco Cessation Through Dental Office Settings, *J. Dent. Educ., 65:* 354, April, 2001.

Mecklenburg, R.E. and Somerman, M.: Cessation of Tobacco Use, in *ADA Guide to Dental Therapeutics*, 2nd ed. Chicago, American Dental Association Publishing, 2000, pp. 569–581.

Mecklenburg, R.E. and Backinger, C.L.: Tobacco and Chemical Dependencies, in Daniel, S. J. and Harfst, S.A., eds.: *Mosby's Dental Hygiene Concepts, Cases, and Competencies.* St. Louis, Mosby, 2002, pp. 228–244.

National Cancer Institute: *State and Local Legislative Action to Reduce Tobacco Use.* Smoking and Tobacco Control Monograph No. 11. Bethesda, MD: U.S. Department of Health and Human Services, National Institutes of Health, National Cancer Institute, NIH Pub. No. 00-4804, August, 2000.

National Cancer Institute: *Population Based Smoking Cessation: Proceedings of a Conference on What Works to Influence Cessation in the General Population,* Smoking and Tobacco Control Monograph No. 12. Bethesda, MD, U.S. Department of Health and Human Services, National Institutes of Health, National Cancer Institute, NIH Pub. No. 00-4892, November, 2000.

Pierce, J.P. and Gilpin, E.A.: Impact of Over-the-Counter Sales on Effectiveness of Pharmaceutical Aids for Smoking Cessation, *JAMA, 288,* 1260, September 11, 2002.

Severson, H.H., Andrews, J.A., Lichtenstein, E., Gordon, J.S., and Barckley, M.F.: Using the Hygiene Visit to Deliver a Tobacco Cessation Program: Results of a Randomized Clinical Trial, *J. Am Dent. Assoc., 129,* 993, July, 1998.

Siegel, M. and Biener, L.: The Impact of an Antismoking Media Campaign on Progression to Established Smoking: Results of a Longitudinal Youth Study, *Am. J. Public Health, 90,* 380, March, 2000.

Diet and Dietary Analysis

Luisa Nappo-Dattoma, RDH, RD, EdD

CHAPTER OUTLINE

Nutrition is an integral part of an individual's general overall health as well as the health status of the oral cavity. The health of oral tissues can be affected by nutrition, diet, and food habits. Box 32-1 outlines relevant terms of standards, diet, nutrition, and oral health.

The existence of the interrelationship between nutritional status, systemic diseases, and oral conditions supports the need for timely and effective diet intervention. Within the scope of practice, the dental hygienist has a responsibility to assess, screen, and deliver nutritional information and instruction to the dental hygiene patient as part of comprehensive education in health promotion and disease prevention and intervention. Dietary and nutritional counseling, as part of a dental caries prevention program and periodontal maintenance, is an essential part of the dental hygiene treatment plan.

■ NUTRIENT STANDARDS FOR DIET ADEQUACY IN HEALTH PROMOTION

Education and instruction center around helping patients learn about the foods that make up an adequate diet and improving their food selection. Achieving an adequate balance in nutrition is a challenging task for all individuals. To facilitate this learning process, multiple standards have been devised; these standards are revised on a regular basis to reflect current research findings.

I. GOVERNMENT AGENCIES

A. Purposes of Standards

1. Facilitate education for individuals about dietary needs and goals for health promotion.

BOX 32-1 KEY WORDS AND ABBREVIATIONS: Diet and Dietary Analysis

A.I.: adequate intake; the recommended nutrient intake utilized when there is not enough information to establish an E.A.R. A.I.s have been established for calcium, vitamin D, and fluoride for all age groups.

Anticariogenic: foods that do not lower the biofilm pH; encourage remineralization.

Cariogenic: foods that do lower the pH and are conducive to dental caries; the degree of cariogenicity depends on many factors, including physical form, texture, and consistency of the carbohydrate-containing food; its retention and clearance time from the oral cavity; and the frequency of use.

Cariogenic exposure: individual ingestion of a cariogenic food that exposes the tooth surface and lowers the pH in the dental biofilm.

Clearance time: the time from the cariogenic exposure until the food is cleared from the oral cavity; influenced by consistency and quantity of saliva; by the action of the tongue, lips, and cheeks; and by the consistency of food.

Diet: customary amount and kind of food and drink taken by an individual from day to day.

Dietary assessment: separation of a dietary food record into individual components of the Food Guide Pyramid; assessment of quality, of whether the individual is using an adequate diet, and of where modifications are needed.

D.R.I.: dietary reference intake; a comprehensive term for categories of reference values that concentrate on maintaining a healthy state for the healthy general population; encompasses the current nutrient recommendations made by the Food and Nutrition Board of the National Academy of Sciences. The categories include the R.D.A., A.I., E.A.R., and U.L.

E.A.R.: estimated average requirement; estimates the nutrient requirements of the average individual; categorized by age and gender; foundation for the R.D.A.

Malnutrition: poor nourishment resulting from improper diet or some defect of metabolism that prevents the body from utilizing its intake of food properly.

Meal plan: a selectively planned or prescribed regimen of food to meet certain needs of the individual.

Noncariogenic food: does not support or promote bacterial growth responsible for caries formation.

Nutrient: a chemical substance in foods that is needed by the body for building and repair; the six classes of nutrients are proteins, fats, carbohydrates, minerals, vitamins, and water.

Nutrient dense: providing a higher nutrient value than calories. Particularly important for those individuals on a low-calorie meal plan to be certain to get adequate nutrients.

Nutrition: sum of processes involved in taking nutrients into the body and assimilating and utilizing them; includes ingestion, digestion, absorption, transport, utilization of nutrients, and excretion of waste products.

Nutritional deficiency: inadequacy of nutrients in the tissues; the result of inadequate dietary intake or impairment of digestion, absorption, transport, or metabolism.

R.D.A.: recommended dietary allowance; recommendations for the average amounts of nutrients that should be consumed daily by healthy people to achieve adequate nutrient intake; categorized by age and gender.

Registered Dietitian: a health professional with a minimum of a bachelor's degree in nutrition or dietetics who has attended an internship program or equivalent and passed the registration exam, all under the approval of the American Dietetic Association (A.D.A.). Continuing education is required to keep credentials current.

U.L.: tolerable upper intake level; maximum intake by an individual that is unlikely to create risks of adverse health effects in almost all healthy individuals. U.L.s were established to avoid toxicity due to excess intake of specific nutrients from food, fortified food, water, and nutrient supplements.

U.S.D.A.: United States Department of Agriculture.

U.S.D.H.H.S.: United States Department of Health and Human Services.

Vegan diet: a diet consisting of only plant foods. Other varieties of the vegan diet are the **fruitarian** (fruits, nuts, honey, and vegetable oils), **lacto-vegetarian** (vegan based with the inclusion of dairy products), and **lacto-ovo-vegetarian** (vegan based with the inclusion of dairy products and eggs).

2. Help achieve diet adequacy of the public.
3. Make recommendations relative to poor food habits such as missed meals, omission of essential foods and nutrients, and illogical dieting.
4. Make specific recommendations for oral health.
5. Motivate for behavior modification.
6. Provide guidelines through printed and web-based educational materials.

II. DIETARY STANDARDS

A. Dietary References Intakes (DRIs)[1]

1. Established for all vitamins and most minerals.
2. Established by the Institute of Medicine for the healthy general population to avoid overconsumption and to prevent chronic disease.

B. Estimated Average Requirements (EARs)[1]

C. Recommended Dietary Allowances (RDAs)[2]

1. Prepared by the National Academy of Sciences, 10th Edition, 1989.
2. Reflect adequate nutrient intake of essential nutrients for healthy individuals to prevent deficiency.
3. Based on gender and age; does not include special needs such as in illness.

C. Adequate Intakes (AIs)[3,4]

D. Tolerable Upper Intake Levels (ULs)[3,4]

III. FOOD GUIDE PYRAMID

A. Developed by the USDA in 1991.
B. Designed as an educational tool for the general public.
C. Five food groups, as illustrated in Figure 32-1.
D. Separate recommendations for different age groups, as illustrated in Figure 32-1.
E. Multiple versions established for different ethnic groups.

IV. US DIETARY GUIDELINES FOR AMERICANS

A. Coordinated with the Food Guide Pyramid.
B. Established by the USDA and the USDHHS.
C. Box 32-2 summarizes the 2000 version.

V. APPLICATION OF STANDARDS

A. Food intake varies with age, gender, activity, and physiological status throughout the life cycle.

B. Nutrient needs are highest for teenage boys and lower for teenage girls, as illustrated in Figure 32-1.
C. Requirements increase with pregnancy and lactation.
D. Requirements decrease with age. With emphasis on nutrient-dense foods, supplementation is highly recommended, particularly with calcium, vitamin D, and vitamin B-12.
E. See Figure 46-8 for requirements for children.

▪ NUTRITION AND ORAL HEALTH RELATIONSHIPS

Nutrition and oral health are closely interrelated. Healthy masticatory function of the oral cavity contributes to proper dietary intake and maintenance of nutritional status. Concurrently, adequate nutrition provides essential nutrients for good health of oral structures and tissues, prevention of oral manifestation of nutritional deficiencies, and proper tooth development and maintenance.

I. SKIN AND MUCOUS MEMBRANE

A. Nutrients and Health of Epithelium

1. Relevant vitamins: vitamin A, B complex, and ascorbic acid.
2. Relevant minerals: zinc and iron.
3. Table 32-1 outlines relevant nutrients, their function, and food sources.

B. Nutritional Deficiencies

1. Nutrient deficiencies produce symptoms of mixed, chronic clinical entities.
2. Influences on clinical manifestations:
   a. Trauma
   b. Local irritation
   c. Systemic factors of chronic disease

C. Oral Manifestations of Nutrient Deficiencies

1. Intraoral lesions and delayed wound healing.
2. Determine vitamin and mineral deficiency.
3. Table 32-2 outlines intraoral manifestations of deficiencies.

D. Extraoral Manifestations of Nutrient Deficiencies

1. Extraoral lesions in skin, nails, and hair.
2. Determine protein, vitamin, and mineral deficiency as etiologic factors.
3. Table 32-2 outlines extraoral manifestations of deficiencies.

Food Guide Pyramid
A Guide to Daily Food Choices

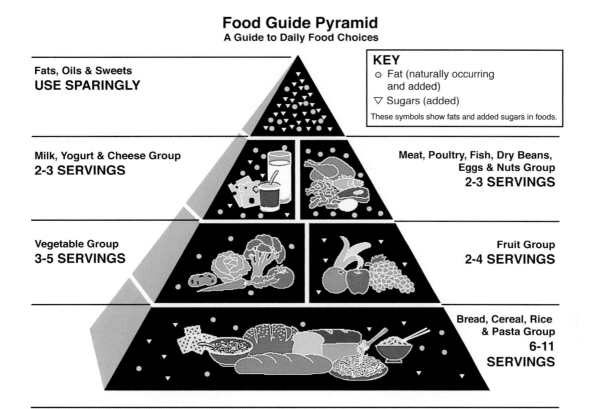

How to Use the USDA Food Guide Pyramid

Food Group	1,600 kcal**	2,200 kcal**	2,800 kcal**
Bread Group 1 slice of bread 1 cup dry cereal 1/2 cup cooked cereal, rice, or pasta	6	9	11
Vegetable Group 1 cup raw leaf vegetables 1/2 cup cooked or raw vegetable 3/4 cup vegetable juice	3	4	5
Fruit Group 1 medium apple, banana, orange 1/2 cup cooked or canned fruit 3/4 cup fruit juice	2	3	4
Milk Group 1 cup milk or yogurt 1 1/2 oz natural cheese 2 oz processed cheese	2 or 3*	2 or 3*	2 or 3*
Meat Group 2-3 oz cooked lean meat, fish, poultry	2, for a total of 5 oz	2, for a total of 6 oz	3, for a total of 7 oz

1,600 kcals is recommended for children ages 2-6 years, most women, and older adults.
2,200 kcals is recommended for older children, teen girls, active women, and most men.
2,800 kcals is recommended for teen boys and active men.
 * Children and teens (9-18) and adults over 50 need 3 servings daily, all others need 2 servings daily.
** kcals stands for kilocalories; the unit of measurement used to express calories in food.

■ **FIGURE 32-1 The USDA Food Guide Pyramid.** Published in the public domain by the US Department of Agriculture and the US Department of Health and Human Services. 5th Edition, 2000. Home and Garden Bulletin No. 232. (*www.usda.gov/cnpp/pyramid.htm*)

BOX 32-2 US Dietary Guidelines for Americans

Aim for Fitness
- Aim for a healthy weight
- Be physically active each day

Build a Healthy Base
- Let the Pyramid guide your food choices
- Choose a variety of grains daily, especially whole grains
- Choose a variety of fruits and vegetables daily
- Keep food safe to eat

Choose Sensibly
- Choose a diet that is low in saturated fat and cholesterol and moderate in total fat
- Choose beverages and foods to moderate your intake of sugars
- Choose and prepare foods with less salt
- If you drink alcoholic beverages, do so in moderation

(Source: *Nutrition and Your Health: Dietary Guidelines for Americans,* 5th Edition, 2000. U.S. Department of Agriculture, U.S. Department of Health and Human Services. Home and Garden Bulletin No. 232, 2000.)

E. Dietary Instruction

1. Educate patient on relevance of nutrient deficiency and extraoral and intraoral lesions.
2. Educate patient on diet adequacy.

II. PERIODONTAL TISSUES

A. Nutrients and Health of Periodontal Tissues

1. Health of gingiva and connective tissues.
2. Wound healing and repair of periodontal tissues and alveolar bone.
3. Relevant vitamins to periodontal health: ascorbic acid, vitamin D.
4. Relevant minerals to periodontal health: zinc, calcium, phosphorus, and magnesium.
5. Table 32-1 outlines relevant nutrients, their function, and food sources.
6. Periodontal infection alters ability of tissue to utilize nutrients and delays healing.
7. Exacerbation of periodontal disease risk linked with smoking and decreased ascorbic acid intake.[5]

8. Decreased intakes of calcium and ascorbic acid linked to increased risk of periodontal disease.[6]

B. Oral Manifestation of Deficiency Related to Periodontal Tissues

1. Incomplete calcification of alveolar bone.
2. Calcium, phosphorus, and vitamin D deficiency.
3. Osteoporosis, osteomalacia, postmenopausal bone alteration.
4. Premature tooth loss secondary to alveolar bone changes.
5. Nutritional deficiencies (Table 32-2).
   a. Protein, ascorbic acid, vitamin B complex, and zinc.
   b. Nutrient deficiency may modify gingival tissue permeability.
   c. Increased susceptibility to dental biofilm associated with periodontal disease.
   d. Increased inflammation and gingivitis.
6. Scurvy
   a. Ascorbic acid deficiency.
   b. Characterized by red, inflamed, friable, bleeding gingiva; diffuse petechiae; and overall sore mouth.

C. Dietary Assessment

1. Periodontal therapy patients need specific instruction in diet selection.
2. Routine maintenance patients.
   a. Regular diet indicated to promote healing.
   b. Firm fibrous foods, such as raw carrots or apples, may stimulate the tissues and improve circulation.
   c. Chewing firm foods increases salivary flow. Saliva acts as a buffer, and increased saliva aids in oral clearance.
3. Surgical intervention patients.
   - May need to alter diet consistency following treatment during the healing period.
   - Soft diet of high-quality protein is indicated for adequate healing of tissues.
   - Puddings, scrambled eggs, milkshakes, yogurt, and cottage cheese have high-quality protein to promote healing.

III. TOOTH STRUCTURE AND INTEGRITY

A. Nutrients and Health of Tooth Structure

1. Adequate nutrition during tooth development is essential for mineralization.

■ TABLE 32-1 NUTRIENTS RELEVANT TO ORAL HEALTH

NUTRIENT	FUNCTION	DEFICIENCY DISEASE	FOOD SOURCE
Vitamin A (retinol, provitamin A carotene)	• Fat soluble • Antioxidant • Bone and tooth development • Skin and mucous membrane integrity • Cell differentiation; essential for reproduction • Vision in dim light • Immune system integrity	• Night blindness • Xerophthalmia • Poor growth • Keratinization of epithelium • Dry, scaly skin • Toxic in large doses: double vision, hair loss, dry mucous membranes, joint pain, liver damage	Egg yolk, liver, fish liver oils, fortified milk, cream, cheeses; green leafy vegetables; orange, red, yellow pigmented fruits and vegetables
Vitamin D (calciferol)	• Fat soluble • Aids in the absorption of calcium and phosphorus • Mineralization of bone	• Rickets in children • Osteomalacia in adults • Osteoporosis • Toxic in large doses: calcification of soft tissues, growth retardation	Exposure to UV sunlight, fortified milk, fish oils
Vitamin E (tocopherol)	• Fat soluble • Antioxidant	• Low incidence of deficiency • Low toxicity	Whole grains, wheat germ, plant oils, margarines, legumes, seeds, nuts, greens
Vitamin K (quinone)	• Fat soluble • Synthesis of prothrombin in blood clotting and bone proteins	• Prolonged clotting time • Hemorrhage • Toxic in large doses (patients on blood thinners need to limit use in diet)	Synthesized by intestinal bacterial flora; dark green leafy vegetables, liver
Thiamin (vitamin B_1)	• Acts as coenzyme in carbohydrate and amino acid metabolism • Essential for synthesis of healthy nerves	• Beri-beri: weight loss, fatigue, edema, depression • Toxicity: not seen	Enriched whole grains and cereals, pork, meats, poultry, nuts, seeds, legumes
Riboflavin (vitamin B_2)	• Coenzyme in energy metabolism of fat, carbohydrate, and protein	• Ariboflavinosis • Angular cheilosis • Growth failure • Eye disorders • Toxicity: not seen	Milk, cheese, enriched and whole grains and cereals, rice, mushrooms, liver
Niacin (vitamin B_3)	• Coenzyme in energy metabolism of fat, carbohydrate, and protein	• Pellagra: diarrhea, dermatitis, dementia, and death • Toxicity: not seen in food sources • Toxicity with large doses of supplements for treatment of hypercholesterolemia (skin redness and flushing, gastric ulcers)	Enriched whole grains and cereals, rice, meat, poultry, fish, green leafy vegetables

■ **TABLE 32-1 NUTRIENTS RELEVANT TO ORAL HEALTH** (Continued)

NUTRIENT	FUNCTION	DEFICIENCY DISEASE	FOOD SOURCE
Pyridoxine (vitamin B_6)	• Coenzyme in amino acid and lipid metabolism • Hemoglobin synthesis • Homocysteine metabolism	• Dermatitis • Depression • Convulsions • Peripheral neuritis • Toxicity not seen in food sources • Toxicity from supplements: neuropathy, irreversible nerve damage	Widespread food sources with the exception of fat and sugar
Cobalamin (vitamin B_{12})	• Maturation of RBC • Requires intrinsic factor from parietal cells for absorption • Cofactor in folate and homocysteine metabolism	• Pernicious anemia secondary to lack of intrinsic factor and total vegan diet • Toxicity: not seen	All animal foods, fortified cereals
Folate (folic acid)	• Maturation of RBC • DNA synthesis • Homocysteine metabolism	• Megaloblastic anemia, • Neural tube defects: spina bifida • Masks B_{12} deficiency • Toxicity: not seen	Green leafy vegetables, fruits, legumes, fortified grains
Ascorbic Acid (vitamin C)	• Antioxidant • Collagen synthesis • Wound healing • Aids in absorption of iron	• Scurvy • Poor wound healing • Petechial hemorrhages • Increased periodontal symptoms • Toxicity: potential for rebound scurvy	Citrus fruits, broccoli, strawberries, peppers, tomatoes, cantaloupe
Calcium	• Muscle contraction • Blood clotting • Nerve impulse transmission • Calcification of bone and tooth structure	• Osteoporosis • Incomplete calcification of hard tissues • Toxicity: not seen	Dairy products, tofu, fortified orange juice, soy milk, green leafy vegetables, canned salmon and sardine bones
Phosphorus	• Required for bone and teeth strength • Acid-base balance • Muscle contraction	• Poor bone maintenance • Incomplete calcification of teeth • Compromised alveolar integrity • Toxicity: skeletal porosity	Dairy products, meat, poultry, processed foods, soft drinks, nuts, legumes, whole grain cereals
Magnesium	• Bone strength and rigidity • Hydroxyapatite crystal formation • Nerve impulse • Muscle contraction	• Muscle weakness • Alveolar bone fragility • Toxicity seen in medications containing magnesium	Wheat bran, whole grains, green leafy vegetables, legumes, nuts, chocolate
Fluoride	• Prevention of caries	• Increased incidence of caries • Toxicity: tooth mottling; enamel hypoplasia	Fluoridated water, tea, seaweed, toothpaste

■ TABLE 32-1 NUTRIENTS RELEVANT TO ORAL HEALTH (Continued)

NUTRIENT	FUNCTION	DEFICIENCY DISEASE	FOOD SOURCE
Iron	• Component of hemo-globin • Carries oxygen to cells • Immune function • Cognitive development	• Anemia: pallor of face, conjunctiva, lips, mucosa, and gingiva • Shortness of breath • Fatigue • Decreased immunity • Toxicity: GI upset; pigmentation; seen in persons with hemochromatosis	Meat, poultry, fish, whole grains, dried fruit, enriched grains
Zinc	• Required for >100 enzymes • Normal growth and development • Taste and smell sensitivity • Sexual development and reproduction • Immune integrity • Wound healing	• Altered taste • Growth retardation • Decreased wound healing • Impaired immunity • Toxicity: rare (stomach irritation, cramps, diarrhea, vomiting)	Seafood, meats, whole grains, greens
Copper	• Aids in iron metabolism • Collagen formation	• Anemia • Poor growth • Low WBC • Bone demineralization • Tissue fragility • Decreased trabeculae of alveolar bone • Toxicity: vomiting, diarrhea	Whole grains, nuts, dried fruits, legumes, shell fish, organ meats

Adapted from Palmer, C.A.: *Diet and Nutrition in Oral Health*, 2003, pp. 96, 100–101, 117–118, 129–132; and Wardlaw, G.M. and Kessel, M.: *Perspectives in Nutrition*, 5th ed, 2002, pp. 355, 402–403, 453, 497.

■ TABLE 32-2 ORAL MANIFESTATIONS OF NUTRITIONAL DEFICIENCIES

ORAL SYMPTOM	NUTRIENT DEFICIENCY
Glossitis	Niacin, folate, riboflavin, vitamins B_6 and B_{12}
Glossodynia	Niacin, vitamins B_6 and B_{12}
Angular cheilosis	Riboflavin, vitamins B_6 and B_{12}, folate, niacin, iron
Inflamed, bleeding gingiva	Vitamin C, vitamin K, vitamin B_{12}, niacin, folate
Stomatitis, mucositis	Niacin, folate, thiamin, vitamin B_{12}
Xerostomia	Zinc, vitamin A, vitamin B_{12}
Sore or burning tongue	Riboflavin, thiamin, niacin, vitamins B_6 and B_{12}, iron
Altered taste	Thiamin, riboflavin, vitamin A, vitamin B_{12}, zinc
↑ Risk candidiasis	Folate, vitamin A, vitamin K, iron, zinc
↓Mineralization of teeth, ↓alveolar integrity	Calcium, phosphorus, magnesium, vitamin D
Delayed wound healing	Vitamin A, vitamin C, riboflavin, zinc
Altered enamel development	Vitamin A, calcium, phosphorus

Adapted from Palmer, C.A.: *Diet and Nutrition in Oral Health*, 2003, pp. 96, 100–101, 117–118, 129–132.

2. Relevant minerals: calcium, phosphorus, magnesium, and fluoride.
3. Relevant vitamin: vitamin A.
4. Table 32-1 outlines relevant nutrients, their function, and food sources.

B. Manifestation of Nutritional Deficiencies

1. Incomplete mineralization of teeth.
2. Deficiency in fluoride associated with decreased resistance to dental caries.
3. Table 32-2 lists oral manifestations of deficiency.

C. Dietary Assessment

1. Diet assessment during early tooth development is essential.
2. The child patient is an excellent candidate for dietary assessment. Anticipatory guidance (instruction) for the parents has special significance.
3. Prevention of demineralization of teeth.

IV. DENTAL CARIES

A. Prevention[7]

1. Fluoride is the essential mineral for dental caries prevention.
2. The complexity of dental caries formation is illustrated in Figure 32-2.

B. Role of Cariogenic Foods[8,9]

1. Caries is a result of excess cariogenic foods not a deficiency disease.
2. Fermentable carbohydrates produce acids when acted on by specific biofilm microorganisms.
3. *Streptococcus mutans* and lactobacilli utilize fermentable carbohydrate for energy.

C. Consistency of Food

1. Soft, sticky foods cling to the teeth and gingiva and encourage food debris accumulation.
2. Microorganisms are protected and nourished, leading to increased acid formation.

D. Dietary Assessment and Counseling

1. Use of dietary assessment and patient instruction relative to dental caries control is paramount.

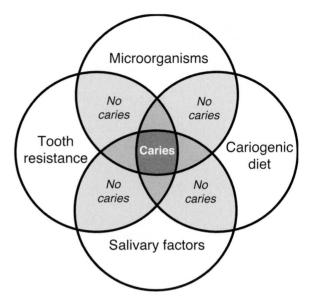

■ **FIGURE 32-2 Dental Caries Process.** Four overlapping circles illustrate the factors involved in the development of dental caries. All four act together, and, as shown by the center, dental caries results. (Adapted from United States Department of Health and Human Services, Public Health Service, National Institute of Dental Research: *Broadening the Scope: Long-Range Research Plan for the 1990s,* NIH Publication No. 90-1188, Washington, D.C., United States Government Printing Office, 1990.)

2. Specified personal recommendations foster behavior modification in disease prevention.

■ COUNSELING FOR DENTAL CARIES CONTROL

Control of dental biofilm and of cariogenic food intake, strengthening of the tooth surface to resist caries activity, and the presence of saliva are essential in the prevention of dental caries. Figure 32-2 illustrates the intricate relationship of all four factors in the development of dental caries.

Control of dental caries by diet accompanies procedures for control of dental biofilm. They are part of the total oral health program that also includes pit and fissure sealants, the restoration of carious teeth, and the implementation of fluoride therapy.

■ THE DIETARY ASSESSMENT

The dietary assessment is an integral part of disease prevention and health promotion in the scope of dental hygiene care. It provides the opportunity for the dental hygienist and patient to collaborate in the evaluation of diet adequacy and in diet intervention.

I. PURPOSES OF A DIETARY ASSESSMENT

A. Identify patients at nutritional and oral health risk and to refer to a physician or Registered Dietitian when intervention is indicated.

B. Provide an opportunity for a patient to study personal dietary habits objectively.

C. Obtain an overall picture of the types of food in the patient's diet, food preferences, and quantity of food eaten.

D. Study the food habits and snacking patterns.

E. Record frequency of use and when the cariogenic food is consumed.

F. Determine the overall consistency of the diet.
   1. Identify fibrous foods regularly consumed.
   2. Identify soft, sticky foods regularly consumed.

G. Identify the nutritional status of an individual with regard to overall requirements and collaborating with the patient on making suggestions for modification in nutritional adequacy of the diet in health promotion.

H. Provide a basis for collaborating with the patient to establish recommendations for changes in the diet important to the health of the oral mucosa and periodontium and to the prevention of dental caries.

II. COMPONENTS OF A DIETARY ASSESSMENT[8]

A. Patient History

1. Information obtained from medical, dental, and social histories is essential in assessing oral health and nutritional status.
   a. Disease states
   b. Medications
   c. Disabilities
   d. Learning limitations
   e. Significant unintentional change in body weight
   f. Factors influencing food use and food intake

2. Dietary influences can be identified by intraoral and extraoral examination revealing oral manifestations of nutritional deficiencies or systemic disease.

3. Table 32-2 lists oral manifestations of deficiency.

B. Clinical Evaluation

1. Evaluation detects high-risk patients by noting factors suggestive of a nutritional problem.

2. Clinical examination and charting of carious lesions and demineralizing areas.

3. Identification of any abnormalities in the patient's overall appearance, weight, skin, nails, and hair.

III. FORMS USED FOR ASSESSMENT

A. 24-Hour Recall (Figure 32-3)

1. A diary of the patient's dietary intake over the previous 24 hours.

2. Obtained by interview with patient.

3. Assesses nutrients, food groups, diet adequacy, form and frequency of the carbohydrate intake, and snacking patterns.

4. Results are reviewed and appropriate education is given at same appointment or a follow-up appointment.

5. It is quick and easy to administer and can be done chairside in one visit.

6. Not necessarily representative of a patient's normal diet.

7. Limited to only one day's intake.

B. Food Diary: 3-7 Days

1. A more accurate account of a patient's intake.

2. Patient completes food diary for 3, 5, or 7 days, inclusive of one weekend day.

3. Affords the patient a more active role in the dietary assessment and a chance to observe areas that require modification.

4. Provide patient with three to seven copies of the food diary and have patient return forms at follow-up visit.

5. At follow-up visit the patient's diary is evaluated for:
   a. Eating patterns
   b. Consumption and frequency of fermentable carbohydrates
   c. Nutritional adequacy

IV. PRESENTATION OF THE FOOD DIARY TO THE PATIENT

A. Explain the Purpose

1. Briefly describe how diet relates to the dental situation.

2. Provide a foundation for the education to follow.

3. Avoid mention of specific foods not to bias patient.

B. Explain the Form

1. Provide written and oral instructions for use of the food diary.

FOOD DIARY

NAME_____   TEL_____

AGE_____   Height_____   Weight_____   BMI_____

Type of foods average	Quality enter, oz	Preparation method
7:30 AM: Orange juice		Bagel Shop
Bagel	whole	
Cream cheese	2 tbsp	
Coffee	16 oz	
Milk and sugar	1/2 cup, 2 packets	
SNACK		
LUNCH		
SNACK		
DINNER		
SNACK		

▪ **FIGURE 32-3 Food Diary.** Sample of a form for patients to use in recording the daily intake of foods eaten. Can be used for the 24-hour recall, or multiple forms can be used in the 3- to 7-day food diary.

2. Provide suggestions for listing various foods and use of household measurements for indicating quantity (Box 32-3).
3. Instruction for completing the food diary encourages the patient to provide a more accurate portrayal of eating behaviors.

C. Complete the Current Day's Food Diary With the Patient

1. Helps illustrate how to itemize and list foods eaten.
2. Provides an example to use at home until next visit.

D. General Directions

1. Emphasize importance of completing the diary for each meal as soon after eating as possible to avoid forgetting.
2. Encourage use of typical days, uncomplicated by illness, dieting, holidays, or other unusual events.
3. Review details of recording the component parts of a combination dish, such as a sandwich:
   a. 2 slices of whole wheat bread
   b. 4 oz of turkey
   c. 1 tablespoon of mustard or light mayo
   d. 2 slices of tomato with lettuce
   e. 1 slice of cheddar cheese

BOX 32-3 Food Diary Instructions

- Write down everything eaten on the food record form provided.

- Record each meal as soon after eating as possible to avoid forgetting.

- Do not choose days when dieting, fasting, or ill.

- Be accurate in determining the amounts eaten, using household measurements (examples: 1/2 cup cereal, 3 oz. fish, 1 tsp. margarine).

- Use brand names whenever possible.

- Record added sauces, gravies, condiments, and all extras (examples: sugar or cream in coffee, mayonnaise, chewing gum, cough drops).

- Record food preparation methods (examples: baked, fried, boiled, grilled).

- Record all fluids; include water and alcoholic beverages.

---

4. Indicate need for recording nutritional supplements and all fluids consumed, including alcoholic beverages.
5. Request that meals eaten other than at home be identified:
   a. Restaurant
   b. Guest at friend's home
   c. Party
6. Instruct patient to select consecutive days and at least one weekend day for a realistic representation of diet pattern.

V. RECEIVING THE COMPLETED FOOD DIARY

A. Obtain Supplemental Data

- The food diary should be received soon after its completion.
- Question the patient to clarify presented information.
- Does food diary represent a typical day or week?
- Identify influences on appetite: illness, stress, etc.
- Identify food likes and dislikes, food preferences, intolerances, food allergies.
- Frequency of dining out.
- Current diet being followed in the home.
- Average alcohol intake.
- Which family member is doing the cooking and food shopping.

B. Review Patient's Food Diary

1. Common omissions
   - Garnishes: frosting, whipped cream, butter or margarine on vegetables, salad dressings, oil.
   - Beverages: quantity, sweetened, decaffeinated.
   - Snacks: type, brand, quantity.
   - Chewing gum or mints: sugarless, quantity.
   - Canned fruit: packed in water or heavy or light syrup.
   - Fruit and vegetables: canned, fresh, frozen.
   - Cereal: brand, type of milk, sugar, quantity.
   - Potato: baked, buttered, fried.
   - Seasonings or sauces: quantity, type.
2. Determine common food habits, such as snacking at night or fast food choices at lunch.

VI. ANALYSIS OF DIETARY ASSESSMENT

Three principal parts of the food diary to analyze are the number of servings in each food group, the frequency of cariogenic foods, and the consistency of the diet.

A. Nutritional Analysis for Adequacy of 24-Hour Recall

1. When time is a factor, a 24-hour analysis is appropriate.
2. Compare food groups represented in the patient's 24-hour food diary with those of the pyramid.
3. Determine nutritional adequacy.
4. Calculate the patient's sweet score, as outlined in Figure 32-4.
5. Cariogenic foods are listed and categorized as solid, liquid, or slowly dissolving (Figure 32-4).
6. Totals for the 1 day are multiplied by respective time factors, and a score determines patient's caries risk.

B. Nutritional Analysis for Adequacy of the Food Diary

1. Comparison of patient's food diary with the Food Guide Pyramid (Figure 32-1).
2. Dietary Analysis Recording Form utilized to analyze adequacy of daily portions of each food group (Figure 32-5).
3. Each food eaten is entered into a food group, with consideration that more than one serving may have been consumed.
4. Totals for the week are added and the average per day is calculated.
5. The average is compared with the recommended servings for each food group.
6. Computerized nutrition analysis programs are available to analyze a 3- or 5-day diary:
   a. Color charts comparing patient's averages with the RDA.
   b. Tables comparing patient with Food Guide Pyramid.
7. Deficiencies easily identified by patient.

C. Analysis of Cariogenic Foods for Caries Incidence[7,8]

1. Identify physical form of carbohydrate.
   a. Liquids: sweetened or unsweetened soft drinks; fruit juice with added sugars.
   b. Soft solid/sticky and retentive: retentive cakes, cookies, chips, pretzels, jellybeans, and caramels.
   c. Hard solid/slowly dissolving: hard candies, mints, and cough drops.
2. Identify frequency of meals and snacks.
   a. Daily or occasionally.
   b. Number of between-meal snacks.
   c. How many snacks include cariogenic foods.

d. Frequency more relevant than quantity in caries incidence.
   e. High frequency of eating events decreases ability of calcium and phosphate to remineralize teeth between episodes.
3. Oral retentiveness of cariogenic foods is relative to length of time food debris remains on teeth and exposure to decreased biofilm pH.[10-12]
   a. Foods assumed to be extremely retentive are actually poorly retained and deliver high load of sugar but for shorter periods of time. Examples: sticky caramels, gummy bears, jellybeans, and chocolate.
   b. Highly retentive fermentable carbohydrates have delayed rate of oral clearance increasing exposure of teeth to a decreased pH and higher potential for demineralization. Examples: crackers, dry cereal, cookies, and chips.
4. Sequence of food consumption related to caries incidence.[13-15]
   • Eating sugar at the end of a meal is considered cariogenic.
   • Eating fermentable carbohydrates at the beginning of a meal or between other noncariogenic foods (protein and fat) is less cumulative in cariogenic potential.
   • Protein and fat are not metabolized by bacteria and should be eaten at the end of a meal.
   • Cheese eaten after sweets or at the end of a meal prevents the decrease in pH and production of acids in the oral cavity.[15]
5. Water aids in rinsing sugars from tooth surface and decreases cariogenic activity.
6. Noncariogenic sweeteners may contribute to caries prevention.[16]
   a. Use of sugar-free gum after meals can be beneficial.
   b. Sugar-free gums decrease lactic acid production and increase salivary flow, potentially buffering acids.
   c. Chewing these gums increases the saliva concentration with mineral ions and aids in the clearance of sugars from the oral cavity.
   d. Sorbitol and xylitol are the most commonly used sugar substitutes.
   e. Xylitol is not fermentable by caries promoting bacteria and is considered nonacidogenic. Sorbitol can be fermented by *S. mutans* at a very slow rate.[17]
7. During counseling appointment, have patient circle in red the cariogenic foods on the food diary.

SCORING THE SWEETS (Caries-Promoting Potential)				
Food Items (From patient's 24-hour recall)	**Reference Foods Considered Cariogenic**	**Frequency** (Place a check for each exposure to cariogenic food)	**Weighted Score**	**Total Points Each Category**
1. 2. 3. 4.	**Liquid** Soft drinks, fruit drinks, cocoa, sugar and honey in beverages, nondiary creamers, ice cream, sherbet, flavored or frozen yogurt, pudding, custard, jello	—— —— —— ——	x1	
1. 2. 3. 4. 5. 6.	**Solid and Sticky** Cakes, cupcakes, doughnuts, sweet rolls, potato chips, pretzels, pastry, canned fruit in syrup, bananas, cookies, chocolate candy, caramel, toffee, jelly beans, other chewy candy, chewing gum, dried fruit, marshmallows, jelly, jam	—— —— —— ——	x2	
1. 2. 3.	**Slowly Dissolving** Hard candies, breath mints, antacid tablets, cough drops	—— —— ——	x3	

TOTAL SCORE _____

Using the 24-hour recall diary:
- Classify each sweet into liquid, solid and sticky, or slowly dissolving. (Use reference food list.)
- For each time a sweet was eaten, either at a meal or between meals (at least 20 minutes apart), place a check in the frequency column.
- In each category tally the number of sweets eaten and multiply by the weighted score. Record the category points in the respective column.
- Tally all the category points to determine the total score.

Sweet score: (Risk for dental caries	**How to lower your risk for caries:**
0-1 **low risk**	1. Cut down on the frequency of between-meal sweets
2-4	2. Don't sip constantly on sweetened beverage
5-7 **moderate risk**	3. Avoid using slowly dissolving items like hard candy, cough drops, etc
8-9	4. Eat more non–decay-promoting foods, such as low-fat cheese, raw
>10 **high risk**	vegetables, crunchy fruits, nuts, popcorn, bottled water

■ **FIGURE 32-4 Sweet Score.** Form to be used to determine patient's caries risk when doing a 24-hour recall at chairside. (Adapted with permission from Carole A. Palmer EdD, RD, Division of Nutrition and Oral Health Promotion, Department of General Dentistry, Tufts University School of Dental Medicine.)

Name _____

Date _____ Age _____

Dietary Analysis

Food Groups	Day 1	2	3	4	5	6	7	Daily Avarage	USDA Various					Adequate	
									Child 2-6 yrs. (1,600)	1,600 Most Females	2,200 Teens	2,800 Most Males	+70 Adults (1,200-1,600)	Yes	No
Grains & Cereals									6	6	9	11	≥6		
Vegetables									3	3	4	5	2-3		
Fruits									2	2	3	4	≥2		
Milk, Yogurt, Cheese									2	2-3	2-3	2-3	3		
Meat, Poultry, Fish									2	2 (5 oz)	2 (6 oz)	2 (7 oz)	≥2 (5 oz)		
Eggs, Dry Beans, Nuts															
Fats and Sweets									"Eat Less"	"Use Sparingly"					

Sweets									Total	
Liquid	With Meal									Total all liquid exposures and multiply by 20 minutes and divide by total numbers of days to equal daily acid attack from liquid. **Total Liquid Minutes** _____
	End of Meal									
	Between Meal									
Soft/Solid	With Meal									Total all liquid exposures and multiply by 40 minutes and divide by total numbers of days to equal daily acid attack from liquid. **Total Liquid Minutes** _____
Sticky/ Retentive	End of Meal									
	Between Meal									
Hard/Solid	With Meal									Add both liquid and solid totals to determine number of minutes per day teeth are under acid attack. *Total Daily Minutes of Acid Attack* _____
Slowly Dissolving	End of Meal									
	Between Meal									

■ **FIGURE 32-5 Dietary Analysis Recording Form.** From the food diary kept by the patient (Figure 32-3), each serving is entered as a check in the space beside the appropriate food group. Each category is totaled, averaged, and compared with the recommendation on the right.

a. Categorizing sweets on Dietary Analysis Recording Form:
Liquid, soft solid, hard solid, and time of eating event.
b. Total the number of sweets for liquid and solids.
c. Multiply total by 20 minutes (liquids) and 40 minutes (solids).
d. Divide by number of days (eg, 3-, 5-, or 7-day diary).
e. Add the liquid and solid scores for total minutes teeth are exposed to sweets and acid attack (Figure 32-5).

D. Analysis of Diet Consistency

1. Types of fibrous foods.
   a. Uncooked, crisp, raw fruits and vegetables
   b. Promote saliva flow
2. Frequency of use; daily, occasionally.
3. Sequence of use; during meal, end of meal, between meals.

E. Benefits of Food Diary Analysis

1. Patient can identify desirable and undesirable practices.
2. Corroborate findings with clinical findings and patient's oral health problems in preparation for counseling session.

■ PREPARATION FOR ADDITIONAL COUNSELING OF PATIENT

I. DEFINE OBJECTIVES

A. To help patient understand the individual oral problems and appreciate the need for changing habits.
B. To explain specific alterations in the diet necessary for improved general and oral health.
C. For dental caries control.
   1. To promote the modification of cariogenic foods, particularly between meals.
   2. To substitute noncariogenic foods into diet.

II. PLANNING FACTORS

A. Patient Attitude

1. Consider patient's willingness and ability to cooperate, as evidenced by keeping appointments and following personal oral care procedures.

2. Consider patient's healthcare beliefs and nutrition and dental knowledge.

B. Possible Barriers

1. Difficulty and resistance to change of normal habits.
2. Patient dissatisfaction with loss of usual or customary foods.
3. Patients may not attempt to make modifications if recommendations are numerous or overwhelming.
4. Lack of appreciation of need for change owing to limited knowledge of diet, nutrition, and oral health relationship.
5. Common misconception about concentrated sugar as indispensable energy source.
6. Social prejudices.
7. Cultural and religious patterns significant to food selection and preparation.
8. Financial considerations in food purchasing.
9. Emotional eating patterns and cravings for sweets.
10. Parental attitude toward sweets in the diet.
    a. Elimination of all sugars would deprive a child of normal childhood pleasures.
    b. All sugars are bad foods for children to have.

III. APPROPRIATE TEACHING MATERIALS

A. Patient's radiographs, charting, and food diary.
B. Diagrams, food models, food labels, or charts of dietary standards and requirements.
C. Educational leaflets to illustrate patient's special dietary or oral health needs.
D. An outline of a realistic diet plan with specific suggestions for food substitutes.
E. A list of snack suggestions.

■ COUNSELING PROCEDURES

I. SETTING

A. An environment free from interruptions and distracting background sounds.
B. Apart from the clinical treatment room.
C. Patient comfort promotes environment conducive to learning.
D. Provide limited but pertinent educational information.
   1. Posters and pamphlets.
   2. Food labels and food models of portion sizes.
   3. Avoid cluttering with new information to minimize confusion.

E. Persons involved in promoting change.
   1. For a younger patient, the primary caregiver should be present since this individual supervises the child's eating.
   2. Person preparing meals and grocery shopping should be present to educate them about appropriate food choices.

II. POINTERS FOR SUCCESS OF A CONFERENCE

A. Be prepared and on time.
B. Plan for only a few simple visual aids.
C. Concentrate on the factors related to the patient's diet-based dental problem.
D. Encourage parents to exclude small children (other than patient) from the conference; they may create distractions.
E. Develop a permissive, friendly atmosphere; establish eye contact with a warm, nonthreatening environment.
F. Take care not to follow a written outline of recommendations so rigidly that the conference lacks spontaneity.
G. Use question format that provides a response filled with information.[18]
   1. Use open-ended questions that elicit information. Examples: "Tell me what was the first thing you ate today?" "How was the omelet prepared?" "What did you put on the bagel?"
   2. Limit closed-ended questions; they provide "yes" or "no" responses and limited information. Example: "Did you eat breakfast today?"
   3. Avoid using "why," it puts the patient on the defensive. Example: "Why do you put sugar in your coffee?"
H. Guide patients to develop their own behavior changes.
   1. Use a patient-centered approach to the counseling session.
   2. Foster greater patient compliance.
   3. Empower the patient to get involved in making the suggestions and recommendation for change.
   4. Put the responsibility for change on the patient.
   5. Keep goals simple, small, and realistic.
I. Use a conversational tone of voice and avoid lecturing.
J. Adequately discuss all questions from patient or parent.
K. Avoid note taking during the conference.
L. Keep session brief, informative, and engaging for the patient.

III. PRESENTATION

A. Review Purposes of the Meeting

1. Provide explanation of the relevance between diet and patient's particular problem.
2. Emphasize health promotion and disease prevention.

B. Clarification of "Cariogenic" Foods

1. Sugar score from 24-Hour Recall or Dietary Analysis Recording Form are powerful tools to emphasize sugars and caries risk.
2. Clarify confusion of hidden sugars, added sugars, and natural sugars.
3. Outline modification of sugar intake and substitutions.

C. Review of Dental Caries Initiation

1. Discuss the role of fermentable carbohydrates in dental caries initiation.
2. Cariogenic food on the tooth surface is changed to acid within 2 to 4 minutes (use Figure 17-6 as an illustration).
3. Acid left undisturbed is not all cleared from the mouth for 20 to 40 minutes.

D. Frequency and Time of Exposure[19]

1. Each exposure of the tooth surface to sucrose or other cariogenic food in a meal or snack increases the amount of acid on the tooth.
2. The pH drops to below 5.5, which is the critical level for demineralization.
3. Figure 32-6 illustrates how the frequent intake of sucrose lowers the pH for several hours in a day.
4. The actual amount of a cariogenic food is not as important as when and how often the tooth is exposed.

E. Retention

1. The texture of cariogenic foods influences the length of time the food stays in the mouth (whether sticky or combined with a sticky food).
2. Vigorous rinsing after eating a cariogenic food may help remove food from the tooth but not the adhered biofilm.
3. Cariogenic foods taken after brushing and flossing before retiring are not cleared readily because salivary flow decreases during sleep.
4. Cariogenic liquids are removed quickly and the enamel will be exposed to an acidic environment for shorter periods of time than retentive or solid foods.

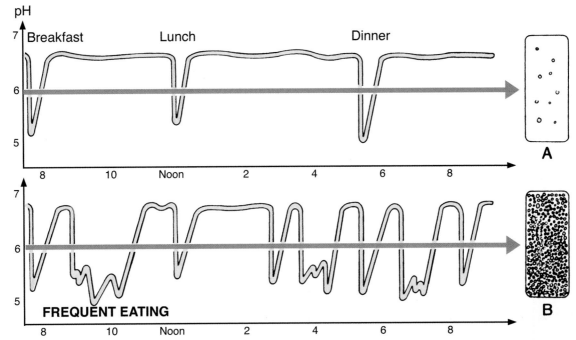

■ **FIGURE 32-6 Cariogenic Foods and Biofilm pH.** The range of pH in the dental biofilm from 5 to 7 pH is shown on the left. Time intervals are shown across the bottom of each graph. The double-line curve represents the variations in biofilm pH throughout a day. Each time sugar or a cariogenic food is taken in, the pH of the dental biofilm drops to or below the critical pH (5.2 to 5.5). As shown in the lower graph, frequent eating keeps the pH at the critical level below which enamel demineralization can occur. **(A)** Bacterial counts are lower. **(B)** Aciduric microorganisms are greatly increased in numbers. The critical pH for the root surfaces is 6.0 to 6.7. (Adapted from Larmas, M.: *Int. Dent. J., 35,* 109, June, 1985.)

IV. SPECIFIC DIETARY RECOMMENDATIONS

A. Examination of the Patient's Food Diary

1. After analyzing the diet, the patient can identify the deficiencies and excesses and suggest alternate choices.
2. Try to retain as many as possible of the patient's present food habits.
3. Make recommendations that can be adapted to the patient's pattern of living.
4. Discuss foods from each food group that are liked by the patient and can be added to the diet.
5. Guide the patient to identify foods in the diary that need changing.
6. Assist patient in finding acceptable substitutions for the cariogenic food choices.
   a. Patients may accept light yogurt as an alternative to ice cream for a snack.
   b. Fruit may be an appealing suggestion.
   c. Patients need to be involved in making changes in their own diets.
7. To enhance compliance, allow patients to create their own meal plans for 1 day (Figure 32-7).

   a. Incorporate the principles discussed during the counseling.
   b. Collaborate on modifications the patient can achieve realistically and is willing to try.
   c. Avoid too many changes that may be overwhelming.
   d. Determine patient comprehension of information presented and patient's motivation level.

B. Basic Principles for Dietary Changes

1. Directions must be simple and specific because interpretation of new ideas can be difficult.
2. Incorporate foods from the food groups to complete the patient's diet to ensure adequacy and balance of nutrients.
3. Limit the use of cariogenic foods to mealtimes.
   a. Evaluate the final food in a meal because it may remain on the teeth if rinsing is not possible.
   b. Recommend chewing a gum containing xylitol at the end of the meal, especially for a caries-susceptible person.

MENU PLANNING RECORD

Instructions: Create a realistic menu for one day.

Time	Meal
_____	Breakfast:
_____	A.M. Snack:
_____	Lunch:
_____	P.M. Snack:
_____	Dinner:
_____	Evening Snack:

Totals in a day: Fruits _____   Vegetables _____
Milk _____   Starch/Bread _____
Fat _____   Protein/Meat _____
Other _____

■ **FIGURE 32-7 Menu Planning Record.** An educational aid to evaluate a patient's understanding of the information discussed in the dietary counseling. Allow the patient to create a menu for 1 day, making realistic modifications as discussed during the counseling session to promote positive oral health. (Adapted from Davis, J.R. and Stegeman, C.A.: *The Dental Hygienist's Guide to Nutritional Care.* 1998, p. 420.)

4. Foods that require chewing increase saliva flow.
   a. Saliva provides additional buffering effects.
   b. Saliva removes cariogenic foods more promptly.
5. Limit between-meal snacking and select snacks from noncariogenic foods.
   a. Nonflavored milk.
   b. Cheese and crackers.
   c. Peanut butter on sliced apples.
   d. Cream cheese on celery.
   e. Sugar-free gelatin or pudding.
6. Use as little concentrated sweet in the preparation of foods as possible.
   a. Decrease the amount of granulated or brown sugar by half when baking.
   b. Observe care in the purchase of prepared foods and include more foods such as unsweetened fruit juice and canned fruits with no sugar added.
   c. Natural sugars are just as detrimental as refined sugars (examples: honey, maple syrup).
7. Encourage daily use of fluoride through water, foods, dentifrices, and rinses.
8. Use of sugar-free chewing gum after or between meals to minimize caries potential.
9. Rinsing with water if toothbrushing is not available.

EVALUATION OF PROGRESS

The success of the dental caries control guidelines and meal plan depends on learning by the patient. Learning implies a change of behavior and progress toward goals that are clearly understood by the learner.

I. IMMEDIATE EVALUATION

A. The patient's expressed interest and demonstration of cooperation in the dietary analysis and counseling session.
B. Patient motivation level of caries control plan.

II. THREE-MONTH FOLLOW-UP

A. Request patient to keep a 3- to 7-day food diary for assessment and evaluation.
B. Review personal oral care procedures and provide suggestions as needed.
C. Collaborate on ideas for further modifications when indicated. Smaller goals may need to be established for greater compliance.
D. Document progress, additional material reviewed, and plan for continued behavior modification.

Everyday Ethics

Ms. Carlson presents with type I diabetes and several significant changes in her oral cavity since her last prophylaxis, including more pronounced angular cheilosis, glossitis, and several proximal carious lesions. The hygienist, Bettina, feels that Ms. Carlson has advanced nutritional needs beyond the scope of practice and, therefore, does not address any chairside dietary assessment with the patient. The appointment continues with routine home care instructions. Bettina mentions her concerns about Ms. Carlson's dietary status to the dentist when the exam is done at the end of the appointment but does not record any recommendations in the chart.

Questions for Consideration

1. What professional protocol for referrals should be followed by the dental hygienist since she feels that giving dietary advice to a patient with diabetes is beyond the scope of practice for a dental hygienist?

2. By eliminating the chairside dietary assessment, did she act nonmaleficently toward the patient? Explain your response.

3. What ethical principles would be ignored if Bettina does not educate the patient about the preventive measures for her dental caries or document this information in the chart?

✔ Factors To Teach The Patient

MEDICATIONS WITH SUCROSE

- The need to avoid liquid or chewable forms containing sucrose or other cariogenic sugar.

- Reasons to avoid frequent daily use of medications with sucrose.

- Advantages of rinsing the mouth of the cariogenic sugar immediately following each dose if the medication cannot be given in a less cariogenic form.

MEDICATIONS WITH SIDE EFFECT OF XEROSTOMIA

- Effect of diuretics, hypertensives, and antidepressants on xerostomia.

- How xerostomia increases the risk of dental caries development.

- Effect of xerostomia on the difficulty in chewing and swallowing and how it compromises nutrient intake.

- The need to avoid the use of slowly dissolving candies to help stimulate saliva. Advantages of using saliva substitutes instead of hard candies.

FACTORS IN DENTAL CARIES

- How dental caries on the tooth surface starts with the microorganisms making acid from the cariogenic foods.

- How the interaction of cariogenic foods, tooth surface, saliva, and microorganisms act together in the role of dental caries process (Figure 32-2).

- How continuous acid production and the pH in the dental biofilm adversely affect the teeth. Need to avoid frequent eating episodes (Figure 32-6).

III. SIX-MONTH FOLLOW-UP

A. Perform examination and clinical procedures.
   1. Scaling as needed.
   2. Topical application of fluoride, depending on self-applied fluoride program.
   3. Charting of carious lesions and demineralized areas.
B. Compare dental caries incidence with previous chartings and completed restorative dentistry.
C. Make collaborative dietary recommendations with patient in accord with new assessment.
D. Document progress, education provided, and plan.

IV. OVERALL EVALUATION

A. Consistent reduction in dental caries rate in the years following the initial counseling shows sustained change in habits.
B. Patient's and parents' attitudes toward maintaining adequate oral health habits.
C. Attempts to maintain a diet containing minimum cariogenic foods.
D. Compliance with keeping regular appointments for professional dental care.

REFERENCES

1. Yates, A.A., Schlicker, S.A., and Suitor, C.W.: Dietary Reference Intakes: The New Basis for Recommendations for Calcium and Related Nutrients, B Vitamins, and Choline, *J. Am. Diet. Assoc.,* 98, 699, June, 1998.
2. National Research Council, Committee on Dietary Allowances, Food and Nutrition Board: *Recommended Dietary Allowances,* 10th ed. Washington, D.C., National Academy of Sciences, Office of Publications, 1989.
3. American Dairy Association and Dairy Council: Dietary Reference Intakes: Calcium and Related Nutrients, *Dairy Council Digest,* 68, 31, November/December, 1997.
4. Institute of Medicine: *DRIs for Thiamin, Riboflavin, Niacin, Vitamin B6, Folate, Panthothenic Acid, Biotin, and Choline.* Washington, D.C., National Academy Press, 1999.
5. Nishida, M., Grossi, S.G., Dunford, R.G., Ho, A.W., Trevison, M., and Genco, R.J.: Dietary Vitamin C and the Risk for Periodontal Disease, *J. Periodontol.,* 71, 1215, August, 2000.
6. Nishida, M., Grossi, S.G. Dunford, R.G., Ho, A.W., Trevison, M., and Genco, R.J.: Calcium and the Risk for Periodontal Disease, *J. Periodontol.,* 71, 1057, July, 2000.
7. Featherstone, J.D.B.: The Science and Practice of Caries Prevention, *J. Am. Dent. Assoc.,* 131, 887, July, 2000.
8. Boyd, L.D. and Dwyer, J.T.: Guidelines for Nutrition Screening, Assessment, and Intervention in the Dental Office, *J. Dent. Hyg.,* 72, 31, Fall, 1998.
9. Burt, B.A. and Satishchandra, P.: Sugar Consumption and Caries Risk: A Systematic Review, *J. Dent.Educ.,* 65, 1017, October, 2001.
10. Kashket, S., Van Houte, J., Lopez, L.R., and Stocks, S.: Lack of Correlation Between Food Retention on the Human Dentition and Consumer Perception of Food Stickiness, *J. Dent. Res.,* 70, 1314, October, 1991.
11. Kashket, S., Zhang, J., and Van Houte, J.: Accumulation of Fermentable Sugars and Metabolic Acids in Food Particles That Become Entrapped on the Dentition, *J. Dent. Res.,* 75, 1885, November, 1996.
12. Lingstrom, P., Birkhed, D., Ruben, J., and Arends, J.: Effects of Frequent Consumption of Starchy Food Items on Enamel and Dentin Demineralization and on Plaque pH In Situ, *J. Dent. Res.,* 73, 652, March, 1994.
13. Linke, H.A.B. and Birkenfeld, L.H.: Clearance and Metabolism of Starch Foods in the Oral Cavity, *Ann. Nutr. Metab.,* 43, 131, May–June, 1999.
14. Rugg-Gunn, A.J., Edgar, W.M., Geddes, D.A.M., and Jenkins, G.N.: The Effect of Different Meal Patterns Upon Plaque pH in Human Subjects, *Br. Dent. J.,* 139, 351, November 4, 1975.
15. Linke, H.A.B. and Riba, H.K.: Oral Clearance and Acid Production of Dairy Products During Interaction With Sweet Foods, *Ann. Nutr. Metab.,* 45, 202, September–October, 2001.
16. Hayes, C.: The Effect of Non-Cariogenic Sweeteners on the Prevention of Dental Caries: A Review of the Evidence, *J. Dent. Educ.,* 65, 1106, October, 2001.
17. Hildebrandt, G.H. and Sparks, B.S.: Maintaining Mutans Streptococci Suppression With Xylitol Chewing Gum, *J. Am. Dent. Assoc.,* 131, 909, July, 2000.
18. Rosal, M.C., Ebbeling, C.B., Lofgren, I., Ockene, J.K., Ockene, I.S., and Hebert, J.R.: Facilitating Dietary Change: The Patient-Centered Counseling Model, *J. Am. Diet. Assoc.,* 101, 332, March, 2001.
19. McBean, L.D.: Diet and Dental Caries: An Overview, *Dairy Council Digest,* 65, 1, January/February, 1994.

SUGGESTED READINGS

Al-Zahrani, M.S., Bissada, N.F., and Borawski, E.A.: Obesity and Periodontal Disease in Young, Middle-Aged, and Older Adults, *J. Periodontol.,* 74, 610, May, 2003.

American Dietetic Association: ADA Reports: Position Paper of the American Dietetic Association: Oral Health and Nutrition, *J. Am. Diet. Assoc.,* 96, 184, February, 1996.

American Dietetic Association: Position of the American Dietetic Association: Dietary Guidance for Healthy Children Aged 2 to 11 Years, *J. Am. Diet. Assoc.,* 99, 93, January, 1999.

Boyd, L.D. and Lampi, K.J.: Importance of Nutrition for Optimum Health of the Periodontium, *J. Contemp. Dent. Pract., 2,* 36, May, 2001 (www.thejcdp.com).

Dorky, R.: Nutrition and Oral Health, *Gen. Dent.,* 49, 576, November–December, 2001.

Dwyer, J.T.: Nutrition Guidelines and Education of the Public, *J. Nutr.,* 131, 3074S, November, 2001.

Hornick, B.: Diet and Nutrition Implications for Oral Health, *J. Dent. Hyg.,*76, 67, Winter, 2002.

Institute of Medicine, Standing Committee on Scientific Evaluation of Dietary Reference Intakes, Food and Nutrition Board: *Dietary Reference Intakes for Calcium, Phosphorus, Magnesium, Vitamin D, and Fluoride,* Washington, D.C., National Academy Press, 1997.

Konig, K.G.: Diet and Oral Health, *Int. Dent. J.,* 50, 162, Number 3, 2000.

Neiva, R.F., Steigenga, J., Al-Shammari, K.F., and Wang, H.L.: Effects of Specific Nutrients on Periodontal Disease Onset, Progression and Treatment, *J. Clin. Periodontol.,* 30, 579, July, 2003.

Russell, R.M., Rasmussen, H., and Lichtenstein, A.H.: Modified Food Guide Pyramid for People Over Seventy Years of Age, *J. Nutr., 129,* 751, March, 1999.

Soderling, E.: Nutrition, Diet, and Oral Health in the 21 Century, *Int. Dent. J., 51,* 389, Supplement, 2001.

Dental Caries and Diet

Gustafsson, B.E., Quensel, C.-E., Lanke, L.S., Lundquist, C., Grahnen, H., Bonow, B.E., and Krasse, B.: The Vipeholm Dental Caries Study: The Effect of Different Levels of Carbohydrate Intake on Caries Activity in 436 Individuals Observed for 5 Years, *Acta. Odontol. Scand., 11,* 232, Numbers 3/4, 1954.

Hargreaves, J.A.: Discussion: Diet and Nutrition in Dental Health and Disease, *Am. J. Clin. Nutr., 61,* 447S, February, 1995.

Jensen, M.E. and Wefel, J.S.: Effects of Processed Cheese on Human Plaque pH and Demineralization and Remineralization, *Am. J. Dent., 3,* 217, October, 1990.

Jensen, M.E., Donly, K., and Wefel, J.S.: Assessment of the Effect of Selected Snack Foods on the Remineralization/Demineralization of Enamel and Dentin, *J. Contemp. Dent. Pract., 1,* 1, August, 2000 (*www.thejcdp.com*).

Papas, A.S., Joshi, A., Palmer, C.A., Giunta, J.L., and Dwyer, J.T.: Relationship of Diet to Root Caries, *Am. J. Clin. Nutr., 61,* 423S, February, 1995.

Peldyak, J. and Makinen, K.K.: Xylitol for Caries Prevention, *J. Dent. Hyg., 76,* 276, Fall, 2002.

Riordan, D.J.: Effects of Orthodontic Treatment on Nutrient Intake, *Am. J. Orthod. Dentofac. Orthop., 111,* 554, May, 1997.

Soderling, E., Makinen, K.K., Chen, C.Y., Pape, H.R., Loesche, W., and Makinen, P.L.: Effect of Sorbitol, Xylitol, and Xylitol/Sorbitol Chewing Gums on Dental Plaque, *Caries Res., 23,* 378, September-October, 1989.

Stegeman, C.A., Carroll, D.K., and Schierling, J.: The Battle of the Fermentable Carbohydrates, *Access, 12,* 38, March, 1998.

Tinanoff, N. and Palmer, C.A.: Dietary Determinants of Dental Caries and Dietary Recommendations for Preschool Children, *J. Public Health Dent, 60,* 197, Summer, 2000.

Fluorides
Durinda J. Mattana, RDH, MS

The use of fluorides provides the most effective method for dental caries prevention and control. Although historically associated primarily with dental caries, the action of fluoride on dental biofilm also has significant effects on the control and maintenance of total oral health.

Fluoride is important for optimum oral health at all ages. Fluoride is made available at the tooth surface by two general means: *systemically,* by way of the circulation to developing teeth, and *topically,* directly to the exposed surfaces of erupted teeth throughout life. Topical uptake of fluoride provides the major caries-inhibiting effect.

Key words associated with fluoride and fluoride therapy are defined in Box 33-1.

■ FLUORIDE METABOLISM[1]

I. FLUORIDE INTAKE

- Fluoride is a systemic nutrient taken in by way of water containing fluoride naturally or by fluoridation, from prescribed dietary supplements, and, in small amounts, from foods.
- Foods and beverages prepared at home or processed commercially using water containing fluoride are also sources of fluoride.
- Varying amounts are ingested from dentifrices, mouthrinses, and other fluoride products used by the individual.

II. ABSORPTION

A. Gastrointestinal Tract

- Fluoride is rapidly taken into the system: the rate and amount of absorption depends on the solubility of the fluoride compound.
- There is less absorption when the fluoride is taken with milk or food.

B. Blood Stream

- Maximum blood levels are reached within 30 minutes of intake. The blood level of fluoride fluctuates with intake.
- Normal plasma levels are very low.
- The fluoride concentration in the saliva ranges from 0.01 to 0.04 ppm, which is less than the plasma level.

III. DISTRIBUTION AND RETENTION

- Fluoride is distributed by the plasma to all tissues and organs. There is a strong affinity for the calcified tissues.
- Approximately 99% of the fluoride in the body is located in the mineralized tissues.
- Concentrations of fluoride are at the surfaces next to the tissue fluid supplying the fluoride.
- The fluoride ion (F) is stored as an integral part of the crystal lattice of teeth and bones. The amount stored varies with the intake, the time of exposure, and the age and stage of the development of the individual. The teeth store small amounts, with highest levels on the tooth surface.

IV. EXCRETION

- Most fluoride is excreted through the kidneys in the urine, with a small amount excreted by the sweat glands and in the feces.
- There is limited transfer from plasma to breast milk for excretion by that route.

■ FLUORIDE AND TOOTH DEVELOPMENT

Fluoride is a nutrient essential to the formation of sound teeth and bones, as are calcium, phosphorus, and other elements obtained from food and water. At this point of study, a review of the histology of tooth development and mineralization can be a helpful supplement to the information included here.[2,3]

I. PRE-ERUPTIVE: MINERALIZATION STAGE

A. Fluoride is deposited during the formation of the enamel, starting at the dentinoenamel junction, after the enamel matrix has been laid down by the ameloblasts (Figure 33-1A).

B. Fluoride is incorporated during mineralization of all of the parts of the teeth.
- Table 46-6 shows the weeks *in utero* when the hard tissue formation begins for the primary teeth.
- The first permanent molars begin to mineralize at birth (Table 15-1, page 262).
- Fluoride is available to the developing teeth by way of the blood plasma to the tissues surrounding the tooth buds.

C. Effect of Excess Fluoride
- The normal activity of the ameloblasts may be inhibited, and a defective enamel matrix can form.
- Dental fluorosis can result.
- Dental fluorosis is a form of hypomineralization that results from ingestion of an excess amount of fluoride during tooth development.

BOX 33-1 KEY WORDS AND ABBREVIATIONS: Fluorides

Abrasive system: substances with cleaning and polishing properties utilized in the formulation of a dentifrice; must be compatible with fluoride compounds and other ingredients and not alter the tooth structure unfavorably.

Acidogenic: producing acid or acidity.

Apatite: a group of minerals of the general formula $Ca_{10}(PO_4)_6X_2$ wherein the X might include hydroxyl (OH), carbonate (CO), fluoride (F), or oxygen (O); crystalline mineral component of hard tissues (bones and teeth).

>   **Hydroxyapatite:** $Ca_{10}(PO_4)_6(OH)_2$; the form of apatite that is the principal mineral component of teeth, bones, and calculus.

>   **Fluorapatite:** the form of hydroxyapatite in which fluoride ions have replaced some of the hydroxyl ions; with fluoride, the apatite is less soluble and therefore more resistant to the acids formed from carbohydrate intake.

>   **Fluorhydroxyapatite:** apatite formed when low concentrations of fluoride react with tooth mineral; at higher concentrations, calcium fluoride is formed.

Cariogenic challenge: exposure of a tooth surface to an acid attack; acid is from the action of dental biofilm and cariogenic food ingested.

Cariostatic: exerting an inhibitory action on the progress of dental caries.

Defluoridation: lowering the amount of fluoride in fluoridated water to an optimum level for the prevention of dental caries and dental fluorosis.

Demineralization: breakdown of the tooth structure with a loss of mineral content, primarily calcium and phosphorus.

Efficacy: with reference to a product: an efficacious product produces a statistically and clinically significant benefit under ideal testing conditions in carefully controlled clinical trials.

Fluoride: a salt of hydrofluoric acid; occurs in many tissues and is stored primarily in bones and teeth.

Fluorosis: form of enamel hypomineralization due to excessive ingestion of fluoride during the development and mineralization of the teeth; depending on the length of exposure and the ppm of the fluoride, the fluorosed area may appear as a small white spot or as severe brown staining with pitting.

Gel: semisolid or solid phase of a colloidal solution.

Glycolysis: process by which sugar is metabolized by bacteria to produce acid.

Hypocalcification: deficient calcification.

>   **Enamel hypocalcification:** defect of enamel maturation caused by hereditary or systemic irregularities.

Maturation: stage or process of becoming mature or attaining maximal development; with respect to tooth development, maturation results from the continuous dynamic exchange of ions into the surface of the enamel from pellicle, dental biofilm, and oral fluids.

O.T.C.: over the counter.

ppm: parts per million; measure used to designate the amount of fluoride used for optimum level in fluoridated water, dentifrice, and other fluoride-containing preparations.

Remineralization: restoration of mineral elements; enhanced by presence of fluoride; remineralized lesions are more resistant to initiation of dental caries than is normal tooth structure.

Subsurface lesion: demineralized area below the surface of the enamel created by acid that has passed through micropores between enamel rods; subject to remineralization by action of fluoride.

Thixotropic: type of gel that sets in a gel-like state but becomes fluid under stress; the fluid form permits the solution to flow into interdental areas.

"White spot": term used to describe a small area on the surface of enamel that contrasts in appearance with the rest of the surface and may be visible only when the tooth is dried; two types of white spots can be differentiated: an area of demineralization and an area of fluorosis (also referred to as an "enamel opacity").

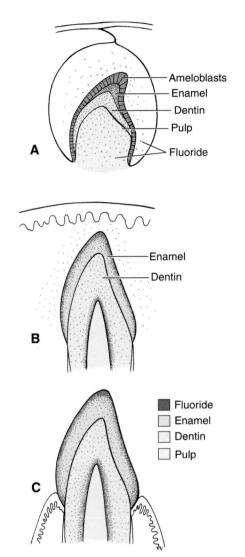

underlying layers of enamel during mineralization.

- Children who are exposed to fluoride for the first time within the 2 years prior to eruption have the greatest amount of fluoride acquired during this pre-eruptive stage.

III. POSTERUPTIVE

A. After eruption and throughout the life span of the teeth
- Fluoride from the drinking water, dentifrice, mouthrinses, and other surface exposures acts to inhibit demineralization and enhance remineralization (Figure 33-2).
- The presence of fluoride on the tooth surfaces can inhibit the initiation and progression of dental caries.

B. Uptake is rapid on the enamel surface during the first years after eruption.
- Uptake is greater at high levels than at low levels of fluoride, especially from supplements

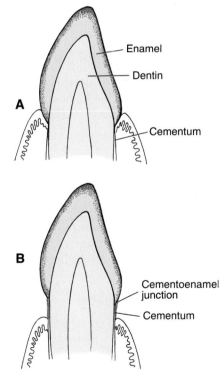

■ **FIGURE 33-1 Systemic Fluoride.** Green dots represent fluoride ions in the tissues and distributed throughout the tooth. **(A)** Developing tooth during mineralization shows fluoride from water and other systemic sources deposited in the enamel and dentin. **(B)** Maturation stage prior to eruption, when fluoride is taken up from tissue fluids around the crown. **(C)** Erupted tooth continues to take up fluoride on the surface from external sources. Note concentrated fluoride deposition on the enamel surface and on the pulpal surface of the dentin.

II. PRE-ERUPTIVE: MATURATION STAGE

A. After mineralization is complete and before eruption, fluoride deposition continues in the surface of the enamel (Figure 33-1B).

B. Fluoride is taken up from the nutrient tissue fluids surrounding the tooth crown.
- Much more fluoride is acquired by the outer surface during this period than in the

■ **FIGURE 33-2 Fluoride Acquisition After Eruption. (A)** Fluoride represented by green dots on the enamel surface is taken up from external sources, including dentifrice, rinse, topical application, and water from fluoridation passing over the tooth. **(B)** Gingival recession exposes the cementum to external sources of fluoride for the prevention of root caries and the alleviation of sensitivity.

used as chewable tablets or a swish-and-swallow liquid.

- Continuing intake of drinking water with fluoride provides a topical source as it washes over the teeth.

▪ TOOTH SURFACE FLUORIDE[4]

Fluoride concentration is greatest on the surface next to the source of fluoride. For the enamel of the erupted tooth, that is the outer surface exposed to the oral cavity. For the dentin, the highest concentration is at the pulpal surface until after recession of the periodontal attachment when the root surface is exposed to the oral cavity.

I. FLUORIDE IN ENAMEL

A. Uptake

- Uptake of fluoride depends on the level of fluoride in the oral environment and the length of time of exposure.
- Hypomineralized enamel absorbs fluoride in greater quantities than sound enamel.

B. Fluoride in the Enamel Surface

- Fluoride is a natural constituent of enamel.
- The outer surface has the highest concentration, and the amount decreases toward the interior of the tooth.

II. FLUORIDE IN DENTIN[4]

- The fluoride level is greater in exposed dentin than in enamel.
- A higher concentration is at the pulpal surface, where exchanges take place.
- Newly formed dentin absorbs fluoride rapidly.

III. FLUORIDE IN CEMENTUM[4]

- The level of fluoride in cementum is high and increases with age.
- With recession of the clinical attachment level in periodontal infection, the root surface is exposed to the fluids of the oral cavity, as shown in Figure 33-2B. Fluoride is then available to the cementum from the saliva and all the sources used by the patient, including drinking water, dentifrice, and mouthrinse.

▪ DEMINERALIZATION– REMINERALIZATION

I. DEMINERALIZATION

A. Initiation

- Demineralization means breakdown of the tooth structure with a loss of mineral content, primarily calcium and phosphorus.
- Breakdown is caused by organic acids produced by acidogenic bacteria after the metabolism of ingested fermentable carbohydrates.
- A shift in the oral equilibrium that favors demineralization over remineralization leads to a subsurface "white spot," the earliest clinically detectable lesion.

B. Progression

- The acids produced in the dental biofilm pass through the microchannels between the enamel rods.
- Demineralization occurs in the subsurface layer.
- Figure 33-3 shows a cross section of enamel with a subsurface demineralized area.
- Eventually the area can be detected on clinical examination when the spot may become chalky or discolored by food or tobacco.
- With further demineralization, the lesion breaks through the tooth surface to form the carious lesion of dental caries.

II. REMINERALIZATION

A. Process of Remineralization

- Remineralization is the recovery of the demineralization process.
- Saliva acts to buffer (neutralize) the acid, and the calcium and phosphorous ions are restored to the crystal structure.
- With the addition of fluoride, the dental carious process is arrested.
- When early remineralization occurs, the white spot will "harden" and the area may be hypermineralized compared with the enamel around it.

B. Role of Fluoride

- Fluoride inhibits demineralization and enhances remineralization
- Dental biofilm may contain 5 to 50 ppm fluoride. The content varies greatly and is constantly changing.

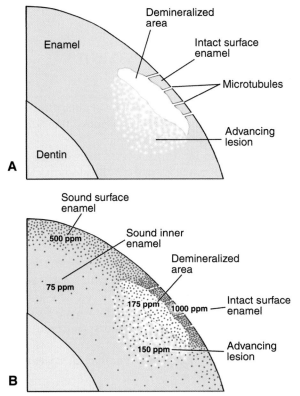

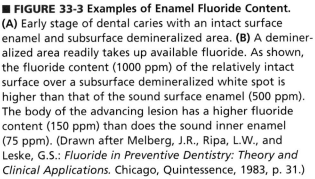

▪ **FIGURE 33-3 Examples of Enamel Fluoride Content. (A)** Early stage of dental caries with an intact surface enamel and subsurface demineralized area. **(B)** A demineralized area readily takes up available fluoride. As shown, the fluoride content (1000 ppm) of the relatively intact surface over a subsurface demineralized white spot is higher than that of the sound surface enamel (500 ppm). The body of the advancing lesion has a higher fluoride content (150 ppm) than does the sound inner enamel (75 ppm). (Drawn after Melberg, J.R., Ripa, L.W., and Leske, G.S.: *Fluoride in Preventive Dentistry: Theory and Clinical Applications.* Chicago, Quintessence, 1983, p. 31.)

- The fluoride in the biofilm may be acquired directly from fluoridated water, dentifrice, and other topical sources, brought by the saliva from the same sources, or from an exchange with the demineralizing tooth surface under the biofilm.
  - Dental biofilm is in direct contact with the tooth surface. The fluid in the biofilm transports the fluoride, other minerals, and the organic acids to the tooth surface.
  - There is a continuous exchange of minerals between biofilm and the enamel crystals at the tooth surface depending on the pH created by the organic acids. The presence of fluoride ions acts to control the demineralization process.

III. SUMMARY OF FLUORIDE ACTION

Having fluoride available to the tooth is key to its effectiveness. Frequent exposure to low-dose fluoride, such as fluoridated water, dentifrice, and mouthrinse, is recommended. There are three basic effects of fluoride to prevent dental caries.

A. Inhibit demineralization.
B. Enhance remineralization of incipient lesions.
C. Inhibit bacterial activity.
- Interferes with enzyme activity.
- Fluoride inhibits *enolase,* an enzyme needed by bacteria to metabolize carbohydrates.

▪ FLUORIDATION

Fluoridation is the adjustment of the fluoride ion content of a domestic municipal water supply to the optimum physiologic concentration that will provide maximum protection against dental caries and enhance the appearance of the teeth with a minimum possibility of producing objectionable enamel fluorosis.[5] Fluoridation has been established as the most efficient, effective, reliable, and inexpensive means for improving and maintaining oral health.

I. HISTORICAL ASPECTS[6]

A. Mottled Enamel and Dental Caries

- **Dr. Frederick S. McKay**
  Early in the 20th century, Dr. McKay began his extensive studies to find the cause of "brown stain," which later was called mottled enamel and now is known as *dental fluorosis.* He observed that people in Colorado Springs, Colorado, with mottled enamel had significantly less dental caries.[7] He associated the condition with the drinking water, but tests were inconclusive.
- **H.V. Churchill**
  In 1931, H.V. Churchill, a chemist, pinpointed fluorine as the specific element related to the tooth changes that Dr. McKay had been observing clinically.[8]

B. Background for Fluoridation

- **Dr. H. Trendley Dean**
  Epidemiologic studies of the 1930s sponsored by the United States Public Health Service and directed by Dr. Dean led to the conclusion that the level of fluoride in the water optimum for dental caries prevention averages 1 ppm in moderate climates. Clinically objectionable dental fluorosis is associated with levels well over 2 ppm.[9]

- From this knowledge and the fact that many healthy people had lived long lives in communities where the fluoride content of the water was much greater than 1 ppm, the concept of adding fluoride to the water developed.
- It was still necessary, however, to show that the benefits from controlled fluoridation could parallel those of natural fluoride.

C. Fluoridation—1945

- The first communities were fluoridated in 1945.
- Research in the communities began before fluoridation was started to obtain baseline information, and it continued over the years with detailed examinations and reports.

D. Control Cities

- Aurora, Illinois, where the natural fluoride level is optimum (1.2 ppm), was used to compare the benefits of natural fluoride in the water supply with those of fluoridation, as well as with a fluoride-free city, Rockford, Illinois.
- Original cities with fluoridation and their control cities in the research are shown in Box 33-2.
- The research conducted in these cities, as well as other research done throughout the world, has documented the influence of fluoride on oral health. The documented effects and benefits are predominantly due to the topical, posteruptive exposure of the teeth and oral environment to fluoride of all sources, particu-

larly the fluoride in fluoridated water, throughout life.

II. WATER SUPPLY ADJUSTMENT

A. Fluoride Level

- Since 1962, the United States Public Health Service has recommended an optimal fluoride concentration of 0.7 to 1.2 ppm.
- The optimum fluoride level for water in temperate climates is 1 ppm. The amount can be adjusted from 0.7 ppm in warmer climates where more water is consumed to 1.2 ppm in colder areas.[5]

B. Chemicals Used

- *Sources.* Compounds from which the fluoride ion is derived are naturally occurring and are mined in various parts of the world. Examples of common sources are fluorspar, cryolite, and apatite.
- *Criteria for acceptance of a fluoride compound for fluoridation*
  - Solubility to permit its regular use in a water plant.
  - Relatively inexpensive.
  - Readily available to prevent interruptions in maintaining the proper fluoride level.
- *Compounds used*
  - Dry compounds: sodium fluoride and sodium silicofluoride.
  - Solution of hydrofluorosilicic acid.

■ EFFECTS AND BENEFITS OF FLUORIDATION

I. APPEARANCE OF TEETH

- Teeth exposed to an optimum or slightly higher level of fluoride frequently are white, shining, opaque, and without blemishes.
- When the level is slightly more than optimum for the individual, white areas, such as bands or flecks, may be apparent. These areas can be seen professionally by drying the teeth and observing them under a dental light. Without such close scrutiny, such spots may blend with the overall appearance.
- Dental fluorosis, associated with higher than optimum fluoride levels, has been classified as shown in Box 33-3.

BOX 33-2 First Fluoridation Research Cities	
Research City	**Control City**
Grand Rapids, Michigan (January, 1945)	Muskegon, Michigan
Newburgh, New York (May, 1945)	Kingston, New York
Brantford, Ontario (June, 1945)	Sarnia, Ontario
Evanston, Illinois (February, 1947)	Oak Park, Illinois

BOX 33-3 Descriptive Criteria and Scoring System for the Tooth Surface Index of Fluorosis (TSIF)

Numerical Score	Descriptive Criteria
0	Enamel shows no evidence of fluorosis.
1	Enamel shows definite evidence of fluorosis, namely, areas with parchment-white color that total less than one third of the visible enamel surface. This category includes fluorosis confined only to incisal edges of anterior teeth and cusp tips of posterior teeth ("snowcapping").
2	Parchment-white fluorosis totals at least one third of the visible surface, but less than two thirds.
3	Parchment-white fluorosis totals at least two thirds of the visible surface.
4	Enamel shows staining in conjunction with any of the preceding levels of fluorosis. Staining is defined as an area of definite discoloration that may range from light to very dark brown.
5	Discrete pitting of the enamel exists, unaccompanied by evidence of staining of intact enamel. A pit is defined as a definite physical defect in the enamel surface with a rough floor that is surrounded by a wall of intact enamel. The pitted area is usually stained or differs in color from the surrounding enamel.
6	Both discrete pitting and staining of the intact enamel exist.
7	Confluent pitting of the enamel surface exists. Large areas of enamel may be missing, and the anatomy of the tooth may be altered. Dark-brown stain is usually present.

From Horowitz, H.S., Driscoll, W.S., Meyers, R.J., Heifetz, S.B., and Kingman, A.K.: A New Method for Assessing the Prevalence of Dental Fluorosis—The Tooth Surface Index of Fluorosis, *J. Am. Dent. Assoc., 109,* 37, July, 1984.

II. DENTAL CARIES: PERMANENT TEETH

A. Overall Benefits

- Continuous use of fluoridated water from birth can result in as many as 40% to 65% fewer carious lesions.
- The effects are similar to those found in communities with optimum levels of natural fluoride in the water.
- Many more individuals are completely caries-free when fluoride is in the water.

B. Distribution

- Anterior teeth, particularly maxillary, receive more protection from fluoride than do posterior teeth.[9] The anterior teeth are contacted by the drinking water as it passes into the mouth.
- Fluoride is added to the surface of the enamel after eruption.

C. Progression

- Not only are the numbers of carious lesions reduced, but the caries rate is slowed.
- Caries progression is also reduced in the surfaces that receive fluoride for the first time after eruption.[10]

III. ROOT CARIES

- Root caries experience of lifelong residents of a community with fluoridated water is in direct proportion to the fluoride concentration in the water compared with the experience of residents of a fluoride-free community.[11]
- The incidence of root caries is approximately 50% less in lifelong residents of a fluoridated community.[12]

IV. DENTAL CARIES: PRIMARY TEETH

- With fluoridation from birth, the caries incidence is reduced up to 50% in the primary teeth.
- For example, children aged 6 to 9 years in Newburgh, New York, had five times as many caries-free primary teeth present as did the children of Kingston, where fluoride was not present in the community drinking water.[13]

V. TOOTH LOSS

Tooth loss is much greater in both primary and permanent teeth without fluoride[13] because of increased dental caries, which progresses more rapidly.

VI. ADULTS

- When a person resides in a fluoride area throughout life, benefits continue.
- In Colorado Springs, adults aged 20 to 44 years who had used water with natural fluoride showed 60% less caries experience than did adults in fluoride-deficient Boulder, Colorado. In Boulder, adults also had had three to four times as many permanent teeth extracted.[14]
- In a survey of adults in Rockford, Illinois (no fluoride), there were about seven times as many edentulous persons as there were in a comparable group in Aurora, Illinois (natural fluoride).[15]

VII. PERIODONTAL DISEASES

- Indirect favorable effects of fluoride on periodontal health can be shown. Improved bone density resulting from fluoride can affect the alveolar bone, along with all bones, and may provide beneficial resistance against bone resorption.
- Dental carious lesions favor dental biofilm retention and, therefore, irritation to gingival tissues, particularly lesions adjacent to the gingival margin and proximal lesions, which favor food impaction. When dental caries, tooth loss, and malocclusion are decreased, a difference can be expected in the periodontal conditions because of lack of retentive areas for dental biofilm.
- The incidence of periodontal diseases increases with age because of the cumulative effects of etiologic factors and the disease processes. With the use of fluorides, particularly fluoridation, fewer teeth are lost because of dental caries at younger ages. Therefore, periodontal disease prevention and control must be emphasized in communities with fluoride in the drinking water.

▪ PARTIAL DEFLUORIDATION

- Several hundred communities in the United States have water supplies that contain more than twice the optimal level of fluoride.
- Water with excess fluoride does not meet the requirements of the United States Public Health Service.
- Defluoridation can be accomplished by one of several chemical systems.[16] The efficacy of the methods has been shown.
- The water supply in Britton, South Dakota, has been reduced from almost 7 ppm to 1.5 ppm

since 1948, and in Bartlett, Texas, from 8 ppm to 1.8 ppm since 1952. Examinations have shown a dramatic reduction in the incidence of objectionable fluorosis in children born since defluoridation.[17,18]

▪ SCHOOL FLUORIDATION

To bring the benefits of fluoridation to children living in rural areas without the possibility for community fluoridation, adding fluoride to a school water supply was an alternative.

- Because of the intermittent use of the school water (5 days each week during the 9-month school year), the amount of fluoride added was increased over the usual 1 ppm.
- Example: After 12 years of fluoride at 5 ppm in the school drinking water of Elk Lake, Pennsylvania, children who had attended that school regularly had 39% fewer decayed, missing, and filled teeth than did those in the control group. The greatest benefits were found on proximal tooth surfaces.[19]
- Example: In the schools of Seagrove, North Carolina, after 12 years with the fluoride level at 6.3 ppm, the children experienced a 47.5% decrease in decayed, missing, and filled surfaces compared with those in the control group.[19]
- School fluoridation has been phased out in several states, and the current extent of this practice is unknown. Operations and maintenance of small fluoridation systems are problematic.[20]
- Such systems have significance in the long history of efforts for fluoridation for all people in the United States.

▪ DISCONTINUED FLUORIDATION

- When fluoride is removed, dental caries control by fluorides is clearly shown in a community.
- Example: In Antigo, Wisconsin, the action of antifluoridationists in 1960 brought about the discontinuance of fluoridation, which had been installed in 1949. Examinations in the years following 1960 revealed the marked drop in the number of children who were caries-free and the steep increases in caries rates. From 1960 to 1966, the number of caries-free children in the second grade decreased by 67%.[21] Fluoridation was reinstated in 1966 by popular demand.

▪ FLUORIDES IN FOODS

I. FOODS[22]

Certain foods contain fluoride, but not enough to constitute a significant part of the day's need for caries prevention. Meat, eggs, vegetables, cereals, and fruits have very small but measurable amounts, whereas fish have larger amounts. Foods cooked in fluoridated water retain fluoride from the cooking water.

II. SALT[23]

- Fluoridated salt has been used, particularly in Switzerland.
- Use of fluoridated salt results in a reduced incidence of dental caries, but effects comparable to those gained by water fluoridation have not been attained.
- The use of salt as it is currently available supplies about one third to one half of the amount of fluoride ingested daily from 1 ppm fluoridated water, when average amounts of water used by individuals are compared.

III. HALO EFFECT

- The "halo effect" refers to the unintentional addition of fluoride to a concentrated beverage that is reconstituted from a water supply containing fluoride in a city other than where it is consumed.
- Many processed beverages such as juices made from concentrate may contain fluoride if the water used to process the juice contains fluoride.
- Juices consumed in one location may contain fluoride from the water of another location in which the juice was reconstituted.[22]

IV. BOTTLED WATER

Bottled water usually does not contain optimal fluoride unless it has a label indicating that it is fluoridated. Patients should be advised to fill their water bottle from a water supply that is fluoridated.

▪ DIETARY FLUORIDE SUPPLEMENTS

Only a percentage of the population receives fluoridated water by fluoridation of the municipal water supply or water containing naturally occurring fluoride. Without fluoride in the drinking water, individuals and communities must resort to other means for making

fluoride available. One method is the use of dietary prescription fluoride supplements. The primary mechanisms of fluoride in caries prevention are topical, posteruptive, but current guidelines call for supplementation of children aged 6 months through 16 years in the following situations:

- People who use a private water supply that does not have natural fluoride and that is not practical to fluoridate.
- When the fluoride in the water is less than optimum level.

I. DETERMINE THE NEED

- Review the patient history to be certain the child is not receiving other fluoride in such preparations as vitamin-fluoride supplements.
- Refer to the list of fluoridated communities available from state or local health departments to determine the patient's fluoride consumption level.
- Request water analysis when the fluoride level in a private water source has not been determined.
- For those whose community water supply has not yet been fluoridated.
- Despite evidence that fluoride passes across the placenta during the fifth and sixth months of pregnancy and enters the prenatal deciduous enamel,[24] administration of prenatal dietary fluoride supplements is not recommended. Use of fluoride supplements by pregnant women has not been shown to benefit their offspring.

II. AVAILABLE FORMS OF SUPPLEMENTS

Products are classified by the American Dental Association, Council on Scientific Affairs. Whenever possible, a supplement that has a topical effect (is chewed, swished, and then swallowed) should be used.

- Available as a pill, chewable tablet, lozenge, drop, or mouthrinse for swallowing after rinsing.
- Prescribed on an individual patient basis for daily use at home, or may be administered to school classroom groups as part of a total public health program.
- Chewing and rinsing with a supplement before swallowing results in a dual action: first, locally on the tooth surface, and second, systemically in unerupted, developing teeth (Figure 33-1A and B).
- After chewing, the mixture should be swished over and between the teeth for 1 minute so that optimal benefit can be obtained.

- The person should not eat or drink for 30 minutes after chewing the tablet. The preferred time for using the tablet is after toothbrushing, before going to bed.
- Maximum topical effect occurs on newly erupted teeth.

A. Tablets and Lozenges

- Tablets may be scored or unscored and may be chewed, rinsed, and swallowed, or dissolved slowly in the mouth as a lozenge.
- The resulting mix with saliva should be swished over and between the teeth for 1 minute.
- For infants, the tablet can be crushed to add to food.

B. Mouthrinse

- A measured amount contains the prescribed daily fluoride.
- Swished for at least 1 minute before swallowing for added topical benefit.

C. Drops

- A liquid concentrate with directions that specify the number of drops for the prescription equivalent.
- Primary use for the child from 6 months to 3 years; a drop can be placed directly into the child's mouth or in food.
- For older children, the tooth contact of the chewable tablet or mouthrinse is important to provide the enamel surface with protective fluoride.

III. PRESCRIPTION

Table 33-1 shows the fluoride dosage necessary to supplement the different levels of fluoride in the drinking water.[25]

- Prescription for breast-fed infant
  - The concentration of fluoride in breast milk is very low, even when the mother uses fluoridated community water. Infants who are totally breast-fed after 6 months need a daily fluoride supplement of 0.25 mg (Table 33-1).
  - In a fluoridated community, an infant who receives other sources of liquid, such as drinking water or supplemental formula feedings made with fluoridated water, does not need the prescription.
- Limitation on total prescription
  - Prescribe no more than 264 mg of sodium fluoride at a time; sufficient for 4 months when 2.2 mg is used daily.
  - The amount (264 mg) is below the toxic or lethal doses and therefore eliminates the hazard of storing large amounts in the home.
- Storage: tablets should be kept out of the reach of children.

▪ PROFESSIONAL TOPICAL FLUORIDE APPLICATIONS

Topical application of fluoride is an essential part of a total preventive program, particularly for patients at risk for dental caries. Topical fluoride applications are both professionally applied and self-applied by the patient. Professionally applied fluorides may be solutions, gels, foams, or varnishes. Professional agents will be described first, followed by self-applied fluorides.

I. INDICATIONS

- The professional application of a high-concentration fluoride preventive agent is a selective procedure for individuals at moderate or high risk for dental caries, such as those listed in Box 33-4.

▪ TABLE 33-1 FLUORIDE SUPPLEMENTS DOSAGE SCHEDULE (mg F/DAY)*			
	WATER FLUORIDE CONCENTRATION (ppm)		
AGE OF CHILD	**LESS THAN 0.3**	**BETWEEN 0.3 AND 0.6**	**GREATER THAN 0.6**
Birth–6 mo	0	0	0
6 mo–3 yr	0.25 mg	0†	0†
3–6 yr	0.50 mg	0.25 mg	0
6–16 yr	1.0 mg	0.5 mg	0

*2.2 mg of sodium fluoride provides 1 mg of fluoride ions.
†Infants receiving their total diet from breast-feeding need a 0.25-mg supplement.
(Recommendations from the American Dental Association, Chicago, IL.)

BOX 33-4 Indications for Professional Topical Fluoride Application: Patients at Risk for Dental Caries

- Primary teeth

    Infant/toddler: prevention of baby bottle tooth decay

    Parental oral care; parental caries pattern

- Posteruptive period

    Rapid uptake of fluoride important for newly exposed enamel

- Active caries (new carious lesions at regular maintenance)

- Secondary/recurrent caries adjacent to previous restorations

- Wearing orthodontic appliances: bands, bonded brackets

- Compromised salivary flow

    Radiation therapy to head and neck

    Sjögren's syndrome or another condition that limits salivary excretion by the glands

    Medication with side effect of xerostomia

- Teeth supporting an overdenture

- Exposed root surfaces following periodontal recession

- Lack of compliance and conscientious efforts for daily dental biofilm removal

- Low or no fluoride in drinking water

- Early carious lesions:

    Pit and fissure: restore caries; sealant for all others

    Proximal surface: need fluoride application

- Routine application after scaling and debridement of exposed root surfaces during dental hygiene periodontal treatments.

II. DEVELOPMENT

- Professionally applied fluoride has been instrumental in the reduction of dental caries in the United States and other industrialized countries since the early 1940s, when Dr. Basil G. Bibby conducted the initial topical sodium fluoride study using Brockton, Massachusetts, schoolchildren.[26]

- More than one-third fewer new carious lesions resulted from a 0.1% aqueous solution applied at 4-month intervals for 2 years.

- The research led to extensive studies by John W. Knutson and others sponsored by the United States Public Health Service. The aim was to determine the most effective concentration of sodium fluoride, the minimum time required for application, and procedural details.[27,28] Their results still provide the basis for the applications currently and described in the following sections.

III. COMPOUNDS

Three high-concentration agents have been evaluated clinically and approved by the American Dental Association and the Food and Drug Administration for professional topical application. Table 33-2 provides a summary of the professionally applied topical agents and the concentrations used.

A. 2.0% Sodium Fluoride (NaF) Gel or Foam for In-office Use

- Sodium fluoride is also called neutral sodium fluoride due to its neutral pH of 7.0.
- Clinical trials demonstrating the efficacy of neutral NaF were based on a series of four or five applications on a weekly basis.[29]
- Quarterly or semi-annual applications are most common in clinical practice.
- Currently available varnish products contain neutral NaF.

B. 1.23% Acidulated Phosphate Fluoride (APF) Gel or Foam for In-office Use

- Effective when used in a 4-minute tray application semi-annually.
- Widely used because of its storage stability, acceptable taste, tissue compatibility, and non-staining characteristic.
- Low pH of 3.5 enhances fluoride uptake. APF preparations with greater than 4.0 pH levels compromise the enamel uptake and should not be used.
- Etches porcelain and composite restorative materials.
    - The hydrofluoride component of APF dissolves the filler particles of the composite resin restorations. Macro-inorganic filler particles of composite materials demonstrate noticeable etched patterns generated by APF, whereas micro-filled materials are not sensitive to the APF agent.[30]

▪ TABLE 33-2 PROFESSIONALLY APPLIED TOPICAL FLUORIDES

AGENT	FORM	CONCENTRATION	APPLICATION MODE	NOTES
Sodium fluoride (NaF) pH = neutral	Aqueous solution 2%	9,040 ppm 0.90% F ion	Paint on	Cotton roll absorbs excess
	Gel 2%	9,040 ppm 0.90% F ion	Tray	Do not overfill: see Figure 33-5 Request patient not to swallow
	Foam 2%	9,040 ppm 0.90% F ion	Tray	Do not overfill: see Figure 33-5 25% the amount of gel is used
	Varnish 5%	22,600 ppm 2.3% F ion	Paint on	Sets promptly to hard yellow film
Acidulated phosphate (APF) pH = 3.5 *Do not use if composite, porcelain, or sealants are present*	Aqueous solution 1.23%	12,300 ppm	Paint on	Cotton roll absorbs excess
	Gel 1.23%	12,300 ppm	Tray	Do not overfill: see Figure 33-5 Request patient not to swallow
	Foam 1.23%	12,300 ppm	Tray	Fill adult and child trays, do not overfill 25% the amount of gel is used
Stannous fluoride (SnF) pH = 2.4–2.8 *No longer used due to disadvantages*	Aqueous solution 8% Freshly mixed daily	19,360 ppm	Paint on	Metallic, bitter taste

- Not to be used for patients with porcelain, composite restorations, and sealants.

C. 8.0% Stannous Fluoride (SnF)

- Only available in solution.
- Seldom used in clinical practice due to its unpleasant taste, instability, tooth staining, and sloughing of gingiva.

IV. CLINICAL PROCEDURES

Benefits from topical application of solution, gel, foam, and varnish are considered within the same general average of 25% to 35% reduction in the incidence of dental caries. Because the caries-preventive effects are similar, the choice of method of application used may be based on ease of application, overall amount of fluoride used, patient age, and acceptance, cost, or clinician's preference.

A. Objectives

1. *Remineralization of demineralized areas*
   - White spots in the cervical third, especially under dental biofilm.
   - Exposed root surfaces after periodontal treatment.
2. *Prevention of dental caries.* Identify special problems, including areas adjacent to restorations, orthodontic appliances; xerostomia; and other risk factors listed in Box 33-4.
3. *Desensitization.* Fluoride aids in blocking dentinal tubules (pages 721 to 722). Varnish covers and protects a sensitive area, and fluoride is

slowly released for uptake. SnF gel and NaF varnish demonstrate a desensitizing effect.

B. Preparation of the Teeth

When fluoride application is to be applied at a time other than following a routine dental hygiene scaling and debridement, rubber cup polishing is not routinely necessary. Fluoride solution or gel application has been shown to provide the same benefits when applied with or without a prior polishing.[31] A toothbrush cleaning is recommended.

1. *Toothbrush preparation.* Use patient instruction time to remove debris and dental biofilm with toothbrush and floss. Patient should learn all methods of caries prevention and how they work together.

2. *Apply principles of selective polishing for stain removal.* After calculus removal when stains must be removed, use the rubber cup with paste selectively on the areas where the stains occur. A fluoride-containing polishing paste may be used. Although only small amounts of fluoride may be added to the tooth surface, the fluoride paste may replace, in part, the fluoride removed by the polishing abrasive.[32]

C. Patient Counseling

1. *Inform patient (and parent).* Let them understand the purposes and benefits as well as the limitation of topical applications. The limitation is that the fluoride is only part of the total prevention program, which includes daily biofilm control and limitation of cariogenic foods.

2. *Appointment sequence*
   a. Schedule appointment to end 30 minutes before the patient's eating time.
   b. Prepare the patient for any discomfort, especially the 4-minute timing.
   c. Explain the need not to swallow but to expectorate immediately after the tray is removed.

3. *After application.* Patient must not rinse, eat, drink, brush, or floss for at least 30 minutes for solution or gel applications and 4 hours after application of varnish. Rinsing immediately after an application has been shown to lessen the benefits.[33]

V. PAINT-ON TECHNIQUE: SOLUTION OR GEL

- Two-step procedure—only one half of the mouth can be completed at one time.
- Requires isolation with cotton roll holders (Figure 34-3).

- Seat patient upright, dry the teeth thoroughly, place the saliva ejector, and apply the solution or gel to the teeth with a cotton tip applicator.
- Teeth must stay wet with the solution or gel for 4 minutes.
- Use a saliva ejector throughout the procedure.
- Wipe excess off teeth after the procedure.

VI. TRAY TECHNIQUE: GEL OR FOAM

- Tray is the most common method of application of gels (Figure 33-4).
- Design of tray: hinged or separated, natural rounded arch shape to hold the gel or foam and prevent ingestion.
- Procedures for a professional gel or foam fluoride application are listed in Table 33-3.

VII. VARNISH

Fluoride varnishes are safe and effective as well as fast and easy to apply. Clinical studies regarding caries reduction are based on applications every 3 to 6 months. Varnishes were introduced in 1964. Fluoride varnishes are of a high concentration (over 20,000 ppm), but only a small amount is used. So the overall amount of fluoride used for a full-mouth application is less than used for gels and foams.[34]

- **Clinical Procedure**
  - Dispense Varnish: If dispensed from a tube (rather than a single-dose packet), discard any clear varnish because the ingredients have separated and will contain only a fraction of the intended amount of fluoride.[35]
  - Dry Each Quadrant: Mandibular first. Wipe teeth dry with gauze square or use gentle compressed air. The procedure is brief, but a saliva ejector may be necessary for selected patients.
  - Apply a thin coat of varnish using a swab or disposable applicator brush; coating is yellow-brown. Apply to cover teeth.
- **Adherence**
  - Sets rapidly in the presence of saliva.
  - Varnish prolongs contact time between the tooth and the fluoride compared with other delivery methods.
- **Instruction for Patient**
  - *Do not disturb.* Instruct patient that the teeth look yellow until the varnish is thoroughly removed.
  - Avoid eating or drinking for 30 minutes and avoid brushing the teeth for at least 4 hours after application; avoid rough foods

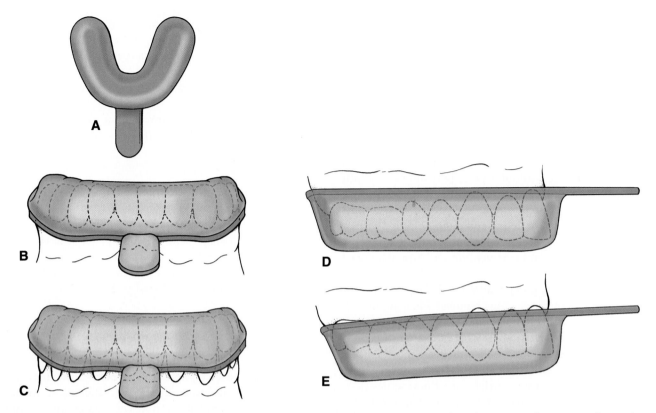

▪ FIGURE 33-4 Tray Selection. (A) Mandibular tray held for try-in. **(B)** Tray over teeth is deep enough to cover the entire exposed enamel above the gingiva. **(C)** In the patient with recession and areas of root surfaces exposed, the same tray is not deep enough to cover the important root surfaces where fluoride is needed for prevention of root caries or hypersensitivity. A custom-made tray is needed. **(D)** Tray adequately covers the distal surface of the most posterior tooth. **(E)** The tray does not cover the distal surface of the most posterior tooth adequately. The tray may need to be repositioned to cover the distal surface, or a larger stock or custom tray is needed.

to allow fluoride uptake to continue undisturbed.

- *Removal.* Patient removes with toothbrush and floss the next day.

- **Infant, Toddler, and Children Under 4 Years**
  - *Position.* Figure 46-5 shows the parent and clinician sitting knee-to-knee with the child held across the knees.
  - *Application.* Treat maxillary anterior teeth first (site of initial baby bottle tooth decay); treat all teeth if possible.
  - *Instruct parent.* Avoid giving food or drink for at least 30 minutes; toothbrush off the coating the next day.

▪ SELF-APPLIED FLUORIDES

Self-applied fluorides include prescription and over-the-counter products. Self-applied products are available as dentifrices, mouthrinses, and gels that may be applied by toothbrushing, rinsing, or trays that are custom made or disposable. A fluoride may also be used as an irrigation agent.

I. METHODS

The three methods for self-application are by mouth tray, rinsing, and toothbrushing.

A. Mouth Tray

- *Custom-made or disposable tray.* The tray should be selected to fit the individual mouth. Instruction is provided not to overfill the tray (Figure 33-5).
- *Overdenture patient.* Gel drops are placed in the impression surface at the location of the natural teeth; denture used as a tray (Figure 29-8).

B. Rinsing

The patient swishes for 1 minute with a measured amount of a fluoride rinse. Except when used as a fluoride supplement in a nonfluoridated community, the fluoride rinse is expectorated.

■ TABLE 33-3 PROCEDURE FOR TOPICAL GEL OR FOAM TRAY APPLICATION

Patient	Seat upright Explain procedure Instruct not to swallow Tilt head forward slightly
Tray coverage	Custom-made or appropriate size with absorptive liners; post-dam border rim Complete dentition must be covered, including anterior and posterior vertical coverage, distal dam depth, and close fit to the teeth Check for areas of recession: may need larger or custom-made tray Proper and improper tray coverage is shown in Figure 33-4
Place gel or foam	Use minimum amount of gel or foam in the trays, as shown in Figure 33-5 Adult: 5 mL maximum (gel = 40% of tray filled; foam = tray completely filled, not overfilled) Child: 4 mL maximum, 2 mL per tray (gel = 30% of tray filled; foam = tray completely filled, not overfilled)
Dry the teeth	Place a saliva ejector in the mouth during the drying procedure Dry the teeth prior to insertion of trays starting with the maxillary teeth; facial, occlusal, and palatal surfaces and then the mandibular teeth; lingual, occlusal, and facial surfaces.
Insert trays	Place both trays in the mouth A two-step procedure (one tray at a time) may be required; if so, patient may not rinse but must expectorate after the removal of each tray to prevent swallowing. Place cotton rolls between the trays on each side of the saliva ejector to prevent dislodging of the trays due to imbalance
Isolation	Use saliva ejector with maximum efficiency suction Garmer cotton-roll holder technique (Figure 34-3): place saliva absorber in cheek, and position holder for stability
Attention	Do not leave patient unattended
Timing	Use a timer; do not estimate (4 minutes) Procedure will take 8 minutes if a two-step procedure is used
Completion	Tilt head forward for removal of tray Request patient to expectorate for several minutes; do not allow swallowing Wipe excess gel or foam from teeth with gauze sponge Use high-power suction to draw out saliva and gel Instruct patient that nothing should be placed in the mouth for 30 minutes; do not rinse, eat, drink, or brush teeth

(Recommendations based on *Oral Health Policies for Children: Protocol for Fluoride Therapy*, American Academy of Pediatric Dentistry, 211 E. Chicago Avenue, Chicago, IL 60611.)

Certain patients will need to learn how to rinse properly to force the solution between the teeth. Box 27-5 lists steps for rinsing.

C. Toothbrushing

- A fluoride gel or paste is used for regular brushing two or three times daily.
- Brush-on gel may be used after regular brushing to provide additional benefits.
- Use an interdental brush to apply fluoride to proximal surfaces or open furcations.

II. INDICATIONS

- Indications for use of mouth tray, rinsing, and/or toothbrushing depend on the individual patient problems.
- Patient needs are determined as part of total care planning.
- Certain patients need multiple procedures combined with professional applications at the regular maintenance appointments. Special indications are suggested as each method is described in the following sections.

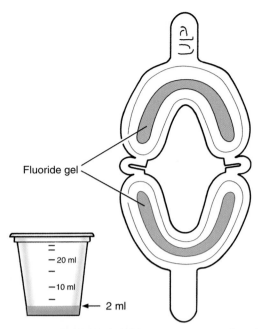

FIGURE 33-5 Measured Gel in Tray. No more than 2 mL of gel should be placed in each tray for small children, and no more than 2.5 mL for larger patients with permanent teeth. A medicine cup can be used to measure the amount once so that the correct level of gel in the tray can be determined. A minimum amount of gel is indicated to prevent ingestion by the patient.

▪ TRAY TECHNIQUE: HOME APPLICATION

The original gel tray studies using custom-fitted polyvinyl mouthpieces compared the use of 1.1% acidulated NaF with plain NaF gel. The gel was applied daily over a 2-year period by schoolchildren aged 11 to 14 years during the school years. Dental caries incidence was reduced up to 80%.[36]

I. INDICATIONS FOR USE

A. Rampant enamel or root caries in persons of any age.
B. Xerostomia from any cause, particularly loss of salivary gland function.
C. Exposure to radiation therapy.
D. Caries prevention under an overdenture.
E. Root surface hypersensitivity.

II. GELS USED

A. Concentrations[37]

APF 0.5%; NaF 1.1%

B. Precautions

1. Do not dispense large quantities. Prescription of 24 to 30 mL of APF 0.5% in a dropper bottle that dispenses drops containing 0.1 mL F is suggested.
2. Do not use acidulated preparations on porcelain, composites, titanium, or sealants.

C. Patient Instructions

1. Brush and floss to remove dental biofilm.
2. Use prepared custom-made polyvinyl tray. A disposable tray can be used if the appropriate fit can be obtained. Load the tray by distributing no more than 5 drops of the gel around each tray. Each drop is equivalent to 0.1 mL.
3. Dry the mouth by swallowing several times.
4. Apply the tray(s) over the teeth and close gently. Hold head upright.
5. Time by a clock for 4 minutes. *Do not swallow.*
6. Expectorate several times when the trays are removed.
7. Do not eat or drink for 30 minutes. Once-daily application should be made just before bedtime.

▪ FLUORIDE MOUTHRINSES

Mouthrinsing is a practical and effective means for self-application of fluoride. Rinsing can be part of an individual care plan or can be included in a group program conducted during school attendance.

I. INDICATIONS

Mouthrinsing with a fluoride preparation may have particular meaning for the following:

A. General prevention of dental caries in:
   • Young persons during the high-risk preteen and adolescent years.
   • Patients with areas of demineralization.
   • Patients with root exposure following recession and periodontal therapy.
   • Participants in a school health group program for all grades.
B. Patients with moderate to rampant dental caries who live in a fluoridated or nonfluoridated community.
C. Patients whose oral health care is complicated by biofilm-retentive appliances, including orthodontics and partial dentures or space maintainers.
D. Patients with xerostomia from any cause, including head and neck radiation and saliva-depressing drug therapy.

E. Patients with hypersensitivity of exposed root surfaces.

II. LIMITATIONS

A. Children under 6 years of age and those of any age who cannot rinse because of oral and/or facial musculature problems or other disability are excluded from the practice of this method.

B. Alcohol Content
- Use of alcohol-based mouthrinses should be discouraged; aqueous solutions are available.
- Alcohol content of commercial preparations is not advisable for children.
- Alcohol-containing preparations should never be recommended for a recovering alcoholic person.

C. Compliance is greater with a daily rinse than with a weekly rinse when practiced on an individual basis at home.

III. PREPARATIONS

Oral rinse supplements are categorized as *low-potency/high-frequency rinses* or *high-potency/low-frequency rinses*.[39] Certain low-potency rinses may be purchased directly over-the-counter (OTC); all others are provided by prescription. Table 33-4 contains the compounds and content.

A. Low-Potency/High-Frequency Over-the-Counter 0.05% NaF, 0.044% APF, or 0.63% SnF

1. *Specifications*
   - Single container must contain no more than 264 mg of NaF (120 mg of fluoride) dispensed at one time.
   - A 500-mL bottle of 0.05% NaF rinse contains 100 mg of fluoride.
   - Bottle must have a child-proof cap.
   - Label must state that the rinse is not to be used by children under 6 years of age or by children with a disability involving oral

and/or facial musculature. Young children do not have sufficient control to expectorate, and they tend to swallow quickly.
   - Label must indicate that the rinse is not to be swallowed.

2. *Procedure for use*
   - Rinse daily (except high-potency rinse is used weekly) with 1 teaspoonful (5 mL) after brushing before retiring.
   - Swish between teeth with lips tightly closed for 60 seconds; expectorate.

B. High-Potency/Low-Frequency Prescription 0.20% NaF; 900 ppm (High Potency)

1. *Use:* Weekly rinse using 5 mL (younger children) or 10 mL (older children) swished for 60 seconds and expectorated.

2. *School group program*
   - The weekly rinse is the most common school-based program in the United States.
   - Advantages are that it requires little time (about 5 minutes once weekly for an entire class), is inexpensive, is easy to learn and is well accepted by participants, and can be carried out by nondental personnel.
   - School officials and a supervising dental hygienist can take responsibility for providing the correctly mixed 0.2% solution and for locking the fluoride in an inaccessible place.

IV. BENEFITS

Benefits from fluoride mouthrinsing have been documented many times since the original research using various percentages of various fluoride preparations.[40,41] Frequent rinsing with low concentrations of fluoride has the following effects:
- A 30% to 40% average reduction in the dental caries incidence.
- Greater benefit for smooth surfaces, but some benefit to pits and fissures.

▪ TABLE 33-4 SELF-APPLIED FLUORIDE MOUTHRINSES

	APF	NaF	SnF
Low potency/high frequency Once daily use	0.044% 440 ppm	0.05% 250 ppm	0.63% Dilute with water to 0.1% 250 ppm
High potency/low frequency Once weekly use		0.2% 900 ppm Used in school-based programs	

- Greatest benefit to newly erupted teeth (thus, the program should be continued through the teenage years to benefit the second and third permanent molars).
- Added benefits for a community with fluoridation.[42]
- Increase in posttreatment benefits as the length of time of rinsing increases.[43]
- Primary teeth present in school-aged children benefit by as much as a 42.5% average reduction in the dental caries incidence.[44]

■ BRUSH-ON GEL

Brush-on gel has been used as an adjunct to the daily application of fluoride in a dentifrice and as a supplement to periodic professional applications. Regular use has been shown to help control demineralization about orthodontic appliances[45] and to provide protection against postirradiation caries in conjunction with other fluoride applications.[46]

I. PREPARATIONS (TABLE 33-5)

A. Sodium fluoride (NaF) 1.1%, neutral pH (5000 ppm).

- Use as a dentifrice: 1.1% neutral NaF with an abrasive system added.
- The rationale for this product is to increase compliance with one step (brushing only) rather than brushing followed by application of the high-concentration gel with a toothbrush.

B. Stannous fluoride (SnF$_2$) 0.4% in glycerin base (1000 ppm)

II. PROCEDURE

- Teeth are cleaned first with thorough brushing and flossing before gel application with a separate toothbrush.
- Use once a day, preferably at night after toothbrushing and flossing.
- Place about 2 mg of the gel over the brush head and spread over all teeth.

■ TABLE 33-5 SELF-APPLIED FLUORIDE GELS: BRUSH-ON OR USE IN CUSTOM TRAYS	
NaF	SnF$_2$
1.1%	0.4%
5,000 ppm	1,000 ppm
Available by prescription only	Available OTC

- Brush 1 minute, then swish before expectorating.

■ FLUORIDE DENTIFRICES

I. DEVELOPMENT

- Historically tried with various compounds, including stannous fluoride, sodium fluoride, sodium monofluorophosphate, and amine fluoride.
- Early research objectives: to find compatible fluoride and abrasive systems and formulations containing available fluoride for uptake by the tooth surface.
- First fluoride dentifrice to gain approval by the American Dental Association, Council on Dental Therapeutics: 0.4% stannous fluoride.[47] A review by Stookey that describes the development of present formulations and the extensive research over past years is recommended for reading.[48]

II. INDICATIONS

A. Dental Caries Prevention

A fluoride dentifrice approved by the American Dental Association should be recommended for all adult patients as part of the complete preventive program.

B. All Patients Regardless of Their Caries Risk

- All patients (except for those under the age of 2 years) benefit from toothbrushing twice per day with a fluoridated toothpaste.
- Patients with moderate to rampant dental caries should be advised to brush several times each day with a fluoride-containing dentifrice.

C. Desensitization

Certain dentifrices containing fluoride also contain a desensitizing agent such as potassium nitrate. These are described on page 725.

III. PREPARATIONS

Fluoride dentifrices are available as gels or pastes. Sodium fluoride and sodium monofluorophosphate dentifrices are approved currently. Amine fluorides have not been developed and promoted in the United States.

A. Current Constituents

1. Sodium fluoride (NaF) 0.24% (1100 ppm).
2. Sodium monofluorophosphate (Na_2PO_3F) 0.76% (1000 ppm). An "extra-strength" Na_2PO_3F contains 1500 ppm.

B. Guidelines for Acceptance

The requirements for acceptance by the American Dental Association are described on page 449. The Seal of Acceptance is illustrated in Figure 27-3.

IV. PATIENT INSTRUCTION: RECOMMENDED PROCEDURES

Instruction in the selection of a dentifrice, the need for frequent use, the method for application to the tooth surfaces, and the effects of fluoride can help the patient appreciate the significant role of fluoride in oral health.

- Select an accepted fluoride-containing dentifrice.
- Place a small amount of dentifrice on the toothbrush.
  - *Toddler (age 2 years).* About one-half the size of a small pea or a tiny touch should be used and spread along the brushing plane as shown in Figure 46-7. The paste should then be spread over all the teeth before starting to brush so that all teeth benefit and large amounts are not available for swallowing.
  - *Older Child (ages 4 and 5 years).* Use only a small amount, the size of a small pea. Demonstrate spreading this amount over the ends of the filaments, and explain that the child should not swallow excess amounts of dentifrice.
  - *Adults.* Use 1/2 inch or less.
- Spread dentifrice over the teeth with a light touch of the brush.
- Proceed with correct brushing for sulcular removal of dental biofilm.
- Keep dentifrice container out of reach of children.

V. BENEFITS

- Dentifrices are used often, at least once or twice each day as recommended.
- Moderate and high caries-risk patients may use a dentifrice several times per day.
- The dentifrice is a continuing source of fluoride for the tooth surface in the control of demineralization and the promotion of remineralization.
- Fluoride is deposited in demineralized white spots, as shown in Figure 33-3.
- Many research studies have shown that the incidence of dental caries can be reduced 20% to 30% when NaF or Na_2PO_3F dentifrices are used regularly.

■ COMBINED FLUORIDE PROGRAM

Most patients can benefit from more than one method of use of fluorides, as listed in Table 33-6. When the preventive program is planned for an individual patient, the fluoride preparations and modes of application selected should provide the greatest possible protection against dental caries.

When self-administered methods are chosen, patient cooperation is a significant factor. Age and eruption pattern influence the method selected. Fluorides must be applied as soon after tooth eruption as possible and continued indefinitely to control demineralization.

Maintenance appointments can be scheduled for frequent topical applications and for continuing instruction and motivation. All methods are supplemented by the use of a dentifrice with fluoride.

■ FLUORIDE SAFETY

Fluoride preparations and fluoridated water have wide margins of safety. Fluoride is beneficial in small amounts, but it can be injurious if used without attention to

■ TABLE 33-6 RECOMMENDATIONS OF FLUORIDE THERAPIES BASED ON CARIES RISK ASSESSMENT

THERAPY	RECOMMENDATION
Use of fluoridated water 1 ppm fluoride	All patients regardless of caries risk assessment
Dentifrice 1,000–1,500 ppm fluoride	All patients regardless of caries risk assessment
Professional fluoride application 9,040–22,600 ppm fluoride	Moderate and high caries risk assessment
Daily low-potency rinses 250 ppm fluoride	Moderate caries risk assessment
Weekly high-potency rinses 900 ppm fluoride	Moderate to high caries risk assessment
Gels (brush-on or trays) 1,000–5,000 ppm fluoride	High caries risk assessment

correct dosage and frequency. All dental personnel should be familiar with recommended approved procedures, know potentials for toxic effects, and be prepared to administer emergency measures should accidental overdoses occur.

I. SUMMARY OF FLUORIDE MANAGEMENT

A. Use and recommend only approved fluoride preparations for patient use. Products have approval from the Food and Drug Administration and the American Dental Association in the United States.

B. Use only researched, recommended amounts and methods for delivery.

C. Know potential toxicity of the various products, and be prepared to administer emergency measures for treating an accidental toxic response.

D. Instruct patients in proper care of fluoride products.

1. Dentist prescribes no more than 264 mg of sodium fluoride at one time. Do not store large quantities in the home.

2. Request parental supervision of a child's brushing or other fluoride administration. Rinses, for example, are not to be used by children under 6 years of age.

3. Fluoride products should have child-proof covers and should be kept out of reach of small children and other persons, such as the mentally challenged, who may not understand limitations.

4. In school health programs, dispensing of the fluoride product must be supervised by responsible adults. Containers must be stored under lock and key when not in active use.

II. ACUTE TOXICITY

- *Acute* refers to rapid intake of an excess dose over a short time.
- *Chronic* applies to long-term ingestion of fluoride in amounts that exceed the approved therapeutic levels.
- *Accidental ingestion* of a concentrated fluoride preparation can lead to a toxic reaction.
- Acute fluoride poisoning is rare.[49]

A. Certainly Lethal Dose (CLD)[50]

A lethal dose is the amount of a drug likely to cause death if not intercepted by antidotal therapy.

1. *Adult CLD:* 5 to 10 g of sodium fluoride taken at one time. The fluoride ion equivalent is 32 to 64 mg of fluoride per kilogram body weight (mg F/kg; Box 33-5A).

2. *Child:* Approximately 0.5 to 1.0 g, variable with size and weight of the child.

B. Safely Tolerated Dose (STD): One Fourth of the CLD

1. *Adult STD:* 1.25 to 2.5 g of sodium fluoride (8 to 16 mg F/kg).

BOX 33-5 Lethal and Safe Doses of Fluoride

A. Lethal and safe dosages of fluoride for a 70-kg adult

Certainly Lethal Dose (CLD)

5–10 g NaF

or

32–64 mg F/kg

Safely Tolerated Dose (STD) = 1/4 CLD

1.25–2.5 g NaF

or

8–16 mg F/kg

B. CLDs and STDs of fluoride for selected ages

Age (years)	Weight (lbs)	CLD (mg)	STD (mg)
2	22	320	80
4	29	422	106
6	37	538	135
8	45	655	164
10	53	771	193
12	64	931	233
14	83	1,206	301
16	92	1,338	334
18	95	1,382	346

(From Heifetz, S.B. and Horowitz, H.S.: The Amounts of Fluoride in Current Fluoride Therapies: Safety Considerations for Children, *ASDC J. Dent. Child.*, 51, 257, July–August, 1984.)

2. *Child:* Box 33-5B shows STDs and CLDs for children.
   - Weights given for each selected age are minimal, and calculations for the doses are conservative.
   - As can be noted from the table, less than 1 g (1000 mg) may be fatal for children 12 years old and younger, and 0.5 g (500 mg) exceeds the STD for all ages shown.
   - For children under 6 years of age, however, 500 mg would be lethal.[50]

III. SIGNS AND SYMPTOMS OF ACUTE TOXIC DOSE

Symptoms begin within 30 minutes of ingestion and may persist for as long as 24 hours.

A. Gastrointestinal Tract

Fluoride in the stomach is acted on by the hydrochloric acid to form hydrofluoric acid, an irritant to the stomach lining. Symptoms include:
1. *Nausea, vomiting, diarrhea.*
2. *Abdominal pain.*
3. *Increased salivation, thirst.*

B. Systemic Involvements

1. *Blood.* Calcium may be bound by the circulating fluoride, thus causing symptoms of hypocalcemia.
2. *Central nervous system.* Hyperreflexia, convulsions, paresthesias.
3. *Cardiovascular and respiratory depression.* If not treated, may lead to death in a few hours from cardiac failure or respiratory paralysis.

IV. EMERGENCY TREATMENT

A. Induce Vomiting

1. *Mechanical.* Digital stimulation at back of tongue or in throat.
2. *Drug.* Ipecac syrup.

B. Second Person

Call emergency service; transport to hospital.

C. Administer Fluoride-Binding Liquid When Patient Is Not Vomiting

1. Milk.
2. Milk of Magnesium.
3. Lime water ($CaOH_2$ solution 0.15%).

D. Support Respiration and Circulation

E. Additional Therapy Indicated at Emergency Room

1. Calcium gluconate for muscle tremors or tetany.
2. Gastric lavage.
3. Cardiac monitoring.
4. Endotracheal intubation.
5. Blood monitoring (calcium, magnesium, potassium, pH).
6. Intravenous feeding to restore blood volume, calcium.

V. CHRONIC TOXICITY

A. Skeletal Fluorosis[49]

Isolated instances of osteosclerosis result from chronic toxicity after long-term (20 or more years) use of water with 10 to 25 ppm fluoride or from industrial exposure. Methods for defluoridation have been developed, as described on page 550.

B. Dental Fluorosis

- Naturally occurring excess fluoride in the drinking water can produce visible fluorosis only when used during the years of development of the crowns of the teeth, namely, from birth until age 12 or 16 years or when the crowns of the third permanent molars are completed.
- No systemic symptoms result from the fluoride, and the individual has protection against dental caries. A classification of fluorosis is found in Box 33-3.

C. Mild Fluorosis

1. *Clinical evaluation*
   - Mild and very mild forms, dental fluorosis appears as white opacities in the enamel surface.
   - No esthetic or health problem is involved. Many such white spots are not visible except when scrutinized under a dental light and the surface is dried.
   - All white spots in the enamel are not related to fluoride intake; distinction must be made by reviewing the patient's dental and fluoride-intake history, by noting the location and distribution of the white spots, and by considering the sequence of tooth development.
2. *Relation to fluoride sources*
   - Mild fluorosis or white spots may result from inadvertent ingestion of excess fluoride by

Everyday Ethics

Daniel was a 4 1/2-year-old boy who was extremely well-behaved and cooperative during his dental hygiene appointment with Nina. When it came time for the fluoride treatment, Nina spent a few extra minutes explaining what the foam would taste like in the "football mouthguard" as she called it. Although Daniel was borderline to receive topical fluoride in a tray because of his age, the hygienist decided it would be important for him, especially since he lived in a community without a fluoridated water supply. Seconds after placing the tray with the fluoride in Daniel's mouth, he gagged, spit out the tray, and vomited.

Questions for Consideration

1. Do you think the benefits of attempting the fluoride treatment outweighed the possible negative experience for Daniel? Why or why not?

2. His mom was upset when Daniel started crying and asked what prompted Nina to give her son the fluoride without permission. Explain the protocol for obtaining informed consent. Would it really be necessary in this situation? Why or why not?

3. What ethical principles support/do not support Nina's decision or course of action with Daniel?

young children during topical procedures both self-applied and professional. No problem exists when care is taken to follow basic steps, such as those listed in Table 33-3 for professional applications and those shown in Figure 46-7 for daily use of dentifrice the size of a small pea. Mouthrinses are not indicated for children under 6 years of age.

- Small amounts of dentifrice may be swallowed incidentally at each brushing. A child of 4 years who lives in a nonfluoridated community, uses a daily supplement (0.5 mg), and swallows two or three small amounts of dentifrice ingests far less than the STD of 106 mg shown in Box 33-5B.

VI. HOW TO CALCULATE AMOUNTS OF FLUORIDE[50-52]

Figure 33-6 is a flowchart that shows the steps necessary to determine the amount of fluoride in a fluoride compound. By doing so, one can then calculate the amount ingested by the patient.

- Multiply the percentage of fluoride ion in the compound by the molecular weight conversion ratio, as shown in Figure 33-6.
- Obtain the ratio by dividing the molecular weight of the compound by the atomic weight of fluoride.
- Example: The molecular weight of sodium fluoride is 42 (Na = 23, F = 19). When divided by 19, a 1 to 2.2 ratio results, as used in the example in Figure 33-6.

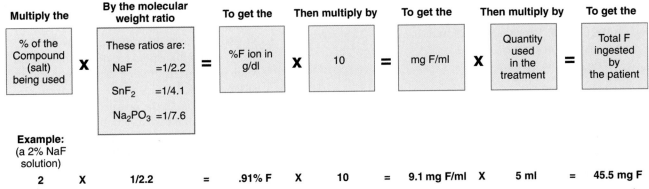

■ **FIGURE 33-6 Fluoride Calculation.** Flowchart shows steps in the calculation of the amount of fluoride in a compound used in treatment. The example shows that 5 mL of a 2% solution of NaF contains 45.5 mg F, an amount slightly greater than half of the safely tolerated dose (STD) for a 2-year-old child (Box 33-5B). (Data from Heifetz, S.B. and Horowitz, H.S.: The Amounts of Fluoride in Current Fluoride Therapies: Safety Considerations for Children, *ASDC J. Dent. Child., 51,* 257, July–August, 1984.)

✔ Factors To Teach The Patient

I. PERSONAL USE OF FLUORIDES

- Purposes, action, and expected benefits relative to the specific forms of fluoride treatment the patient will receive.

- Specific instruction concerning self-applied techniques that will be performed at home. Prepared printed instruction materials can be especially useful.

II. NEED FOR PARENTAL SUPERVISION

- Supervise daily care of child's teeth and mouth, including brushing of teeth using small, pea-sized quantity of dentifrice to prevent excess ingestion of fluoride.

- Keep fluoride products out of reach of small children.

- Brush teeth before using chewable dietary supplements. Avoid eating and drinking after use. Preferred time for use is just before going to bed.

III. DETERMINING NEED FOR FLUORIDE SUPPLEMENTS

- Reference to list of communities with fluoride in the drinking water at optimum level.

- Where to call to obtain information about fluoride in drinking water: health department, water department, or other community source.

- Where to send private water source sample for fluoride analysis.

IV. FLUORIDES ARE PART OF THE TOTAL PREVENTIVE PROGRAM

- Control of cariogenic foods in the diet, particularly between meals.

- Regular professional supervision and care.

V. FLUORIDATION

- In a nonfluoridated community, information concerning the significance of fluoridation.

- How drinking fluoridated water helps people of all ages.

VI. BOTTLED DRINKING WATER

- Use fluoridated water.

- When bottled water does not have a label indicating that it is fluoridated, how the water bottle can best be filled from a water supply that is fluoridated.

REFERENCES

1. **Ekstrand**, J.: Fluoride Metabolism, in Fejerskov, O., Ekstrand, J., and Burt, B.A., eds.: *Fluoride in Dentistry*, 2nd ed. Copenhagen, Munksgaard, 1996, pp. 55–67.

2. **Bhaskar**, S.N., ed.: *Orban's Oral Histology and Embryology*, 11th ed. St. Louis, Mosby, 1990, pp. 28–48, 75–105.

3. **Melfi**, R.C. and Alley, K.E.: *Permar's Oral Embryology and Microscopic Anatomy*, 10th ed. Philadelphia, Lippincott Williams & Wilkins, 2000, pp. 43–87.

4. **Yoon**, S.H., Brudevold, F., Gardner, D.E., and Smith, F.A.: Distribution of Fluoride in Teeth From Areas With Different Levels of Fluoride in the Water Supply, *J. Dent. Res., 39,* 845, July–August, 1960.

5. **Richards**, L.F., Westmoreland, W.W., Tashiro, M., McKay, C.H., and Morrison, J.T.: Determining Optimum Fluoride Levels for Community Water Supplies in Relation to Temperature, *J. Am. Dent. Assoc., 74,* 389, February, 1967.

6. **Herschfeld**, J.J.: Classics in Dental History: Frederick S. McKay and the "Colorado Brown Stain," *Bull. Hist. Dent., 26,* 118, October, 1978.

7. **McKay**, F.S.: The Relation of Mottled Enamel to Caries, *J. Am. Dent. Assoc., 15,* 1429, August, 1928.

8. **Churchill**, H.V.: Occurrence of Fluorides in Some Waters of United States, *J. Indust. Engin. Chem., 23,* 996, 1931.

9. **Dean**, H.T., Arnold, F.A., Jr., and Elvove, E.: Domestic Water and Dental Caries. V. Additional Studies of the Relation of Fluoride Domestic Waters to Dental Caries Experience in 4425 White Children, Aged 12 to 14 Years, of 13 Cities in 4 States, *Public Health Rep., 57,* 1155, August 7, 1942.

10. **Backer Dirks**, O., Houwink, B., and Kwant, G.W.: Some Special Features of the Caries Preventive Effect of Water Fluoridation, *Arch. Oral Biol., 4,* 187, August, 1961.

11. **Burt**, B.A., Ismail, A.I., and Eklund, S.A.: Root Caries in an Optimally Fluoridated and a High-fluoride Community, *J. Dent. Res., 65,* 1154, September, 1986.

12. **Stamm**, J.W., Banting, D.W., and Imrey, P.B.: Adult Root Caries Survey of Two Similar Communities With Contrasting Natural Water Fluoride Levels, *J. Am. Dent. Assoc., 120,* 143, February, 1990.

13. **Ast**, D.B. and Fitzgerald, B.: Effectiveness of Water Fluoridation, *J. Am. Dent. Assoc., 65,* 581, November, 1962.

14. **Russell**, A.L. and Elvove, E.: Domestic Water and Dental Caries. VII. A Study of the Fluoride-Dental Caries Relationship in an Adult Population, *Public Health Rep., 66,* 1389, October 26, 1951.

15. **Englander**, H.R. and Wallace, D.A.: Effects of Naturally Fluoridated Water on Dental Caries in Adults, *Public Health Rep., 77,* 887, October, 1962.

16. **Murray**, J.J., Rugg-Gunn, A.J., and Jenkins, G.N.: *Fluorides in Caries Prevention*, 3rd ed. Oxford, Wright, Butterworth-Heinemann, 1991, pp. 94–99.

17. **Horowitz**, H.S., Maier, F.J., and Law, F.E.: Partial Defluoridation of a Community Water Supply and Dental Fluorosis, *Public Health Rep., 82,* 965, November, 1967.

18. **Horowitz**, H.S. and Heifetz, S.B.: The Effect of Partial Defluoridation of a Water Supply on Dental Fluorosis—Final Results in Bartlett, Texas, After 17 Years, *Am. J. Public Health, 62,* 767, June 1972.

19. **Horowitz**, H.S.: Effectiveness of School Water Fluoridation and Dietary Fluoride Supplements in School-aged Children, *J. Public Health Dent., 49,* 290, Special Issue, 1989.

20. **United States Centers for Disease Control and Prevention:** Recommendations for Using Fluoride to Prevent and Control Dental Caries in the United States, *MMWR 50,* No. RR-14, 16, August 17, 2001.

21. **Lemke**, C.W., Doherty, J.M., and Arra, M.C.: Controlled Fluoridation: The Dental Effects of Discontinuation in Antigo, Wisconsin, *J. Am. Dent. Assoc., 80,* 782, April, 1970.

22. **Jackson**, R.D., Brizendine, E.J., Kelly, S.A., Hinesley, R., Stookey, G.K., and Dunipace, A.J.: The Fluoride Content of Foods and Beverages From Negligibly and Optimally Fluoridated Communities, *Community Dent. Oral Epidemiol., 30,* 382, October, 2002.

23. **Burt**, B.A. and Marthaler, T.M.: Fluoride Tablets, Salt Fluoridation, and Milk Fluoridation, in Fejerskov, O., Ekstrand, J., and Burt, B.A., eds.: *Fluoride in Dentistry,* 2nd ed. Copenhagen, Munksgaard, 1996, pp. 291–310.

24. **Toyama**, Y., Nakagaki H., Kato, S., Huang S., Mizutani, Y., Kojima, S., Toyama, A., Ohno N., Tsuchiya, T., Kirkham, J., and Robinson, C.: Fluoride Concentrations at and Near the Neonatal Line in Human Deciduous Tooth Enamel Obtained From a Naturally Fluoridated and a Non-fluoridated Area, *Arch. Oral Biol., 46,* 147, February, 2001.

25. **Burrell**, K.H. and Chan, J.T.: Systemic and Topical Fluorides, in American Dental Association, Council on Scientific Affairs: *ADA Guide to Dental Therapeutics,* 2nd ed. Chicago, ADA Publishing Co., 2000, p. 231.

26. **Bibby**, B.G.: Use of Fluorine in the Prevention of Dental Caries. II. The Effects of Sodium Fluoride Applications, *J. Am. Dent. Assoc., 31,* 317, March 1, 1944.

27. **Knutson**, J.W.: Sodium Fluoride Solutions: Technique for Application to the Teeth, *J. Am. Dent. Assoc., 36,* 37, January, 1948.

28. **Galagan**, D.J. and Knutson, J.W.: The Effect of Topically Applied Fluorides on Dental Caries Experience. VI. Experiments With Sodium Fluoride and Calcium Chloride . . . Widely Spaced Applications . . . Use of Different Solution Concentrations, *Public Health Rep., 63,* 1215, September 17, 1948.

29. **Warren**, D.P. and Chan, J.T.: Topical Fluorides: Efficacy, Administration, and Safety, *Gen. Dent., 45,* 134, March–April, 1997.

30. **Soeno**, K., Matsumura, H., Atsuta, M., and Kawasaki, K.: Influence of Acidulated Fluoride Agents and Effectiveness of Subsequent Polishing on Composite Material Surfaces, *Oper. Dent., 27,* 305, May–June, 2002.

31. **Ripa**, L.W.: Need for Prior Toothcleaning When Performing a Professional Topical Fluoride Application: Review and Recommendations for Change, *J. Am. Dent. Assoc., 109,* 281, August, 1984.

32. **Vrbic**, V., Brudevold, F., and McCann, H.G.: Acquisition of Fluoride by Enamel From Fluoride Pumice Pastes, *Helv. Odontol. Acta., 11,* 21, April, 1967.

33. **Stookey**, G.K., Schemehorn, B.R., Drook, C.A., and Cheetham, B.L.: The Effect of Rinsing With Water Immediately After a Professional Fluoride Gel Application on Fluoride Uptake in Demineralized Enamel: An *In Vivo* Study, *Pediatr. Dent., 8,* 153, June, 1986.

34. **Strohmenger**, L. and Brambilla, E.: The Use of Fluoride Varnishes in the Prevention of Dental Caries: A Short Review, *Oral Diseases, 7,* 71, March, 2001.

35. **Shen**, C. and Autio-Gold, J.: Assessing Fluoride Concentration Uniformity and Fluoride Release From Three Varnishes, *J. Am. Dent. Assoc., 133,* 176, February, 2002.

36. **Englander**, H.R., Keyes, P.H., and Gestwicki, M.: Clinical Anticaries Effect of Repeated Topical Sodium Fluoride Applications by Mouthpieces, *J. Am. Dent. Assoc., 75,* 638, September, 1967.

37. **Burrell** and Chan: op. cit., pp. 236–241.

38. **American Dental Association,** Council on Dental Materials, Instruments, and Equipment and Council on Dental Therapeutics: Status Report: Effect of Acidulated Phosphate Fluoride on Porcelain and Composite Restorations, *J. Am. Dent. Assoc., 116,* 115, January, 1988.

39. **Ripa**, L.W.: Fluoride Rinsing: What Dentists Should Know, *J. Am. Dent. Assoc., 102,* 477, April, 1981.

40. **Torell**, P. and Ericsson, Y.: The Potential Benefits Derived From Fluoride Mouth Rinses, in Forrester, D.J. and Schulz, E.M., eds.: *International Workshop on Fluorides and Dental Caries Reductions.* Baltimore, University of Maryland School of Dentistry, 1974, pp. 114–176.

41. **Birkeland**, J.M. and Torell, P.: Caries-Preventive Fluoride Mouthrinses, *Caries Res., 12,* 38, Supplement 1, 1978.

42. **Driscoll**, W.S., Swango, P.A., Horowitz, A.M., and Kingman, A.: Caries-Preventive Effects of Daily and Weekly Fluoride Mouthrinsing in a Fluoridated Community: Final Results After 30 Months, *J. Am. Dent. Assoc., 105,* 1010, December, 1982.

43. **Leske**, G.S., Ripa, L.W., and Green, E.: Posttreatment Benefits in a School-Based Fluoride Mouthrinsing Program: Final Results After 7 Years of Rinsing by All Participants, *Clin. Prev. Dent., 8,* 19, September–October, 1986.

44. **Ripa**, L.W., Leske, G.S., and Varma, A.: Effect of Mouthrinsing With a 0.2 Percent Neutral NaF Solution on the Deciduous Dentition of First to Third Grade School Children, *Pediatr. Dent., 6,* 93, June, 1984.

45. **Stratemann**, M.W. and Shannon, I.L.: Control of Decalcification in Orthodontic Patients by Daily Self-administrated Application of a Water-free 0.4 Per Cent Stannous Fluoride Gel, *Am. J. Orthod., 66,* 273, September, 1974.

46. **Wescott**, W.B., Starcke, E.N., and Shannon, I.L.: Chemical Protection Against Postirradiation Dental Caries, *Oral Surg. Oral Med. Oral Pathol., 40,* 709, December, 1975.

47. **American Dental Association,** Council on Dental Therapeutics: Evaluation of Crest Toothpaste, *J. Am. Dent. Assoc., 61,* 272, August, 1960.

48. **Stookey**, G.K.: Are All Fluoride Dentifrices the Same? in Wei, S.H.Y., ed.: *Clinical Uses of Fluorides.* Philadelphia, Lea & Febiger, 1985, pp. 105–131.

49. **Hodge**, H.C. and Smith, F.A.: Fluoride Toxicology, in Newbrun, E., ed.: *Fluorides and Dental Caries,* 3rd ed. Springfield, IL, Charles C Thomas, 1986, pp. 199–220.

50. **Heifetz**, S.B. and Horowitz, H.S.: The Amounts of Fluoride in Current Fluoride Therapies: Safety Considerations for Children, *ASDC J. Dent. Child., 51,* 257, July–August, 1984.

51. **Bayless**, J.M. and Tinanoff, N.: Diagnosis and Treatment of Acute Fluoride Toxicity, *J. Am. Dent. Assoc., 110,* 209, February, 1985.

52. **Lyon**, T.C.: Topical Fluorides: How Much Are You Using? *Dent. Hyg., 59,* 58, February, 1985.

SUGGESTED READINGS

Cirincione, U.K.: The Safe Use of Fluorides in Dental Hygiene Practice, *J. Dent. Hyg., 66,* 319, September, 1992.

Clarkson, J.J.: International Collaborative Research on Fluoride, *J. Dent. Res., 79,* 893, April, 2000.

Featherstone, J.D.B.: Prevention and Reversal of Dental Caries: Role of Low Level Fluoride, *Community Dent. Oral Epidemiol., 27,* 31, February, 1999.

Levy, S.M., Kiritsy, M.C., and Warren, J.J.: Sources of Fluoride Intake in Children, *J. Public Health Dent., 55,* 39, Winter, 1995.

Fluoridation

Burt, B.A., Keels, M.A., and Heller, K.E.: The Effects of a Break in Water Fluoridation on the Development of Dental Caries and Fluorosis, *J. Dent. Res., 79,* 761, February, 2000.

Edelstein, B.L., Cottrel, D., O'Sullivan, D., and Tinanoff, N.: Comparison of Colorimeter and Electrode Analysis of Water Fluoride, *Pediatr. Dent., 14,* 47, January/February, 1992.

Grembowski, D., Fiset, L., and Spadafora, A.: How Fluoridation Affects Adult Dental Caries: Systemic and Topical Effects Are Explored, *J. Am. Dent. Assoc., 123,* 49, February, 1992.

Hayward, K.: Promotion of Water Fluoridation, *Contemporary Oral Hyg., 2,* 36, January/February, 2002.

Heilman, J.R., Kiritsy, M.C., Levy, S.M., and Wefel, J.S.: Assessing Fluoride Levels of Carbonated Soft Drinks, *J. Am.. Dent. Assoc., 130,* 1593, November, 1999.

Horowitz, H.S.: Grand Rapids: The Public Health Story, *J. Public Health Dent., 49,* 62, Winter, 1989.

Horowitz, H.S.: The Effectiveness of Community Water Fluoridation in the United States, *J. Public Health Dent., 56,* 253, Special Issue, 1996.

Ong, Y.S., Williams, B., and Holt, R.: The Effect of Domestic Water Filters on Water Fluoride Content, *Br. Dent. J., 181,* 59, July 20, 1996.

Supplements

British Dental Association, the British Society of Paediatric Dentistry and the British Association for the Study of Community Dentistry: Fluoride Supplement Dosage, *Br. Dent. J., 182,* 6, January 11, 1997.

Ismail, A.I.: Fluoride Supplements: Current Effectiveness, Side Effects, and Recommendations, *Community Dent. Oral Epidemiol., 22,* 164, June, 1994.

Johnson, S.A. and DeBiase, C.: Concentration Levels of Fluoride in Bottled Drinking Water, *J. Dent. Hyg., 77,* 161, Summer, 2003.

Stannard, J., Rovero, J., Tsamtsouris, A., and Gavris, V.: Fluoride Content of Some Bottled Waters and Recommendations for Fluoride Supplementation, *J. Pedod., 14,* 103, Number 2, 1990.

Toumba, K.J., Levy, S., and Curzon, M.E.J.: The Fluoride Content of Bottled Drinking Water, *Br. Dent. J., 176,* 266, April 9, 1994.

Dental Fluorosis

Bowen, W.H.: Fluorosis. Is it Really a Problem?, *J. Am. Dent. Assoc., 133,* 1405, October 2002.

Driscoll, W.S., Horowitz, H.S., Meyers, R.J., Heifetz, S.B., Kingman, A., and Zimmerman, E.R.: Prevalence of Dental Caries and Dental Fluorosis in Areas With Negligible, Optimal, and Above-Optimal Fluoride Concentrations in Drinking Water, *J. Am. Dent. Assoc., 113,* 29, July, 1986.

Lalumandier, J.A. and Rozier, R.G.: Parents' Satisfaction With Children's Tooth Color: Fluorosis as a Contributing Factor, *J. Am. Dent. Assoc., 129,* 1000, July, 1998.

Lewis, D.W. and Banting, D.W.: Water Fluoridation: Current Effectiveness and Dental Fluorosis, *Community Dent. Oral Epidemiol., 22,* 153, June, 1994.

Nowjack-Raymer, R.E., Selwitz, R.H., Kingman, A., and Driscoll, W.S.: The Prevalence of Dental Fluorosis in a School-Based Program of Mouthrinsing, Fluoride Tablets, and Both Procedures Combined, *J. Public Health Dent., 55,* 165, Summer, 1995.

Pendrys, D.G.: Risk of Enamel Fluorosis in Nonfluoridated and Optimally Fluoridated Populations: Considerations for the Dental Professional, *J. Am. Dent. Assoc., 131,* 746, June, 2000.

Skotowski, M.C., Hunt, R.J., and Levy, S.M.: Risk Factors for Dental Fluorosis in Pediatric Dental Patients, *J. Public Health Dent., 55,* 154, Summer, 1995.

Stookey, G.K.: Review of Fluorosis Risk of Self-applied Topical Fluorides: Dentifrices, Mouthrinses and Gels, *Community Dent. Oral Epidemiol., 22,* 181, June, 1994.

Topical Fluorides

American Dental Association Division of Science: Topical Fluoride for Office Use, *J. Am. Dent. Assoc., 133,* 502, April 2002.

Heath, K., Singh, V., Logan, R., and McIntyre, J.: Analysis of Fluoride Levels Retained Intraorally or Ingested Following Routine Clinical Applications of Topical Fluoride Products, *Aust. Dent. J. 46,* 24, March, 2001.

Lavigne, S.: Not All Trays Are Created Equal: An Analysis of Fluoride Tray Fit, *J. Can. Dent. Hyg. Assoc. (Probe), 34,* 217, November/December, 2000.

Pimlott, J.: Professionally Applied Topical Fluorides: Providing Optimal Patient Care Using an Evidence-Based Approach, *J. Can. Dent. Hyg. Assoc. (Probe), 33,* 175, November–December, 1999.

Ripa, L.W.: A Critique of Topical Fluoride Methods (Dentifrices, Mouthrinses, Operator-, and Self-applied Gels) in an Era of Decreased Caries and Increased Fluorosis Prevalence, *J. Public Health Dent., 51,* 23, Winter, 1991.

Ripa, L.W.: Review of the Anticaries Effectiveness of Professionally Applied and Self-applied Topical Fluoride Gels, *J. Public Health Dent., 49,* 297, Special Issue, 1989.

Van Horn, R.: A Review of Professional and Home Fluorides, *J. Pract. Hyg., 9,* 30, March/April, 2000.

Van Horn, R.: Fluoride Therapy—Not Just for Kids, *J. Pract. Hyg., 9,* 51, May/June, 2000.

Warren, D.P., Henson, H.A., and Chan, J.T.: Dental Hygienist and Patient Comparisons of Fluoride Varnishes to Fluoride Gels, *J. Dent. Hyg., 74,* 94, Spring, 2000.

Wei, S.H.Y. and Chik, F.F.: Fluoride Retention Following Topical Fluoride Foam and Gel Application, *Pediatr. Dent., 12,* 368, November/December, 1990.

Varnish

Arends, J., Duschner, H., and Ruben, J.L.: Penetration of Varnishes into Demineralized Root Dentine *in vitro, Caries Res., 31,* 201, May–June, 1997.

Bravo, M., Baca, P., Llodra, J.C., and Osorio, E.: A 24-month Study Comparing Sealant and Fluoride Varnish in Caries Reduction on Different Permanent First Molar Surfaces, *J. Public Health Dent., 57,* 184, Summer, 1997.

Mandel, I.D.: Guest Editorial: Fluoride Varnishes—A Welcome Addition, *J. Public Health Dent., 54,* 67, Spring, 1994.

Seppä, L., Leppänen, T., and Hausen, H.: Fluoride Varnish Versus Acidulated Phosphate Fluoride Gel: A 3-Year Clinical Trial, *Caries Res., 29,* 327, September–October, 1995.

Dentifrices

Davies, R.M., Ellwood, R.P., and Davies, G.M.: The Rational Use of Fluoride Toothpaste, *Int. J. Dent. Hyg., 1,* 3, February, 2003.

Horowitz, H.S.: The Need for Toothpastes With Lower Than Conventional Fluoride Concentrations for Preschool-Aged Children, *J. Public Health Dent., 52,* 216, Summer, 1992.

Levy, S.M.: A Review of Fluoride Intake From Fluoride Dentifrice, *ASDC J. Dent. Child., 60,* 115, March–April, 1993.

Rolla, G., Øgaard, B., and deAlmeida Cruz, R.: Clinical Effect and Mechanism of Cariostatic Action of Fluoride-Containing Toothpastes: A Review, *Int. Dent. J., 41,* 171, June, 1991.

Triratana, R., Rustogi, K.N., Volpe, A.R., DeVizio, W., Petrone, M., and Giniger, M: Clinical Effect of a New Liquid Dentifrice Containing Triclosan/Copolymer and Existing Plaque and Gingivitis, *J. Am. Dent. Assoc., 133,* 219, February, 2002.

Warren, J.J. and Levy, S.M.: A Review of Fluoride Dentifrice Related to Dental Fluorosis, *Pediatr. Dent., 21,* 265, July/August, 1999.

Periodontal Relationship

Grembowski, D., Fiset, L., Spadafora, A., and Milgrom, P.: Fluoridation Effects on Periodontal Disease Among Adults, *J. Periodont. Res., 28,* 166, May, 1993.

Paine, M.L., Slots, J., and Rich, S.K.: Fluoride Use in Periodontal Therapy: A Review of the Literature, *J. Am. Dent. Assoc., 129,* 69, January, 1998.

Ravald, N. and Birkhed, D.: Factors Associated With Active and Inactive Root Caries in Patients With Periodontal Disease, *Caries Res., 25,* 377, September–October, 1991.

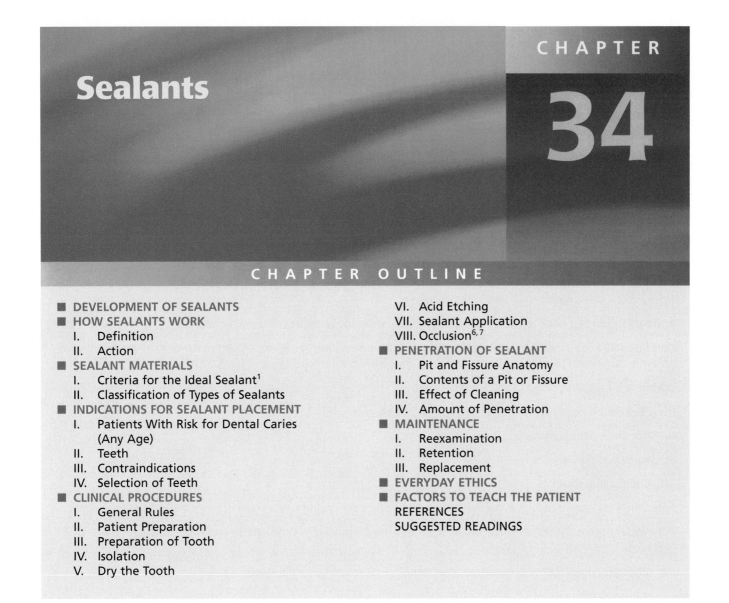

Sealants

CHAPTER 34

CHAPTER OUTLINE

As part of a complete preventive program, pit and fissure sealants are indicated for selected patients. Because topically or systemically applied fluorides protect smooth tooth surfaces more than occlusal surfaces, a method to reduce the incidence of occlusal dental caries is needed. The incidence of new pit and fissure caries can be lowered significantly by the application of adhesive sealants. Box 34-1 provides definitions and terminology relative to sealants and their application.

Other preventive measures used for and by the patient are necessary. Sealant application should be part of a complete prevention program, not an isolated procedure. As an isolated procedure, patient (and parent) may misunderstand the selected area of prevention that this measure represents. Other surfaces and other teeth still need other methods of preventive protection.

■ DEVELOPMENT OF SEALANTS

Sealants were developed by Dr. Michael Buonocore and the group of dental scientists at the Eastman Dental Center in Rochester, New York. The focus of the early research was on the need to prepare the enamel surface so that a dental material would adhere. They demonstrated that by using an acid etch process, the enamel could be altered to increase retention. The research proved to be a major breakthrough, particularly in esthetic and preventive dentistry.[1,2]

BOX 34-1 KEY WORDS AND ABBREVIATIONS: Pit and Fissure Sealants

Acid etchant: in sealant placement, the enamel surface is prepared by the application of phosphoric acid, which etches the surface to provide mechanical retention for the sealant.

Articulating paper: an inked ribbon held between teeth to determine tooth contacts.

Bibulous: absorbent; a flat bibulous pad, placed in the cheek over the opening of Stensen's duct, is used to aid in maintaining a dry field while placing sealants.

Biocompatibility: the ability of things to exist together without harm.

Bis-GMA: bisphenol A-glycidyl methylacrylate; plastic material used for dental sealants.

Bonding (mechanical): physical adherence of one substance to another; the adherence of a sealant to the enamel surface is accomplished by an acid-etching technique that leaves microspaces between the enamel rods; the sealant becomes mechanically locked (bonded) in these microspaces.

Bond strength: expression of the degree of adherence between the tooth surface and the sealant.

Conditioner: a substance added to another substance to increase its usability; in sealant placement, the acid etchant is added to the enamel to prepare it for bonding with the sealant.

Curing: the process by which plastic becomes rigid.

Incipient caries: beginning caries, caries limited to the enamel.

In vitro: under laboratory conditions.

In vivo: within the living body.

Micropores: tiny openings.

Polymer: a compound of high molecular weight formed by a combination of a chain of simpler molecules (monomers).

Polymerization: a reaction in which a high-molecular-weight product is produced by successive additions of a simpler compound.

    Photopolymerization: polymerization with the use of an external light source.

    Autopolymerization: self-curing; a reaction in which a high-molecular-weight product is produced by successive additions of a simpler compound; hardening process of pit and fissure sealants.

Sealant: organic polymer that bonds to an enamel surface by mechanical retention accommodated by projections of the sealant into micropores created in the enamel by etching; the two types of sealants, filled and unfilled, both are composed of Bis-GMA.

    Filled sealant: contains, in addition to Bis-GMA, microparticles of glass, quartz, silica, and other fillers used in composite restorations; fillers make the sealant more resistant to abrasion.

Viscosity: in general, the resistance to flow or alteration of shape by any substance as a result of molecular cohesion.

■ HOW SEALANTS WORK

I. DEFINITION

A pit and fissure sealant is an organic polymer (resin) that flows into the pit or fissure and bonds to the enamel surface mainly by mechanical retention.

II. ACTION

A. Purpose of the Sealant

1. To provide a physical barrier to "seal off" the pit or fissure.
2. To prevent oral bacteria and their nutrients from collecting within the pit or fissure to create the

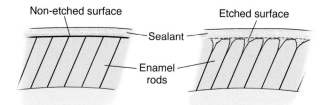

Non-etched surface   Etched surface

Sealant

Enamel rods

■ **FIGURE 34-1 Enamel–Sealant Interface.** Diagram of enamel–sealant interface to compare nonetched surface with etched surface. Etching produces microscopic porosities in the enamel to increase the area of retention. The unpolymerized resin flows into the porosities and hardens in tag-like projections, as shown on the right. (Adapted from Buonocore, M.G., Matsui, A., and Gwinnett, A.J.: Penetration of Resin Dental Materials Into Enamel Surfaces With Reference to Bonding, *Arch. Oral Biol., 13,* 61, 1968.)

acid environment necessary for the initiation of dental caries.

3. To fill the pit or fissure as deep as possible. When sealant material is worn or cracked away on the surface around the pit or fissure, the sealant in the depth of the micropore can remain and provide continued protection.

B. Purpose of the Acid Etch

1. To produce irregularities or micropores in the enamel.
2. To allow the liquid resin to penetrate into the micropores and create a bond or mechanical locking. Figure 34-1 illustrates the sealant placed on a smooth enamel surface in contrast with placement on an etched surface with retention.

■ SEALANT MATERIALS

I. CRITERIA FOR THE IDEAL SEALANT[1]

A. Achieve prolonged bonding to enamel.
B. Be biocompatible with oral tissues.
C. Offer a simple application procedure.
D. Be a free-flowing, low-viscosity material capable of entering narrow fissures.
E. Have low solubility in the oral environment.

II. CLASSIFICATION OF TYPES OF SEALANTS

A majority of sealants in clinical use are made of Bis-GMA (bisphenol A–glycidyl methylacrylate). The techniques of application vary slightly among available products.

The American Dental Association has a program for evaluation and acceptance of pit and fissure sealants.[3] The three types of sealants currently available are filled,

unfilled, and fluoride-releasing filled. Sealants are also identified by the method required for polymerization.

A. Classification by Method of Polymerization

1. *Self-cured or Autopolymerized*
   a. Preparation: the material is supplied in two parts. When the two are mixed they quickly polymerize (harden).
   b. Advantages: no special equipment required.
   c. Disadvantages: mixing required; working time limited because polymerization begins when the material is mixed.
2. *Visible-Light–Cured or Photopolymerized*
   a. Preparation: the material hardens when exposed to a special curing light.
   b. Advantages: no mixing required; increased working time due to control over start of polymerization.
   c. Disadvantages: extra costs and disinfection time required for curing light, protective shields, and/or glasses.

B. Classification by Filler Content

1. *Filled*
   a. Purpose of filler: to increase abrasion resistance, bond strength, and wear.
   b. Fillers: glass and quartz particles.
   c. Effect: viscosity of the sealant is increased. Flow into the depth of a fissure varies.
2. *Unfilled*
3. *Fluoride-Releasing*
   a. Purpose: enhance caries resistance.
   b. Action: remineralization of incipient caries at base of pit or fissure.

D. Classification by Color

1. Available: clear, tinted, and opaque.
2. Purpose: quick identification for evaluation during maintenance assessment.
3. Effect: clear, tinted, or opaque sealants do not differ in retention.

■ INDICATIONS FOR SEALANT PLACEMENT

I. PATIENTS WITH RISK FOR DENTAL CARIES (ANY AGE)

A. Xerostomia: from medications or other reasons.
B. Patient undergoing orthodontics.
C. Incipient caries: when the caries is limited to the enamel.

II. TEETH

A. Newly erupted: as soon after eruption as possible.
B. Occlusal contour: when pit or fissure is deep and irregular.
C. Caries history: other teeth restored or have carious lesions.

III. CONTRAINDICATIONS

A. Radiographic evidence of proximal dental caries.
B. Pit and fissures are well coalesced and self-cleansing; low caries risk.

IV. SELECTION OF TEETH

Figure 34-2 is a flowchart to assist in decision making.

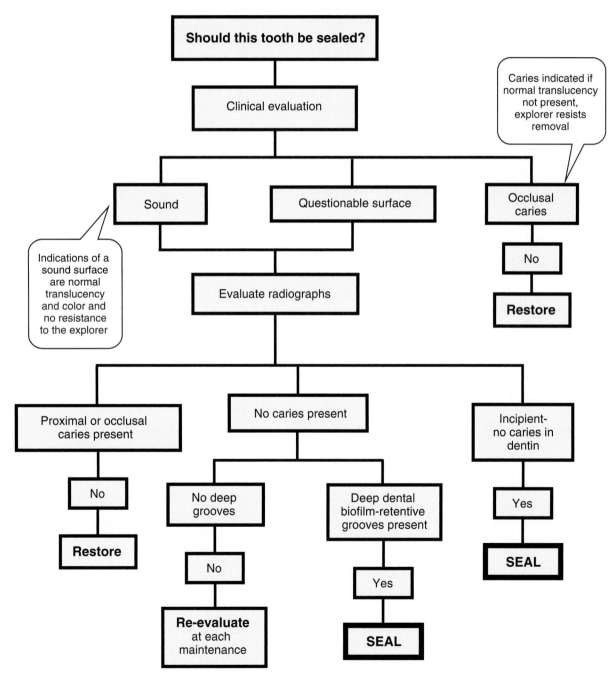

■ **FIGURE 34-2 Tooth Selection for Sealant Placement.** Flow chart to assist in decision making for placement of sealants.

▪ CLINICAL PROCEDURES

I. GENERAL RULES

A. Treat each quadrant separately.

B. Use four-handed method with assistant
1. To ensure moisture control.
2. To work efficiently and save time.

C. Follow manufacturer's directions for each product.

D. Success of treatment (retention) depends on the precision in each step of the application.

E. Retention of sealant depends on maintaining a dry field during etching and sealant placement.

F. Steps in procedure: follow the outline in Table 34-1.

▪ TABLE 34-1 SEALANT APPLICATION PROCEDURES

PROCEDURE: WHAT TO DO	INSTRUMENTS AND EQUIPMENT: WHAT IS NEEDED
Preparation • Set up tray • Seat patient comfortably • **Debride** occlusal surface • Use toothbrush, air-powder polisher device or prophy brush and pumice • **Rinse** for 20 to 30 seconds • **Evaluate** teeth to be sealed clinically (Figure 34-2)	• Safety glasses for the patient • Prophy angle and brushes, toothbrush, or an air-powder polishing unit • Mirror, explorer, and cotton pliers
Etching • **Isolate** area • **Dry** area for 20 to 30 seconds with tri-syringe • **Etch** for 30 to 60 seconds • Gel: brush on surface and leave in contact without disturbing it • Liquid: cover surface and continue to keep surface wet by adding • *Do not rub* • **Rinse** until surface is free of etch • Gel: 60 seconds • Liquid: 30 seconds • **Re-isolate** area • **Dry** for 20 seconds and check for chalky appearance • *If not chalky, re-etch*	• Isolation materials: Rubber dam setup or Cotton rolls and Garmer holders, bibulous pads • Brushes or cotton pellets to dispense etch • Acid etch material (15%–50%) phosphoric acid additional etch throughout etch time • Tri-syringe • High-speed suction • Saliva ejector
Application • **Apply** sealant material • Mix autopolymerized sealant material prior to placement • Light cured needs no mixing • **Cure** while maintaining a dry field	• Sealant material • Brushes or flow tubes or cannulas to dispense sealant material • Mixing sticks (if using self-cured) • Material tray or waxed paper pad • Ultraviolet safety glasses or shield for clinician • Timer or watch with a second hand
Evaluation • Evaluate the placed sealant for voids and air bubbles • Add additional sealant if necessary • Re-etch prior to placement of material if salivary contamination occurs • Check occlusion with articulating paper, adjust if sealant interferes with occlusion • Floss contact areas	• Articulation paper • Dental floss
Follow-up • Educate the patient • Administer fluoride treatment • Re-evaluate at each subsequent appointment	• Fluoride gel and trays

II. PATIENT PREPARATION

- Explain the procedure and steps to be performed.
- The patient must wear safety eyewear for both protection from the chemicals of etching and sealant, but also from the light of the curing lamp.

III. PREPARATION OF TOOTH

A. Purposes

1. Remove deposits and debris.
2. Permit maximum contact of the etch and the sealant with the enamel surface.
3. Encourage sealant penetration into the pit or fissure.

B. Examine the Surfaces: Remove calculus and heavy stains.

C. Patient With No Stain or Calculus

1. Request patient to brush; apply filaments straight into occlusal pits and fissures (see Figure 25-14A).
2. Suction the pits and fissures with high-velocity evacuator.
3. Use sharp explorer tip to dig out debris and bacteria from the pit or fissure.
4. Suction again to remove loosened material.
5. Evaluate for additional cleaning; the brushing may be sufficient.

D. Cleansing Procedure: Choices:

1. Polishing cup and brush with pumice; low-speed handpiece
   a. Disadvantage: pumice particles become lodged in the pits and not rinsed out.
   b. Alternative: use bristle brush with clear water.
2. Air-powder polisher[4,5]

IV. ISOLATION

A. Purposes of Isolation

1. Keep the tooth clean and dry for optimal action and bonding of the sealant.
2. Eliminate possible contamination by saliva and moisture from the breath.
3. Keep the materials from contacting the oral tissues, being swallowed accidentally, or being unpleasant to the patient because of flavor.

B. Rubber Dam

1. Rubber dam application is the method of choice because the most complete isolation is obtained. This method is especially helpful when more than one tooth must be sealed.
2. Rubber dam is essential when profuse saliva flow and overactive tongue and oral muscles make retraction and consistent maintenance of a dry, clean field impossible.
3. Combined treatment should be planned. When a quadrant has a rubber dam and anesthesia for restoration of other teeth, teeth indicated for sealant may be treated.
4. Use anesthesia when application of the clamp cannot be tolerated by the patient.
5. Rubber dam may not be possible when a tooth that is essential for holding the clamp is not fully erupted.

C. Cotton-Roll Isolation

1. Patient position: tilt head to allow saliva to pool on the opposite side of the mouth.
2. Position cotton-roll holder (Garmer holder, Figure 34-3).

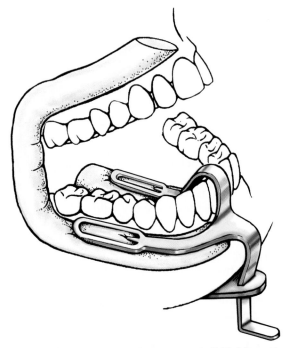

■ **FIGURE 34-3 Isolation Using Cotton-Roll Holders.** One half of the teeth are treated simultaneously. A continuous cotton roll extends from the mandibular anterior vestibule to the maxillary anterior vestibule. Bevel end of cotton rolls to facilitate retention. Lingual prong holds cotton roll adjacent to tongue over floor of the mouth.

3. Place saliva ejector.
4. Apply triangular saliva absorber over the opening of the parotid duct in the cheek (bibulous pad).
5. Take great care to prevent contamination from entering the area to be etched.

V. DRY THE TOOTH

A. Purposes

1. Prepare the tooth for acid etch.
2. Eliminate moisture and contamination.

B. Use Clean Air

1. Clear the air by releasing the spray into a sink.
2. Test for absence of moisture by blowing on a mirror or other dry surface.

C. Time: Air dry the tooth for at least 10 seconds.

VI. ACID ETCHING

A. Action

1. Create micropores to increase the surface area and provide retention for the sealant.
2. Remove contamination from enamel surface.
3. Provide antibacterial action.

B. Etch Forms

1. *Phosphoric acid:* 15% to 50%, depends on product and manufacturer.
2. *Liquid:* Low viscosity allows good flow into pit or fissure but may be difficult to control.
3. *Gel:* Tinted gel with thick consistency allows increased visibility and control but may be difficult to rinse off the tooth surface.
4. *Semi-gel:* Tinted, with viscosity between the gel form and the liquid allows good visibility, control, and rinsing ease.

C. Etch Timing: varies from 15 to 60 seconds. Follow manufacturer's instructions for each product.

D. Etch Delivery

1. Liquid etch
   a. Use a small brush, sponge, or cotton pellet.
   b. Apply continuously throughout the etch time to keep the surface moist.
2. Gel and semi-gel: use a syringe, brush, or manufacturer-supplied single-use cannula.

E. Completion of Etching

1. Rinse thoroughly; apply suction to prevent saliva from reaching the etched surface.
2. Dry, and examine the etched surface.
3. Repeat etching process if the surface does not appear white and chalky.
4. Dry for 15 to 20 seconds; maintain isolation ready for sealant application.

VII. SEALANT APPLICATION

A. Follow Manufacturer's Instructions

B. General Instructions

1. Avoid overmanipulation to prevent producing air bubbles.
2. Use disposable implement supplied.
3. Cover all pits and fissures but do not overfill to a high, flat surface.
4. After placement: leave in place for 10 seconds to allow for optimum penetration.

C. Curing

1. *Timing:* 20 to 30 seconds in accord with manufacturer's instructions. Longer curing time is related to increased retention.
2. *Apply curing light:* Use eye protection. Cover entire tooth surface to allow complete polymerization.
3. *Check for voids:* Material can be added if surface has not been contaminated or wet.

VIII. OCCLUSION[6,7]

A. Use articulating paper to locate high spots; adjust as required.
B. Occlusal wear: unfilled sealants wear down to correct height; filled sealants require occlusal adjustment.

■ PENETRATION OF SEALANT

The penetration of a sealant depends on the configuration of the pit or fissure, the presence of deposits and debris within the pit or fissure, and the properties of the sealant itself.

I. PIT AND FISSURE ANATOMY

A review of the anatomy of pits and fissures may be helpful in understanding the effects of sealants in the prevention of dental caries. The shape and depth of pits and fissures vary considerably even within one tooth.

Long narrow pits and grooves reach to, or nearly to, the dentinoenamel junction. Others are *wide V-shaped* or *narrow V-shaped,* whereas still others may have a *long constricted form with a bulbous terminal portion* (Figure 34-4). The pit or fissure may take a wavy course; thus, it may not lead directly from the outer surface to the dentinoenamel junction.

II. CONTENTS OF A PIT OR FISSURE

A pit or fissure contains dental biofilm, pellicle, debris, and sometimes relatively intact remnants of tooth development.

III. EFFECT OF CLEANING

The narrow, long fissures are difficult to clean completely. Retained cleaning material can block the sealant from filling the fissure and can also become mixed with the sealant. Removal of pumice used for cleaning and thorough washing are necessary to the success of the sealant.

IV. AMOUNT OF PENETRATION

Wide V-shaped and shallow fissures are more apt to be filled by sealant (Figure 34-5B). Although ideally the sealant should penetrate to the bottom of a pit or fissure, such penetration is frequently impossible. Microscopic examination of pits and fissures after sealant application has shown that the sealant does not penetrate to the bottom because residual debris, cleansing agents, and trapped air prevent passage of the material (Figure 34-5C and D).

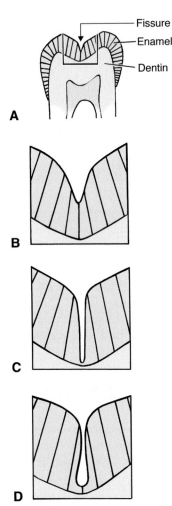

■ **FIGURE 34-4 Occlusal Fissures.** Drawings made from microscopic slides show variations in shape and depth of fissures. **(A)** Tooth with section enlarged for B, C, and D. **(B)** Wide V-shaped fissure. **(C)** Long narrow groove that reaches nearly to the dentinoenamel junction. **(D)** Long constricted form with a bulbous terminal portion.

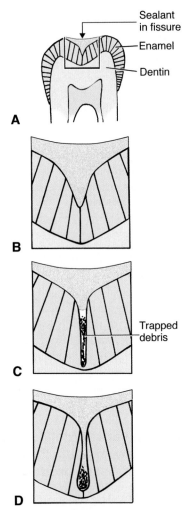

■ **FIGURE 34-5 Pit and Fissure Sealant in Fissures.** Drawings made from microscopic slides show extent to which sealant fills a fissure. **(A)** Tooth with section enlarged for B, C, and D. **(B)** Sealant fills wide V-shaped fissure and extends a short way up the slopes of surrounding cusps. **(C)** and **(D)** Fissures partially filled as a result of narrow constriction of the groove and blockage by trapped debris.

Everyday Ethics

Lillian had always enjoyed doing sealants when she was in dental hygiene school. They had been required to do quite a few, and as students they got to participate in "Sealant Day," a volunteer program carried out by the local dental hygienists every spring.

Now, when she came back from the state dental hygiene meeting, she was all excited about the new interpretation of the practice act by the Dental Board and greeted her employer, Dr. Fine, with the news the first thing Monday morning. The Board had voted that the dental hygienist who had been in practice for 2 years full-time (or part-time equivalent) could make the decision whether a pit or fissure needed a sealant. There was a continuing education course and an examination required.

Lillian added: "Remember Jack—that teenager that was here last week? He had some really deep fissures that I was sure would benefit from sealants. Can I go ahead and schedule him? I told him he needed them. He has an appointment with you to have a few cavities filled, but that wouldn't fit in your book until nearly the end of the month."

Dr. Fine continued quietly to tie on his gown for the first patient, and then he smiled and said, "Well, Lil, let's wait until he comes in for his appointment with me and I'll look at them."

Questions for Consideration

1. Professionally, what action(s) can Lillian take to initiate a system of collaboration between her and Dr. Fine to pursue the new practice protocols?

2. What ethical issues may be involved here?

3. Which of the core values describe the current relationship between Lillian and Dr. Fine? And which core values describe Lillian's wishes to extend the services for Jack's (the patient's) benefit?

■ MAINTENANCE

I. REEXAMINATION

At each maintenance appointment, or at least every 6 months, each sealant should be examined for deficiencies that may have developed.

Factors To Teach The Patient

- Sealants are part of a total preventive program. Sealants are not substitutes for other preventive measures. Limitations of dietary sucrose, use of fluorides, and dental biofilm control are major factors with sealants for prevention of dental caries.

- What a sealant is and why such a meticulous application procedure is required.

- What can be expected from a sealant; how long it lasts, how it prevents dental caries.

- Need for examination of the sealant at frequent, scheduled appointments, and need for replacement when indicated.

II. RETENTION

A. Retention Time

Sealants can be retained for many years.[8] Although surface sealant may be lost, sealant in the pits and fissures and sealant that penetrated into the microspaces of the enamel still remain and provide protection.[9]

B. Retention Factors

1. *During placement*
   a. Precision of technique.
   b. Exclusion of moisture and contamination during placement.
2. *Care of existing restorations.* Avoid using an air-powder polisher on intact existing sealants during maintenance appointments. Sealant wear increases with time of exposure to air-powder polisher abrasion.[10]

III. REPLACEMENT

A. Consult the manufacturer's instructions.
B. Tooth preparation: same as for original application.
C. Removal of sections of retained sealant is not usually necessary.
D. Re-etching of the tooth surface is always essential.

REFERENCES

1. **Handleman**, S.L. and Shey, Z.: Michael Buonocore and the East-man Dental Center: A Historic Perspective on Sealants, *J. Dent. Res.*, 75, 529, January, 1996.

2. **Cueto**, E.I. and Buonocore, M.G.: Sealing of Pits and Fissures With an Adhesive Resin: Its Use in Caries Prevention, *J. Am. Dent. Assoc.*, 75, 121, July, 1967.

3. **American Dental Association**, Division of Science: Pit and Fissure Sealants: Product Names and Manufacturers, *J. Am. Dent. Assoc.*, 133, 1274, September, 2002.

4. **Scott**, L., Brockmann, S., Houston, G., and Tira, D.: Retention of Dental Sealants Following the Use of Airpolishing and Traditional Cleaning, *Dent. Hyg.*, 62, 402, September, 1988.

5. **Brockmann**, S.L., Scott, R.L., and Eick, J.D.: A Scanning Electron Microscopic Study of the Effect of Air Polishing on the Enamel-Sealant Surface, *Quintessence Int.*, 21, 201, March, 1990.

6. **Stach**, D.J., Hatch, R.A., Tilliss, T.S., and Cross-Poline, G.N.: Change in Occlusal Height Resulting From Placement of Pit and Fissure Sealants, *J. Prosthet. Dent.*, 68, 750, November, 1992.

7. **Tilliss**, T.S.I., Stach, D.J., Hatch, R.A., and Cross-Poline, G.N.: Occlusal Discrepancies After Sealant Therapy, *J. Prosthet. Dent.*, 68, 223, August, 1992.

8. **Simonsen**, R.J.: Retention and Effectiveness of Dental Sealant After 15 years, *J. Am. Dent. Assoc.*, 122, 34, October, 1991.

9. **Buonocore**, M.G.: Pit and Fissure Sealing, *Dent. Clin. North Am.*, 19, 367, April, 1975.

10. **Huennekens**, S.C., Daniel, S.J., and Bayne, S.C.: Effects of Air Polishing on the Abrasion of Occlusal Sealants, *Quintessence Int.*, 22, 581, July, 1991.

SUGGESTED READINGS

American Dental Association, Council on Access, Prevention and Interprofessional Relations: Caries Diagnosis and Risk Assessment, *J. Am. Dent. Assoc.*, 126, 1S, Supplement, June, 1995.

Daniel, S.J., Scruggs, R.R., and Grady, J.J.: The Accuracy of Student Self-evaluations of Dental Sealants, *J. Dent. Hyg.*, 64, 339, September, 1990.

Llodra, J.C., Bravo, M., Delagado-Rodriguez, M., Baca, P., and Galvez, R.: Factors Influencing the Effectiveness of Sealants: A Meta-analysis, *Community Dent. Oral Epidemiol.*, 21, 261, October, 1993.

Nathanson, D., Lertpitayaklin, P., Lamkin, M.S., Edalatpour, M., and Chou, L.C.: In Vitro Elution of Leachable Components From Dental Sealants, *J. Am. Dent. Assoc.*, 128, 1517, November, 1997.

Ripa, L.W.: Sealants Revisited: An Update of the Effectiveness of Pit-and-Fissure Sealants, *Caries Res.*, 27, 77, Supplement 1, 1993.

Simonsen, R.J.: Pit and Fissure Sealants: Review of the Literature, *Pediatr. Dent.*, 24, 393, September/October, 2002.

Clinical Procedures

Carstensen, W.: The Effects of Different Phosphoric Acid Concentrations on Surface Enamel, *Angle Orthod.*, 62, 51, Spring, 1992.

Feigal, R.J., Hitt, J., and Splieth, C.: Retaining Sealant on Salivary Contaminated Enamel, *J. Am. Dent. Assoc.*, 124, 88, March, 1993.

Lehtinen, R. and Kuusilehto, A.: Absorption of UVA Light by Latex and Vinyl Gloves, *Scand. J. Dent. Res.*, 98, 186, April, 1990.

Marcushamer, M., Neuman, E., and Garcia-Godoy, F.: Fluoridated and Nonfluoridated Unfilled Sealants Show Similar Shear Strength, *Pediatr. Dent.*, 19, 289, May/June, 1997.

Poulos, J.G. and Styner, D.L.: Curing Lights: Changes in Intensity Output With Use Over Time, *Gen. Dent.*, 45, 70, January–February, 1997.

Waggoner, W.F. and Siegal, M.: Pit and Fissure Sealant Application: Updating the Technique, *J. Am. Dent. Assoc.*, 127, 351, March, 1996.

Other Sealant Techniques

Croll, T.P.: The Quintessential Sealant? *Quintessence Int.*, 27, 729, November, 1996.

DeCraene, G.P., Martens, C., and Dermaut, R.: The Invasive Pit-and-Fissure Sealing Technique in Pediatric Dentistry: An SEM Study of a Preventive Restoration, *ASDC J. Dent. Child.*, 55, 34, January–February, 1988.

doRego, M.A. and deAraújo, M.A.M.: A 2-Year Clinical Evaluation of Fluoride-Containing Pit and Fissure Sealants Placed With an Invasive Technique, *Quintessence, Int.*, 27, 99, February, 1996.

Feldens, E.G., Feldens, C.A., deAraújo, F., and Souza, M.A.L.: Invasive Technique of Pit and Fissure Sealants in Primary Molars: A SEM Study, *J. Clin. Pediatr. Dent.*, 18, 187, Spring, 1994.

Garcia-Godoy, F., Summitt, J.B., and Donly, K.J.: Caries Progression of White Spot Lesions Sealed With an Unfilled Resin, *J. Clin. Pediatr. Dent.*, 21, 141, Winter, 1997.

Kramer, P.F., Zelante, F., and Simionato, M.R.L.: The Immediate and Long-term Effects of Invasive and Noninvasive Pit and Fissure Sealing Techniques on the Microflora in Occlusal Fissures of Human Teeth, *Pediatr. Dent.*, 16, 108, March/April, 1993.

Mertz-Fairhurst, E.J., Curtis, J.W., Ergle, J.W., Rueggeberg, F.A., and Adair, S.M.: Ultraconservative and Cariostatic Sealed Restorations: Results at Year 10, *J. Am. Dent. Assoc.*, 129, 55, January, 1998.

Treatment

■ INTRODUCTION

Instrumentation for scaling, root planing, extrinsic stain removal, care of dental restorations, and postcare procedures are included in Section VI. Placement and removal of dressings, removal of sutures, and treatment of hypersensitive teeth are described. Immediate evaluation of techniques and their effects, short-term follow-up, and maintenance assessment follow instrumentation. These procedures are all part of *nonsurgical periodontal therapy*.

The first objective of treatment is to create an environment in which the tissues can return to health. In the sequence of patient treatment, introduction to preventive measures occurs first, before professional instrumentation.

After health has been attained, the patient's self-care on a daily basis is essential to keep the teeth and gingival tissues free from new or recurrent disease caused by the microorganisms of dental biofilm. Professional instrumentation makes a limited contribution to arresting the progression of disease without daily biofilm control measures performed by the patient.

■ ORAL PROPHYLAXIS: DEFINITION DILEMMA

The term *oral prophylaxis* refers to those specific treatment procedures aimed at removing local irritants to the gingiva, including complete calculus removal with bacte-

rial debridement. A smooth tooth surface resists the retention of dental deposits. The oral prophylaxis performed with these objectives is truly a *preventive periodontal treatment procedure*.[1]

There is a definite need for clarification and new terminology for the various services performed under the title "oral prophylaxis." Through common usage, oral prophylaxis has taken on a variety of meanings.

Because *prophylaxis* means *prevention of disease*, then *oral prophylaxis*, as the *prevention of oral disease*, should include such preventive procedures as restoring individual teeth, replacing missing teeth, adjusting the occlusion, correcting faulty proximal contacts, and many other procedures, the basic purposes of which are preventive.[2]

Unfortunately, the term "oral prophylaxis" also is sometimes used to mean a superficial 5- to 10-minute application of a rubber polishing cup with an abrasive paste to the enamel surfaces that appear above the gingival margin. The term "oral prophylaxis" obviously must be carefully and specifically defined if it is to be applied to the comprehensive treatment services of a dental hygienist.

In the development of a meaningful concept of the oral prophylaxis upon which the procedures and anticipated outcomes described in this book are based, the only acceptable definition is based on the preventive aspects of periodontal infections.

■ OBJECTIVES OF TREATMENT

Specific objectives for each type of instrumentation are included in the chapter that describes the details of the technique. General objectives of dental hygiene instrumentation are to

A. Create an environment in which the tissues can return to health and then be maintained in health.
B. Eliminate or suppress periodontal pathogenic microorganisms and control reinfection.
C. Aid in the prevention and control of gingival and periodontal infections by removal of factors that predispose to the retention of dental biofilm. Factors particularly implicated are dental calculus and irregular and overhanging restorations.
D. Compose the total treatment needed for certain patients with uncomplicated disease and the initial preparatory phase of treatment for others with more advanced disease.
E. Assist in the maintenance phase of care to prevent recurrence of disease.
F. Provide the patient with smooth tooth surfaces, which are easier to clean and to keep biofilm-free by daily self-care procedures.
G. Assist in instructing the patient in the appearance and feeling of a thoroughly clean mouth as

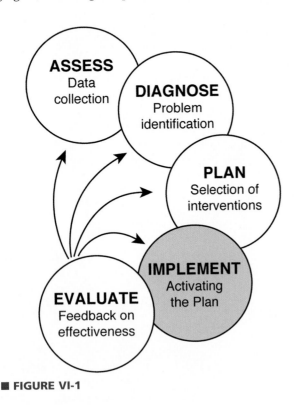

■ **FIGURE VI-1**

▪ TABLE VI-1 ETHICAL AND PROFESSIONAL ISSUES

PROFESSIONAL ISSUES	EXPLANATION	APPLICATION
Expressed or Implied Contracts	An agreement to perform tasks that can be written (third-party payment) or oral (between provider and patient) for a course of treatment.	Coding of dental hygiene services based on current edition of Current Dental Terminology (CDT) guidelines. Documenting a code for a gingivitis diagnosis versus periodontal maintenance.
Whistle-Blowing	The disclosure of illegal or immoral wrongs that are under the control of the individual practitioner. May involve negligent acts.	Reporting the lack of infection control procedures to a state dental board or the actions of an impaired colleague.
Privacy Rights	Involves the reform of health information through protection of privacy, insurance access, preventing fraud and abuse, and standardization within the healthcare industry.	Health Insurance Portability & Accountability Act (HIPAA) is a federal mandate affecting the confidentiality of dental records, especially where computers are used to document patient data.
Supervision	The ethical and legal working relationship between the dentist, dental hygienist, and other dental personnel.	A dental hygienist rendering treatment to patients of record from the dental practice who now reside in a nursing home in a neighboring community.

a motivation toward the development of adequate habits of personal oral care.

H.   Prepare the teeth and gingiva for dental procedures, including those performed by the restorative dentist, prosthodontist, orthodontist, pedodontist, and oral surgeon.

I.   Improve oral esthetics and sanitation.

▪ ETHICAL APPLICATIONS

Many facets of dental hygiene care relate directly to the provider-patient relationship and surrounding professional issues. Concerns such as insurance contracts, whistle-blowing, and maintaining privacy rights of patients affect the overall delivery of dental services. The dental hygienist must acknowledge the ethical implications of providing care beyond the treatment alone.

Thus, the conduct of the professional dental hygienist prior to, during, and following the dental hygiene appointment is subject to moral assessment.

Both rights and duties are important in the ongoing relationship between the patient and the dental hygienist. A responsibility exists to treat patients equitably, aware of their best interest at all times. Practicing a consistent and professional demeanor with all patients and all members of the dental team can be achieved and will uphold high standards and quality of care. Several ethical and professional issues to be considered are found in Table VI-1.

REFERENCES

1.   *World Workshop in Periodontics.* Ann Arbor, University of Michigan, 1966, p. 450.
2.   **Bunting**, R.W.: *Oral Hygiene*, 3rd ed. Philadelphia, Lea & Febiger, 1957, p. 233.

Anxiety and Pain Control

Donna J. Stach, BS, RDH, MEd

Concern for patient anxiety and pain is an integral part of a dental hygiene appointment. Recognizing and managing a patient's anxiety and pain is an essential part of dental hygiene care planning. The decision to use a pharmacologic agent for management of anxiety and pain is dependent upon a number of factors. Periodontal health status, the treatment being rendered, and the patient's pain threshold must all be considered. Pain threshold is highly individual and variable. Box 35-1 provides terminology and definitions relative to anxiety and pain and to their management.

▪ COMPONENTS OF PAIN

There are two components of pain. *Pain perception* is primarily a neurologic experience of pain; *pain reaction* is the personal interpretation and response to the pain message. Pain may occur during or following treatment.

I. PAIN PERCEPTION

A. Relates to the physical process of receiving a painful stimulus and transmitting the information through the nervous system to the brain.
B. In the brain it is interpreted as pain.
C. There is little variability in pain perception between individuals with intact nervous systems.

II. PAIN REACTION

A. The reaction is a combination of the interpretation and the response to the pain message.
B. The reaction is highly variable between individuals and even in the same individual at different times.
C. Accounts for much of the variability seen between patients in personal pain management needs.
D. Many factors influence pain reaction. Factors included are age, fatigue, emotional state, and both cultural and ethnic learned behaviors.

E. The presence of anxiety has special significance because with anxiety the patient is predisposed to feel pain.
F. People with a strong or rapid reaction to pain are said to have a low pain threshold.

▪ PAIN CONTROL MECHANISMS

Five pain control mechanisms are available. They are often combined for optimum effect. Decisions about anxiety and pain management are included during dental hygiene care planning and written into the care plan. It is important to match the pain control method to the patient's treatment needs and medical status. All pain management techniques are more effective if utilized before the patient experiences pain.

The five categories of pain control mechanisms are the following:

I. REMOVE THE PAINFUL STIMULUS

A. Affects pain perception.
B. Examples: patient avoids dental appointment; clinician corrects faulty, pain-causing instrument technique.

II. BLOCK THE PATHWAY OF THE PAIN MESSAGE

A. Affects pain perception.
B. Examples: use of local anesthetic, topical anesthetic.

III. PREVENT PAIN REACTION BY RAISING PAIN REACTION THRESHOLD

A. Affects pain reaction.
B. Examples: use of nitrous oxide–oxygen conscious sedation; nonopioid analgesics such as nonsteroidal anti-inflammatory drugs (NSAIDs).

BOX 35-1 KEY WORDS: Anxiety and Pain Control

Ambient air: surrounding atmosphere.

Analgesia: diminution or elimination of pain in the conscious patient.

Anesthesia: loss of feeling or sensation, especially loss of tactile sensitivity, with or without loss of consciousness.

>**Block anesthesia:** induced by injecting the anesthetic close to a nerve trunk; may be at some distance from the area to be treated.

>**General anesthesia:** the elimination of all sensations, accompanied by the loss of consciousness.

>**Infiltration anesthesia:** induced by injecting the anesthetic directly into or around the tissues to be anesthetized.

>**Local anesthesia:** loss of sensation, especially pain, in a circumscribed area without loss of consciousness; also called regional anesthesia.

>**Topical anesthesia:** a form of local anesthesia whereby free nerve endings in accessible structures are rendered incapable of stimulation by the application of an anesthetic drug directly to the surface of the area.

Anxiety: a negative, emotional response to an anticipated event, the outcome of which is unknown. This is a learned response from personal experience or the stories of others.

Aspiration: recommended technique for preventing injection of local anesthetic directly into circulatory system. Negative pressure is created in anesthetic cartridge. If needle tip is in artery or vein, blood will be visible in cartridge.

Conscious: state in which patient is capable of rational response to commands and protective reflexes are intact, including the ability to maintain a patent airway independently and continuously.

Conscious sedation: the calming or allaying of nervous excitement while maintaining a conscious state by pharmacologic, nonpharmacologic, or combined methods.

Epinephrine: a hormone secreted by the adrenal medulla that, among many functions, causes vasodilation of blood vessels of skeletal muscles, vasoconstriction of arterioles of skin and mucous membranes, and stimulation of heart action; used in local anesthetics for its vasoconstrictive action.

Hypoxia: diminished availability of oxygen to body tissues.

>**Diffusion hypoxia:** lack of adequate amounts of oxygen that can result from the rapid diffusion of nitrous oxide molecules from the blood stream into the lungs. Occurs if 100% oxygen is not administered at the conclusion of a nitrous oxide–oxygen sedation procedure.

Iatrosedation: reduction of anxiety as a result of the clinician's behavior or actions. A psychosomatic method of pain control.

Metered spray: a method for dispensing topical anesthetic that administers a fixed volume of drug and then stops automatically.

Occupational exposure: subject to an action or influence, usually negative, as a result of one's occupation or work environment.

Pain: a sensation in which a person experiences discomfort, distress, or suffering; may vary in intensity from mild discomfort to intolerable agony.

Pain threshold: point at which a sensation starts to be painful and a response results. Varies between individuals based on interpretation of sensation. May be altered by some drugs.

>**High pain threshold:** a greater than average tolerance to a painful stimulus.

>**Low pain threshold:** a strong or rapid reaction to a painful stimulus.

KEY WORDS: Anxiety and Pain Control, continued

Potency: strength of a drug. Amount of a medication or drug necessary to achieve a desired effect.

Psychosomatic method: any nonpharmacologic technique that reduces anxiety and improves pain control. Effective because the mind influences the body's perception and interpretation of pain.

Scavenging device: that part of the nitrous oxide equipment that collects exhaled nitrous oxide and removes it. The main component is the scavenging nasal hood. Since 1980 the American Dental Association has recommended that effective scavenging devices be installed whenever nitrous oxide is used to reduce occupational exposure.

Sedation: one of the stages of anesthesia in which the patient is still conscious but is under the influence of a central nervous system depressant drug.

Titration: a technique for individualization of drug dose. Administration of small, incremental dose of a drug until the desired clinical action is observed.

Vasoconstrictor: a drug that constricts blood vessels. An additive to most local anesthetic solutions to offset the vasodilating actions of the local anesthetic.

IV. DEPRESS CENTRAL NERVOUS SYSTEM

A. Affects pain reaction.
B. Example: general anesthesia.

V. USE PSYCHOSEDATION METHODS (ALSO CALLED IATROSEDATION)

A. Affects both pain perception and pain reaction.
B. Includes any nonpharmacologic technique that reduces patient anxiety, builds a trust relationship, or lets the patient feel more in control.
C. May be used alone or may be combined with pharmacologic pain management.
D. Examples: explain procedures carefully; allow patient to express concerns; use relaxation or distraction techniques.

▪ NONOPIOID ANALGESICS

Over-the-counter (OTC) analgesics are an effective adjunct for preventing or reducing the mild to moderate discomfort that patients experience during dental hygiene therapy or postoperatively.

I. DRUGS

A. Nonsteroidal anti-inflammatory drugs (NSAIDs).

1. The drugs of choice for dental pain.
2. Ibuprofen: Details are shown in Box 35-2.

B. Acetaminophen

II. ACTION OF NSAIDS

A. Blocks prostaglandin synthesis at peripheral nerve endings to inhibit generation of pain message.[1]
B. Suppresses onset of pain.
C. Decreases pain severity.

III. INDICATIONS

A. Mild to moderate pain during treatment.
B. Mild to moderate pain postoperatively.

BOX 35-2 Ibuprofen*

Analgesic Activity
Onset: 30 minutes after administration.

Peak analgesic: 2–3 hours after administration.

Maintenance analgesia: Administer second dose 4 hours after initial dose.

Suggestions for Time of Administration
For treatment pain: Take 2 hours before.

For postoperative pain without local anesthetic: Take immediately before treatment.

For postoperative pain with local anesthetic: Take at completion of treatment.

*Ibuprofen is considered drug of choice for dental pain.

▪ NITROUS OXIDE–OXYGEN SEDATION

The gases nitrous oxide and oxygen, in combination, are widely used in dental and dental hygiene practice settings. A state of conscious sedation is produced with the patient awake, relaxed, responsive to commands, able to cooperate with treatment, and having intact protective reflexes. The patient has some degree of analgesia and a higher pain reaction threshold.

▪ CHARACTERISTICS OF NITROUS OXIDE

I. ANESTHETIC AND ANALGESIC PROPERTIES

A. Produces analgesia.
B. Achieves optimum analgesia and patient cooperation at 30% to 40% nitrous oxide for most patients. The need for higher or lower concentrations depends on individual biologic variability.
C. Reduces the intensity of pain but does not block it; only mildly potent as an anesthetic gas.
D. Combines with local anesthetic when the patient experiences significant discomfort.

II. CHEMICAL AND PHYSICAL PROPERTIES

A. Gas at room temperature and pressure.
B. Heavier than air.
C. Colorless; sweet smelling.
D. Nonirritating and nonallergenic.
E. Nonflammable but will support the combustion of flammable substances.

III. BLOOD SOLUBILITY

A. Relatively insoluble in blood; primary saturation of blood occurs in 3 to 5 minutes.[2]
B. The gas molecules at the alveoli-blood interface and blood-brain interface pass readily to the tissue with the lowest concentration of nitrous oxide.
   1. Results in rapid onset and recovery.
   2. Results in potential diffusion hypoxia at completion of sedation procedure if 100% oxygen is not administered.

IV. PHARMACOLOGY OF NITROUS OXIDE

A. Is not metabolized in the body; remains unchanged in blood and tissues.
B. Enters and exits almost entirely through the lungs.

▪ EQUIPMENT FOR NITROUS OXIDE–OXYGEN

The equipment for nitrous oxide–oxygen conscious sedation is available as a portable unit or a central storage system with gas piped to individual treatment rooms. Currently available units have several built-in safety features to ensure that a minimal level of oxygen is always delivered and that the two gases could not be reversed inadvertently in delivery. The equipment can be divided into three basic parts: gas storage cylinders, a gas delivery system, and a scavenger system with the nasal hood (mask) having components of both the gas delivery and scavenger portions.

I. COMPRESSED GAS CYLINDERS

A. Nitrous Oxide

1. *Color code*: Light blue.
2. *Physical state*: Gas and liquid.
3. *Pressure*: Constant at 750 pounds per square inch (psi) until almost empty.

B. Oxygen

1. *Color code*: Green (international = white).
2. *Physical state*: Gas.
3. *Pressure:* Falls at a uniform rate with use from a full pressure of 2,000 psi or 2,200 psi for size E or H cylinders, respectively.
4. *Use ratio*: About 2.5 cylinders of oxygen are used for each comparably sized cylinder of nitrous oxide.

C. Handle Carefully

1. Use no grease, oil, lubricant, or hand cream around the cylinder valves or any fittings that come in contact with the gases.
2. Store vertically on a rack or in another stable and secure manner.
3. Open cylinder valves slowly in a counterclockwise direction.

II. GAS DELIVERY SYSTEM

A. Regulator or Reducing Valve

1. Converts high pressure of gas in the cylinders to a usable, lower level.
2. Subject to extreme high temperature if compressed gas cylinders are opened quickly.

B. Flow Meter

1. Visual indicator of liters per minute (L/min) flow of oxygen and nitrous oxide.
2. Flow meter comes in two designs:
   a. Gas flow rates of nitrous oxide and oxygen are adjusted independently. The sum of the two is the total gas flow rate.
   b. A total combined gas flow rate is established and the respective concentrations of the two gases are adjusted concurrently.

C. Reservoir Bag

1. Reservoir of gases to accommodate an exceptionally deep breath.
2. Allows for visualization of respirations for monitoring.
3. Degree of inflation can be used to help establish total flow rate of gas needed by the patient for comfortable respirations.
4. May be used to provide oxygen in assisted ventilation if attached to a full face mask with relief valve.

D. Conducting or Breathing Tubes

III. NASAL HOOD, NOSE PIECE, MASK

A. Deliver gas for patient inhalation.
B. Collect exhaled gas and direct it into scavenger system.
C. Good fit and seal around patient's nose are essential in size selection.
D. Ideally a disposable item, or sterilize before each use.

IV. SCAVENGER SYSTEM

A. Removes exhaled gas to keep nitrous oxide levels low in the ambient air of the treatment room.
B. Connects to the office central evacuation system.
C. Vents to outside of building and away from windows and air intakes.

V. SAFETY FEATURES

A. **Universal color coding** of cylinders, hoses, flow controls for each gas.
B. **Pin index** and **diameter index** safety systems physically prevent gas cylinders or hoses from being mistakenly interchanged between the gases due to incompatible placement of pins (projections) and diameter differences in the couplings.
C. **Minimum oxygen flow**, 30% or 3 L/min.
D. **Oxygen fail-safe** system automatically shuts off nitrous oxide if the oxygen falls below a minimum level.

E. **Emergency air inlet** to provide room air if system shuts down.
F. **Oxygen flush button** to supply 100% oxygen quickly.

VI. EQUIPMENT MAINTENANCE

A. **Function Checks**
   Maintain working order and safe practice by periodic checking of equipment.
B. **Gas Leaks**
   All equipment connections and rubber goods are subject to leaking. Figure 35-1 shows the places that should be examined for tight connections, defects, and wear. Apply soapy water to connections; bubbles will form if leaks are present.

▪ PATIENT SELECTION

I. INDICATIONS

A. Patient with mild to moderate anxiety.
B. Medically compromised patient who would benefit from additional oxygen and/or anxiety reduction. Examples: patient with a cardiovascular or cerebrovascular disease, or with stress-induced bronchial asthma.
C. Procedures that are short in duration and cause a low level of pain. The analgesic effect is most pronounced on the soft tissues, making it especially useful during dental hygiene procedures.
D. Patient with strong gag reflex.

II. CONTRAINDICATIONS

The gas is nonirritating to the respiratory system and does not interact chemically or biotransform within the body. There are no known allergies.

Individuals with the following conditions should be evaluated carefully before nitrous oxide–oxygen sedation:

A. Recent ophthalmic surgery using intraocular gases.
   1. Absolute contraindication following surgery with:
      a. Perfluoropropane for 8 weeks.
      b. Sulfur hexafluoride for 2 weeks.
   2. Vision damage could result from increased pressure on the eye during healing.[3]
B. Unable to cooperate and/or communicate.
   1. Unwilling to breathe through nose and/or leave nasal hood in place.
   2. Claustrophobia.
C. Moderate to severe chronic obstructive pulmonary disease (COPD). Examples: emphysema, chronic bronchitis.

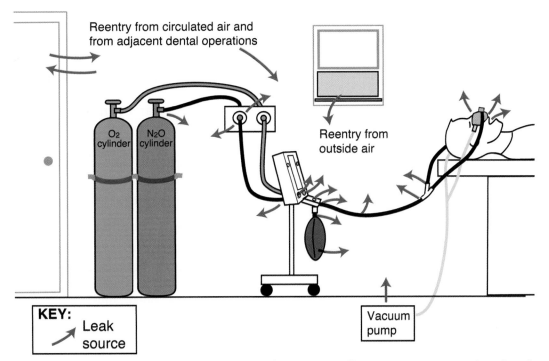

■ FIGURE 35-1 Potential Sources of Leaks From Nitrous Oxide–Oxygen Delivery Systems. Arrows show locations where regular inspection and testing is necessary. The most common sites of leakage are: *High-pressure connections*: from the gas delivery cylinders, the wall connectors, the hoses connecting to the anesthetic machine, and the anesthesia machine itself (especially the on-demand valve). *Low-pressure connections*: from the anesthetic flow meter and the scavenging mask. Look for loose-fitting connections, loosely assembled or deformed slip joints and threaded connections, defective or worn seals, and gaskets. *Rubber goods*: hoses and reservoir bag. Look for cracks and tears. (Adapted from **NIOSH:** *Alert: Controlling Exposures to Nitrous Oxide During Anesthetic Administration.* [NIOSH Publication No. 94-100]. Cincinnati, U.S. Department of Health, Education, and Welfare, Public Health Service, Centers for Disease Control and Prevention, National Institute for Occupational Safety and Health, 1994, p. 5.)

D. Upper respiratory tract obstruction or infection if nose breathing would be difficult or breathing apparatus cannot be sterilized or replaced.

E. Conditions of confined air spaces within the body that would be adversely affected by increased pressure, such as middle ear or tympanic membrane problems, blockage of Eustachian tube or sinuses, bowel obstruction.

F. Severe personality disorders characterized by a tenuous grasp on reality.

G. Compulsive personalities who do not like the feeling of "losing control."

H. Patients who do not want nitrous oxide–oxygen sedation for any of a variety of personal reasons.

I. Pregnancy
   1. Prudent practice would suggest that no elective drugs be administered during pregnancy, especially during the first trimester.
   2. Consultation with the patient's obstetrician is advisable.
   3. 2nd and 3rd Trimester: Dose and exposure should be kept to a minimum.

4. May be sedation method of choice because of lack of effect in most organ systems, rapid removal from body, and lack of metabolism in the body.[4]

■ CLINICAL PROCEDURES FOR NITROUS OXIDE–OXYGEN ADMINISTRATION

Box 35-3 lists the sequence of steps for nitrous oxide–oxygen administration.

I. PATIENT PREPARATION

A. Inform

1. Prior to appointment
   a. No specific food limitations but generally avoid fasting or heavy meals just before the appointment.
   b. Wear comfortable clothing and loosen tight collars.

BOX 35-3 Steps in Nitrous Oxide-Oxygen Administration

1. Assess patient's medical status.

2. Take and record pretreatment vital signs.

3. Educate patient and secure informed consent.

4. Prepare delivery equipment (open tanks, select nasal hood).*

5. Activate scavenger system.

6. Turn on oxygen to a flow rate of 5–7 L/min.

7. Place nasal hood and adjust to fit.

8. Adjust gas flow rate.

9. Begin nitrous oxide at about 10%–20%.

10. Titrate to optimum level.

11. Monitor throughout treatment.

12. Return to 100% oxygen.

13. Take and record posttreatment vital signs.

14. Remove nasal hood when patient feels fully recovered.

15. Record progress notes.

*Sequence may vary. Equipment preparation may precede patient assessment steps if treatment planned in advance.

---

2. At time of appointment
   a. Explain procedure in positive terms. Stress the pleasant sense of relaxation; the patient will be aware and in control at all times.
   b. Establish informed consent.

B. Assess

1. Evaluate patient's medical status.
2. Take and record vital signs.

II. EQUIPMENT PREPARATION

A. Nasal Hood

1. Select the appropriate size for optimum comfort and minimum gas leakage.
2. Attach to tubing.

B. Scavenger System

1. Connect, usually to high-speed volume evacuation, and activate system.
2. Adjust setting of scavenger system.

C. Turn on Gas Cylinders

1. Open slowly, first oxygen, then nitrous oxide.
2. Centralized gas systems are turned on at the beginning of the day.

III. TECHNIQUE FOR GAS DELIVERY

A. Establish Volume of Gas Flow

1. 100% oxygen.
2. Gas flow rate between 5 and 7 L/min for adults, 3 and 4 L/min for children.
3. Place nasal hood, adjust for comfort; patient may assist in positioning.
4. Adjust flow using the inflation of the reservoir bag and feedback from the patient.

B. Titration

Individualized drug dose is determined by increasing the percentage of nitrous oxide in small increments until the optimum sedation level is achieved based on clinical signs and symptoms.

1. *Initial Concentration.* Start titration at about 20% concentration of nitrous oxide. Because of the rapid uptake of nitrous oxide in the lungs and distribution through the body, the effect of each dose can be assessed after 1 to 2 minutes.

2. *Patient Response.* Observe the patient for signs of relaxation or other changes. Ask the patient what is felt. Use the patient's signs and symptoms to determine when the optimum level of sedation has been reached. Table 35-1 lists signs and symptoms for various levels of nitrous oxide–oxygen sedation.

3. *Adjust Dose.* Increase or decrease the nitrous oxide by 5% to 10% when the optimum individual dose has not been achieved. Wait 1 to 2 minutes and reassess. Repeat as needed.
   a. Distribution of optimum sedation dose for different individuals follows a bell curve. For about 70% of patients, the ideal is in the 30% to 40% nitrous oxide range.[5]
   b. At high altitudes, greater nitrous oxide concentrations will be needed because of the change in the partial pressure of the gases.

4. *Time.* Allow approximately 5 minutes for titration.

5. *Monitor.* Continue to monitor and adjust the concentration throughout the appointment. As

■ TABLE 35-1 CORRELATION OF SIGNS AND SYMPTOMS TO LEVELS OF NITROUS OXIDE–OXYGEN SEDATION

LEVELS	SYMPTOMS	SIGNS
1. Early to ideal sedation	Light-headedness (dizziness) Tingling of hands and feet Body warmth Feeling of vibration throughout body Numbness of hands and feet Numbness of soft tissues of oral cavity Feeling of euphoria Feeling of lightness or heaviness in extremities Analgesia	Blood pressure, heart rate slightly elevated early in procedure, then return to baseline values Respirations are normal Peripheral vasodilation Flushing of extremities, face Decreased muscle tone as anxiety decreases (arms and legs relax)
2. Heavier sedation/slight oversedation	Hearing, especially of distant sounds, becomes more acute Visual images become confused (patterns on ceiling begin to move) Sleepiness Laughing, crying Dreaming Nausea	Movement increases Heart rate, blood pressure increase Rate of respiration increases Sweating increases Possible tearing
3. Oversedation	Nausea	Vomiting Loss of consciousness

Adapted from Malamed, S.F.: *Sedation, A Guide to Patient Management,* 4th ed. St. Louis, Mosby, 2003, pp. 198.

the appointment proceeds or during less anxiety-producing parts of the appointment, a lower dose may be more comfortable. Avoid excessive fluctuations.

6. *Attend Patient.* Never leave a sedated patient unattended; sedation can become deeper without some stimulation or interaction.

7. *Outcome.* Titration increases clinical success rate of nitrous oxide–oxygen conscious sedation and decreases adverse responses.

IV. COMPLETION OF SEDATION

A. Recovery

1. *Procedure.* At the completion of sedation, return the patient to 100% oxygen for at least 3 to 5 minutes or longer if needed for full recovery.

2. *Factors Affecting Recovery Time.* Biologic variation, duration of sedation procedure, and concentration of nitrous oxide administration. Generally, the more nitrous oxide administered, the longer the recovery time.

3. *Signs of Recovery.* Patient's report of feeling "back to normal," comparable presedation and postsedation vital signs.

B. Diffusion Hypoxia

If patient is returned directly to room air rather than 100% oxygen, diffusion hypoxia can result.

1. Nitrous oxide diffuses into an area of lower concentration more rapidly than oxygen, causing inadequate oxygen in the alveoli if the patient is not given supplemental oxygen at the completion of sedation.

2. Hypoxia can result in patient discomfort or syncope.

3. Inadequate postsedation oxygen may result in a feeling of lethargy or headache.

C. Dismissal Follows Full Recovery

Usually the patient is able to return to all normal activities, including driving.

D. Record Keeping

The following items should be included in the patient's record:

1. Presedation and postsedation vital signs.

2. Concentrations of both nitrous oxide and oxygen administered.

3. Total gas flow rate (L/min).

BOX 35-4 Example Progress Notes: Nitrous Oxide–Oxygen Conscious Sedation

Patient presented with a pronounced gag reflex that caused anxiety about dental treatment. Medical history is nonsignificant. Total gas flow rate: 5 L/min; 35% nitrous oxide and 65% oxygen (OR 2 L/min nitrous oxide and 4 L/min oxygen) for 40 min. Patient reported tingling in extremities and a relaxed feeling. Full-mouth debridement completed without incident. After treatment, 100% oxygen was administered for 5 min; patient said he felt fully recovered.

Vital Signs	Pretreatment	Posttreatment
Blood pressure	124/84	120/82
Pulse	75	70
Respirations	12	12

4. Length of time for sedation procedure.
5. Length of time on recovery oxygen.
6. Statement of patient's recovery status and any postcare instructions given.
7. Summary of patient's response to nitrous oxide can be helpful for subsequent appointments.
8. An example of progress notes is shown in Box 35-4.

▪ POTENTIAL HAZARDS OF OCCUPATIONAL EXPOSURE

Chronic occupational exposure to nitrous oxide may have deleterious effects on health. Overexposure must be prevented.[6,7]

I. ISSUES OF OCCUPATIONAL EXPOSURE

A. Potential Health Problems

1. Reduced fertility with as little as 3 to 5 hours of unscavenged nitrous oxide exposure per week.[8]
2. Spontaneous abortion.[9]
3. Increased rate of neurologic, renal, and liver disease.[9]
4. Decreased mental performance, audiovisual ability, and manual dexterity.[6]

B. Recommended Exposure Levels

1. Consensus has not been reached on occupational exposure limits; there is currently no exposure standard.

2. National Institute of Occupational Safety and Health (NIOSH) recommends no more than 25 parts per million (ppm) during administration.

II. METHODS FOR MINIMIZING OCCUPATIONAL EXPOSURE

A. Use an effective scavenging system that can move 45 L/min of air.
B. Maintain equipment and inspect regularly for gas leaks, especially at the locations shown in Figure 35-1. Shut off and secure equipment at the end of each day's use.
C. Improve general air quality: introduce fresh air, use a nonrecycling air-conditioning system, or open a window. Vent the scavenger system gases outside the building and away from windows and air intakes.
D. Use an air sweep fan to direct nitrous oxide away from the clinicians' breathing zone; periodically monitor air quality in the clinicians' breathing zone.
E. Minimize patient conversations and mouth breathing; fit the nasal hood carefully to avoid leaks.
F. Set conservative limits on the duration and concentration of nitrous oxide use per patient.

▪ ADVANTAGES AND DISADVANTAGES OF CONSCIOUS SEDATION ANESTHESIA

I. ADVANTAGES

A. Both a mild analgesic and sedative: reduces patient's reaction to pain by raising pain threshold.
B. Increases relaxation and cooperation during treatment.
C. Reduces the gag reflex.
D. Very safe with few side effects and few medical contraindications.
E. Excellent for management of many medically compromised patients:
   1. Provides oxygen enrichment as well as stress reduction.
   2. Helps prevent emergencies because of anxiety and pain management.
F. Readily absorbed and excreted from the body; rapid onset and recovery from drug effect.
   1. Able to titrate to optimum level.
   2. Recovery complete so patient can be dismissed to return to normal activities.

G. Appointments less stressful for clinician because of relaxed, conscious, cooperative patient.

II. DISADVANTAGES

A. A low-potency analgesic drug.
1. Not effective with all patients because of low potency; does not block all perception.
2. Severely distressed or phobic patient may need a more potent drug or combination of drugs.
B. Patient must be able and willing to breathe through the nose.
C. Equipment and gases are expensive.
D. Use of poor techniques such as failure to titrate or use a scavenger system results in undesirable patient experiences and potential staff health risks.
E. Potential for recreational abuse by health professionals.
F. May stimulate sexual fantasies in some patients, and any resulting accusations can result in embarrassment, loss of reputation, and/or license.

■ LOCAL ANESTHESIA

Local anesthesia is the main modality for the management of dental pain. It blocks sensations, especially of pain, from teeth, soft tissues, and bone in the anesthetized area. Root instrumentation without discomfort requires a profound pulpal and periodontal tissue level of anesthesia.[10]

Dental hygiene treatment provided with the use of local anesthesia is a more comfortable and satisfying treatment for both the patient and clinician. Instrumentation can be comprehensive and definitive, and patient compliance can increase.

■ PHARMACOLOGY OF LOCAL ANESTHETICS

Local anesthetics are the most frequently used drugs for dental and dental hygiene treatment. They are safe when administered in the recommended manner and amounts.

I. CONTENTS OF A LOCAL ANESTHETIC CARTRIDGE

A dental cartridge is prefilled by the manufacturer to include the following:
A. *Amide anesthetic*: Blocks the transfer of ions across the nerve membrane, which stops the transmission of pain messages.
B. *Vasoconstrictor*: Constricts local blood vessels to offset the vasodilation caused by the amide anesthetic. Cartridges without vasoconstrictor are available.
C. *Antioxidant*: Preservative for the vasoconstrictor, usually sodium metabisulfite or sodium bisulfite.
D. *Sterile water*: Diluent.
E. *Sodium chloride*: Creates an isotonic match with the body.

II. ESTER AND AMIDE ANESTHETIC DRUGS

Dental local anesthetic drugs can be divided chemically into two major groups: esters and amides. The first dental anesthetic was procaine (Novocain), an ester, which has not been available in dental cartridges in the United States since 1996. Except for topicals, all currently used local anesthetic agents are amides. There are a number of available drugs in this group that are similar for safety and effectiveness.[11,12]

A. General Characteristics of Ester Anesthetics

1. Widely used in topical anesthetic agents.
2. Have a higher incidence of allergic reactions; are less effective and shorter acting compared with amides.
3. Metabolized in the blood plasma by the enzyme cholinesterase. The medical condition atypical plasma cholinesterase may result in the slow removal of the drug from the body.

B. General Characteristics of Amide Anesthetics

1. Extremely low incidence of allergic reactions.
2. Potential for toxicity or drug overdose make attention to detail in technique of administration and total drug dose critical.
3. Metabolized by the liver (see specific medical considerations, page 596).
4. Cause vasodilation of local blood vessels.

III. CHARACTERISTICS OF SPECIFIC SHORT- AND MEDIUM-ACTING AMIDE DRUGS

A. Lidocaine

1. Proprietary names include Xylocaine, Octocaine, Lignospan.
2. First amide and still most widely used dental anesthetic; also available as a topical.
3. Used with vasoconstrictor to give adequate working time.

B. Mepivacaine

1. Proprietary names include Carbocaine, Polocaine, Isocaine.
2. Causes less vasodilation than lidocaine; therefore, can be used for short procedures without vasoconstrictor.
3. Mepivacaine 3%, also called Mepivacaine Plain, is often the drug of choice when vasoconstrictors or their sulfite antioxidants are contraindicated.

C. Prilocaine

1. Proprietary names are Citanest Plain and Citanest Forte.
2. Metabolic by-products can cause transient methemoglobinemia, a condition that reduces the blood's oxygen-carrying capacity (see specific medical considerations, page 596)
3. Can be used without vasoconstrictor because it causes limited vasodilation.
4. When injected into tissues with limited vascularity, the duration of action is similar with and without vasoconstrictor. Example: inferior alveolar nerve block injection.

D. Articaine

1. Proprietary names are Septocaine, Septanest and Ultracaine.
2. Reported to diffuse through soft and hard tissues better than other amides.
3. Metabolic by-products can cause transient methemoglobinemia.
4. Metabolized primarily in plasma; has shorter half-life so reinjection may occur sooner.

IV. CHARACTERISTICS OF SPECIFIC LONG-ACTING AMIDE DRUGS

A. Bupivacaine

1. Proprietary name: Marcaine
2. Long-lasting anesthetic with an extended period of analgesia for postcare pain management.
3. May have delayed onset of action.

B. Etidocaine

1. Proprietary name: Duranest
2. Long-lasting anesthetic with an extended period of analgesia for postcare pain management.

V. VASOCONSTRICTORS

A. Reasons for Use

1. *Safety.* Potential for toxic reaction (overdose) to anesthetic is reduced by slowing the rate at which it enters circulation.
2. *Longevity.* Duration of anesthetic effect is increased.
3. *Effectiveness.* Depth and profoundness of anesthetic is increased.
4. *Hemostasis.* Only if drug is locally injected directly into the area.

B. Potential Risks With Use of Vasoconstrictors

1. Hypersensitivity to the drugs.
2. Medical problems (see specific medical considerations, page 596).
3. Drug interactions (see potential drug interactions, page 597).
4. Degree of risk to medically compromised patients, including those with heart disease, varies. Use of vasoconstrictors in low doses is considered safe.[13]

C. Drugs Used

1. *Epinephrine*
   a. Potent sympathomimetic amine.
   b. Used in low concentrations, usually 1:100,000 or 1:200,000.
   c. Maximum recommended doses (MRDs) for healthy patients and for medically compromised, especially those with cardiac disease, are given in Table 35-2.
2. *Levonordefrin* (Neo-Cobefren)
   a. Half as potent as equal doses of epinephrine and with less cardiac effect.
   b. Used at higher concentration (1:20,000) to accomplish adequate vasoconstriction.
   c. Higher doses may result in greater increase in blood pressure than epinephrine.
   d. Maximum recommended doses (MRDs) for healthy patients and for medically compromised, especially those with cardiac disease, are given in Table 35-2.

VI. CRITERIA FOR DRUG SELECTION

Amide local anesthetics are safe and effective when employed properly.[14]

    A. Length of time pain control is needed is a primary criterion for drug selection. Table 35-3 shows the typical duration of action for common local anesthetics.

■ TABLE 35-2 VASOCONSTRICTORS: CONCENTRATIONS AND MAXIMUM RECOMMENDED DOSE (MRD)

VASOCONSTRICTORS AND CONCENTRATIONS	MRD IN HEALTHY PATIENTS		MRD IN MEDICALLY COMPROMISED PATIENTS	
	MG/APPT	CARTRIDGES/APPT	MG/APPT	CARTRIDGES/APPT
Epinephrine				
1:50,000	Use not recommended		Use not recommended	
1:100,000 (0.018 mg/cart.)	0.2	10	0.04	2
1:200,000 (0.009 mg/cart.)	0.2	*	0.04	4
Levonordefrin				
1:20,000 (0.09 mg/cart.)	1.0	10	0.2	2

*Local anesthesia is the limiting drug.
Adapted from Biron, C.R.: Vasoconstrictors, *RDH, 13,* 40, May, 1993.

■ TABLE 35-3 DURATION OF ACTION OF COMMON LOCAL ANESTHETICS

DRUG NAME	DURATION OF ACTION	
GENERIC NAME	SOFT TISSUE	PULPAL
Short Acting		
3% mepivacaine	2–3 hr	Infiltration: 20 min Block: 40 min
4% prilocaine	Infiltration: 1½ hr	Infiltration: 10 min
Medium Acting		
2% lidocaine w/epinephrine 1:100,000	3–5 hr	60 min
2% mepivacaine w/levonordefrin 1:20,000x	3–5 hr	60–90 min
4% prilocaine	Block: 2–4 hr	Block: 60 min
4% prilocaine w/epinephrine 1:200,000	3–8 hr	60–90 min
4% articaine w/epinephrine 1:100,000	3–6 hr	60–75 min
Long Acting		
0.5% bupivacaine w/epinephrine 1:200,000	4–9+ hr	90–180 min
1.5% etidocaine w/epinephrine 1:200,000	4–9 hr	90–180 min

Adapted from Malamed, S.F.: *Handbook of Local Anesthesia,* 4th ed. St. Louis, Mosby, 1997, pp. 55–67.

B. Medical status of the patient.
C. Potential for prolonged discomfort after treatment.
D. Potential for self-inflicted injury before anesthetic wears off.

■ INDICATIONS FOR LOCAL ANESTHESIA

Local anesthesia is indicated for treatment that has the potential to cause discomfort or pain. Anesthesia prevents both the patient and the clinician from the anticipation of discomfort, thus allowing both to relax and to make treatment comfortable.

I. DENTAL HYGIENE PROCEDURES

A. Scaling and root planing in areas with probing depths of 4 mm or greater.
B. Extensive instrumentation with either manual or power-driven instruments.
C. Treatment in areas of challenging pocket topography, furcations, or other difficult root anatomy.
D. Instrumentation of sensitive root surfaces.
E. Instrumentation in areas of painful, inflamed soft tissue.
F. Treatments that involve soft tissue manipulation.
   1. Gingival curettage.
   2. Suture removal.
   3. Removal of subgingival overhang.
G. Treatment in areas of excessive hemorrhage.

II. PATIENT FACTORS

A. Extent of patient's disease and deposits directly influence the extent or rigor of the needed treatment.
B. Patient's pain reaction or pain threshold.

▪ PATIENT ASSESSMENT

The goal of patient assessment is to ensure an effective and safe local anesthesia experience. Pretreatment evaluation is the first and most important step for avoiding a medical emergency.

I. SOURCES OF INFORMATION FOR COMPLETE PREANESTHETIC ASSESSMENT

A. Vital signs.
B. Medical history; ASA status (Table 21-1, page 354).
C. Current medications.
D. Emotional status/anxiety level.
E. Dental history related to local anesthesia.
F. Chief complaint and presence of inflammation.

II. TREATMENT OPTIONS BASED ON ASSESSMENT FINDINGS

Amide local anesthetics and the small amount of vasoconstrictor normally incorporated into the dental anesthetic cartridge can be administered safely to almost all patients.

A. Use local anesthetic without special precaution.
B. Avoid use of local anesthetic or of a specific local anesthetic because of high medical risk.
C. Select an alternative drug that will minimize or avoid risk.
D. Limit the dose of drug given at any specific appointment.
E. Use local anesthesia combined with maximum stress management; use in combination with nitrous oxide–oxygen conscious sedation.
F. Seek medical intervention, consult, or additional testing before proceeding.
G. Increase drug dose for an infiltration or give block or regional injections rather than infiltration in inflamed tissue as low pH inhibits drug distribution and effectiveness.

III. GENERAL MEDICAL CONSIDERATIONS

A. ASA IV patients and some ASA III patients (especially those who are anxious about injections) may not have the functional reserve to tolerate the injection procedure and the subsequent treatment (ASA, Table 21-1).
B. Patients who are too medically compromised for local anesthesia may not be appropriate for any elective dental therapy.

C. When performing a risk-benefit analysis for use of local anesthesia, consider the potential for medical distress that can result from inadequate pain control.
D. Seek a medical consult when there is doubt about the safety of a local anesthetic choice.

IV. SPECIFIC MEDICAL CONSIDERATIONS

Most contraindications are relative, meaning that a case-specific evaluation needs to focus on the severity of the condition and treatment needs.

A. Allergy

1. *Amide anesthetics.* True allergy is rare. If confirmed, avoid all amide anesthetics.
2. *Ester anesthetics.* Allergy is fairly common. If confirmed, avoid all ester anesthetics, including topical anesthetics; and para-aminobenzoic acid (PABA) preservatives, such as methylparaben.
3. *Bisulfites.* Sodium metabisulfite, acetone sodium bisulfite, and sodium or potassium bisulfite are used as the preservatives for the vasoconstrictor. If allergy is known, avoid anesthetics containing vasoconstrictors.

B. Hyperthyroidism

1. *Uncontrolled:* Avoid vasoconstrictor.
2. *Controlled:* Normal local anesthesia.

C. Impaired Liver or Kidney Function

1. Only severe impairment is clinically relevant.
2. Half-life of amide anesthetic could be prolonged, which could result in overdose.

D. Malignant Hyperthermia

1. Trend is to consider amide anesthetics used in dentistry as safe.
2. Medical consult is indicated as this could be a life-threatening condition.

E. Methemoglobinemia

1. A congenital or acquired condition; hemoglobin molecule is converted to methemoglobin, which has less oxygen-carrying capacity. A cyanosis-like state may develop if a high percentage of molecules convert.
2. Prilocaine and articaine cause a dose-related methemoglobinemia. Avoid their use in patients with a preexisting condition.

F. Heart Failure

1. Reduced circulation resulting from heart failure slows elimination of amide anesthetic, which increases potential for anesthetic overdose.
2. Patient is stress intolerant: pain and anxiety must be carefully managed. Consider use of nitrous oxide–oxygen sedation alone or in combination with local anesthesia.

G. Coronary Disease, Heart Attack, Recent Heart Surgery, Angina Pectoris, Hypertension, and Stroke

1. Concern is for use and amount of vasoconstrictor.
2. Decision based on patient ASA category, treatment, and treatment time needs; possible medical consultation.
3. Usual treatment decision is to limit total amount of vasoconstrictor or, in some cases, to eliminate its use.

H. Hemophilia

1. Excessive bleeding may result from needle contact with blood vessel.
2. Decision, based on severity of condition, can range from treatment in hospital to avoiding injections into highly vascularized areas (example: the posterior superior alveolar [PSA]).

I. Pregnancy

1. Local anesthetic and vasoconstrictors are not teratogens and may be safely administered.
2. It is prudent practice to limit any elective drug administration, especially during the first trimester.

J. Potential Drug Interactions

All medications reported in a patient's medical history need to be checked for potential drug interactions before selecting the pain control plan. Following are examples of frequently prescribed or otherwise used drugs that interact with an anesthetic or a vasoconstrictor. Precaution is needed.
1. Cimetidine and lidocaine.
2. Nonselective beta blockers and vasoconstrictors.
3. Tricyclic antidepressants and vasoconstrictors.
4. Phenothiazines and vasoconstrictors.
5. Cocaine and vasoconstrictors.

▪ ARMAMENTARIUM FOR LOCAL ANESTHESIA

I. SYRINGE

A. Design Features

1. Durable metal or plastic can be sterilized and reused with the addition of a new needle and cartridge.
2. Single-use, disposable syringes have safety features to prevent inadvertent needle stick after use.
3. Provide good visibility of the cartridge.

B. Promote Easy Aspiration

1. Manual aspiration is the traditional design.
2. Self-aspirating syringe works well for small hands.

II. NEEDLE

A. Disposable

Intended for single patient use.

B. Parts and Lengths of the Needle (Figure 35-2)

1. *Long needle*: Approximately 1 1/2 inches or 40 mm.
2. *Short needle*: Approximately 1 inch or 25 mm. Used for most injections.
3. *Ultra-short needle*: Approximately ½ inch or 12 mm.

C. Gauge or Needle Diameter

1. *Size*: Ranked from largest to smallest, 25-, 27-, and 30-gauge needles are used in dentistry.
2. *Rigidity*: 25-gauge needles are stiffer and deflect less as they penetrate the tissue. They are preferred for accuracy when a long needle is needed.
3. *Aspiration*: Larger-gauge needles provide easier and more accurate aspiration.

III. CARTRIDGE OR CARPULE

A. Volume: 1.8 mL of solution in the United States.
B. Storage
  1. Store at cool room temperature and away from the light.
  2. Do not store in an alcohol or disinfectant solution.

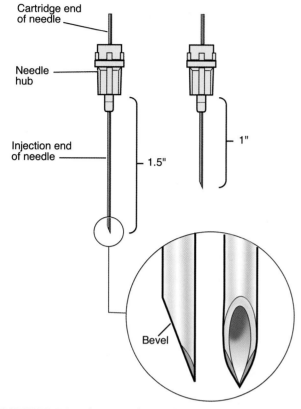

■ FIGURE 35-2 The Dental Anesthetic Needle. Dental needles are available in two lengths, *long* and *short.* Lengths vary slightly between manufacturers. The components of the needle are *cartridge end,* which penetrates the rubber diaphragm of the dental cartridge; *hub,* which attaches the needle to the syringe (made of plastic or metal); *injection end* or shank or shaft, which penetrates the oral tissue so that anesthetic solution is deposited at the desired site. **INSERT:** Shows an enlargement of the tip of the needle with sharp terminus and bevel. When giving an injection, the needle is oriented so that the bevel is parallel to the bone to help prevent the needle from catching the periosteum, the sensitive covering over the bone.

C. Label each cartridge: drug, manufacturer, and expiration date information.

D. Color coding: local anesthetic drug is identified by color on cartridge. Color codes are shown in Box 35-5.

IV. ADDITIONAL ARMAMENTARIUM

A. Topical antiseptic to prevent postinjection infections.

B. Topical anesthetic to increase patient comfort.

C. Cotton gauze to wipe the injection site to clean, dry, and remove the topical anesthetic. May also be used to improve grasp for lip or cheek retraction.

BOX 35-5 Anesthesia Color Code

Anesthesia color codes

Newly mandated uniform system for local anesthesia cartridges bearing the ADA Seal of Acceptance.

PRODUCT	COLOR
Lidocaine 2% with Epinephrine 1:100,000	
Lidocaine 2% with Epinephrine 1:50,000	
Lidocaine Plain	
Mepivacaine 2% with Levonordefrin 1:20,000	
Mepivacaine 3% Plain	
Prilocaine 4% with Epinephrine 1:200,000	
Prilocaine 4% Plain	
Bupivacaine 0.5% with Epinephrine 1:200,000	
Articaine 4% with Epinephrine 1:100,000	

D. Needle recapping device, if self-recapping needle is not used.

E. Sharps disposal system to meet safe practice standards for used needle disposal.

V. SEQUENCE OF SYRINGE ASSEMBLY

Figure 35-3 illustrates the assembly of the conventional anesthetic syringe; sequence makes the attachment between the harpoon and rubber stopper easier without applying excess force to the glass cartridge.

VI. COMPUTER-CONTROLLED ANESTHESIA DELIVERY SYSTEM (COMPUDENT™)

A. Pressure, volume, and rate of speed of local anesthetic delivery are precisely regulated by a computer.

B. Device includes a light, pen-like hand piece attached to a computer-controlled, 2-speed motor that is activated by a foot control. Any gauge Luer-lock needle and standard anesthetic cartridge may be used.

C. Slow, controlled delivery of anesthesia solution promotes more comfortable injections, especially

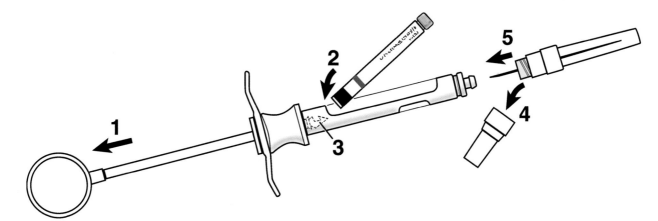

■ **FIGURE 35-3 Sequence for Assembling a Breech-Loading Aspirating Syringe. 1.** Pull back on thumb ring. **2.** Insert anesthetic cartridge, rubber stopper end first, toward the thumb ring, then the diaphragm end toward the needle opening. **3.** Set harpoon and test for lock into rubber stopper. **4.** Remove safety cap from needle. **5.** Screw needle onto the syringe.

palatal and periodontal ligament (PDL) injections; allows unique injections, the anterior middle superior alveolar (AMSA) and the palatal anterior superior alveolar (P-ASA), as well as all traditional dental injections.

■ CLINICAL PROCEDURES FOR LOCAL ANESTHETIC ADMINISTRATION

Administer the most comfortable injections possible by using gentle tissue manipulation, careful needle penetration, slow deposition of solution, and good patient communication.

I. INJECTION(S) SELECTION

A. Basic Injections

Table 35-4 lists injections with hard and soft tissues anesthetized, and the branches of the trigeminal nerve involved.

B. Areas Anesthetized: Shown in Figure 35-4

C. Steps and Procedures

Box 35-6 outlines the sequence and procedures for the administration of local anesthesia.

II. ASPIRATION

A. Purpose

To determine that the tip of the needle is not within a blood vessel. An anesthetic solution must be deposited extravascularly to be effective and to prevent toxicity.

B. When to Aspirate

*   Before depositing anesthetic solution.
*   Periodically throughout injection.

C. Procedure

1. Hold the needle steady so that the tip does not change position.
2. Create negative pressure within the dental cartridge.
    a. *Standard harpoon-style syringe.* Pull back gently on the thumb ring. Movement is small, only 1 to 2 mm.
    b. *Self-aspirating syringe.* Stop applying positive pressure to the thumb ring.
3. Rotate the syringe by a quarter turn and repeat aspiration (prevent a false negative).

D. Interpretation

Any fluid at the tip of the needle will be drawn into the cartridge. If the tip of the needle is in an artery or vein, blood will become visible; it may only be a small amount at the needle end of the cartridge.
1. *Negative aspiration.* No blood in cartridge; proceed with injection.
2. *Positive aspiration.* Blood in the cartridge.
    a. A small amount of blood with most of the cartridge clear: move to a new location and reaspirate.
    b. Cartridge generally bloody: withdraw needle, replace cartridge, and repeat injection.

■ TABLE 35-4 COMMON LOCAL ANESTHETIC INJECTIONS FOR DENTAL HYGIENE PROCEDURES

INJECTION	TISSUES ANESTHETIZED	BRANCH OF THE TRIGEMINAL NERVE
Maxillary Arch		**Maxillary Division**
Posterior superior alveolar (PSA)	*Hard tissue*: second and third molars; first molar excluding mesiobuccal root; associated supporting structures	Posterior superior alveolar
	Soft tissue: overlying facial tissues	
Middle superior alveolar (MSA)	*Hard tissue*: first and second premolars, mesiobuccal root of first molar, and associated supporting structures	Middle superior alveolar
	Soft tissue: overlying facial tissues	
Anterior superior alveolar (ASA)	*Hard tissue*: canine and incisors and associated supporting structures	Anterior superior alveolar
	Soft tissue: overlying facial tissues and lip	
Infraorbital (IO)	*Hard tissue*: premolars, canine, incisors, and associated supporting structures	Infraorbital (includes both anterior and middle superior alveolar)
	Soft tissue: overlying facial tissues, cheek, and lip	
Greater palatine (GP)	*Hard tissue*: none	Greater palatine
	Soft tissue: palatal tissue from teeth to midline from distal of third molar to canine	
Nasopalatine (NP)	*Hard tissue*: none	Nasopalatine
	Soft tissue: palatal tissues from left canine to right canine	
Infiltration (Inf)	*Hard tissue*: individual teeth associated supporting structures	Individual terminal branches
	Soft tissue: facial tissue overlying individual teeth	
Mandibular Arch		
Long buccal (LB)	*Hard tissue*: none	Buccal (long buccal)
	Soft tissue: facial tissue of molars	
Inferior alveolar with lingual (mandibular block) (IA)	*Hard tissue*: molars, premolars, canine, and incisors to midline, as well as associated supporting structures	Inferior alveolar (includes dental, mental, and incisive branches)
	Soft tissue: facial tissue anterior to mental foramen, including lip	
	Hard tissue: none	Lingual
	Soft tissue: lingual tissue from molar to midline, including anterior two thirds of tongue; floor of mouth	
Gow-Gates technique (GG)	*Hard tissue*: mandibular teeth to midline; body of mandible; inferior portion of ramus	Third division nerve block (includes inferior alveolar, mental, incisive, lingual, mylohyoid, auriculotemporal, and buccal nerves)
	Soft tissue: facial and lingual tissue; anterior two thirds of tongue and floor of mouth; skin over the zygoma; posterior portion of the cheek and temporal regions	

■ TABLE 35-4 COMMON LOCAL ANESTHETIC INJECTIONS FOR DENTAL HYGIENE PROCEDURES (Continued)		
Mental and incisive (M/I)	*Hard tissue*: premolars, canine, incisors, and associated supporting structures	Mental and incisive branch of inferior alveolar
	Soft tissue: facial tissue and lip anterior to mental foramen	
Either Arch		
Interpapillary	*Hard tissue*: none	Free nerve endings
	Soft tissue: individual papilla	
Periodontal ligament (PDL)	*Hard tissue*: individual tooth	Terminal nerve endings
	Soft tissue: adjacent	

Adapted from Stach, D.J.: Pain and Pain Control: Topical and Local Anesthesia, in Woodall, I.R.: *Comprehensive Dental Hygiene Care,* 4th ed. St. Louis, Mosby, 1993, p. 688.

III. SHARPS MANAGEMENT[15-17]

A. Needle Recapping

1. Needles with engineered sharps injury protection are preferred, such as a self-sheathing safety needle or safety syringe. An example of a devise that meets these requirements is shown in Figure 35-5.

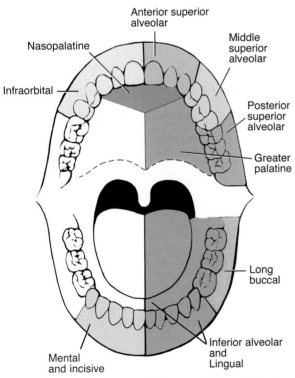

■ **FIGURE 35-4 Diagrammatic Representation of Teeth and Soft Tissues Anesthetized by Common Dental Injections.**

2. Also acceptable:
   - One-handed "scoop" technique (Figure 35-6A)
   - Mechanical device to hold the needle sheath (Figure 35-6B)

B. No Manipulation

Do not manipulate needles; do not bend, break, or shear.

C. Needle Removal

Disposal containers for contaminated sharps should be readily accessible and located as close as possible to the area of use.

IV. TREATMENT RECORD: ANESTHESIA ENTRY

Goal is to have a clear but brief medical/legal record.

A. Medical Status and Vital Signs

B. Choice of Injection(s)

1. Reason for use of anesthesia if not otherwise clear.
2. Injection(s) given with location. Examples: (1) infiltration over no. 8; (2) right inferior alveolar.

C. Drug

1. Topical, local anesthetic and vasoconstrictor.
2. Concentration of drugs. Example: 2% lidocaine with 1:100,000 epinephrine.
3. Dose can be recorded in cartridges, milliliters, or milligrams.

BOX 35-6 Steps in the Administration of Local Anesthesia

1. Assess patient medical status, treatment, and pain control needs in order to select injection(s) and anesthetic drug.

2. Assemble and test the syringe set-up (Figure 35-3).

   a. Orient the needle so that the bevel will be toward the bone during the injection.

   b. Test the assembled syringe.

3. Position patient for good visibility and to prevent syncope with head level with or lower than heart.

4. Use topical anesthetic.

   a. Apply topical to dry tissue at the injection site for the appropriate time. For benzocaine 1 to 2 minutes is optimal.

   b. Remove residual topical anesthetic.

5. Wipe injection site with gauze to dry and clean surface bacteria, saliva, and topical anesthetic from the area before injection.

6. Retract the lip or cheek for good visibility; stretch the tissue for easier needle penetration.

7. Keep the syringe out of the patient's sight.

8. Establish a fulcrum or hand rest for stability during the injection.

9. Insert the needle into the tissue and gently advance to desired site for administration of anesthetic.

10. Aspirate before depositing solution; reaspirate as needed throughout procedure.

11. Deposit the anesthetic solution slowly (1 to 2 min for full cartridge) to prevent patient discomfort and to reduce potential for a toxic reaction.

12. Withdraw the needle carefully at the completion of the injection, and recap the needle using a safe technique.

13. Remain with and observe the patient. Adverse drug reactions are most likely to occur during or shortly after the injection.

14. Record injection information in patient chart.

15. Use positive, supportive communication with the patient throughout the procedure.

D. Effects/Reactions

1. Effect or profoundness of anesthesia; anesthetic duration if unusual.
2. Patient acceptance or response, if significant.
3. Adverse drug reaction, if any.

E. Comments as Appropriate

1. Instructions to patient.
2. Atypical occurrence or finding; positive aspiration.
3. Future alert or plan.

F. Example of Progress Notes

An example of progress notes is shown in Box 35-7.

G. Abbreviations

May be used and are acceptable when they are clearly understood and standardized in the dental practice or clinic.

▪ POTENTIAL ADVERSE REACTIONS TO LOCAL ANESTHESIA PROCEDURES

Local anesthetics, like all drugs, have both desirable and potentially undesirable effects. Additional information on managing anesthetic reactions is listed in Table 66-4.

I. ADVERSE DRUG REACTIONS

A. Toxic Drug Overdose

1. Overdose is the most common adverse drug reaction with amide anesthetics.
2. Occurs when the circulating blood level of the drug becomes too high and reaches a toxic level for the individual.
3. Typical causes of overdose.

   a. *Intravascular injection*: Prevented by aspiration prior to deposition of the anesthetic drug.

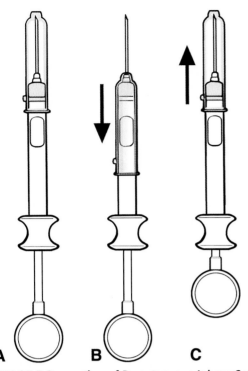

■ **FIGURE 35-5 Prevention of Percutaneous Injury: Self-sheathing Safety Needle. (A)** Syringe with protective sheath over the needle. **(B)** As the injection is made, the sheath slides back. **(C)** After injection, the sheath returns to cover the needle and protect the clinician during disposal.

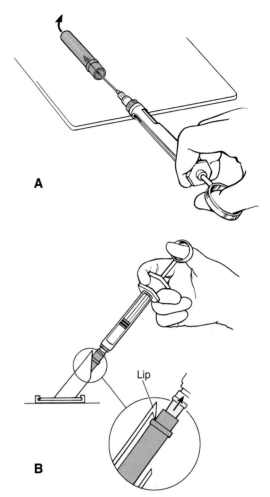

■ **FIGURE 35-6 Prevention of Percutaneous Injury: Alternative Needle Recapping Methods.** One-handed recapping or recapping with a safety mechanical device to hold the needle sheath is acceptable. **(A)** "Scoop" technique. Cap is placed on the tray and the needle is guided into it. **(B)** Example of commercially available holder for cap. Device is fastened to the tray, and cap is removed and recapped by directing the needle into the cap holder. Needles must be discarded in a puncture-resistant container.

    b. *Excessive total drug dose*: Affected by drug volumes; drug choice; patient's lean weight, age, physical/medical status.

    c. *Rapid absorption into the circulatory system*: Affected by rate of injection, presence or absence of a vasoconstrictor, or vascularity of injection site.

    d. *Reduced elimination and/or metabolism of drug*: Reduced kidney or liver function or reduced circulation as a result of congestive heart failure may reduce the rate at which the drug is removed from circulation.

B. Allergy

1. *Incidence*: Although often reported, incidence is rare with amide drugs. (Review allergy under specific medical considerations [page 596].)

2. *Definition*: Allergy is a hypersensitive state where a subsequent exposure to an allergen results in an exaggerated response. In local anesthesia, the most common allergens are the bisulfite antioxidant or ester topical anesthetic.

3. *Symptoms*: Response may range from mild, such as localized erythema or itching, to life threatening,

---

BOX 35-7 Example Progress Notes: Local Anesthesia

Nonsignificant medical history, BP 120/80, pulse 68. Patient reported general root sensitivity. For periodontal debridement of max. right quadrant, administered 3.6 ml 2% lidocaine (lido) with epinephrine (epi) 1:100,000 for right anterior superior alveolar (ASA), middle superior alveolar (MSA), posterior superior alveolar (PSA), inferior alveolar (IA). Benzocaine topical. Anesthesia profound; procedure well tolerated.

such as generalized anaphylaxis or laryngeal edema.

4. *Onset*: May range from a few seconds to many hours.

5. *Management*: Table 66-4 presents procedures for managing an allergic reaction.

II. PSYCHOGENIC REACTIONS

A. Cause

Anxiety response to the injection procedure.

B. Symptoms

1. Vasodepressor syncope (fainting) and hyperventilation are most common.

2. Symptoms can be highly varied and may mimic drug reactions or other medical conditions.

3. Reactions reported by patients as allergies are often psychogenic in nature.

III. LOCAL COMPLICATIONS

The problems and symptoms vary with each situation.

A. Symptoms

1. *Trismus*: Spasm of the jaw muscles that restricts opening or makes it uncomfortable.

2. *Hematoma* (bruise): Blood from a breached artery or vein leaks into the surrounding tissue.

3. *Paresthesia*: Trauma to nerve results in persistent anesthesia, usually lasting a few days to weeks.

4. *Epithelial desquamation* (tissue sloughing): May follow prolonged application of topical anesthetic.

B. Primary Prevention

Use of excellent injection technique.

▪ ADVANTAGES AND DISADVANTAGES OF LOCAL ANESTHESIA

I. ADVANTAGES

A. Patient experiences no pain or discomfort during treatment procedure.

B. Clinician has increased confidence to provide complete treatment when the patient is pain free.

C. Local effect results in loss of sensation in area of treatment without a change in level of consciousness or patient cooperation.

D. Completely reversible without residual side effects.

E. Rapid onset of action.

F. Adequate duration of clinical action that is reasonably predictable and that can be varied by choice of commercially available drugs.

G. Relatively free of allergic reactions.

H. Hemostasis if injected directly into area of desired hemorrhage control.

II. DISADVANTAGES

A. Anticipating and receiving dental injections may cause high anxiety for patient. Effects may include:
1. Need for special anxiety reduction technique.
2. Undesirable psychogenic reactions.
3. Avoidance of needed care.

B. Significant potential exists for toxicity (overdose) with amide drugs.

C. There are systemic side effects from both the local anesthetic drug and vasoconstrictor.

D. Where state law or skill levels preclude the dental hygienist from administering local anesthesia, it may be inconvenient or time consuming for the dentist to provide the injections.

▪ TOPICAL ANESTHESIA

A topical anesthetic is a drug applied directly to the surface of the mucous membrane to produce a loss of sensation. A topical anesthetic is used with varying degrees of success for short-duration desensitization of the gingiva, but it does not influence sensations in the teeth. It is not a substitute for local anesthetic administered by injection.

Topical anesthetic applied to the tissue using the transoral patch method provides a profound level of anesthesia to the soft tissues. It may provide slight loss of sensation to the teeth as well.

I. INDICATIONS FOR USE

A topical anesthetic can be used conservatively for selected dental hygiene and dental services, including the following:

A. Preparation for local anesthesia injection.

B. Prevention of gagging in radiographic techniques and impression taking.

C. Temporary relief of pain from localized diseased areas, such as oral ulcers, wounds, or inflammation.

D. During instrumentation for probing and scaling. When discomfort involves the teeth as well as gingiva, a local anesthetic usually is indicated.

E. Suture removal.

II. ACTION OF A TOPICAL ANESTHETIC

A. Purpose

The purpose of a topical anesthetic is to desensitize the mucous membrane by anesthetizing the terminal nerve endings. The superficial anesthesia produced is related to the amount of absorption of the drug by the tissue.

B. Absorption of Drug

1. Varies with:
   - Thickness of stratified squamous epithelial covering.
   - Degree of keratinization.
2. Tissue absorption
   - Highly resistant: skin, lips, palatal mucosa.
   - Absorb slowly: attached gingiva, buccal mucosa.
   - Prompt absorption: tissue without keratinization, such as vestibular mucosa or over the pterygomandibular space.

III. AGENTS USED IN SURFACE ANESTHETIC PREPARATIONS

Table 35-5 provides onset and duration of topical anesthetics.

A. Benzocaine or Ethyl Aminobenzoate (Ester Type)

1. Used in 20% formulation; most widely used topical agent.
2. Available as liquid, gel, ointment, and spray.
3. Not readily absorbed into circulation; potential for toxicity is minimal.
4. May cause allergic reaction, especially with prolonged or repeated application.

B. Tetracaine Hydrochloride (Ester Type)

1. Available as part of a combination of drugs in liquid, gel, and controlled-dose spray.

2. Most toxic of the dental topical anesthetics; rapidly absorbed.

C. Lidocaine and Lidocaine Hydrochloride (Amide Type)

1. The only amide used as a topical.
2. Available in ointment and transoral patch.
3. Toxicity unlikely from topical alone but would be additive with other amide anesthetics.

D. Lidocaine: Transoral Patch

1. A delivery system that uses a bioadhesive patch to improve the duration of contact between the topical and oral soft tissue.
2. Provides profound soft tissue anesthesia as well as minimal pulpal anesthesia in some cases.

▪ APPLICATION OF TOPICAL ANESTHETIC

I. PATIENT PREPARATION

A. Consult history and other records for pertinent information concerning a patient's previous experiences with anesthetics. A patient with an allergy to a local anesthetic may also be allergic to a topical anesthetic.

B. Determine the most appropriate anesthetic agent and method of application.

C. Explain purpose and anticipated effect to the patient.

II. APPLICATION TECHNIQUES

Several application techniques are available. Not all methods are applicable to all products. Select the most appropriate method from the following:

▪ TABLE 35-5 TOPICAL ANESTHETIC APPLICATION TIMES

DRUG	INITIAL ONSET	OPTIMUM APPLICATION*	DURATION
Benzocaine	30 sec	1–2 min	5–15 min
Tetracaine (combined with other drugs)	2 min		20–60 min
Lidocaine ointment	1–2 min	3–5 min	15 min
Lidocaine transoral patch	2½–5 min	Varies by procedure** (maximum 15 min after application)	45 min (after 15-min application)

*Optimum depth and intensity.
**See application technique transoral patch (see text).

Everyday Ethics

(?) Mr. Denver, in for a dental hygiene appointment, stated that he has not been to a dental office for the past 5 years because he is fearful of oral treatment owing to past painful experiences. Oral examination revealed bleeding on probing, generalized 5- to 6-mm pockets, and heavy biofilm and calculus deposits. Proposed treatment is four appointments for periodontal debridement with patient instruction, followed by a reevaluation.

Questions for Consideration

1. What anxiety and pain management methods could be used for this patient, and which methods are legal for a dental hygienist to administer in your state or province?

2. What are the ethical issues of providing treatment that would predictably cause pain without at least offering adequate pain management?

3. Is the "standard of care" for pain management different if a dentist or a dental hygienist provides the deep scaling? Explain.

A. Surface Application

1. May be used with liquid, gel, or ointment formulations of any of the available topical agents.
2. Topical is applied with a cotton-tipped swab or cotton roll.

✔ Factors To Teach The Patient

I. NITROUS OXIDE–OXYGEN CONSCIOUS SEDATION

- Inform the clinician if the sedation becomes too strong or is too weak so that adjustments can be made. The level of sedation should be adjusted individually for optimum relaxation and comfort.

- The gas will not result in unusual or undesirable behavior; the patient will maintain control of all personal actions.

- Eat normally before treatment; avoid fasting or heavy meals.

II. LOCAL AND TOPICAL ANESTHESIA

- Be careful not to bite lip, cheek, or tongue while tissues are without normal sensations. Warn and watch children to prevent injury. Do not test anesthesia by biting the lip.

- Avoid chewing hard foods and avoid hot food and drinks until normal sensation has returned.

3. Time before becoming effective varies with the drug used.
4. After application, excess topical is removed by rinsing or gentle wiping.

B. Aerosol Spray

1. Prevent inhalation by avoiding spray preparations when another method would be as effective. A spray must never be directed toward the throat.
2. Use metered- or controlled-dose spray dispensers to prevent inadvertent overdose.

C. Transoral Patch[18]

1. Air dry the tissue for 30 seconds, apply the patch, and hold in place with firm finger pressure for an additional 30 seconds.
2. Apply for 5 to 10 minutes prior to most procedures; may be left in place for up to 15 minutes. Suggested application times for typical procedures are:
   a. 5 minutes for most injections.
   b. 8 to 10 minutes for palatal injections.
   c. 15 minutes for most instrumentation (may be able to begin after 5 minutes).
3. Test tissue to confirm level of anesthesia after an appropriate application time. If adequate, remove the patch.
   a. Periodontal instrumentation may be started while the patch is in place if anesthesia is adequate; remove after 15 minutes.
   b. Injections should not be given through a patch.
4. Typical patch placement for scaling of the mandibular incisors is shown in Figure 35-7.

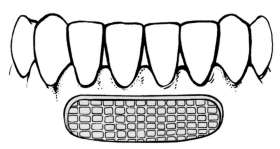

■ **FIGURE 35-7 Transoral Lidocaine Patch Placement.** In this example, for topical anesthesia to the mandibular incisors and facial tissues, patch is placed over the roots of the incisors with the upper edge 2 to 4 mm apical to the free gingival margin. Patch may be left in place during scaling and root planing for up to 15 minutes.

III. COMPLETION OF TOPICAL ANESTHETIC APPLICATION

A. Wait appropriate length of time for anesthetic to take effect before proceeding.

B. Limit drug exposure.

   1. Apply only to the area of need.

   2. Use the smallest effective amount.

   3. Remove residual drug after application time.

C. Apply to a limited area at a time when using a drug with a short duration of action for a long procedure such as scaling.

D. Record topical anesthetic drug information in the patient's record.

REFERENCES

1. **Dionne**, R.A., Phero, J.C., and Becker, D.E.: *Management of Pain and Anxiety in the Dental Office.* Philadelphia, W.B. Saunders Co, 2002, p. 27.

2. **Malamed**, S.F.: *Sedation: A Guide to Patient Management,* 4th ed. St. Louis, Mosby, 2003, p. 198.

3. **Berthold**, M.: Safety Alert: Nitrous Oxide. *ADA News, 33,* 20, May 6, 2002.

4. **Malamed:** op. cit., pp. 191–192.

5. **Malamed:** op. cit., pp. 253–254.

6. **NIOSH:** *Alert: Controlling Exposures to Nitrous Oxide During Anesthetic Administration.* (NIOSH Publication No.94-100). Cincinnati, U.S. Department of Health, Education, and Welfare, Public Health Service, Centers for Disease Control, National Institute for Occupational Safety and Health, 1994, pp. 1–11.

7. **ADA Council on Scientific Affairs, ADA Council on Dental Practice:** Nitrous Oxide in the Dental Office, *J. Am. Dent. Assoc., 128,* 364, March, 1997.

8. **Rowland**, A.S., Baird, D.D., Weinberg, C.R., Shore, D.L., Shy, C.M., and Wilcox, A.J.: Reduced Fertility Among Women Employed as Dental Assistants Exposed to High Levels of Nitrous Oxide, *N. Engl. J. Med., 327,* 993, October 1, 1992.

9. **Cohen**, E.N., Gift, H.C., Brown, B.W., Greenfield, W., Wu, M.L., Jones, T.W., Whitcher, C.E., Driscoll, E.J., and Brodsky, J.B.: Occupational Disease in Dentistry and Chronic Exposure to Trace Anesthetic Gases, *J. Am. Dent. Assoc., 101,* 21, July, 1980.

10. **Sisty-LePeau**, N., Nielson-Thompson, N., and Lutjen, D.: Use, Need and Desire for Pain Control Procedures by Iowa Hygienists, *J. Dent. Hyg., 66,* 137, March, 1992.

11. **Malamed**, S.F.: *Handbook of Local Anesthesia,* 4th ed. St. Louis, Mosby, 1997, pp. 37–67.

12. **Requa-Clark**, B.S. and Holroyd, S.V.: *Applied Pharmacology for the Dental Hygienist,* 4th ed. St. Louis, Mosby, 2000, pp. 222–225.

13. **Jastak**, J.T., Yagiela, J.A., and Donaldson, D.: *Local Anesthesia of the Oral Cavity,* Philadelphia, W.B. Saunders Co., 1995, pp. 69–78.

14. **Malamed**, S.F., Sykes, P., Kubota, Y., Matsuura, H., and Lipp, M.: Local Anesthesia: A Review, *Anesth. Pain Control Dent., 1,* 11, Winter, 1992.

15. **United States Occupational Safety and Health Administration:** Rules and Regulations, *Fed. Reg., 56,* 64175, December 6, 1991.

16. **United States Occupational Safety and Health Administration:** Rules and Regulations, *Fed. Reg., 66,* 5317, January 18, 2001.

17. **Organization for Safety and Asepsis Procedures:** Devices With Sharps Safety Features, *Infect. Control Practice, 1,* 1, November, 2002.

18. **Noven Pharmaceuticals, Inc.,** Miami, Fla, 33186.

SUGGESTED READINGS

Bowen, D.M. and Paarmann, C.S.: Use of Pain Control Modalities, in Hodges, K.O.: *Concepts in Nonsurgical Periodontal Therapy.* New York, Delmar Publishers, 1997, pp. 227–252.

Dionne, R.A., Gordon, S.M., McCullagh, L.M., and Phero, J.C.: Assessing the Need for Anesthesia and Sedation in the General Population, *J. Am. Dent. Assoc., 129,* 167, February, 1998.

Gadbury-Amyot, C.C., Overman, P.R., Carter-Hanson, C., and Mayberry, W.: An Investigation of Dental Hygiene Treatment Fear. *J. Dent. Hyg., 70,* 115, May–June, 1996.

Karadottir, H., Lenoir, L., Barbierato, B., Bogle, M., Riggs, M., Sigurdsson, T., Crigger, M., and Egelberg, J.: Pain Experience by Patients During Periodontal Maintenance Treatment, *J. Periodontol., 73,* 536, May, 2002.

McCarthy, F.M., Pallasch, T.J., and Gates, R.: Documenting Safe Treatment of the Medical-Risk Patient, *J. Am. Dent. Assoc., 119,* 383, September, 1989.

Milgrom, P., Coldwell, S.E., Getz, T., Weinstein, P., and Ramsay, D.S.: Four Dimensions of Fear of Dental Injections, *J. Am. Dent. Assoc., 128,* 756, June, 1997.

Pihlstrom, B.L., Hargreaves, K.M., Bouwsma, O.J., Myers, W.R., Goodale, M.B., and Doyle, M.J.: Pain After Periodontal Scaling and Root Planing, *J. Am. Dent. Assoc., 130,* 801, June, 1999.

Raab, F.J., Schaffer, E.M., Guillaume-Cornelissen, G., and Halberg, F.: Interpreting Vital Sign Profiles for Maximizing Patient Safety During Dental Visits, *J. Am. Dent. Assoc., 129,* 461, April, 1998.

Tripp, D.A., Neish, N.R., and Sullivan, M.J.L.: What Hurts During Dental Hygiene Treatment, *J. Dent. Hyg., 72,* 25, Fall, 1998.

Weinberg, M.A. and Fine, J.D.: Common Analgesics in the Treatment of Acute Dental Pain, *J. Pract. Hyg., 11,* 39, November/December, 2002.

Nitrous Oxide–Oxygen Conscious Sedation

ADA Council on Scientific Affairs, ADA Council on Dental Practice: Nitrous Oxide in the Dental Office, Appendix G, in *ADA Guide to Dental Therapeutics.* Chicago, ADA Publishing Co., Inc., 1998, pp. 554–556.

Campagna, J.A., Miller, K.W., and Forman, S.A.: Mechanisms of Actions of Inhaled Anesthetics. *N. Engl. J. Med., 348,* 2110, May 22, 2003.

Clark, M.S. and Brunick, A.L.: *Handbook of Nitrous Oxide and Oxygen Sedation.* St. Louis, Mosby, 1999, pp. 1–242.

Clark, M.S., Renehan, B.W., and Jeffers, B.W.: Clinical Use and Potential Biohazards of Nitrous Oxide/Oxygen, *Gen. Dent., 45,* 486, September–October, 1997.

Howard, W.R.: Nitrous Oxide in the Dental Environment: Assessing the Risk, Reducing the Exposure, *J. Am. Dent. Assoc., 128,* 356, March, 1997.

Peretz, B., Katz, J., Zilburg, I., and Shemer, J.: Response to Nitrous Oxide and Oxygen Among Dental Phobic Patients, *Internat. Dent. J., 48,* 17, February, 1998.

Rohlfing, G.K., Dilley, D.C., Lucas, W.J., and Van, Jr, W.F.: The Effect of Supplemental Oxygen on Apnea and Oxygen Saturation During Pediatric Conscious Sedation, *Pediatr. Dent., 20,* 8, January/February, 1998.

Stach, D.J.: Nitrous Oxide Sedation: Understanding the Benefits and Risks, *Am. J. Dent., 8,* 47, February, 1995.

Zacny, J.P., Hurst, R.J., Graham, L., and Janiszewski, D.J.: Preoperative Dental Anxiety and Mood Changes During Nitrous Oxide Inhalation, *J. Am. Dent. Assoc., 133,* 82, January, 2002.

Local and Topical Anesthesia

Clancy, M.S.: Clinical Overview of Anesthetic Use in Dentistry, *J. Pract. Hyg., 7,* 36, March/April, 1998.

Goulet, J.-P., Pérusse, R., and Turcotte, J.-Y.: Contraindications to Vasoconstrictors in Dentistry: Part III. Pharmacologic Interactions, *Oral Surg. Oral Med. Oral Pathol., 74,* 692, November, 1992.

Hersh, E.V.: Local Anesthetics in Dentistry: Clinical Considerations, Drug Interactions, and Novel Formulations, *Compend. Cont. Educ. Dent., 14,* 1020, August, 1993.

Houpt, M.I., Heins, P., Lamster, I., Stone, C., and Wolff, M.S.: An Evaluation of Intraoral Lidocaine Patches in Reducing Needle-Insertion Pain, *Compend. Cont. Educ. Dent., 18,* 309, April, 1997.

Malamed, S.F., Gagnon, S., and Leblanc, D.: Articaine Hydrochloride: A Study of the Safety of a New Amide Local Anesthetic, *J. Am. Dent. Assoc., 132,* 177, February, 2001.

Malamed, S.F., Gagnon, S., and Leblanc, D.: Efficacy of Articaine: A New Amide Local Anesthetic, *J. Am. Dent. Assoc., 131,* 635, May, 2000.

Malamed, S.F.: Calculation of Local Anesthetic and Vasopressor Dosages, Appendix J, in *ADA Guide to Dental Therapeutics.* Chicago, ADA Publishing Co., Inc., 1998, p. 562.

Pallasch, T.J.: Anesthetic Management of the Chemically Dependent Patient, *Anesth. Prog., 39,* 157, Number 4/5, 1992.

Perry, D.A. and Loomer, P.M.: Maximizing Pain Control, *Dimensions Dent. Hyg., 1,* 28, April/May, 2003

Pérusse, R., Goulet, J.-P., and Turcotte, J.-Y.: Contraindications to Vasoconstrictors in Dentistry: Part I. Cardiovascular Diseases, *Oral Surg. Oral Med. Oral Pathol., 74,* 679, November, 1992.

Pérusse, R., Goulet, J.-P., and Turcotte, J.Y.: Contraindications to Vasoconstrictors in Dentistry: Part II. Hyperthyroidism, Diabetes, Sulfite Sensitivity, Cortico-dependent Asthma, and Pheochromocytoma, *Oral Surg. Oral Med. Oral Pathol., 74,* 687, November, 1992.

Rethman, J.: Local Anesthetic Administration. General Guidelines for Success, *J. Pract. Hyg., 7,* 40, March/April, 1998.

Webber, B., Orlansky, H., Lipton, C., and Stevens, M.: Complications of an Intra-arterial Injection From an Inferior Alveolar Nerve Block. *J. Am. Dent. Assoc., 132,* 1702, December, 2001.

Yagiela, J. and Malamed, S.F.: Injectable and Topical Local Anesthetics, in *ADA Guide to Dental Therapeutics.* Chicago, ADA Publishing Co., Inc., 1998, pp. 1–16.

Computer-Controlled Anesthesia

Friedman, M.J. and Hochman, M.N.: A 21st Century Computerized Injection System for Local Pain Control, *Compend. Cont. Educ. Dent., 18,* 995, October, 1997.

Krochak, M. and Friedman, N.: Using a Precision-Metered Injection System to Minimize Dental Injection Anxiety, *Compend. Cont. Educ. Dent., 19,* 137, February, 1998.

Instruments and Principles for Instrumentation

Stacy A. Matsuda, RDH, BS

Instrumentation begins with the identification of the various types of instruments for specific services to be performed and knowledge of the parts of those instruments. The requirements for putting the instruments into action to accomplish a particular task are stabilization by means of a correct grasp and finger rest, adaptation, angulation, lateral pressure, and stroke. Key words related to basic instrumentation are defined in Box 36-1.

A study of oral and dental anatomy and histology necessarily accompanies learning instrumentation procedures and skills. Development of a thorough, efficient, and safe procedure for treatment depends on an understanding of the normal, healthy, and diseased characteristics of the dental and periodontal tissues being treated.

A high degree of skill in the care and use of the fine instruments is required. Skill depends on knowledge and understanding of the goals of therapy and of how the goals can be reached through application of the fundamental principles of instrumentation.

▪ INSTRUMENT IDENTIFICATION

The instruments needed for examination and evaluation were described on pages 223, 225 to 227, and 235 to 237 instruments for scaling and related procedures are described in this chapter.

I. RECOGNITION OF INSTRUMENTS

Each instrument must be recognized by sight and distinguished at a glance by the profile of the instrument. The clinician must be able to designate the names and numbers, and to associate each instrument promptly with the various phases of instrumentation. Such spot identification contributes to neatness of tray arrangement and efficiency of service rendered through prompt selection of the proper instrument for the service to be performed.

BOX 36-1 KEY WORDS: Principles for Instrumentation

Adaptation: relationship between the working end of an instrument and the tooth surface being treated.

Angulation: the angle formed by the working end of an instrument with the surface to which the instrument is applied for treatment.

Blade: working end of an instrument with special design for a particular clinical treatment.

Curet: a curved, rounded dental instrument utilized for scaling, root planing, and gingival curettage.

> **Area-specific curet:** a specialized instrument designed with specific angles in the shank for adaptation to a certain group of tooth surfaces.

> **Universal curet:** a curet designed for use on any tooth surface where the adaptation, angulation, and other principles of instrument used can be correctly and effectively accomplished.

Curettage: removal of inflamed soft tissue lining of a pocket wall.

Dominant hand: the hand generally used for performing fine tasks such as writing and holding instruments for scaling.

Finger rest: for an intraoral rest, the place on a tooth or teeth where the third or ring finger of the hand holding the instrument is placed to provide stabilization and control during activation of the instrument.

Fulcrum: the support upon which a lever rests while force intended to produce motion is exerted.

Indirect vision: use of a dental mouth mirror to view the area of instrumentation. Indirect lighting is provided by the mirror.

Lateral pressure: the minimal pressure that is required of an instrument against the tooth or soft tissue to accomplish the objective of the designated treatment.

Offset blade: the blade of an area-specific Gracey curet in which the lower shank is at a 70° angle to the face of the blade; contrasts with a universal curet blade, which is at a 90° angle with the lower shank (Figure 36-6).

Scaler: instrument with two cutting edges that meet at a point; designed for supragingival **scaling** (the removal of calculus).

Scaling: instrumentation of a tooth surface to remove supragingival and subgingival calculus.

Shank: the part of the instrument between the handle and the working end.

> **Lower or terminal shank:** the part of the shank next to the blade.

Stroke: a single unbroken movement made by an instrument against a tooth surface during an examination or treatment procedure to accomplish a particular objective; the motion made for activation of an instrument.

II. CLASSIFICATION BY PURPOSE AND USE

- *Examination Instruments*: Probe, explorer.
- *Treatment Instruments*: Curets, scalers (scaler, file, hoe, chisel).

III. DESCRIPTION ON THE INSTRUMENT HANDLE

- *Design Name*: The school or individual responsible for the design or development.
- *Design Number*: The traditional number used to identify the specific instrument. The same instrument may be made by various manufacturers using the same number.

▪ INSTRUMENT PARTS

The three major parts are the *working end*, the *shank*, and the *handle* or shaft. The relationship of these parts is illustrated by the curet in Figure 36-1.

I. WORKING END

- The working end refers to that part used to carry out the purpose and function of the instrument. Each working end is unique to the particular instrument.
- The working end of a sharp instrument is called a blade.

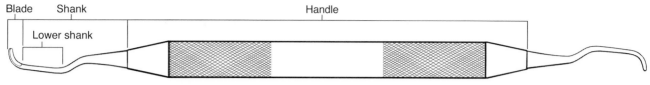

▪ **FIGURE 36-1 Parts of an Instrument.** Curet shows the relationship of the working end (blade), shank, and handle. The section of the shank next to the blade is referred to as the terminal or lower shank.

- The parts of a sharp blade are:
  1. *Cutting Edge*: A very fine line where two surfaces meet. For example, the face and the lateral surfaces meet to form the sharp cutting edge of a curet (see Figure 36-4).
  2. *Lateral Surfaces*: The lateral surfaces meet or are continuous (as in the round back of a curet) to form the back of the instrument.

II. SHANK

The shank connects the working end with the handle, as shown in Figure 36-1. The shape and rigidity of the shank govern the access of the working end to accomplish the intended purpose for which the instrument was designed.

A. Shape

1. *Straight*: For adaptation to tooth surfaces with unrestricted access, such as for anterior teeth. With many instruments, the straight shank can aid in correct positioning for treatment.
2. *Angled*: For adaptation to tooth surfaces with restricted access, such as proximal surfaces of posterior teeth. In general, the more restricted the access, the more angulated a shank must be and the sharper the bends of the angles.
   - Examples are the Gracey curets nos. 11 and 12 and nos. 13 and 14, each of which has three bends.
   - Because the *distal* surfaces of molars and premolars are much less accessible than are the mesial surfaces, the shank angles of the nos. 13 and 14 are designed with deeper bends to make access possible.

B. Lower or Terminal Shank

The section of the shank adjacent to the blade is called the lower or terminal shank.
1. *Instrument Positioning*. During positioning of a curet for treatment, the terminal shank is utilized to provide the clue to the appropriate blade adaptation and angulation for scaling and root planing.

2. *Elongated Terminal Shank*. Special instruments have been designed with terminal shanks longer than the traditional lengths. The purpose is to give better access to deep pockets.

C. Shank Flexibility

Instruments are made with shanks of varying degrees of thickness and rigidity that relate to the purpose for which they are used.
1. *Rigid, Thick Shank*. A thick shank is stronger and is able to withstand pressure without flexing when applied during instrumentation. Strong instruments are needed for removal of heavy calculus deposits.
2. *Less Rigid, More Flexible Shank*. A thinner shank may provide more tactile sensitivity and is used, for example, for removal of fine deposits of calculus and for maintenance root debridement.

III. HANDLE

The handle is the part of the instrument that is held (grasped) during activation of the working end.

A. Overall Design

1. *Single-ended instrument*: Has one working end.
2. *Double-ended instrument*: May have paired (mirror image) or complementary working ends. Paired working ends are used for access to proximal surfaces from the facial or lingual aspects.
3. *Cone socket handles*: Are separable from the shank and working end. They permit instrument exchanges and replacements.

B. Weight

Hollow handles are lighter and are preferred to solid handles because the lighter weight enhances tactile sensitivity and lessens fatigue.

C. Diameter

In general, four diameters of instrument handles are available. As shown in Figure 36-2, the most common

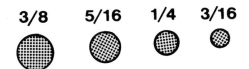

3/8 5/16 1/4 3/16

■ **FIGURE 36-2 Diameters of Instrument Handles.** The most common diameters are 3/8, 5/16, 1/4, and 3/16 inch. For comfort and tactile sensitivity, the widest diameter with a lightweight, hollow handle is recommended.

diameters available from manufacturers are 3\8, 5\16, 1\4, and 3\16 inch.

The ideal instrument for comfort and best tactile sensitivity has a lightweight, serrated, hollow handle with a 3\8- or 5\16-inch diameter.

D. Surface Texture: Serrations

Instrument handles may be smooth, ribbed, or knurled. For control and comfort without muscle fatigue, a smooth handle should be avoided.

■ INSTRUMENT FEATURES

I. INSTRUMENT BALANCE

A. Definition

The working end of a balanced instrument is centered in line with the long axis of the handle (Figure 36-3).

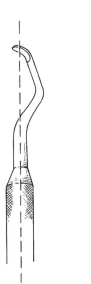

■ **FIGURE 36-3 Instrument Balance.** The working end of a balanced instrument is centered in line with the long axis of the instrument handle.

B. Effect of Shank Length

The distance from the cutting edge (working end) of the blade to the junction of the shank and handle should not be greater than 35 to 40 mm (1 1/2 inches). Too short a distance limits action; too long a distance may result in an unbalanced instrument.

II. FABRICATION MATERIALS

A. Working Ends

1. **Metal**
The type of steel used at the working end can affect the performance of the instrument.
    a. Stainless Steel
Maintains its finish without corrosion.
    b. Carbon Steel
Known for its hardness, strength, and ability to hold an edge longer.
2. **Nonmetal**
Alternative plastic working ends are available for restorative work that cannot withstand scratching from metal, such as implant abutments.
    a. Material: Plastic, Nylon, Graphite
    b. Uses
      • Probes and debriding instruments for dental implants.
      • Probes and mirrors for screening and surveys.

B. Handle

1. **Metal**
Traditionally, all handles were composed of stainless steel. Handles are largely a preference choice for the clinician.
2. **Nonmetal**
Some manufacturers offer handles composed of alternate materials in addition to stainless steel.
    a. Resin
    b. Nylon

■ THE INSTRUMENTS

Each instrument is designed for a specific type of application during treatment procedures. An instrument first can be categorized by whether it is designed primarily for supragingival treatment procedures (scalers) or for subgingival treatment (curets). Scalers and curets are then subdivided by their blade anatomy.

I. CATEGORIES

A. Curets

1. Universal
2. Area specific

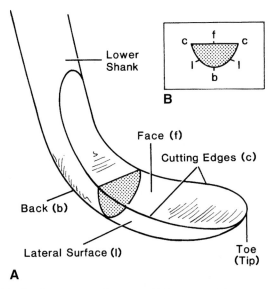

■ **FIGURE 36-4 Parts of a Curet. (A)** Curet with parts labeled. Lower shank is also called the terminal shank. The curet has a round toe, whereas the scaler has a pointed tip. **(B)** Cross section of a curet labeled *f* (face), *c* (cutting edges), *l* (lateral surfaces), and *b* (back).

B. Scalers

1. Scaler
   a. Curved scaler
   b. Straight scaler
2. File scaler
3. Hoe scaler
4. Chisel scaler

II. INSTRUMENT BLADE ANATOMY

The parts of the blade of a scaler or a curet are the *face* (inner surface), *lateral surfaces, back, tip* (scaler) or *toe* (curet), and *cutting edges*. A cutting edge is formed by the junction of the face and the lateral surface.

Figure 36-4 shows a curet with each part labeled. The parts of a scaler are the same. The differences are the pointed tip and the V-shaped back, shown in Figure 36-9. Each type of instrument is described in the next sections.

■ CURETS

I. CHARACTERISTICS

A. Blade

1. *Cutting Edges*
   • Two cutting edges on a curved blade (Figure 36-4A).
   • The two cutting edges curve around to meet at the toe.

• In reality, a curet has one continuous cutting edge because the two sides are united without interruption by the rounded toe.
2. *Face:* Flat in cross section (Figure 36-4B) and curved lengthwise.
3. *Back or Undersurface:* Rounded.
4. *Cross Section of the Blade:* Shaped like a half circle.
5. *Internal Angles*
   • Angles of 70° to 80° are formed where the lateral surfaces meet the face.
   • Figure 36-5 shows the cross section of a curet with the internal angles marked.

B. Shank

1. *Anterior Teeth.* Shank, blade, and handle may be in a relatively flat plane for curets primarily adaptable to anterior teeth.
2. *Posterior Teeth.* The shank is contra-angled for access to proximal surfaces.

C. Universal Curet

A universal curet can be adapted for instrumentation on any tooth surface.
1. *Working ends:* paired mirror-image, usually placed on a single handle.
2. *Face:* perpendicular (at a 90° angle) to the lower shank (Figure 36-6A).
3. *Cutting edge:* continuous around the face; used on both sides and around the toe.
4. *Angulation and adaptation:* determine the side that is correct for the surface being treated.

D. Area-Specific Curet

The Gracey curets are area specific, which means that each curet is designed for adaptation to specific surfaces.
1. *Working ends:* paired mirror-image, usually placed on a single handle. The original seven pairs are numbers 1–2, 3–4, 5–6, 7–8, 9–10, 11–12, and 13–14.

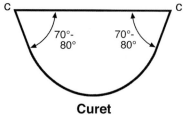

Curet

■ **FIGURE 36-5 Internal Angles of a Curet.** Cross section of a curet shows the 70° to 80° internal angles at the cutting edges. These angles are restored by sharpening techniques.

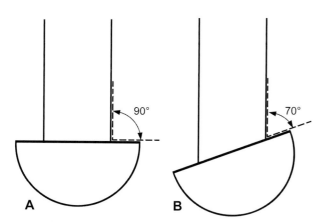

■ FIGURE 36-6 Curet Design. (A) A universal curet with the blade at a 90° angle to the lower shank. **(B)** Offset blade of an area-specific curet at a 70° angle to the lower shank.

2. *Face*: "offset" (at an angle of approximately 70°) in relation to the lower shank (Figure 36-6B).
3. *Cutting edge*: continuous around the face.
4. Only the longer, outer cutting edge that is lower when the handle is held vertically is used during instrumentation.

E. Variations

Variations of area-specific curets provide clinicians with greater opportunities to complete subgingival instrumentation with improved skills.

1. **Objectives**
   - To facilitate access to the base of deeper pockets.
   - To conform to the curvatures of roots on multi-rooted teeth and single-rooted teeth with moderate to severe loss of attachment.
2. *Shank*: Terminal (lower) shank elongated by 3 mm to adapt in deeper pockets. The total length of the shank from blade to handle is not changed.
3. *Blade*: Reduced length, half the length of a standard Gracey blade, for special adaptation to the curved features of root morphology otherwise difficult to access.
   a. Concavities: Longitudinal depressions on proximal surfaces; Depressions associated with furcations: coronal to the furcation entrance and interradicular.
   b. Convexities: Narrow root surfaces and line angles.
   c. Facilitates adaptation to deep narrow pockets and furcation areas.

II. PURPOSES AND USES

A. Standard instrument for subgingival scaling and root planing.

B. After ultrasonic or sonic scaling to complete the procedure as needed.
C. Removal of supragingival calculus, especially the fine supragingival calculus close to the gingival margin. The rounded instrument is best adapted to the cervical area; round back does not traumatize the gingival margin.
D. Curettage of the inflamed lining of the gingival wall of a pocket.
E. Useful for obtaining a sample of subgingival plaque to place on a glass slide for the phase microscope or for microbiologic tests.

III. APPLICATION

A. Angulation

Blade is applied to the tooth so that the face forms a 70° angle with the tooth surface to be treated.

B. Adaptation

Principles of adaptation are described on page 623 in this chapter.
- Toe third or lower third of the cutting edge is maintained on the tooth surface at all times.
- Minimize soft tissue trauma caused by toe extending away from the tooth in the narrow pocket.
- Changes in tooth surface contour require constant attention so that safe contact is maintained.
- On line angles, only 1 or 2 mm near the toe may be used (see Figure 37-5).

C. Curet Selection

Universal curets are used for subgingival scaling for removal of as much of the calculus as possible, followed by area-specific curets for fine scaling and root planing.

D. Design

- The design of the curet allows easy entrance into the sulcus or pocket.
- The curved blade with rounded end permits access to the base of the sulcus or pocket.
- The slender shank permits entrance to the sulcus with minimal tissue distention.
- The rounded back minimizes possible trauma at the base of the sulcus or pocket.

E. Stroke

Pull stroke only; applied in vertical, horizontal, or oblique directions (see Figure 36-18).

▪ SCALERS

I. SCALERS

The "sickle" scaler (Figure 36-7) and the "Jacquette" scaler (Figure 36-9) are referred to simply as "scalers," either curved or straight, respectively. Scalers may have a straight or contra-angled shank. The blades and cutting edges may be straight or curved.

A. Curved Scaler

*   Two cutting edges on a curved blade (Figure 36-7).
*   Face is flat in cross section and curved lengthwise.
*   The face converges with the two lateral surfaces to form the *tip* of the scaler, which is a sharp point.
*   In cross section, some blades are triangular (Figure 36-7B), whereas others are trapezoidal.
*   Internal angles of 70° to 80° are formed where the lateral surfaces meet the face at the cutting edges. Figure 36-8 shows the cross section of a scaler with the internal angles marked.

B. Straight Scaler

*   Two cutting edges on a straight blade (Figure 36-9).
*   Face (between the cutting edges) is flat.

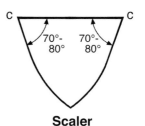

Scaler

▪ **FIGURE 36-8 Internal Angles of a Scaler.** Cross section of a scaler shows the 70° to 80° internal angles. These angles are restored by sharpening techniques.

*   The face converges with the two lateral surfaces to form the tip of the scaler, which is a sharp point.
*   Cross section of the blade is triangular (Figure 36-9B).
*   Internal angles of 70° to 80° are formed where the lateral surfaces meet the face at the cutting edges (Figure 36-8).

C. Angulation of the Shank

Both curved and straight scalers are available with angulated or straight shanks.

1. *Straight*: Single instrument in which the relationships of the shank, blade, and handle are in a flat plane; adaptable primarily for anterior teeth, although may be used for scaling premolars when the lips and cheeks permit retraction for correct angulation.

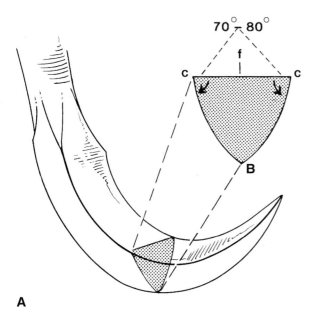

A

▪ **FIGURE 36-7 Curved Scaler. (A)** The curved blade terminates in a point. **(B)** Cross section shows the face *(f)* and the two cutting edges *(c)* formed where the lateral surfaces meet the face at 70° to 80° angles. This type of scaler is also called a sickle scaler.

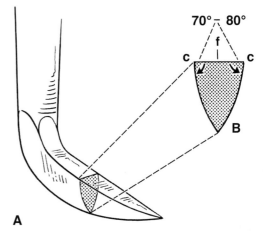

A

▪ **FIGURE 36-9 Straight Scaler. (A)** The straight blade converges to a point where the two cutting edges meet at the tip. **(B)** Cross section of the scaler shows the face *(f)*, the two cutting edges *(c)*, and the 70° to 80° internal angles. This type of scaler is also known as the Jacquette scaler.

2. *Modified or Contra-Angle*: Paired instruments that are mirror images of each other to provide access to the proximal surfaces of posterior teeth; one adapts from the facial and the other from the lingual and palatal aspects.

D. Purposes and Uses of Scalers

1. Principally for the removal of supragingival calculus.
2. May be useful for removal of gross calculus that is slightly below the gingival margin when the calculus is continuous with the supragingival calculus, and when the gingival tissue is spongy and flexible to permit easy insertion of the instrument.
3. Contraindications for use of scalers subgingivally:
    a. Cause undue trauma to the gingival tissue because of the large size, thickness, and length of the blade.
    b. Pointed tip and straight cutting edges cannot be adapted to the curved tooth surfaces. Risk of grooving or scratching the cemental surface is greater.
    c. Tactile sensitivity decreased with larger, heavier blades.
4. Small scalers can be useful for removal of fine supragingival deposits directly under contact areas and between overlapping teeth.

E. Application

1. *Angulation*. The face of the blade is adapted to the tooth surface at an angle of approximately 70° (60° to 80°).
2. *Stroke*. Pull stroke only for this type of blade.

II. FILE SCALER

A. Characteristics

*   Multiple cutting edges lined up as a series of miniature hoes on a round, oval, or rectangular base (Figure 36-10A).
*   The multiple blades are at a 90° angle with the shank (Figure 36-10B).
*   Shanks are variously angulated: most are paired instruments.
*   Reduced tactile sensitivity because of the series of blades.

B. Purposes and Uses of a File Scaler

1. Removal of calculus
    *   Crushes and fragments calculus prior to use of curets.

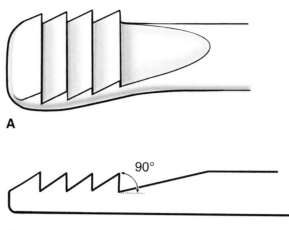

■ **FIGURE 36-10 File Scaler. (A)** A file has multiple cutting edges. **(B)** Each blade is at a 90° angle with the shank.

*   Burnished calculus that is impervious to removal with other bladed instruments can be removed with the file scaler.
*   Gross deposits of calculus on patients for whom ultrasonic use is contraindicated.
*   Calculus embedded in cementum in initial root planing prior to definitive instrumentation with Gracey curets.
2. Smoothing of the tooth at the cementoenamel junction.
3. Smoothing down of overextended or rough amalgam restorations, particularly on proximal surfaces or in the cervical areas.

C. Application

1. Adaptation
    Entire working surface is placed flat against the area to be treated. Flat blade adapted to the curved tooth surfaces is difficult. In certain relationships the file has only a tangential contact.
2. Pressure applied permits the cutting edges to grasp the surface.
3. Stroke: pull only, using a linear motion.
4. File use: must always be followed with curet(s) to leave a smooth surface on roots.

III. HOE SCALER

A. Characteristics

1. Single straight cutting edge (Figure 36-11).
2. *Blade*: turned at a 99° angle to the shank.
3. *Cutting edge*: beveled at a 45° angle to the end of the blade (Figure 36-11B).
4. *Shank*: variously angulated for adaptation of cutting edges to accessible tooth surfaces; some are paired.

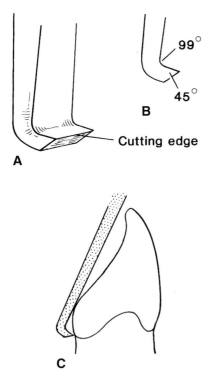

■ **FIGURE 36-11 Hoe Scaler. (A)** The hoe has a single cutting edge. **(B)** The blade is turned at an angle of 99° to the shank, and the cutting edge is beveled at a 45° angle. **(C)** Adaptation to a tooth for removal of calculus is with a two-point contact where possible.

B. Purposes and Uses of a Hoe Scaler

1. Removes supragingival calculus, particularly large, accessible, tenacious pieces.
2. Contraindications for use subgingivally:
   • Insertion of the thick-bladed instrument into the sulcus can cause unnecessary distention of the pocket wall.
   • Lack of adaptability of the wide straight cutting edge to the curved root surface.
   • Difficulty of use without gouging the cemental surface. The sharp "corners" should be rounded (as shown in Figure 36-35).
   • Lack of sensitivity because of the bulk of the instrument and the marked angulation of the shanks of some hoes.
   • Impossibility of reaching the bottom of the pocket without stretching and tearing the gingival pocket wall unnecessarily because of the size and shape of the blade.

C. Application

• Full width of the cutting edge is in contact with the calculus.

• Two-point contact is maintained with the tooth to stabilize the instrument during the positioning and activation.
• Two-point contact means contact of the cutting edge and the side of the shank with the tooth (Figure 36-11C).
• Hoes are not generally applied to proximal surfaces except the surface adjacent to an edentulous area.
• **Pull stroke** is used toward occlusal or incisal surfaces.

IV. CHISEL SCALER

A. Characteristics

1. Single straight cutting edge (Figure 36-12).
2. Blade is continuous with a slightly curved shank.
3. End of blade is flat and beveled at 45° (Figure 36-12B).

B. Purposes and Uses of a Chisel Scaler

• Removal of supragingival calculus from exposed proximal surfaces of anterior teeth where interdental gingiva is missing.
• Dislodgement of heavy calculus from the proximal areas of mandibular anterior teeth. When the calculus on the lingual surfaces forms a continuous bridge across several teeth, the chisel can be pushed horizontally from the facial aspect to break up the large masses of calculus.
• Proximal surfaces of premolars when flexibility of the lips and cheeks permits retraction for proper positioning of the cutting edge.

C. Application

1. Apply full width of cutting edge: sharp corners can nick and groove the tooth surface. The sharp

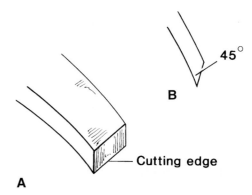
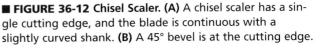

■ **FIGURE 36-12 Chisel Scaler. (A)** A chisel scaler has a single cutting edge, and the blade is continuous with a slightly curved shank. **(B)** A 45° bevel is at the cutting edge.

"corners" should be rounded during sharpening (Figure 36-35).

2. *Stroke:* horizontal only, from facial to lingual on proximal surfaces of anterior, particularly mandibular, teeth.

▪ PRINCIPLES FOR INSTRUMENT USE

Understanding the purpose of each instrument and developing dexterity in the effective use of the instruments are basic to clinical dental hygiene practice. The clinical results obtained for the patient depend in part on the proficiency and thoroughness with which the instrumentation is accomplished.

Stability is essential for effective, controlled action of an instrument. The correct use depends on maintaining *control* of the movement of the instrument through use of an effective *grasp* and the establishment and maintenance of an appropriate, firm, fulcrum *finger rest*.

▪ INSTRUMENT GRASP

I. FUNCTIONS OF THE INSTRUMENT GRASP

A. Dominant Hand

The right hand is the dominant hand for the right-handed clinician. A few rare people are completely ambidextrous, and others are partially dexterous with the nondominant hand, a useful capability when carrying out dental and dental hygiene procedures. Exercises for developing dexterity are provided on pages 627 to 629.

The dominant hand is used to hold and activate the treatment instrument. The manner in which the instrument is held influences the entire procedure.

B. Nondominant Hand

The right-handed clinician uses the left hand and the left-handed clinician uses the right hand for essential supplementary functions to assist the dominant hand. Figure 36-13 shows the recommended modified pen grasp (described later) for each hand. The mouth mirror is held by the nondominant hand. With the appropriate grasp and finger rest, the following effects can be provided:

1. Control of the position of the mirror for indirect vision, indirect lighting, and retraction.
2. Assistance in providing the dominant hand with an auxiliary finger rest.

C. Grasp Dynamics

A rigid grasp, in which the instrument is gripped tightly, lessens the tactile sensitivity and, hence, the effectiveness of instrumentation. The appropriate grasp is controlled, displays the confidence of the clinician in the work being done, and provides the following effects:

1. Increased fingertip tactile sensitivity.
2. Positive control of the instrument with balance and flexibility during motion.
3. Decreased hazard of trauma to the dental and periodontal tissues, which in turn results in less postcare discomfort for the patient.
4. Prevention of fatigue to clinician's fingers, hand, and arm.

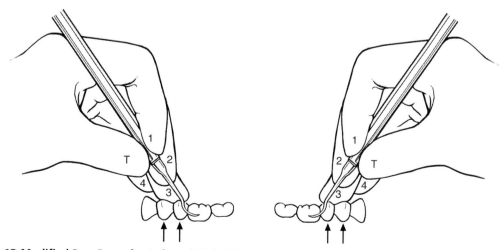

▪ **FIGURE 36-13 Modified Pen Grasp for Left and Right Hands.** An instrument is held by the thumb *(T)*, index finger *(1)*, and the second, or "middle," finger *(2)*, which also provides support. The third, or "ring," finger *(3)* serves as the finger rest, and the fourth, or "little," finger *(4)* is positioned beside the ring finger to supplement the finger rest.

II. TYPES

A. Modified Pen Grasp

1. *Description.* The modified pen grasp is a three-finger grasp with specific target points of the thumb, index finger, and middle (second) finger all in contact with the instrument.
   a. Thumb: the center of the upper aspect of the pad.
   b. Index finger: the center of the upper aspect of the pad.
   c. Middle finger: the inside upper corner of the pad, behind the upper corner of the nail.
2. *Location on Handle.* The instrument is held by the thumb and index finger on the handle, near the junction of the shank. The upper corner of the middle finger is placed on the upper portion of the shank to hold and guide the movement (Figure 36-13).
3. *Role of Middle Finger*
   • The shank of the instrument is held against the inside upper corner of the pad of the middle finger.
   • The instrument is not held across the nail or the side of the middle finger, as in a pen grasp usually used for writing.
   • The specific position of the middle finger is extremely important to instrument control in preventing the instrument from slipping during adaptation and activation.
4. *Role of Ring Finger.* The ring finger is used to establish a finger rest, or fulcrum.
5. *Additional Support.* The side-to-side contact of index, middle, and ring fingers allows for greater stability, strength, and control during instrumentation.

B. Palm Grasp

1. *Description.* The handle of the instrument is held in the palm by cupped index, middle, ring, and little fingers. The thumb is free to serve as the fulcrum (Figure 36-14).
2. *Limitations of Use.* Instruments for calculus removal, root planing, and maintenance root debridement are not used with a palm grasp. The possible exception is a chisel scaler when it is used to remove gross calculus by a push stroke (pages 618 to 619).
3. *Examples of Uses for Palm Grasp*
   a. Air syringe.
   b. Rubber dam clamp holder.
   c. Neivert whittler for instrument sharpening (Figure 36-31).

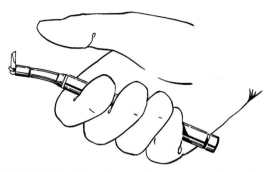

■ **FIGURE 36-14 Palm Grasp of Instrument.** The instrument handle is held in the palm by cupped index, middle, ring, and little fingers. Thumb is free and serves as the finger rest.

   d. Nondominant hand stabilizing the instrument for sharpening (Figure 36-25A).

■ NEUTRAL POSITIONS

Neutral positions for the wrist, forearm, elbow, and shoulder are basic to:
   • Efficient performance directed at the prevention of occupational pain risks, particularly those risks related to cumulative trauma disorders.
   • Clinical activities to prevent cumulative trauma disorders, particularly prevention of carpal tunnel syndrome, are considered in Chapter 5 and encouraged later in this chapter.
      General clinician and dental chair positioning are described in Chapter 5.
   • Principles of the 90°-90°-90° body position for the clinician are illustrated in Figures 5-1 and 5-2 (page 86).
   • Correct seating includes a right angle at each of the hips, knees, and ankles.
   • In this section, the neutral positions for the hand, wrist, elbow, and shoulder can be related directly to the grasp and finger rest for instrumentation.[1]

I. WRIST

   • The wrist is straight, and the forearm and the hand are in the same horizontal plane when in the neutral position.
   • Figure 36-15 illustrates the straight wrist and the effect of a bent wrist.
   • Carpal tunnel syndrome, brought on by pressure on the median nerve in the carpal tunnel, is one of the nerve entrapment conditions that results

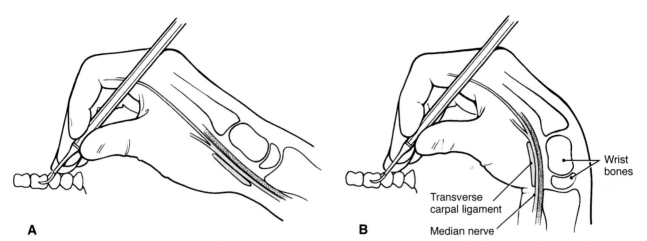

■ **FIGURE 36-15 Effect of Wrist Position. (A)** Wrist in neutral position in straight line with forearm. **(B)** Bent wrist shows cramping of median nerve in the carpal tunnel of the wrist. Repeated pressure on the median nerve can cause carpal tunnel syndrome.

from inappropriate work habits, such as working with a bent wrist.

II. ELBOW

The neutral elbow is at 90°, the forearm is positioned horizontally, and the hand is straight ahead.

III. SHOULDER

In neutral, both shoulders are level and relaxed to their lowest position. From a lateral position, each shoulder should be vertically in line with, and beneath, each ear. The upper arms are straight down to the elbow.

■ FULCRUM: FINGER REST

A fulcrum must always be used when instruments are applied to the teeth and gingiva.

I. DEFINITION

A. Fulcrum

The support, or point of rest, on which a lever turns in moving a body.

B. Finger Rest

The support, or point of finger rest on the tooth surface, on which the hand turns in moving an instrument.

II. OBJECTIVES

An effective, well-established finger rest is essential to the following:

A. Stability

For controlled action of the instrument.

B. Unit Control

Provides a focal point from which the whole hand can move as a unit.

C. Prevention of Injury

Injury to the patient's oral tissues can result from irregular pressure and uncontrolled movement.

D. Comfort for the Patient

Confidence in the clinician's ability, which results from the feeling of securely applied instruments.

E. Control of Length of Stroke

With instrument grasp, the finger rest limits the instrumentation to where it is needed.

III. INTRAORAL RESTS

The intraoral finger rest is essentially a total hand-coordinated effort to provide stabilization. Figure 36-13 shows the fingers grouped together with the fulcrum where the ring finger (no. 3 in Figure 36-13) maintains its position on a tooth near the tooth being treated.

A. Digits Used for Finger Rest

1. *Modified Pen Grasp*:
   a. Ring finger. Little finger is held close beside ring finger (finger nos. 3 and 4 in Figure 36-13).

b. Supplementary. Middle finger is held beside ring finger to provide total hand unity; ring finger maintains regular fulcrum position, and middle finger maintains its grasp on the instrument.

2. *Palm Grasp*: Thumb.

B. Location of Finger Rest

1. *Purposes*. The location of a finger rest is selected for the following reasons:
   a. Convenience to area of instrumentation.
   b. Ease in instrument adaptation.
   c. Maintenance of an effective grasp.
   d. Application of the appropriate angulation.
   e. Stability and control of instrument during the activation (strokes).
   f. Safety of the clinician. A finger rest placed in line of the stroke direction could result in a rubber glove puncture and/or a finger stab if the patient moved suddenly or the instrument slipped for any reason.

2. *Principles*
   a. The first choice for a finger rest is usually the tooth adjacent to the tooth being treated.
   b. Maintain the rest on firm stable tooth or teeth. The patient's chin, lips, and cheeks are mobile and flexible and therefore less reliable for stability.
   c. Where possible, the rest should be on the same arch, maxillary or mandibular, as the instrumentation; also, where possible, the rest should be in the same quadrant.

IV. VARIATIONS OF FINGER REST

A basic fulcrum location cannot always be used or may require supplementation.

A. Problems

1. A patient's facial musculature; oral anatomic features, such as size of tongue or mouth opening (microstomia); arrangement of the teeth or malocclusions of individual teeth; or physical disability affecting the oral cavity indirectly may interfere with customary positioning for instrumentation.
2. Tenacious calculus in difficult-access areas may not be removed and root surfaces may not be planed by the usual procedures. Greater support and pressure to the instrument are required.
3. When the problem in instrumentation seems to be related to space and accessibility, the height and position of the patient's oral cavity should be checked. Also, a change in the clinician's working position may be necessary.

B. General Categories of Variations[2]

When a variation in finger rest is used, basic rules for stability and control are applied, and rests on movable tissues are avoided. Three types of variations are suggested here: *substitute, supplementary,* and *reinforced* finger rests. Any of these variations may require an external position.

1. **Substitute**
   a. Missing teeth where finger rest is usually applied.
      • For an edentulous area, a cotton roll or gauze sponge may be packed into the area to provide a dry finger rest.
      • Otherwise, a rest across the dental arch or in the opposite arch may be required to provide stability.
   b. Mobile teeth, or teeth with inadequate bony support.
      • Avoid mobile teeth for finger rests or use only with minimal pressure for brief periods.
      • Not only would the rest on a mobile tooth be unstable, but pressure, movement, and undue stress on the tooth could traumatize and tear the periodontal ligament fibers.
   c. Index finger of nondominant hand may be placed in the vestibule over a cotton roll or a dry gauze square.
      • The usual finger rest can be placed on the index finger to aid retraction and visibility, particularly in the mouth of a small child.

2. **Supplementary**
   Place the index finger of the nondominant hand on the occlusal surfaces of teeth adjacent to the working area. The finger rest can then be applied to the nondominant index finger.
   • This is known as a "finger-on-finger" rest.
   • Such supplements are very useful for achieving a parallel orientation of the terminal shank to proximal surfaces.
   • This serves to establish and maintain working angulation in areas that are difficult to achieve.
   • They are not useful for certain distal surfaces where the mouth mirror is essential for vision.

3. **Reinforced**
   a. In this type, a support is placed between the instrument handle and the working end to provide additional strength and force, particularly for hard, tenacious calculus in pockets.
      • Greater control of the instrument can result and, when applied correctly, reduce the danger of instrument breakage.

- A definite rest for both hands is needed to distribute the pressure.

b. Index finger of nondominant hand can be rested on the tooth adjacent to the one being scaled, while the thumb is placed on the instrument shank (or handle) for a reinforcement.

V. TOUCH OR PRESSURE APPLIED TO FINGER REST

A. Balance

The fulcrum finger maintains a secure hold with variable pressure to balance the action of the instrument being applied. A balance must also exist between the pressure exerted against the tooth and the pressure into the fulcrum. These pressures will be described under Activation.

B. Effects of Excess Pressure

1. Decreased stability.
2. Diminished control.
3. Overtightened grasp to accommodate.
4. Fatigue of patient caused by use of mandibular fulcrums. Heavy pressure on the movable mandible can cause fatigue in the temporomandibular joint and related muscles and, thus, discomfort for the patient.
5. Fatigue in clinician's fingers and hand.

■ ADAPTATION

With an appropriate grasp and finger rest, the instrument is next ready for application. The working end of the instrument is adapted to the surface of the tooth or tissue where instrumentation is to take place.

I. RELATION TO TOOTH SURFACE

The side of the tip or toe is maintained in close approximation to the surface being examined or treated. The blade of an instrument is divided into thirds referred to as the shank third, the middle third, and the toe (or tip) third, as shown in Figure 37-4.

II. CHARACTERISTICS OF A WELL-ADAPTED INSTRUMENT

A. Working End

1. The working end of the instrument is correctly positioned for the task to be accomplished. For example, when scaling, the angle formed by the face of the instrument and the tooth surface is crucial for effective calculus removal. Angulation is described in a following section.

2. The instrument is adapted for maximum usefulness of the working end. For example, 2 to 3 mm of the toe third of a curet may be adaptable when on a "flat" surface, whereas at a line angle or convex surface of a narrow root, less than 2 mm may be adaptable.

3. The working end is applied to conform to the contour of the tooth surface.

4. As the instrument is activated, it can be adjusted to changes required by variations in the surface topography.

B. Soft Tissue

A properly adapted instrument harms neither the tissue being treated nor the surrounding or adjacent tissues.

III. PROBLEM AREAS

Areas where instrument adaptation is most difficult and requires more attention, time, and careful application of skill include the following:

A. Line Angles

All line angles require that the instrument be rolled between the fingers to turn the working end as the instrument is activated. At each change of direction around a line angle, the instrument must be rolled to keep it adapted to the surface. Figure 36-16 shows the adaptation of an explorer tip to a line angle.

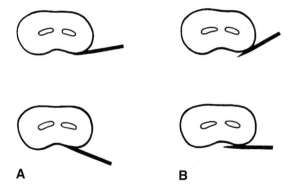

A   **B**

■ **FIGURE 36-16 Instrument Adaptation.** Cross section of maxillary first permanent premolar to show adaptation of the tip of an explorer. **(A)** Appropriate adaptation in which the tip of the explorer is maintained on the tooth surface in a series of strokes to explore around a line angle. **(B)** Incorrect adaptation with the tip of the explorer extended away from the tooth surface.

B. Convex and Rounded Surfaces

Particularly of narrow roots.

C. Cervical Area

Where the root is constricted.

D. Proximal Root Surfaces

Root surfaces may be concave, have longitudinal grooves, or have open furcations.

■ ANGULATION

A factor closely related to and directly influencing instrument adaptation is angulation. Angulation refers to the angle formed by the working end of an instrument with the surface to which the instrument is applied. Each instrument is applied to a surface in a specific manner for optimum adaptation and angulation.

I. PROBE

The usual adaptation of a probe is to maintain the side of the working tip on the tooth, with the long axis of the working end nearly parallel with the tooth surface.

As used for a bleeding index, the tip is placed inside the pocket wall and pressed lightly on the wall as the probe is moved horizontally around the tooth (see Figure 20-9, page 338).

II. EXPLORER

An explorer is held with the tip at a right angle to the occlusal surface when detecting occlusal pit or fissure caries. On other surfaces, the side of the tip is kept on the tooth at all times. The angle is 5° or less. Figure 13-15 (page 239) illustrates the use of the subgingival explorer.

III. SCALERS AND CURETS

Angulation for a scaler or a curet means the angle formed by the face of the instrument with the surface to which the instrument is applied. Figure 36-17 shows the various angles for curet adaptation. At zero angulation the curet face is flat against the tooth surface (Figure 36-17A).

A. Scaling and Root Planing

- For curets and scalers, an angle of 70° between the face of the instrument and the tooth surface permits effective calculus removal (Figure 36-17B).
- Markedly closed angulation uses only the side of a sharp cutting edge and can result in burnishing.

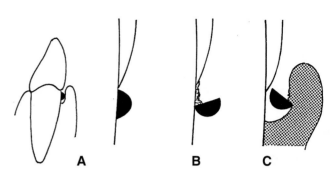

■ **FIGURE 36-17 Instrument Angulation.** Enlargement of pocket area from the tooth on the left shows cross section of a curet blade in black. **(A)** The curet is angulated at 0° with the tooth surface when used in an exploratory or insertion stroke. At 0° the face of the blade is flat against the tooth surface. **(B)** Blade angulated at approximately 70° with the tooth surface for scaling and root planing. **(C)** Open blade angulated toward the pocket wall in position for gingival curettage. The face of the blade forms an angle of approximately 70° with the soft tissue pocket wall.

- Burnishing produces a smooth veneer, making the calculus difficult or impossible to detect with an explorer.

B. Gingival Curettage

The face is turned toward the soft tissue wall of the pocket. The angle formed by the face of the curet blade and the soft tissue pocket wall being treated is approximately 70° (Figure 36-17C).

■ LATERAL PRESSURE

Lateral pressure means the pressure of the instrument against the tooth surface during activation. It is described as light, moderate, or heavy pressure.

I. DETECTION INSTRUMENTS

Explorers and probes are used with a light pressure to maximize the sense of touch in detecting irregularities.

II. TREATMENT INSTRUMENTS

A. Assessment Stroke

A light pressure equal to that used by an explorer is applied as the curet blade is moved across the tooth surface. The purpose of the assessment stroke is to:
1. Assess the surface texture of the root.
2. Confirm the positioning of the curet at the soft tissue attachment.

3. Rehearse an intended movement of the curet prior to activating a working stroke to confirm correct adaptation.

B. Scaling Stroke or Working Stroke

A definite, well-controlled, firm stroke of moderate to heavy pressure is used for calculus removal.

C. Root Planing Stroke

A varying amount of pressure is applied, dependent upon the surface textures of the root surface. Lateral pressure begins as moderately firm if deposits are present. As strokes continue, a lighter pressure is applied progressively as the root surface becomes smooth.

D. Root Debridement Stroke

A lighter pressure is applied as a curet disrupts and removes dental biofilm from the root surface of a previously root planed tooth.

III. ERRORS IN TECHNIQUE

A. Effects of Insufficient Pressure

1. Burnishing of calculus.
2. Loss of control when both fulcrum and lateral pressure are insufficient.

B. Effects of Excessive Pressure

1. Excess removal of tooth structure; gouging of root surfaces.
2. Loss of instrument control.
3. Patient discomfort.
4. Clinician fatigue.

▪ ACTIVATION: STROKE

A stroke is an unbroken movement made by an instrument; it is the action of an instrument in the performance of the task for which it was designed.

Strokes may be identified by the instrumentation being performed. Examples are the "probing stroke," "scaling stroke," or "root planing stroke." Technique for each type is described in the chapters covering the specific procedures.

I. CHARACTERISTICS OF STROKES

A. Types of Strokes by Action

1. *Pull*. Example: scaler removing calculus.
2. *Placement*. Example: exploratory stroke when a curet is being positioned.

3. *Combined Push and Pull*. Example: explorer in a walking stroke, which is moving the instrument up and down with equal pressure on the surface (see Figure 13-15, page 239).
4. *Walking Stroke*. Example: probe is moved up and down, touching the coronal border of the periodontal attachment with each down stroke (see Figure 13-6, page 231).

B. Types of Strokes by Function

1. *Assessment Stroke*
   • Used to detect irregularities of the tooth surface such as the presence of calculus, a carious lesion, or a rough overhanging margin.
   • The assessment stroke is also called an exploratory stroke. The grasp pressure is light so that tactile sense is magnified.
   • Examples:
   a. Probe is used to locate the attachment at the bottom of the periodontal pocket (pages 229 to 230) and to estimate the amount of deposit present on the root surfaces while probing.
   b. Explorer is used to evaluate for smoothness following treatment.
   c. Ultrasonic tip is used with the power turned off only to confirm the soft tissue attachment for adequate access to the base of the pocket.
2. *Working Stroke*
   The stroke applied to accomplish a task such as calculus removal or reshaping an overhanging margin.

C. Types of Strokes by Direction (Figure 36-18)

1. *Diagonal or Oblique*: Stroke that is diagonal across the surface being treated (Figure 36-18A).
2. *Vertical*: Strokes parallel with the long axis of the tooth being treated (Figure 36-18B).
3. *Horizontal*: Strokes parallel with the occlusal surface of the tooth being treated (Figure 36-18C).

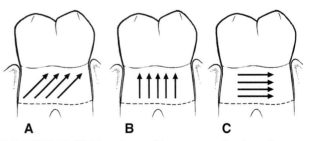

▪ **FIGURE 36-18 Directions of Instrument Strokes.** Arrows on root surface represent **(A)** diagonal or oblique strokes, **(B)** vertical strokes, and **(C)** horizontal strokes.

They are sometimes called circumferential, which should not be interpreted to mean that a stroke can be made to go around a tooth or large segment of a tooth. A horizontal stroke necessarily must be a short stroke because of the constant changes in the topography of the tooth surface.

4. *Circular:* Stroke used with a handpiece. A small circular stroke is used with varying pressure to:
   • Apply polishing agent with a rubber cup (pages 734 to 735).
   • Polish amalgams using stones, burs, rubber cups, and points (pages 750 to 751).

II. FACTORS THAT INFLUENCE SELECTION OF STROKE

A. Size, contour, and position of gingiva.
B. Surface and section of surface where the instrument is used.
C. Probing depth.
D. Size and shape of instrument used.
E. Procedure objective, for example, nature of the deposit to be removed.

III. NATURE OF STROKE

A. Grasp

The grasp of a scaler or curet is light while the working end is positioned for the stroke, and then the instrument is held more firmly during movement. An explorer and a probe should be held lightly for tactile sensitivity at all times.

B. Hand Stability

During a stroke, the whole hand pivots or rotates on the fulcrum.

C. Motion

The motion for a stroke is generated by a unified action of the shoulder, arm, wrist, and hand.

D. Length

1. The length of the scaling stroke is limited by the extent of calculus deposit and by the anatomic features of the area where the deposit is located.
2. The stroke is short, controlled, decisive, and directed to protect the tissues from trauma.
3. Instrumentation should be applied to the section of the tooth where treatment is indicated. This section is called the *instrumentation zone.* Strokes should not be long enough to pass over the whole crown when the calculus represents only a small area at the cervical third of the tooth.
4. The length of a stroke varies with each instrument and purpose. A description of strokes for each instrument is included in the respective chapters. The probe is described on pages 230 to 231; the explorer, pages 238 to 240; scalers and curets, pages 625, 658 to 659; and the ultrasonic scaler, page 668.

IV. BALANCE OF PRESSURE

A balance or equalization of pressure must exist between the instrument blade against the tooth surface and the pressure on the fulcrum. Keeping the two forces equal will facilitate a stable, intentional control of the instrument as it is activated.

A. Assessment

1. When exploring the tooth surface, the pressure of the instrument on the tooth is light.
2. The grasp pressure of the fingers holding the instrument is also light, in order to achieve tactile sensitivity.
3. The pressure of the fulcrum finger is light but secure and stable.

B. Calculus Removal

1. When moving from assessment to activation of a working stroke, the pressure on the tooth and into the fulcrum increases dramatically.
2. As the working stroke is initiated to remove calculus on a tooth surface, the pressure of the instrument against the tooth is very strong.
3. The pressure of the grasp finger(s) supplying lateral pressure to the handle of the instrument in order to engage the blade for the working stroke is of equal strength to the pressure of the instrument against the tooth.
4. The pressure of the fulcrum finger must be equally firm to achieve stability and control of the instrument as it is activated.

C. Maintenance Root Debridement

1. When removing dental biofilm from a tooth surface with minimal deposit, the pressure of the instrument on the tooth is light to moderate.
2. The pressure of the specific grasp finger(s) supplying lateral pressure to the handle of the instrument equals the pressure of the blade on the tooth.
3. The pressure of the fulcrum finger is similarly moderate.

4. The pressures are somewhat variable according to the textures encountered.
   • When the texture changes from grainy to rough, the pressure of both fulcrum finger and blade must increase in order to remove the deposit on the tooth surface.
   • Pressure is, therefore, responsive to the tactile information transmitted as the instrument progresses along the tooth surface.

■ VISIBILITY AND ACCESSIBILITY

I. EFFECTS OF ADEQUATE VISION AND ACCESSIBILITY

A. Instrumentation is more thorough with minimal trauma to the oral tissues.
B. Length of time required may be lessened, thereby lessening fatigue for patient and clinician.
C. Patient cooperation can be increased because of shortened treatment time and less discomfort.

II. CONTRIBUTING FACTORS

A. Patient and clinician positions.
B. Efficient use of direct or reflected (by mouth mirror) illumination for each tooth surface.
C. Adequate, yet gentle, retraction of lips, cheeks, and tongue with consideration for the patient's comfort and clinician's convenience.

■ DEXTERITY DEVELOPMENT

The dental hygiene student and the dental hygienist returning to practice after a temporary leave of absence can appreciate the need for exercises to develop dexterity and strength for the efficient and effective use of instruments. In addition, all students, returning retirees, and dental hygienists continuing in practice need an understanding of preventive measures that can preserve the health of their hands, arms, shoulders, and all muscles and joints involved when undertaking patient care.

However generally dexterous a person may be, the use of new or unusual instruments requires different procedures for coordination. Control is essential, and guided strength contributes to control.

Proficiency during procedures comes from repeated correct use of the instruments. Exercises for the fingers, hands, and arms supplement experience. Directed exercises are needed for both hands, separately and together. A regular period of time each day **during the training period** should be set aside for exercises.

I. SQUEEZING THERAPY PUTTY OR A SOFT BALL

A. Purpose

To develop strength and control.

B. Procedure

1. Hold putty in palm of hand; grip with thumb and all fingers (Figure 36-19A).
2. Tighten and release grip at regular intervals.
3. One hand rests while other is exercising.
4. Use a ball in each hand at the same time.

II. STRETCHING

A. Purposes

1. To strengthen finger and hand muscles.
2. To develop control of finger movements.

B. Rubber Band on Finger Joints

1. Place band at joint between first phalanx and second phalanx.

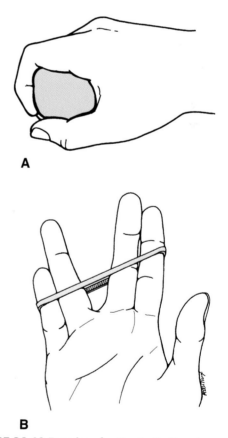

A

B

■ **FIGURE 36-19 Exercises for Dexterity Development. (A)** Squeezing therapy putty can aid in developing strength and control. **(B)** Stretching a rubber band can be applied at each group of finger and thumb joints.

2. Stretch band by separating middle and ring fingers (Figure 36-19B).
3. Place band at joint between second phalanx and third phalanx and proceed as before.
4. Place bands on both hands and do exercises together.

C. Rubber Band on Finger Joints With Use of Fulcrum

1. Place band on joint between first phalanx and second phalanx.
2. Establish fulcrum (ring finger) on tabletop with little finger closely adjacent to it; elbow and forearm are free, as they are during instrumentation. Keep wrist straight, in same horizontal line as the forearm, and hold elbow at 90°. Stretch band by separating middle and ring fingers.
3. Touch thumb and index and middle fingers to simulate a modified pen grasp for holding an instrument. Stretch band by separating middle and ring fingers.
4. Variations
   a. Hold instrument in modified pen grasp while doing the exercise.
   b. Do writing exercise with rubber band in place.
5. Rest one hand while other is being exercised.

III. WRITING

A. Purposes

1. To develop correct modified pen grasp.
2. To propel instrument by activation from wrist and arm, without moving fingers.
3. To practice use of instruments when mouth mirror is required.
4. To develop control and precision.

B. Circles and Vertical Lines

1. Hold long, well-sharpened pencil with modified pen grasp.
2. Establish fulcrum (ring finger) on a piece of paper on tabletop. Keep wrist straight in line with forearm; elbow is at 90°, and shoulder is in neutral position. Forearm and elbow are free.
3. Inscribe counterclockwise small circles and vertical lines on paper, rapidly and lightly at first, slowly and with more pressure later.
4. Accomplish writing by activation of the hand by the upper arm, without flexing or extending the thumb and fingers holding the pencil.
5. Practice with each hand separately at first; then use a pencil in each hand at the same time, alternating

writing action to simulate adaptation of the mirror first and then the explorer or scaler.

C. Using Mouth Mirror

1. Hold mouth mirror with modified pen grasp in nondominant hand close to pencil while practicing writing exercises (previous section) through the mirror. Reverse hands.
2. Using engineer's graph paper and modified pen grasp with fulcrum as described earlier, follow the lines of the small squares while looking in mirror held with opposite hand.

D. Everyday Penmanship

1. Use modified pen grasp whenever possible for writing.
2. Practice word writing with the left hand (with the right hand for left-handed person) to increase dexterity for handling instruments.

IV. MOUTH MIRROR, COTTON PLIERS, AND EXPLORER

A. Purposes

1. To develop ability to turn mouth mirror at various angles.
2. To develop dexterity in holding objects with cotton pliers.
3. To establish desired grasp of explorer to ensure maximum touch sensitivity.

B. Mouth Mirror

1. Hold mouth mirror with modified pen grasp, ring finger on tabletop as fulcrum finger with little finger closely adjacent to it; elbow and forearm are free. The mirror is used most frequently in the nondominant hand.
2. Practice turning mirror with fingers, adjusting as to the several surfaces of the tooth.
3. Hold a small object in the dominant hand for viewing in mirror held in nondominant hand.
4. Practice crossing the mirror over fulcrum finger as in position for retracting lower lip while viewing lingual surfaces of mandibular anterior teeth in mouth mirror.

C. Cotton Pliers

1. Make small, tight cotton pellets with thumb and index and middle fingers of each hand; then make one in each hand simultaneously.

2. Hold cotton pliers with modified pen grasp and establish fulcrum finger on tabletop; elbow and forearm are free.
3. Practice picking up cotton pellets using mirror vision (right hand, then left).
   a. Use in wiping motion on tabletop or other object.
   b. Move to different area to release pellet.

V. TACTILE SENSITIVITY

A. Explorer

1. Mount small pieces of various grades of fine-grain sandpaper on a card.
2. Hold explorer with modified pen grasp, and establish fulcrum finger on tabletop, with upper arm and forearm free. With eyes closed, compare roughness of the various grades of sandpaper. Use a light, exploring stroke.
3. Use extracted teeth to feel with explorer tip until a light grasp permits maximum security of grasp and maximum sense of touch. Extracted teeth can be used to provide a contrast between exploring enamel, cementum, calculus, or other rough area of tooth surface.

B. Probe

1. Repeat exercises described for explorer.
2. Compare with explorer.

■ PREVENTION OF CUMULATIVE TRAUMA

Hand in hand with learning the instruments and attaining dexterity in their use for the treatment of patients is the well-being of the dental hygienist. Primary occupational hazards are related to personal everyday habits during chairside practice. The symptoms of carpal tunnel syndrome are caused by compression of the median nerve within the carpal tunnel as shown in Figure 36-15 (page 621).

Along with the exercises for the development of strength and control in the hands, other types of exercises are needed for maintaining general musculoskeletal health. Problems of posture, extended periods of time spent in the same work position, and repetitive movements during actual instrumentation, point to areas that need study and planning for action in advance, before serious disability can occur.

I. EXERCISES

• Stretching exercises for stress release, improvement of posture, and counteracting repetitive

movements used during instrumentation are suggested in Figure 36-20.
• Other exercises are shown in Figure 5-6 (page 85).

II. CLINICAL APPLICATIONS

• Exercises performed chairside, between appointments, can contribute greatly to long-range prevention.
• One idea for an exercise during patient treatment is shown in Figure 36-21. Each time an instrument is returned to the tray, fingers and wrists can be stretched before picking up the next instrument needed.

■ INSTRUMENT SHARPENING

Objectives for techniques of sharpening emphasize the preservation of the original shape of the instrument while restoring a sharp cutting edge. Instruments designed for a particular purpose should continue to be used in the manner for which they were designed and should not be distorted by inaccurate sharpening techniques.

Sharpening procedures are not easy to learn and require skill and patience to accomplish. While the process may seem tedious and time consuming, sharpening is an essential and integral part of instrumentation that cannot be overlooked. Successful clinical outcomes using bladed instruments are dependent upon correctly contoured and sharpened instruments.

This chapter includes sharpening procedures for the scaler, file, hoe, chisel, curet, and explorer, using various sharpening stones and devices. The principles of sharpening that are outlined and illustrated here may be applied to various types of sharpening stones and instruments. Terms related to instrument sharpening are defined in Box 36-2.

I. BENEFITS FROM USE OF SHARP MANUAL INSTRUMENTS

Instruments must be sharp if scaling, root planing, and maintenance root debridement are to be completed efficiently with minimal trauma to the tissues. When the instrument blade is maintained with its original contour and sharp cutting edges, the following may be expected:

• Greater precision of treatment, improved quality of results, and less working time involved.
• Increased tactile sensitivity during instrumentation. A sharp instrument does not have to be gripped as firmly as a dull one.

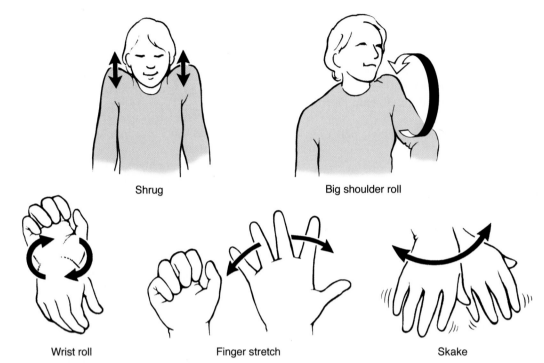

■ **FIGURE 36-20 Chairside Stretching Exercises.** Stretching exercises to relax the back, shoulders, and neck are shown with the shrug and rolling the head around with the big shoulder roll. Hand and finger rolls, stretches, and shaking can be performed anytime, even while attending a patient.

- Greater control of the instrument because of the lighter grasp needed; less pressure on the tooth being scaled or planed and decreased pressure on the finger rest are required.
- Fewer strokes required.

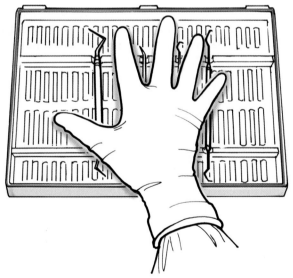

■ **FIGURE 36-21 Stretching Fingers Prior to Instrument Retrieval.** One of the exercises that can be used during actual clinical practice.

- Less possibility of burnishing rather than removing the calculus.
- Prevention of unnecessary trauma to gingival tissues and, therefore, less discomfort experienced by the patient.
- Decreased possibility of nicking, grooving, or scratching the tooth surfaces.
- Less fatigue for the clinician.

II. CONSEQUENCES OF USING DULL MANUAL INSTRUMENTS

- Stress and frustration of using ineffective instruments.
- Wasted time, effort, and energy.
- Loss of control and increased likelihood of slipping with instrument and lacerating the gingival tissue.
- Loss of patient confidence in clinician's ability.
- Increased likelihood of developing work-related musculoskeletal disorders (WMDs) from excessive muscle strain and increased number of stroke repetitions.

III. SHARPENING STONES

A. Materials and Their Sources

1. *Natural Abrasive Stones.* Quarried from mineral deposits, the hard Arkansas stone is used for

BOX 36-2 KEY WORDS: Sharpening

Arkansas stone: fine-grained sharpening stone quarried from natural mineral deposits.

Burnish: to smooth and polish; an effect that can result when a dull scaler or curet is passed over tenacious calculus in an attempt to remove the deposit.

Cutting edge: the fine line formed where the face and lateral surfaces of a scaler or curet meet when the instrument is sharp; when the instrument is dull, the line has thickness and may even reflect light.

Hone: a sharpening stone (noun). **Honing:** sharpening (verb).

Rotary stone: a sharpening stone mounted on a metal mandrel for use in a dental hand piece.

Sharpness: when a scaler or curet is sharp, the cutting edge is a fine line that does not reflect light.

Testing stick: plastic 1/4-inch rod, 3 inches long, used to test the sharpness of a scaler or a curet.

---

dental instruments because of its fine abrasive particle size.

2. *Artificial Materials*
   a. Hard, nonmetallic substances impregnated with aluminum oxide, silicon carbide, or diamond particles. Examples: ruby stone, carborundum stones, and the diamond hone.
   b. Ceramic aluminum oxide.
   c. Steel alloys are metals that are harder than most dental instrument steel and, therefore, are capable of sharpening the instrument. Example: tungsten carbide steel used in the Neivert whittler.

B. Categories

Sharpening stones as they are manufactured for use may be classified into two general groups: those for manual (unmounted) sharpening and those for power-driven (mandrel-mounted) sharpening. Examples of procedures using both unmounted and mounted stones are supplied in this chapter.

1. Unmounted
   a. **Flat stones**: Rectangular stones with square or rounded edges, or with one side grooved for the special adaptation of curved blades.
   b. **Cylindrical** (tapered or straight) or rectangular with rounded edges.
   c. **Other types**: Sharpening devices, such as the Neivert whittler.
2. Mandrel Mounted
   Cylindrical (straight or tapered) small stones of various diameters designed to fit the various sizes of instrument blades.

IV. DYNAMICS OF SHARPENING

A. Sharpening Stone Surface

A sharpening stone acts as an abrasive to reshape a dulled blade by grinding the surface until the cutting edge is restored. The surface of the stone is made up of masses of minute crystals, which are the abrasive particles that accomplish the grinding of the instrument. A smaller particle size or a finer grain, as it is generally called, abrades or reduces more slowly and produces a finer cutting edge.

B. Cutting Edge

1. The cutting edge is a very fine *line* formed where the face and lateral surface meet at an angle.
2. The edge is a line and, therefore, has length but no thickness.
3. The edge becomes dull when pressed against a hard surface (the tooth), or it may be nicked when drawn over a rough surface.
4. A dull edge is rounded and therefore has thickness. *The object in sharpening is to reshape the cutting edge to a fine line.*

C. Sharpening

Sharpening is accomplished by grinding the surface or surfaces that form the cutting edge.

V. TESTS FOR INSTRUMENT SHARPNESS

A. Visual or Glare Test

1. Examine the cutting edge under adequate light using magnification.

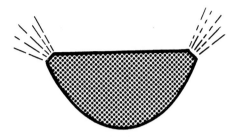

■ **FIGURE 36-22 Cross Section of a Dull Curet.** A sharp curet has a fine line at the cutting edge that will not reflect light. A dull cutting edge is like a small surface and reflects light as shown.

2. Because the sharp cutting edge is a fine *line,* it does not reflect light.
3. The dull cutting edge presents a rounded, shiny *surface,* which reflects light. Figure 36-22 shows the cross section of a dull universal curet. The cutting edges are tiny surfaces that reflect light. Compare the cutting edges with Figure 36-5, which shows the sharp cutting edges, at the points labeled "c," of a universal curet.

B. Plastic Testing Stick

1. Use a sterile plastic or acrylic 1/4-inch rod, 3 inches long.
2. Place the fulcrum finger on the end of the stick.
3. Apply the heel end of the instrument blade to the plastic stick, first at 90°, then closed to the correct angle for scaling (70°).
4. Press lightly but firmly.
5. Roll the blade forward from heel to toe by turning or rolling the instrument handle in the fingers.

C. Confirming Sharpness Using the Plastic Test Stick

1. The **sharp** cutting edge engages or grips the plastic as the length of the blade is tested. Each portion of the cutting edge will engage the plastic uniformly as the blade advances.
2. The **dull** cutting edge does not catch without undue pressure and slides easily over the surface of the stick.
3. Because the edge is not uniformly dulled during use, there will be portions of the blade that exhibit varying degrees of sharpness or dullness.
4. As the instrument blade is rolled along the test stick, the degree of slipping vs. engagement will indicate the degree of sharpness or dullness. If only limited portions of the blade exhibit dull-

ness, attempt to note the segments that slip as the blade is rolled along the test stick.
   a. The entire length of the cutting edge is always sharpened to maintain the original form.
   • Awareness of the portion(s) exhibiting dullness can guide pressure and the number of strokes.
   • This helps to minimize oversharpening.
   b. Careful evaluation will increase efficiency and raise the likelihood that dull portions of the blade are restored to sharpness.

VI. EVALUATION OF TECHNIQUE

A. Observe closely the stabilization of both the instrument and stone, each kept aligned in a single plane.
   1. Self-check: as the stone is activated for sharpening, observe the top of the instrument to ensure it is secure and not moving.
   2. Self-check: observe stone to ensure it remains in a single plane of movement back and forth as it is activated.
B. Evaluate by turning the instrument over to examine the back of the lateral surfaces under well-lit magnification.
   • A solid, consistent bevel results from:
      • Instrument and stone positioned at the correct angle.
      • Movement occurring in a single plane.
   • Irregular bevel is revealed by:
      • Breaks in the fine line of the blade edge.
      • Varying facets indicating the improper stone placement/movement.

■ SOME BASIC SHARPENING PRINCIPLES

I. STERILIZATION OF THE SHARPENING STONE

• A sterile sharpening stone and testing stick are parts of a basic clinic set up for a scaling appointment.
• Instruments then may be sharpened throughout the procedure as they show signs of dullness.
• Efficiency increases, and the patient benefits from receiving a more thorough treatment in less time.
• Sterilization of stones may be accomplished using any of the acceptable sterilization methods described on pages 69 to 72, in accord with specific manufacturer's recommendations.

- Over time, the steam autoclave may dry out an Arkansas stone and lead to chipping or breakage.

II. INSTRUMENT HANDLING

All instruments must be handled with care to preserve sharpness and prevent accidental damage to the cutting edges.

III. PREPARATION OF STONE FOR SHARPENING

A. Dry Stone

Because of the problems related to maintaining a sterile stone and preventing contamination when oil, tap water, or a lubricant is applied, the use of a dry stone provides a particular advantage.

A dry stone contributes to the following effects:
1. Sharpens the cutting edge without nicks in the blade; nicks can be created from particles of metal suspended in a lubricant.
2. Allows the stone to be completely sterilized without the problem of interference by the oil left in and on the stone.

B. Water on Stone

Ceramic stones may be used dry or with water.

C. Lubricated Stone

Certain quarried stones need lubrication to prevent drying out. Instruments are autoclaved before sharpening, and then stone and instruments are sterilized again after nonsterile lubricant is used.

The lubricant can provide the following effects:
1. Facilitate the movement of the instrument blade over the stone and prevent scratching of the stone.
2. Suspend the metallic particles removed during sharpening and so help to prevent clogging of the pores of the stone (glazing).

IV. SHARPENING

A. Objectives

The objectives during sharpening are twofold:
1. To produce a sharp cutting edge.
2. To preserve the original shape of the instrument.
   - Instrument shape is also known as contour.
   - The contour of a curet toe is a smooth, continuous curvature with no points or flat edges.

B. When to Sharpen

- Sharpen at the first sign of dullness during an appointment.

- When instruments become grossly dulled, recontouring wastes the instrument. Restoration of the original contour while maintaining a strong blade is difficult to achieve.

C. Angulation

- Before starting to sharpen, analyze the cutting edge and establish the proper angle between the stone and the blade surface.
- Maintain the angle through the firm grasp, secure finger rest, moderate pressure, short stroke, and other features of the technique appropriate to the individual instrument.

D. Maintain Control

- Maintain control so that the entire surface is reduced evenly.
- Care must be taken not to create a new bevel at the cutting edge.

E. Prevent Grooving

- Prevent grooving of the sharpening stone by varying the areas for instrument placement.
- Cleaning and stain removal procedures are described on page 643.

V. AFTER SHARPENING

Gently hone or burnish the nonbeveled surface adjacent to the cutting edge.

A. Honing

Honing means sharpening, but in common usage, honing has been applied to the process whereby the "bur" or "wire edge" is removed from the side of the cutting edge that was not reduced.

B. How the Wire Edge Is Produced

- During sharpening, some of the metal particles removed during grinding remain attached to the edge of the instrument and create the wire edge.
- If allowed to remain, the tiny particles may be removed when the instrument is applied to the tooth surface during treatment.
- By sharpening into, toward, or against the cutting edge, the production of a wire edge is minimized.

C. Removal of Wire Edge

- Pass a sharpening stone along the side of the cutting edge using an even and light pressure.

- One or two strokes are usually sufficient.
- If heavy pressure is applied, the bevel of the cutting edge can be altered.

VI. INSTRUMENT WEAR

As curets are used, they wear down at the cutting edge, leaving a narrower face and shorter length over a period of time. Sharpening also contributes to this size reduction. At some point in time, when their size has been reduced sufficiently, they must be retired and discarded because their blades will no longer access or adapt to the tooth surface.

Instruments that have become excessively narrow are sometimes reserved for patients with minimal deposit. Exert care when using overly thinned curets. If strong lateral pressure is applied, they may break off at the tip, leaving the last few millimeters embedded in the sulcus or pocket. Protocol for retrieving a broken instrument tip is included in Box 37-5, page 674.

Evaluation during sharpening procedures provides the opportunity for proper attention to instrument maintenance.

- Consider usefulness and suitability of instruments for various procedures as they are sharpened and assigned to tray setups.
- Assign thinner-bladed instruments to procedures that do not require moderate or heavy calculus removal, such as maintenance appointments.
- Discard or recycle instruments that have outlived their usefulness with shortened blades that cannot access proximal surfaces sufficiently.

▪ SHARPENING CURETS AND SCALERS

In the sections following, procedures for a variety of sharpening techniques are outlined. In general, manual sharpening procedures are the methods of choice so that the blade is not reduced unnecessarily by a rapid-cutting mounted stone.

I. TECHNIQUE OBJECTIVES

- Preserve the original contour of the blade.
- Sharpen frequently to prevent need for excessive recontouring of the blade.

II. SELECTION OF CUTTING EDGES TO SHARPEN

A. Scalers

- Most scalers are universal instruments.
- Cutting edges on both sides of the face are sharpened (Figure 36-23).

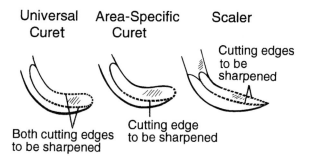

■ **FIGURE 36-23 Selection of Cutting Edge to Sharpen.** Both cutting edges and the rounded toe are sharpened for a universal curet. An area-specific curet is sharpened on the longer cutting edge and the rounded toe. A scaler is sharpened on the two sides, and the tip is brought to a point.

B. Curets: Universal

- Cutting edges on both sides of the face and the toe are sharpened (Figure 36-23).
- A three-step sharpening procedure is used.

C. Curets: Area Specific

- Cutting edge on one side of the face and the toe are sharpened.
- Sharpen the longer cutting edge, generally it will be the one farthest from the handle. In Figure 36-23, it is shown with a dotted line.
- A two-step sharpening procedure is used.

▪ MOVING FLAT STONE: STATIONARY INSTRUMENT

The side of the cutting edge formed by the lateral surface is reduced by this method. The technique described applies to both curets and scalers. Because the scaler has a pointed tip and the curet has a round toe end, a variation is necessary in the adaptation of the sharpening stone to that portion of the blade.

I. EXAMINE THE CUTTING EDGE TO BE SHARPENED

Test for sharpness to determine specific areas that are dull, but plan to sharpen the whole cutting edge(s) to maintain original contour.

II. REVIEW THE ANGULATION TO BE RESTORED AT THE DULL CUTTING EDGE

- Internal angle of the blade at the cutting edge(s) is 70° to 80° (Figures 36-5 and 36-8).

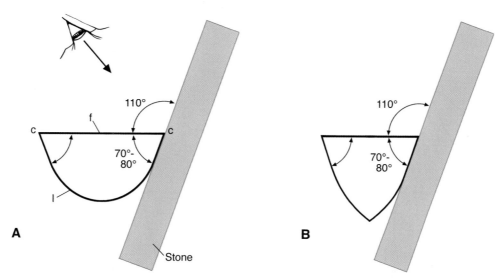

■ **FIGURE 36-24 Angulation for Sharpening.** Cross sections of a curet **(A)** and a scaler **(B)** show correct angulation of the face *(f)* of the blade with the flat sharpening stone to reproduce the internal angle of the instrument at 70°. Note the cutting edges *(c)* and the lateral surfaces *(1)*.

- Visible angle at which the stone will be placed will be 110°, as shown in Figure 36-24.

III. STABILIZE AND POSITION THE INSTRUMENT

- Grasp the instrument in the nondominant hand in a palm grasp.
- Lean the hand against the edge of an immovable workbench or table under bright light (Figure 36-25A).
- The instrument should be low enough to allow the clinician to see clearly the cutting edges.
- Turn the face of the instrument up and parallel with the floor. Point the curet toe (or scaler tip) toward the clinician to provide better access for moving the stone.
- Note the shape of the face from above as outlined in Figure 36-26.
  - The cutting edges begin at the lower shank.
  - The cutting edges are parallel, until they converge.
- For the curet, they curve to form the toe.
- For the scaler, they taper to make the pointed tip.

IV. APPLY THE SHARPENING STONE

- Hold the stone perpendicular to the floor, at the end of the cutting edge nearest the lower shank.
- From that 90° angle with the face of the instrument, open the stone to make an angle of 110° (Figure 36-24).

V. ACTIVATE THE SHARPENING STONE

A. Steps One and Two

- Maintain the stone in contact with the blade and at the proper angle throughout the procedure.
- Tighten the grasp on the instrument (nondominant fist) while applying a smooth even pressure to the cutting edge to keep the instrument stable and motionless.
- Move the stone up and down with short rhythmical strokes about 1/2 inch high. Place more pressure on the down stroke. Maintain the 110° angle precisely. Finish each area with a down stroke.
- *For the universal curet*:
  1. Follow the cutting edge to where the curvature for the toe begins, applying 3 or 4 down strokes overlapping at each millimeter of the cutting edge.
  2. Proceed to the opposite side to sharpen, repeating the steps just described (Figure 36-25).
  3. Next, proceed to the third step to sharpen the toe.
- *For the Area-specific curet*: Apply sharpening strokes **only** to the one selected side: proceed to the third step to sharpen all around the toe.
- *For the scaler*: Follow the same procedure to where the cutting edge tapers to form the sharp tip and continue in that direction to finish that side of the blade. Proceed to the other side to sharpen the opposite cutting edge.

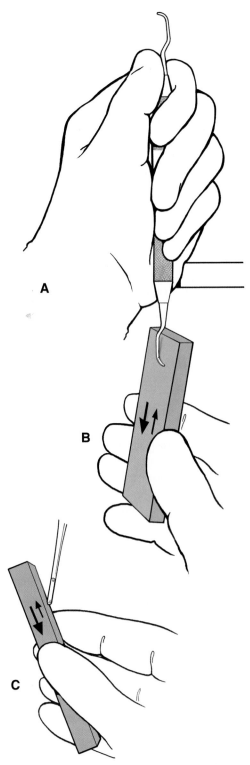

■ **FIGURE 36-25 Stationary Instrument—Moving Stone Technique. (A)** Grasp the instrument with the nondominant hand. Stabilize the hand on the edge of a stationary table or bench and provide good light on the instrument. **(B)** The stone is angled with the face of the instrument at 110° (Figure 36-24) to maintain the internal angle of the blade at 70° to 80°. **(C)** Stone reversed to sharpen the opposite cutting edge of a universal curet.

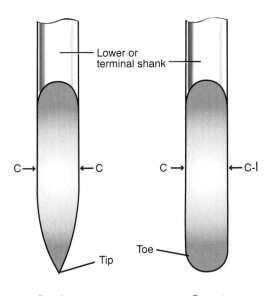

■ **FIGURE 36-26 View of a Scaler and a Curet Looking Into the Face.** The cutting edges (*c* and *c-1*) are parallel until they curve in to form the pointed tip (scaler) or the round toe (curet).

B. Step Three: The Toe of a Curet

- Tip curet down to make the toe parallel with floor.
- Apply stone to make a 90° angle with the toe.
- Open the stone to make a 110° angle.
- Apply strokes for sharpening as described for the sides of the face.

VI. TEST FOR SHARPNESS

- Apply testing stick along the entire cutting edges.
- Repeat sharpening procedures as necessary to retain clean sharp cutting edges.

▪ STATIONARY FLAT STONE: MOVING INSTRUMENT

I. CURET

A. Place the stone flat on a steady surface.
B. Examine the cutting edges to be sharpened. Test for sharpness.
C. Hold the instrument in a modified pen grasp, and establish a secure finger rest (Figure 36-27A).
D. Apply the cutting edge to the stone. An angle of 110° is formed by the stone and face.
   1. Because the curet is curved, only a small section of the cutting edge can be applied at one time.

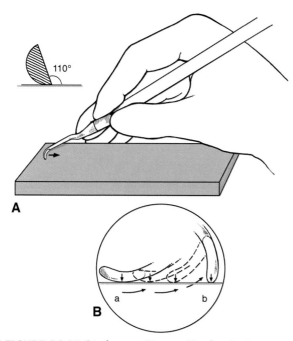

■ **FIGURE 36-27 Stationary Stone—Moving Instrument Technique. (A)** Stone placed flat with blade in position at the beginning of the sharpening stroke. With the finger rest stabilized on the edge of the stone, the cutting edge is maintained at the proper angulation (110°) as the instrument is drawn along the stone with an even, moderate pressure. **(B)** The movement of the blade is shown by the arrows, which indicate each portion of the cutting edge as the blade is turned on the stone from the beginning *(a)* to the completion *(b)* of the stroke at the center of the round toe of the curet. For a universal curet, the instrument is turned over and the opposite cutting edge is sharpened.

Universal curets are sharpened on both sides and around the toe. Gracey curets are sharpened on one side only and around the toe (see Figure 36-23).

    J. Use the manual sharpening cone (described in the next section) or the Neivert whittler (page 639) for removing the wire edge or for sharpening from the facial aspect.

II. SCALER

    A. Place the stone flat on a firm table or bench top under adequate light. Do not tilt the stone while sharpening.

    B. Examine cutting edges to be sharpened. Test for sharpness.

    C. Hold the instrument with a firm pen grasp, using thumb, index, and middle (second) fingers to prevent the instrument from rotating or changing angles during sharpening (Figure 36-28A).

    D. Establish finger rest on side of stone using ring and little fingers.

    E. Stabilize stone with fingers of opposite hand.

    F. Apply cutting edge to be sharpened to the stone. Maintain 70° to 80° internal angle of the instrument (Figure 36-28B). The portion of the cutting edge nearest the shank is applied first.

    G. Apply moderate to light but firm pressure while instrument is in motion. Heavy pressure can reduce control of instrument, cause scratching of

    2. Sharpening is performed in a *series* of applications of the cutting edge to the stone, each overlapping the previous, as the instrument is turned and drawn steadily along the stone.

    3. The portion of the cutting edge nearest the shank is applied first (Figure 36-27B, a).

    E. Apply moderate to light but firm pressure while the instrument is activated.

    F. Use a slow, steady stroke to maintain control and to ensure that each portion of the cutting edge receives equal treatment.

    G. Move the blade forward into the cutting edge. Turn the instrument continuously until the center of the round end of the blade is reached (Figure 36-27B, b).

    H. Test for sharpness along the entire cutting edge; reapply to stone as necessary for ideal sharpness.

    I. Turn the instrument to sharpen the second cutting edge. Overlap at the center of the round toe.

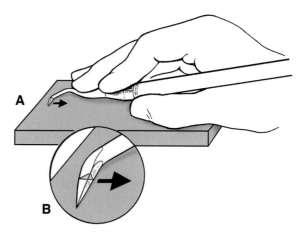

■ **FIGURE 36-28 Stationary Stone Technique for a Straight Scaler. (A)** With a modified pen grasp and a finger rest established on the side of the stone, the scaler is positioned for sharpening. **(B)** The portion of the cutting edge nearest the lower shank is applied first with an angle of 110° between the face and the stone. The instrument is turned continuously to follow the arclike shape of the blade. The cutting edges are sharpened to the pointed tip.

the stone, and produce an unfavorable bevel at the cutting edge.

H. Use a short, slow stroke to maintain the exact relation of the cutting edge to the stone.
    1. Pull blade forward, toward the cutting edge.
    2. All fingers move with the arm as a unit.
    3. Use a slow, steady stroke to maintain control and to ensure that each portion of the cutting edge receives equal treatment.
    4. Turn the instrument continually to follow the shape of the blade to the pointed tip.
I. Test for sharpness after one or two strokes. Repeat as needed for ideal sharpness.
J. Turn instrument and proceed to sharpen other lateral surface. When instrument placement is awkward for a modified contra-angle scaler, use a narrow side of the stone.

■ SHARPENING CONE

I. DESCRIPTION

A. Types

Stones are cylindrical Arkansas cones (tapered or straight), or rectangular with rounded edges, and tapered carborundum stones.

B. Uses

1. *Arkansas.* Tapered cone is recommended for curved cutting edges of scalers and curets.
2. *Carborundum.* Coarser grain is useful for preliminary shaping or sharpening of excessively dulled instruments. Use of a finer stone follows to refine the cutting edge.

II. SHARPENING PROCEDURE

A. Position

1. Hold instrument in nondominant hand across palm, with fingers and thumb grasping firmly. Direct blade toward self, with face of the blade up and parallel with the floor.
2. For additional support, place instrument over the edge of a firm hard block and maintain rigidly (Figure 36-29).
3. Stabilize arms between the wrists and elbows on the edge of a solid table or bench top.
4. Use the following procedure for a tapered cone:
    a. With a firm grasp of the sharpening cone, position the appropriate diameter of the cone to fit the curvature of the surface to be sharpened.

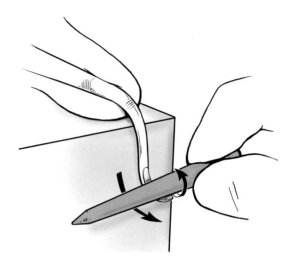

■ FIGURE 36-29 Sharpening Cone. A cylindrical stone is applied to the face of a curet. The instrument is stabilized over a firm block, and the stone is positioned to fit the curvature of the surface to be sharpened. An even pressure is applied across the face of the instrument so that both cutting edges will be sharpened on the same plane.

    b. Apply the stone straight across the face so that an even pressure can be applied to both cutting edges simultaneously to produce an evenly sharpened instrument (Figure 36-29).

B. Motion

1. Rotate stone counterclockwise over the instrument with even, firm pressure.
2. Continue rotation of stone upward (as in a circle) when approaching the end of the curet to prevent tapering off and reshaping (flattening) the curvature of the tip. (Figure 36-32B illustrates this motion for the mounted stone.)

C. Test for Sharpness

Test for sharpness after a few applications. Repeat as necessary to obtain ideal sharpness.

■ THE NEIVERT WHITTLER

I. DESCRIPTION

A. Working End

The working end consists of five sharpening edges and a rounded burnishing edge of tungsten carbide steel.

B. Handle

The handle, which is made of stainless steel, is bulky and hexagonal for comfortable grasping (Figure 36-30).

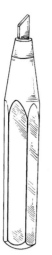

■ **FIGURE 36-30 The Neivert Whittler.** The working end is made of tungsten carbide steel and the handle is made of stainless steel.

II. USES

A. Manufacturer's instructions describe the procedure used for sharpening straight and curved blades, including those of dental instruments, scissors, and knives.

B. Particularly useful for the face of a curved scaler or curet.

C. The outer rounded edge is designed for honing.

III. SHARPENING PROCEDURE

A. Position

Stability and control are most important.

1. Hold instrument to be sharpened firmly in the nondominant hand, across palm, grasping with all fingers and the thumb, with the surface to be sharpened turned toward self. The instrument can also be stabilized over the edge of a firm, hard surface, as shown for the cone in Figure 36-29.

2. Stabilize arms between the wrists and the elbows on the edge of an immovable table or bench top.

3. Whittler is held in a palm grasp with thumb under handle adjacent to the working end. At the same time, the thumb rest is applied beneath the instrument blade on the nondominant hand (Figure 36-31A).

4. Apply working end to the curvature of the surface to be sharpened straight across so that even pressure can be applied to both cutting edges simultaneously, thereby producing an evenly sharpened instrument (Figure 36-31B).

B. Motion

1. Draw the whittler edge across the length of the face with a moderate, even pressure.

2. As the end is approached, continue in an upward motion to prevent tapering off and reshaping curvature of the toe.

C. Test for Sharpness

Test for sharpness after a few applications.

D. Hone

Hone the lateral surfaces of blade next to cutting edges.

■ MANDREL-MOUNTED STONES

I. DESCRIPTION

A. Types

1. *Arkansas*: Fine grain.

2. *Ruby Stone*: Coarser grain, especially useful for recontouring excessively dull instrument. When

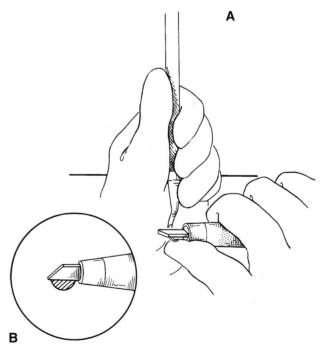

■ **FIGURE 36-31 Sharpening With a Neivert Whittler. (A)** The instrument is stabilized in the nondominant hand, and the whittler is held in a palm grasp with the thumb rest close to the instrument to be sharpened. **(B)** Close-up shows position of the blade of the sharpener across the face of the curet.

used for routine sharpening, the ruby stone should be applied conservatively.

B. Shapes

The stones are cylindrical with flat end or cone shape.

C. Use

1. Applicable to most cutting edges. Various sizes and grains of stones are selectively utilized.
2. Coarse-grained ruby stone may be useful for reshaping.
3. Stones are sterilized and may be used with water for cooling.

II. SHARPENING PROCEDURE

A. Select Stone

Select a sharpening stone with a diameter appropriate to fit the blade of the instrument to be sharpened.

B. Position

1. Hold instrument to be sharpened in a palm grasp with blade face up.
2. Hold handpiece in other hand using a palm grasp with the thumb securely placed against the thumb of the hand holding the instrument (Figure 36-32A).
3. Stabilize arms between wrists and elbows on the edge of a solid table or bench top.

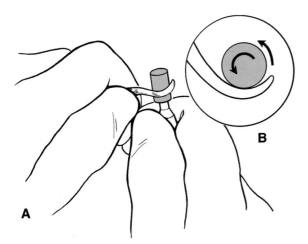

▪ **FIGURE 36-32 Mandrel-Mounted Sharpening Stone. (A)** A mounted stone with a diameter appropriate for the curved blade to be sharpened is positioned across the face for even sharpening of the cutting edges. Hands and arms are stabilized for precision and control. **(B)** With low speed to minimize heat production, the rotating stone is passed along the face of the instrument. Near the toe, the stone is moved upward to prevent flattening of a curved instrument.

4. Apply stone to surface to be sharpened straight across so that light, even pressure can be applied to both cutting edges simultaneously, thereby producing an evenly sharpened instrument.

C. Motion

1. Use low speed to:
   a. Minimize heat production (alteration of the temper of the steel can result with repeated use).
   b. Allow complete control of position of sharpening stone on blade.
2. Apply light pressure to prevent undue reduction of instrument. Pressure, however, should be sufficiently heavy to create a smooth surface.
3. Maintain blade shape. Pass the rotating stone upward when approaching the end of the blade to prevent tapering off and reshaping the tip (Figure 36-32B).

D. Test for Sharpness

Test for sharpness after one or two applications. Repeat when necessary.

E. Hone

Hone the lateral borders of the cutting edges.

III. DISADVANTAGES OF POWER-DRIVEN SHARPENING

A. Inconsistent results because of variations in speed and difficulty of stabilization of instrument and sharpening stone.
B. Excess reduction of instrument during shorter period of use; less conservation of instruments than by manual methods.
C. Frictional heat may affect the temper of the steel.

▪ SHARPENING THE FILE SCALER

Files are sharpened with an instrument called a tang file. Use of magnification and good illumination are necessary when sharpening files to ensure correct placement of the tang file.

Use a test stick to check for the degree of sharpness to determine whether the file will need to be sharpened. If the file blades do not grasp the plastic test stick when adapted lightly, they will need to be sharpened.

I. SURFACE TO BE GROUND

Examine the file closely with the head of the working end positioned outward (Figure 36-10A). Note the two angular surfaces that meet to form a "V" shape (Figure 36-10B). The surface to be contacted with the tang file and ground during sharpening is the surface of the "V" that is furthest away from you.

II. SHARPENING PROCEDURE

A. Place the sterile file on a clean surface with good illumination and some means of magnification. Secure it with the back of the head facing down and the series of teeth facing up.

B. Position the right end of the tang file in the channel as shown in the illustration (Figure 36-33A). (Left-handed clinicians reverse the process, positioning the left end of the tang file in the channel.)

C. With light to moderate steady pressure, pull the tang file through the channel, moving in a straight line from one end to the other in just one direction.

D. Release pressure and reposition the tang file back at the starting point. Repeat the process. Two or three passes with the tang file are usually sufficient to bring the edges back to sharpness.

E. Sharpen the remaining blades using the same technique.

F. Test for sharpness and repeat the sharpening stroke as needed for ideal edge sharpness.

▪ SHARPENING THE HOE SCALER

The hoe has only one surface to be ground. Because placement of the small surface on the flat stone is difficult to visualize, magnification is needed.

I. SURFACE TO BE GROUND

Examine surface to be ground (Figure 36-34A). Test for sharpness.

II. SHARPENING PROCEDURE

A. Hold instrument in modified pen grasp. Establish finger rest on the stone.

B. Apply the surface to be ground to the stone in correct relationship to maintain the 45° bevel (Figure 36-34B).

C. With moderate, steady pressure, pull the instrument toward the cutting edge a short distance. Allow the whole hand to move with the arm as a unit.

D. Release pressure and slide the instrument back. Repeat.

E. Test for sharpness and reapply as needed for ideal sharpness.

F. Hone the undersurface of the blade adjacent to the cutting edge.

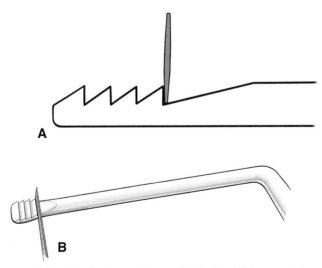

▪ **FIGURE 36-33 Sharpening a File Scaler. (A)** Tang file in position against one of the several surfaces to be ground. **(B)** With the file scaler stabilized to prevent movement, the Tang file is pulled through the channel using a moderate, steady pressure against the surface to be ground.

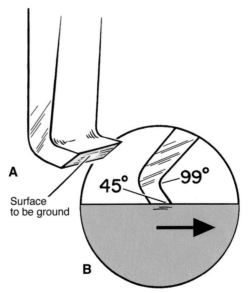

▪ **FIGURE 36-34 Sharpening a Hoe Scaler. (A)** Surface to be ground. **(B)** Hoe adapted to the surface of a stationary flat stone at the proper angle to maintain the original bevel of 45°. Arrow indicates direction of the sharpening stroke leading into the cutting edge.

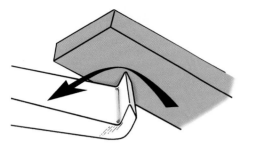

■ **FIGURE 36-35 Rounding a Hoe Scaler.** To round the sharp corners of the hoe scaler, a flat stone is rubbed over the instrument with a gentle rolling motion.

III. ROUND CORNERS

Corners should be rounded at each end of the cutting edge.
A. Rounded corners help to prevent laceration of soft tissue or grooving of tooth surface.
B. Hold instrument in nondominant hand with corners of cutting edge directed inward.
C. Rub the surface of the sharpening stone across each corner with a gentle rolling motion (Figure 36-35). Two or three applications are usually sufficient.

■ SHARPENING THE CHISEL SCALER

Sharpening procedures for the chisel are similar to those for the hoe. Again, the surface is small, the angulation is difficult to visualize, and the use of magnification is needed.

I. SURFACE TO BE GROUND

Examine surface to be ground (Figure 36-36A). Test for sharpness.

II. SHARPENING PROCEDURE

A. Hold instrument with a modified pen grasp, establish finger rest, and apply the surface to be ground to the stone in the correct relationship to maintain the 45° bevel (Figure 36-36B).
B. With moderate, steady pressure, push the instrument forward, toward the cutting edge, without changing the relationship with the stone.
C. After two or three applications, test for sharpness and reapply as necessary for an ideal cutting edge.
D. Hone the nonbeveled surface.

III. ROUND CORNERS

Round the corners at each end of the cutting edge. In a manner similar to that shown in Figure 36-35 for the hoe scaler, rub the surface of the flat stone across each corner of the chisel with a gentle, even, rolling motion. Two or three applications are usually sufficient.

■ SHARPENING EXPLORERS

I. TESTS FOR SHARPNESS

A. Visual

When examined under concentrated light, a dull explorer tip appears rounded.

B. Plastic Testing Stick

A sharp explorer grips the plastic tester on light pressure and moves with resistance when pulled over the surface. A dull explorer does not catch. It slides.

II. RECONTOUR

Small-nosed pliers can be used to straighten a bent tip.

III. SHARPENING PROCEDURE

A. Use flat stone.
B. Instrument is held with a modified pen grasp. Finger rest is established on side of stone.
C. Placement and movement of the tip over the stone resemble somewhat the procedure for the curet on the stone (see Figure 36-27B).

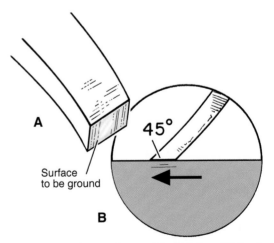

■ **FIGURE 36-36 Sharpening a Chisel Scaler. (A)** Surface to be ground. **(B)** Chisel is adapted to the surface of a stationary flat stone at the proper angle to maintain the original bevel of 45°. Arrow indicates direction of the sharpening stroke leading into the cutting edge.

Everyday Ethics

Diane just finished practicing her first month as a registered dental hygienist. She takes a moment to reflect on the challenges of seeing a full schedule of patients each day. Overall, Dr. Dakin has been pleased with her work, but Diane recounts one day when she missed two obvious subgingival pieces of calculus on teeth #27 distally and #28 mesially. It wasn't enough that she accidentally skipped that area, but Dr. Dakin made a few negative comments jokingly that embarrassed Diane. He smiled at the patient and said, "You'll be fine."

After he left, the patient turned to Diane and said, "What was that all about?"

Diane simply answered, "Oh, he likes to tease me sometimes."

Diane pondered what she would do if this situation occurred in the future.

Questions for Consideration

1. Given the hygienist's neophyte status as a clinician, how could she address Dr. Dakin's negative comments? Include the terms beneficence and nonmaleficence in the discussion.

2. What should be said to the patient regarding what occurred?

3. Describe Diane's alternatives to prevent a recurrence.

---

1. Place side of tip on stone at approximately a 15° to 20° angle of stone with shank of explorer.
2. As tip is moved over the surface, the handle is rotated so that even pressure can be applied to each part of the tip.

■ CARE OF SHARPENING EQUIPMENT

I. FLAT ARKANSAS STONE

A. Prepare for Sterilization

Submerge in ultrasonic cleaner or scrub with soap and hot water to remove metal particles left from sharpening.

B. Stain Removal

Periodically clean with ammonia, gasoline, or kerosene when stone becomes discolored. If the stone becomes "glazed" by metal particles ground into the surface, rub the stone over emery paper placed on a flat, solid surface.

C. Storage

Keep in sealed, sterilized package until needed for sharpening.

II. MOUNTED STONES

A. Arkansas Mounted Stones

Same basic procedures as those for the flat stone.

B. Ruby Stone

1. Clean by scrubbing with soap and water.
2. Maintain an ungrooved surface by frequently applying the stone to a Joe Dandy disc (Figure 36-37). A sandpaper disc is too flexible for this purpose.
3. Sterilize in a sealed bag.

III. CARE OF THE TANG FILE

Because the tang file corrodes easily when exposed to moisture, it requires special handling.

- Wipe the tang file with a sterile gauze 2×2 soaked with isopropyl alcohol after use.

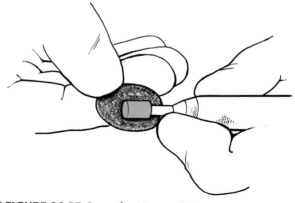

■ **FIGURE 36-37 Care of a Mounted Stone.** A Joe Dandy disc is used to maintain a smooth surface on the mounted stone. Repeated sharpenings tend to make grooves in a stone.

Factors To Teach The Patient

- Why it is necessary to use a variety of instruments for scaling.

- When and why there is a need for several appointments.

- Benefits of using a finely sharpened instrument for calculus removal.

- Harmful effects of using dull instruments.

- The relationship of personal daily care using dental floss and a toothbrush to the need for frequent appointments with the dental hygienist.

- Sterilize in a dry heat oven or chemical vapor sterilizer (pages 71 to 72).

IV. MANUFACTURER'S DIRECTIONS

Follow manufacturer's directions for all artificial stones.

REFERENCES

1. Meador, H.L.: The Biocentric Technique: A Guide to Avoiding Occupational Pain, *J. Dent. Hyg., 67,* 38, January, 1993.
2. Pattison, A.M. and Pattison, G.L.: *Periodontal Instrumentation,* 2nd ed. Norwalk, CT, Appleton & Lange, 1992, pp. 166, 232, 371.

SUGGESTED READINGS

Hard, D.: Oral Prophylaxis, in Bunting, R.W.: *Oral Hygiene,* 3rd ed. Philadelphia, Lea & Febiger, 1957, pp. 249–258.

Hirschfeld, L.: Subgingival Curettage in Periodontal Treatment, *J. Am. Dent. Assoc., 44,* 301, March, 1952.

MacDonald, G., Wilson, S.G., and Waldman, K.B.: Physical Characteristics of the Hand and Early Clinical Skill: Their Relationship in a Group of Dental Hygiene Students, *J. Dent. Hyg., 65,* 380, October, 1991.

Tondrowski, V.E.: Preclinical Procedures for the Dental Hygiene Student, *J. Dent. Educ., 20,* 321, November, 1956.

Instruments

Balevi, B.: Engineering Specifics of the Periodontal Curet's Cutting Edge, *J. Periodontol., 67,* 374, April, 1996.

Fredekind, R. and Cuny, E.: Instruments Used in Dentistry, in Murphy, D.C., ed.: *Ergonomics and the Dental Care Worker,* Washington, D.C., American Public Health Association, 1998, pp 169-189.

Glenner, R.A.: The Scaler, *Bull. Hist. Dent., 38,* 31, April, 1990.

Kunselman, B., Mann, G.B., and Mauriello, S.M.: Task Analysis of the Gracey 17/18 Curet, *J. Pract. Hyg., 8,* 11, November/December, 1999.

Long, B.A. and Singer, D.L.: A New Curet Series: The Gracey Curvettes, *RDH, 12,* 46, February, 1992.

Tal, H., Kozlovsky, A., Green, E., and Gabbay, M.: Scanning Electron Microscope Evaluation of Wear of Stainless Steel and High Carbon Steel Curettes, *J. Periodontol., 60,* 320, June, 1989.

Sharpening Procedures

Glasscoe, D.D.: The Cutting Edge, *RDH, 22,* 82, November, 2002.

Green, E. and Seyer, P.C.: *Sharpening Curets and Sickle Scalers,* 2nd ed. Berkeley, CA, Praxis Publishing Co., 1972, 40 pp.

Marquam, B.J.: Keep Eye on Sharpening Techniques to Prevent Disease Transmission, *RDH, 12,* 20, August, 1992.

Murray, G.H., Lubow, R.M., Mayhew, R.B., Summitt, J.B., and Usseglio, R.J.: The Effects of Two Sharpening Methods on the Strength of a Periodontal Scaling Instrument, *J. Periodontol., 55,* 410, July, 1984.

Nield-Gehrig, J.S.: *Fundamentals of Periodontal Instrumentation,* 4th ed. Philadelphia, Lippincott Williams & Wilkins, 2000, pp. 407–428.

Parkes, R.B. and Kolstad, R.A.: Effects of Sterilization on Periodontal Instruments, *J. Periodontol., 53,* 434, July, 1982.

Rossi, R. and Smukler, H.: A Scanning Electron Microscope Study Comparing the Effectiveness of Different Types of Sharpening Stones and Curets, *J. Periodontol., 66,* 956, November, 1995.

Sasse, J.: Cutting Edges of Curets: Effect of Repeated Sterilization, *Dent. Hyg., 61,* 14, January, 1987.

Schulze, M.B.: Instrument Sharpening—"The Flat Stone in Motion," *DentalHygienistNews, 3,* 7, Summer, 1990.

Shepherd, K.R.: Instrument Sharpening: An Essential Aspect of Periodontal Therapy, *J. Pract. Hyg., 8,* 41, November/December, 1999.

Nonsurgical Periodontal Instrumentation

Stacy A. Matsuda, RDH, BS

Basic treatment for inflammatory gingival and periodontal infections is the removal of dental biofilm, bacterial toxic materials (endotoxins), and supragingival and subgingival calculus. The term *debridement* has been applied to the group of procedures involved and includes professional intervention by the clinician as well as the procedures carried out by the patient daily, when using a toothbrush and proximal biofilm-removal devices. **Periodontal debridement** includes all of the following therapeutic interventions:

- Scaling (manual and power-driven) to remove calculus and all soft deposits.
- Root planing to eliminate subgingival calculus and smooth the tooth surface.
- Root debridement to eliminate subgingival biofilm and lightly mineralized deposits.

Periodontal debridement can provide the definitive or complete treatment for many patients with less advanced infections. For those with more advanced disease, debridement is the preparatory or initial therapy. The progress and success of treatment can be influenced by innate or acquired host factors.

Dental hygiene care aims to *prevent, arrest, control,* or *eliminate* the infection in the gingiva (Case type I) or periodontal tissues (Case types II, III, IV). The ultimate goals of the instrumentation are to eliminate pathogenic microorganisms that cause the infection and to promote continuing health in the periodontal tissues. Box 37-1 contains key words related to nonsurgical therapy.

The long-range success of treatment depends on the *control* of the dental biofilm by the patient on a daily basis. Therefore, instruction and monitoring biofilm-control procedures must precede, continue simultaneously with, and follow professional mechanical instrumentation.

▪ THE SCOPE OF NONSURGICAL THERAPY

The current chapter is devoted to techniques for the removal of supragingival and subgingival deposits using manual and power-driven scaling procedures. Chapter 38 includes a variety of adjunctive interventions also considered within the scope of nonsurgical periodontal therapy. The indication for each procedure is assessed on an individual patient basis that includes periodontal risk assessment. Nonsurgical therapy may include a combination of the following procedures:

   I. Removal of dental biofilm, endotoxins, other bacterial products, and calculus.
   II. Root planing to remove residual calculus and create a smoother tooth surface.
   III. Irrigation using an antimicrobial agent.
   IV. Sustained-release antibiotic or antimicrobial agent particularly for refractory infections.
   V. Removal of iatrogenic biofilm retainers.
     - Overhanging margins of restorations.
     - Unfinished, poorly contoured, or unpolished restorations.
   VI. Concurrent dental therapeutic interventions. Examples include:
     - Restore to arrest advanced carious lesions to aid gingival healing by preventing food impaction and making personal biofilm removal possible.
     - Analysis and correction of occlusal irregularities.

BOX 37-1 KEY WORDS: Nonsurgical Instrumentation

Bacteremia : presence of bacteria in the blood.

Endotoxin: lipopolysaccharide (LPS) complex found in the cell wall of many gram-negative microorganisms; contained superficially within periodontally involved cementum.

Furcation: anatomic area between the roots of a multirooted tooth.

   Furcation invasion: pathologic resorption of bone within a furcation.

Instrumentation zone: area on tooth where instrumentation is confined; area where calculus and altered cementum are located and treatment is required.

Nonsurgical periodontal therapy: dental biofilm removal and control, supragingival and subgingival scaling, root planing, and adjunctive treatments such as the use of chemotherapy; the basic objectives are to restore periodontal health; arrest or slow the progression of early periodontal disease; or, for more advanced disease, to prepare the tissues for more complex periodontal therapy.

Root planing: a definitive treatment procedure designed to remove altered cementum or surface dentin that is rough, impregnated with calculus, or contaminated with toxins or microorganisms. Also termed **debridement** or **root preparation.**

Scaling: instrumentation of the crown or root surfaces to remove dental biofilm and calculus.

■ PREPARATION OF THE CLINICIAN

Skill in procedures for disease control for a patient requires more than the development of manual procedures for applying instruments to the tooth surfaces. In these refined and exacting techniques, knowledge of the anatomic, histopathologic, and physiologic characteristics of the teeth and supporting tissues is necessary. Such knowledge must be tied together with recognition of the clinical manifestations of the tissues in disease and then in health as the effects of treatment become apparent.

■ FOCUS OF TREATMENT

The focus of clinical treatment is on the elimination of the causes of the infection. Dental biofilm, endotoxins and other bacterial products, cementum, and calculus are all involved, but the primary sources of infection are periodontal pathogenic microorganisms in the biofilm.

I. DENTAL BIOFILM

A. Gingival inflammation and periodontal destruction result from the action of pathogenic microorganisms in dental biofilm.

B. Dental biofilm attaches to the surfaces of the gingiva and the teeth. Dental calculus is calcified dental biofilm.

II. ENDOTOXIN

A. Lipopolysaccharides or endotoxins, derived from the cell walls of gram-negative pathogenic microorganisms, are toxic to human tissue and cause inflammation and destruction of the periodontal attachment.

B. Endotoxins are embedded in the cemental surface and in the superficial biofilm and can be removed readily.[1-4]

III. CEMENTUM

A. The cementum is thin at the cervical third of the root. Some or even complete removal of the cementum during instrumentation for calculus removal is inevitable.

B. Excess removal of the cementum and vigorous root planing is not necessary.[5,6] However, a smooth surface is significant, since the microorganisms collect and colonize on a rough surface much more rapidly than on a smooth surface.[7,8]

IV. CALCULUS

A. Calculus is not directly a cause of gingival inflammation, but the irregular surface provides a nidus for bacteria of the biofilm to collect and multiply.

B. Calculus must be removed to provide a healing environment for the periodontal tissues.

▪ AIMS AND EXPECTED OUTCOMES

The effects and benefits of complete, carefully performed nonsurgical periodontal therapy are summarized here.

I. INTERRUPT OR STOP THE PROGRESS OF DISEASE

A. Reduce formation of dental biofilm.
B. Delay repopulation of pathogenic microorganisms.
C. Change behavioral and lifestyle habits of the patient to reduce risk factors for periodontal infections.

II. CREATE AN ENVIRONMENT THAT ENCOURAGES THE TISSUE TO HEAL AND THE INFLAMMATION TO BE RESOLVED

A. Convert pocket (disease) to sulcus (health).
B. Shrink previously enlarged spongy tissue.
C. Reduce probing depths.
D. Eliminate bleeding on probing.
E. Regenerate the gingival tissues to normal color, size, and contour.
F. Change the quality of the tissues from spongy to firm.
G. Improve the integrity of the clinical attachment.
H. Remove calculus and restorative dentistry irregularities to reduce biofilm retention.

III. INDUCE POSITIVE CHANGES IN THE QUALITY AND QUANTITY OF THE SUBGINGIVAL BACTERIAL FLORA

A. Before instrumentation, the predominant microorganisms are anaerobic, gram-negative, motile forms with many spirochetes and rods, high counts of all types of microorganisms, and many leukocytes.

B. After instrumentation, the composition of the bacterial flora shifts to a predominance of aerobic, gram-positive, nonmotile, coccoid forms with lowered total counts and fewer leukocytes (Table 37-1).

IV. PROVIDE INITIAL PREPARATION (TISSUE CONDITIONING) FOR COMPLICATED PERIODONTAL THERAPY REQUIRED FOR ADVANCED DISEASE

A. Reduce or eliminate etiologic and predisposing factors.
B. Permit reevaluation. Surgical procedures may be lessened in extent.

V. EDUCATE AND MOTIVATE THE PATIENT

A. To appreciate the values of a healthy mouth.
B. To assume a co-therapist role in maintaining the health established in the treatment phase.
C. To make a commitment to perform daily personal biofilm control measures.
D. To continue with periodic maintenance appointments at the recommended interval for ongoing monitoring of periodontal health.

▪ CARE PLAN FOR INSTRUMENTATION

The needs of the individual patient are identified through **patient assessment**. The course of treatment is defined by the dental hygiene diagnosis and care plan. Included in the care plan are the following:

- The special management required for the individual patient.
- The distribution and severity of the periodontal infection.
- The treatment sequence needed for the individual.
- The length and number of appointments required to fulfill the need.
- A plan for reevaluation and continuing care.

▪ TABLE 37-1 EFFECT OF INSTRUMENTATION ON POCKET MICROFLORA

PERIODONTAL INFECTION BEFORE TREATMENT	PERIODONTAL HEALTH AFTER TREATMENT
Predominant flora is:	**Predominant flora is:**
Anaerobic	Aerobic
Gram-negative	Gram-positive
Motile	Nonmotile
Spirochetes, motile rods; pathogenic	Coccoid forms; nonpathogenic
Very high total count of all types of microorganisms	Much lower total counts of all types of microorganisms
Many leukocytes	Lower leukocyte counts

■ OVERALL APPOINTMENT SYSTEMS

Whether a single or multiple appointment plan is required, the initial step is patient instruction. The overall care plan must be described and the informed consent of the patient, parent, or guardian obtained. Treatment begins with the patient's own treatment. In this chapter, the segment of the appointments devoted to instrumentation for the removal of calculus, dental biofilm, and endotoxins are described.

I. WHEN A SINGLE APPOINTMENT MAY BE ADEQUATE

A. The diagnosis is Case type I or even Case type II with small areas of deposits readily accessible; anesthesia usually is not needed.

B. Only a few teeth present; limited areas of anesthesia may be needed.

C. Patient presents with an acceptable biofilm score, and evidence of reasonable personal care without need for time for extended instruction and motivation.

D. Patient acts responsibly in keeping appointments for maintenance and continued monitoring for disease control.

II. PLANNED MULTIPLE APPOINTMENTS

The extent of periodontal involvement (Case types II, III, IV), probing measurements, distribution and extent of calculus deposits, and oral cleanliness that shows evidence of the patient's personal care or lack of it are major determinants in the number of appointments needed. The patient should never be promised that the treatment will be completed in a given number of appointments.

A. Quadrant Scaling Appointments

• One efficient system for appointment planning is by quadrants with anesthesia, at 1-week intervals to permit patient learning and progressive healing.

• With less severe periodontitis and a compliant patient, two quadrants of the same side (maxillary and mandibular arches) may be completed at an appointment.

• The patient is informed that after the scaling is completed, an appointment for evaluation will be needed.

B. Tissue Conditioning

• At the initial appointment, basic dental biofilm removal is introduced.

• Interdental devices to complement the use of a toothbrush can be added as the patient demonstrates readiness.

• At each successive appointment, a biofilm score is shown to the patient, and procedures are reviewed.

• Each week, the tissues will show changes toward a healthy state.

• The patient is self-treating and at the same time is *conditioning* the tissue for the clinician. As a result, there is less debris and less bleeding during instrumentation and fewer bacteria for the aerosol contamination created during instrumentation.

• The effect is a cleaner environment in which the clinician can carry out the treatment procedures.

C. Evaluation

• At each appointment, the quadrants previously treated are examined for evidence of healing.

• Calculus left inadvertently can be removed by remedial scaling procedures.

• Evaluation: at least 2 weeks after the scaling series, healing of the tissues is expected to be well under way. Restoration of the clinical attachment permits probing.

III. "FULL-MOUTH DISINFECTION"

A. Definition

• System of scaling in two long appointments completed within a 24-hour period.

• The procedures are best accomplished under anesthesia practicing with a chairside assistant.

• Original research combined the concentrated deposit removal with professional and personal multiple treatments with chlorhexidine for additional oral disinfection.[9,10] Follow-up research showed no significant difference with or without the intense disinfection using chlorhexidine.[11,12]

B. Rationale

• Periodontal diseases are infections: ridding the mouth of as many of the pathogens as possible at one time can encourage healing.

• In the quadrant system, it is possible for the scaled quadrant to become reinfected from pathogens left in untreated quadrants.

C. Limitations

• Case selection: many patients would not be able to withstand such intense treatment.

- Patient instruction: opportunities for review and repeated instruction at the patient's learning pace are not available without a series of extra appointments.
- Reevaluation by the clinician has advantages after a period of time. Completed increments can be evaluated and tissue response can be monitored.

IV. PRELIMINARY PARTIAL SCALING

One system used by some clinicians involved an initial or full-mouth debridement or "gross scaling," usually with an ultrasonic scaling device.

- A series of appointments was then planned for deep scaling by quadrants to complete the instrumentation.
- This approach was abandoned many years ago due to the potential for problems.
- These problems could ultimately compromise the patient's health and interfere with favorable outcomes.

V. PROBLEMS OF INCOMPLETE SCALING

Removing the coronal-most portion of the deposit while leaving pathogenic bacteria beneath the soft tissues is not recommended for a number of reasons. Before using such a plan, the following should be considered:

A. Healing at the Gingival Margin: Limited Access

- When the irritants are removed around the opening of the pocket, the tissue heals and the gingival margin can close tight around the tooth.
- The marginal tissue may take on a color and shape that appears normal to the patient, but deep calculus and adherent biofilm remain undisturbed on the root surfaces.
- Despite the appearance of improvement, the probing depth and bleeding on probing have not changed.
- With tightening of the opening of the pocket, insertion of curets for additional deep instrumentation at subsequent appointments can be difficult. This access limitation compromises the thoroughness of instrumentation that is necessary for healing and resolution of infection.

B. Potential for Abscess Formation[13]

1. *Predisposing factors:*
   - Deep suppurating pockets; advanced periodontal infection.
   - Pockets extending into furcation areas or intrabony defects.

- Patient susceptible to infection, such as with uncontrolled diabetes, with an immunodeficiency disease, or being treated with an immunosuppressive drug.

2. *Sequence: With partial scaling,*
   - Healing can begin.
   - The tissue at the gingival margin tightens.
   - The pocket closes.
   - Microorganisms multiply within.
   - An abscess develops.

C. Patient Instruction

- When supragingival calculus and dental biofilm are removed from the crowns of the teeth, the "visible lesson" is taken away.
- As gingival swelling, sensitivity, and bleeding subside, the patient may be less motivated to return for the completion of treatment.
- When treatment is carried out quadrant by quadrant, the patient has unscaled areas with which to compare the healing quadrants. The patient can see and feel changes and improvements that contrast with untreated areas.

D. Roughened Calculus

- Calculus roughened by partial removal can be a source of increased subgingival biofilm collections. The surface of calculus is highly porous microscopically, allowing bacteria to collect and colonize.
- The rough surface thus provides more sources for infection by holding pathogenic microorganisms and their inflammatory byproducts in intimate contact with the surrounding gingival tissues.[7,8]

E. Patient Misunderstanding

- For the patient with limited understanding of the seriousness and extent of periodontal infection, the mouth may feel good and look good after a gross "cleaning."
- As a result, the patient may not appreciate the need to return for the continuing appointments to complete the deep scaling. The personal objective of "clean teeth" had been fulfilled.
- Later, when severe periodontitis develops, the patient may claim that incomplete treatment was provided originally.
- By receiving repeated information at each successive quadrant treatment and by seeing the changes, the patient can gain a better understanding of the seriousness of the disease in the periodontal tissues.

VI. SCALING TO COMPLETION

A. Segmental Approach

1. Quadrant or sextant treatments are recommended to prevent the aforementioned problems associated with incomplete scaling.
2. Decisions are made according to what can reasonably be completed by the individual clinician within the time frame of a given appointment.
3. Treatment appointments are scheduled accordingly.

B. Care Planning Factors to Consider

1. *Access:* the relative ease of insertion to base of the soft tissue pocket.
   - Fibrosity and tissue tone of the free gingiva.
   - Probing depths: attachment pattern around the full circumference of each tooth.
2. *Deposit on tooth surfaces*
   - Extent and distribution of calculus.
   - Tenacity of calculus.
3. *Root anatomy*
   - Multirooted teeth with furcation involvement.
   - Deep concavities.
4. *Patient factors*
   - Need for local anesthetic or nitrous oxide/oxygen sedation.
   - Limited capacity for opening mouth.
   - Behavioral factors such as apprehension.

■ PREPARATION FOR INSTRUMENTATION

I. REVIEW THE PATIENT'S ASSESSMENT RECORD

A. **Note Special Needs:** from medical history and previous appointment experiences.
B. **Identify:** systemic or physical problems with potential for emergency.

II. REVIEW RADIOGRAPHIC FINDINGS

A. Findings Applicable During Instrumentation

- Anatomic features of roots, furcations, and bone level, which may need special adaptations of curets.
- Overhanging restorations that must be removed.

B. Use Radiographs as Guide

Keep radiographs on lighted viewbox throughout the treatment for reference.

III. REVIEW CARE PLAN AND RECORD NOTES

A. Note flow and sequence of planned appointments.
B. Note findings that apply to the instrumentation process.
   - Examine periodontal probings to review attachment topography and access limitations.
   - Assemble procedure tray setup to include appropriate instruments.
C. Review previous appointment notes.
   - Read details of prior treatment, noting segments completed, which will be reassessed for healing.
   - Ascertain how previous treatment appointments have been tolerated by the patient.
   - Anticipate anesthesia requirements.
D. Keep periodontal probing chart prominently displayed throughout the treatment for reference.

IV. PATIENT PREPARATION

A. **Premedication Requirements for Patient at Risk**
   - Transient bacteremia can occur during and immediately after scaling procedures.
   - Frequency and duration of bacteremia depends on severity of periodontal infection and inflammation and the degree of trauma during the instrumentation.[14,15]
   - Check that the patient has taken the medication as prescribed.
B. **Provide Preprocedural Bactericidal Rinse**
C. **Prepare for Anesthesia as Indicated**

V. SUPRAGINGIVAL EXAMINATION

A. Visual

- Gross deposits and tooth surface irregularities can be seen by direct vision. Fine, unstained, white or yellowish calculus is frequently invisible when wet with saliva.
- Observe tooth surfaces closely while a gentle stream of compressed air is applied. Dry calculus is seen more readily than wet calculus.

B. Tactile

- Without deposits or anatomical irregularities, the enamel surface is smooth.
- An explorer tip passed over the surface slides freely, smoothly, and quietly.
- When rough calculus deposits are present, the explorer tip does not slide freely but meets with resistance over varying textures.
- Deposits can produce a scratchy sound or an audible click as the explorer passes over them.

VI. SUBGINGIVAL EXAMINATION

A. Visual

1. *Gingiva.* The clinical appearance suggestive of underlying calculus may be:
   - Soft, spongy, bluish-red gingiva, with enlargement of the interdental papillae over proximal surface calculus.
   - Dark-colored area beneath relatively translucent marginal gingiva.
2. *Calculus*
   - A loose, resilient pocket wall can be deflected from the tooth surface with a gentle stream of compressed air.
   - Dark, subgingival calculus can be seen within the pocket on the root.

B. Tactile

1. *Periodontal charting*
   - Use probing depth recordings as a basic guide.
   - Confirm recorded probing depths of segment to be instrumented.
   - Study the soft tissue attachment pattern to select effective procedures.
2. *Identify shallow pockets (sulci)*
   - Scaling in shallow pockets of fewer than 3 mm can lead to loss of periodontal attachment.[16-18]
   - Research has shown that repeated use of a curet when no calculus is present can result in detachment of periodontal ligament fibers and that healing does not bring them back.[18]
   - Root surfaces free of calculus may require biofilm removal.
   - Confine instrumentation to light-pressured but comprehensive biofilm debridement.
3. *Determine distribution and extent of deposits*
   - Figure 37-1 illustrates probing. As the probe passes over the surface it may be intercepted by calculus (Figure 37-1B).
   - Use an explorer for distinction of fine hard deposits.
4. *Evaluate tooth topography*
   - Detect grooves and furcations using a horizontal stroke (Figure 37-1C).
   - Use a furcation probe to examine furcations.
   - Note root and furcation variations (Figure 37-2).

VII. FORMULATE STRATEGY FOR INSTRUMENTATION

A. Combine clinical findings with information in the patient's documented record.

B. Determine a strategy for instrumentation.

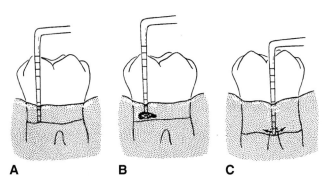

■ **FIGURE 37-1 Subgingival Examination Using a Probe. (A)** Probe inserted to the bottom of a pocket for complete examination prior to subgingival scaling. **(B)** As the probe passes over the root surface, it may be intercepted by a hard mass of calculus. **(C)** Using a horizontal probe stroke to examine the topography of a furcation area. Keep the side of the tip of the probe on the tooth surface and slide over one root, into the furcation, and across to the other root.

■ CALCULUS REMOVAL

I. PREREQUISITES

A. Position of clinician to prevent cumulative trauma.

B. Clear visibility with excellent lighting.

C. Sharp instruments.

II. LOCATION OF INSTRUMENTATION

Figure 37-3 illustrates the location of instrumentation. Instrumentation and the selection of the correct instrument depend on:

A. Type of pocket (gingival or periodontal).

B. Location of calculus (on crown or root surface).

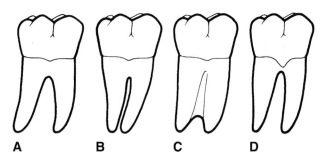

■ **FIGURE 37-2 Anatomic Variations of Furcations. (A)** Widely separated. **(B)** Separated but close together. **(C)** Fused roots separated only in the apical portion. **(D)** Presence of an enamel projection that may be conducive to an early furcation involvement. (From Carranza, F.A. and Newman, M.G.: *Clinical Periodontology,* 8th ed. W.B. Saunders Co., 1996, p. 641.)

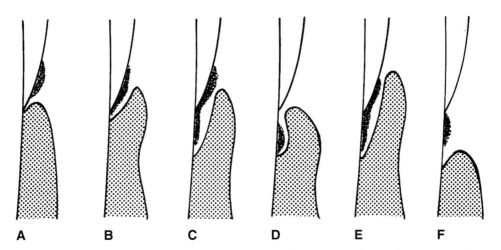

■ **FIGURE 37-3 Location of Instrumentation.** The location of calculus deposits, level of periodontal attachment, depth of pocket, and position of the gingival margin determine the site of instrumentation. **(A)** Supragingival calculus on the enamel. **(B)** Gingival pocket with both supragingival and subgingival calculus on enamel. **(C)** Periodontal pocket with both supragingival and subgingival calculus. **(D)** Periodontal pocket with subgingival calculus only on root surface. **(E)** Periodontal pocket with subgingival calculus on both enamel and root surface. **(F)** Calculus on root surface exposed by gingival recession.

C. Position of gingival margin (recession or covering cementoenamel junction).
D. Level of clinical attachment (no loss of attachment or on root).

III. THE SCALING PROCESS

The process is the series of procedures and events that lead to achievement of a specific result.

A. Definitions

*   *Scaling:* removal of calculus and dental biofilm from the supragingival and subgingival exposed tooth surfaces.
*   *Root Planing:* removal of all residual calculus and toxic materials from the root to produce a clean, smooth tooth surface. Other names include *debridement, root detoxification,* and *root preparation.*

B. Instrumentation Zone[19]

*   Area of the tooth where instrumentation is performed for scaling and root planing.
*   Location: above the clinical attachment of the periodontal fibers; extends the height and width of the hard and soft deposits of calculus and biofilm to be removed.
*   Scaling and root planing strokes for deposit removal must be limited to the instrumentation zone. Extending the strokes to clean areas where

no deposits exist can be harmful to the tooth, allow the clinician to lose control, dull the instrument, and waste time.

C. Systematic Deposit Removal

1. Tooth to tooth.
2. Section to section of deposit on each tooth surface.
3. Strokes overlap.
    *   Each stroke overlaps the previous stroke in channels.
    *   The instrument is positioned progressively along the area of the deposit, within the *instrumentation zone.*
4. Nature of the deposit
    *   The oldest calculus, located next to the tooth surface, is the hardest calculus.
    *   The outermost calculus is covered with a layer of dental biofilm that has not yet started to mineralize.

IV. SPECIAL SUBGINGIVAL CONSIDERATIONS

Although the basic steps described for calculus removal apply to both supragingival and subgingival deposits, subgingival techniques are unique and complicated by several significant factors. The instrumentation is more complex and difficult than supragingival calculus removal. Some of the variables are included here.

A. Subgingival Anatomy

1. *Tooth Surface Pocket Wall*
   - As shown in Figure 37-3B, C, and E, some subgingival instrumentation is on the crown (enamel), and some on the root (cementum or dentin).
   - In the cervical third of the root, the cementum is thin (0.03 to 0.06 mm) and may have been removed during previous instrumentation.
2. *Soft Tissue Pocket Wall*
   - The pocket wall hugs closely to the tooth surface covered with rough calculus, which in turn is covered with bacterial biofilm.
   - Only a narrow area is available for manipulation of instruments.
   - The pocket narrows in the deeper area next to the clinical attachment.
   - Bleeding during instrumentation is inevitable because of the inflammation in the wall of the pocket.
3. *Variations in Probing Depths*
   - The periodontal charting is a primary guide to subgingival instrumentation and will serve as a road map to guide instrument depth of insertion.
   - Probing depths must be recorded about each tooth because the depths can vary on a single surface.

B. Accessibility and Visibility

- Pocket is a confined area; instrumentation is necessary in areas where access is difficult.
- Instrumentation must depend almost entirely on tactile sensitivity.
- Soft tissue pocket wall limits freedom of movement. Careful adaptation to tooth surface configurations is essential.

C. Subgingival Calculus

1. *Location:* Subgingival calculus may be located on the enamel, the root, or both (Figure 37-3B, C, D, E).
2. *Attachment*
   - Calculus attaches to the cementum in minute irregularities and in areas of cemental resorption.
   - It is more tenacious than on the enamel and requires a different technique for removal.
   - On the enamel it is attached primarily by means of an acquired pellicle, which makes calculus removal much easier.

3. *Morphology of Calculus*
   - Subgingival calculus is irregularly deposited. It occurs in nodular, ledge, smooth veneer, and other forms.
   - Previously scaled or burnished calculus: subgingival calculus that has been partially scaled and left after incomplete instrumentation is usually smooth and may not be detected when an explorer is used to check the area.

■ MANUAL SCALING STEPS

Types of instruments and the basic principles for their use are included in Chapter 36. This chapter continues from Chapter 36 to describe the use of the instruments for deposits removal. Box 37-2 summarizes the steps.

I. SELECT CORRECT CUTTING EDGE

A. Curets are paired and usually mounted on double-ended handles. Single-ended handles may be selected for certain patients or procedures.
B. Correct blade for scaling: when positioned on the tooth surface, only the back of the blade can be seen.
C. Incorrect blade adaptation: the open face of the blade will be seen.
   - It would be impossible to angulate at 70° for scaling.
   - The *open* blade is in the correct position for gingival curettage to remove the inner soft tissue lining of the pocket wall.

II. INSTRUMENT GRASP

A. **Apply a Modified Pen Grasp** (Figure 36-13).
   - Thumb and index and middle fingers make up the grasp points.
B. **Use a Light Grasp** for:
   - Instrument insertion and positioning.
   - Assessment strokes.
   - Root debridement strokes to remove biofilm.
C. **Keep the Grasp Firm and Secure** during calculus removal.
D. **Apply a Light Grasp With Light Lateral Pressure After Calculus Removal.**
   1. To remove small irregularities.
   2. To leave the treated area smooth.

III. STABILIZATION: ESTABLISH THE FINGER REST

A. Primary Rest Fingers

1. Ring and little fingers (numbers 3 and 4 in Figure 36-13).

BOX 37-2 Steps for Calculus Removal Using Manual Instruments

Assessment

1. Probe to determine pocket/sulcus characteristics and confirm soft tissue attachment topography.

2. Explore to determine location and extent of deposits and tooth surface irregularities.

3. Select correct instruments that will adapt and conform to concavities and other root morphology characteristics for areas being treated.

Preparation: Instrument Control

4. Hold instrument with a modified pen grasp.

5. Identify correct cutting edge of blade for surface being scaled.

   • For area-specific curets: terminal shank parallel with surface being scaled.

   • For universal curets: terminal shank *less* than parallel with surface being scaled (approximately 20°).

6. Establish a light hand rest for instrument placement to allow for adjustment and repositioning.

7. Insert: use placement or exploratory stroke to locate apical edge of deposit.

8. Adjust working angulation (average at 70°).

Action: Strokes

9. Secure a stable, functional extraoral hand rest or intraoral finger rest that can support instrument placement and activation at correct working stroke angulation.

   • Pressure into the fulcrum must equal the pressure against the tooth.

   • Balance fulcrum pressure with lateral pressure of the strokes.

10. Activate for working stroke.

    a. Apply firm lateral pressure for calculus removal.

    b. Apply moderate lateral pressure to smooth the surface.

    c. Apply light lateral pressure for biofilm debridement.

    d. Control length and direction of stroke: respect the Instrumentation Zone.

    e. Maintain continuous adaptation throughout the stroke.

Channels: Overlap to Completion

11. Continue channel scaling with overlapping multidirectional strokes.

    a. Apply placement stroke to reposition blade for next stroke.

    b. Activate instrument circumferentially around tooth

    c. Keep toe adapted around line angles by rolling handle.

    d. Cover all surfaces comprehensively to remove all traces of calculus and biofilm.

Evaluation

12. Use explorer to determine end point of treatment.

2. Rest fingers are kept close to the middle finger (number 2) and join the total hand motion during activation.

B. Location

1. *Intraoral rests:*
   - Placed on the tooth adjacent to the one being scaled, or as near as convenient.
   - Avoid position in the path of the strokes to protect from accidental glove and finger cut.
   - Distance rests: long stretches between the rest and the point of instrument application can decrease control.
2. *Variations:* substitute, supplementary, and reinforced rests are described on page 622.

C. Dry the Rest Position

- Biofilm and saliva make tooth surfaces slippery.
- Use compressed air or dry with gauze sponge.

IV. ADAPTATION OF THE CUTTING EDGE

A. Apply Blade to Conform to Tooth Surface Being Treated

- Because of tooth contours, only a portion of a blade can be adapted.
- The toe and middle thirds of a curet blade are used most frequently (Figure 37-4).

B. Maintain Adaptation

- Roll the handle around line angles and other tooth convexities.

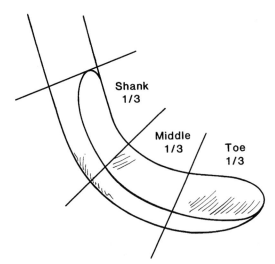

■ FIGURE 37-4 Curet Divided Into Thirds. The toe third is kept in contact with the tooth surface during instrumentation. Because of tooth contours, most strokes for scaling and root planing are accomplished using the toe third. Adaptation of the toe third is shown in Figure 37-5.

- Maintain close adaptation of the cutting edge to prevent trauma of the adjacent soft tissue (Figure 37-5B).

V. ANGULATION

A. Insertion

Close the angle to nearly flat against the tooth surface (0°) as the instrument is inserted to the base of a pocket (Figure 37-6A and B).

B. Establish Optimal Angle for Scaling

A 70° angle is effective for deposit removal using a scaler or a curet.

VI. LATERAL PRESSURE

A. Degree of Pressure of Blade Against Tooth

Whether a light, moderate, or heavy pressure is needed will depend on the nature of the deposit and the type of therapy being performed.

1. *Light Pressure*
   - Assessment.
   - Instrument insertion.
   - Confirmation of the soft tissue attachment.
2. *Moderate to Heavy Pressure*
   - For calculus removal.
   - Working strokes require strong to moderate lateral pressure depending on the degree of mineralization of the calculus.
   - Recently formed calculus can be removed more readily than calculus present on the root for many years.
3. *Biofilm Debridement*
   - When the root surface is free of calculus, confine instrumentation to light-pressured debridement.
   - The tactile sense transmits vibrations felt from any irregularities present.
   - Lateral pressure against the tooth can be increased for removal.
   - Unnecessary and unwarranted tooth structure removal can be minimized.

B. Balance of Pressure During Stroke

Careful control is accomplished by a balance of pressure between:

1. The grasp of the instrument.
2. The pressure on the finger rest.
3. The lateral pressure against the tooth.

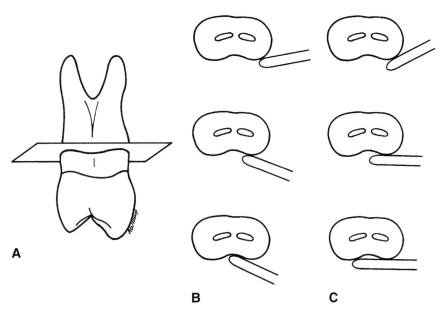

■ **FIGURE 37-5 Instrument Adaptation. (A)** Maxillary first premolar shows cross section of root drawn for (B) and (C). **(B)** Diagram of three positions of a curet shows correct adaptation at a line angle and on the concave mesial surface with toe third of the instrument maintained on the tooth as the instrument is adapted. **(C)** Diagram shows incorrect adaptation with toe of curet extended away from the tooth surface.

C. Factors Affecting Lateral Pressure

1. *Sharp Instrument*
   • A minimum degree of pressure allows the cutting edge to "grab" the calculus.

• Engaging the deposit provides clean leverage and effective removal.
• Less time is required.
• Fewer strokes are necessary.
• Fatigue is kept to a minimum.

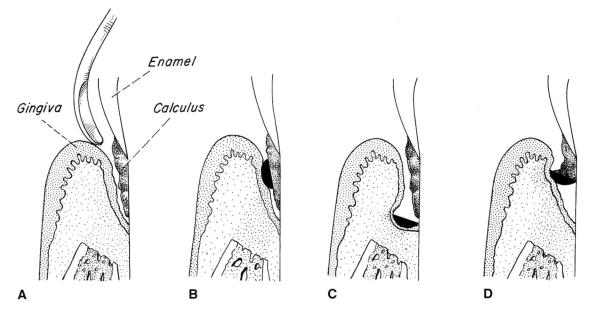

■ **FIGURE 37-6 Subgingival Scaling and Root Planing. (A)** The curet is inserted gently under the gingival margin. **(B)** With a placement stroke, the blade is passed over the surface of the tooth or calculus. Note 0° angle of the face of the curet with the calculus. **(C)** The curet is lowered to the base of the pocket until the tension of the soft tissue is felt with the rounded back of the curet. The curet then is positioned at an angle of 70° to 80° with the tooth surface beneath the calculus deposit. **(D)** The blade is moved along the root surface in a scaling stroke to remove the calculus.

2. *Dull Instrument*
   - When dull, the blade cannot engage the deposit and will slide over it, burnishing it on the tooth surface.
   - The more the deposit is burnished with repeated strokes, the more difficult it becomes to remove.
   - More strokes are taken, causing increased fatigue.
   - Inefficiency increases treatment time.
   - Grasp and lateral pressures must increase to compensate for the sliding effect.
   - Stroke control is reduced with the heavier pressure needed for a dull blade; this can lead to instrument slippage and trauma to the patient's soft tissues.
   - Loss of confidence for the clinician.

VII. ACTIVATION: STROKE

A. Tighten the Grasp

1. Renew the stability of the rest position; whether an intraoral finger rest or an extraoral hand rest, the pressure of the rest will equal the pressure against the tooth.
2. Move the instrument firmly and deliberately, making each stroke intentional.
3. Wrist and arm bear the weight during the stroke, rather than flexing the fingers in the grasp.

B. Maintain Cutting Edge Evenly During the Stroke

1. *Angulation:* Maintain blade position by observing lower shank from beginning to end of each stroke.
   - Relationship of the angle of the lower shank to the tooth surface stays consistent for the full length of the stroke.
   - Parallel orientation of shank to surface being scaled for Gracey curets; less than parallel orientation of shank to surface being scaled for universal curets.
   - Guard against blade closure. Changing the angulation at the cutting edge can lead to burnishing.
     - Wrist motion activations that pivot on the fulcrum finger move the instrument handle from side to side.
     - Side to side handle movement is often indicative of blade closure during stroke.
2. *Maintain the adaptation:* handle is rolled between fingers to keep the cutting edge adapted correctly.

C. Motion Control

Without independent finger movement, the hand, wrist, and arm act as a continuum to activate the instrument.

D. Direction of Strokes

1. Select overlapping vertical, oblique (diagonal), or horizontal strokes to accommodate the anatomical features of the tooth surfaces.
2. Strokes are applied systematically, not haphazardly.
3. Avoid horizontal strokes at the bottom of a pocket to avoid damage to the clinical attachment.

E. Length of Stroke: Within Instrumentation Zone

1. Short, smooth, decisive strokes permit accommodation of the cutting edges to changes in the topography of the tooth surface.
2. Confine the strokes within a pocket to prevent the need for repeated removal and reinsertion of the curet; prevent trauma to the gingival margin.

VIII. CHANNELS OF STROKES: COVERAGE

A. Make Strokes in Channels (Figure 37-7)

- At the completion of each stroke, move the instrument laterally to the adjacent part of the deposit.
- Maintain the same finger rest.

B. Overlap Strokes in Channels

- Ensure complete coverage of every square millimeter of subgingival surface for thorough removal of deposits.

C. Repeat Strokes

- Continue until surface has been completely debrided.

IX. PLANE THE ROOT SURFACE

A. Finishing Techniques

- Purpose: smoothing the tooth surfaces to lessen immediate recolonization of bacteria.
- Procedure: instrumentation is basically the same as for scaling.
- Application: only where deemed necessary after exploration with a fine subgingival explorer.

B. Touch and Pressure

1. Specific differences in technique are related to touch and pressure.

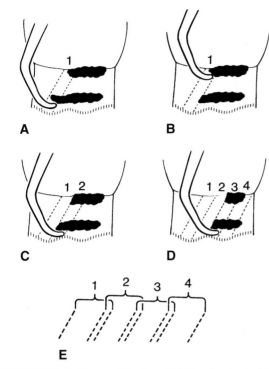

■ **FIGURE 37-7 Channel Scaling. (A)** Curet adapted in position for channel 1 stroke from the base of the pocket under the calculus deposit. **(B)** Completion of stroke for channel 1. **(C)** Using an exploratory stroke, the curet is lowered into the pocket and is positioned for calculus removal in channel 2. **(D)** Curet positioned for channel 3. Several strokes in each channel may be needed to ensure complete calculus removal. **(E)** Strokes of each channel must overlap strokes of the previous channel. (Adapted from Parr, R.W., Green, E., Madsen, L., and Miller, S.: *Subgingival Scaling and Root Planing*. Berkeley, CA, Praxis Publishing Co., 1976.)

- A lighter grasp will increase tactile sensitivity.
- Light lateral pressure is applied for maximum sensitivity to minute irregularities of the surface.
- A lighter stroke can be used for final smoothing of the root surface; increased pressure is not needed.

2. Sharp instruments are essential for tactile transmission.

C. Strokes

1. Use smooth strokes that overlap systematically.
2. As the surface becomes smoother, longer strokes with reduced pressure help to remove small lines, scratches, or grooves without gouging the surface.
3. Stroke direction
   - Vertical and then oblique strokes are used (Figure 37-8).

- Keep horizontal strokes away from the attachment epithelium.

4. Adaptation
   - Careful adaptation of the curet to the unique anatomic features of the roots is needed.
   - Convex surfaces, constricted cervical areas, concavities and grooves of the proximal surfaces, and the variations in furcations all require precise adaptation.
   - Minibladed Gracey curets are designed specifically to access and adapt to concavities and convexities where standard-length blades either can span across or protrude beyond (Figure 37-5C).
   - As a surface area becomes smooth, a gradual change in the sound of the instrument may occur. At completion, the instrument may be as quiet as when used on polished enamel.

X. EVALUATION

A. Use a subgingival explorer to examine for completion of calculus removal and smoothness of the treated surfaces.

B. Apply explorer in both vertical and diagonal strokes to detect irregularities (Figure 37-8).

C. Refine slight spots of roughness with a sharp curet.

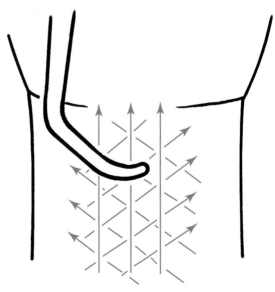

■ **FIGURE 37-8 Root Surface Strokes.** The use of strokes in vertical and oblique directions with light lateral pressure can help to eliminate grooves left after scaling. A smooth surface results. (Adapted from Parr, R.W., Green, E., Madsen, L., and Miller, S.: *Subgingival Scaling and Root Planing*. Berkeley, CA, Praxis Publishing Co., 1976, p. 42.)

D. Adapt curet with light lateral pressure for maximum sensitivity to minute irregularities of the surface. Avoid grooving the treated surface.

E. Postcare patient instructions are described on page 670.

▪ ULTRASONIC AND SONIC SCALING

Manual instrumentation was the only method available for the safe removal of supragingival and subgingival calculus until the ultrasonic scaling device was introduced in the 1950s.[20,21] The power-driven scaling device converted high-frequency electrical energy into mechanical energy in the form of rapid vibrations.

Technologic advances in ultrasonics allowed for rapid calculus removal and resulted in much less hand fatigue for the clinician. Later, sonic scalers were developed that worked on the same principle but utilized an air turbine as an energy source. Terminology related to power-driven instrumentation is defined in Box 37-3.

For many years, power-driven scaling devices were recommended for supragingival scaling only. Because of advances in design and efficiency of the devices, they are now recommended for both supragingival and subgingival treatment. Slimmer ultrasonic instrument tips have been designed to provide better access to deeper areas created by clinical attachment loss.

▪ MODE OF ACTION

Although the main action of the ultrasonic and sonic scalers is mechanical, cavitation and irrigation also play important roles in debridement.

I. MECHANICAL VIBRATION

A. Power-driven scaling devices convert electrical energy (ultrasonic) or air pressure (sonic) into high-frequency sound waves.

B. Sound waves produce rapid vibrations in the specially designed scaling tips.

BOX 37-3 KEY WORDS: Ultrasonic and Sonic Instrumentation

Acoustic turbulence: agitation in the fluids surrounding a rapidly vibrating ultrasonic tip; has potential to disrupt the bacterial matrix.

Cavitation: action created by the formation and collapse of bubbles in the water by high-frequency sound waves surrounding an ultrasonic tip.

Ferromagnetic: type of rod with unusually high magnetic permeability used in magnetostrictive ultrasonic unit inserts.

Kilohertz (kHz): a unit of energy equal to 1000 cycles per second.

Lavage: the therapeutic washing of the pocket and root surface to remove endotoxins and loose debris.

Magnetic field: space occupied by magnetic lines of force.

Magnetostrictive: ultrasonic scaling device that generates a magnetic field and produces tip vibrations by the expansion and contraction of a metal stack or rod.

Piezoelectric: ultrasonic scaling device activated by dimensional changes in crystals housed in the handpiece.

Sonic scaler: type of mechanical power-driven scaler that functions from energy delivered by a vibrating working tip in the frequency of 2500 to 7000 cycles per second; driven by compressed air, the handpiece connects directly to a conventional rotary handpiece tubing.

Stack: magnetostrictive inserts made of flat metal strips stacked, or sandwiched, together; metal in stack acts like an antenna to pick up magnetic field and cause vibration.

Transducer: a device that converts energy or power from one form to another.

Ultrasonic scaler: power-driven scaling instrument that operates in a frequency range between 25,000 to 50,000 cycles per second to convert a high-frequency electrical current into mechanical vibrations.

C. Calculus is incrementally shattered from the tooth surface when the vibrations are applied to the deposit.

II. CAVITATION

A. Water is required to dissipate the heat produced at the vibrating tip.
B. Cavitation occurs when the water meets the vibrating tip. Minute bubbles are created that collapse and release energy.[22]
C. Effect of cavitation. Although the cavitation has little influence on hard deposit removal, it is capable of destroying surface bacteria[23] and can remove endotoxin from the root surface.[24]

III. IRRIGATION

- The water spray penetrates to the base of the pocket[25] to provide a continuous flushing of debris, bacteria, and endotoxin.
- Oscillation of the ultrasonic tip causes hydrodynamic waves to surround the tip. This acoustic turbulence is believed to have a disruptive effect on surface bacteria.[26,27]
- Ultrasonic debridement following manual instrumentation provides cleansing and rinsing of scaled and root planed surfaces, which can promote healing of soft tissues.

IV. VARIABLE ELEMENTS

Power-driven scaling devices feature varying elements but are mainly distinguished by their frequency output and the direction and pattern of tip motion, as shown in Box 37-4.
A. **Amplitude:** distance of tip movement
- Distance of tip movement determines power output of the instrument.

- Adjustable component on all ultrasonic devices.
- Measured in micrometers.
B. **Frequency:** speed of movement
- Number of cycles per second (cps) the tip moves.
- Adjustable component available only on manually tuned ultrasonic devices.
- Majority of available devices have tuning preset, or "automatic."

■ ULTRASONIC SCALING DEVICES

I. TWO TYPES

A. Magnetostrictive ultrasonic scalers.
B. Piezoelectric ultrasonic scalers.

II. EQUIPMENT

Ultrasonic scaling devices share certain attributes and are differentiated by others.

A. Unit Parts

- Electric generator.
- Handpiece assembly.
- Set of interchangeable scaling tip inserts.
- Foot control to activate the handpiece.

B. Tip Activation

- Vibrations in the tip occur when electric current is applied to the handpiece.

C. Water Source

- Necessary for delivery of water to the handpiece.

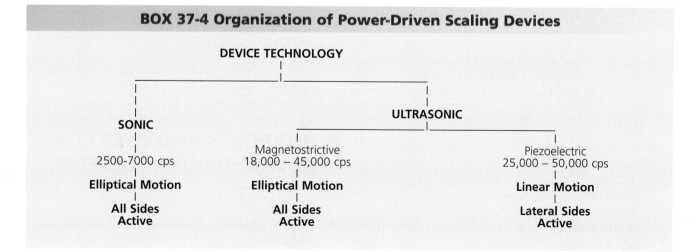

BOX 37-4 Organization of Power-Driven Scaling Devices

DEVICE TECHNOLOGY

SONIC

2500-7000 cps

Elliptical Motion

All Sides Active

ULTRASONIC

Magnetostrictive
18,000 – 45,000 cps

Elliptical Motion

All Sides Active

Piezoelectric
25,000 – 50,000 cps

Linear Motion

Lateral Sides Active

- Water is carried through or around the instrument tip.
- Cools tip. Rapid tip movement creates friction and/or temperature increase in the tooth.
- Flushes subgingival debris.

III. MAGNETOSTRICTIVE ULTRASONIC SCALERS

A. Composition

1. Conventional magnetostrictive units: utilize a longitudinal stack of metal strips in the handpiece.
2. Ferromagnetic units: utilize a fragile ferric rod that generates less heat than the conventional metal stack.

B. Activation

1. Vibrations in the tip occur when electric current is applied to the handpiece.
2. A magnetic field is created; with expansion and contraction of metal strips in the handpiece.

C. Tip Motion

1. Conventional tip moves in an elliptical pattern; all surfaces of the tip are active.
2. Ferromagnetic tip rotates 360° in three different planes; equal effectiveness on all sides of the tip.

D. Tip Shape

Cross section of tip is round.

E. Frequency

1. Conventional units range from 18,000 to 45,000 cycles per second (cps).
   - Older units are designed to operate at 25,000 cps and are called 25-kilohertz (kHz) machines.
   - Newer units are designed to operate at 30,000 cps and are called 30-kHz machines.
2. Ferromagnetic units operate at 42,000 cps.

IV. PIEZOELECTRIC ULTRASONIC SCALERS

A. **Composition:** scaler devices feature a ceramic rod in the handpiece.
B. **Activation:** by dimensional changes in quartz or metal alloy crystal transducers housed in the handpiece.
C. **Tip Motion:** moves in a linear pattern, forward and backward.

- Only the lateral surfaces of the tip are active.
- Handpiece position must be adjusted at each line angle to maintain adaptation of the lateral surface of the tip to the tooth; accomplished by pivoting the wrist to approximate a 90° turn of the instrument to move from facial or lingual surfaces to proximal surfaces and back again.

D. **Tip Shape:** cross section of tip is trapezoidal with angular edges.
E. **Frequency:**
   1. Varies according to manufacturer.
   2. Ranges from 25,000 to 50,000 cps.

■ SONIC SCALING DEVICES

I. EQUIPMENT: UNIT PARTS

- Handpiece
- Interchangeable scaling tips.
- Handpiece attaches directly to the dental unit and is activated with the conventional handpiece foot control.

II. TIP ACTIVATION

A. Tip Motion

- Driven by compressed air from the dental unit rather than electrical energy.
- Moves in an elliptical pattern.
- All surfaces of the tip are active.

B. Amplitude

- Less powerful than ultrasonic scalers.

C. Frequency

- Producing vibrations at the tip; range between 2,500 and 7,000 cps.
- Because of fewer vibrations produced, calculus removal is more difficult.

D. Water Source

- Water is required to cool the friction between the instrument tip and the tooth surface.
- Heat is not generated by the scaling tip.

■ PURPOSES AND USES FOR POWER-DRIVEN SCALERS

I. INDICATIONS FOR USE

A. Removal of supragingival calculus and tenacious stains.

B. Subgingival periodontal debridement, including:
- Removal of calculus, attached biofilm, and endotoxins from the root surface.
- Removal of unattached biofilm from the sulcular space.[28]

C. Initial debridement
- For a patient with necrotizing ulcerative gingivitis or other conditions that can be relieved by removal of deposits.
- Loose debris and microorganisms must first be removed by rinsing, brushing, and flossing during patient instruction to prevent contaminated aerosol production.

D. Debridement of furcation areas following manual instrumentation.[29,30]

E. Debridement of deposits prior to oral surgery.

F. Removal of orthodontic cement; debonding.

G. Removal of overhanging margins of restorations.

II. CONTRAINDICATIONS

A. General Health Conditions

1. *Communicable Disease.* Patient with a communicable disease that can be transmitted by aerosols, such as tuberculosis.

2. *Susceptibility to Infection.* Compromised patient with marked susceptibility to infection.
Examples: immunosuppression from disease or chemotherapy, uncontrolled diabetes, debilitation, or kidney or other organ transplant.

3. *Respiratory Risk.* Patient with a respiratory risk. Septic material and microorganisms from biofilm and periodontal pockets can be aspirated into the lungs.[31]
- History of chronic pulmonary disease, including asthma, emphysema, or cystic fibrosis.
- History of cardiovascular disease with secondary pulmonary disease or breathing problem.

4. *Swallowing Difficulty.* Patient with a swallowing problem or prone to gagging.
Examples: amyotrophic lateral sclerosis, muscular dystrophy, paralysis, multiple sclerosis.

5. *Cardiac Pacemaker.*
- Although no case has ever been reported in which an ultrasonic scaler disrupted a pacemaker, theoretically it is possible.
- Some newer devices have protective coverings. Consultation with the patient's cardiologist is necessary.

B. Oral Conditions

1. *Demineralized Areas*
- Ultrasonic vibrations can remove the delicate remineralizing cover of a demineralized area.

2. *Exposed Dentinal Surfaces*
- Tooth structure can be removed in excess and create sensitivity.
- The smear layer can be removed and dentinal tubules uncovered, which can increase sensitivity or aggravate existing sensitivity.

3. *Children*
- Young, growing, developing tissues are sensitive to ultrasonic vibrations.
- Primary and newly erupted permanent teeth have large pulp chambers. The vibrations and heat from the ultrasonic scaler may damage pulp tissue.

III. PRECAUTIONS

A. Damage to the Integrity of Restorations

- Porcelain: fracturing; loss of marginal integrity.[32,33]
- Amalgam: surface defects; loss of marginal integrity.[34,35]
- Composites: surface alterations.[36]

B. Titanium Implant Abutments

Ultrasonic instrumentation will damage titanium surfaces unless the tip insert is covered with a specially designed plastic sheath.[37,38]

IV. RISK CONSIDERATIONS

A. Clinician

1. *Cumulative Trauma*
- It has been estimated that dental hygienists apply over 32 tons of scaling forces per year using over 25,000 scaling strokes for calculus removal.[39,40]
- Many dental hygienists suffer from symptoms related to cumulative trauma.
- Powered scaling actually reduces the force needed to remove deposits, and it can reduce the risk of carpal tunnel syndrome and other musculoskeletal disorders.

2. *Magnetic Fields*
- Ultrasonic scalers produce weak, time-varying magnetic fields similar to those produced by common household appliances.

- There is no scientific evidence that cumulative exposure to weak, time-varying magnetic fields has caused any biological harm to any dental personnel.[41]

B. Patient

1. *Heat Production*
   - Potential damage to the pulp tissue should be kept in mind during instrumentation.[42]
   - Constant motion of the instrument, correct angulation, and ample water for cooling are essential to operation.
2. *Hearing Shifts*
   - Extended exposure to noises above a certain level, such as the noise of a high-speed handpiece or an ultrasonic scaler, may be potentially damaging.
   - Temporary hearing shifts have been demonstrated for a group of patients.[43]

▪ INSTRUMENT TIP DESIGN

I. PARTS

The parts are illustrated in Figure 37-9. The design of the instrument tip will vary according to the intended use. Figure 37-10 shows examples of various tip designs.

II. SIZE AND TYPE

A. Conventional or Standard Tip

- Traditional ultrasonic and sonic tips, bulkier than most curet tips. Also called **universal** tips.
- Generally used for moderate to heavy deposit removal from supragingival or relatively shallow subgingival surfaces.
- Standard tips for both magnetostrictive and piezoelectric devices may be used on any power setting.

B. Periodontal or Narrow-Profile Tip

- Thinner and longer tips provide better access to subgingival surfaces.

- Allow superior coverage of deep pockets and furcations.
- Most magnetostrictive thin tips must be used on low to medium power only.
- Piezoelectric thin tips may be used on high power, which will not burnish calculus.
- Tip design innovations continue to emerge in answer to the demands of advanced nonsurgical therapy.
  - Bladed and beveled tips are capable of removing calculus rapidly.
  - Diamond-coated tips used on low power are effective for fine scaling and root planing.

C. Plastic or Carbon Composite Tip[37,44]

- A close-fitting plastic sheath fits over the metal working end to protect vulnerable restorative surfaces such as titanium abutments of implants, or esthetic materials surfaces.
- Dentin and titanium surfaces can be safely instrumented with the plastic tip. A light, gentle activation is all that is needed to remove soft and mineralizing deposits.

III. SHAPE

A. **Straight:** Tip slightly curved in only one direction; designed to be used throughout the mouth. Also called universal.
B. **Contra-Angled:** Instrument tips have curvatures to left and right designed to adapt to posterior surfaces of the teeth.
C. **Beavertail:** Designed to be used on supragingival surfaces for the removal of heavy calculus and stain and orthodontic cement.
D. **Thin Periodontal:** Straight or contra-angled tip designed for subgingival instrumentation.
E. **Ball Point:** An 0.8-mm sphere found on the tip designed for final flushing in furcations.[25] Use for smoothing following manual instrumentation since the ball point has a noted tendency to burnish calculus.

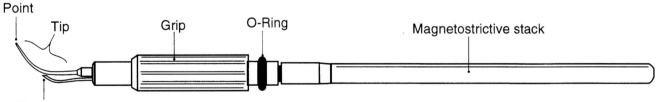

■ **FIGURE 37-9 Ultrasonic Handpiece Insert.** With parts labeled, showing design with external water delivery tube.

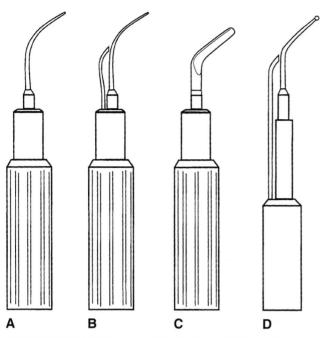

■ **FIGURE 37-10 Ultrasonic Tip Designs. (A)** Straight tip with internal flow water delivery. **(B)** Thinner tip with external water delivery. **(C)** Beavertail for supragingival surfaces needing removal of heavy calculus or cement. **(D)** 0.8-mm ball-end design for adaptation in furcation areas.

IV. WATER DELIVERY

A. **External Tube.** An external tube delivers the water to the tip of the instrument (Figure 37-10 B and D).

B. **Internal Tube.** Water is delivered from the unit to cool the tip through the internal structure of the insert.

■ CLINICAL PREPARATION

I. DENTAL HYGIENE CARE PLAN

A. **Review Patient's Medical History and Treatment Records**

B. **Oral Examination**

Obtain current periodontal probings. Review the care plan, radiographs, and chart to determine the following:
- Location of deposits.
- Depth of pockets and soft tissue attachment topography.
- Presence of exposed furcations.

C. **Instrumentation Plan**
- Plan a systematic sequence.
- Complete one quadrant before starting another, instrumenting each tooth to completion.

II. INFECTION CONTROL MEASURES

A. Personal Protective Equipment

1. The clinician and assistant must wear protective eyewear, high-efficiency bacterial face mask, gloves, and protective outerwear.
   - Use of a face shield as well as a regular mask is needed for added protection against aerosols.
   - Use of a surgical cap to prevent contamination of hair is recommended.
2. Masks should be changed often: a maximum of 20 minutes, or at the first sign of moisture.

B. Flush Water Lines[45]

1. Biofilm forms on the internal surfaces of dental tubing, as found in the dental unit and ultrasonic unit.
2. Opportunistic pathogens can colonize and replicate on these internal surfaces.
   - Risk of exposure to dental personnel through the aerosol emerging in the vicinity of the treatment area to beyond 20 feet.
   - Risk of exposure to the patient through aspiration and/or bacteremia.
3. To reduce bacterial contamination, water lines must be flushed.
   - Flush for 2 to 3 minutes at the beginning of each day.
   - Flush for 20 to 30 seconds between patients.
   - Flush before sterile insert is placed in the handpiece.

C. High-Volume Evacuation

1. Deposition of tooth-associated materials into the pulmonary system during ultrasonic scaling can result in pulmonary infection.[31]
2. Use of high-volume evacuation will reduce aspiration of contaminated aerosols by both the patient and the clinician.
3. An assistant is required when a high-volume evacuator is used.
4. A special high-volume evacuator attachment provides suction around the handpiece tip and reduces aerosol contamination in the treatment room.[46,47]

III. ULTRASONIC UNIT PREPARATION

A. Establish Power and Water Connections

B. Fill Ultrasonic Handpiece With Water

- Hold upright as handpiece is filled and insert is placed.

- Fill with water before placing the insert to eliminate trapped air and reduce heat.
- To prevent sterile insert from being flushed with stagnant water in pipes.

C. Select Insert

1. Insert must be compatible with ultrasonic unit available.
2. The metal stacks in the 30-kHz inserts are much shorter than the 25-kHz inserts.
3. The tip should be appropriate for the intended use.
   - Standard tip for calculus removal.
   - Slender profile elongated thin tips for biofilm debridement during maintenance phase.

D. Set Power Level

1. Select the power setting according to the task at hand.
   - Calculus: medium-high to high power is needed.
   - Soft deposit: low to medium power is sufficient for removal of attached and unattached biofilm.
2. Consistent use of the unit on the lowest power setting for all case types will burnish the calculus present.

E. Adjust Water

1. Water provides cooling and irrigation.
2. Proper water setting should create a fine mist at the tip of the instrument.
3. Increase water if heat is produced.

F. Use of an Antimicrobial Solution

1. Some ultrasonic units have reservoirs so an antimicrobial solution can be used as the coolant since the lavage of ultrasonics can penetrate to the base of the pocket.[25]
2. When 0.12% chlorhexidine is used as the coolant/irrigant, there is a greater reduction in clinical probing depth.[48,49]
3. Antimicrobial solutions will reduce the number of pathogens present in the contaminated aerosol.

IV. SONIC UNIT PREPARATION

A. Flush water lines in slow-speed-handpiece line for 2 minutes.
B. Attach sonic handpiece to slow-speed-handpiece line.
C. Select and screw sonic tip into handpiece.

V. PATIENT PREPARATION

A. Review Health History

1. Check to ensure that any patient requiring preprocedural antibiotic has taken the prescribed medication. Bacteremia is produced in a high percentage of patients treated by powered instrumentation, as well as manual instrumentation.[50]
2. Identify any contraindications to ultrasonic instrumentation.

B. Explain Procedure

1. Describe and demonstrate sound and spray, vibration, and the purpose for use.
2. Hearing-impaired patient should turn off a hearing aid.

C. Provide Protection for Patient

1. Safety glasses to prevent eye infections or injury.
2. Fluid-resistant drape over patient to keep moisture from skin and clothing.

D. Preprocedural Rinse

- Ultrasonic and sonic instrumentation generates aerosols that are heavily contaminated by microorganisms.[51]
- Prior to treatment, patients are directed to rinse with an antimicrobial mouthrinse for 30 seconds to decrease incidence of bacteremia.[52]
- The use of chlorhexidine is preferred for the preprocedural rinse because of its substantivity.

E. Patient Position

Place the patient in a supine position for maximum visibility.

F. Patient Breathing

- Explain to the patient, and request breathing/air exchange through the nose only.
- Reduces potential for aspiration of oral pathogens into lung tissue.
- Allows water to pool for evacuation with saliva ejector.
- Less fogging of mouth mirror.
- More comfort for patient.

G. Pain Control

Prepare to use topical or local anesthetic as necessary.

H. Water Control

- Prepare to use evacuation with saliva ejector or high-volume evacuator with assistant as indicated by the severity and degree of sepsis and communicability of infection from the patient.
- Evacuation system must be properly disinfected before use.
- Shape and position saliva ejector so that the patient can hold it in place to collect water that is pooling in the mouth.

■ INSTRUMENTATION

As with manual instrumentation, power instrumentation depends on skill and technique. Because tactile sensitivity is reduced or absent when power instrumentation is used, knowledge and awareness of tooth morphology assists the clinician in debriding periodontal pockets efficiently and safely.

Ultrasonic instrumentation is technique dependent. Care in adapting the working end to the tooth surface and methodical activation using sufficient power to disrupt the mineralized deposit are necessary.

I. PRINCIPLES FOR TECHNIQUE

A. Power Setting

1. *Low Power*
   - While more comfortable for the patient, low power is not capable of removing calculus completely.
   - Deposit can become burnished on the root surface and leave a polished exterior surface that is difficult to detect and remove.
   - Remnants of burnished calculus can harbor pathogenic contaminants.
   - Pathogenic contaminants remain despite cavitation and lavage provided through the ultrasonic tip.
2. *High to Medium Power*
   - Calculus can be removed using higher power settings, provided the proper technique is employed.
   - Use of anesthesia permits maximum thoroughness while keeping the patient comfortable.

B. Transfer of Energy

- The full length of the tip is vibrating, but only the terminal few millimeters will transfer maximum energy capable of disrupting calculus.

C. Adaptation

- Position side of tip against tooth, with the few millimeters nearest the end of the tip closely adapted on the surface at all times (Figure 37-11A).
- May be difficult to accomplish, since the end segment of the tip is generally straight in contrast to anatomical curvatures of the tooth anatomy.

D. Activation

- For energy to transfer from active tip to deposit, it must be moved at a speed that allows the transfer.
- The tip is moved constantly at a slow to moderate pace.

II. ULTRASONIC SCALING

A. Grasp

1. Use a modified pen grasp.
2. A light grasp will increase tactile sensitivity.

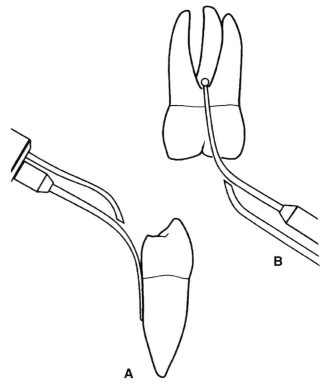

■ **FIGURE 37-11 Adaptation of Ultrasonic Tip. (A)** The side of the point of a tip is placed parallel to the tooth surface to prevent damage to the tooth structure. Damage occurs when the point is held perpendicular to the surface. **(B)** Ball end of tip designed for adaptation in furcation areas.

3. The weight of the cord tends to pull on the handpiece and place additional strain on the wrist. Manage cord drag by the following:
   - Loop the cord and hold it between the ring finger and little finger.
   - Drape the cord over the shoulder.

B. Fulcrum

1. A hard tissue fulcrum is not required because force and pressure against the tooth surface are not indicated.
2. A gentle finger rest is used to stabilize and guide the instrument tip in anterior segments.
3. Extraoral and soft tissue rests allow for proper access and adaptation to deeper posterior segments.

C. Adaptation

1. Keep the side of the instrument tip closely adapted to the tooth surface (Figure 37-11A).
2. Do not hold the tip perpendicular to the tooth surface at any time because damage to the tooth surface can result.
3. *Narrow Periodontal Pockets*
   - Narrow subgingival pockets interfere with proper adaptation and impede visibility.
   - When instrumenting narrow pockets use an insert with appropriate length and limited width.
   - Direct the tip apically and confirm access to the attachment prior to activating the tip.

D. Stroke

1. Keep the instrument tip moving at a moderate to slow pace with a feather-light touch at all times to prevent the following:
   - Scratches or gouging on the tooth surface.
   - Excessive heat build-up.
   - A shock-like effect to the patient.
2. Use featherlike pressure to prevent tooth damage. Excessive lateral pressure can result in the following:
   - Damage to the tooth surface.
   - Dampening and deactivation of the tip vibrations.
   - Burnishing of calculus.
3. Overlap strokes.
   - For comprehensive coverage of all surfaces.
   - Strokes may be horizontal, vertical, oblique, or a combination.
4. Instrument tip may bind when inserted interproximally.

- If so, deactivate the power, remove the instrument tip.
- Reactivate the instrument.

III. WATER CONTROL

A. Foot pedal

- Release the foot pedal at regular intervals to aid in water control.
- Stop periodically to evaluate tooth surfaces.

B. Mirror Use

- Water is continuously sprayed onto the mirror surface, making indirect vision difficult.
- Wipe the wet surface of the mirror with a gloved finger to coalesce the drops into a clear wet surface. When water is allowed to pool on the surface in this manner, a clearer image of the working area can be seen through the water.

IV. MANUAL SCALING

- Complete the procedure with manual instruments directly following ultrasonic instrumentation.
- Check subgingival areas with a subgingival explorer.
- Remove remaining subgingival irregularities and smooth the surface with curets.
- Manual scaling is especially important following the use of conventional ultrasonic tips, which are bulky and provide limited application subgingivally.

V. EVALUATION

A. Use a Periodontal Subgingival Explorer

- To evaluate the effectiveness of instrumentation periodically during treatment.
- There may be areas of root contour where it is not possible to adapt the insert tip, thus leaving portions of the root surface untreated.
- Portions of the root that cannot be accessed by the ultrasonic tip must be instrumented using curets that can be adapted.

B. The Ultrasonic Tip Without Power Can Be Used as a Probe Only

- To confirm access to the soft tissue attachment.
- DO NOT use the insert tip to evaluate the tooth surface.

- There is insufficient tactile sensitivity to accomplish a careful assessment of the root surface smoothness with the insert.

VI. TROUBLESHOOTING

There may be a number of reasons for the ultrasonic instrument to produce unacceptable instrumentation. The causative factor must be analyzed in order to remedy the problem.

A. Tip Wear

- As an ultrasonic tip is used over a period of time, the length of the tip is reduced. With each millimeter of tip length lost, there is a corresponding loss of power.
- Tips must be checked periodically for wear and replaced when length has reached a point beyond which the tip is incapable of producing sufficient vibration.

B. Improper Adaptation

- Failure to adapt the terminal few millimeters of the tip to the tooth surface.
- Root morphology has many curvatures featuring convex and concave surfaces.
- Straight instruments do not adapt well to curved surfaces.
- Curets, specifically mini-bladed curets, are designed to conform to root contours.
- Supplement ultrasonic instrumentation with manual instrumentation to access the highly curved portions of the root.

C. Stroke Too Rapid

- Moving the tip too quickly across the tooth surface.
- Keep tip moving slowly and methodically.
- Brisk tip movement is ineffective on deposit removal.

D. Inadequate Coverage

- Failure to keep strokes confined to close, overlapping channels.
- Moving the tip in a random, scribbling pattern can treat effectively only those limited portions of the root surface that were contacted by the moving tip.
- Move the tip in overlapping segments or channels that comprehensively cover every square millimeter of root surface.

E. Tip Pressure

- Exerting pressure with the tip against the tooth surface.
- The tip must be held with only a light but secure contact and close adaptation against the tooth surface.
- Lateral pressure will render the vibrations ineffective due to a dampening effect.

■ COMPLETION OF INITIAL THERAPY

After each treatment using nonsurgical instrumentation, an immediate evaluation is made and special instructions are given to the patient for the initial tissue healing period. A follow-up telephone call to the patient during the evening after the appointment can be a welcome gesture that conveys professional responsibility and concern.

A short-term follow-up appointment is scheduled in a minimum of 2 weeks when initial healing will be in progress. After health has been attained, it must be maintained. Planning for a long-term maintenance program is described on pages 757 to 759.

I. IMMEDIATE EVALUATION

A. Teeth

- Observation and exploration reveal the immediate effects of instrumentation on the teeth.
- An objective has been to produce smooth tooth surfaces, free from deposits.
- The effect of specific instrumentation is to facilitate the patient's self-care by removing local factors, particularly calculus and overhanging fillings, that encourage dental biofilm retention.

B. Gingiva

- The gingival changes are not apparent immediately after instrumentation.
- Tissue regeneration and initial healing begin in a few days, and by 2 weeks, the area can be gently probed. Maturation of connective tissue and keratinization of epithelium take much longer.
- The objective of treatment is to *create an environment in which the gingival tissue can heal and be maintained in health by the patient.*

II. EXAMINATION

When scaling is accomplished over a series of appointments, each previously scaled quadrant or area is examined and rescaled as needed at each appointment. Visual and tactile methods are applied carefully to each tooth surface.

A. Visual

- Compressed air should be used with a mouth mirror and adequate lighting to examine the supragingival areas and just below the gingival margins.
- Transillumination methods are applied.

B. Tactile

- An evaluation by exploring immediately after completion of instrumentation is made to ascertain that the tooth surfaces are smooth and that all detectable calculus has been removed.

III. INSTRUCTION AFTER SCALING AND ROOT PLANING

Personalized instructions are provided for each patient at the end of each dental hygiene and periodontal appointment. Instruction pertaining to periodontal dressings and sutures is outlined in Table 40-1. Many of the same principles can be applied for postcare instruction when a dressing has not been applied.

IV. PRINTED TAKE-HOME INSTRUCTIONS

Personalized printed instructions help to give the patient a handy reference. Verbal instructions alone can be forgotten or misinterpreted by even the most conscientious patient.

An added personal note or underlining of significant parts of the printed materials can let a patient sense the caring attitude of the professional team.

A. Information to Include

1. Possible discomfort to expect.
2. Rinsing.
3. Toothbrushing.
4. Eating.
5. Where to call in case of problem or question.

B. Rinsing

A warm solution is soothing to the tissues and improves the circulation, thereby helping healing.
1. **Solutions Suggested for Use**
   - *Hypertonic Salt Solution:* Level 1/2 teaspoonful of table salt in 1/2 cup (4 ounces) of warm water; provides 3 or 4 mouthfuls for holding and swishing thoroughly.

- *Sodium Bicarbonate Solution:* Level 1/2 teaspoonful of baking soda in 1 cup (8 ounces) of warm water.
   - Directions for Salt or Bicarbonate Solutions: Every 2 hours; after eating; after toothbrushing; before retiring.
2. **Chlorhexidine 0.12%.** Following instrumentation for NUG, NUP, and advanced periodontitis, chlorhexidine rinsing is advised.
   - Directions: twice daily, after breakfast and before going to bed, without eating after rinsing to take advantage of the substantivity property of chlorhexidine.
   - It must be made clear that it is not a substitute for personal biofilm removal with toothbrush and interdental aids.

C. Toothbrushing

The use of a soft brush is recommended after scaling and root planing. The patient must clearly understand the importance of daily biofilm removal.

D. Eating

Dietary and nutritional factors are discussed.
- Patients who are anesthetized must avoid chewing solid food until the anesthetic has worn off to avoid trauma to the tongue, cheek, and lips.
- If the tissues are tender during healing, use bland foods lacking in strong, spicy seasonings, as well as continuing use of nutritional foods to promote healing.
- Foods for a liquid or a soft diet are suggested on page 861.

▪ FOLLOW-UP EVALUATION

The real evaluation, the true test of successful treatment, cannot be made until at least 2 weeks after the initial scaling and root planing has been completed. At that time, the response of the gingival tissue to therapy is apparent.

I. ASSESSMENT PROCEDURE

A. Periodontal Probing

1. Complete probing is performed and documented.
2. Bleeding points are noted as probings are made and documented in the periodontal charting record.
3. Patient biofilm control efforts are evaluated.
   - Obtain biofilm score after the soft tissue visual inspection has been completed.

- Provide feedback for the patient's efforts and the degree of improvement noted as well as areas needing further attention.

B. Tactile Evaluation

1. Areas demonstrating bleeding points are carefully assessed with a periodontal explorer for residual calculus deposits.
   - For areas of clinical attachment loss greater than 5 millimeters, use a periodontal explorer.
   - Residual calculus can be expected on any subgingival surface that demonstrates bleeding on gentle probing.
2. Special checks for difficult-to-access areas
   - Concavities and depressions of the root anatomy.
   - Furcation invasions.

II. REINSTRUMENTATION

A. Remove Remaining Calculus

- Use only optimally sharpened instruments.

B. Anticipate Effects

- Smooth root surfaces that are free of calculus create a biologically compatible root surface that can support healing in the overlying tissues.

III. MAINTENANCE INTERVAL DETERMINED

A. Assessment findings indicate the relative success of therapy delivered.
B. Based upon the findings, a determination is made as to recommended intervals for subsequent maintenance appointments.
C. Factors taken into account include the following:
   - Soft tissue response to instrumentation and degree of healing.
   - Changes and/or stabilization in probing depth.
   - Patient factors: use of tobacco.
   - Currently demonstrated biofilm control efforts; level of skill.
   - Motivation and responsibility assumed for daily personal oral self-care.
   - Psychosocial factors; stress.

▪ EFFECTS OF NONSURGICAL INSTRUMENTATION

The essential components of successful nonsurgical instrumentation are thorough subgingival debridement by the clinician and effective dental biofilm control by the patient. The focus of treatment and the aims and expected outcomes are specified at the beginning of this chapter.

Tissue response is the most significant measure of success in periodontal debridement. Tissue response is manifested by clinical features commonly referred to as the endpoints of therapy.

I. CLINICAL ENDPOINTS

A. Bleeding on probing: eliminated.
B. Probing depths: reduced.
C. Attachment levels: same or improved.
D. Inflammation: resolved.
E. Gingival appearance: size reduced, color normal.
F. Subgingival microflora: lowered in numbers, delay in repopulation.
G. Dental biofilm control record: improvement in scores approaching 100% biofilm-free.
H. Tooth surface: smooth; no biofilm-retentive irregularities.
I. Quality of life factors: oral comfort with freedom from pain.

II. HEALING

A. Factors Affecting Healing

1. Severity of the infection and clinical features at the start of treatment.
2. Noncompliance of the patient
   a. To dental biofilm control.
   b. To follow the complete treatment plan.
3. Tobacco use: smoking.[53]
4. Systemic influences
   a. Diabetes.
   b. Lowered defense: immunocompromised as, for example, in HIV/AIDS, cancer chemotherapy.
5. Root surface irregularities from incomplete debridement: retained calculus, endotoxins, and microorganisms.

B. Healing Process

1. *Resolution of Inflammation.* Edema recedes, necrotic cells are cleared away, and tissue regenerates.
2. *Clinical Attachment.* A long epithelial attachment can be expected.

III. EFFECT ON MICROORGANISMS

A. Changes in Pocket Flora[54,55]

- The subgingival bacterial flora is changed after debridement, as shown in Table 37-1.

- Prior to instrumentation for treatment of periodontitis, the subgingival microorganisms are primarily anaerobic, gram-negative, motile forms.
- After scaling and root planing, the total number of subgingival organisms decreases substantially. A shift to aerobic, gram-positive, nonmotile forms occurs.

B. Effect of Conversion of Microorganisms

- The disease-producing gram-negative pocket microorganisms are changed to a health-producing gram-positive flora.
- The gingiva reflects the changes. Gingival bleeding on probing is lessened, and the color, size, shape, and other characteristics assume a normal appearance.

C. Repopulation

- Without personal daily biofilm control, the microorganisms can return to pretreatment levels within an average of 42 days.[56]
- With biofilm control, the repopulation of the pocket takes longer, even in susceptible patients.

- In many patients, nonsurgical periodontal therapy results in a gingival condition that can be maintained free from reinfection.

D. Endotoxins

- Endotoxins are lipopolysaccharides (LPSs) released from gram-negative bacterial cell walls.
- They occur in the bacteria covering the cementum and superficially in the cementum itself. Endotoxins have been shown to be toxic to human cells.[57] Endotoxins do not penetrate deeply into cemental surfaces.[1,2]
- Retained endotoxins are held by calculus not removed during instrumentation as well as by new microorganisms recolonizing on the surfaces.

IV. COMPARISON OF MANUAL AND POWER-DRIVEN INSTRUMENTATION

Ultrasonic and manual nonsurgical instrumentation produce equivalent results in calculus and dental biofilm removal. Long-term goals of therapy are accomplished by both.[17,28,58,59] A blended approach that utilizes both methods of instrumentation is preferred. The patient benefits from therapy incorporating the strengths of each approach.

Everyday Ethics

? Lorna and Sommer both practice as hygienists in the same office approximately 2 1/2 days per week. Lorna graduated from dental hygiene school about 15 years ago, while Sommer was licensed just 3 years ago. They generally had their select patients that were routinely scheduled with the same hygienist. One day Mrs. Border shows up in Lorna's appointment book because she wanted to fit in her regular maintenance appointment before going to stay with her daughter.

Since she was going to be gone all winter, the receptionist scheduled her with the first available hygienist. Lorna reviewed the patient's medical history and made a mental note that she suffered seasonal asthma attacks. Following the oral examination, Lorna began to explore, finding rough areas that she assumed was the tooth surface. Upon further instrumentation, the areas turned out to be

deep calculus. Lorna worked diligently but needed to re-appoint Mrs. Border for a second visit. The patient was outraged and complained that Lorna should have used the 'sprayer-machine' like Sommer usually does.

Questions for Consideration

1. While respecting both the patient's autonomy and Sommer's role as a professional, how should Lorna proceed to address this dilemma?

2. What action needs to be taken to ensure that the patient's rights and that Lorna's duties are being fulfilled?

3. Realizing that this calculus could not have formed since the previous appointment, should Lorna be paternalistic toward the patient? Why or why not?

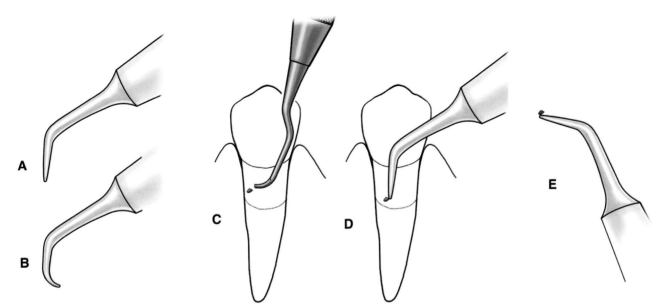

■ **FIGURE 37-12 Broken Instrument Tip Retrieval. (A)** and **(B)** Two shapes of the "Periotriever" Magnetic instruments: **(A)** for straight entrance to pocket and **(B)** shaped to enter furcations. **(C)** Curet in pocket with broken tip. **(D)** Magnetized Retriever in pocket searching for broken tip. **(E)** Curet tip removed from pocket attached to the Retriever. (Modified from Schwartz, M.: The Prevention and Management of the Broken Curet, *Compend. Cont. Educ. Dent., 19,* 418, April, 1998.)

■ INSTRUMENT MAINTENANCE

I. MANUAL SCALERS AND CURETS

A. Examine for Wear While Sharpening

- Reserve thinned or shortened curets to use for conscientious, motivated maintenance patients with shallow sulci and minimal calculus.
- Heavier bladed, newer curets are indicated for application of strong lateral pressure necessary for initial therapy, root preparation, and moderate to heavy accumulations of calculus.
- Handle all instruments with care. Avoid damage, breakage, and dulling of sharp cutting edges.

II. ULTRASONIC TIPS

- Avoid dry heat sterilization; use steam or chemical vapor autoclave.
- Insert tips wear with use and must be monitored.
  - Worn out tips are incapable of removing deposit; calculus is merely burnished.
  - Worn out tips can cause damage to tooth surfaces.
  - Check at intervals (appropriate to extent of use) and replace.

III. BROKEN INSTRUMENTS

The procedure to follow when an instrument blade tip breaks in a patient's mouth during treatment will be in accord with the dentist's own policy. The principal objective in the location of a broken instrument tip is to know positively that the tip has been removed (Figure 37-12). A general procedure is suggested in Box 37-5.

✔ **Factors To Teach The Patient**

- The nature, occurrence, and etiology of calculus.
- The importance of and necessity for complete removal of calculus to the health of the oral tissues in the prevention of periodontal infections.
- The relationship of the accumulation of dental biofilm to the patient's personal oral hygiene procedures.
- Basic reasons for need and the advantages of multiple appointments to complete the scaling and root planing.
- Needed frequency of maintenance appointments in relation to oral health.

BOX 37-5 Care of a Broken Instrument

PREPARATORY PLANNING

—Discuss with dentist during early practice days

—Determine practice policy

OBJECTIVE

Know positively that the broken segment (i.e., tip of scaler) has been completely removed

IMMEDIATE ACTION

1. Cease procedure, retain retraction

2. Do not move patient's head

3. Isolate with gauze sponge

4. Do not use air/water syringe

5. Adjust saliva ejector to opposite side

6. Do not alarm the patient by describing what happened

EXAMINATION OF AREA

1. Do not dry with air

2. Use careful, gentle retraction to examine the immediate area

   —Floor of mouth

   —Mucobuccal fold

3. Blot the gingival tissue dry with a cotton roll to examine around the tooth

4. Use transilluminating light or mouth light

5. Examine gingival sulcus

   —Use a curet applied gently with a spoon-like stroke

   —Take great care not to push the tip into the base of the pocket (in case the broken segment is there)

TREATMENT

1. Apply a magnetized retrieving instrument (Figure 37-12)**

2. Consult with dentist for assistance in accord with previously discussed policy

3. Prepare a radiograph of the area

4. When not found during any of above procedures:

   Arrange for a periodontal surgical procedure

**Adapted from Schwartz, M.: The Prevention and Management of the Broken Curet, *Compend. Cont. Educ. Dent., 19,* 418, April, 1998.

REFERENCES

1. **Nakib**, N.M., Bissada, N.F., Simmelink, J.W., and Goldstine, S.N.: Endotoxin Penetration Into Root Cementum of Periodontally Healthy and Diseased Human Teeth, *J. Periodontol., 53,* 368, June, 1982.

2. **Moore**, J., Wilson, M., and Kieser, J.B.: The Distribution of Bacterial Lipopolysaccharide (Endotoxin) in Relation to Periodontally Involved Root Surfaces, *J. Clin. Periodontol., 13,* 748, September, 1986.

3. **Smart**, G.J., Wilson, M., Davies, E.H., and Kieser, J.B.: The Assessment of Ultrasonic Root Surface Debridement by Determination of Residual Endotoxin Levels, *J. Clin. Periodontol., 17,* 174, March, 1990.

4. **Chiew**, S.Y.T., Wilson, M., Davies, E.H., and Kieser, J.B.: Assessment of Ultrasonic Debridement of Calculus-Associated Periodontally Involved Root Surfaces by the Limulus Amoebocyte Lysate Assay: An *in vitro* Study, *J. Clin. Periodontol., 18,* 240, April, 1991.

5. **Nyman**, S., Westfelt, E., Sarhed, G., and Karring, T.: Role of "Diseased" Root Cementum in Healing Following Treatment of Periodontal Disease: A Clinical Study, *J. Clin. Periodontol., 15,* 464, August, 1988.

6. **Corbet**, E.F., Vaughan, A.J., and Kieser, J.B.: The Periodontally-Involved Root Surface, *J. Clin. Periodontol., 20,* 402, July, 1993.

7. **Quirynen**, M. and Bollen, C.M.L.: The Influence of Surface Roughness and Surface-Free Energy on Supra- and Subgingival Plaque Formation in Man: A Review of the Literature, *J. Clin. Periodontol., 22,* 1, January, 1995.

8. **Leknes**, K.N.: The Influence of Anatomic and Iatrogenic Root Surface Characteristics on Bacterial Colonization and Periodontal Destruction: A Review, *J. Periodontol., 68,* 507, June, 1997.

9. **Vandekerckhove**, B.N.A., Bollen, C.M.L., Dekeyser, C., Darius, P., and Quirynen, M.: Full- Versus Partial-Mouth Disinfection in the Treatment of Periodontal Infections. Long-term Clinical Observations of a Pilot Study, *J. Periodontol., 67,* 1251, December, 1996.

10. **Mongardini**, C., van Steenberghe, D., Dekeyser, C., and Quirynen, M.: One Stage Full- Versus Partial-Mouth Disinfection in the Treatment of Chronic Adult or Generalized Early-onset Periodontitis in Long-term Clinical Observations, *J. Periodontol., 70,* 632, June 1999.

11. **Quirynen**, M., Mongardini, C., DeSoete, M., Pauwels, M., Coucke, W., van Eldere, J., and van Steenberghe, D.: The Role of Chlorhexidine in the One-Stage Full-Mouth Disinfection Treatment of Patients With Advanced Adult Periodontitis, *J. Clin. Periodontol., 27,* 578, August, 2000.

12. **Greenstein**, G.: Full-Mouth Therapy Versus Individual Quadrant Root Planing: A Critical Commentary, *J. Periodontol., 73,* 797, July, 2002.

13. **Perry**, D.A. and Taggart, E.J.: Occurrence Rate of Acute Periodontal Abscess Following Scaling Procedures, *J. Dent. Res., 76,* 335, Abstract 2569, Special Issue, 1997.

14. **Bender**, I.B., Naidorf, I.J., and Garvey, G.J.: Bacterial Endocarditis: A Consideration for Physician and Dentist, *J. Am. Dent. Assoc., 109,* 415, September, 1984.

15. **Pallasch**, T.J. and Slots, J.: Antibiotic Prophylaxis and the Medically Compromised Patient, *Periodontol. 2000, 10,* 107, 1996.

16. **Ramfjord**, S.P., Caffesse, R.G., Morrison, E.C., Hill, R.W., Kerry, G.J., Appleberry, E.A., Nissle, R.R., and Stults, D.L.: Four Modalities of Periodontal Treatment Compared Over Five Years, *J. Periodontal Res., 22,* 222, May, 1987.

17. **Badersten**, A., Nilvéus, R., and Egelberg, J.: Effect of Nonsurgical Periodontal Therapy. I. Moderately Advanced Periodontitis, *J. Clin. Periodontol., 8,* 57, February, 1981.

18. **Lindhe**, J., Nyman, S., and Karring, T.: Scaling and Root Planing in Shallow Pockets, *J. Clin. Periodontol., 9,* 415, September, 1982.

19. **Glickman**, I.: *Clinical Periodontology*, 4th ed. Philadelphia, W.B. Saunders, 1972, p. 625.
20. **Zinner**, D.D.: Ultrasonic Studies in Dentistry: A Preliminary Report, American Institute of Ultrasonics in Medicine; Proceedings of the Fourth Annual Conference on Ultrasonic Therapy; Library of Congress Number 55-12257, August 27, 1955, pp. 6–16.
21. **Johnson**, W.N. and Wilson, J.R.: The Application of the Ultrasonic Dental Unit to Scaling Procedures, *J. Periodontol., 28,* 264, October, 1957.
22. **Walmsley**, A.D., Laird, W.R.E., and Williams, A.R.: A Model System to Demonstrate the Role of Cavitational Activity in Ultrasonic Scaling, *J. Dent. Res., 63,* 1162, September, 1984.
23. **Baehni**, P., Thilo, B., Chapuis, B., and Pernet, D.: Effects of Ultrasonic and Sonic Scalers on Dental Plaque Microflora In Vitro and In Vivo, *J. Clin. Periodontol., 19,* 455, August, 1992.
24. **Walmsley**, A.D., Walsh, T.F., Laird, W.R.E., and Williams, A.R.: Effects of Cavitational Activity on the Root Surface of Teeth During Ultrasonic Scaling, *J. Clin. Periodontol., 17,* 306, May, 1990.
25. **Nosal**, G., Scheidt, M.J., O'Neal, R., and Van Dyke, T.E.: The Penetration of Lavage Solution Into the Periodontal Pocket During Ultrasonic Instrumentation, *J. Periodontol., 62,* 554, September, 1991.
26. **McInnes**, C., Engel, D., and Martin, R.W.: Fimbria Damage and Removal of Adherent Bacteria After Exposure to Acoustic Energy, *Oral Microbiol. Immunol., 8,* 277, October, 1993.
27. **McInnes**, C., Engel, D., Moncla, B.J., and Martin, R.W.: Reduction in Adherence of *Actinomyces viscosus* After Exposure to Low-Frequency Acoustic Energy, *Oral Microbiol. Immunol., 7,* 171, June, 1992.
28. **Copulos**, T.A., Low, S.B., Walker, C.B., Trebilcock, Y.Y., and Hefti, A.F.: Comparative Analysis Between a Modified Ultrasonic Tip and Hand Instruments on Clinical Parameters of Periodontal Disease, *J. Periodontol., 64,* 694, August, 1993.
29. **Takacs**, V.J., Lie, T., Perala, D.G., and Adams, D.F.: Efficacy of 5 Machining Instruments in Scaling of Molar Furcations, *J. Periodontol., 64,* 228, March, 1993.
30. **Leon**, L.E. and Vogel, R.I.: A Comparison of the Effectiveness of Hand Scaling and Ultrasonic Debridement in Furcations as Evaluated by Differential Dark-field Microscopy, *J. Periodontol., 58,* 86, February, 1987.
31. **Suzuki**, J.B. and Delisle, A.L.: Pulmonary Actinomycosis of Periodontal Origin, *J. Periodontol., 55,* 581, October, 1984.
32. **Lee**, S.-Y., Lai, Y.-L., and Morgano, S.M.: Effects of Ultrasonic Scaling and Periodontal Curettage on Surface Roughness of Porcelain, *J. Prosthet. Dent., 73,* 227, March, 1995.
33. **Vermilyea**, S.G., Prasanna, M.K., and Agar, J.R.: Effect of Ultrasonic Cleaning and Air Polishing on Porcelain Labial Margin Restorations, *J. Prosthet. Dent., 71,* 447, May, 1994.
34. **Rajstein**, J. and Tal, M.: The Effects of Ultrasonic Scaling on the Surface of Class V Amalgam Restorations—A Scanning Electron Microscope Study, *J. Oral Rehabil., 11,* 299, May, 1984.
35. **Sivers**, J.E. and Johnson, G.K.: Comparison of Effects of Ultrasonic and Sonic Instrumentation on Amalgam Restorations, *Gen. Dent., 37,* 130, March–April, 1989.
36. **Bjornson**, E.J., Collins, D.E., and Engler, W.O.: Surface Alteration of Composite Resins After Curette, Ultrasonic, and Sonic Instrumentation: An *in vitro* Study, *Quintessence Int., 21,* 381, May, 1990.
37. **Gantes**, B.G. and Nilvéus, R.: The Effects of Different Hygiene Instruments on Titanium Surfaces: SEM Observations, *Int. J. Periodontics Restorative Dent., 11,* 225, Number 3, 1991.
38. **Rapley**, J.W., Swan, R.H., Hallmon, W.W., and Mills, M.P.: The Surface Characteristics Produced by Various Oral Hygiene Instruments and Materials on Titanium Implant Abutments, *Int. J. Oral Maxillofac. Implants, 5,* 47, Number 1, 1990.
39. **White**, D.J., Cox, E.R., Arends, J., Nieborg, J.H., Leydsman, H., Wieringa, D.W., Dijkman, A.G., and Ruben, J.R.: Instruments and Methods for the Quantitative Measurement of Factors Affecting Hygienist/Dentist Efforts During Scaling and Root Planing of the Teeth, *J. Clin. Dent., 7,* 32, Number 2, 1996.
40. **Liskiewicz**, S.T. and Kerschbaum, W.E.: Cumulative Trauma Disorders: An Ergonomic Approach for Prevention, *J. Dent. Hyg., 71,* 162, Summer, 1997.
41. **Bohay**, R.N., Bencak, J., Kavaliers, M., and MacLean, D.: A Survey of Magnetic Fields in the Dental Operatory, *J. Can. Dent. Assoc., 60,* 835, September, 1994.
42. **Abrams**, H., Barkmeier, W.W., and Cooley, R.L.: Temperature Changes in the Pulp Chamber Produced by Ultrasonic Instrumentation, *Gen. Dent., 27,* 62, September–October, 1979.
43. **Möller**, P., Grevstad, A.O., and Kristoffersen, T.: Ultrasonic Scaling of Maxillary Teeth Causing Tinnitus and Temporary Hearing Shifts, *J. Clin. Periodontol., 3,* 123, May, 1976.
44. **Gantes**, B.G., Nilvéus, R., Lie, T., and Leknes, K.N.: The Effect of Hygiene Instruments on Dentin Surfaces: Scanning Electron Microscopic Observations, *J. Periodontol., 63,* 151, March, 1992.
45. **Barbeau**, J., Tanguay, R., Faucher, E., Avezard, C., Trudel, L., Cote, L., and Prevost, A.P.: Multiparametric Analysis of Waterline Contamination in Dental Units, *Appl. Environ. Microbiol., 62,* 3954, November, 1996.
46. **Harrel**, S.K., Barnes, J.B., and Rivera-Hidalgo, F.: Reduction of Aerosols Produced by Ultrasonic Scalers, *J. Periodontol., 67,* 28, January, 1996.
47. **King**, T.B., Muzzin, K.B., Berry, C.W., and Anders, L.M.: The Effectiveness of an Aerosol Reduction Device for Ultrasonic Scalers, *J. Periodontol., 68,* 45, January, 1997.
48. **Reynolds**, M.A., Lavigne, C.K., Minah, G.E., and Suzuki, J.B.: Clinical Effects of Simultaneous Ultrasonic Scaling and Subgingival Irrigation With Chlorhexidine. Mediating Influence of Periodontal Probing Depth, *J. Clin. Periodontol., 19,* 595, September, 1992.
49. **Taggart**, J.A., Palmer, R.M., and Wilson, R.F.: A Clinical and Microbiological Comparison of the Effects of Water and 0.02% Chlorhexidine as Coolants During Ultrasonic Scaling and Root Planing, *J. Clin. Periodontol., 17,* 32, January, 1990.
50. **Bandt**, C.L., Korn, N.A., and Schaffer, E.M.: Bacteremias from Ultrasonic and Hand Instrumentation, *J. Periodontol., 35,* 214, May–June, 1964.
51. **Legnani**, P., Checchi, L., Pelliccioni, G.A., and D'Achille, C.: Atmospheric Contamination During Dental Procedures, *Quintessence Int., 25,* 435, June, 1994.
52. **Fine**, D.H., Mendieta, C., Barnett, M.L., Furgang, D., Meyers, R., Olshan, A., and Vincent, J.: Efficacy of Preprocedural Rinsing With an Antiseptic in Reducing Viable Bacteria in Dental Aerosols, *J. Periodontol., 63,* 821, October, 1992.
53. **Preber**, H. and Bergström, J.: The Effect of Non-surgical Treatment on Periodontal Pockets in Smokers and Non-smokers, *J. Clin. Periodontol., 13,* 319, April, 1996.
54. **Listgarten**, M.A. and Helldén, L.: Relative Distribution of Bacteria at Clinically Healthy and Periodontally Diseased Sites in Humans, *J. Clin. Periodontol., 5,* 115, May, 1978.
55. **Slots**, J., Mashimo, P., Levine, M.J., and Genco, R.J.: Periodontal Therapy in Humans. I. Microbiologic and Clinical Effects of a Single Course of Periodontal Scaling and Root Planing, and of Adjunctive Tetracycline Therapy, *J. Periodontol., 50,* 495, October, 1979.
56. **Mousqués**, T., Listgarten, M.A., and Phillips, R.W.: Effects of Scaling and Root Planing on the Composition of the Human Subgingival Microbial Flora, *J. Periodont. Res., 15,* 144, March, 1980.
57. **Aleo**, J.J., DeRenzis, F.A., Farber, P.A., and Varboncoeur, A.P.: The Presence and Biologic Activity of Cementum-Bound Endotoxin, *J. Periodontol., 45,* 672, September, 1974.

58. **Oosterwaal,** P.J.M., Matee M.I., Mikx, F.H.M., van't Hof, M.A., and Renggli, H.H.: The Effect of Subgingival Debridement With Hand and Ultrasonic Instruments on the Subgingival Microflora, *J. Clin. Periodontol., 14,* 528, October, 1987.

59. **Badersten,** A., Nilvéus, R., and Egelberg, J.: Effect of Nonsurgical Periodontal Therapy. II. Severely Advanced Periodontitis, *J. Clin. Periodontol., 11,* 63, January, 1984.

SUGGESTED READINGS

American Academy of Periodontology, Research, Science and Therapy Committee: Position Paper: Sonic and Ultrasonic Scalers in Periodontics, *J. Periodontol., 71,* 1792, November, 2000.

Cobb, C.M.: Non-surgical Pocket Therapy: Mechanical, *Ann. Periodontol., 1,* 443, November, 1996.

Greenstein, G.: Periodontal Diseases Are Curable, *J. Periodontol., 73,* 950, August, 2002.

Lowenguth, R.A. and Greenstein, G.: Clinical and Microbiological Response to Nonsurgical Mechanical Periodontal Therapy, *Periodontol. 2000, 9,* 14, 1995.

Miller, C.S., Leonelli, F.M., and Latham, E.: Selective Interference With Pacemaker Activity by Electrical Dental Devices, *Oral Surg. Oral Med. Oral Pathol. Oral Radiol. Endod., 85,* 33, January, 1998.

Paolantonio, M., diPlacido, G., Scarano, A., and Piatteli, A.: Molar Root Furcation: Morphometric and Morphologic Analysis, *Int. J. Periodont. Restorative Dent., 18,* 489, October, 2000.

Reed, K.L.: Sonic Scalers: A Review, *Gen. Dent., 40,* 34, January–February, 1992.

Manual Scaling

Hoang, T., Jorgensen, M.G., Keim, R.G., Pattison, A.M., and Slots, J.: Povidone-iodine as a Periodontal Pocket Disinfectant, *J. Periodont. Res., 38,* 311, June, 2003.

Kocher, T., König, J., Hansen, P., and Rühling, A.: Subgingival Polishing Compared to Scaling With Steel Curettes: A Clinical Pilot Study, *J. Clin. Periodontol, 28,* 194, February, 2001.

Landry, C., Long, B., Singer, D., and Senthilselvan, A.: Comparison Between a Short and a Conventional Blade Periodontal Curet: An *in vitro* Study, *J. Clin. Periodontol., 26,* 548, August, 1999.

Lux, G.: The Use of Scaling and Root Planing in Long-term Management of Advanced Periodontitis: A Case Report, *Canad. Dent. Hyg. Assoc. (PROBE), 33,* 94, July/August, 1999.

Magnusson, I., Geurs, N.C., Harris, P.A., Hefti, A.F., Mariotti, A.J., Mauriello, S.M., Soler, L., and Offenbacher, S.: Intrapocket Anesthesia for Scaling and Root Planing in Pain-Sensitive Patients, *J. Periodontol., 74,* 597, May, 2003.

Mann, G.B. and Wilder, R.S.: An Update on Hand Instruments for Use in Nonsurgical Periodontal Therapy, *Access, 13,* 24, December, 1999.

Pattison, A.M. and Matsuda, S.: The Influence of Endoscopy on Periodontal Instrumentation. Part II. Hand Instrument Selection for Initial Therapy, *Dimens. Dent. Hyg., 1,* 4, November, Supplement, 2003.

Pihlstrom, B.L., Hargreaves, K.M., Bouwsma, O.J., Myers, W.R., Goodale, M.B., and Doyle, M.J.: Pain After Periodontal Scaling and Root Planing, *J. Am. Dent. Assoc., 130,* 801, June, 1999.

Ultrasonic Scaling

Busslinger, A., Lampe, K., Beuchat, M., and Lehmann, B.: A Comparative in vitro Study of a Magnetostrictive and a Piezoelectric Ultrasonic Scaling Instrument, *J., Clin. Periodontol., 28,* 642, July, 2001.

Carr, M.: Ultrasonics, *Access, 13,* May–June, *Special Supplement,* 1999.

Clifford, L.R., Needleman, I.G., and Chan, Y.K.: Comparison of Periodontal Pocket Penetration by Conventional and Microultrasonic Inserts, *J. Clin. Periodontol., 26,* 124, February, 1999.

Fong, C.: Ultrasonics—Part I. Clinical Applications, *Contemporary Oral Hyg., 2,* 13, March/April, 2002.

Fong, C.: Ultrasonics—Part II. Clinical Applications, *Contemporary Oral Hyg., 2,* 18, May/June, 2002.

Khambay, B.S. and Walmsley, A.D.: Acoustic Microstreaming: Detection and Measurement Around Ultrasonic Scalers, *J. Periodontol., 70,* 626, June, 1999.

Lea, S.C., Landini, G., and Walmsley, A.D.: Displacement Amplitude of Ultrasonic Scaler Inserts, *J. Clin. Periodontol., 30,* 505, June, 2003.

Low, S.B.: Technology and Ultrasonic Debridement, *Compend. Cont. Educ. Oral Hyg., 7,* 3, Number 3, 2000.

Pattison, A.M., Matsuda, S.A., and Pattison, G.L.: Clinical Observations on Ultrasonic Tip Selection for Initial Periodontol Therapy, *Dimens. Dent. Hyg., 1,* 32, June/July, 2003.

Ultrasonics/Aerosol Production

Barnes, J.B., Harrel, S.K., and Rivera-Hidalgo, F.: Blood Contamination of the Aerosols Produced by *in vivo* Use of Ultrasonic Scalers, *J. Periodontol., 69,* 434, April, 1998.

Gross, K.B.W., Overman, P.R., Cobb, C., and Brockman, S.: Aerosol Generation by Two Ultrasonic Scalers and One Sonic Scaler: A Comparative Study, *J. Dent. Hyg., 66,* 314, September, 1992.

Harrel, S.K.: Contaminated Dental Aerosols, *Dimens. Dent. Hyg., 1,* 16, October, 2003.

Rivera-Hidalgo, F., Barnes, J.B., and Harrel, S.K.: Aerosol and Splatter Production by Focused Spray and Standard Ultrasonic Inserts, *J. Periodontol., 70,* 473, May, 1999.

Effects of Treatment

American Academy of Periodontology: Position Paper: Treatment of Plaque-induced Gingivitis, Chronic Periodontitis, and Other Clinical Conditions, *J. Periodontol., 72,* 1790, December, 2001.

Aukhil, I.: Biology of Wound Healing, *Periodontology 2000, 22,* 44, 2000.

Cobb, C.M.: Clinical Significance of Non-surgical Periodontal Therapy: An Evidence-Based Perspective of Scaling and Root Planing, *J. Clin. Periodontol., 29,* 6, Supplement 2, May, 2002.

Cugini, M.A., Haffajee, A.D., Smith, C., Kent, R.L., and Socransky, S.S.: The Effect of Scaling and Root Planing on the Clinical and Microbiological Parameters of Periodontal Diseases: 12-Month Results, *J. Clin. Periodontol., 27,* 30, January, 2000.

Dufour, L.A. and Bissell, H.S.: Periodontal Attachment Loss Induced by Mechanical Subgingival Instrumentation in Shallow Sulci, *J. Dent. Hyg., 76,* 207, Summer, 2002.

Fujise, O., Hamachi, T., Inoue, K., Miura, M., and Maeda, K.: Microbiological Markers for Prediction and Assessment of Treatment Outcome Following Non-surgical Periodontal Therapy, *J. Periodontol., 73,* 1253, November, 2002.

Izumi, Y., Hiwatashi-Horinouchi, K., Furuichi, Y., and Sueda, T.: Influence of Different Curette Insertion Depths on the Outcome of Nonsurgical Periodontal Treatment, *J. Clin. Periodontol., 26,* 716, November, 1999.

Loesche, W.J., Giordano, J.R., Soehren, S., and Kaciroti, N.: The Nonsurgical Treatment of Patients With Periodontal Disease: Results After Five Years, *J. Am. Dent. Assoc., 133,* 311, March, 2002.

Petersilka, G.J., Ehmke, B., and Flemmig, T.F.: Antimicrobial Effects of Mechanical Debridement, *Periodontol. 2000, 28,* 56, 2002.

Nonsurgical Periodontal Therapy: Supplemental Care Procedures

The two essential components of successful nonsurgical therapy are complete subgingival scaling with root debridement and effective dental biofilm control. The objective is to eliminate or at least suppress the pathologic microorganisms in the subgingival area to promote healing and hence control the infection.

Supplemental care procedures are selected in accord with the special needs of the patient. The need, the procedures, and the expected outcomes are carefully explained to the patient. The patient must accept responsibility and understand that the success of all periodontal therapy depends on the daily personal biofilm control by the patient.

In this chapter, purposes and procedures for professional irrigation and local delivery of antimicrobials are described. Box 38-1 defines key words and related terminology.

I. PATIENT NEEDS

For the patient with uncomplicated gingivitis, complete scaling and patient compliance in personal daily biofilm removal usually can bring about a reversal of inflammation, and health can be maintained. Likewise, for the patient with early periodontitis, control of infection also may be attained through nonsurgical periodontal therapy. Maintaining the healthy state requires continuing routine appointments for professional scaling and supervision of the patient's biofilm removal methods.

On the other hand, for patients with moderate to advanced periodontal conditions, or refractory patients with poor response to routine therapy, supplemental therapeutic measures usually are required. Certain periodontal conditions of patients of all

BOX 38-1 KEY WORDS: Nonsurgical Periodontal Therapy

Antibiotic: a form of antimicrobial agent produced by or obtained from microorganisms that can kill other microorganisms or inhibit their growth; may be specific for certain organisms or may cover a broad spectrum.

Antimicrobial therapy: use of specific chemical or pharmaceutical agents for the control or destruction of microorganisms, either systemically or at specific sites.

Attachment: with reference to the *clinical attachment level,* which is the position of the periodontal attached tissue at the base of a sulcus or pocket as measured from a fixed point.

> **New attachment:** the union of connective tissue or epithelium with a root surface that has been deprived of its original attachment apparatus; the new attachment may be epithelial adhesion and/or connective tissue adaptation or attachment, and it may include new cementum.

> **Reattachment:** the reunion of epithelial and connective tissues with root surfaces and bone such as occurs after an incision or injury.

Biodegradable: susceptible of degradation by biological processes, as by bacterial or other enzymatic action.

Cannula: tubular instrument placed in a cavity to introduce or withdraw fluid.

Chemotherapy: treatment by means of chemical or pharmaceutical agents.

Controlled release: local delivery of a chemotherapeutic agent to a site-specific area; may be a patch to be worn on the skin or a polymeric fiber, such as that used to deliver an agent to a periodontal pocket.

Infection: invasion and multiplication of microorganisms in body tissues.

> **Endogenous infection:** caused by microorganisms that are part of the normal microbiota of the skin, nose, mouth, and intestinal and urogenital tracts.

> **Exogenous infection:** caused by organisms acquired from outside the oral cavity or the host.

> **Opportunistic infection:** occurs in a systemically or locally impaired host; opportunistic pathogens may not be highly virulent, but they can cause disease when the host defense is altered.

Open scaling and root planing: instrumentation performed after the area has been exposed by tissue removal or the tissue is separated and laid back as a flap; visibility and accessibility allow more thorough treatment.

Refractory periodontitis: clinical attachment loss despite optimal subgingival debridement and performance of acceptable oral hygiene by the patient.

---

degrees of disease severity will require surgical or other advanced therapeutic procedures and will be referred to a periodontist.

II. SUPPLEMENTAL CARE PROCEDURES

Examples of supplemental care procedures that are carried out by the dental hygienist described in other chapters of this book include:

A. Smoking cessation assistance.
B. Desensitization of teeth.
C. At-home rinsing, irrigation, use of dentifrice, and other selective use of antimicrobials.
D. Care for dental implants.
E. Dental caries prevention: fluoride applications and other preventive measures, especially for root caries prevention for the patient with periodontal recession.
F. Correction of biofilm-retaining irregularities; overhang removal when not included in the routine tooth preparation procedures.
G. Dietary analysis for all special needs.
H. Personal counseling for patients with systemic conditions for which periodontal infection is a risk factor (pregnancy, cardiovascular disease, diabetes).

■ ANTIMICROBIAL TREATMENT

The use of antimicrobial agents for supplemental or adjunctive treatment of gingival and periodontal infections may be local or systemic.

I. OBJECTIVES OF ANTIMICROBIAL THERAPY

By arresting the infection using antimicrobial drugs, further loss of periodontal attachment and other periodontal tissue destruction caused by microorganisms can be prevented. Treatment using antimicrobials aims to suppress and eliminate pathogenic microorganisms to allow the recolonization of the microbiota that are compatible with health.

II. TYPES OF DELIVERY OF ANTIMICROBIALS

The types will be described in the following order in this chapter.

A. Systemic Administration

Systemic administration of antibiotics is well known and highly successful in the world of medical care. Antibiotics have saved the lives of many people with generalized infectious diseases.

B. Local Delivery

The knowledge that periodontal diseases are site-specific infections has led to the development of methods for placing antimicrobials directly at the site of the infection—the pocket. Irrigation and controlled-release methods will be described.

▪ SYSTEMIC

I. ACTION OF SYSTEMICALLY ADMINISTERED ANTIBIOTIC

In contrast to locally applied agents placed directly into a pocket, antibiotics administered systemically reach the pathogenic organisms in the pocket through the circulation. The antibiotic is absorbed into the circulation from the intestine. From the bloodstream, the drug is passed into the body tissues. It enters the periodontal tissues and passes into the pocket by way of the gingival sulcus fluid. The systemically administered drug is in a diluted form by the time it reaches the pathogenic microorganisms, where the destruction is taking place.

II. SELECTION OF ANTIBIOTIC

Ideally, the specific microorganism that is causing a certain periodontal disease should be determined first, and the antibiotic that is selected should be specific for that organism.[1] Microbiological testing is available and can be used to guide clinical decisions. Examples of specific treatment in current practice are the use of tetracyclines and metronidazole in combination with mechanical debridement to treat *Actinobacillus actinomycetemcomitans* in juvenile periodontitis and refractory periodontal conditions.[2,3]

Periodontal diseases are caused by mixed infections of microorganisms. The pathogens tend to work in clusters, that is, in combination with other organisms. Selective identification of specific organisms that match with specific antibiotics has been accomplished only to a limited degree.

III. LIMITATIONS

The precautions and adverse effects, as well as the acquisition of antibiotic resistance by the organisms, preclude the widespread use of systemic antibiotics for periodontal problems. Limitations include the following:
A. Side effects of certain antibiotics.
B. Potential for the development of resistant strains.
C. Local concentration diluted by the time the drug reaches the pathogens; drug is "wasted" in that it covers a large area not needing the treatment.
D. Superimposed infection can develop, such as candidiasis.
E. Low compliance of the patient in following the prescription for the required number of days.

IV. USE OF SYSTEMIC THERAPY

Most periodontal infection does not require systemic therapy except when there is systemic involvement shown by generalized symptoms such as fever. Examples are an acute inflammation in necrotizing ulcerative gingivitis or abscess formation. Treatment using systemic antibiotics is a selective procedure.[1]

▪ PROFESSIONAL SUBGINGIVAL IRRIGATION

Professional subgingival irrigation is based on the premise that delivery of antimicrobial agents may enhance the effects of treatment by scaling and root planing. Irrigation into a pocket can disrupt the numbers of microorganisms left behind following instrumentation.

Studies have shown that repopulation of the subgingival microflora can occur within weeks after treatment.[4] In addition, the reduction of the subgingival flora depends on the ability of the clinician to remove subgingival biofilm and calculus definitively; clearly, total removal is difficult in deep pockets.

Irrigation with an antimicrobial agent provides a supplemental therapeutic step and results in additional clinical benefits.[5]

I. DELIVERY METHOD

A presterilized disposable cannula, with a side port, multiple side ports, or end release (Figure 38-1A), is used with one of the following:

- Disposable hand syringe.
- Specially designed jet irrigator.
- Air-driven irrigation handpiece.

II. PROCEDURE

A. Prepare the cannula by bending it slightly as it is uncovered (Figure 38-1B).
B. Insert the cannula subgingivally (Figure 38-1C).
C. Allow the irrigant to fill the pocket.
D. Apply circumferentially, releasing solution at three points on the facial surface and three on the lingual surface.
E. Irrigate all teeth, quadrants, or specific selected sites as dictated by the patient's need.

III. RECOMMENDATIONS FOR USE

A. Preprocedural Delivery

An antimicrobial agent can aid in reducing the numbers of microorganisms to prevent aerosol contamination during instrumentation.

B. Preanesthesia Application

Used to reduce microorganisms before application of topical anesthetic in preparation for local anesthetic injection.

C. Maintenance Phase: Postprocedure Irrigation

1. Patient with site(s) not responding to traditional periodontal care.
2. Patient with gingivitis superimposed on periodontitis.
3. Patient with areas inaccessible to mechanical instrumentation because of root contour, furcations, or depth of pocket where open scaling and root planing are not alternatives.

IV. ANTIMICROBIAL AGENTS

A variety of antimicrobial agents, saline solution, and water have been researched for professional irrigation with varying results. Products used include chlorhexidine gluconate and stannous fluoride.[5-8]

V. SPECIAL CONSIDERATIONS

A. Antibiotic Premedication

Subgingival irrigation can produce a bacteremia. Professional irrigation requires premedication in patients susceptible to the effects of bacteremia. When irrigation is selected as a specific form of treatment for a patient susceptible to bacterial endocarditis, the periodontal tissues should be brought to health first. The usual procedure for all dental appointments should be followed.

B. Irrigation Pressure

Professional irrigation systems usually control the amount of pressure. Caution must be exercised, however, when irrigating with a disposable syringe because pressure may exceed the safety level for the oral tissues.

▪ LOCAL DELIVERY OF ANTIMICROBIALS

Local delivery means that the medication used to treat the periodontal infection is concentrated at the site of the infection. The infecting pathogenic microorganisms are located in the depths of the pockets and the surrounding tissue. Irrigation does deliver the medication to the pocket, but the action is temporary because of the constant turnover and cleansing that is going on in the pocket.

Controlled delivery refers to providing the medication over an extended period of time by being held in the pocket and released slowly. Slow-release methods are used in a variety of ways. The nicotine patch, used to assist a person trying to break a smoking addiction, is an example.

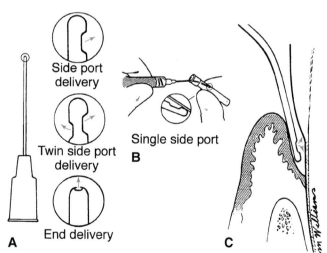

■ **FIGURE 38-1 Professional Irrigation. (A)** Types of cannula tips with side-port or end-delivery openings. **(B)** Prepare the cannula for use by bending the sterile tip within the encasement to make the insertion easier. **(C)** With knowledge of each probing depth, insert the cannula gently to near the bottom of a pocket. No force should be used.

I. REQUIREMENTS

A local delivery method can place high concentrations of the antimicrobial in an infected pocket. To be successful the medication must[9]:

A. Be of a concentration that will act on the microorganisms causing the infection.

B. Reach all areas of the pocket to the very bottom and into furcations.

C. Stay in contact long enough at the effective concentration for the antimicrobial action to take place.

D. Comparison with systemic: When systemic treatment is used, much less of the antimicrobial medication reaches the actual site of the infection where the pathogens are concentrated because the agent becomes diluted as it passes through the system.

II. USES FOR SLOW-RELEASE LOCAL DELIVERY[10]

A. At Initial Therapy

Periodontal diseases result from local infection with a pathogenic microflora. The periodontal pocket is generally teeming with microorganisms and may also contain subgingival calculus, which further adds to harbor bacteria. Scaling and root planing are highly effective procedures for controlling periodontal infections, reducing inflammation, and reducing probing depths.

The adjunctive use of local antimicrobials may enhance the effect of the mechanical instrumentation. Research has shown that the adjunctive use of a controlled-release antimicrobial increases the effect of scaling and root planing.[11]

B. Adjunctive Treatment: At Reevaluation

For the minority of sites that do not respond to basic therapy and may be classified as refractory periodontal disease, a local delivery method can be selected. At the completion of periodontal therapy, a reevaluation is made at the first maintenance appointment, and areas that do not respond to additional scaling and root planing may be selected for a local drug delivery treatment.

C. Recurrent Disease

Over time during the maintenance phase of therapy, pockets can recolonize. Recurrence of periodontal infection usually occurs in localized pockets, particularly in areas most difficult for the patient to carry out complete dental biofilm removal on a daily basis.

D. Peri-Implantitis

The ailing or failing implant may respond to a localized slow-release antimicrobial.

E. Periodontal Abscess

After incision and drainage has been established, a locally delivered, sustained-release antimicrobial may aid the healing process. When a tetracycline fiber is used, it may serve as a wick in the drainage of the abscess.

F. Preparation for Periodontal Surgery

Preconditioning the tissue and lessening the severity of the infection can contribute to less bleeding during surgery and smoother, more rapid healing.

III. TYPES OF LOCAL DELIVERY AGENTS

Available for treatment of periodontal infections are a tetracycline fiber; a chlorhexidine chip; and antibiotic gels, metronidazole, minocycline, and doxycycline.

Subgingival drug therapy should always be applied as a supplement or adjunctive procedure after meticulous scaling and root debridement has been completed and the results evaluated. Special features of each type and procedures for clinical application are presented. For all products, the manufacturer's advice and directions should be followed.

■ TETRACYCLINE FIBER

The concept of a controlled local delivery for treatment of periodontal pathogens in a pocket infection was developed over many years by Goodson and coworkers.[12]

Use of the fiber has shown significant clinical improvement in probing depth, clinical attachment level, and bleeding on probing[13-15] and reduction of sites with periodontal pathogenic microorganisms.[16]

I. DESCRIPTION

A. Monolithic fiber: 9 inches (23 cm) long, 0.5 mm diameter; flexible.

B. Composition of fiber: ethylene/vinyl acetate, biocompatible copolymer.

C. Contents: 12.7 mg tetracycline hydrochloride (25%) mixed with the polymer; imparts a yellow color to the fiber.

D. Controlled delivery; nonbiodegradable; maintains high concentration over full 10-day period of application.

II. ACTION

A. Slow-Release

The pocket moisture dissolves the drug from the fiber.

B. Amount Released

Depends on the length of fiber used; higher dose in deep pockets where more fiber length is used.

C. Comparison With Systemically Administered Antibiotic

1. *Prescription:* 250-mg tablets taken four times per day for 10 days results in a total dose of 10,000 mg.
2. *Fiber:* a total dose of 12.7 mg is possible when a whole fiber is used.

D. Suggested Contraindications

1. Sensitivities or allergies to tetracycline or the cyanoacrylate used for dressings.
2. Immunocompromised patient susceptible to infection related to overgrowth of fiber-resistant bacteria or *Candida.*
3. Pregnant or breast-feeding women. The amount of tetracycline is small, but prudent practice suggests that no elective drugs be administered during pregnancy or lactation.
4. Patient with inadequate self-care who does not comply with routine maintenance must be informed of the potential for limited success.

III. PLACEMENT PROCEDURES

A. Site Selection

Probing depth of 5 mm or more is best for fiber retention.

B. Fiber Preparation

1. *Length needed.* Depends on probing depth; more efficient to work with 2- to 3-inch lengths.
2. *Number of teeth treated.* More than one pocket can be treated in the same appointment on the same side, preferably the same quadrant for convenience and comfort of patient's postcare. Chewing, brushing, and other disturbances increase chances of displacement.
3. *Sterility of the fiber.* Once the package is opened, extra fiber not used cannot be kept for a future appointment.

C. Steps in Placement

1. *Anesthesia.* Anesthesia is not usually needed for fiber placement. When scaling is performed at the same appointment, anesthesia may have been administered already.
2. *Isolation.* Cotton rolls and saliva ejector are indicated.
3. *Fiber placement*
   a. Place fiber around the tooth first to aid retention; thread under contact areas by looping fiber with dental floss or using a floss threader.
   b. Use a gingival retraction cord packing instrument or other dull instrument to pack the fiber down; pass the fiber to the bottom of the pocket.
   c. Fold the fiber back and forth on itself (Figure 38-2A).
   d. Furcation area. Use a small piece of fiber to pack the furca first; then fill the rest of the pocket.
   e. Interdental pocket. Pack from either or both facial and lingual or palatal.
   f. Fill to within 1 mm of the gingival margin. Anticipate that the tissue will shrink.
   g. When the pocket is filled, trim ends of fiber that extend above gingival margin and pack down (Figure 38-2B).
4. *Place adhesive dressing*
   a. Isolate, dry gently with gauze square or light air blast.
   b. Apply the adhesive dressing all around the margin in small amounts to hold the fiber in place.

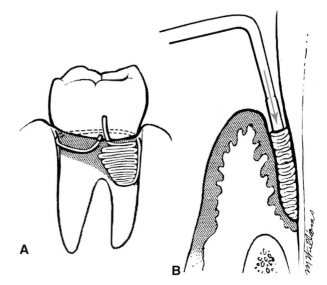

▪ **FIGURE 38-2 Tetracycline Fiber. (A)** The fiber is first placed around the tooth to provide retention. Then, starting at the very bottom of the pocket, the fiber is layered on itself until the pocket is filled. **(B)** Pack the fiber down with a dull instrument.

c.   Adhesive sets rapidly. May cover with water-soluble lubricant to smooth the surface and prevent sticking.

5.   *Additional recommendation.* Cover with periodontal dressing to ensure that the fiber cannot be displaced.

6.   Make appointment for fiber removal in 7 to 14 days.

D. Patient Instruction

1.   Prevent accidental removal:
     a.   Do not touch with fingers or tongue.
     b.   Avoid coarse, rough, or sticky foods.
     c.   Brush and floss all other teeth; avoid area of fiber.

2.   Rinse with chlorhexidine 0.12% twice daily.

3.   Call for appointment if fiber is lost before 7 days; must be replaced for complete treatment.

E. Fiber Removal

1.   Provide patient with preprocedural antimicrobial mouthrinse.

2.   Isolate, dry the surface, tease the fiber out using a curet; cut the fiber that crosses through the interdental area.

3.   Examine tissue. There may be a small gap between margin and tooth; it will close in a short time. Check for and remove any newly formed calculus.

4.   Instruct patient to resume regular self-care procedures to control dental biofilm; advise patient to continue chlorhexidine rinsing for a few more days.

F.   EVALUATION

Examine in 2 to 3 weeks to ensure that tissue has responded and that the patient is maintaining the area. Proceed to 3-month maintenance.

■ CHLORHEXIDINE CHIP

The chlorhexidine chip benefits periodontal health by significant improvements in probing depths, gain of clinical attachment, and reduced subgingival bacteria.[17]

The chlorhexidine chip is intended for use as an adjunctive therapy with scaling and root debridement. Chlorhexidine as an agent for local delivery has the advantage over the antibiotics in that there is no potential for the development of bacterial resistance.

I.   DESCRIPTION

A.   Size: 4 by 5 mm and 0.35 mm thick (Figure 38-3A).
B.   Shape: rectangular, rounded at one end (resembling a baby's fingernail).[10]

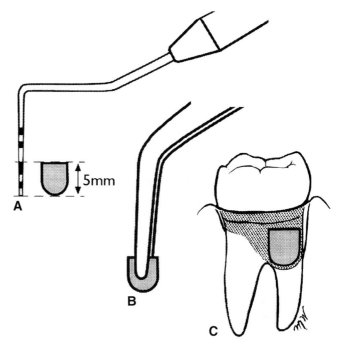

■ **FIGURE 38-3 Chlorhexidine Chip. (A)** The chip is 5 mm × 4 mm rounded at one end. **(B)** For insertion, the chip is grasped by cotton pliers on the square side. **(C)** The chip is inserted to the very base of the pocket where the periodontal pathogens are concentrated.

C.   Contents: matrix of hydrolyzed gelatin with 2.5 mg chlorhexidine gluconate incorporated; color is orange-brown.
D.   Controlled delivery; biodegradable; maintains a high level of chlorhexidine for 7 to 10 days. The gingival sulcus fluid concentration is greater than 125 µg/mL for 8 days.

II. PLACEMENT PROCEDURE

A. Site Selection

1.   *Pocket Depth.* The chip should be contained within the pocket, so since the chip is 5 mm long, pockets of more than 5 mm are indicated for treatment.

2.   *Chips Placed.* More than one pocket can be treated in the same appointment on the same side, preferably in the same quadrant for the comfort and convenience of the patient's postcare.

B. Chip Care and Preparation

1.   Store chips in a refrigerator (2° to 8°C, 36° to 46°F).

2.   Package contains 10 chips. Each chip is packaged individually in a separate compartment of an aluminum blister pack.

C. Steps in Placement

1. *Isolation*
   a. Position cotton rolls and saliva ejector.
   b. Dry the area with a sponge to prevent wetting chip during placement. Chip may start to soften and become more difficult to place if it gets wet before placement in the pocket.
2. *Insertion*
   a. Hold chip with cotton pliers; position chip with round side away from the cotton pliers (Figure 38-3*B*).
   b. Insert the chip to the bottom of the pocket; position at the deepest part (Figure 38-3*C*).

C. Action

1. Chip biodegrades in 7 to 10 days.
2. Approximately 40% of the chlorhexidine may be released within the first 24 hours, and the rest over the following 7 to 10 days.

D. Patient Instructions

1. Avoid disturbing the area. Do not use dental floss at the site of the insertion for 10 days.
2. Brush all other teeth and clean interdentally as usual.
3. Although some mild to moderate sensitivity may be expected during the first week after placement, contact the clinic or office promptly if pain, swelling, or other problem occurs.

E. Maintenance Appointments

1. Place a chip in pockets 5 mm or deeper at each 3-month maintenance appointment.
2. Evaluate probing depth and clinical attachment levels.
3. Ascertain that patient is maintaining a high level of dental biofilm control.

▪ DOXYCYCLINE POLYMER

Biodegradable doxycycline polymer in liquid form is delivered by cannula into a pocket and solidifies on contact with the dampness of the sulcus fluid. Beneficial effects include reduction of probing depths, gain of attachment, and destruction of periodontal pathogenic microorganisms.[18,19]

I. DESCRIPTION

A. Equipment

1. *Syringe.* Containing liquid 10% doxycycline hyclate.
2. *Cannula.* Blunt ended, 23 gauge, narrow diameter.

B. Preparation of Agent

1. *Mixing.* Two syringes are coupled and the substances are passed back and forth until mixed (Figure 38-4*A*). The manufacturer's instructions should be followed with care.
2. *Adapt cannula.* Attach 23-gauge cannula to syringe. As the cap is removed, the cannula is held part way and bent against the wall of the cover to provide an angle appropriate for insertion into the periodontal pocket (Figure 38-4*B*).

II. DELIVERY

A. Insert Cannula to Base of Pocket

Express the agent to just over the gingival margin; withdraw cannula (Figure 38-4*C*).

B. Packing

Use a blunt instrument to pack the agent down. Add more if necessary to fill the pocket. Wet the instrument to prevent sticking to the agent.

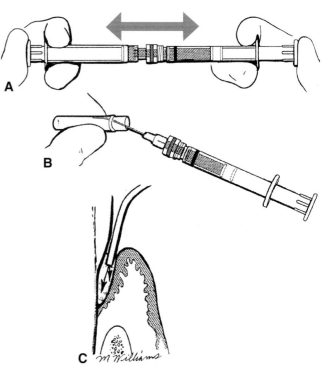

▪ **FIGURE 38-4 Doxycycline Polymer Gel. (A)** Syringes are coupled and the contents passed back and forth until mixed. **(B)** The cannula is attached to the syringe with the agent; as the cap is removed, the cannula is pressed against the side to bend it to an angle appropriate for accessing the pocket to be treated. **(C)** The cannula is inserted to the base of the pocket, and the agent is released to fill the pocket.

Everyday Ethics

At the first 3-month maintenance appointment for Mrs. Orban, who had had a series of six sextant appointments of deep scaling and root planing with anesthesia, the tissue still showed many areas of inflammation, with probing depths over 4 mm and bleeding on probing. She had received repeated personal instruction with each of the appointments, and she had never achieved a truly favorable score on her biofilm disclosing tests.

Elta, the dental hygienist, showed her maintenance charting and oral tissue review to Dr. Finley, and they both examined the original radiographs. Elta had made two vertical bitewings for the molars at this current appointment.

Elta told Dr. Finley that she thought the best procedure was for Mrs. Orban to see the periodontist. "I think she will take her condition more seriously. She never acts as though she believes what I tell her,"

Elta said. "She still talks as though she just came to have her teeth 'cleaned.'" Dr. Finley agreed to recommend the periodontist, and he personally explained the choice of treatment to Mrs. Orban. Mrs. Orban definitely told them she was not going to a periodontist under any circumstance and asked for further treatment from Dr. Finley.

Questions for Consideration

1. What ethical issues may be involved when a patient asks for the general practitioner to take over treatment that is customarily carried out by the dental hygienist?

2. Is this an ethical issue or dilemma for Dr. Finley? Explain the rationale.

3. Select terms from the core values to help in the discussion of this problem.

C. Hardening of Agent

On contact with the moisture of the pocket, the agent will harden.

D. Periodontal Dressing

Placing a dressing over the area aids retention.

E. Patient Instruction

- Prevent accidental removal.
- Routine brushing and other self-care on all other areas.

F. Appointment for Removal of Dressing

- Evaluate tissue; evaluate biofilm removal.
- Plan routine maintenance.

■ METRONIDAZOLE GEL

Metronidazole in the form of a suspension is delivered by cannula for periodontal pocket therapy. As a biodegradable product with sustained release, its benefits have been shown to include probing depth and bleeding on probing reduction, clinical attachment gain, and reduced incidence of periodontal pathogenic organisms.[20-22] An advantage that metronidazole has is a specific activity against anaerobic microorganisms without generalized destruction of all aerobes as well.

I. DESCRIPTION

A. Composition: oil-based gel with 25% metronidazole in glyceryl mono-oleate and sesame oil.
B. Sustained release: 24 to 36 hours.

II. DELIVERY

A. Delivered by cannula in a viscous consistency; liquefies by body heat, and then hardens when in contact with fluids of the pocket to form crystals.
B. Two applications 1 week apart are recommended.

 Factors To Teach The Patient

- What a periodontal pocket is and why it needs to be treated.

- How the treatment using tetracycline fiber, chlorhexidine chip, or doxycycline polymer (whichever is being used to treat the patient) affects the infection in the pocket.

- How to use the home irrigator; relation between home irrigation and the irrigation in the dental office.

- The success of all periodontal therapy depends on the daily personal dental biofilm control by the patient.

▪ MINOCYCLINE HYDROCHLORIDE

Bioresorbable minocycline hydrochloride is delivered in powdered microsphere form to be placed in periodontal pockets to aid in pocket depth reduction. The treatment is used in conjunction with scaling and root planing.

I. DESCRIPTION

A. Unit dose cartridge contains 1 mg minocycline.
B. Sustained release 14 days.
C. Refrigeration not needed.
D. Contraindications
   - Do not use for patients sensitive to tetracycline.
   - Do not use for women who are pregnant.

II. DELIVERY

A. Insert unit cartridge into dispenser handle.
B. Place saliva ejector and keep the mouth dry.
C. Insert the cannula tip into the base of the pocket and deposit the powder.
D. The bioadhesive microspheres activate and adhere on contact with moisture.

III. MAINTENANCE

A. Probe carefully to test results of treatments.
B. Repeat treatment as needed.

REFERENCES

1. van Winkelhoff, A.J., Rams, T.E., and Slots, J.: Systemic Antibiotic Therapy in Periodontics, *Periodontol. 2000, 10,* 45, 1996.
2. Slots, J. and Rosling, B.G.: Suppression of the Periodontopathic Microflora in Localized Juvenile Periodontitis by Systemic Tetracycline, *J. Clin. Periodontol., 10,* 465, September, 1983.
3. Loesche, W.J., Schmidt, E., Smith, B.A., Morrison, E.C., Caffesse, R., and Hujoel, P.P.: Effect of Metronidazole on Periodontal Treatment Needs, *J. Periodontol., 62,* 247, April, 1991.
4. Mousquès, T., Listgarten, M.A., and Phillips, R.W.: Effect of Scaling and Root Planing on the Composition of the Human Subgingival Microbial Flora, *J. Periodont. Res., 15,* 144, March, 1980.
5. Southard, S.R., Drisko, C.L., Killoy, W.J., Cobb, C.M., and Tira, D.E.: The Effect of 2% Chlorhexidine Digluconate Irrigation on Clinical Parameters and the Level of *Bacteroides gingivalis* in Periodontal Pockets, *J. Periodontol., 60,* 302, June, 1989.
6. Schmid, E., Kornman, K.S., and Tinanoff, N.: Changes of Subgingival Total Colony Forming Units and Black Pigmented Bacteroides after a Single Irrigation of Periodontal Pockets with 1.64% SnF2, *J. Periodontol., 56,* 330, June, 1985.
7. Mazza, J.E., Newman, M.G., and Sims, T.N.: Clinical and Antimicrobial Effect of Stannous Fluoride on Periodontitis, *J. Clin. Periodontol., 8,* 203, June, 1981.
8. Schlagenhauf, U., Stellwag, P., and Fiedler, A.: Subgingival Irrigation in the Maintenance Phase of Periodontal Therapy, *J. Clin. Periodontol., 17,* 650, October, 1990.
9. Goodson, J.M.: Controlled Drug Delivery: A New Means of Treatment of Dental Diseases, *Compend. Cont. Educ. Dent., 6,* 27, January, 1985.
10. Killoy, W.J. and Polson, A.M.: Controlled Local Delivery of Antimicrobials in the Treatment of Periodontitis, *Dent. Clin. North Am., 42,* 263, April, 1998.
11. Greenstein, G. and Polson, A.: The Role of Local Drug Delivery in the Management of Periodontal Diseases: A Comprehensive Review, *J. Periodontol., 69,* 507, May, 1998.
12. Goodson, J.M., Haffajee, A., and Socransky, S.S.: Periodontal Therapy by Local Delivery of Tetracycline, *J. Clin. Periodontol., 6,* 83, April, 1979.
13. Newman, M.G., Kornman, K.S., and Doherty, F.M.: A 6-Month Multicenter Evaluation of Adjunctive Tetracycline Fiber Therapy Used in Conjunction With Scaling and Root Planing in Maintenance Patients: Clinical Results, *J. Periodontol., 65,* 685, July, 1994.
14. Kerry, G.: Tetracycline-Loaded Fibers as Adjunctive Treatment in Periodontal Disease, *J. Am. Dent. Assoc., 125,* 1199, September, 1994.
15. Vandekerckhove, B.N.A., Quirynen, M., and van Steenberghe, D.: The Use of Tetracycline-Containing Controlled-Release Fibers in the Treatment of Refractory Periodontitis, *J. Periodontol., 68,* 353, April, 1997.
16. Lowenguth, R.A., Chin, I., Caton, J.G., Cobb, C.M., Drisko, C.L., Killoy, W.J., Michalowicz, B.S., Pihlstrom, B.L., and Goodson, J.M.: Evaluation of Periodontal Treatments Using Controlled-Release Tetracycline Fibers: Microbiological Response, *J. Periodontol., 66,* 700, August, 1995.
17. Stabholz, A., Sela, M.N., Friedman, M., Golomb, G., and Soskolne, A.: Clinical and Microbiological Effects of Sustained Release Chlorhexidine in Periodontal Pockets, *J. Clin. Periodontol., 13,* 783, September, 1986.
18. Polson, A.M., Garrett, S., Stoller, N.H., Bandt, C.L., Hanes, P.J., Killoy, W.J., Southard, G.L., Duke, S.P., Bogle, G.C., Drisko, C.H., and Friesen, L.R.: Multi-center Comparative Evaluation of Subgingivally Delivered Sanguinarine and Doxycycline in the Treatment of Periodontitis. II. Clinical Results, *J. Periodontol., 68,* 119, February, 1997.
19. Garrett, S., Adams, D., Bandt, C., Beiswanger, B., Bogle, G., Caton, J., Donly, K., Drisko, C., Hallmon, W., Hancock, B., Hanes, P., Hawley, C., Johnson, L., Kiger, R., Killoy, W., Mellonig, J., Polson, A., Ryder, M., Wang, H., Wolinsky, L., and Yukna, R.: Two Multi-center Clinical Trials of Subgingival Doxycycline in the Treatment of Periodontitis, *J. Dent. Res., 76,* 153 (Abstract no. 1113), Special Issue, 1997.
20. Klinge, B., Attström, R., Karring, T., Kisch, J., Lewin, B., and Stoltze, K.: 3 Regimens of Topical Metronidazole, Compared With Subgingival Scaling on Periodontal Pathology in Adults, *J. Clin. Periodontol., 19,* 708, October, Part II, 1992.
21. Ainamo, J., Lie, T., Ellingsen, B.H., Hansen, B.F., Johansson, L.-A., Karring, T., Kisch, J., Paunio, K., and Stoltze, K.: Clinical Responses to Subgingival Application of a Metronidazole 25% Gel Compared to the Effect of Subgingival Scaling in Adult Periodontitis, *J. Clin. Periodontol., 19,* 723, October, Part II, 1992.
22. Lie, T., Bruun, G., and Böe, O.E.: Effects of Topical Metronidazole and Tetracycline in Treatment of Adult Periodontitis, *J. Periodontol., 69,* 819, July, 1998.

SUGGESTED READINGS

Drisko, C.H.: Non-surgical Pocket Therapy: Pharmacotherapeutics, *Ann. Periodontol., 1,* 491–506, November, 1996.
Finkelman, R.D. and Williams, R.C.: Local Delivery of Chemotherapeutic Agents in Periodontal Therapy: Has Its Time Arrived? *J. Clin. Periodontol., 25,* 943, November, 1998 (Part II).

Goodson, J.M.: Antimicrobial Strategies for Treatment of Periodontal Diseases, *Periodontol. 2000, 5,* 142, 1994.

Killoy, W.J.: Chemical Treatment of Periodontitis: Local Delivery of Antimicrobials, *Int. Dent. J., 48,* 305, June, Supplement 1, 1998.

Larsen, T. and Fiehn, N.-E.: Development of Resistance to Metronidazole and Minocycline *in vitro, J. Clin. Periodontol., 24,* 254, April, 1997.

Systemic Antibiotics

American Academy of Periodontology: Position Paper: Systemic Antibiotics in Periodontics, *J. Periodontol., 67,* 831, August, 1996.

Greenstein, G.: Clinical Significance of Bacterial Resistance to Tetracyclines in the Treatment of Periodontal Diseases, *J. Periodontol., 66,* 925, November, 1995.

Pallasch, T.J.: Pharmacokinetic Principles of Antimicrobial Therapy, *Periodontol. 2000, 10,* 5, 1996.

Walker, C.B.: Selected Antimicrobial Agents: Mechanisms of Action, Side Effects and Drug Interactions, *Periodontol. 2000, 10,* 12, 1996.

Walker, C.: Antibiotics, in American Dental Association: *ADA Guide to Dental Therapeutics.* Chicago, ADA Publishing Co., 1998, pp. 134–163.

Walker, C.B.: The Acquisition of Antibiotic Resistance in the Periodontal Microflora, *Periodontol. 2000, 10,* 79, 1996.

Professional Irrigation

Allison, C., Simor, A.E., Mock, D., and Tenenbaum, H.C.: Prosol-Chlorhexidine Irrigation Reduces the Incidence of Bacteremia During Ultrasonic Scaling With the Cavi-Med.: A Pilot Investigation, *J. Can. Dent. Assoc., 59,* 673, August, 1993.

Chapple, I.L.C., Walmsley, A.D., Saxby, M.S., and Moscrop, H.: Effect of Subgingival Irrigation With Chlorhexidine During Ultrasonic Scaling, *J. Periodontol., 63,* 812, October, 1992.

Chaves, E.S., Kornman, K.S., Manwell, M.A., Jones, A.A., Newbold, D.A., and Wood, R.C.: Mechanism of Irrigation Effects on Gingivitis, *J. Periodontol., 65,* 1016, November, 1994.

Fine, J.B., Harper, D.S., Gordon, J.M., Hovliaras, C.A., and Charles, C.H.: Short-term Microbiological and Clinical Effects of Subgingival Irrigation With an Antimicrobial Mouthrinse, *J. Periodontol., 65,* 30, January, 1994.

Greenstein, G.: Supragingival and Subgingival Irrigation: Practical Application in the Treatment of Periodontal Diseases, *Compend. Cont. Educ. Dent., 13,* 1098, December, 1992.

Lofthus, J.E., Waki, M.Y., Jolkovsky, D.L., Otomo-Corgel, J., Newman, M.G., Flemmig, T., and Nachnani, S.: Bacteremia Following Subgingival Irrigation and Scaling and Root Planing, *J. Periodontol., 62,* 602, October, 1991.

Rams, T.E. and Slots, J.: Local Delivery of Antimicrobial Agents in the Periodontal Pocket, *Periodontol. 2000, 10,* 139, 1996.

Reynolds, M.A., Lavigne, C.K., Minah, G.E., and Suzuki, J.B.: Clinical Effects of Simultaneous Ultrasonic Scaling and Subgingival Irrigation With Chlorhexidine: Mediating Influence of Periodontal Probing Depth, *J. Clin. Periodontol., 19,* 595, September, 1992.

Schlagenhauf, U., Horlacher, V., Netuschil, L., and Brecx, M.: Repeated Subgingival Oxygen Irrigations in Untreated Periodontal Patients, *J. Clin. Periodontol., 21,* 48, January, 1994.

Shiloah, J. and Patters, M.R.: DNA Probe Analysis of the Survival of Selected Periodontal Pathogens Following Scaling, Root Planing, and Intra-pocket Irrigation, *J. Periodontol., 65,* 568, June, 1994.

Stabholz, A., Kettering, J., Aprecio, R., Zimmerman, G., Baker, P.J., and Wikesjö, U.M.E.: Retention of Antimicrobial Activity by Human Root Surfaces After *in situ* Subgingival Irrigation With Tetracycline HCL or Chlorhexidine, *J. Periodontol., 64,* 137, February, 1993.

Tetracycline Fiber

Carlson-Mann, L.D.: Use of Tetracycline Fibre to Treat Localized Unstable Periodontitis, *Can. Dent. Hyg. Assoc./PROBE, 29,* 150, July/August, 1995.

Ciancio, S.G., Cobb, C.M., and Leung, M.: Tissue Concentration and Localization of Tetracycline Following Site-Specific Tetracycline Fiber Therapy, *J. Periodontol., 63,* 849, October, 1992.

Davis, M.W.: Techniques to Enhance Success in Placement of Tetracycline Fibers as a Periodontal Therapy, *Gen. Dent. 46,* 62, January–February, 1998.

Latner, L.: Patient Selection and Clinical Applications of Periodontal Tetracycline Fibers, *Gen. Dent., 46,* 58, January–February, 1998.

Mombelli, A., Lehmann, B., Tonetti, M., and Lang, N.P.: Clinical Response to Local Delivery of Tetracycline in Relation to Overall and Local Periodontal Conditions, *J. Clin. Periodontol., 24,* 470, July, 1997.

Morrison, S.L., Cobb, C.M., Kazakos, G.M., and Killoy, W.J.: Root Surface Characteristics Associated With Subgingival Placement of Monolithic Tetracycline-Impregnated Fibers, *J. Periodontol., 63,* 137, February, 1992.

Radvar, M., Pourtaghi, N., and Kinane, D.F.: Comparison of 3 Periodontal Local Antibiotic Therapies in Persistent Periodontal Pockets, *J. Periodontol., 67,* 860, September, 1996.

Rapley, J.W., Cobb, C.M., Killoy, W.J., and Williams, D.R.: Serum Levels of Tetracycline During Treatment With Tetracycline-Containing Fibers, *J. Periodontol., 63,* 817, October, 1992.

Tonetti, M.S.: Local Delivery of Tetracycline: From Concept to Clinical Application, *J. Clin. Periodontol., 25,* 969, November, 1998 (Part II).

Tonetti, M., Cugini, M.A., and Goodson, J.M.: Zero-order Delivery With Periodontal Placement of Tetracycline-Loaded Ethylene Vinyl Acetate Fibers, *J. Periodont. Res., 25,* 243, July, 1990.

Tonetti, M.S., Pini-Prato, G., and Cortellini, P.: Principles and Clinical Applications of Periodontal Controlled Drug Delivery With Tetracycline Fibers, *Int. J. Periodont. Restorative Dent., 14,* 421, October, 1994.

Wilson, T.G., McGuire, M.K., Greenstein, G., and Nunn, M.: Tetracycline Fibers Plus Scaling and Root Planing Versus Scaling and Root Planing Alone: Similar Results After 5 Years, *J. Periodontol, 68,* 1029, November, 1997.

Chlorhexidine Chip

Friedman, M. and Golomb, G.: New Sustained Release Dosage Form of Chlorhexidine for Dental Use. I. Development and Kinetics of Release, *J. Periodont. Res., 17,* 323, Number 3, 1982.

Jeffcoat, M.K., Bray, K.S., Ciancio, S.G., Dentino, A.R., Fine, D.H., Gordon, J.M., Gunsolley, J.C., Killoy, W.J., Lowenguth, R.A., Magnusson, N.I., Offenbacher, S., Palcanis, K.G., Proskin, H.M., Finkelman, R.D., and Flashner, M.: Adjunctive Use of a Subgingival Controlled-Release Chlorhexidine Chip Reduces Probing Depth and Improves Attachment Level Compared With Scaling and Root Planing Alone, *J. Periodontol., 69,* 989, September, 1998.

Killoy, W.J.: The Use of Locally Delivered Chlorhexidine in the Treatment of Periodontitis: Clinical Results, *J. Clin. Periodontol., 25,* 953, November, 1998 (Part II).

Soskolne, W.A., Heasman, P.A., Stabholz, A., Smart, G.J., Palmer, M., Flashner, M., and Newman, H.N.: Sustained Local Delivery of Chlorhexidine in the Treatment of Periodontitis: A Multi-center Study, *J. Periodontol., 68,* 32, January, 1997.

Soskolne, A., Golomb, G., Friedman, M., and Sela, M.N.: New Sustained Release Dosage Form of Chlorhexidine for Dental Use. II. Use in Periodontal Therapy, *J. Periodont. Res., 18,* 330, May, 1983.

Stabholz, A., Soskolne, W.A., Friedman, M., and Sela, M.N.: The Use of Sustained Release Delivery of Chlorhexidine for the Maintenance of Periodontal Pockets: 2-Year Clinical Trial, *J. Periodontol.*, *62*, 429, July, 1991.

Metronidazole

Greenstein, G.: The Role of Metronidazole in the Treatment of Periodontal Diseases, *J. Periodontol.*, *64*, 1, January, 1993.

Hitzig, C., Charbit, Y., Bitton, C., Fosse, T., Teboul, M., Hannoun, L., and Varonne, R.: Topical Metronidazole as an Adjunct to Subgingival Debridement in the Treatment of Chronic Periodontitis, *J. Clin. Periodontol.*, *21*, 146, February, 1994.

Magnusson, I.: The Use of Locally Delivered Metronidazole in the Treatment of Periodontitis. Clinical Results, *J. Clin. Periodontol.*, *25*, 959, November, 1998 (Part II).

Pedrazzoli, V., Kilian, M., and Karring, T.: Comparative Clinical and Microbiological Effects of Topical Subgingival Application of Metronidazole 25% Dental Gel and Scaling in the Treatment of Adult Periodontitis, *J. Clin. Periodontol.*, *19*, 715, October, Part II, 1992.

Somayaji, B.V., Jariwala, U., Jayachandran, P., Vidyalakshmi, K., and Dudhani, R.V.: Evaluation of Antimicrobial Efficacy and Release Pattern of Tetracycline and Metronidazole Using a Local Delivery System, *J. Periodontol.*, *69*, 409, April, 1998.

Stelzel, M. and Flores-de-Jacoby, L.: Topical Metronidazole Application Compared With Subgingival Scaling: A Clinical and Microbiological Study on Recall Patients, *J. Clin. Periodontol.*, *23*, 24, January, 1996.

Minocycline Gel

Jones, A.A., Kornman, K.S., Newbold, D.A., and Manwell, M.A.: Clinical and Microbiological Effects of Controlled-Release Locally Delivered Minocycline in Periodontitis, *J. Periodontol.*, *65*, 1058, November, 1994.

Preus, H.R., Lassen, J., Aass, A.M., and Ciancio, S.G.: Bacterial Resistance Following Subgingival and Systemic Administration of Minocycline, *J. Clin. Periodontol.*, *22*, 380, May, 1995.

Saito, A., Hosaka, Y., Nakagawa, T., Seida, K., Yamada, S., and Okuda, K.: Locally Delivered Minocycline and Guided Tissue Regeneration to Treat Post-juvenile Periodontitis: A Case Report, *J. Periodontol.*, *65*, 835, September, 1994.

Vandekerckhove, B.N.A., Quirynen, M., and van Steenberghe, D.: The Use of Locally Delivered Minocycline in the Treatment of Chronic Periodontitis: A Review of the Literature, *J. Clin. Periodontol.*, *25*, 964, November, 1998 (Part II).

Acute Periodontal Conditions

The dental hygienist frequently participates in clinical treatment procedures for acute gingival lesions. Key words for acute conditions are defined in Box 39-1.

NECROTIZING ULCERATIVE GINGIVITIS/PERIODONTITIS

Necrotizing ulcerative gingivitis (NUG) and necrotizing ulcerative periodontitis (NUP) are acute, inflammatory, destructive diseases of the periodontium. Other names that have been used include necrotizing gingivitis (NG), acute necrotizing ulcerative gingivitis (ANUG), trench mouth, Vincent's infection, Vincent's disease, and ulceromembranous gingivitis. The condition may be superimposed over existing periodontitis.

Although NUG may occur at any age, it is usually seen among young people between ages 15 and 30 years. It is rare in children under 10 years of age in the United States, but it is not uncommon in young children from low socioeconomic groups studied in South America and in some developing countries.[1,2] Malnutrition and lowered resistance to infection are significant predisposing factors. Individuals with Down's syndrome have been shown to have an increased incidence of NUG.

TYPES OF NECROTIZING PERIODONTAL CONDITIONS

I. NECROTIZING ULCERATIVE GINGIVITIS (NUG)

A. Basic Characteristics

Gingival inflammation limited to the free gingiva with ulceration of one or more interdental papilla tips. Other clinical signs include pain and bleeding.

689

BOX 39-1 KEY WORDS: Acute Periodontal Conditions

Abscess: localized collection of pus in a circumscribed or walled-off area formed by the disintegration of tissues.

Acute: runs a relatively short course; produces pain and local inflammation.

Chronic: slow development with little evidence of inflammation; usually an intermittent pus discharge; may follow an acute abscess.

Periapical: circumscribed collection of pus around the apex of a tooth root; results from pulpal necrosis.

Periodontal: localized in the periodontal tissues; also called **lateral** or **parietal.**

Fetor oris: foul, offensive odor from the mouth; halitosis.

Fistula: a pathologic sinus or abnormal passage that leads from an abscess to the surface of the gingiva or mucosa.

Gum boil: a lay term for a circumscribed swelling in the tissue over the alveolar process, usually at the level of the root apices; may break and drain periodically, thus preventing pain.

Linear gingival erythema: gingivitis in the HIV-positive patient; characterized by a well-demarcated band of intense erythema at the gingival margin, not associated with bacterial plaque, and which does not respond to conventional plaque-removal procedures.*

Malaise: feeling of general indisposition, uneasiness, discomfort; may be early indication of illness.

Necrosis: death of tissue; morphologic changes indicative of cell death caused by enzymatic degradation.

Necrotizing ulcerative periodontitis (NUP): severe and rapidly progressive disease that has a distinctive erythema of the free gingiva, attached gingiva, and the alveolar mucosa; extensive soft tissue necrosis that usually starts with the interdental papillae; marked loss of periodontal attachment; deep probing depths may not be evident because of marked recession.

Parenteral: not administered by way of the alimentary canal, but, for example, subcutaneous, intramuscular, or intravenous.

Pericoronitis: gingival inflammation around the crown of an incompletely erupted tooth; most frequently occurs about a mandibular third molar.

Pseudomembrane: false membrane; false layer of tissue that covers a surface.

Purulent: accompanied by or containing pus.

Sinus tract: a channel that connects with an abscess or suppurating area.

Ulceration: formation or development of an ulcer with loss of epithelial surface and sloughing of necrotic inflammatory tissue.

*From Greenspan, J.S.: Periodontal Complications of HIV Infection, *Compend. Cont. Educ. Dent., 15,* S694, Suppl. Nov. 18, 1994.

B. HIV-Positive Patient

Linear gingival erythema with ulceration of tips of interdental papillae.[3]

II. NECROTIZING ULCERATIVE PERIODONTITIS

A. Basic Characteristics

Destructive infection of periodontal tissues with ulceration of interdental papillae, cratering of inter-

dental bone and soft tissue, and clinical attachment loss.

B. HIV-Positive Patient

An increased incidence of NUG/NUP has been diagnosed in HIV-positive patients. A more severe, rapidly progressive breakdown of the periodontium occurs with ulceration of interdental papillae, cratering of interdental bone, clinical attachment loss, and presence of exposed bone with sequestration in the most severe involvement. Because of the rapid breakdown, necrosis, and tissue recession with severe attachment loss, the condition usually is not associated with deep pockets.[3]

III. NECROTIZING STOMATITIS

Necrosis may extend beyond the tooth-supporting tissues and cause bone destruction and sequestration. Severe disease may resemble noma or cancrum oris.

IV. CANCRUM ORIS (NOMA)

Orofacial gangrenous necrosis is believed to be an extension of untreated NUP. It is predisposed by malnutrition and debilitating systemic illness.[1,2]

■ CLINICAL RECOGNITION

I. INITIAL SIGNS AND SYMPTOMS

The patient with NUG or NUP reports
 A. Sudden onset.
 B. Pain and soreness caused by slight pressure, such as during chewing and toothbrushing; may be intensified by hot or highly seasoned foods. Gentle probing may produce an exaggerated pain response.
 C. Bleeding that occurs spontaneously or on slight pressure.
 D. Poor appetite.
 E. Metallic or other unpleasant taste.
 F. Fetid odor.

II. CHARACTERISTIC CLINICAL FINDINGS

A. Interdental Necrosis

Ulceration of the papillae produces craterlike defects in the col area. In early disease, only the tips of papillae are involved, followed by progressive destruction of entire papillae and extension to the marginal gingiva facially and lingually (Figure 39-1).

B. Pseudomembrane

Forms over the necrotic area. It is a gray, loose, necrotic slough that, when wiped off, exposes a red and shiny hemorrhagic gingiva. The pseudomembrane consists primarily of fibrin, necrotic tissue, leukocytes, and masses of microorganisms.

C. Extent

The membranous ulceration may be seen locally, that is, between two or three teeth, or it may be generalized throughout both maxillary and mandibular arches.

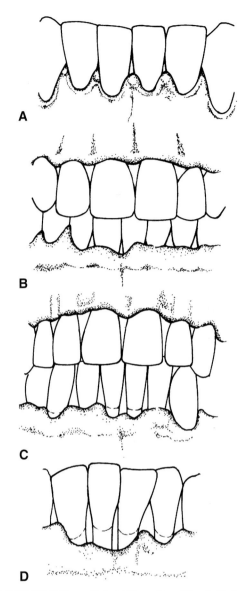

■ **FIGURE 39-1 Necrotizing Ulcerative Gingivitis/ Periodontitis. (A)** Early lesion with blunted papillae and interdental necrosis. **(B)** Increased destruction with loss of interdental tissue; rolled margins of the gingiva. **(C)** More advanced destruction with recession and interdental cratering. **(D)** Very advanced lesions, with loss of attached gingiva, recession, and tooth mobility.

D. Other Clinical Findings

 1. Debris, materia alba, and biofilm that collect profusely because the patient avoids brushing the sensitive teeth and gingiva.
 2. Fetor oris (bad breath) that is often severe. It is caused by necrotic tissue, stagnant saliva, and breakdown products of blood and debris.
 3. Increased salivation.

E. Signs of Systemic Involvement

Examination should always be made to detect the presence of the following:
1. Malaise.
2. Lymphadenopathy of submandibular and cervical nodes.
3. Possible slight elevation of body temperature.

▪ RISK FACTORS

NUG is an infectious disease caused by a fusospirochetal complex of microbes that develops and increases in association with predisposing factors that have lowered the body's defenses. Major predisposing factors are stress, neglected oral hygiene, inadequate diet, and tobacco smoking.

I. LOCAL FACTORS

NUG is rarely, if ever, seen in a clean, healthy, cared-for, and professionally supervised mouth. Many of the factors that can be considered predisposing are the same as those that predispose to chronic marginal gingivitis.

Predisposing factors include
A. Preexisting gingivitis and/or periodontitis.
B. Inadequate personal oral care with general neglect.
C. Tobacco use.
D. Factors related to retention of microorganisms and deposits.

II. STRESS FACTORS

A. Acute anxiety related to life situations is a common characteristic of patients with NUG. In susceptible people, the condition has been found to occur or recur during periods of stress. Examples include students during examination periods, military men in combat, and people during important decision-making times.
B. Emotional stress is frequently accompanied by poor oral care, improper diet, excessive smoking, overexertion, interrupted sleep, and other deviations in health habits.

III. SYSTEMIC: DISEASE-RESISTANCE FACTORS

A. Dietary and nutritional inadequacies; vitamin deficiencies.
B. Recent illnesses; frequent upper respiratory infections, infectious mononucleosis, pernicious anemia, hepatitis, and HIV infection.
C. Side effects of chemotherapy and radiation.
D. Fatigue; insufficient sleep.

▪ ETIOLOGY

Bacteriologic and immunologic factors are implicated. For many years, bacteriologic smears were made from the NUG lesion and examined by microscope for the presence of fusiform bacilli and spirochetes. The smear test is no longer considered significant for making a diagnosis.

I. MICROBIOLOGY[4]

Of the many types of organisms found in NUG lesions, fusiform bacilli and medium-sized spirochetes predominate. The constant flora has been shown to include *Treponema* and *Selenomonas* species, *Prevotella intermedia*, *Porphyromonas gingivalis*, and *Fusobacterium* species.

II. COURSE OF DEVELOPMENT

A. Description of the Lesion

1. NUG is superimposed on gingivitis or periodontitis.
2. Ulceration and necrosis begin in the col area.
3. Both epithelial tissue and connective tissue are involved.
4. The disease process progresses to involve the entire papilla and, eventually, the marginal gingiva on the facial and lingual surfaces.
5. The pseudomembrane covering the lesion is a necrotic slough of the surface epithelium. It contains leukocytes, bacteria, epithelial cells, and fibrin.
6. Connective tissue shows the signs of acute inflammation. It is hyperemic and filled with leukocytes, and its capillaries are engorged. When the pseudomembrane is lifted, the red inflamed connective tissue can be seen.

B. Microscopic Examination

Four layers in the lesion have been described from observations made by electron microscopy.[5] All layers contain spirochetes.
1. *Bacterial Zone.* The most superficial zone consists primarily of a mass of varied bacteria, including a few spirochetes.
2. *Neutrophil-rich Zone.* Under the bacterial zone is a layer of leukocytes, predominantly neutrophils. Microorganisms, including many spirochetes, are found among the leukocytes.
3. *Necrotic Zone.* This zone contains disintegrating tissue cells, many spirochetes, and other bacteria.
4. *Spirochetal Infiltration Zone.* In this nonnecrotized layer where tissue components are still preserved, spirochetes have invaded, but other microorganisms have not.

■ DENTAL HYGIENE CARE

Patient instruction and motivation for self-care are needed along with skillful subgingival instrumentation. After the initial symptoms have subsided, complete therapy must be carried out. The tissue destruction usually has left the gingiva deformed, with interdental flattening or cratering. Surgical treatment may be needed to restore a physiologic form that can be maintained by the patient in the plan to prevent recurrence of the disease.

I. PREPARATION FOR DIAGNOSIS

Initially, certain data must be collected for making the diagnosis and care plan. Basic information needed is suggested by the steps described here.

A. History

1. *Record the Chief Complaint.* The history of the current disease is described by date of onset, duration, symptoms as reported, and what self-treatment the patient has already performed.
2. *Record Whether This Is a Recurrence.* If so, note details of previous episodes and the treatment given.
3. *Obtain Information Needed for Preliminary Treatment*
   a. Conditions needing medical consultation.
   b. Need for premedication for prevention of infective endocarditis.
   c. Allergies.
4. *Use Knowledge of Predisposing Factors for NUG to Gather Pertinent Information*
   a. Tobacco habits.
   b. Recent illnesses or types of therapy may explain a lowered resistance.
   c. Record of immediately previous 24-hour food intake. When the mouth has been sore and eating has been painful, a diet recording may not be typical of the patient's usual intake. Later, a 5-day or week-long food record will be requested as part of the continuing prevention program.
   d. Variations of normal sleeping hours and routine.

B. Examination

1. *Record the Patient's Temperature*
2. *Extraoral Examination*
   a. Palpate submandibular and cervical nodes.
   b. Observe face and skin to determine whether flushed, damp.
   c. Observe signs of malaise.

3. *Oral Examination.* Without instrumentation, a preliminary examination can be made and the overall appearance of the gingival tissue recorded. The dentist may prefer to see the gingiva as it appears initially, before instrumentation or rinsing, to make the diagnosis and prepare the treatment plan. Instrumentation will be temporarily delayed for patients requiring premedication.

II. CARE PLAN

The dental hygiene care plan is formulated within the total treatment plan. Only a partial treatment plan is made until after the acute phase of the disease has passed.

A. Systemic Treatment

1. Directions concerning diet, rest, and other systemic influences.
2. Multivitamin supplements are sometimes prescribed.
3. After the diagnosis is made, the dentist determines whether systemic antibiotic therapy is indicated. Except for a patient who requires antibiotic coverage to prevent infective endocarditis, antibiotics are prescribed conservatively.

B. Relief of Acute Symptoms

1. Personal care instructions for rinsing, brushing, and limiting use of tobacco.
2. Debridement of teeth and gingiva.
3. Subgingival scaling started.
4. Chlorhexidine 0.12% rinse twice daily.

C. Basic Therapy

1. *Preventive program*
   a. Instruction for prevention of recurrence of NUG; eliminate tobacco use.
   b. Dietary analysis and counseling.
   c. Self-care fluoride, professional application when indicated.
2. *Complete scaling and debridement.*
3. *Reduction or elimination of predisposing factors to NUG*
   a. Removal of overhanging margins and other biofilm retention factors.
   b. Restoration of teeth and contact areas.
4. *Evaluation for periodontal surgery.* Need for restoration of tissue contour and elimination of craters.
5. *Restoration of occlusion.* Prosthetic replacements and all other dental needs.

▪ CARE FOR THE ACUTE STAGE

A series of appointments for a typical patient with NUG is outlined here. The number of appointments and the exact procedure at each appointment depend on the severity of the disease and the response of the gingiva as treatment progresses.

Four or five appointments may be needed during the acute stage, depending on the probing depths and the extent of calculus deposits. The basic objective is to debride the teeth thoroughly to encourage soft tissue healing. When the acute stage has subsided, a regular appointment plan is established for continued supervision.

I. ACUTE PHASE: FIRST APPOINTMENT

A. Patient Instruction

1. Explain local causes and control measures.
2. Demonstrate biofilm with a disclosing agent.
3. Show biofilm removal procedures, using a soft brush moistened with warm water.

B. General Debridement

1. Apply hydrogen peroxide (3% solution mixed with equal parts of water) with cotton pellets at proximal areas; request patient to rinse. Avoid use of compressed air or water spray to prevent dispersion of contaminated aerosols.
2. Apply topical anesthetic, or when painful, treat by quadrants, using block anesthesia.
3. Use manual instruments for scaling to prevent aerosols. Use warm water for frequent irrigation while scaling.

C. Subgingival Instrumentation

The gingiva responds sooner when scaling can be started at the first visit.
1. Perform instrumentation carefully to prevent tissue damage.
2. Have assistant evacuate continuously to prevent contaminated aerosols and to protect the patient from inhaling microorganisms.
3. Irrigate and evacuate frequently to clear all debris and calculus removed during instrumentation.

D. Patient Instruction

1. *Instructions for Home Use.* Instructions for home procedures must be carefully explained. Written directions are needed.

2. *Instructions for Continuing Care.* Inform the patient that treatment will not be complete when the pain is eliminated. Explain the underlying gingival or periodontal infection and how NUG recurs if the periodontal condition is not treated.
3. *Rinsing Directions.* Vigorous rinsing with warm water or weak saline solution is necessary every hour during the period of acute symptoms. Using 3% hydrogen peroxide with equal parts of water is preferred by some clinicians. If used, it should be recommended for only a few days and then discontinued.

    Rinsing with chlorhexidine (0.12%) twice daily continues: use 0.5 ounce after brushing after breakfast, and after brushing and flossing before retiring; swish between the teeth for 1 minute.
4. *Toothbrushing.* Use a soft nylon brush gently, but thoroughly. Clean the teeth as much as possible especially before going to bed. When a softbrush is not given the patient at the clinic or office, write down the names of specific brushes for the patient to purchase.

F. Introduce Tobacco Cessation

1. *Inform Patient.* Describe the effect of smoked or smokeless tobacco on the oral cavity, with special emphasis on facts about the gingival tissues.
2. *Avoiding Tobacco Products.* The heavy smoker who is not ready for cessation can be requested to limit the use while treatment for NUG is under way.

G. Diet[6]

1. Recommend frequent, small, nutritious meals that incorporate daily requirements from the Food Guide Pyramid (page 523).
2. A liquid or soft bland diet is advised for the first day, particularly for the patient with systemic symptoms or pronounced sensitivity when chewing. A diet of soft solids can be used on the second day.
3. The choice of foods should include increased amounts of meat and milk groups and of fruits and juices.
4. Avoid highly seasoned foods and alcoholic beverages.

II. ACUTE PHASE: SECOND APPOINTMENT

A. Patient Examination

1. *Changes.* A remarkable improvement usually can be seen within 24 hours, with pain and discomfort

lessened, the pseudomembrane gone, and tissue enlargement reduced.
2. *Toothbrushing.* Apply disclosing agent and show patient missed areas. Emphasize thorough coverage of the entire dentition, using sulcular brushing.

B. Scaling and Root Debridement

Continue procedures from the previous appointment after checking areas previously treated. The objective is to be as thorough as possible because biofilm retained over residual calculus and altered cementum can keep the tissues from healing completely.

C. Instruction: Second Day

1. *Rinsing.* When healing is progressing favorably, change rinsing schedule to every 2 hours.
2. *Proximal Surfaces.* The use of floss is advised and should be emphasized at this or the third appointment, depending on the readiness of the patient and the tissue. Other proximal cleaning devices may be useful. When the interdental embrasures are open as a result of papillary necrosis (Figure 39-1*C* and *D*), an interdental brush or other device is indicated. The importance of complete biofilm removal must be explained.
3. *Diet.* A liquid diet is not usually indicated after the first day, and the patient can use the soft solids diet or a regular diet adapted with bland foods that will not irritate the healing tissues.
4. *Instructions.* Provide specific written instructions.

III. SUCCESSIVE APPOINTMENTS

After the acute stage, regular appointments for basic treatment are planned. The gingiva is evaluated, and repeated scaling and debridement are performed as needed to complete that part of the treatment.

A. Complete Assessment

The complete plan for dental care is prepared, and the patient is instructed for continued treatment.

B. Recurrence of NUG/NUP

When the gingival and bony craters that remain after the initial healing phase are not treated, they are vulnerable to continuing disease and recurrence of NUG. Biofilm and debris can collect readily in the misshapen proximal areas, and these areas are difficult to clean with biofilm control techniques. Gingival craters invite further tissue breakdown, leading to periodontal pocket formation.

Surgical treatment is explained to the patient. When bony craters exist, treatment may involve flap surgery with osseous reshaping.

▪ PERIODONTAL ABSCESS

Gingival and periodontal abscesses occur within the periodontal tissues. An abscess is called *gingival* when it is located in the marginal area and *periodontal* when it is in the deeper periodontal tissues. They may also be known as *lateral abscesses* because they occur along the lateral surfaces of a tooth, in contrast to a periapical abscess, which is associated with the apex.

I. DEVELOPMENT OF A PERIODONTAL ABSCESS

Pus collects in the tissue as a result of bacterial infection. The infection may be a complication of an existing periodontal disease, or it may be an immediate result of microorganisms forced into the tissue by some form of trauma. The body's reaction is to send large numbers of defense cells to the area, particularly polymorphonuclear leukocytes (PMNs), which are major constituents of the purulent exudate (pus) that collects.

Pus is a thick fluid product of inflammation. It contains many living and dead PMNs mixed with debris from cells and tissues that have been destroyed by the enzymes released by the PMNs. Unless there is a means for drainage, the pus collects and forms an abscess.

A sinus or fistula may form. Drainage may occur through the sinus and release the pressure within the abscess, thereby relieving the pain the patient may experience.

II. ETIOLOGIC FACTORS

A. Periodontal Pockets

Deep pockets of chronic inflammatory periodontal infection provide an environment for abscess formation. Special anatomic variations predispose to abscess formation. Instrumentation applied within the pocket and the effects of the instrumentation may be the precipitating factors that initiate abscess formation.

1. *Anatomic Features.* Intrabony pockets, pockets that extend into bifurcation or trifurcation areas, and complex pockets that develop in winding or irregular shapes are particularly susceptible to becoming closed and, therefore, susceptible to abscess formation.
2. *Instrumentation.*[7] Incomplete scaling in the depth of a pocket may allow the tissue at the opening of the pocket to heal, tighten, and prevent

drainage from the infectious material deep in the pocket. Biofilm and calculus remaining in the sealed off part of the pocket attract the collection of more bacteria and PMNs, and an abscess develops.

B. Trauma

Foreign objects may enter by way of the sulcus or pocket and become embedded along with microorganisms. The infection leads to abscess formation.
1. *Implanted or Impacted Material*[8]
    a. Popcorn husk, small fish bone or shellfish fragment, seeds, seed coverings, or other material from food.
    b. Oral hygiene devices include toothbrush bristle or filament or a sliver from a toothpick.
2. *Instrumentation.* Trauma during subgingival instrumentation may force infectious material into the pocket wall.

C. Patient Susceptibility to Infection

The possibility for abscess formation within the gingival tissue is increased from any of the etiologic factors that have been mentioned when the patient's resistance to infection is lowered. Patients with uncontrolled diabetes or who are receiving immunosuppressive medication are examples of those at greater risk.

III. CLINICAL SIGNS AND SYMPTOMS

Even though clinical manifestations may vary, the classic signs and symptoms are listed here.

A. Clinical Appearance

The area of the abscess is enlarged, with a red, shiny, smooth surface. It may appear domelike or pointed, and on slight digital pressure, pus may appear.

B. The Tooth

1. *Sensitivity.* The tooth may be sensitive to percussion. When extruded, it may be sensitive to touching the tooth in the opposing jaw. It may be slightly mobile.
2. *Pulp Vitality Test.* Pulp testing usually reveals a vital tooth, responding within the normal range.
3. *Radiographs.* A radiolucency may be noted along the lateral wall beside the tooth, but such a finding is variable. No bone loss shows in early lesions. The amount of bone destruction and the location of the abscess influence the possible radiographic findings.

C. General Physical Condition

Occasionally, a patient shows evidence of systemic involvement, such as a slight elevation in body temperature, malaise, and lymphadenopathy.

D. Chronic Abscess

In the chronic state, a sinus tract usually opens on the gingival surface and drains periodically. Before drainage, the patient may have a dull pain from the pressure of the fluid within the abscess area. Acute symptoms may be expected from time to time unless definitive periodontal therapy is completed.

IV. COMPARISON OF PERIAPICAL AND PERIODONTAL ABSCESSES

The dentist must often differentiate between a periapical and a periodontal abscess. Certain signs and symptoms are nearly the same for both. A few of the potentially distinguishing findings are noted here.

A. Pulp Test

The tooth with a periapical lesion does not respond normally to a pulp tester.

B. Sinus Tract Formation

The opening of a sinus tract from a periapical abscess usually is positioned more apically, whereas the opening from a periodontal abscess is more coronal.

C. Pain

Sharp steady pain is typical of a periapical lesion, whereas the pain from a periodontal abscess varies.

D. Periodontal Examination

A tooth with a periapical lesion is not necessarily periodontally involved. Probing may reveal no probing depth of note, and no bone loss may be apparent in the radiograph.

Occasionally, a combined periodontic and endodontic lesion occurs. Communication between a deep periodontal pocket and an apical lesion is not unusual. Communication may also exist from a periodontal pocket into the pulp by way of a lateral or accessory canal through the dentin.

E. Dental Caries

A diseased pulp leading to a periapical abscess is caused by either trauma to the tooth or dental caries extending inward until the pulp becomes infected. A carious lesion may also be present with a periodontal abscess and may complicate the differential diagnosis.

F. Radiographic Examination

Early stages of either a periapical or a periodontal abscess are not evident in a radiograph. A widening of the periodontal ligament space may appear.

V. CARE PLAN

Two phases of treatment are used for the patient with a periodontal abscess. The first is for immediate relief of acute symptoms, and the second is the definitive treatment followed by preventive maintenance. The entire plan should be explained to the patient at the outset.

A. Objectives of Emergency Treatment

1. Relieve pain.
2. Establish drainage.
3. Determine need for systemic antibiotic therapy.

B. Review Medical History

Determine necessary preappointment precautions, such as the need for antibiotic premedication.

C. Examination for Systemic Involvement

Antibiotic medication is frequently prescribed by the dentist when systemic involvement is definite.

1. Determine and record the patient's body temperature.
2. Examine submandibular and neck nodes for lymphadenopathy.

D. Provide Anesthesia

When the abscess is confined to the gingival area, and the drainage may be expected to cause little if any discomfort, a topical anesthetic may suffice. Usually, block anesthesia is indicated.

E. Methods for Drainage

1. *Via Pocket or Sulcus Opening.* Isolate the area, swab with a topical antiseptic, and use a probe to gain admission into the sulcus or pocket. Gently probe circumferentially until an opening into the abscess is found. Drainage usually begins promptly.
2. *Curet Area.* Use a curet to open the area, and locate and remove a foreign body irritant when it is known to be present from the history obtained from the patient. Scaling and debridement are performed as needed.

F. Postoperative Instructions

Rinsing with hot saline solution every 2 hours is advised. The patient should return for observation in 24 to 48 hours. Relief from pain and discomfort can be expected and appointments for definitive treatment

---

Everyday Ethics

 Sue has not seen Mr. Rufus for over a year. He called requesting an appointment because he is overdue and is suddenly having mouth pain and a "horrible metallic taste." When he arrives, Mr. Rufus says "Hello," and Sue is overtaken by a strong mouth odor.

Upon review of his medical history, Mr. Rufus appears to be quite healthy, but he describes the heart-breaking details of his divorce proceedings. His dental problems started about the same time. He confides in Sue that he has hardly eaten or brushed his teeth for the past 2 days.

Sue begins an extraoral and intraoral examination, but Mr. Rufus says it is too painful for her to retract his cheeks and lips. During the brief examination, she noticed punched out papillae and pseudomembrane formation over much of his gingiva. She immediately suspects necrotizing ulcerative gingivitis (NUG), or perhaps necrotizing ulcerative periodontitis (NUP).

Questions for Consideration

1. At what point should Sue consult with the dentist to confirm diagnosis of NUG or NUP before discussing the details with the patient?

2. Sue has empathy for all that Mr. Rufus has gone through personally, but she feels it is her duty to mention the offensive mouth odor. How can she do this without offending or embarrassing him?

3. Is it ethical for Sue to ask questions about the patient's personal life with particular reference to his divorce? Why or why not?

✔ **Factors To Teach The Patient**

- Premature discontinuation of treatment for NUG because acute signs have subsided can lead to recurrence of the infection.

- The role of diet, rest, and dental biofilm control in the prevention of NUG.

- The avoidance of an oral irrigating device in the presence of acute inflammatory conditions. Microorganisms may be forced into the tissues beneath a pocket, and bacteremia can be produced.

planned. Biofilm control instruction is initiated or continued, and scaling and debridement are completed.

G. Anticipated Results

1. Acute symptoms are resolved.
2. Pain relief occurs within a short time following the initiation of drainage because the pressure is released from within the abscessed area.
3. Extruded tooth returns to its normal position.
4. Swelling is reduced.
5. Temporary comfort is obtained for the patient; the lesion is reduced to a standard chronic lesion that requires additional treatment.
6. If drainage is not complete, an acute lesion may develop into a lesion with a chronic sinus.

VI. DEFINITIVE THERAPY

Whatever pocket elimination procedures are indicated should be completed within a reasonable time to prevent further complications. Careful and regular dental biofilm control with scaling and debridement are usually needed.

REFERENCES

1. Enwonwu, C.O.: Infectious Oral Necrosis (cancrum oris) in Nigerian Children: A Review, *Community Dent. Oral Epidemiol., 13,* 190, June, 1985.
2. Taiwo, J.O.: Oral Hygiene Status and Necrotizing Ulcerative Gingivitis in Nigerian Children, *J. Periodontol., 64,* 1071, November, 1993.
3. Greenspan, J.S.: Periodontal Complications of HIV Infection, *Compend. Cont. Educ. Dent., 15,* S694, Supplement Number 18, 1994.
4. Loesche, W.J., Syed, S.A., Laughon, B.E., and Stoll, J.: The Bacteriology of Acute Necrotizing Ulcerative Gingivitis, *J. Periodontol., 53,* 223, April, 1982.
5. Listgarten, M.A.: Electron Microscopic Observations on the Bacterial Flora of Acute Necrotizing Ulcerative Gingivitis, *J. Periodontol., 36,* 328, July–August, 1965.
6. Davis, J.R. and Stegeman, C.A.: *The Dental Hygienist's Guide to Nutritional Care.* Philadelphia, W.B. Saunders Co., 1998, pp. 382–386.
7. Armitage, G.C.: *Biologic Basis of Periodontal Maintenance Therapy.* Berkeley, CA, Praxis Publishing Co., 1980, pp. 154–159.
8. Gillette, W.B. and Van House, R.L.: Ill Effects of Improper Oral Hygiene Procedures, *J. Am. Dent. Assoc., 101,* 476, September, 1980.

SUGGESTED READINGS
Necrotizing Ulcerative Gingivitis

Barr, C.E. and Robbins, M.R.: Clinical and Radiographic Presentations of HIV-1 Necrotizing Ulcerative Periodontitis, *Spec. Care Dentist., 16,* 237, November/December, 1996.

Cutler, C.W., Wasfy, M.O., Ghaffar, K., Hosni, M., and Lloyd, D.R.: Impaired Bactericidal Activity of PMN From Two Brothers With Necrotizing Ulcerative Gingivo-periodontitis, *J. Periodontol., 65,* 357, April, 1994.

Glick, M., Muzyka, B.C., Salkin, L.M., and Lurie, D.: Necrotizing Ulcerative Periodontitis: A Marker for Immune Deterioration and a Predictor for the Diagnosis of AIDS, *J. Periodontol., 65,* 393, May, 1994.

Haring, J.I.: Case #1 Acute Necrotizing Ulcerative Gingivitis, *RDH, 15,* 13, January, 1995.

Horning, G.M.: Necrotizing Gingivostomatitis: NUG to Noma, *Compend. Cont. Educ. Dent., 17,* 951, October, 1996.

Horning, G.M. and Cohen, M.E.: Necrotizing Ulcerative Gingivitis, Periodontitis, and Stomatitis: Clinical Staging and Predisposing Factors, *J. Periodontol., 66,* 990, November, 1995.

Murayama, Y., Kurihara, H., Nagai, A., Dompkowski, D., and Van Dyke, T.E.: Acute Necrotizing Ulcerative Gingivitis: Risk Factors Involving Host Defense Mechanisms, *Periodontol. 2000, 6,* 116, 1994.

Osuji, O.O.: Necrotizing Ulcerative Gingivitis and Cancrum Oris (Noma) in Ibadan, Nigeria, *J. Periodontol., 61,* 769, December, 1990.

Riviere, G.R., Weisz, K.S., Simonson, L.G., and Lukehart, S.A.: Pathogen-related Spirochetes Identified Within Gingival Tissue from Patients with Acute Necrotizing Ulcerative Gingivitis, *Infect. Immun., 59,* 2653, August, 1991.

Robinson, P.G., Winkler, J.R., Palmer, G., Westenhouse, J., Hilton, J.F., and Greenspan, J.S.: The Diagnosis of Periodontal Conditions Associated With HIV Infection, *J. Periodontol., 65,* 236, March, 1994.

Rowland, R.W., Mestecky, J., Gunsolley, J.C., and Cogen, R.B.: Serum IgG and IgM Levels to Bacterial Antigens in Necrotizing Ulcerative Gingivitis, *J. Periodontol., 64,* 195, March, 1993.

Tolle-Watts, L.: ANUG—Dental Hygiene Intervention, *DentalHygienistNews, 4,* 1, Summer, 1991.

Periodontal Abscess

Carranza, F.A. and Newman, M.G.: *Clinical Periodontology,* 8th ed. Philadelphia, W.B. Saunders Co., 1996, pp. 292–294, 483–485.

Dello Russo, N.M.: The Post-prophylaxis Periodontal Abscess: Etiology and Treatment, *Int. J. Periodontics Restorative Dent., 5,* 28, Number 1, 1985.

Fedi, P.F. and Vernino, A.R.: *The Periodontic Syllabus,* 3rd ed. Baltimore, Williams & Wilkins, 1995, pp. 187–189.

Flood, T.R., Samaranayake, L.P., MacFarlane, T.W., McLennan, A., MacKenzie, D., and Carmichael, F.: Bacteremia Following Incision and Drainage of Dento-alveolar Abscesses, *Br. Dent. J., 169,* 51, July 21, 1990.

Hafström, C.A., Wikstrom, M.B., Renvert, S.N., and Dahlén, G.G.: Effect of Treatment on Some Periodontopathogens and Their Antibody Levels in Periodontal Abscesses, *J. Periodontol., 65,* 1022, November, 1994.

Haring, J.I.: Case #4 Periodontal Abscess, *RDH, 16,* 12, April, 1996.

McLeod, D.E., Lainson, P.A., and Spivey, J.D.: Tooth Loss Due to Periodontal Abscess: A Retrospective Study, *J. Periodontol., 68,* 963, October, 1997.

Taani, D.S.Q.: An Effective Treatment for Chronic Periodontal Abscesses, *Quintessence Int., 27,* 697, October, 1996.

Sutures and Dressings

Marilyn Cortell, RDH, MS

Many periodontal surgical procedures require sutures and dressings. The dental hygienist will often participate in the patient's initial preparation and postcare; therefore, knowledge of the surgical and posttreatment procedures will support continuity of treatment. Key words related to sutures and dressings are defined in Box 40-1.

■ SUTURES

A suture is a strand of material used to ligate blood vessels and approximate tissue. Sutures are necessary in many oral surgical procedures when a surgical wound must be closed, a flap positioned, or tissue grafted.

Through the centuries, a wide range of suture materials has been used, including silk, cotton, linen, and animal tendons and intestines. Today's suture materials are designed for specific procedures, thus decreasing poten-

tial for postsurgical infections while providing patient comfort and convenience.

I. FUNCTIONS OF SUTURES

A. Close periodontal wounds and secure grafts in position.
B. Assist in maintaining hemostasis.
C. Reduce posttreatment discomfort.
D. Promote primary intention healing.
E. Prevent underlying bone exposure.
F. Protect healing surgical wound from foreign debris and trauma.

II. CHARACTERISTICS OF SUTURE MATERIALS

A. Sterile.
B. Handle comfortably and easily.

BOX 40-1 KEY WORDS: Sutures and Dressings

Border mold: the shaping of the peripheries of a dressing by manual manipulation of the tissue adjacent to the borders (for example, lips, cheeks) to duplicate the contour and size of the vestibule.

Chemical cure: mode of self-cure or setting of a dressing in which the ingredients unite in a chemical process that starts as soon as the blending is complete; the setting time is influenced by warm temperature and the addition of an accelerator.

Coapt: to approximate, as the edges of a wound; bring edge to edge with no overlap.

Dressing: any of various materials used for covering and protecting a wound; in dentistry, may sometimes be called a pack.

> **Pressure dressing:** for maintaining pressure to control bleeding or to hold a particular flap or graft in position.

> **Protective dressing:** to shield an area from injury or trauma.

Eugenol: constituent of clove oil; used in early periodontal dressings with zinc oxide for its alleged antiseptic and anodyne properties; more recently found to be toxic, to elicit allergic reactions, and to hinder, more than promote, healing.

Hemostasis: the termination of bleeding by mechanical or chemical means or by the complex coagulation process of the body that consists of vasoconstriction, platelet aggregation, and thrombin and fibrin synthesis.

Hydrolysis: a process in which water slowly penetrates the suture filaments, causing breakdown of the suture's polymer chain. Hydrolyzation yields a lesser degree of tissue reaction.

Ligation: application of a wire or thread (suture) to hold or constrict tissue.

Suture: a stitch or series of stitches made to secure apposition of the edges of a surgical or traumatic wound.

> **Suture apposition:** a suture that holds the margins of an incision close together.

Swage: the fusion of a suture material to the needle, which allows for a smooth eyeless attachment. The suture will then pass through the tissue as smoothly as possible.

Tensile strength: amount of strength the suture material will retain throughout the healing period. As the wound gains strength, the suture loses strength.

Visible-light cure: light activation using a photocure system; shorter curing time than self-cure (chemical cure); does not start setting until the light is activated, thereby allowing longer working time for adapting the dressing material.

C. Pass through tissue with minimal trauma.
D. Cause little or no tissue reaction throughout healing.
E. Possess a high tensile strength.

III. CLASSIFICATION OF SUTURE MATERIALS

A. By Number of Strands

1. *Monofilament suture*: Single strand of material.
2. *Multifilament suture*: Several strands twisted or braided together.

B. By Material Used

1. *Natural*: Capable of causing adverse tissue reaction.

2. *Synthetic*: Developed to reduce tissue reactions and unpredictable rates of absorption commonly found in natural sutures.

C. By Absorption Properties

1. *Absorbable sutures*: Approximate tissue until wound heals sufficiently to endure normal stress.
   a. Natural absorbable sutures: digested by body enzymes.
      Examples: surgical gut, chromic gut.
   b. Synthetic absorbable sutures: broken down by hydrolysis, a process in which water slowly penetrates the suture filaments, causing a breakdown of the suture's polymer chain. Hydrolyzation yields a lesser degree of tissue reaction.

Examples: polyglactin (Vicryl™), poliglecaprone (Monocryl™), polydioxanone (PDS™ II).

2. *Nonabsorbable sutures*: Not digested by body enzymes or hydrolyzation. Must be removed within specific time period.
   a. Natural nonabsorbable.
      Example: silk.
   b. Synthetic nonabsorbable.
      Examples: nylon (Ethilon™), polyester (Ethibond™), polypropylene (Prolene™) polytetrafluoroethylene (ePTFE) (Gore-Tex™)

D. By Diameter of Suture Material

1. Diameters range from 1-0 to 11-0.
2. More zeros, smaller the diameter.
3. Fewer zeros, larger the diameter.
   Example: 3-0 is larger than 5-0.

■ NEEDLES

Many types of suturing needles are available. Their use and selection are primarily based on specific procedures, location for use, and clinician's preference.

I. NEEDLE COMPONENTS

A. Swaged End (Eyeless)

Swaged (eyeless) allows suture material and needle to act as one unit (Figure 40-1).

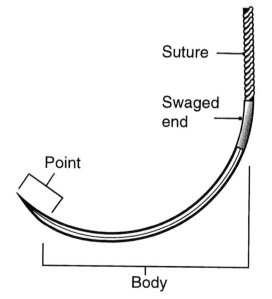

■ **FIGURE 40-1 Suture Needle Components.**

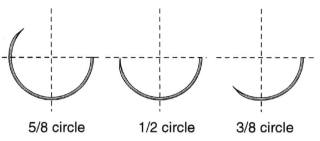

5/8 circle   1/2 circle   3/8 circle

■ **FIGURE 40-2 Suture Needles.** A curved needle is manipulated with a needleholder. The 3/8 curve is most effective for closure of skin and mucous membranes and is a needle of choice in many dental and periodontal surgeries.

B. Body

1. Shape/curvature:
   a. Straight.
   b. Half-curved.
   c. Curved 1\4, 3\8, 1\2, 5\8 (Figure 40-2).
2. *Diameter*: Gauge or size: finer for delicate surgeries.
3. The body is the strongest part of the needle that is grasped with the needleholder during the surgical procedure. The swaged end is the weakest part of the body.

C. Point

1. The point of the needle extends from the extreme tip of the needle to the widest part of the body.
2. Each needle point is designed and manufactured to penetrate tissue with the highest degree of sharpness.

II. NEEDLE CHARACTERISTICS

A. Material

Most needles are made of stainless steel formulated and sterilized for surgical use.

B. Attachment

Majority of needles are permanently attached to suture material; eliminates need for threading and unnecessary handling.

C. Cutting Edge (Figure 40-3)

1. *Reverse cut*: Has two opposing cutting edges, with a third located on outer convex curve of needle.
2. *Conventional cut*: Consists of two opposing cutting edges and a third within the concave curvature of the needle.

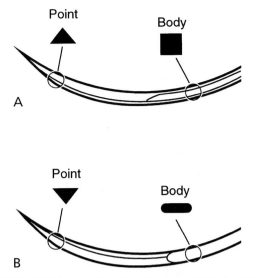

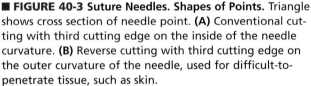

■ **FIGURE 40-3 Suture Needles. Shapes of Points.** Triangle shows cross section of needle point. **(A)** Conventional cutting with third cutting edge on the inside of the needle curvature. **(B)** Reverse cutting with third cutting edge on the outer curvature of the needle, used for difficult-to-penetrate tissue, such as skin.

D. Requirements

1. Needle point design to meet the needs of specific surgical procedures.
2. Surgical needles are intended to carry suture material through tissues with minimal trauma.
3. Must be sharp enough to penetrate tissues with minimal resistance.
4. Must be rigid enough to resist bending, yet still flexible.
5. Must be **sterile** and corrosion resistant.

■ KNOTS

The Encyclopedia of Knots describes more than 1,400 knots. Only a few are used in dentistry. The type of knot used will depend on the specific procedure, the location of the incision, and the amount of stress the wound will endure. Surgeons and square knots are most frequently used in dentistry, with the square knot being the easiest and most reliable.

I. KNOT CHARACTERISTICS

A. A knot should be tied as small as possible.
B. Completed knot should be firm to reduce slipping.
C. Excessive tension should be avoided so the suture material will not break or further traumatize the tissue.

II. KNOT MANAGEMENT

A. Tie knots on facial aspect for easier access in removal.
B. Leave 2-to 3-mm suture "tail" to assist in locating at the time of removal.

III. SUTURING PROCEDURES

Many different patterns of suturing are used. Assisting and observing during the surgical procedure can be an educational experience for the dental hygienist.

General types of sutures frequently used in the oral cavity are described here briefly.

A. Blanket

Each stitch is brought over a loop of the preceding one, thus forming a series of loops on one side of the incision and a series of stitches over the incision (Figure 40-4A). It is also called a continuous lock. This stitch is used, for example, to approximate the gingival margins after alveolectomy.

B. Interrupted

Figure 40-4B show a series of interrupted sutures.

C. Continuous Uninterrupted

A series of stitches tied at one or both ends. Examples of sutures that may be applied in a series are the sling or suspension and the blanket.

D. Circumferential

A term applied to a suture that encircles a tooth for suspension and retention of a flap.

E. Interdental

Where the flaps are on both the lingual and facial sides, interdental ligation joins the two by passing the suture through each interdental area (Figure 40-4C). Coverage for the interdental area can be accomplished by coapting the edges of the papillae.

F. Sling or Suspension

When a flap is only on one side, facial or lingual, the sutures are passed through the interdental papilla, through the interdental area, around the tooth, and then into the adjacent papilla (Figure 40-4D). The suture is adjusted so that the flap can be positioned for correct healing.

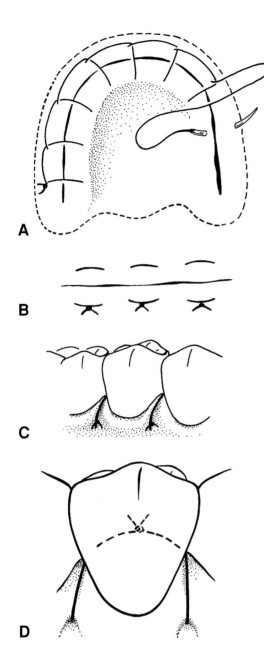

■ **FIGURE 40-4 Types of Sutures. (A)** Blanket stitch. **(B)** Interrupted, individual sutures. **(C)** Interdental individual sutures. **(D)** Sling or suspension suture tied on the lingual (*dotted line*).

■ PROCEDURE FOR SUTURE REMOVAL

I. SUPPLIES FOR SUTURE REMOVAL

- Mouth mirror.
- Cotton pliers.
- Curved sharp scissors with pointed tip (suture scissors).

- Gauze sponge.
- Topical antiseptic.
- Topical anesthetic: Use type that can be applied safely on an abraded or incompletely healed area.
- Cotton pellets.
- Saliva ejector tip.

II. PREPARATION OF PATIENT

A. Patient History Check

Suture removal can cause bacteremia.[1,2] High-risk patients need antibiotic premedication for suture removal (page 122).

B. Patient Examination

1. Observe healing tissue around the suture(s).
2. Record any deviations in color, size, shape of the tissue, adaptation of a flap, or coaptation of an incision healing by first intention.

C. Preparation of the Sutured Area

1. Sutures placed without a dressing may have a crust over them at the time of removal. Apply a water-based gel with a cotton swab or pellet, and in a short time, the crust will soften and can be wiped away. If the suture is removed with the crust it can cause unnecessary patient discomfort.
2. Debride and rinse the area to remove debris particles, using a cotton-tipped applicator or a cotton pellet dipped in 3% peroxide. Follow with another rinse, or wipe gently with a gauze sponge.
3. Place and adjust saliva ejector.
4. Retract and pat area with gauze sponge to remove surface moisture.
5. Swab area with topical antiseptic. Maintain retraction to prevent dilution.
6. Apply topical anesthetic.

D. Retraction

Three hands are really needed: one for retraction, one for cotton pliers to hold and remove the suture, and one for cutting the suture. When an assistant is not available, a cotton roll placed in the vestibule may provide enough retraction along with the finger rest and little finger of the nondominant hand holding the cotton pliers.

III. STEPS FOR REMOVAL

The suture removal procedure described here and illustrated in Figure 40-5 is for a single interrupted suture.

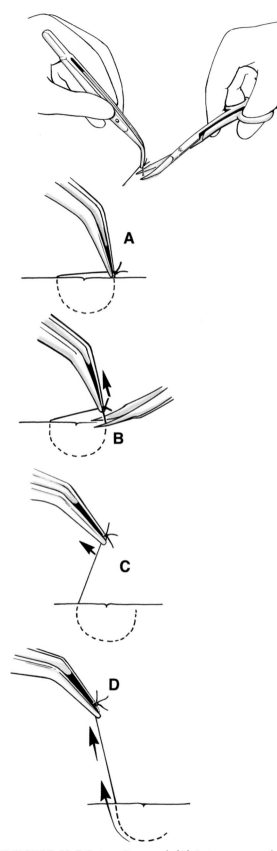

The same principles apply for the ends and each segment of a continuous suture, wherever septic suture material can pass through the soft tissue.

A. Grasp the suture knot with the cotton plier held in the nondominant hand. Gently draw the suture up about 2 mm and hold with slight tension (Figure 40-5A). A finger rest is needed for control.

B. Insert tip of sharp scissors under the suture, slightly depress the tissue with the back of the scissor blade, and cut the suture in the part that was previously buried in the tissue (Figure 40-5B).

C. Hold knot end up with the cotton plier and pull gently to allow suture to exit through the side opposite where it was cut (Figure 40-5C). This prevents any part of the exposed contaminated segment of the suture from passing through the tissue and introducing infectious material.

D. Withdraw gently and steadily (Figure 40-5D).

E. Place each suture on a sponge for final counting, and proceed to remove the next suture.

F. Count the total number of sutures removed. The number of sutures removed should correspond to the number of sutures placed.

    1. During healing, sutures can become loosened, misplaced, or occasionally covered by tissue.

    2. The effect of a remaining suture can lead to infection and possible abscess around the suture left behind.

G. Apply gauze sponge with slight pressure on bleeding spots.

H. Request patient to close on the sponge while dressing is readied (when a dressing replacement is indicated).

IV. SAFETY MEASURES

A. Count sutures; record number placed and number removed.

B. Observe all tissue and record observations, noting any adverse reactions or bleeding.

C. Record patient's comments.

D. Sutures should not be left longer than 7 to 14 days.

E. Use caution when removing a periodontal dressing to prevent tearing a suture that may have become embedded in the dressing.

▪ **FIGURE 40-5 Suture Removal. (A)** Suture grasped by pliers near the entrance into tissue. **(B)** Suture pulled gently up while scissor is inserted close to the tissue. Suture is cut in the part previously buried in the tissue. **(C)** Suture is held up for vertical removal. **(D)** Suture is pulled gently to bring it out on the side opposite from where it was cut. The object is to prevent the external part of the suture from passing through the tissue and introducing infectious material.

F. Provide proper postappointment instructions both verbally and in writing.

V. RECORD KEEPING

A. At the Time of Surgical Treatment

1. Record the number of sutures placed.
2. Location of the suture placement.
3. Type and description of sutures.
4. Indicate dressing type.

B. At the Suture Removal Appointment

1. Note presence and condition of dressing.
2. Indicate if no dressing remains.
3. Place removed sutures on a gauze pad.
4. The number of sutures removed should correspond with the number placed.

C. Documentation Examples

Date: placed 4 interdental sutures, between #13 & 14, 4-0 Ethicon™ silk. Coe-Pak™ dressing applied.
  Complete Signature: dentist
  Date of removal: dressing fragmented, little protection remains. Removed 4 interdental silk sutures, minimal bleeding, tissue appearance consistent with normal healing.
  Complete signature: dental hygienist and dentist

■ PERIODONTAL DRESSINGS

A dressing may be placed over the surgical wound following periodontal surgery. Dressings are used for all surgical procedures by some clinicians, occasionally by others, and rarely by others.

I. PURPOSES AND USES

A. Provide protection for a surgical wound against external irritation or trauma.
B. Help prevent posttreatment bleeding by securing initial clot formation.
C. Support mobile teeth during healing.
D. Assist in shaping or molding newly formed tissue, in securing a flap, or in immobilizing a graft.
E. Retain site-specific materials for slow-release chemotherapy within pockets (pages 682 to 683).

II. CHARACTERISTICS OF ACCEPTABLE DRESSING MATERIAL

An acceptable dressing material has the following characteristics:
A. Preparation, placement, and removal will take place with minimal discomfort to the patient.
B. Material adheres to itself, teeth, and adjacent tissues, and maintains retention within interdental areas.
C. Provides stability and flexibility to withstand distortion and displacement without fracturing.
D. Be nontoxic and nonirritating to oral tissues.
E. Possesses a smooth surface that will resist accumulation of dental biofilm.
F. Will not traumatize tissue or stain teeth and restorative materials.
G. Possesses an aesthetically acceptable appearance.

■ TYPES OF DRESSINGS

Traditionally, dressings were classified into two groups: those that contained eugenol and those that did not. With the development of new products, "noneugenol-containing" dressings have been reclassified into chemical-cure and visible-light-cure materials. They are available as ready-mix, paste-paste, or paste-gel preparations.

The American Dental Association Council on Scientific Affairs reviews products. Approved products use the ADA seal (Figure 27-3).

I. ZINC OXIDE WITH EUGENOL DRESSING

A. Basic Ingredients

1. *Powder*: Zinc oxide, powdered rosin, and tannic acid. In the past, some formulas used asbestos fiber as a binder. Because airborne asbestos is a recognized pulmonary health hazard, dental team members responsible for mixing periodontal dressings frequently may become overexposed. Asbestos fiber is no longer an acceptable ingredient of dressings.
2. *Liquid*: Eugenol, with oil, such as peanut or cottonseed, and thymol.

B. Examples

Well-known dressings are Wards Wondrpack™ and Kirkland Periodontal Pack™.

C. Advantages

1. *Consistency*: Firm and heavy, provides support for tissues and flaps.
2. *Slow setting*: Extended working time.
3. *Preparation and storage*: Can be prepared in quantity and stored (frozen) in work-size pieces.

D. Disadvantages

1. *Taste*: Sharp, unpleasant taste.
2. *Tissue reaction*: Irritating; hypersensitivity reactions can occur.
3. *Consistency*: Dressing is hard, brittle, and breaks easily. Rough surface encourages dental biofilm retention.

II. CHEMICAL-CURED DRESSING

The ingredients of commercial products are trade secrets, but some general information about available dressings can be found. Two examples of chemical-cured dressings are PerioCare™ and Coe-Pak™.

A. Basic Ingredients[3]

1. *PerioCare™*: Paste-gel.
   a. Paste: zinc oxide, magnesium oxide, calcium hydroxide, and vegetable oils.
   b. Gel: resins, fatty acids, ethyl cellulose, lanolin, calcium hydroxide.
2. *Coe-Pak™*: Paste-paste.
   a. Base: rosin, cellulose, natural gums and waxes, fatty acid, chlorothymol, zinc acetate, alcohol.
   b. Accelerator: zinc oxide, vegetable oil, chlorothymol, magnesium oxide, silica, synthetic resin, and coumarin.

B. Advantages

1. *Consistency*: Pliable, easy to place with light pressure.
2. *Smooth surface*: Comfortable to patient; resists biofilm and debris deposits.
3. *Taste*: Acceptable.
4. *Removal*: Easy, often comes off in one piece.

III. VISIBLE-LIGHT-CURED DRESSING

Visible-light-cured (VIC) dressing (*Barricaid™*) is available in a syringe for direct application or from a mixing pad for indirect application. The same light-curing unit used for composite restorations and sealants is also used for this curing process.

A. Basic Ingredients[3]

Gel ingredients include polyester urethane dimethacrylate resin, silanated silica, visible-light-cure photoinitiator and accelerator, stabilizer, and colorant.

B. Advantages

1. *Color*: More like gingiva than most other dressings.
2. *Setting*: Does not begin until activated by the light-curing unit. Exposure before placement

should be limited as daylight in a room may begin the activation process.
3. *Removal*: Easy, often comes off in one piece.

IV. COLLAGEN DRESSINGS

- Absorbable collagen dressings used to promote wound healing.
- Special use in periodontal surgery for a collagen patch dressing: For protection of graft sites of the palate during healing.
- One form prepared in a bullet shape to use for deep biopsy sites.
- Available in individual unit sterile packages.
- Collagen dressing may be placed on clean moist or bleeding wounds.

▪ CLINICAL APPLICATION

I. DRESSING PLACEMENT

A. General Procedure

For all types of dressing, follow the manufacturer's instructions. Each product has unique properties that require special handling.

B. Retention

1. Mold the dressing by pressing at each interproximal site. Do not extend over the height of contour of each tooth.
2. Border mold to prevent displacement by the tongue, cheeks, lips, or frena.
3. Check the occlusion and remove areas of contact.

II. CHARACTERISTICS OF A WELL-PLACED DRESSING (FIGURE 40-6)

Dressings placed in keeping with biologic principles contribute to healing and are tolerated more comfortably by

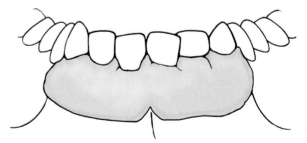

▪ **FIGURE 40-6 Periodontal Dressing.** A dressing must cover the surgical wound without unnecessary overextension and fill interdental areas to lock the dressing between the teeth. It should be molded in the vestibule and around frena to allow movement of the lips, cheeks, and tongue with no displacement of the dressing.

the patient. A satisfactory dressing has the following characteristics:

A. Is secure and rigid. A movable dressing is an irritant and can promote bleeding.

B. Has as little bulk as possible, yet is bulky enough to give strength.

C. Locks mechanically interdentally and cannot be displaced by action of tongue, cheek, or lips.

D. Covers the entire surgical wound without unnecessary overextension.

E. Fills interdental area and adequately covers the treated area to discourage retention of debris and dental biofilm.

F. Possesses a smooth surface to prevent irritation to cheeks and lips while resisting debris and biofilm retention.

III. PATIENT DISMISSAL AND INSTRUCTIONS

A. Patient must not be dismissed until bleeding or oozing from under the dressing has ceased.

B. Written instructions are more effective than verbal. Table 40-1 lists items for which instructions should be given to a patient who has a periodontal dressing. Printed instructions can be prepared from these items. Other instructions for the patient after general oral surgery or tooth removal may be found on page 854.

▪ DRESSING REMOVAL AND REPLACEMENT

During healing, epithelium covers a wound in 5 to 6 days, and complete restoration of epithelium and connective tissue can be expected by 21 days. The dressing may be left in place from 7 to 10 days, as determined by the surgeon.

Keep the following factors relative to dressings in mind:

• If the dressing becomes dislodged before the removal appointment, the healing tissue should be evaluated.

• When the dressing remains intact for 4 or 5 days, replacement may not be necessary.

• When replacement is indicated, the dressing should be replaced in its entirety rather than patched.

• Instruct the patient to proceed with daily frequent biofilm removal and rinsing using an antimicrobial agent.

I. PATIENT EXAMINATION

A. Question patient about and record posttreatment effects or discomfort. Record length of time the dressing remained in place.

B. Examine the mucosa around the dressing and record its appearance.

Everyday Ethics

Miss Osgood arrives for a suture removal appointment with Agnes, the dental hygienist, and immediately explains the discomfort she is feeling. When asked why she didn't come in sooner to have the area observed, she said it was so close to the removal appointment she might as well wait. Agnes notes from the record that no dressing was placed. The area appears inflamed, with a slight cyanotic appearance circumscribing the suture area. The patient prerinsed with a 0.12% chlorhexidine, and Agnes began removing the sutures. Moderate bleeding and discomfort were present.

Upon removal, Agnes noted that only three sutures could be found, but four had been placed. When she conferred with the dentist, Agnes was told to dismiss the patient and to prepare a prescription for penicillin V to "take care of the infection. Eventually the suture will be absorbed by body tissues."

Questions for Consideration

1. Given the sequence of events, what issues of professionalism are exhibited in the working relationship between the dentist and the dental hygienist?

2. Was the treatment provided within an acceptable standard of care for this patient? Why or why not?

3. What information needs to be documented in the progress notes concerning the services rendered and dialogue that occurred with the patient?

■ TABLE 40-1 INSTRUCTIONS FOR POSTTREATMENT CARE

FACTOR	INSTRUCTIONS TO PATIENT	PURPOSE OF INSTRUCTION
Information specific for patient about the dressing	• Dressing will protect the surgical wound • Do not disturb the dressing • Allow it to remain until the next appointment	• An informed patient is more likely to be more compliant
Care during the first few hours	• Dressing will not set for a few hours • Do not eat anything that requires chewing • Use only cool liquids • Stay quiet and rest	• Dressing must become hard and be left undisturbed
Anesthesia	• Be careful not to bite lip or cheek • Avoid foods that require chewing until anesthesia has worn off	• Prevent trauma to cheek and lips
Discomfort after anesthesia wears off	• Have the prescription filled and follow the directions • Do not take more than directed • Avoid aspirin	• Pain control • Aspirin can interfere with blood-clotting mechanism
Ice pack or cold compress	• Use as directed only • Common protocol is: Apply every 30 minutes for 15 minutes; or 15 minutes on and 15 minutes off	• Prevent swelling from edema
Bleeding	• Slight bleeding within the first few hours is not unusual • Do not suck on the area or use straws • Blood clot should be left undisturbed for as long as possible	• Alleviate patient concern over small amounts of bleeding; however, persistent or excessive bleeding should be reported to the dentist immediately
Dressing care and retention	• Avoid disturbing the dressing with the tongue or trying to clean under it • Small particles may chip off, which is no problem unless sharp edges irritate the tongue or the dressing becomes loose • Call the dentist if the entire dressing or a large portion falls off before the 5th day • Rinse with a saline solution; rinse with chlorhexidine 0.12% morning and evening after brushing teeth	• Dressing is needed for wound protection • Epithelium covers wound by 5th or 6th day in normal healing
Use of tobacco and tobacco products	• Do not smoke; avoid all tobacco products • A heavy smoker should make every effort to decrease quantity of tobacco used	• Heat and smoke irritate the gingiva and delay healing
Rinsing	• Do not rinse on the day of the treatment • Second day: use saline solution made with 1/2 teaspoon (measured) in 1/2 cup of warm water every 2 to 3 hours • Begin chlorhexidine 0.12% twice daily	• Might disturb blood clot • Saline cleanses and aids healing

■ TABLE 40-1 INSTRUCTIONS FOR POSTTREATMENT CARE (Continued)		
FACTOR	**INSTRUCTIONS TO PATIENT**	**PURPOSE OF INSTRUCTION**
Toothbrushing and flossing	• Continue to maintain optimal home care in untreated areas • Lightly brush occlusal surface over dressing material • Use soft brush with water, and carefully clean film from dressing • Clean the tongue	• Dental biofilm control essential to reduce the number of oral microorganisms • Odor and taste control • Oral sanitation
Eating	• Use highly nutritious foods for healing • Food guide pyramid (Figure 32-1) • Use soft-textured diet • Avoid highly seasoned, spicy, hot, sticky, crunchy, and coarse foods	• Healing tissue requires a healthy diet and specific comfort foods • Protects dressing from breakage or displacement
Mastication	• Avoid foods that require excessive chewing • Chew only on untreated side • Use ground meat or cut meat into small, bite-sized pieces	• To protect the dressing while it protects the surgical site

II. PROCEDURE FOR REMOVAL

A. Insert a scaler or plastic instrument under the border of the dressing and apply lateral pressure.

B. Watch for sutures that can get lodged in the dressing. They may need to be cut for release. Use principles for suture removal as described on pages 703 to 705.

C. Remove fragments of dressing gently with cotton pliers to avoid scratching the thin epithelial covering of the healing tissue.

D. Observe tissue and record its appearance. Note any deviations from normal healing.

E. Use a scaler for removal of fragments adhering to tooth surfaces; use a curet for particles near the gingival margin. All calculus and roughness should be eliminated to prevent new dental biofilm retention.

F. Syringe with a gentle stream of *warm* water. W*arm* diluted mouthrinse may soothe the traumatized area.

III. PROCEDURAL SUGGESTIONS FOR DRESSING REPLACEMENT

A. Use a topical anesthetic to prevent patient discomfort.

B. Use a soft dressing with minimal pressure during application.

IV. DENTAL BIOFILM CONTROL FOLLOW-UP

Biofilm control follow-up is essential after final dressing removal.

A. Use a soft brush on the treated area, paying careful attention to biofilm removal at the gingival margin. Use usual methods for all other areas of the mouth.

B. Increase intensity of care on the treated area each day, with a return to uncompromised oral hygiene procedures by 3 or 4 days.

C. Rinse with chlorhexidine 0.12% during the healing period twice daily and gently force liquid between the teeth.

D. Recommend a dentifrice with sodium fluoride for root caries prevention to be used regularly and indefinitely.

✔ **Factors To Teach The Patient**

• Explanations for the items in Table 40-1.

• Care of the mouth during the period after treatment while wearing a periodontal dressing.

• Reasons for not using aspirin for pain relief.

• Tobacco use is detrimental and delays healing.

• Why regular maintenance is critical after treatment is formally over.

E. Should the patient experience postsurgical sensitivity recommend a dentifrice containing a desensitizing agent. Other suggestions for coping with sensitivity may be found on pages 720 to 723.

V. FOLLOW-UP

Return for observation of complete healing in 1 week to 1 month, depending on individual patient's progress and total treatment plan.

REFERENCES

1. **King**, R.C., Crawford, J.J., and Small, E.W.: Bacteremia Following Intraoral Suture Removal, *Oral Surg. Oral Med. Oral Pathol., 65,* 23, January, 1988.
2. **Giglio**, J.A., Rowland, R.W., Dalton, H.P., and Laskin, D.M.: Suture Removal-Induced Bacteremia: A Possible Endocarditis Risk, *J. Am. Dent. Assoc., 123,* 65, August, 1992.
3. **von Fraunhofer**, J.A. and Argyropoulos, D.C.: Properties of Periodontal Dressings, *Dent. Materials, 6,* 51, January, 1990.

SUGGESTED READINGS

Newman, M.G., Takei, H.H., and Carranza, F.A.: *Carranza's Clinical Periodontology,* 9th ed. Philadelphia, WB Saunders Co., 2002, pp. 729–733 (Dressings) and 767–773 (Suture Techniques).
Pattison, A.M. and Pattison, G.L.: *Periodontal Instrumentation,* 2nd ed. Norwalk, CT, Appleton & Lange, 1992, pp. 441–451, 452–457.
Vernino, A.R.: Principles of Periodontal Surgery, in Fedi, P.F., Vernino, A.R., and Gray, J.L.: *The Periodontic Syllabus,* 4th ed. Philadelphia, Lippincott Williams & Wilkins, 2000, pp. 113–121.

Sutures

Hutchens, L.H.: Periodontal Suturing: A Review of Needles, Materials, and Techniques, *Postgrad. Dent., 2,* 3, Number 4, 1995.

Selvig, K.A., Biagiotti, G.R., Leknes, K.N., and Wikesjo, U.M.E.: Oral Tissue Reactions to Suture Materials, *Internat. J. Periodont. Restorative Dent., 18,* 475, Number 5, 1998.
Shaw, R.J., Negus, T.W., and Mellor, T.K.: A Prospective Clinical Evaluation of the Longevity of Resorbable Sutures in Oral Mucosa, *Br. J. Oral Maxillofac. Surg., 34,* 252, June, 1996.

Dressings

Checchi, L. and Trombelli, L.: Postoperative Pain and Discomfort With and Without Periodontal Dressing in Conjunction With 0.2% Chlorhexidine Mouthwash After Apically Positioned Flap Procedure, *J. Periodontol., 64,* 1238, December, 1993.
Cheshire, P.D., Griffiths, G.S., Griffiths, B.M., and Newman, H.N.: Evaluation of the Healing Response Following Placement of Coe-Pak and an Experimental Pack After Periodontal Flap Surgery, *J. Clin. Periodontol., 23,* 188, March, 1996.
Gilbert, A.D., Lloyd, C.H., and Scrimgeour, S.N.: The Effect of a Light-Cured Periodontal Dressing Material on HeLa Cells and Fibroblasts in Vitro, *J. Periodontol., 65,* 324, April, 1994.
Jorkjend, L. and Skoglund, L.A.: Effect of Non-eugenol- and Eugenol-containing Periodontal Dressings on the Incidence and Severity of Pain After Periodontal Soft Tissue Surgery, *J. Clin. Periodontol., 17,* 341, July, 1990.
Samuelson, G., Rakes, G., and Aiello, A.: Visible-light-polymerized Periodontal Dressing for Treatment of Trauma From Orthodontic Appliances, *J. Clin. Orthod., 24,* 564, September, 1990.
Skoglund, L.A. and Jorkjend, L.: Postoperative Pain Experience After Gingivectomies Using Different Combinations of Local Anaesthetic Agents and Periodontal Dressings, *J. Clin. Periodontol., 18,* 204, March, 1991.
Smeekens, J.P.A.M., Maltha, J.C., and Renggli, H.H.: Histological Evaluation of Surgically Treated Oral Tissues After Application of a Photocuring Periodontal Dressing Material: An Animal Study, *J. Clin. Periodontol., 19,* 641, October, 1992.
Thorstensen, A.E.R., Duguid, R., and Lloyd, C.H.: The Effects of Adding Chlorhexidine and Polyhexamethylene Bisguanide to a Light-Cured Periodontal Dressing Material, *J. Oral Rehabil., 23,* 729, November, 1996.

CHAPTER 41

Dentin Hypersensitivity

Terri S. I. Tilliss, RDH, MS, MA
Janis G. Keating, RDH, MA

CHAPTER OUTLINE

When a patient presents for care, the dental hygienist is often the first oral health professional to encounter the presence of hypersensitive teeth. Individuals who suffer from hypersensitivity may be clearly uncomfortable during dental hygiene treatment, since exposure to stimuli such as the cold water spray and contact with the instruments can elicit the pain of hypersensitive teeth. Experiences of hypersensitivity outside the dental setting may also be reported. Activities of daily living such as eating or drinking cold foods or beverages may cause pain. Patients will look to the dental hygienist to provide relief from the pain they experience and to understand how this condition impacts their quality of life.

Hypersensitivity can be challenging to diagnose because the presenting symptoms can be confused with other forms of dental pain with a differing etiology. Managing hypersensitivity can be complex owing to the availability of numerous treatment approaches that vary in the degree of relief they provide for different individuals.

Understanding the predisposing factors leading to gingival recession and to cementum and enamel loss is necessary to prevent further soft and hard tissue loss and to decrease the potential for development of additional hypersensitivity. Box 41-1 provides definitions for terms relating to hypersensitivity.

■ DEFINING HYPERSENSITIVITY

There are several definitive characteristics that are associated with dentin hypersensitivity. Numerous stimuli are known to elicit the pain response in individuals with exposed dentin surfaces.

711

BOX 41-1 KEY WORDS AND ABBREVIATIONS: Dentin Hypersensitivity

Abfraction: wedge-or v-shaped cervical lesion located where the stresses caused by lateral or eccentric tooth movements during occlusal function, bruxing, or parafunctional activity results in enamel microfractures.

ADA: American Dental Association.

Dentin hypersensitivity: transient pain arising from exposed dentin, typically in response to a variety of stimuli, that cannot be explained as arising from any other form of dental defect or pathology and that subsides quickly when stimulus is removed.

FDA: Food and Drug Administration.

Hydrodynamic theory: currently accepted mechanism for pain impulse transmission to the pulp resulting from fluid movement within the dentin tubule, which stimulates the nerve endings at the dentinopulpal interface.

Intertubular dentin: dentin that is located between dentinal tubules.

Intratubular or peritubular dentin: lining of the dentinal tubules that becomes mineralized with increasing age, resulting in thicker, sclerotic dentin.

Iontophoresis: a means of applying medications with the assistance of a small electric current to impregnate with ions of soluble salts; used in dentistry to transfer fluoride ions into the tooth.

Neural depolarization mechanism: reduction of the resting potential of the nerve membrane so that a nerve impulse is fired. At rest, the inner surface of the nerve fiber is negatively charged and impermeable to sodium ions. A stimulus temporarily alters the membrane, making it permeable so that potassium leaks out and sodium rushes into the nerve fiber. This mechanism is known as the sodium-potassium pump. This reversal of electrical charge, or **depolarization**, creates the nerve impulse. The process then reverses, and the membrane potential is restored, or **repolarized.**

Osmosis: the passage of fluids and solutions of lesser concentration through a selective membrane to one of greater solute concentration.

OTC: over the counter.

Patent: open, unobstructed.

Secondary dentin: dentin that is secreted slowly over time after root formation to 'wall off' the pulp from fluid flow within dentinal tubules following a stimulus; results in narrower pulp chamber and root canals.

Smear layer: has been referred to as 'grinding debris' from instrumentation or other devices that are applied to the tooth; consists of microcrystalline particles of cementum, dentin, tissue, and cellular debris; serves to plug tubule orifices.

Tertiary/reparative dentin: a type of dentin formed along the pulpal wall or root canal as a protective mechanism in response to trauma or irritation, as from caries or a traumatic cavity preparation.

I. IDENTIFYING CHARACTERISTICS

- Sharp, short, or transient pain of rapid onset.
- Presents as a chronic condition with acute episodes.
- Discomfort that cannot be ascribed to any other dental defect or pathology.[1]
- Cessation from pain upon removal of stimulus.
- Pain in response to a non-noxious stimulus, one that would not normally cause pain or discomfort.

II. ELICITING STIMULI

A. *Tactile or mechanical*: contact with toothbrush or other oral hygiene devices, eating utensils, periodontal and dental instruments, and friction from prosthetic devices such as denture clasps.

B. *Thermal*: temperature change caused by hot and cold foods and beverages, and cold air as it contacts the teeth.

C. *Evaporative*: dehydration of oral fluids as from high-volume evacuation or use of air syringe to dry teeth during intraoral procedures.

D. *Osmotic*: alteration of osmotic pressure in tubules due to isotonic solutions of sugar and salt.

E. *Chemical*: acids in foods and beverages such as citrus fruits, condiments, spices, wine and carbonated beverages; also acids from acidogenic bacteria following carbohydrate exposure; from acidic gastric regurgitation.

▪ ETIOLOGY OF DENTIN HYPERSENSITIVITY

Dentin hypersensitivity is preceded by gingival recession. When gingiva is no longer covering the root portion of the tooth and cemental loss has exposed the dentin, then the exposed tooth surface is susceptible to hypersensitivity.

Although less common, loss of enamel and subsequent dentin exposure on the crown of the tooth can also lead to hypersensitivity. Both enamel and cementum may be lost either gradually or suddenly. Enamel is less susceptible to demineralization than cementum since it has a higher mineral content. A more acute hypersensitivity will develop with sudden dentin exposure since gradual exposure would allow for the development of protective measures such as smear layer, sclerosis, and proliferation of secondary or reparative dentin. There are a number of predisposing factors that contribute to hypersensitivity, with rarely one single cause. A review of tooth biology contributes to an understanding of the mechanism of hypersensitivity.

I. BIOLOGY OF TOOTH STRUCTURES

A. Dentin

- The portion of the tooth covered by enamel on the crown and cementum on the root.
- Composed of a series of fluid-filled tubules, which become narrower in diameter and branch as they extend from the pulp to the dentinoenamel junction, as shown in Figure 41-1.
- Dentinal tubules are the portals through which stimuli are transmitted to the pulp.
- Innervated with nerve fibers from the pulp chamber; the odontoblastic processes extend only a short distance into the dentin tubules, as shown in Figure 41-1.

B. Pulp

- Highly innervated with nerve fiber endings that extend just beyond the dentinopulpal interface of the dentinal tubules; nerve fibers intertwine around the odontoblastic processes.[2]
- Odontoblasts (dentin-producing cells) located adjacent to the pulp extend their processes from the dentinopulpal interface about one-third of the way through the dentinal tubule. The processes are not thought to be responsible for transmission of the pain response from the stimulus to the pulpal nerve fibers due to their limited length.[3]
- Nerves exhibit excitability via the same neural depolarization mechanism (sodium-potassium pump), which characterizes the response of any nerve to a stimulus.

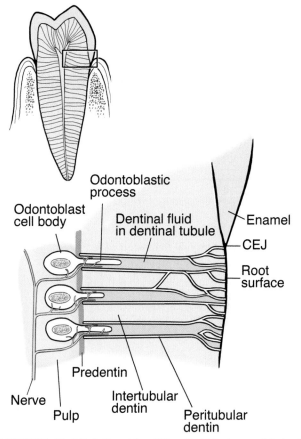

▪ **FIGURE 41-1 Relationship of Dentin Tubules and Pulpal Nerve Endings.** Nerve endings from the pulp wrap themselves around the odontoblasts that extend only a short distance into the tubule. Fluid-filled dentin tubules transmit fluid disturbances through the mechanism known as hydraulic conductance.

II. MECHANISMS OF DENTIN EXPOSURE

Ideally, gingival tissue provides a protective covering over the root surface. If the gingiva no longer covers the root, the cemental surface is vulnerable to wear and subsequent dentin exposure. It is this process of gingival recession, cemental loss, and subsequent dentin exposure that sets the stage for the development of hypersensitivity, as seen in Figure 41-2. The development of gingival recession has a multifactorial etiology.[4,5]

A. Factors Contributing to Gingival Recession and Subsequent Root Exposure

- Effects of oral hygiene self-care:
  - Use of medium or hard filament toothbrush.
  - Frequent or aggressive toothbrushing and/or other oral hygiene devices.

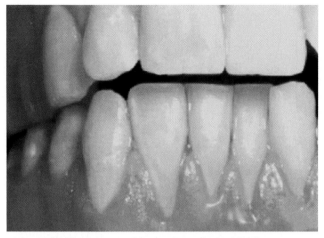

■ FIGURE 41-2 Gingival Recession of Mandibular Incisors. Note severe recession on the left central incisor and moderate recession on the right central and lateral incisors. If the thin cemental layer of the exposed root surface is lost, dentin hypersensitivity can develop.

- An anatomic narrow zone of attached gingiva that is more susceptible to abrasion.
- A thin labial plate of bone that is often consistent with a labial orientation of one or more teeth.
- A tight and short frenum attachment that can pull on gingival tissues during oral movement.
- Tissue destructive patterns of periodontal diseases, including periodontitis and necrotizing ulcerative gingivitis (NUG); junctional epithelium migrates apically in response to inflammatory factors, leading to connective tissue breakdown and loss of periodontal attachment.
- Periodontal surgical procedures to alter the architecture of gingival tissues.
- Debridement procedures that resolve tissue inflammation with the objective of tissue shrinkage.
- Oral surgery procedures such as crown lengthening, repositioning of gingival tissues, or tooth extraction that can affect remaining teeth.
- Orthodontic tooth movement may result in apical migration of the junctional epithelium.
- Subgingival instrumentation involving scaling and root planing of shallow sulci.[6]
- Restorative procedures, such as crown preparation, that abrade marginal gingival tissues.
- The aging process, along with the contribution of lifetime periodontal infections and misuse of oral hygiene devices.

B. Loss of Enamel and Cementum

Loss of tooth structure rarely develops from a single cause but rather from a combination of contributing factors.
- Cementum at the cervical area is thin (0.05 mm) and is subject to wear.
- Enamel and cementum do not meet at the CEJ in about 10% of teeth, leaving an area of exposed dentin, as shown in Figure 14-2.
- Attrition and abrasion cause loss of tooth structure, but over time these gradual traumatic processes also stimulate natural protective measures such as secondary dentin and sclerosis.
- Erosion from dietary acids, such as citrus fruits/juices, wine, and cola drinks, especially combined with abrasion from toothbrushing and toothpaste.[7,8]
  - Brushing with toothpaste immediately after consumption of acidic food or drink should be avoided.[1]
  - Gastric acids from such conditions as gastric reflux, morning sickness, or self-induced vomiting (bulimia) frequently exposing teeth to a highly acidic environment.
- Abfraction, a cervical lesion caused by occlusal stresses or tooth flexure from bruxing, can lead to loss of tooth structure due to enamel chipping away from the cervical portion of the tooth, as shown in Figure 41-3.
  - Lesion appears as a wedge- or V-shaped cervical notch.
  - A co-factor with abrasion.
- Crown preparation procedures that remove enamel or cementum can expose dentin at the cervical area.
- Instrumentation during scaling or root debridement procedures.
- Frequent or improper stain removal techniques, where abrasive particles abrade and wear away the cementum.
- Root caries that disrupts the intact cementum to expose the dentin.

■ NATURAL DESENSITIZATION

Hypersensitivity can decrease over time, even without treatment interventions, because nature provides several mechanisms that gradually reduce hypersensitivity. When conducting clinical research trials, it can be challenging to determine the effects of treatment regimens, since natural desensitizing is also occurring. Many of the commercial desensitization agents have been designed to

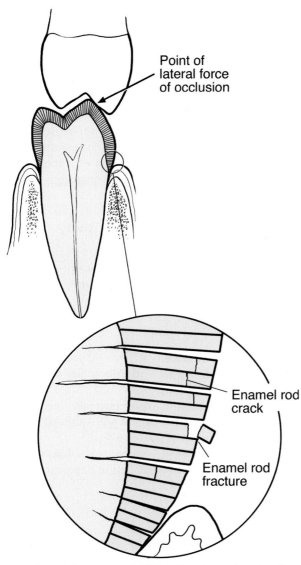

• Results in a smaller-diameter tubule that is less able to transmit stimuli through the dentinal fluid to the nerve fibers at the dentinopulpal interface.

II. SECONDARY DENTIN

• Deposited over time after teeth are fully developed, secreted more slowly than primary dentin that formed prior to tooth eruption; both types of dentin are created by odontoblasts.
• Deposited on the floor and roof of the pulp chamber, which decreases the size of pulp tissue over time.
• Creates a "walling off" effect between the dentinal tubules and the pulp to insulate the pulp from dentin fluid disturbances caused by a stimulus.

III. TERTIARY DENTIN/REPARATIVE DENTIN

• Formed in the area where exposed dentin has been traumatized by a stimulus such as dental caries.
• Similar to secondary dentin.
• Tertiary dentin insulates the pulp from dentinal tubule fluid disturbances.

IV. SMEAR LAYER

• Consists of a combination of organic and inorganic microcrystalline shavings of cementum, dentin, and also contains tissue debris, odontoblastic processes, and other microbial elements.[9]
• Occludes the dentinal tubule orifices, forming a "smear plug" or a "natural bandage" that blocks stimuli; toothpaste abrasives help to create the smear layer.
• Occurs from scaling and root instrumentation, cutting with a bur attrition, or burnishing with a toothbrush, toothpick, or other device.
• Dynamic nature of the smear layer is subject to dissolution by acids or mechanical disruption, such as from ultrasonic debridement.
• Smear layer may have a positive or negative effect. It protects from hypersensitivity, but may interfere with reattachment of periodontal tissues.

V. CALCULUS FORMATION

Provides a protective coating to shield exposed dentin from stimuli and explains postdebridement sensitivity that can occur after removal of heavy calculus.

■ **FIGURE 41-3 Process of Abfraction.** Lateral occlusal forces stress the enamel rods at the cervical area, resulting in enamel rod fracture over time. In an advanced stage, a wedge- or V-shaped cervical lesion is visible. Although minute cracks in the enamel rods may not be clinically evident, the tooth can exhibit hypersensitivity.

simulate the natural methods of desensitization. There are several mechanisms by which desensitization can naturally occur over time.

I. SCLEROSIS OF DENTIN

• Occurs by mineral deposition within tubules as a result of traumatic stimuli, such as attrition or dental caries.
• Creates a thicker, highly mineralized layer of *peritubular* dentin (deposited within the periphery of the tubules).

■ IMPULSE TRANSMISSION

I. HYDRODYNAMIC THEORY

Hydrodynamic theory is the currently accepted explanation for transmission of stimuli from the outer surface of dentin to the pulp.

   A. Developed by Brannstrom in the 1960s,[10] who theorized that a stimulus at the outer aspect of dentin will cause fluid movement within the dentinal tubule, which signals the nerves in the pulp.

   B. Credibility for this theory is supported by the larger number of widened dentin tubules seen with hypersensitive teeth compared with non-sensitive teeth.[11] Figure 41-4 depicts open dentinal tubules at the microscopic level.

II. NEURAL ACTIVITY

Pain is registered by the depolarization/neural discharge mechanism that characterizes all nerve activity. The sodium-potassium pump is responsible for depolarizing the nerve as potassium leaves the nerve cell and sodium enters it.

■ CHARACTERIZING PATIENTS AND THEIR PAIN

Different individuals react differently to pain based upon factors such as age, gender, situation and context, previous experiences, present expectations, and other psychological and physiological parameters.

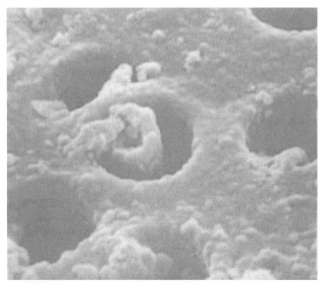

■ **FIGURE 41-4 Open Dentin Tubules.** Open dentin tubules as seen in dentin hypersensitivity surround a partially occluded tubule (center) viewed with scanning electron microscopy.

I. PATIENT PROFILE

The reported prevalence of hypersensitivity varies due to differences in the stimulus, and how it was applied, and whether data are gathered by patient report or clinical examination. Patient accounts may not represent true hypersensitivity since the pain can be confused with other conditions. Therefore, selection of a standardized clinical examination technique is advantageous for identifying hypersensitivity.

A. Prevalence of Hypersensitivity

   • It has been reported that 8% to 30% of the adult population experiences hypersensitivity.[12]
   • Higher prevalence has been reported in periodontally involved populations.[13]

B. Age

   • Greatest incidence is at 20 to 40 years of age.[12]
   • Incidence and severity declines after the 4th and 5th decades of life.[4]
   • Gingival recession, loss of enamel/cementum is more prevalent among the aged, although dentin hypersensitivity is not.
   • Natural mechanisms of desensitization, such as sclerosis and secondary dentin deposition, occur with aging.

C. Gender

Although hypersensitivity apparently occurs equally between men and women,[12,14] women report more hypersensitivity and report pain differently than men.[15]

D. Teeth Affected

   • Teeth with gingival recession are most likely to exhibit dentin sensitivity.
   • Hypersensitivity occurs on any tooth; primarily at the cervical one-third of the buccal/facial surfaces of premolars and canines.

II. THE PAIN EXPERIENCE

A. Pain Perception

   • Stimuli that affect the fluid flow within the dentinal tubules can activate the receptors of terminal nerve endings near to or surrounding the dentinal tubules; activation of these nerve fibers elicits the pain reception.

- Pain experience is not always in direct proportion to the degree of recession, the amount of tooth structure loss, or to the quality or quantity of stimulus.
- Pain, a subjective phenomenon, is experienced differently by individuals (page 584). Many variables, such as stress, fatigue, and health beliefs, impact pain perception.

B. Impact of Pain

- Individuals with hypersensitivity may experience elements of both acute and chronic pain; acute pain may lead to anxiety, whereas chronic pain may be associated with depression.
- Stress may exacerbate the pain response and is a consideration in the dental hygiene care plan.
- The persistent discomfort from dentin hypersensitivity may affect one's daily life.

■ DIFFERENTIAL DIAGNOSIS

When a patient presents with pain, a differential diagnosis is conducted prior to treating for hypersensitivity. Etiology of pain can be systemic, pulpal, periapical, restorative, degenerative, or neoplastic. Effective interviewing combined with diagnostic techniques and tests will assist in the differential diagnosis. The dental hygienist may conduct several of the diagnostic tests to provide the data needed for appropriate diagnosis. When other probable causes of pain have been ruled out, hypersensitivity can be discussed with the patient and treatment options explored.

I. DESCRIBING THE PAIN OF DENTIN HYPERSENSITIVITY

- Hypersensitivity pain experienced from a non-noxious stimulus, such as cold water, can mimic pain experienced from a noxious agent, such as dental caries.
- Hypersensitivity and other types of pain are reported by the patient as being in the mild-to-moderate range and can be intensified by thermal, sweet, and sour stimuli.
- Pulpal pain is from deep dental caries, pulpal inflammation, or infection and is severe, intermittent, and throbbing; it may occur without provocation and persist after stimulus is removed.
  - Pain of hypersensitivity subsides after stimulus removal.
  - Hot and/or cold stimuli can elicit both the pain of hypersensitivity and pulpal pain.

- Chewing (occlusal pressure) elicits only a pulpal pain response.

II. DATA COLLECTION BY INTERVIEW

- A. Direct, Open-Ended Questions
  - Help to establish the location, degree of pain, onset/duration, stimuli, intensity, and relieving factors related to the painful response; patients may have difficulty characterizing the pain.
  - Trigger questions as suggested in Box 41-2 can elicit detailed information to help characterize the pain and assist in the dental hygiene diagnosis.
- B. Establishing rapport and utilizing effective listening and counseling skills are essential for developing treatment/management strategies.
- C. Dental history, including pain chronology, nature, location, aggravating and alleviating factors, and history of dental treatment/restorations.

BOX 41-2 Trigger Questions for Data Collection

- Which tooth or teeth is/are sensitive and on which aspect?

- On a scale from 1 to 10, how much does it hurt, with 10 being the most painful?

- How long does the pain last?

- Can the pain be characterized as sharp, dull, shooting, throbbing, persistent, constant, pressure, burning, intermittent?

- Does it hurt when you bite down (pressure)?

- Does the discomfort linger or stop immediately after a stimulus such as cold water is removed?

- On a scale from 1 to 10, how much does the pain impact your daily life?

- Is the pain stimulated by certain foods? Sweet? Sour? Acidic?

- Does sensitivity result from hot or cold food or beverages?

- Does discomfort stop immediately upon removal of the painful stimuli, such as cold food or beverage?

- How effectively are you managing the stress in your life?

III. DIAGNOSTIC TECHNIQUES AND TESTS

Patients may have difficulty in describing and localizing their pain; therefore, diagnostic techniques and tests can assist in differentiating among the numerous causes of tooth pain.

A. Clinical examination of the teeth and palpation of surrounding tissues.

B. Evaluation of nasal congestion, drainage, or sinus pressure may indicate sinus infection that is expressed as tooth pain.

C. Occlusal examination utilizing marking paper to detect existing premature contact or hyperfunction created by placement of a new restoration or crown.

D. Radiographic examination to indicate possible pulpal pathology or other irregularities of the teeth or surrounding structures.

E. Percussion or tapping of teeth with instrument handle; a pain response may be indicative of pulpitis.

F. Mobility testing to detect trauma or periodontal pathology (page 240).

G. Pain from biting pressure as assessed with a bite stick may indicate tooth fracture.

H. Transillumination with a high-intensity focused light enhances visualization of a cracked tooth; dyes may also be useful to indicate a fracture line.

I. Thermal and electric pulp tests may indicate pulpal pathology (page 273).

Signs, symptoms, and specific clinical assessments utilized to differentiate a variety of conditions characterized as tooth pain are detailed in Table 41-1.

■ HYPERSENSITIVITY MANAGEMENT

When the differential diagnosis reveals dentinal hypersensitivity, the dental hygiene care plan includes further assessment and patient education in conjunction with treatment interventions.

I. ASSESSMENT COMPONENTS

A. Determine Extent and Severity of Pain

*   Self-report of symptoms, including the eliciting stimuli.

*   Establish a baseline of pain intensity using objective measures such as the Visual Analog Scale (VAS) and/or the Verbal Rating Scale (VRS) to quantify the subjective phenomenon of pain, as described in Box 41-3.

*   Maintain the VAS/VRS assessment form in the patient record.

B. Evaluate inappropriate oral hygiene self-care procedures that may contribute to loss of gingiva or tooth structure.

C. Assess the degree of acidic food and beverage intake utilizing a diet analysis (pages 528 to 530); correlate with timing of toothbrushing.

D. Determine prevalence of parafunctional habits, such as bruxing, that may contribute to abfraction.

E. Assess stress levels and stress-reduction efforts.

II. EDUCATIONAL CONSIDERATIONS

A. Provide education regarding etiology and contributing factors. Explain time-dependent natural improvement in sensitivity.

B. Encourage patients to select realistic self-care practices to increase commitment.

C. Utilize effective communication to increase compliance and to decrease patient anxiety.

D. Describe and teach self-care measures; involve the patient in technique demonstrations.

III. TREATMENT HIERARCHY

A. Treatment goals include pain relief and modification or elimination of contributing factors.

B. Mild to moderate pain can be addressed with conservative, but slower-acting, activities or agents; more severe pain will require an aggressive approach.

C. Proceed from the most conservative and least invasive measures to more aggressive modalities.

D. Pain resolution is difficult to predict due to variable success with different treatment options among individuals.

*   Historically, a vast array of treatment approaches have been utilized with varying degrees of success; no one best method has been identified.

*   Characteristics of an ideal desensitizing agent are listed in Box 41-4 and are useful evaluation criteria when selecting a desensitizing agent.

*   A trial-and-error approach may be necessary until a particular treatment option is found to be most effective.

E. Treatment options consist of self-care measures and professional interventions or a combination; these approaches have synergistic effects with the same objective of reducing hypersensitivity.

■ TABLE 41-1 DIFFERENTIAL DIAGNOSIS OF TOOTH PAIN

CONDITION	SIGNS AND SYMPTOMS	CLINICAL ASSESSMENT
Dentinal hypersensitivity	Thermal, mechanical, evaporative, osmotic, chemical sensitivity Sharp, sudden, transient pain	Clinical examination: gingival recession and loss of tooth structure
Caries extending into dentin	Thermal sensitivity Pain upon pressure Pain with sweets	Clinical examination Radiographic examination
Pulpal caries	Thermal stimuli Severe, intermittent, throbbing pain on chewing	Clinical examination Radiographic examination
Fractured restoration	Thermal sensitivity Pain upon pressure	Clinical examination
Fractured tooth	Thermal sensitivity Pain upon pressure	Occlusal examination Transillumination
Recently placed restoration	Thermal sensitivity Pain upon pressure	Dental history Clinical examination Occlusal examination
Occlusal trauma	Chemical sensitivity Thermal sensitivity Pain upon pressure Mobility	Occlusal examination
Pulpitis	Severe, intermittent throbbing pain	Percussion Thermal and electric pulp tests
Sinus infection	"Nondescript" tooth pain Nasal congestion (drainage) Sinus pressure	Clinical examination, including extraoral sinus palpation Radiographic examination
Galvanic pain	Sudden stabbing pain upon tooth to tooth contact	Examination for contact between restoration of dissimilar, nonprecious metals
Periodontal ligament inflammation	Pain on chewing	Percussion Clinical examination, including palpation for apical tenderness
Abfraction	"Cratered" areas of enamel or dentin at CEJ in the shape of a wedge- or V-shaped notch Thermal, mechanical, evaporative, osmotic, chemical sensitivity Sharp, sudden, transient pain	Clinical examination Occlusal examination

IV. REASSESSMENT

A. Evaluate Treatment Interventions

- Allow sufficient time to elapse to evaluate effectiveness of treatment recommendations and effects of natural desensitization.
- Repeat the VAS and/or the VRS to compare changes in pain perceptions from baseline.

B. Persistent pain may require systematic use of various desensitizing interventions and agents, comparing outcomes.

■ DENTAL HYGIENE CARE AND TREATMENT INTERVENTIONS

I. MECHANISMS OF DESENSITIZATION

Treatment for hypersensitivity is based on the principles of the hydrodynamic theory with the aim of interrupting pain transmission in several ways.

A. Nerve depolarization by interfering with the sodium-potassium pump mechanism.

BOX 41-3 Subjective Pain Assessment Form

Name: _____

Date: _____

Teeth: _____

VAS—Visual Analog Scale

Please place an 'X' on the line at a position between the two extremes to represent the level of pain that you experience.

No Discomfort |————————————————| Severe Discomfort

VRS—Verbal Rating Scale

Please describe the pain you experience on a scale from 0 to 3:

0 = No discomfort/pain, but aware of stimulus

1 = Mild discomfort/pain

2 = Marked discomfort/pain

3 = Marked discomfort/pain that lasted more than 10 seconds

Adapted from Melzach, R.: *Pain Measurement and Assessment*. New York, Raven Press, 1983.

- Potassium based products are believed to depolarize the nerve fiber membrane.[16]
- The potassium may maintain the nerve fibers in a depolarized state in which the pain response does not occur.

BOX 41-4 Ideal Desensitizing Agents

- Easy application procedure
- Minimal application time
- Does not endanger the soft tissues
- Inexpensive
- Requires few dental appointments
- Does not cause pulpal irritation or pain
- Rapid and lasting effect
- Causes no staining
- Consistently effective
- Acceptable taste

Adapted from Grossman, L.I.: A Systematic Method for Treatment of Hypersensitive Dentin, *J. Am. Dent. Assoc., 22*, 592, 1935.

B. Occlusion of dentin tubule orifices to prevent fluid disturbance from a stimulus.

C. Sclerosis of the dentin tubule lumen, decreasing the inner diameter and resulting in reduced fluid flow.

D. Tubule sealing, bonding, or placing a physical barrier between the dentin and stimulus.

E. Eliminate pain stimulus; allow time for natural desensitization mechanisms to decrease sensitivity.

II. SELF-CARE MEASURES

- Institute self-care measures prior to or with self-applied or professional desensitizing measures.
- Encourage behavioral change from risky to protective habits.
- Inform the patient that it may take 2 to 4 weeks to notice a decrease in sensitivity.

A. Dietary Modifications

- Limit foods and beverages that incite a pain response, including citrus fruits and juices, acidic soda/cola beverages, sharp flavors and spices, pickled foods, wine, and ciders; these dissolve the smear layer, resulting in dentinal tubules open to effects of a stimulus.
- Discourage brushing immediately after ingesting acidic foods to eliminate the combined effects of

erosion and abrasion, which can accelerate tooth structure loss.

- Eliminate extremes of hot and cold foods and beverages.
- Refer for treatment those patients with eating disorders or systemic conditions that repeatedly create an acidic oral environment.

B. Dental Biofilm Control

- In the presence of dental biofilms, the dentinal tubule orifice increases to three times the original size; subsequent reestablishment of biofilm control measures results in a 20% decrease in the size of the dentinal tubule orifice, suggesting a deleterious role of biofilm acids.[17]
- Clinical evidence indicates that the presence of dental biofilm on exposed root surfaces does not always correlate with dentin sensitivity.[4]
- Meticulous, gentle dental biofilm control measures that do not abrade gingival tissues or cervical hard tooth structure are recommended.

C. Toothbrush Type and Technique

- Use of a soft or ultra-soft toothbrush and focused brushing of one or two teeth, rather than one long horizontal stroke over several teeth, may prevent further recession and loss of tooth structure.
- Professional observation of brushing technique allows for correction of unsafe brushing techniques and reinforcement of safe and effective dental biofilm removal; simple alterations can reduce and prevent dentin hypersensitivity.
- Toothbrushing is sequenced by beginning in least sensitive areas and ending with more sensitive areas; the filaments are stiffer and brushing is more aggressive in the initial phases of brushing.
- Using the nondominant hand exerts less pressure than with the dominant hand.
- A modified pen grasp rather than a traditional palm grasp will reduce the amount of pressure applied.
- Use of a power toothbrush removes dental biofilm effectively using less than half the pressure of a manual toothbrush; a manual brush exerts 200 to 400 grams/pressure while power brushes require 70 to 150 grams/pressure.[18] Additionally, some power toothbrushes have a self-limiting mechanism to reduce filament action if too much pressure is applied.

D. Burnishing

- Repeated rubbing of the tooth with a toothpick or wood stick is referred to as burnishing; see

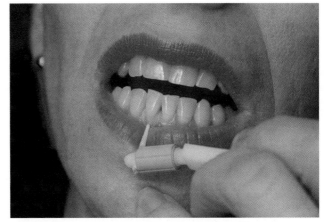

■ **FIGURE 41-5 Burnishing Sensitive Root Surface.** A small amount of a fluoride agent or fluoride dentifrice can be burnished into the sensitive area with a toothpick or wooden point. Moderate pressure with a "rubbing" or circular stroke is applied. A toothpick holder facilitates effective use of a toothpick to burnish an exposed root surface.

Figure 41-5 for placement of toothpick. This contributes to the formation of a smear layer that occludes the dentinal tubules.
- Use of a toothpick and fluoride dentifrice for burnishing can reduce sensitivity by occluding tubule openings with fluoride or dentifrice particles.[19]
- Burnishing activity of the toothpick itself may result in increased production of secondary or reparative dentin, which is produced to counteract the physical irritation.

III. SELF-APPLIED AGENTS

A. Desensitizing Agents Used in Dentifrices

- 5% potassium nitrate is the primary ingredient in OTC sensitivity-reducing dentifrices and has been approved by the FDA and ADA.
- Fluoride is also contained in desensitizing dentifrice formulations.
  - Sodium, stannous, and monofluorophosphate particles provide some occlusion of dentin tubules.[20]
  - Sodium fluoride also precipitates calcium fluoride crystals to decrease the lumen size.[21]
- Use of dentifrices containing abrasive particles occludes dentinal tubules.[22]
- Tartar control dentifrices can result in increased tooth sensitivity for some individuals, although the mechanism is unknown.

B. Concentrated Fluoride Desensitizing Agents

- Stannous fluoride gel (0.4%)
  - Occludes dentinal tubules.
  - Scleroses the lumen with tin and fluoride particles.[23]
- Sodium fluoride (1.1%)
  - Creates a barrier by precipitating calcium fluoride at the dentin surface.
  - Precipitate is soluble in saliva, which explains the transitory nature of fluoride, requiring continued daily application.[21]
- OTC or prescription high-dose fluoride gels or pastes are brushed onto the affected teeth or applied with a tray technique after removal of dental biofilm.
- Application is recommended just prior to bed or when eating, drinking, and rinsing has concluded for the day.

C. Mouthrinses

When many teeth are affected, concentrated neutral sodium fluoride prescription mouthrinse can be utilized for desensitization. Acidic mouthrinses are discouraged due to exacerbation of hypersensitivity, particularly when immediately followed by toothbrushing.

IV. PROFESSIONAL MEASURES

A. Periodontal Debridement Considerations

- Prior to debridement, the possibility of postprocedure sensitivity is explained; patients respond more favorably to treatment when they know what to expect.
- For patients who present with hypersensitivity, comfort during treatment can be facilitated with use of the following:
  - 5% Sodium fluoride varnishes.
  - 0.4% Stannous fluoride, 1.09% sodium fluoride, and 0.14% hydrogen fluoride combined.
  - 2.7% Potassium oxalate, 6% ferric oxalate, or aluminum oxalate.
  - 5% Gluteraldehyde and 35% hydroxyethylmethacrylate (HEMA).
  - Nitrous oxide sedation.
  - Local anesthesia (for severe or pervasive hypersensitivity).
- Following periodontal debridement:
  - Apply sodium fluoride varnish.
  - Instruct patient in daily use of self-applied agents.

B. Sclerosing Agents

- Sodium fluoride varnish creates a precipitate of calcium fluoride-like globules that form a precipitate[24]; the varnish vehicle prolongs the contact between fluoride and the dentin, which is likely to promote precipitation within the dentin tubule lumen. The use of fluoride varnish for the treatment of dentin hypersensitivity was approved by the FDA in 1994.
  - Application does not require drying the tooth with air, since the material sets in the presence of moisture. The surface is blotted with gauze; a microbrush is utilized to paint the exposed dentin surface with the varnish (page 555).
  - Daily oral hygiene self-care is not resumed until the next day to allow the fluoride to fully impregnate the tooth surface.
- Stannous fluoride (0.4%) is applied utilizing tray delivery. In-office therapy is often followed by daily applications by the patient.
- 5% Gluteraldehyde preparations coagulate proteins and amino acids within the dentinal tubule to decrease the lumen size. 5% Gluteraldehyde combined with HEMA, a hydrophilic resin, acts to seal tubules in combination with the sclerosing property of gluteraldehyde for a stronger desensitizing effect.
  - Application requires cotton roll isolation; minimal amounts are applied to the surface with a microbrush excess.
  - Prevent excess flow into soft tissues since gluteraldehyde may cause gingival irritation.
- Dibasic calcium phosphate and calcium hydroxide create calcium crystals or stimulate reparative dentin to reduce dentin sensitivity. However, calcium hydroxide can be readily dissolved by dietary and biofilm acids.

C. Occluding Agents

- Stannous fluoride.
- Strontium chloride, which precipitates to occlude tubule openings.
- Oxalates such as ferric oxalate and potassium oxalate, which form insoluble calcium oxalate crystals that occlude the tubules.[25,26]

D. Tubule Sealing or Bonding Agents

The tubule openings are sealed over to prevent stimuli from signaling the nerves at the dentinopulpal interface.

- Resins are applied following an acid etch step, which may remove the smear layer, often creating

Everyday Ethics

? Marcy practices in a dental practice where the dentist, Dr. Goldman, sees the patient at every other dental hygiene visit unless requested for special needs.

Mrs. Stuart arrives for her dental hygiene appointment but is not scheduled to see Dr. Goldman until her next visit. She is complaining of discomfort "on the lower back teeth" when she chews and when she eats or drinks something cold. The pain may last up to an hour.

At the completion of the scaling and debridement, Marcy gives Mrs. Stuart a sample of desensitizing toothpaste and suggests they will see how it is at the next appointment. Marcy then advised Mrs. Stuart to "Call if it gives you more trouble." The patient is not classified as having a peri-odontal condition, and she is not particularly dental caries prone, so her next visit will be in 6 months.

Questions for Consideration

1. What obligation, if any, do Marcy and Dr. Goldman have to this patient to conduct an oral/dental exam during this appointment to establish a differential diagnosis?

2. Discuss several aspects of informed consent that apply to this patient's right-to-know about dental sensitivity.

3. How should the maintenance recall interval be structured to meet the needs of this patient? Explain the rationale.

---

discomfort. The tooth surface must be dehydrated prior to resin application, which can also create discomfort and may require the use of local anesthetic to control pain.
- Dentin sealers obturate the tubule opening and do not require use of an acid etch step or dehydration.
- Methylmethacrylate polymer seals the tubule opening.

E. Physical Blocking

- Periodontal soft tissue grafts cover the sensitive dentinal surface, yet often with unpredictable results.
- Composite/glass ionomer restorations.
- Crown placement.

F. Iontophoresis

- A low-voltage electric current is used to impregnate the tooth with ions from fluoride.
- Two to six times more fluoride can be incorporated into dentin than when treated with traditional delivery of topical sodium fluoride.[27]

G. Lasers

- Lasers such as the Nd:Yag have been used in conjunction with sodium fluoride varnish.[28] Laser-applied fluoride can close previously open dentinal tubules.[29] Long-term in-vivo studies are

needed to establish safety and efficacy. FDA approval of such devices for this therapeutic modality has not been obtained.

H. Eliminate Parafunctional Habits

Interruption of bruxing and clenching behaviors in combination with other self-care interventions can reduce dentinal hypersensitivity.[30] Occlusal adjustments to eliminate abfractive forces may also be considered. Stress reduction protocols can be discussed and utilized to reduce subconscious parafunctional behaviors.

I. Tooth Whitening–Induced Sensitivity

Tooth whitening agents may contribute to increased dentinal hypersensitivity, although this effect dissipates over time. Individuals with exposed dentin and existing dentin hypersensitivity are at increased risk for hypersensitivity secondary to tooth whitening.
- As many as 1/4 of individuals who use whitening agents in prefabricated trays develop dentin hypersensitivity.[31]
- Recommendations to prevent or reduce tooth whitening–induced sensitivity:
  - Concurrent use of a potassium nitrate dentifrice.
  - Lower concentration of carbamide peroxide.
  - Desensitizing agents with occluding properties may block tubules from receiving the whitening agent.

✔ **Factors To Teach The Patient**

- Etiology of gingival recession.

- Activities and habits that may contribute to dentin hypersensitivity.

- Mechanisms of dentin tubule exposure, allowing various stimuli to trigger pain response that is transmitted to the nerve of the tooth.

- Natural desensitization mechanisms that can improve sensitivity over time.

- Importance of appropriate oral hygiene self-care techniques, such as using a soft toothbrush and avoiding a vigorous brushing technique that may contribute to gingival recession and subsequent abrasion of root surface.

- Connection between an acidic diet and dentin sensitivity; specific foods and beverages that should be limited.

- Toothbrushing should not immediately follow consumption of acidic foods or beverages or use of acidic mouthwashes.

- Why all agents available for treatment do not reduce dentin hypersensitivity equally for all teeth.

- The challenges of managing hypersensitivity, hierarchy of treatment measures, and variability in resolution of pain.

REFERENCES

1. Addy, M.: Etiology and Clinical Implications of Dentine Hypersensitivity, *Dent. Clin. North Am., 34,* 503, July, 1990.

2. Frank, R.M.: Attachment Sites Between Odontoblast Process and the Intradentinal Nerve Fibre, *Arch. Oral Biol., 13,* 833, July, 1968.

3. Thomas, H.F. and Cavrella, P.: Correlation of Scanning and Transmission Electron Microscopy of Human Dentinal Tubules, *Arch. Oral. Biol., 29,* 641, August, 1984.

4. Addy, M. and Pearce, N.: Aetiological, Predisposing and Environmental Factors in Dentine Hypersensitivity, *Arch. Oral. Biol., 39,* 33S, Supplement, 1994.

5. Dababneh, R.H., Khouri, A.T., and Addy, M.: Dentine Hypersensitivity: An Enigma? A Review of Terminology, Epidemiology, Mechanisms, Aetiology, and Management, *Br. Dent. J., 187,* 606, December 11, 1999.

6. Dufour, L.A. and Bissell, H.S.: Periodontal Attachment Loss Induced by Mechanical Subgingival Instrumentation in Shallow Sulci, *J. Dent. Hyg., 76,* 207, Summer, 2002.

7. Prati, C., Montebugnoli, L., Suppa, P., Valdre, G., and Mongiorgi, R.: Permeability and Morphology of Dentin After Erosion Induced by Acidic Drinks, *J. Periodontol., 74,* 428, April, 2003.

8. Absi, E.G., Addy, M., and Adams, D.: Dentine Hypersensitivity: The Effect of Toothbrushing and Dietary Compounds on Dentine In Vitro, *J. Oral Rehabil., 19,* 101, March, 1992.

9. Cohen, S. and Burns, R.C., eds: *Pathways of the Pulp,* 8th ed. St. Louis, Mosby, 2002, p. 305.

10. Brannstrom, M., Linden, L. A., and Astrom, A.: The Hydrodynamics of the Dental Tubule and of Pulp Fluid: A Discussion of Its Significance in Relation to Dentinal Sensitivity, *Caries Res., 1,* 310, No. 4, 1967.

11. Absi, E.G., Addy, M., and Adams, D.: Dentine Hypersensitivity: The Development and Evaluation of a Replica Technique to Study Sensitive and Non-Sensitive Cervical Dentine, *J. Clin. Periodontol., 16,* 190, March, 1989.

12. Flynn, J., Galloway, R., and Orchardson, R.: The Incidence of 'Hypersensitive' Teeth in the West of Scotland, *J. Dent., 13,* 230, September, 1985.

13. Taani, Q. and Awartani, F: Clinical Evaluation of Cervical Dentin Sensitivity (CDS) in Patients Attending General Dental Clinics and Periodontal Specialty Clinics (PSC), *J. Clin. Periodontol., 29,* 118, February, 2002.

14. Fischer, C., Fischer, R.G., and Wennberg, A.: Prevalence and Distribution of Cervical Dentine Hypersensitivity in a Population in Rio De Janeiro, Brazil, *J. Dent., 20,* 272, October, 1992.

15. Zakrzewska, J.M.: Women as Dental Patients: Are There Any Gender Differences, *Int. Dent. J., 46,* 548, December, 1996.

16. Orchardson, R. and Gillam, D.G.: The Efficacy of Potassium Salts as Agents for Treating Dentin Hypersensitivity, *J. Orofac. Pain, 14,* 9, Winter, 2000.

17. Kawasaki, A., Ishikawa, K., Suge, T., Shimizu, H., Suzuki, K., Matsuo, T., and Ebisu, S.: Effects of Plaque Control on the Patency and Occlusion of Dentine Tubules In Situ, *J. Oral Rehabil., 28,* 439, May, 2001.

18. van der Weijden, G.A., Timmerman, M.F., Reijerse, E., Snoek, C.M., and van der Velden, U.: Toothbrushing Force in Relation to Plaque Removal, *J. Clin. Periodontol., 23,* 724, August, 1996.

19. Pashley, D.H., Leibach, J.G., and Horner, J.A.: The Effects of Burnishing F/kaolin/glycerin Paste on Dentin Permeability, *J. Periodontol., 58,* 19, January, 1987.

20. Addy, M. and Mostafa, P.: Dentine Hypersensitivity: I. Effects Produced by the Uptake In Vitro of Metal Ions, Fluoride, and Formaldehyde Onto Dentine, *J. Oral Rehab., 15,* 575, November, 1988.

21. Tal, M., Oran, M., Gedalia, I., and Ehrlich, J.: X-ray Diffraction and Scanning Electron Microscopy Investigations of Fluoride-Treated Dentine in Man, *Arch. Oral Biol., 21,* 285, May, 1976.

22. Pratti, C., Venturi, L., Valdre, G., and Mongiorgi, R.: Dentin Morphology and Permeability After Brushing With Different Toothpastes in the Presence or Absence of Smear Layer, *J. Periodontol., 73,* 183, February, 2003.

23. Ellingson, J.E. and Rolla, G.: Treatment of Dentin With Stannous Fluoride: SEM and Electron Microprobe Study, *Scand. J. Dent. Res., 15,* 281, August, 1987.

24. Dijkman, T.G. and Arends, J.: The Role of 'CaF2' Like Material in Topical Fluoridation of Enamel In Situ, *Acta Odontol. Scand., 46,* 391, December, l988.

25. Cooley, R.L. and Sandoval, V.A.: Effectiveness of Potassium Oxalate Treatment on Dentin Hypersensitivity. *Gen. Dent., 37,* 330, July/August, 1989.

26. Johnson, R.and Muzzin, K.B.: Effects of Potassium Oxalate on Dentin Hypersensitivity In Vivo, *J. Periodontol., 60,* 151, March, 1989.

27. McBride, M. A., Gilpatrick, R. O., and Fowler, W. L.: The Effectiveness of Sodium Fluoride Iontophoresis in Patients With Sensitive Teeth, *Quintessence Int., 22,* 637, August, 1991.

28. **Lin, W.H.**, Liu, H.C., Lin, C.P.: The Combined Occluding Effect of Sodium Fluoride Varnish and Ng: YAG Laser Irradiation on Human Dentinal Tubules, *J. Endod., 25,* 424, June, l999.

29. **Moritz, A.**, Schoop, U., Goharkhay, K., Aoid, M., Reichenbach, P., Lothaller, M.A., Wernisch, J., and Sperr, W.: Long-term Effects of CO_2 Laser Irradiation on Treatment of Hypersensitive Dental Necks: Results of an In Vivo Study, *J. Clin. Laser Med. Surg., 16,* 211, August, 1998.

30. **Spranger, H.**: Investigation Into the Genesis of Angular Lesions at the Cervical Region, *Quintessence Int., 26,* 149, February, 1995.

31. **Frazier, K.B.** and Haywood, V.B.: Teaching Nightguard Bleaching and Other Tooth-Whitening Procedures in North American Dental Schools, *J. Dent. Educ., 64,* 357, May, 2000.

SUGGESTED READINGS

General

Addy, M.: Dentine Hypersensitivity: New Perspectives on an Old Problem, *Int. Dent. J., 52,* 367, Supplement 1, May, 2002.

Jacobsen, P.L. and Bruce, G.: Clinical Dentin Hypersensitivity: Understanding the Causes and Prescribing a Treatment, *J. Contemp. Dent. Pract., 2,* 1, Winter, 2001. Available at: www.jcdp.com. Accessed July 29, 2003.

Scherman, A. and Jacobsen, P.L.: Managing Dentin Hypersensitivity: What Treatment to Recommend to Patients, *J. Am. Dent. Assoc., 123,* 57, April, 1992.

Tilliss, T.S.I. and Keating, J.G.: Understanding and Managing Dentin Hypersensitivity, *J. Dent. Hyg., 76,* 296, Fall, 2002.

Biology of Tooth Structure

Addy, M., Loyn, T., and Adams, D.: Dentine Hypersensitivity: Effects of Some Proprietary Mouthwashes on the Dentine Smear Layer: A SEM Study, *J. Dent., 19,* 148, June, 1991.

Aw, T.C., Lepe, X., Johnson, G.H., and Mancl, L.: Characteristics of Noncarious Cervical Lesions: A Clinical Investigation, *J. Am. Dent. Assoc., 133,* 725, June, 2002.

Hardgreaves, K.M., Goodis, H.E., eds.: *Seltzer and Bender's The Dental Pulp,* 4th ed. Chicago, Quintessence, 2002, pp. 75–80.

Holland, G.R.: Morphological Features of Dentine and Pulp Related to Dentine Sensitivity, *Arch. Oral Biol., 39,* 3S, Supplement, 1994.

Dentin Hypersensitivity Management

Absi, E.G., Addy, J., and Adam, D.: Dentin Hypersensitivity: Uptake of Toothpastes on to Dentin and Effect of Brushing, Washing, and Dietary Acid SEM In Vivo Study, *J. Oral. Rehabil., 22,* 175, March, 1995.

Cuesta Frechoso, S., Menendez, M., Guisasola, C., Arregui, I., Tejerina, J.M., and Sicilia, A.: Evaluation of the Efficacy of Two Potassium Nitrate Bioadhesive Gels (5% and 10%) in the Treatment on Dentine Hypersensitivity: A Randomised Clinical Trial, *J. Clin. Periodontol., 30,* 315, April, 2003.

Hoyt, W.H. and Bibby, B. G.: Use of Sodium Fluoride for Densensitizing Dentin, *J. Am Dent. Assoc., 30,* 1372, September 1, 1943.

Ide, M., Wilson, R.F., and Ashley, F.P.: The Reproducibility of Assessment for Cervical Dentine Hypersensitivity, *J. Clin. Periodontol., 28,* 16, January, 2001.

Kimura, Y., Wilder-Smith, P., Yonaga, K., and Matsumoto, K.: Treatment of Dentine Hypersensitivity by Lasers: A Review, *J. Clin. Periodontol., 27,* 715, October, 2000.

Kuriowa, M., Kodaka T., Muroiwa, M., and Abe, M.: Dentin Hypersensitivity: Occlusion of Dentinal Tubules by Brushing With and Without Abrasive Dentifrice, *J. Periodontol., 65,* 291, April, 1994.

Lavigne, S.E., Gutenkunst, L.S., and Williams, K.B.: Effects of Tartar-Control Dentifrice on Tooth Sensitivity: A Pilot Study, *J. Dent. Hyg., 71,* 105, May–June, 1997.

Muzzin, K.B and Johnson, R.: Effects of Potassium Oxalate on Dentin Hypersensitivity In Vivo, *J. Periodontol., 60,* 151, March, 1989.

Pereira, R. and Chava, V.K.: Efficacy of a 3% Potassium Nitrate Desensitizing Mouthwash in the Treatment of Dentinal Hypersensitivity, *J. Periodontol., 72,* 1720, December, 2001.

Sommerman, M. and Chan, J.T.: Desensitizing Agents, in *ADA Guide to Dental Therapeutics,* 2nd ed. Chicago, ADA Publishing, 2000, pp. 242–249.

Periodontal Debridement Considerations

Tammaro, S., Wennstrom, J.L., and Bergenholtz, G.: Root-Dentin Sensitivity Following Non-Surgical Periodontal Treatment, *J. Clin. Periodontol., 27,* 690, September, 2000.

Tooth Whitening

Haywood, V.B.: Dentin Hypersensitivity: Bleaching and Restorative Considerations for Successful Management, *Int. Dent. J. 52,* 367, Supplement 1, May, 2002.

Nathanson, D.: Vital Tooth Bleaching: Sensitivity and Pulpal Considerations, *J. Am. Dent. Assoc., 128:* 41S, Supplement, April 1997.

Clinical Research

Gillam, D.G.: Clinical Trial Designs for Testing of Products for Dentine Hypersensitivity: A Review, *Periodontal Abstr., 45,* 37, February, 1997.

Holland, G.R., Narhi, M.N., Addy, M., Gangarosa, L., and Orchardson, R.: Guidelines for the Design and Conduct of Clinical Trials on Dentine Hypersensitivity, *J. Clin. Periodontol., 24,* 808, November, 1997.

Extrinsic Stain Removal

Esther M. Wilkins, RDH, BS, DMD and
Caren M. Barnes, RDH, BS, MS

CHAPTER OUTLINE

After treatment by scaling, root planing, and other dental hygiene care, the teeth are assessed for the presence of remaining dental stains. The use of polishing agents for stain removal is a selective procedure that not every patient needs, especially on a routine basis.

Stains on the teeth are not etiologic factors for any disease or destructive process. Therefore, the removal of stains is for esthetic, not for health, reasons. The term "selective polishing" is used to indicate that polishing procedures are to be included where there is a *need* just as all dental hygiene care is selected for the patient. Key words related to stain removal, instruments, coronal polishing, and air-powder polishing are defined in Box 42-1.

■ EFFECTS OF POLISHING

Attention must be given to the positive and negative effects of polishing so that scientific decisions can be made for the treatment of each patient. *Professional judgment based on a patient's needs determines when a service is to be included in a dental hygiene care plan.*

I. BACTEREMIA

- Bacteremia can be created during the use of power-driven stain removal instruments; the *medical history* must be recorded initially.

BOX 42-1 KEY WORDS AND ABBREVIATIONS: Extrinsic Stain Removal

Abrasion: wearing away of surface material by friction.

Abrasive: a material composed of particles of sufficient hardness and sharpness to cut or scratch a softer material when drawn across its surface; available in various particle sizes.

Air-powder polisher: air-powered device using air and water pressure to deliver a controlled stream of specially processed sodium bicarbonate slurry through the handpiece nozzle; also called air abrasive, air polishing, air-powered abrasive, or airbrasive.

Binder: substance used to hold abrasive particles together; examples are ceramic bonding used for mounted abrasive points, electroplating for binding diamond chips for rotary instruments, and rubber or shellac for soft discs.

Coronal polishing: polishing of the anatomic crowns of the teeth to remove dental biofilm and extrinsic stains; does not involve calculus removal.

Glycerin: clear, colorless, syrupy fluid used as a vehicle and sweetening agent for drugs and as a solvent and vehicle for abrasive agents.

Grit: with reference to abrasive agents, grit is the particle size.

Polishing: the production, especially by friction, of a smooth, glossy, mirrorlike surface that reflects light; a very fine agent is used for polishing after a coarser agent is used for cleaning.

p.s.i: pounds per square inch.

r.p.m.: revolutions per minute.

Slurry: thin, semifluid suspension of a solid in a liquid.

- Review and update the medical history at each succeeding appointment.
- Bacteremias result from manipulation of the gingival tissues.
- Occurrence of bacteremias: In one research study, 11 of 39 children (mean age, 9 years) developed bacteremia following application of a rubber cup with a prophylaxis paste.[1]
- Other research: Children undergoing dental treatment were evaluated for bacteremia following toothbrushing alone, professional polishing with a rubber cup, or scaling. The results showed the presence of positive blood cultures in each group, with no difference in the intensity of the bacteremia between groups.[2]
- For patients at risk, particularly those with damaged or abnormal heart valves, prosthetic valves, joint replacements, rheumatic heart disease, and other conditions listed on pages 123 to 125, antibiotic prophylaxis as outlined by the American Heart Association is needed.

II. ENVIRONMENTAL FACTORS

A. Aerosol Production

- Aerosols are created during the use of all rotary instruments, including a prophylaxis handpiece with a polishing paste and the air and water sprays used during rinsing.[3]
- The biologic contaminants of aerosols stay suspended for long periods and provide a means for disease transmission to dental personnel, as well as to succeeding patients.
- Use of power-driven instruments should be limited when a patient is known to have a communicable disease.
- Standard precautions are routine.

B. Spatter

- Protective eyewear is needed for all dental team members and for the patient.
- Serious eye damage has occurred as a result of spatter in the eye from a polishing paste or from instruments.
- Constituents of commercial prophylaxis pastes may include various chemicals, such as oils, that can aggravate a severe inflammatory response.[4]

III. EFFECT ON TEETH

A. Removal of Tooth Structure

- Polishing for 30 seconds with a pumice paste may remove as much as 4 μm of the outer enamel.[5]

- The outermost layer of tooth structure contains the greatest amounts of fluoride.[6] The surface fluoride protects against dental caries. The concentration of fluoride drops quickly inward toward the dentin, so if the surface layer is polished away, the protection is greatly diminished.
- The *fluoride-rich surface* is important and should not be removed.
- Surface enamel can be readily removed with polishing instruments.

B. Areas of Demineralization

- Demineralization Areas: More surface enamel is lost from abrasive polishing over demineralized white spots than over intact enamel.[7]
- Remineralization of a demineralized area can be interrupted when the surface enamel is removed. As shown in Figure 33-3 (page 547), the enamel surface layer is thin over a subsurface demineralized zone.

C. Areas of Thin Enamel, Cementum, or Dentin

- Amelogenesis imperfecta is an example of thin enamel resulting from imperfect tooth development (page 319).
- Exposure of Dentinal Tubules: cementum and dentin are softer and more porous, so greater amounts of these can be removed during polishing than of the enamel.[5,6] When cementum is exposed because of gingival recession, polishing of the exposed surfaces should be avoided.
- Smear layer can be removed and dentinal tubules exposed.[8]
- When surface structure is removed, unnecessary tooth sensitivity can result.

D. Surface Roughness of Teeth and Restorations

- A coarse abrasive may create a rougher tooth surface than existed before polishing.
- Microorganisms collect and colonize on a rough surface much more rapidly than on a smooth surface.[9,10]
- Certain polishing pastes can roughen the surfaces of restorative materials.[11,12]

E. Heat Production

- Steady pressure with a rapidly revolving rubber cup or bristle brush and a minimum of wet abrasive agent can create sufficient heat to cause pain and discomfort for the patient.

- Damage to the pulp by the heat has not been documented, but the pulps of children are large and may be more susceptible to heat.
- The rule is light pressure, a slow-motion instrument, and plenty of moisture mixed with the abrasive agent.

IV. EFFECT ON GINGIVA

- Trauma to the gingival tissue can result, especially when the prophylaxis angle is run at a high speed and the rubber cup is applied for an extended period.
- In one study, a rubber cup with pumice rotated for 2 minutes caused total removal of the epithelium inside the crest of the free gingiva.[13] Complete healing from such a wound takes 8 to 14 days.
- The soreness and sensitivity of the tissues could prevent adequate biofilm removal by the patient during that time, and a severe inflammation could result, along with calculus reformation.
- With the fast rotation of a rubber cup, particles of a polishing agent can be forced into the subepithelial tissues and create a source of irritation.
- Stain removal after gingival and periodontal treatments, including scaling and root planing, is not recommended on the same day. The diseased lining of the pocket usually has been removed, and the pocket wall is wide open and can receive particles that may become embedded out of reach of the most careful irrigation and rinsing.
- Rotation of the rubber cup can force microorganisms into the tissues. An inflammatory response can be expected, and bacteria may gain access to the bloodstream to create a bacteremia.
- Foreign-body reactions to abrasives have been tested. Several agents have been shown to have potential for creating reactions. Some explanation for delayed healing following tissue trauma may be found in this concept.[14]

▪ INDICATIONS FOR STAIN REMOVAL

I. TO REMOVE EXTRINSIC STAINS NOT OTHERWISE REMOVED DURING TOOTHBRUSHING AND SCALING

A. Patient Instruction

- Discuss source of stain and how it can be prevented.
- Encourage patient to make necessary habit changes.

- Practice toothbrushing to remove stains incorporated in dental biofilm.
- Example of patient's own stain removal: brown stain of chlorhexidine rinsing removed using a toothpick.[15] The toothpick holder is shown in Figure 26-12.

B. Scaling and Root Planing

- Stains can be removed during scaling, root planing, and debridement of dental biofilm
- Example: black line stain has been identified as a type of calculus. It is described on pages 316 to 317.[16] If polishing procedures were to be applied before scaling the black line stain, much tooth surface structure could be removed because of the firm attachment of the black line stain.

II. TO PREPARE THE TEETH FOR CARIES-PREVENTIVE AGENTS

A. Pit and Fissure Sealant

- Follow manufacturer's directions. Sealants vary in their requirements.
- Research has shown that sealants have been successfully placed without the initial cleaning of the teeth.
- Commercial prophylactic pastes contain oils, flavoring substances, or other agents that may interfere with the integrity of the sealant.
- A plain, fine pumice mixed with water is indicated when precleaning is determined to be necessary (page 574).

B. Professional Application of Fluoride Solutions or Gels

- Complete tooth polishing is not necessary before fluoride application.
- Research has since shown that biofilm and debris removal can be accomplished adequately by the patient using a toothbrush and dental floss, after complete calculus removal.
- The pellicle on the tooth surface does not act as a barrier to fluoride, and fluoride uptake in the enamel from a fluoride application is similar whether the teeth are brushed by the patient or polished with pumice.[17]

III. TO CONTRIBUTE TO PATIENT MOTIVATION

Removal of biofilm must be a *daily* procedure carried out *by the patient*. It must be accomplished thoroughly at least twice daily, and for some patients three times daily, if infection is to be controlled and the sanitation of the mouth maintained.

A. Development of Biofilm

- A one-time removal of soft deposits from the teeth at a dental hygiene appointment does not accomplish any long-range preventive purpose because deposits return promptly.
- It is known that pellicle returns to cover the teeth within minutes after complete polishing.
- Biofilm begins to collect on the pellicle within 1 or 2 hours, increasing in thickness until, by 12 to 24 hours, biofilm is thick enough to show clearly when a disclosing agent is applied.
- Undisturbed, biofilm may begin to calcify within a few days in a calculus-susceptible patient (pages 306, 308).

B. Motivation

The effect of stain removal as a preventive measure for gingival disease or dental caries has not been proven. Smooth polished tooth surfaces may contribute in part to the following effects:

- Help the instructed patient to obtain more satisfactory results from self-care procedures. A smooth surface should be easier to clean.
- Show the patient the appearance and feeling of a clean mouth for motivational purposes. The greatest change in behavior, or the true learning, however, usually can be obtained through patient participation in the use of a disclosing agent and personal removal of biofilm with floss and toothbrush.

■ CLINICAL APPLICATION OF SELECTIVE STAIN REMOVAL

Because of the numbers of health and safety factors involved, the decision to "polish" should be based on consideration for the individual patient. Instruction for stain prevention is important for all patients.

I. SUMMARY OF CONTRAINDICATIONS FOR POLISHING

The following list suggests some of the specific instances in which polishing either should be postponed or is contraindicated indefinitely.

A. No Unsightly Stain

- The principle of selective polishing is not to polish unless necessary.

- Appearance is important to patients, but maintaining the integrity of the tooth surface for disease prevention is more important.
- When stain is noted on specific tooth surfaces, a stain removal procedure can be applied to selected areas without having to cover all the teeth in a generalized procedure.

B. Characteristics of Patients at Risk for Dental Caries

Patients at risk for dental caries need extra fluoride to protect their tooth surfaces. Chances cannot be taken on the loss of the fluoride-rich enamel and root surfaces by unnecessary abrasive polishing. Examples include:

1. Rampant caries, nursing caries, root caries, all ages.
2. Demineralized areas.
3. Xerostomia for any reason.

C. Patients With Respiratory Problems

Power-driven instruments are contraindicated for such conditions as asthma or emphysema when breathing is a problem.

D. Tooth Sensitivity

Abrasive agent uncovers ends of dentinal tubules in areas of thin cementum or dentin.

E. Restorations

Restorations and titanium implants may be scratched by polishing abrasive.

F. Newly Erupted Teeth

Incomplete mineralization of surface.

G. Conditions Requiring Postponement for Later Evaluation

1. When instruction for personal biofilm removal (daily care) has not yet been given or when the patient has not demonstrated adequate biofilm control.
2. Soft spongy tissue that bleeds on brushing or gentle instrumentation.
3. Immediately following deep subgingival scaling and root planing because abrasive particles can become embedded in the pocket wall and interfere with healing.
4. Communicable disease potentially disseminated by aerosol.

II. SUGGESTIONS FOR CLINIC PROCEDURE

A. Give Instruction First

1. Daily dental biofilm removal to assist in dental stain control.
2. Tobacco cessation introduction when stain is primarily from tobacco use (page 513).

B. Remove Stain by Scaling

Whenever possible, stains can be removed during scaling, root planing, and debridement. Unsightly stains can be removed for the new patient initially. At that time, an explanation of the selective polishing principle can be presented and assistance given for a preventive plan for stain control.

C. Use Minimal Polishing Techniques

- Low-abrasion paste.
- Low-speed handpiece.
- Minimal heat production.
- Rubber cup at 90° to tooth surface with intermittent light applications.

▪ CLEANING AND POLISHING AGENTS

Traditionally, abrasive agents have been applied with polishing instruments to remove extrinsic dental stains. Abrasives selected are expected to produce a clean tooth surface free of extrinsic stains but to "do no harm" to the tooth surface, existing restorations, or gingiva.

I. FACTORS AFFECTING ABRASIVE ACTION

During polishing, sharp edges of abrasive particles are moved along the surface of a material, abrading it by producing microscopic scratches or grooves. The rate of abrasion, or speed with which structural material is removed from the surface being polished, is governed by characteristics of the abrasive particles, as well as by the manner in which they are applied.

A. Characteristics of Abrasive Particles

1. *Shape*. Irregularly shaped particles with sharp edges produce deeper grooves and thus abrade faster than do rounded particles with dull edges.
2. *Hardness*. Particles must be harder than the surface to be abraded; harder particles abrade faster.
3. *Body Strength*. Particles that fracture into smaller sharp-edged particles during use are more

abrasive than are those that wear down with use and become dull and rounded.

4. *Attrition Resistance.* Effective abrasive particles do not dull or become embedded in the surface being abraded; particles with greater attrition resistance abrade faster.

5. *Particle Size (Grit)*
   - The larger the particles, the more abrasive they are and the less polishing ability they have.
   - Finer abrasive particles achieve a glossier finish.
   - Abrasive and polishing agents are graded from coarse to fine based on the size of the holes in a standard sieve through which the particles will pass.
   - The finer abrasives are called powders or flours and are graded in order of increasing fineness as F, FF, FFF, and so on.
   - Particles embedded in papers are graded 0, 00, 000, and so on.

B. Principles for Application of Abrasives

1. *Quantity Applied.* The more particles applied per unit time, the faster the rate of abrasion.
   - Particles suspended in water or other vehicles for frictional heat reduction.
   - Dry powders or flours represent the greatest quantity that can be applied per unit of time.
   - Frictional heat produced is proportional to the rate of abrasion; therefore, the use of *dry agents* is *contraindicated* for polishing natural teeth because of the potential danger of thermal injury to the dental pulp.

2. *Speed of Application.* The greater the speed of application, the faster the rate of abrasion.
   - With increased speed of application, pressure must be reduced.
   - *Rapid abrasion* is *contraindicated* because it increases frictional heat.

3. *Pressure of Application.* The heavier the pressure applied, the faster the rate of abrasion.
   - *Heavy pressure* is *contraindicated* because it increases frictional heat.

4. *Summary.* When cleaning and polishing are indicated after patient evaluation, the following should be observed:
   - Use wet agents.
   - Apply a rubber polishing cup, using low speed.
   - Use a light, intermittent touch.

II. ABRASIVE AGENTS

The abrasives listed here are examples of commonly used agents. Some are available in several grades, and the specific use varies with the grade. For example, while a superfine grade might be used for polishing enamel surfaces and metallic restorations, a coarser grade would be used for laboratory purposes only.

Abrasives for use daily in a dentifrice necessarily are of a finer grade than those used for professional polishing accomplished a few times each year.

A. Silex (Silicon Dioxide)

- *XXX Silex:* Fairly abrasive.
- *Superfine Silex:* Can be used for heavy stain removal from enamel.

B. Pumice

Powdered pumice is of volcanic origin and consists chiefly of complex silicates of aluminum, potassium, and sodium. The specifications for particle size are listed in the *National Formulary*[18] as follows:
- *Pumice Flour or Superfine Pumice:* Least abrasive, and may be used to remove heavy stains from enamel.
- *Fine Pumice:* Mildly abrasive.
- *Coarse Pumice:* Not for use on natural teeth.

C. Calcium Carbonate (Whiting, Calcite, Chalk)

- Various grades are used for different polishing techniques.

D. Tin Oxide (Putty Powder, Stannic Oxide)

- Polishing agent for teeth and metallic restorations.

E. Emery (Corundum)

Not used directly on the enamel.
- *Aluminum Oxide (Alumina):* The pure form of emery. Used for composite restorations and margins of porcelain restorations.
- *Levigated Alumina:* Consists of extremely fine particles of aluminum oxide, which may be used for polishing metals but are destructive to tooth surfaces.

F. Rouge (Jeweler's Rouge)

- Iron oxide is a fine red powder sometimes impregnated on paper discs.
- It is useful for polishing gold and precious metal alloys in the laboratory.

G. Diamond Particles

- Constituent of diamond polishing paste for porcelain surfaces.

■ CLINICAL APPLICATIONS

I. PREPARATION OF POLISHING AGENT

Agents used for stain removal from the natural teeth and for polishing restorations are mixed with water or other lubricant to facilitate particle movement across the tooth surface and to reduce frictional heat. A quantity of paste can be prepared in advance and kept in a closed jar. Glycerin is added to help as a spreading factor and to prevent splashing during application of the polishing cup.

A. Preparation of Single Quantity

- Place water or flavored mouthrinse in a dappen dish. Some agents require a specific amount of water.
- Add the dry agent to saturation and stir.

B. Consistency

The paste should be as moist as possible, but transportable between dappen dish and the teeth.

II. COMMERCIAL PREPARATIONS

Numerous dental prophylactic cleaning and polishing preparations are available. Clinicians need more than one type available to meet the requirements of individual restorative materials.

A. Constituents

Most commercially prepared polishing pastes contain an abrasive; water; a humectant; a binder; and agents for sweetening, flavoring, and color. Approximate proportions and purposes of each constituent with examples are as follows:
1. *Abrasive:* 50% to 60%, main ingredient. Examples: pumice, silicon dioxide.
2. *Water:* 10% to 20%, solvent, provides desired consistency.
3. *Humectant:* 20% to 25%, moisture retainer, stabilizes the ingredients. Examples: glycerin, sorbitol.
4. *Binder:* 1.5% to 2.0%, prevents separation, non-spatter. Examples: agar, sodium silicate powder.
5. *Sweetener:* Artificial, noncariogenic.
6. *Flavoring and Coloring Agents.*

B. Packaging

- Commercial preparations are in the forms of pastes, powders, or tablets.
- Some are available in measured amounts contained in small plastic or other individual packets that contribute to the cleanliness and sterility of the procedure.
- Selection of a preparation has been based on its qualities of abrasiveness, consistency for convenient use, or flavor for patient pleasure.

C. Fluoride Prophylaxis Pastes

1. *Limited Caries Prevention.*
   - Application of fluoride by pastes cannot be considered a substitute for conventional topical application on the basis of present-day research.
   - Although reviews of the research show that moderate caries-preventive effects have been demonstrated, other studies have had minimal or no statistically significant results.[19,20]
2. *Enamel Surface.* A limitation of the paste preparations is that certain abrasives can remove a thin layer of enamel during polishing.[4,21] With the removal of the enamel, the outer layer of fluoride is also removed, possibly as fast as it is added from the paste, but this concept has not been researched.
3. *Clinical Application.* Use only an amount sufficient to accomplish stain removal to prevent a child patient from swallowing unnecessary fluoride. The paste may contain 4,000 to 20,000 ppm fluoride ion.[22]

■ PROCEDURES FOR STAIN REMOVAL (CORONAL POLISHING)

I. PATIENT PREPARATION FOR STAIN REMOVAL

A. Instruction and Clinical Procedures

- Practice biofilm control.
- Complete scaling, root planing, and overhang removal.
- Inform the patient that polishing is a cosmetic procedure, not a therapeutic one.

B. Evaluation

- After scaling and other periodontal treatment, an evaluation is made to determine the need for stain removal of teeth, polishing restorations, and dental prostheses.

- Review medical history to determine premedication requirements for the patient.
- Determine the time that the patient had taken the prescription. When the initial part of the appointment (scaling and related procedures) has been lengthy, the benefit from the premedication may have passed.
- Check all restorations to ensure that the correct polishing agent has been selected.

II. ENVIRONMENTAL PREPARATION

Environmental factors are described in Chapters 2, 3, and 4. A topical summary is provided here.

A. Procedures to Lessen the Extent of Contaminated Aerosols

1. Clear the water that will be used for rinsing. Flush water through the tubing for 2 minutes at the beginning of each work period and for 30 seconds after each appointment.
2. Request that the patient rinse with an antimicrobial mouthrinse to reduce the numbers of oral microorganisms before starting instrumentation.
3. Use high-velocity evacuation.

B. Protective Barriers

Protective eyewear and coverall are necessary for the patient. The clinician wears the usual barrier protection, namely, eyewear, mask, gloves, and clinic gown to cover clothing.

III. INSTRUMENTS

- Both power-driven and manual instruments may be useful when polishing.
- All instruments should be used with discretion and in a manner requiring minimal abrasion of the tooth surface.
- Because tooth structure is removed when an abrasive is used on the enamel, and still more is removed when it is used on dentin or cementum, only a mild abrasive agent is appropriate.

▪ THE PORTE POLISHER

The porte polisher is a prophylactic manual instrument designed especially for extrinsic stain removal or application of treatment agents such as for hypersensitive areas.

It is constructed to hold a wood point at a contra-angle. The wood points may be cone or wedge shaped

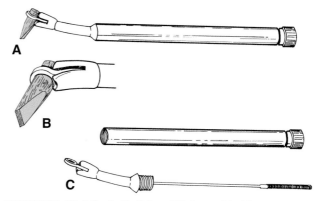

▪ **FIGURE 42-1 Porte Polisher. (A)** Assembled instrument shows position of wood point ready for instrumentation. **(B)** Disassembled, ready for autoclave. **(C)** Working end shows wedge-shaped wood point inserted.

and made of various kinds of wood, preferably orange-wood. Figure 42-1 illustrates a typical porte polisher.

The instrument frequently is held in a palm grasp, as shown in Figure 36-14. The wood point is applied to the tooth surface using firm, carefully directed, massaging circular or linear strokes to accommodate the anatomy of each tooth. A firm finger rest and moderate pressure of the wood point provide protection for the gingival margin and efficiency in technique.

The porte polisher is useful for instrumentation of difficult-to access surfaces of the teeth, especially malpositioned teeth. Other features are no heat generation, no noise compared with powered handpieces, and minimal production of aerosols. In addition, the porte polisher is readily portable and therefore is useful in any location, for example, for a bedridden patient.

▪ THE POWER-DRIVEN INSTRUMENTS

I. HANDPIECE

A handpiece is used to hold rotary instruments in the dental unit. The three basic designs are straight, contra-angle, and right angle. Rotary instruments have been classified according to their rotational speeds, designated by revolutions per minute (r.p.m.) as high speed and low (or slow) speed.

A. Ultra or High Speed

1. *Speed:* 100,000 to 800,000 r.p.m.
2. *Uses:* For cavity preparation and other restorative preparations.
3. *Fiberoptic Light:* Better visibility is provided when a fiberoptic light is built into the head of the

handpiece. The beam of light is projected onto the field of operation when the handpiece is activated.

B. Low Speed

Typical range is 6,000 to 10,000 r.p.m. Lowest speeds are used for polishing and finishing procedures.

II. PROPHYLAXIS ANGLE

Contra- or right-angle attachment for the handpiece to which polishing devices (rubber cup, bristle brush) are attached.

Many types of prophylaxis angles are available. Some are disposable and others are made of stainless steel and may have hard chrome, carbon steel, or brass bearings. Unless they are disposable, only instruments that can be sterilized should be selected.

III. PROPHYLAXIS ANGLE ATTACHMENTS

A. Rubber Polishing Cups

1. *Types* (Figure 42-2)
   a. Slip-on: With ribbed cup to aid in holding polishing agent.
   b. Slip-on: With bristles inside cup.
   c. Threaded (screw type): With plain ribbed cup or flange (webbed) type.
   d. Mandrel mounted.
2. *Materials*
   a. Natural rubber: More resilient; adapts readily to fit the contours of the teeth.
   b. Synthetic: Stiffer than natural rubber.

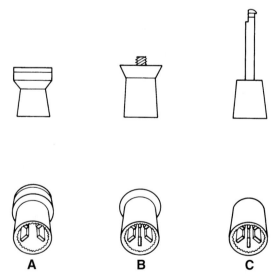

■ **FIGURE 42-2 Rubber Cup Attachments. (A)** Slip-on or snap-on for button-end prophylaxis angle. **(B)** Threaded for direct insertion in right angle. **(C)** Mandrel stem for latch-type angle.

B. Bristle Brushes

1. *Types*
   a. For prophylaxis angle: Slip-on or screw type.
   b. For handpiece: Mandrel mounted.
2. *Materials:* Synthetic.

IV. USES FOR ATTACHMENTS

A. Handpiece With Straight Mandrel

1. Dixon bristle brush (type C, soft) for polishing removable dentures.
2. Mounted stone for sharpening instruments.
3. Rubber cup on mandrel for polishing facial surfaces of anterior teeth.

B. Prophylaxis Angle With Rubber Cup or Brush

1. *Rubber Cup:* For removal of stains from the tooth surfaces and polishing restorations.
2. *Brush*
   a. For removing stains from deep pits and fissures and enamel surfaces away from the gingival margin. A brush is not recommended for use on exposed cementum or dentin because they are easily grooved by such an instrument.
   b. For preliminary polishing of amalgam restorations.

■ USE OF THE PROPHYLAXIS ANGLE

I. EFFECTS ON TISSUES: PRECAUTIONS

- Can cause discomfort for the patient if care and consideration for the oral tissues are not exercised to prevent unnecessary trauma.
- Tactile sensitivity of the clinician while using a thick, bulky handpiece is diminished, and unnecessary pressure may be applied inadvertently.
- Some loss of tooth structure occurs during polishing when an abrasive agent is used. Research on the effects on tooth structure are reviewed on pages 727 to 728.
- The greater the speed of application of a polishing agent, the faster the rate of abrasion. Therefore, the handpiece should be operated at a low r.p.m.
- Trauma to the gingival tissue can result from too high a speed, extended application of the rubber cup, or use of an abrasive polishing agent.

- Tissue damage and the need for antibiotic premedication for risk patients are described on pages 726 to 727.

II. PROPHYLAXIS ANGLE PROCEDURE

- Apply the polishing agent only where it is needed, that is, where there is unsightly stain. Contraindications are listed on pages 729 to 730.
- As with all oral procedures, a systematic order should be followed.

A. Instrument Grasp

Modified pen grasp (Figure 36-13, page 619).

B. Finger Rest

1. Establish firmly on tooth structure.
2. Use a wide fulcrum area when practical to aid in the balance of the large instrument. For example, place cushion of fulcrum finger across occlusal surfaces of premolars while polishing the molars.
3. Avoid use of mobile teeth as finger rests.

C. Speed of Handpiece

1. Use lowest available speed to minimize frictional heat.
2. Adjust r.p.m. by changing the position of the rheostat foot pedal.

D. Use of Rheostat Pedal

1. Apply steady pressure with foot to produce an even, low speed.
2. Keep sole of the foot that activates rheostat pedal flat on the floor. Use toe to activate rheostat pedal.

E. Rubber Cup: Stroke and Procedure

1. Observe where stain removal is needed to prevent unnecessary rubber cup application.
2. Fill rubber cup with polishing agent, and distribute agent over tooth surfaces to be polished.
3. Establish finger rest and bring rubber cup almost in contact with tooth surface before activating power source.
4. Using slowest r.p.m., apply revolving cup at a 90° angle lightly to tooth surface for 1 or 2 seconds. Use a light pressure so that the edges of the rubber cup flare slightly.
5. Move cup to adjacent area on tooth surface; use a patting or brushing motion.
6. Replenish supply of polishing agent frequently.

7. Turn handpiece to adapt rubber cup to fit each surface of the tooth, including proximal surfaces and gingival surfaces of fixed partial dentures.
8. Start with the distal surface of the most posterior tooth of a quadrant and move forward toward the anterior. For each tooth, work from the gingival third toward the incisal third of the tooth.
9. When two polishing agents of different abrasiveness are to be applied, use a separate rubber cup for each.
10. Cups that cannot be sterilized are used only once. Disposable one-use cups are preferred.

F. Bristle Brush

Bristle brushes should be used selectively and limited to occlusal surfaces. Lacerations of the gingiva and grooves and scratches in the tooth surface, particularly the roots, can result.

1. Soak stiff brush in hot water to soften bristles.
2. Distribute mild abrasive polishing agent over occlusal surfaces of teeth to be polished.
3. Place fingers of nondominant hand in a position that both retracts and protects cheek and tongue from the revolving brush.
4. Establish a firm finger rest and bring brush almost in contact with the tooth before activating power source.
5. Using slowest r.p.m., apply revolving brush lightly to the occlusal surface only, avoiding contact of bristles with soft tissues.
6. Use a short stroke in a brushing motion; follow the inclined planes of the cusps.
7. Move from tooth to tooth to prevent generation of excessive frictional heat. Avoid overuse of the brush unnecessarily. Replenish supply of polishing agent frequently.

G. Irrigation

Teeth and interdental areas should be irrigated thoroughly several times with water from the syringe to remove abrasive particles. The rotary movement of the rubber cup or bristle brush tends to force the abrasive into the gingival sulci, thereby creating a potential source of irritation to the soft tissues.

■ POLISHING PROXIMAL SURFACES

Considerable care must be exercised in the use of floss, tape, and finishing strips. Understanding the anatomy of the interdental papillae and their relationship to the contact areas and proximal surfaces of the teeth is prerequisite to the prevention of tissue damage. Inadequate contacts between teeth provide potential areas of food impaction and biofilm retention. Chart the contacts for consideration by the dentist during treatment planning.

As much polishing as possible of accessible proximal surfaces is accomplished during the use of the rubber cup in the prophylaxis angle. This is followed by the use of dental tape with polishing agent when necessary. Finishing strips are used only in selected instances, when all other techniques fail to remove a stain.

The use of dental floss or tape for dental biofilm control on proximal tooth surfaces is an essential part of self-care by the patient.

I. DENTAL TAPE AND FLOSS

A. Features

- Floss and tape are described on pages 429 to 432.
- The wax covering affords some protection for the tissues, facilitates the movement of the floss or tape, prevents excessive absorption of moisture, and helps prevent shredding.
- Tape is flat and has relatively sharp edges, whereas floss is round. Either floss or tape may injure the tissue when used incorrectly or carelessly.

B. Uses

1. *Tape for Polishing*
   - Proximal tooth surfaces.
   - Gingival surface of fixed partial denture.
2. *Floss for Removing*
   - Debris and food particles. Patient instruction with toothbrush and floss at the beginning of the appointment prepares the teeth for scaling.
   - Particles of polishing agents at the completion of polishing procedures from interproximal areas, gingival sulci, and gingival surface of fixed partial dentures.
   - Retained abrasive particles after use of finishing strips.

C. Technique for Dental Floss and Tape

- Techniques for tape and floss application are described on pages 430 to 432 and illustrated in Figures 26-3, 26-4, and 26-5.
- The same principles apply whether the patient or the clinician is using the floss.
- Finger rests must be used to prevent snapping through contact areas.
1. *Polishing With Dental Tape*. Polishing agent is applied to the tooth, and the tape is moved gently back and forth over the area where stain was observed.

2. *Polishing Gingival Surface of a Fixed Partial Denture*. A floss threader is used to position the floss or tape over the gingival surface. Floss threaders are described and illustrated on pages 472 and 473. Polishing agent is applied under the pontic, and the floss or tape is moved back and forth.
3. *Flossing After Polishing*. Particles of abrasive agent should be removed by irrigation and by using a clean length of floss applied in the usual manner.
4. *Rinsing and Irrigation*. Irrigate with water-spray syringe to clean out all abrasive agent.

II. FINISHING STRIPS

A. Description

- Finishing strips are also known as linen abrasive strips.
- They are thin, flexible, and tape-shaped.
- Available in four widths: extra narrow, narrow, medium, and wide.
- Made of linen or plastic, with one smooth side and the other side that serves as a carrier for abrasive agents bonded to that side.
- "Gapped" strips are available with an abrasive-free portion to permit sliding the strip through a contact area without abrading the enamel.
- Available in extra fine, fine, medium, and coarse grit. *Only extra narrow or narrow strips with fine grit are suggested for stain removal, and then only with discretion.*

B. Use

1. *For Stain Removal on Proximal Surfaces of Anterior Teeth.* When other polishing techniques are unsuccessful.
2. *Precautions for Use*
   a. Edge of strip is sharp and may cut gingival tissue or lip.
   b. Rough working side of strip is capable of removing tooth structure and may make nicks or grooves, particularly in the cementum.
   c. Use of a finishing strip should be limited to enamel surfaces.

C. Technique for Finishing Strip

1. *Grasp and Finger Rest*
   - A strip no longer than 6 inches is most conveniently applied.
   - Grasp and fulcrum must be well controlled.
   - Protection of the lip by retraction with the thumb and index finger holding the strip is mandatory.

2. *Positioning*
   - Direct the abrasive side of the strip toward the proximal surface to be treated, as the strip is worked slowly and gently between the teeth with a slight sawing motion.
   - Bring strip just through the contact area. If the strip breaks, immediately use floss to remove particles of abrasive.
   - When a space is clearly visible through an interproximal area and the interdental papilla is missing, a narrow finishing strip may be threaded through. Prepare strip by cutting the end on a diagonal to facilitate threading.
3. *Stain Removal*
   - Press abrasive side of strip against tooth. Draw back and forth in a 1/8-inch arc two or three times, rocking on the established fulcrum.
   - Remove strip. Do not attempt to turn the strip while it is in the interdental area.
4. *Dental Floss*. Follow each application of a finishing strip with dental floss to remove abrasive particles.

■ AIR-POWDER POLISHING

Principles of selective stain removal are applied to the use of the air-powder polishing system. After biofilm control instruction, instrumentation, and periodontal debridement are completed, follow with an evaluation of a need for stain removal.

I. PRINCIPLES OF APPLICATION

Air-powder polishing is an efficient and effective method for mechanical removal of stain and biofilm.[23] Air-powder polishing systems use air, water, and sodium bicarbonate or aluminum trihydroxide to deliver a controlled spray that propels the polishing particles to the tooth surface.[24] The equipment, manufactured by several companies, is operated using inlet air pressure between 40 and 100 psi and inlet water pressure between 20 and 60 psi.

The orifice of the handpiece nozzle should be kept in a constant circular motion, with the nozzle tip 4 to 5 mm away from the enamel surface. The spray is angled away from the gingival margin. The periphery of the spray may be near the gingival margin, but the center should be directed at an angle less than 90° away from the margin.

Complete directions for care of equipment and preparation for use of the device are provided by the various manufacturers.

II. USES OF AIR-POWDER POLISHING

A. Requires less time, is ergonomically favorable to the clinician, and generates no heat.[25]

B. Sodium bicarbonate is less abrasive than traditional prophylaxis pastes, which makes the air-powder polisher ideal for stain and biofilm removal.

C. Removal of heavy, tenacious tobacco stain and chlorhexidine-induced staining.[23]

D. Stain and biofilm removal from orthodontically banded and bracketed teeth[26] and dental implants.[27]

E. Prior to bonding procedures.[28]

F. Root detoxification for periodontally diseased roots.[29]

III. TECHNIQUE

Proper angulation of the air-powder polishing handpiece is essential to reduce the amount of inherent aerosols created[30-32] and to remove stain and biofilm without iatrogenic soft tissue trauma.

A. For Anterior Teeth

The handpiece nozzle should be placed at a 60° angle to the facial and lingual surfaces of anterior teeth (Figure 42-3A).

B. For Posterior Teeth

The handpiece nozzle should be placed at an 80° angle to the facial and lingual surfaces (Figure 42-3B).

C. For Occlusal Surfaces

The handpiece nozzle should be placed at a 90° angle to the occlusal plane (Figure 42-3C).

D. Incorrect Angulation

Incorrect angulation of the handpiece is probably the single most common cause of excess aerosol production. When a clinician directs the handpiece at a 90° angle toward a facial, buccal, and some lingual surfaces, the result is an immediate reflux of the aerosolized spray back onto the clinician. Changing the angle of incidence to the proper angulations of 60° and 80° will result in a change in the angle of the reflection, thus reducing the amount of reflux of aerosolized spray.

IV. RECOMMENDATIONS AND PRECAUTIONS

A. Aerosol Production

A copious spray containing oral debris and microorganisms is produced. As with all contaminated

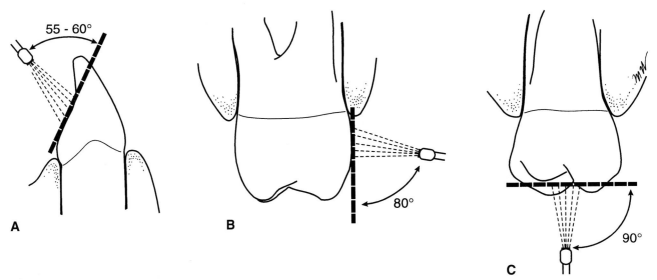

■ FIGURE 42-3 Air-Powder Polishing. Direct the aerosolized spray for **(A)** the anterior teeth at a 60° angle, **(B)** the posterior teeth facial and lingual or palatal at an 80° angle, and **(C)** the occlusal surfaces at a 90° angle to the occlusal plane.

aerosols, a health hazard can exist. Suggestions for minimizing contamination and the effects of the aerosols include the following:

1. Patient uses a preprocedural antibacterial mouthrinse.[33]
2. High-volume evacuation is needed, using a wide tip held near the tooth where the spray is released from the nozzle or using a high-volume scavenger attachment for a high-volume evacuation suction tip or saliva ejector.[31]

B. Protective Patient and Clinician Procedures

1. Use protective eyewear, protective gown, and hair cover.
2. Lubricate patient's lips to prevent drying effect of the sodium bicarbonate using a nonpetroleum lip lubricant.
3. Do not direct the spray on the gingiva, directly into the gingival sulcus or other soft tissues, which creates patient discomfort and undue tissue trauma.

Everyday Ethics

? Miss Dean, a new patient, 57 years old, was in for her second appointment. Her first one included her complete examination and treatment plan with the dentist. Her record shows generalized recession and a variety of tooth-color restorations, which Polly, the dental hygienist, now notes to guide her dental hygiene procedures. Since there were few calculus deposits and it was apparent that Miss Dean was conscientious about her daily personal oral hygiene, Polly completed the scaling and proceeded to prepare the gel-tray for a fluoride application. This was a routine procedure for patients with recession.

Miss Dean watched for a minute and then said, "Aren't you going to polish my teeth? My other hygienist always finished with a good polishing." Polly started to explain. Miss Dean seemed perturbed.

Questions for Consideration

1. How is it an ethical issue when a patient wants a service that the hygienist deems not needed or even detrimental?

2. What choices of procedure does Polly have? Which of the alternatives should she select?

3. Describe how this episode should be documented in the patient's record.

Factors To Teach The Patient

- How dental biofilm and stains form on the natural teeth and their replacements.

- The meaning of selective polishing and why it is not necessary to polish all teeth at every appointment when daily care is effective.

- Stains and biofilm removed by polishing can return promptly if biofilm is not removed faithfully on a schedule of two or three times each day.

- Polishing agents utilized during professional coronal polishing are too abrasive for daily home use.

4. Avoid directing the spray into periodontal pockets with bone loss or into extraction sites as a facial emphysema can be induced.[34]

V. RISK PATIENTS: AIR-POWDER POLISHING CONTRAINDICATED

The information from the patient's medical history must be reviewed and appropriate applications made. Antibiotic premedication is indicated for all the same patients who are at risk for any dental hygiene procedure (pages 122 to 125).

A. Contraindications

1. Physician-directed sodium-restricted diet (for sodium bicarbonate powder only)
2. Respiratory disease or other condition that limits swallowing or breathing.
3. Patients with end-stage renal disease.
4. Communicable infection that can contaminate the aerosols produced.

B. Other Contraindications

1. *Root Surfaces.* Routine polishing of cementum and dentin should be avoided. They can be removed readily during air-powder polishing.[29]
2. *Soft, Spongy Gingiva.* The air-powder can irritate the free gingival tissue, especially if not used with the recommended technique. When heavy stain calls for the use of an air-powder polisher, the patient should be instructed in daily bacterial biofilm removal, scaling and periodontal debridement should be completed, and the stain removal should be postponed until soft tissue has healed.
3. *Restorative Materials.* The use of air-powder polishing on composite resins, cements, and other nonmetallic materials can cause removal or pitting.[35] Table 42-1 provides a guide as to which restorative materials can be safely treated with air-powder polishing agents, the sodium bicarbonate powder, and the aluminum trihydroxide powder.[24] Significant damage to margins of dental castings has been shown.[36]

■ TABLE 42-1 RECOMMENDATIONS OF USE OF AIR POLISHING WITH SODIUM BICARBONATE OR ALUMINUM TRIHYDROXIDE POLISHING POWDER ON RESTORATIVE MATERIALS

RESTORATIVE MATERIAL	SPECIALLY PROCESSED SODIUM BICARBONATE AIR POLISHING POWDER	ALUMINUM TRIHYDROXIDE AIR POLISHING POWDER
Amalgam	Yes	No
Gold	Yes*	No
Porcelain	Yes*	No
Hybrid composite	No	No
Microfilled composite	No	No
Glass ionomer	No	No
Compomer	No	No
Luting agents	No	No

*Only if margin is avoided.

REFERENCES

1. **De Leo**, A.A.: The Incidence of Bacteremia Following Oral Prophylaxis on Pediatric Patients, *Oral Surg., 37,* 36, January, 1974.
2. **Lucas**, V. and Roberts, G.J.: Odontogenic Bacteremia Following Tooth Cleaning Procedures in Children, *Pediatr. Dent., 22,* 96, March/April, 2000.
3. **Micik**, R.E., Miller, R.L., Mazzarella, M.A., and Ryge, G.: Studies on Dental Aerobiology: I. Bacterial Aerosols Generated During Dental Procedures, *J. Dent. Res., 48,* 49, January–February, 1969.
4. **Hartley**, J.L.: Eye and Facial Injuries Resulting From Dental Procedures, *Dent. Clin. North Am., 22,* 505, July, 1978.
5. **Vrbic**, V., Brudevold, F., and McCann, H.G.: Acquisition of Fluoride by Enamel From Fluoride Pumice Pastes, *Helv. Odontol. Acta, 11,* 21, April, 1967.
6. **Brudevold**, F., Gardner, D.E., and Smith, F.A.: The Distribution of Fluoride in Human Enamel, *J. Dent. Res., 35,* 420, June, 1956.
7. **Zuniga**, M.A. and Caldwell, R.C.: The Effect of Fluoride-Containing Prophylaxis Pastes on Normal and "White-Spot" Enamel, *ASDC J. Dent. Child., 36,* 345, September–October, 1969.
8. **Kontturi-Närhi**, V., Markkanen, S., and Markkanen, H.: Effects of Airpolishing on Dental Plaque Removal and Hard Tissues as Evaluated by Scanning Electron Microscopy, *J. Periodontol., 61,* 334, June, 1990.
9. **Leknes**, K.N.: The Influence of Anatomic and Iatrogenic Root Surface Characteristics on Bacterial Colonization and Periodontal Destruction: A Review, *J. Periodontol., 68,* 507, June, 1997.
10. **Quirynen**, M. and Bollen, C.M.L.: The Influence of Surface Roughness and Surface-Free Energy on Supra- and Subgingival Plaque Formation in Man: A Review of the Literature, *J. Clin. Periodontol., 22,* 1, January, 1995.
11. **Roulet**, J.F. and Roulet-Mehrens, T.K.: The Surface Roughness of Restorative Materials and Dental Tissues After Polishing With Prophylaxis and Polishing Pastes, *J. Periodontol., 53,* 257, April, 1982.
12. **Serio**, F.G., Strassler, H.E., Litkowski, L.J., Moffitt, W.C., and Krupa, C.M.: The Effect of Polishing Pastes on Composite Resin Surfaces: A SEM Study, *J Periodontol. 59,* 837, December, 1988.
13. **Löe**, H.: Reactions of Marginal Periodontal Tissues to Restorative Procedures, *Int. Dent. J., 18,* 759, December, 1968.
14. **Miller**, W.A.: Experimental Foreign Body Reactions to Toothpaste Abrasives, *J. Periodontol., 47,* 101, February, 1976.
15. **Tilliss**, T.S.I., Stach, D.J., and Cross-Poline, G.N.: Use of Toothpicks for Chlorhexidine Staining, *J. Clin. Periodontol., 19,* 398, July, 1992.
16. **Theilade**, J., Slots, J., and Fejerskov, O.: The Ultrastructure of Black Stain on Human Primary Teeth, *Scand. J. Dent. Res., 81,* 528, Number 7, 1973.
17. **Tinanoff**, N., Wei, S.H.Y., and Parkins, F.M.: Effect of a Pumice Prophylaxis on Fluoride Uptake in Tooth Enamel, *J. Am. Dent. Assoc., 88,* 384, February, 1974.
18. **United States Pharmacopeia:** *The National Formulary,* January 1, 1995. United States Pharmacopeial Convention, Inc., 12601 Twinbrook Parkway, Rockville, MD 20852, p. 1342.
19. **Wei**, S.H., Ngan, P.W.K., Wefel, J.S., and Kerber, P.: Evaluation of Fluoride Prophylaxis Pastes, *J. Dent. Res., 60,* 1297, July, 1981.
20. **Ripa**, L.W.: The Roles of Prophylaxis and Dental Prophylaxis Pastes in Caries Prevention, in Wei, S.H.Y., ed.: *Clinical Uses of Fluorides.* Philadelphia, Lea & Febiger, 1985, pp. 45–49.
21. **Vrbic**, V. and Brudevold, F.: Fluoride Uptake From Treatment With Different Fluoride Prophylaxis Pastes and From the Use of Pastes Containing a Soluble Aluminum Salt Followed by Topical Application, *Caries Res., 4,* 158, Number 2, 1970.
22. **Burrell**, K.H. and Chan, J.T.: Systemic and Topical Fluorides, in American Dental Association, Council on Scientific Affairs: *ADA Guide to Dental Therapeutics,* 2nd ed., Chicago, ADA Publishing Co., 2000, p. 236.
23. **Weaks**, L.M., Lescher, N.B., Barnes, C.M., and Holroyd, S.V.: Clinical Evaluation of the Prophy-jet as an Instrument for Routine Removal of Tooth Stain and Plaque, *J. Periodontol., 55,* 486, August, 1984.
24. **Barnes**, C.M., Covey, D.A., Walker, M.P., and Ross, J.A.: An in vitro Evaluation of the Effects of Aluminum Trihydroxide Delivered via the Prophy Jet on Dental Restorative Materials, In Press, *J. Prosthet. Dent.* 90, September, 2004.
25. **Orton**, G.S.: Clinical Use of an Air-Powder Abrasive System, *Dent. Hyg., 61,* 513, November, 1987.
26. **Barnes**, C.M., Russell, C.M., Gerbo, L.R., Wells, B.R., and Barnes, D.W.: Effects of an Air-Powder Polishing System on Orthodontically Bracketed and Banded Teeth, *Am. J. Orthod. Dentofac. Orthop., 97,* 74, January, 1990.
27. **Barnes**, C.M., Fleming, L.S., and Mueninghoff, L.A.: An SEM Evaluation of the In-vitro Effects of an Air-Abrasive System on Various Implant Surfaces, *Int. J. Oral Maxillofac. Implants, 6,* 463, Number 4, 1991.
28. **Scott**, L. and Greer, D.: The Effect of an Air Polishing Device on Sealant Bond Strength, *J. Prosthet. Dent., 58,* 384, September, 1987.
29. **Atkinson**, D.R., Cobb, C.M., and Killoy, W.J.: The Effect of an Air-Powder Abrasive System on *in vitro* Root Surfaces, *J. Periodontol., 55,* 13, January, 1984.
30. **Barnes**, C.M.: The Management of Aerosols With Airpolishing Delivery Systems, *J. Dent. Hyg., 65,* 280, July–August, 1991.
31. **Harrel**, S.K., Barnes, J.B., and Rivera-Hidalgo, F.: Aerosol Reduction During Air Polishing, *Quintessence Int., 30,* 623, September, 1999.
32. **Worrall**, S.F., Knibbs, P.J., and Glenwright, H.D.: Methods of Reducing Bacterial Contamination of the Atmosphere Arising From Use of an Air-Polisher, *Br. Dent. J., 163,* 118, August 22, 1987.
33. **Fine**, D.H., Mendieta, C., Barnett, M.L., Furgang, D., Meyers, R., Olshan, A., and Vincent, J.: Efficacy of Preprocedural Rinsing With an Antiseptic in Reducing Viable Bacteria in Dental Aerosols, *J. Periodontol., 63,* 821, October, 1992.
34. **Finlayson**, R.S. and Stevens, F.D.: Subcutaneous Facial Emphysema Secondary to Use of the Cavi-jet, *J. Periodontol., 59,* 315, May, 1988.
35. **Barnes**, C.M., Hayes, E.F., and Leinfelder, K.F.: Effects of an Airabrasive Polishing System on Restored Surfaces, *Gen. Dent., 35,* 186, May–June, 1987.
36. **Felton**, D.A., Bayne, S.C., Kanoy, B.E., and White, J.T.: Effect of Air Abrasives on Marginal Configurations of Porcelain-Fused-to-Metal Alloys: An SEM Analysis, *J. Prosthet. Dent., 65,* 38, January, 1991.

SUGGESTED READINGS

American Dental Hygienists' Association: Position on Polishing Procedures, *Access, 11,* 29, August, 1997.

Barnes, C.M., Fleming, L.S., and Russell, C.M.: An *in vitro* Evaluation of Commercially Available Disposable Prophylaxis Angles, *J. Dent. Hyg., 65,* 438, November–December, 1991.

Barnes, C.M., Fleming, L.S., and Russell, C.M.: Evaluation of Performance Characteristics of Four Commercially Available Disposable Prophylaxis Angles, *J. Pract. Hyg., 2,* 18, March/April, 1993.

Dean, M.-C., Barnes, D.M., and Blank, L.W.: A Comparison of Two Prophylaxis Angles: Disposable and Autoclavable, *J. Am. Dent. Assoc., 128,* 444, April, 1997.

Nordstrom, N.K., Uldricks, J.M., and Beck, F.M.: Selective Polishing: An Educational Trend in Dental Hygiene, *J. Dent. Hyg., 65,* 428, November–December, 1991.

Nunn, P.F.: "Selective Polishing"—Time for a Change? *Access, 11,* 38, January, 1997.

Air-Powder Polishing

Bay, N.L., Overman, P.R., Krust-Bray, K., Cobb, C., and Gross, K.B.W.: Effectiveness of Antimicrobial Mouthrinses on Aerosols Produced by an Air Polisher, *J. Dent. Hyg., 67,* 312, September–October, 1993.

Boyde, A.: Airpolishing Effects on Enamel, Dentine, Cement, and Bone, *Br. Dent. J., 156,* 287, April 21, 1984.

Brown, F.H., Ogletree, R.C., and Houston, G.D.: Pneumoparotitis Associated With the Use of an Air-Powder Prophylaxis Unit, *J. Periodontol., 63,* 642, July, 1992.

Gerbo, L.R., Lacefield, W.R., Barnes, C.M., and Russell, C.M.: Enamel Roughness After Air-Powder Polishing, *Am. J. Dent., 6,* 98, April, 1993.

Gutmann, M.E.: Air Polishing: A Comprehensive Review of the Literature, *J. Dent. Hyg., 72,* 47, Summer, 1998.

Logothetis, D.D., Gross, K.B.W., Eberhart, A., and Drisko, C.: Bacterial Airborne Contamination With an Air-Polishing Device, *Gen. Dent., 36,* 496, November–December, 1988.

Mishkin, D.J., Engler, W.O., Javed, T., Darby, T.D., Cobb, R.L., and Coffman, M.A.: A Clinical Comparison of the Effect on the Gingiva of the Prophy-jet and the Rubber Cup and Paste Techniques, *J. Periodontol., 57,* 151, March, 1986.

Restorative Materials

Cooley, R.L. and Lubow, R.M.: Effect of Air-Powder Abrasive on Glass Ionomer Microleakage, *Gen. Dent., 37,* 16, January–February, 1989.

Cooley, R.L., Lubow, R.M., and Brown, F.H.: Effects of Air-Power Abrasive Instrument on Porcelain, *J. Prosthet. Dent., 60,* 440, October, 1988.

Elaides, G.C., Tzoutzas, J.G., and Vougiouklakis, G.J.: Surface Alterations on Dental Restorative Materials Subjected to an Air-Powder Abrasive Instrument, *J. Prosthet. Dent., 65,* 27, January, 1991.

Gutmann, M.S.E., Marker, V.A., and Gutmann, J.L.: Restoration Surface Roughness After Air-Powder Polishing, *Am. J. Dent., 6,* 99, April, 1993.

Homiak, A.W., Cook, P.A., and DeBoer, J.: Effect of Hygiene Instrumentation on Titanium Abutments: A Scanning Electron Microscopy Study, *J. Prosthet. Dent., 67,* 364, March, 1992.

Huennekens, S.C., Daniel, S.J., and Bayne, S.C.: Effects of Air Polishing on the Abrasion of Occlusal Sealants, *Quintessence Int., 22,* 581, July, 1991.

Koka, S., Han, J.-S., Razzoog, M.E., and Bloem, T.J.: The Effects of Two Air-Powder Abrasive Prophylaxis Systems on the Surface of Machined Titanium: A Pilot Study, *Implant Dent., 1,* 259, Number 2, 1992.

Vermilyea, S.G., Prasanna, M.K., and Agar, J.R.: Effect of Ultrasonic Cleaning and Air Polishing on Porcelain Labial Margin Restorations, *J. Prosthet. Dent., 71,* 447, May, 1994.

Care of Dental Restorations

Joan C. Gibson-Howell, RDH, MSEd, EdD

The longevity, esthetic appearance, and smooth surfaces of dental restorations depend on appropriate care by the dental hygienist and the daily personal care by the patient. It is the responsibility of the dental hygienist to be current in knowledge and techniques to prevent damaging the restorations during the professional oral health care appointment procedures. In addition, the dental hygienist is responsible for educating the patient about proper home care techniques that contribute to the maintenance of the dental material. Key words related to the care of restorations are defined in Box 43-1.

I. DENTAL HYGIENE CARE PLANNING

Radiographs and clinical examination with charting are basic to knowing individual patient requirements as each care plan is selected and implemented.

BOX 43-1 KEY WORDS: Care of Restorations

Abrasion: a wear process.

Abrasive discs: abrasive particles are bonded to paper, metal, or plastic backing to form discs.

Burnishing: a process of smoothing a surface by rubbing lightly with a specially designed instrument or cotton pellet. The effects are improved marginal adaptation and increased hardness.

Carving: the removal of excess filling material, using special instruments. The goal is to produce accurate anatomic contours and restore form and function to the tooth.

Cavosurface junction: the junction of any wall of a cavity preparation with the unprepared tooth structure.

Corrosion: chemical and electrochemical deterioration on the surface and the subsurface of an amalgam restoration that usually begins as tarnish. Caused by environmental factors, such as, air, moisture, acid or alkaline solutions, or other chemicals. Corrosion at the margin can cause deterioration and fracturing, resulting in biofilm accumulation. By-products can be carried to the dentin and show a discoloration around the restoration.

Direct restoration: placed and formed in the cavity preparation; includes amalgam, composite resins, and glass ionomer cement.

Ditching: formation of a gap or groove between the cavity preparation margin and the restorative material.

Finishing: process that involves removing marginal irregularities, defining anatomic contours, and smoothing away surface roughness of a restoration.

Flash: type of overhang in which a thin layer of restoration extends beyond the cavosurface junction: also called a feather ledge.

Grit: the size of the abrasive particle.

Indirect restoration: formed on a die reproduction of a prepared tooth and then cemented into place: includes porcelain, gold inlays, and porcelain crowns.

Margination: process of removing excess restorative material and applying finishing techniques to reestablish a smooth, well-adapted cavosurface margin. The resultant junction should conform in shape and normal anatomic characteristics.

Overcontour: an excess of restorative material such that the normal anatomic form is altered.

Overhang: area of a restoration where the restorative material extends outward past the cavosurface margin of the cavity preparation; associated with gingival and periodontal disease, due to mechanical impingement and biofilm retention.

Polishing: process carried out after placement of a restoration to remove minute scratches from the surface of a restoration and obtain a smooth, shiny luster. Also applied after other refinishing techniques to produce an unscratched homogeneous surface. Uses abrasive agents to remove roughness, eliminate pits or grooves, and make the surface more resistant to bacterial accumulation.

Prophylactic paste: a paste containing polishing agents that is applied to teeth with a rubber cup and handpiece for cleaning purposes.

Recontour: instrumentation to reshape and remove marginal excess and to restore the natural anatomic form.

Tarnish: a discoloration of the surface of a metal restoration, usually from sulfides. Caused by lack of cleanliness, biofilm accumulation, and certain foods.

A. New Patient to the Practice

- Identify and document the type of dental material placed and irregularities of existing restorations.
- Determine an accurate dental hygiene diagnosis and care plan that includes appropriate finishing and polishing agents for the preservation of each restoration.
- Outline and present the care plan to the dentist and the patient.

B. Patient for Continuing Care

- Provide and monitor maintenance care.
- Maintain an accurate record of restorative materials and the appropriate finishing and polishing agents to be used for each during treatment procedures.
- Identify and document irregularities of restorations for care planning.
- Use appropriate finishing and polishing procedures for each dental material.

II. SUPPORTIVE CARE OF RESTORATIVE MATERIALS

Characteristics of a properly finished and polished restoration are listed in Box 43-2. With such characteristics together with conscientious personal daily care by the patient, the restoration can be expected to contribute to the patient's oral health for a very long time. Finishing and polishing of restorations contribute to the following effects:

- Improved gingival health due to less biofilm retention by restorative irregularities.

BOX 43-2 Characteristics of an Acceptable Finished and Polished Restoration

- Smooth anatomic contours
- Contact areas intact with normal form
- Embrasures spaced correctly
- Refined margins
- Smooth resistant surfaces
- Functional effectiveness
- Acceptable appearance
- No biofilm-retaining irregularities
- Restored health of the gingival tissues

- Improved compatibility of the restorative material with the gingival and oral soft tissues.
- Increased integrity of the junction of the tooth surface and the restoration.
- Improved maintenance by the patient; biofilm is more readily removed from smooth surfaces than from rough surfaces.
- Increased longevity of the serviceable life of the restoration due to the removal of factors that lead to surface changes and recurrent dental caries.
- Improved appearance of the restoration.

III. LONGEVITY OF A RESTORATION

The following factors influence the length of time a restoration maintains its original form and function:

A. **Initial Preparation and Placement of the Restoration**
- Design of the cavity preparation.
- Mix and manipulation of the dental material.
- Prevention of contamination during the insertion.
- Finishing and polishing.

B. **Patient Care of Completed Restoration:** daily biofilm control procedures

C. **Professional Care by the Dental Hygienist at Maintenance Appointments**

IV. RESPONSIBILITIES OF THE DENTAL HYGIENIST

- Learn/apply current information and techniques about the properties and uses of new dental materials.
- Service/treat restorations to maintain their original marginal integrity and surface finish.
- Teach/inform patients about restorative materials and methods to use for proper personal care and continued maintenance.

V. RISK FACTORS: POORLY MAINTAINED RESTORATIVE MATERIALS

- Dental hygienists' lack of current information concerning materials and their maintenance.
- Patients' lack of information concerning the value of proper daily care; compliance in the care of their restorations.
- Patients' lack of understanding regarding the benefits of well-maintained restorations.
- Patients' lack of knowledge about their own dental caries risk: high, medium, or low, based on *Mutans streptococci* and *Lactobacilli* counts and the high acid/sugar diet intake.

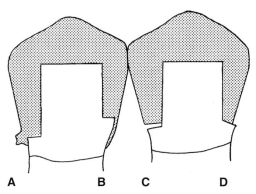

■ **FIGURE 43-1 Proximal Surface Irregularities. (A)** Overhang. **(B)** Flash. **(C)** Open or deficient margin. **(D)** Undercontoured margin that can result from an improperly placed matrix band or misdirected carving.

■ MARGINAL IRREGULARITIES

A restoration should follow the normal contours of the natural tooth. Certain deficiencies must be corrected by replacement of the restoration.

I. OVERHANGING MARGINS

An overhang is illustrated in Figure 43-1A. Overhangs may occur on any tooth surface, supragingivally or subgingivally, or in any class of cavity preparation. Proximal overhangs result primarily from:

- Improper placement of the matrix band and/or wedge.
- Incorrect manipulation of the dental material.
- Finishing errors.

II. FLASH

A. Occlusal

- Figure 43-2A illustrates an occlusal ledge or flash that was left during carving.

- When performed correctly, carving brings the prepared cavosurface margin into view and makes the filling material flush with the enamel.

B. Proximal-Gingival

- Can result when restorative material is packed between a matrix band and the tooth surface below the cavity preparation (Figure 43-1B).
- The flash can occur when a wedge is not used or not positioned to adapt the matrix tightly against the tooth surface.
- A tooth with a concave proximal surface is vulnerable to flash.

III. OPEN MARGIN

There is a distinct space between the restoration and the wall of the cavity preparation, as shown in Figure 43-1C.

IV. UNDERCONTOURED (Figure 43-1D)

- Opposite of an overhang: deficiency of dental material between the margin and the cavity wall.
- On a proximal surface: deficiency from improper placement of the matrix and/or wedge.
- Other examples: missing contact area, flattened cervical ridge, incomplete marginal ridge, or incomplete filling of the cavity preparation.

V. OVERCONTOURED

- Excess of dental material changes the normal anatomic form of the restoration.
- Proximal overcontoured surfaces may widen the contact area or narrow the embrasure.
- Overcontoured crown can cause biofilm retention with subsequent gingival inflammation.

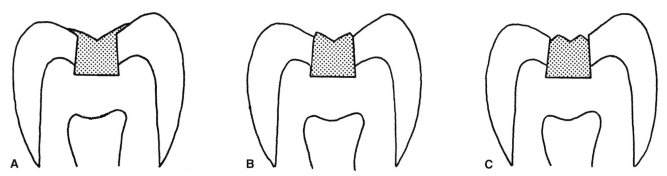

■ **FIGURE 43-2 Marginal Irregularities. (A)** Flash on the occlusal surface related to a Class I restoration. Flash refers to a thin layer of restoration that extends over the margin of the cavity preparation. **(B)** Irregular margin results when the flash breaks off. **(C)** Ditching results from broken off flash.

- Example: In Figure 30-1C, overcontoured crowns of a double abutment have narrowed the embrasure. Problems of biofilm control around overcontoured crown margins are shown in Figure 30-4 (page 489).

VI. DITCHING OR GROOVING

Figure 43-2C shows a gap on the occlusal surface where either the flash broke off or contraction of the material caused the restoration to pull away from the tooth structure. The retention of biofilm with resultant recurrent dental caries can occur in the area.

▪ OVERHANGING RESTORATIONS

Recontouring overhanging restorations is an essential part of dental and periodontal treatment. Initial therapy or Phase 1 periodontal therapy must include the correction of overhangs if periodontal health is to be restored.[1]

I. IDENTIFICATION

A. **Clinical.** An overhang is identified by the:
  - Relation to the gingival margin (supragingival or subgingival).
  - Location on specific tooth surface: enamel, cementum, or dentin.
  - Size or extent.
  - Information from the patient relative to floss breakage and food impaction.
B. **Radiographic**
  - Limited to proximal surfaces viewed in the radiograph.
  - Visibility changed by angulation of the x-ray.
  - Must be supplemented by a clinical examination with an explorer.
  - Use magnification to detect dental caries adjacent to an overhang.

II. EFFECTS OF OVERHANGING RESTORATIONS

A. Relationship to Periodontal Disease and Dental Caries

An overhang or marginal irregularity is a significant iatrogenic contributing factor because it can:
- Provide a niche where microorganisms that cause periodontal diseases and dental caries can proliferate.
- Catch and tear dental floss.
- Render the area inaccessible to a toothbrush and other dental biofilm-removing aids; hinder the patient from disease control procedures.
- Increase the severity of existing inflammation.[1-3]
- Increase the chance of adjacent bone loss.[1,4]
- Retain debris and microorganisms contributing to halitosis and a general lack of oral sanitation.

B. Benefits of Overhang Removal

- Efficient use of dental floss and other interdental cleaning devices.
- Improvement in periodontal health when combined with scaling, root planing, and dental biofilm control.[2,5]

III. INDICATIONS TO MAINTAIN OR REPLACE THE RESTORATION

All overhanging restorations need to be corrected or removed and replaced for the health of the periodontium. Whether an overhang can be recontoured or needs to be replaced with a new restoration requires a professional decision.

A. Indications for Continued Maintenance of the Restoration

- The tooth anatomy can be maintained or improved to conform to normal contour.
- The overhang is small or moderate in size.
- The proximal contact is intact.
- No adjacent secondary dental caries or fractures of the margin are present.
- The overhang is accessible for necessary instrumentation to finish and polish without damaging the adjacent tooth structure or traumatizing the gingival tissues.

B. Indications for Removal and Replacement of the Restoration

- The overhang is extensive and would require excessive appointment time.
- Secondary marginal or recurrent dental caries is present.
- The contact area must be restored.
- Fractures, chips, cracks, or broken margins are apparent.
- When replacement is delayed, a gross overhang should be reshaped and smoothed to enable the patient to remove dental biofilm more completely.

■ AMALGAM RESTORATIONS

Amalgam is a leading restorative material. The type of amalgam alloy used and the amount of carving completed at the time of placement dictates the extent of finishing needed for a recently placed restoration prior to polishing. Descriptive characteristics of amalgam are included in Table 43-1.

I. PROPERTIES AND CHANGES

A. Surface Changes

1. Tarnish
   - A surface discoloration resulting from sulfides; caused by lack of cleanliness, dental biofilm accumulation, and certain foods and acidic beverages.
   - Occurs less frequently on properly finished and polished restorations.
2. Corrosion
   - Deterioration caused by chemical or electrochemical reaction; environmental factors in the dark, warm, acidic environment of the mouth.
   - Polished amalgam restorations resist corrosion.
   - Marginal corrosion can lead to recurrent dental caries.
   - Products of corrosion may pass into the dentinal tubules and the area around the restoration will appear bluish-black.

B. Dimensional Changes

1. Expansion
   - May appear extruded above the cavosurface margin.
   - Caused by incomplete trituration and condensation, or moisture contamination during mixing and placing.
2. Contraction
   - Amalgam pulls away from cavosurface margin.
   - Figure 43-2C depicts ditching or grooving from contraction.

C. Strength Changes

- Fractures from insufficient strength.
- Due to occlusal pressures; improper finishing and carving.

II. FINISHING SYSTEMS

- Placement, carving, and finishing completed at one appointment; subsequent appointment for complete finishing and polishing at least 24 hours later.

- Newer spherical, fast-setting amalgam can be placed, carved, finished, and polished at the same appointment.
- Figure 43-3 displays a decision-making flow chart to assist in selecting appropriate procedures.

■ MARGINATION OF AN AMALGAM RESTORATION

I. PROCEDURES SUMMARIZED

A. Remove excess amalgam.
B. Finish all cavosurface margins to ensure they are continuous and smooth.
C. Smooth all surfaces of the restoration.

II. MANUAL INSTRUMENTS

A. General Suggestions for Use

1. Select on basis of accessibility of the filling, amount of reduction required, and surface finish indicated.
2. Instruments: amalgam knife, file, cleoid and discoid carvers, scalers, curets, finishing strips.
3. Technique
   - Maintain sharp instruments.
   - Remove excess amalgam in small increments to prevent fracture.
   - Work deliberately to prevent damage to gingival tissue and surrounding tooth surfaces, especially cementum.
   - Maintain tooth anatomy; use the tooth surface as a guide to contour the restoration.
   - Move a bladed instrument parallel to, or slightly toward, the margin of the prepared tooth.
   - Keep carver in contact with the tooth surface to reduce risk of ditching.

B. Amalgam Knife (Figure 43-4)

- Hold the blade across the tooth structure and amalgam; activate knife diagonally across the junction.
- Use short, overlapping shaving strokes; remove amalgam in small increments to prevent fracture risk.
- For proximal adaptation, move knife away from gingiva to prevent pushing bits of amalgam into the tissue; evacuate continuously.

C. File (Figure 43-4)

- Determine file design (push or pull); position file accordingly.

■ TABLE 43-1 COMPARISON OF RESTORATIVE DENTAL MATERIALS

LEAKAGE AND RECURRENT DENTAL CARIES	AMALGAM	COMPOSITES	GLASS IONOMERS	PORCELAIN	GOLD ALLOY
Description and Uses	• Mercury and silver alloy • Hardens at mouth temperature	• Glass filler forms a solid tooth-colored restoration • Self or light cure	• Fluoride with glass powder and organic acid • Forms a solid esthetic restoration	• Glass-like esthetic restoration	• Alloy of gold, copper, and other metals
Leakage and Recurrent Caries	• Moderate • Recurrent caries is similar to other materials	• Low when bonded to a tooth • Recurrent caries depends on continued care	• Low • Recurrent caries is similar to other materials • Fluoride may benefit	• Seal depends on material, tooth structure, and procedure	• Good seal • Recurrent caries is similar to other materials
Resistance to Wear and Fracture	• Highly resistant • Good strength in high-stress areas • Brittle and subject to chipping	• Moderate, but less than amalgam • Moderately resistant to fracture	• Highly resistant on chewing surfaces • Low to moderate resistance to fracture	• High resistance, but can wear opposing teeth • Prone to fracture under impact	• High resistance, yet gentle to opposing teeth • High resistance to fracture
Clinical Considerations	• Moderately tolerant to placement conditions	• Very little tolerance to moisture • Must be placed in a dry field	• Very little tolerance to moisture • Must be placed in a dry field	• Multiple procedural steps • Highly accurate clinic and lab process	• Multiple procedural steps • Highly accurate clinic and lab process
Durability	• Good to excellent in large restorations	• Good in small to moderate-sized restorations	• Moderate to good in non-stress restorations • Poor in high-stress areas	• Brittle • May fracture under heavy biting stress	• High strength to resist fracture and wear
Esthetics	• Gray to silver • Does not mimic natural tooth color	• Mimics natural tooth color • Subject to stain over time	• Mimics natural tooth color • Lacks natural translucency of enamel	• Mimics natural tooth color	• Metals do not mimic natural tooth color
Sensitivity	• Possible early sensitivity to hots and colds	• Depends on adequate bonding to tooth	• Low • Depends on adequate bonding to tooth	• Low	• High
Cost and Number of Visits	• Depends on size • Generally lower • One or two visits	• Moderate • Depends on size and technique • One or two visits depending on technique	• Moderate • Depends on size and technique • One visit	• Higher • At least two visits	• Higher • At least two visits

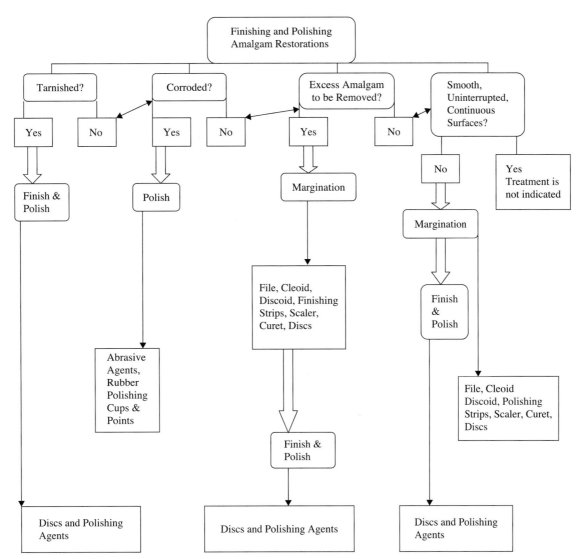

■ FIGURE 43-3 Finishing and Polishing an Amalgam Restoration Flow Chart. Follow the flow of steps according to questions and responses.

- Use coarser file for bulk of amalgam; refine margin smoothness with finer file.
- Extend strokes across amalgam and tooth to prevent leaving a defect.
- Use short, controlled strokes with light to moderate pressure.

D. Cleoid and Discoid Carvers (Figure 43-4)

- Refine fossae and fissures with small sharp cleoid; avoid discoid in occlusal fissures to prevent rounding.
- Use the discoid as an aid for redefining margins.

E. Finishing Strips

- Use narrow, fine, or medium strips after gross amalgam has been removed.

- Avoid a finishing strip on a contact area.
- Prepare to thread the strip through an embrasure: cut the end on a diagonal, or use a strip with a gap or clear middle area.
- Avoid pressure on adjacent tooth surface: cementum can be easily grooved.

F. Scaler

- Use only a strong scaler: tip can be broken when extra force is applied.
- Using a metal cutting edge on metal dulls the instrument.

G. Curet

- Universal curet: an aid for smoothing proximal surface.

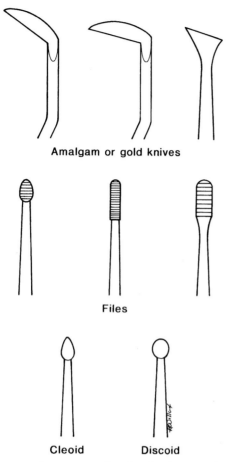

Amalgam or gold knives

Files

Cleoid   Discoid

■ **FIGURE 43-4 Instruments for Margination.** Amalgam and gold foil knives; various shapes of files; and the amalgam carvers, cleoid and discoid, especially useful for margination.

- Cross oblique strokes over the junction of the material and the tooth.

III. POWER-DRIVEN INSTRUMENTS

A. General Suggestions

1. Effect of overheating
   - Irreversible pulp damage.
   - Alteration of chemical structure of restorative material.
   - Patient discomfort: tooth sensitivity.
2. Use low speed: intermittent light strokes in multidirectional motion.

B. Finishing Burs and Stones

1. Selection: shape for accessibility: flame, round, pear.
2. Select color for abrasivity
   - Green stones to remove excess.
   - White stones to reduce fine limited surfaces and marginal discrepancies.

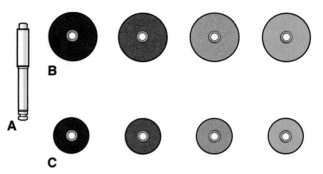

■ **FIGURE 43-5 Use of Discs.** Discs are available in several sizes, some with moisture-resistant backings. Abrasive devices are used in sequence in descending order of abrasiveness, coarse to fine. The mildest possible should be selected at the start to prevent unnecessary removal of material or tooth structure. **(A)** Mandrel for holding discs. **(B)** and **(C)** Two sizes of discs shaded to represent coarse to fine.

3. Adaptation
   - Remaining enamel will guide the contour.
   - Hold the instrument across the cavosurface margin and move diagonally to prevent fracture or ditching.
   - Keep bur or stone in constant motion with a light sweeping stroke to prevent leaving marks and grooves.

C. Discs (Figure 43-5)

1. Selection: garnet (coarse); cuttle (fine)
   - Coarse: remove bulk readily; may be more damaging to soft tissues and tooth structure.
   - Proximal surface: activate disc to prevent flattening of the restoration and to avoid contact area.
   - Use short, diagonal, overlapping strokes with a sweeping motion across cavosurface margin; rotate disc from tooth structure to restoration to reduce chance of ditching.
   - Direct strokes away from gingival tissues.

▪ POLISHING AN AMALGAM RESTORATION

After margination and finishing, the amalgam is polished. Figure 43-3 provides a decision-making flow chart to assist in selection of procedures.

I. GENERAL SUGGESTIONS

A. Use Wet Polishing Agents
- Avoid dry polishing with powders or discs; heat production.

- Use separate polishing cups and points for different abrasive agents.
B. **Use Low Speed.** Use light intermittent strokes.
C. **Avoid Cementum.** Do not extend brushes or cups over the cementum. Abrasive polishing agent can groove and scratch the cementum.
D. **Do Not Overpolish.** Overpolishing can:
  - Alter the contour of the restoration and destroy the contact area.
  - Remove surrounding tooth structure, especially cementum.

II. POLISHING PROCEDURES

A. Rubber Cups and Points

- Brown and green rubber cups and points have abrasive incorporated; for use after conventional burs, stones, or discs.
- Points for occlusal; cups for proximal surfaces.
- Use brown first, follow with green: with light, intermittent strokes under wet conditions.
- Some cups and points can be sterilized; others are disposable.

B. Mounted Brushes: Pointed or Cup Shaped

- Soften brushes by soaking in warm water.
- Use a fine pumice or fine silex in a wet, water slurry.
- Apply agent over the area before starting power-driven instrument.
- Use a slow to moderate speed; keep brush or cup in constant motion with light, intermittent strokes to prevent heat.
- Use dental tape to apply agent to proximal surface not reached by other instruments; avoid contact area.
- With each succeeding change of abrasive from coarse to fine, rinse all previous agents from the area; use a fresh cup or point.
- Rinse and evaluate frequently to prevent overpolishing.

C. Final Polish

- Apply tin oxide in a thin, wet slurry with water; use a new rubber cup.
- Apply with light intermittent strokes.
- Rinse and evaluate.

D. Manufacturer's Instructions

Always consult manufacturer's instructions for use of all dental materials.

III. EVALUATION

- Periodontal tissues are examined 4 to 6 weeks after margination and polishing procedures.
- Complete Records: to show treatment outcome, patient disposition, follow-up recommendations, patient compliance with personal care of the teeth and the supporting structures as well as the care of the restorations.

■ ESTHETIC RESTORATIONS

The older composite restorations were usually unfilled resins or silicates that were chemically cured, light cured, or light activated and chemically cured. They contained an organic resin matrix and an inorganic filler of differing particle sizes. As a result, chipping, staining, and breakdown of the margins were more likely to occur.

Current composite materials consist of complex blends of polymerized resins with glass powder fillers. Unlike the older unfilled resins, there is an additive to supply an opaque characteristic. Composites require careful consideration when a polishing agent is selected for dental hygiene care.

Composite resins have a smoother surface and are highly polishable compared with previous direct esthetic restorative materials. Both glass ionomer and compomer restorative materials provide the benefit of fluoride release yet have limited stress ability and do not produce as smooth a surface compared with composite resins.

Table 43-1 provides a comparison of composite resin, glass ionomer, and porcelain esthetic restorations.

■ COMPOSITE RESINS

Composites are esthetic restorative materials composed of two or more materials. They are commonly made of glass filler and an acrylic combined to enhance the properties of each material.

I. USES

- Class I and II posterior direct restorations.
- Class III, IV, and V anterior direct restorations.
- Veneers for teeth that have been intrinsically stained by drugs or chemicals.
- Fill spaces, such as diastemas.
- Improve the size or contour of small or misshapen teeth.
- Pit and fissure sealants.

II. CHARACTERISTICS

- Softer to an explorer than enamel or porcelain.
- Esthetic, tooth colored, but may stain.
- Highly polishable.
- Must individualize which polishing agent to use.

■ MICROFILLED COMPOSITE RESINS

Microfilled composite resins are composed of very fine silica filler. They polish very smooth, possess excellent polishing qualities, and have a higher luster (compared with hybrid composite resins).

I. USES

- Anterior esthetic restorations.
- Diastema closures.
- Hand-sculpted composite veneers.
- Class III and V restorations.

II. CHARACTERISTICS

- Easy to regain surface luster.
- High surface shine using rubber polishing cups, wheels, and points.
- Easy to ditch or scratch upon margination.
- Chips can be modified and stains can be removed with a sequence of finishing discs and strips.

■ HYBRID COMPOSITE RESINS

Hybrid composite resins are a mix of glass and silica with large, different-sized filler particles. They can be used where strength and wear resistance are more important than surface luster.

I. USES

- Class IV anterior restorations.
- Incisal edges of anterior teeth.
- Class I or II posterior restorations where there is a moderate stress chewing load.

II. CHARACTERISTICS

- More difficult to achieve and maintain a high luster polish.
- Best strength of all resin categories.
- Polishable using a diamond-impregnated polisher.
- Do not polish as smoothly or with as much shine as the microfill composite resins.

■ COMPOMER

Compomer is a direct esthetic restorative material that is a combination of glass ionomer and composite.

I. USES

- Class I, II, III, and V restorations in low stress-bearing areas of patients with moderate risk for dental caries.
- Buildups or cores for cast crowns.
- Esthetic repair for fractured or chipped porcelain restorations.

II. CHARACTERISTICS

- Smoother surface than glass ionomer, yet not as smooth as composite resin materials.
- Best translucency of any of the direct esthetic restorative materials.
- Releases fluoride similar to glass ionomers.
- Less wear resistant than composites.
- Good handling characteristics.

■ GLASS IONOMER RESINS

Glass ionomer restorative materials are composed of a polyacrylic matrix filled with aluminosilicate particles. A significant benefit of using glass ionomer restorative cements is the release of fluoride to reduce dental caries.

I. USES

- Cements or low stress-bearing restorations.
- Limited use as Class I and II restorations in the primary dentition.
- Class I, II, and V restorations on a high caries risk patient where esthetics are not critical.

II. CHARACTERISTICS

- Cannot be polished to the same smoothness as composite resin.
- Minimal shine.
- Brittle, experience higher incidence of fracture and wear.
- Use is limited to low stress or surface abrasion areas.
- More opaque, therefore, may be less desirable than other composite resin materials.

■ PORCELAIN

A ceramic or porcelain restoration is completed in the laboratory prior to cementation into the patient's mouth.

Porcelain restorations are the longest lasting cosmetic restoration.

When consistently and properly maintained, a porcelain restoration can last for many years. Yet, if not, the restoration may become rough on the occlusal/incisal surface and increase wear of the opposing dentition. In addition, roughness may increase the susceptibility to stain and dental caries. If the gingival margins are not adequately polished, there can be increased gingival and periodontal inflammation.[7]

I. TYPES AND USES

- High-fusing material is used for denture teeth.
- Medium-fusing material is used for anterior porcelain jacket crowns, ceramic restorations, inlays, onlays, and crowns.
- Low-fusing material is used in porcelain-fused-to-metal crowns.

II. CHARACTERISTICS

- Mimics tooth color.
- More esthetic appearance than composite resins.
- Retains luster over time if appropriate porcelain abrasive system is used to maintain.
- Subject to fracture.
- Susceptible to staining if margins are inadequately maintained.
- Brittle nature may require it to be fused to metal for strength.

■ DENTAL HYGIENE CARE

Tooth-colored restorations require special attention and care during dental hygiene appointments. Commercially available polishing pastes are available to remove stain. Yet, it is the abrasive agents in the pastes that can be detrimental to the composite and/or porcelain material.

The term "selective polish" takes on special meaning. In customary use, stain removal is selectively performed when there is unsightly stain that has not been removed by toothbrushing and other oral hygiene procedures or during the scaling and debridement portion of the appointment. Now, the dental hygienist must also determine what specific polishing agent is required for specific types of restorations.

I. IDENTIFICATION OF THE RESTORATIVE MATERIAL

Recognizing the presence of a restoration can be difficult when the dental material is nearly a perfect match for the natural tooth. A margin between the restoration and the tooth substance may be invisible. Methods to assist in the identification of an esthetic restoration include:

- **Review the Patient Record:** The practice in which the restoration was placed should document accurately and chart the types of esthetic restorations.
- **Gather Patient Information:** Although it may not be appropriate to rely on patient information regarding the specific type of material that makes up an esthetic restoration, it is wise to question the patient about the restorative material and learn as much as possible.
- **Use Tactile Detection:** Composite restorations have a distinct tactile feel with a dental explorer that contrasts with a natural tooth or a ceramic or porcelain restoration. A black line of metal may also be apparent when an explorer is used on the material.
- **Use of Air:** Esthetic restorations may reveal a dry, chalky appearance when air is applied. The air may assist in differentiating between the restoration and natural tooth.

II. CARE OF COMPOSITE RESIN RESTORATIONS

Most composite resin restorations are finished and polished at the time of placement. The objective, therefore, is to "do no harm" and to maintain the original finish of the material at future appointments without change. Table 43-2 suggests products and materials that can be used safely on composite type restorations.

A. POLISHING COMPOSITE RESTORATIONS

- Examine and identify the dental material.
- Follow manufacturers' instructions: use recommended polishing agents, armamentarium, sequence, and procedures.
- Consult Table 43-2.
- Avoid use of:

  Conventional polishing pastes
  Air polishers
  Ultrasonic and sonic scalers

B. POSTCARE

- Apply a topical neutral sodium fluoride.
- Avoid the use of acidulated phosphate or stannous fluoride since they may cause alteration of the filler particles and discoloration of the resin.
- Avoid recommending mouthrinses containing alcohol. Alcohol may act as a solvent for the BIS-GMA resin resulting in softening of the material, making it rougher and easier to stain.

▪ TABLE 43-2 RECOMMENDATIONS FOR POLISHING ESTHETIC RESTORATIVE MATERIALS

MATERIAL	PRODUCT	DIRECTIONS	DISCS
Porcelain	D Porcelain Polishers™ Proxyt™ (Ivoclar-Vivident)	Use dry; low speed, moderate pressure; coarse to medium to fine abrasives	Sof-lex™ discs (3 M)
Glass ionomers	Proxyt™ (Ivoclar-Vivident)	Use water-soluble lubricant to prevent dessication; coarse to medium to fine abrasives	Sof-lex™ discs (3 M); PoGo Polishing Disc™ (Dentsply Caulk)
Microfilled composites	Prisma Gloss™ (Dentsply Caulk)	Prophy cup, water, aluminum oxide paste; rubber polisher; coarse to medium to fine abrasives	Sof-lex™ discs (3 M); PoGo Polishing Disc™ (Dentsply Caulk)
Hybrid composites	Prisma Gloss™ rubber polisher (Dentsply Caulk); D Fine Rubber Polishing Points™	Prophy cup, water, aluminum oxide paste; coarse to medium to fine abrasives	PoGo Polishing Disc™ (Dentsply Caulk)
	Prisma Gloss™ Extrafine (Dentsply Caulk)	Prophy cup, water, aluminum oxide paste; coarse to medium to fine abrasives	Sof-lex™ discs (3 M)

Recommendations based on Barnes, C.M., Covey, D.A., Walker, M.P.: Maintenance of the Esthetic Integrity of Dental Restorations, *RDH, 23,* 74, March, 2003.

III. DENTAL HYGIENE CARE FOR PORCELAIN

A. Debridement

- Gently debride deposits with sharp curets.
- Avoid the use of a sickle, ultrasonic, or sonic scaler, air polisher, or air abrasive unit.
- Consider the use of a plastic instrument as an adjunct.

B. Polishing

- Consult Table 43-2.

C. Routine Care Procedures

- Use a low-speed handpiece and a special paste for porcelain.
- Put a drop of water in a soft, flexible rubber cup or felt disc or wheel. Polish for 15-30 seconds

Everyday Ethics

A new patient makes an appointment in the office having just moved across country from a distant city. Mrs. Wilhelm brings a duplicate copy of bitewings that were taken 14 months ago. Ramona, the dental hygienist, proceeds with a complete medical history, full mouth radiographs, and a thorough intraoral and extraoral examination.

The patient raves about her previous dentist and how only he did the "cleaning" appointments for her even though "there were girls" in the office. Mrs. Wilhelm also indicates that she was on a 5-month interval for recalls. Ramona is pleased by the patient's positive view of dentistry until she begins to probe and chart the hard tissue. On proximal tooth surfaces, several overhangs were evident. Mrs. Wilhelm offers that some fillings had to be replaced but that her previous dentist never charged her for them.

Questions for Consideration

1. How should Ramona proceed to educate Mrs. Wilhelm, careful that all of the oral findings have not been definitively confirmed with current radiographs or by the dentist?

2. Explain how the principles of veracity and role fidelity relate to this scenario?

3. How is Ramona's "duty" to Mrs. Wilhelm different since she is a new patient in the practice? What conflicts might be anticipated in dealing with this patient?

per surface. Dilute the paste with water as the polishing progresses.

D. Neutral Sodium Fluoride Topical Application

- Avoid the use of acidulated phosphate fluoride or stannous fluoride.

■ THE MAINTENANCE APPOINTMENT

Continuing care for all types of restorations is a constant concern. The patient expects restorations to last a long time and the esthetic features be maintained.

I. ASSESSMENT

A. Review Dental History

B. Study Previous Patient Charts/Records

1. *Tooth-Colored Restorations:* Identify locations and specific materials.

Factors To Teach The Patient

- The importance of the patient's continued self-care in maintaining restorations.

- The advantages of proper and regular use of a soft brush in a sulcular technique, dental floss, and a mild, fluoridated, nonabrasive dentifrice.

- The advantages of limiting cariogenic foods.

- The harmful effects of rough and defective restorations on gingival disease and dental caries.

- Causes of discoloration of plastic and porcelain restorative materials.

- The need to quit the use of tobacco.

- The adverse effects of oral habits that may cause chipping or fracturing of restorations.

- The advantages of having finished and polished restorations.

- The need for daily and/or professional applications of neutral sodium fluoride to promote remineralization on the periphery of restorations.

2. *Instruments and Agents:* Identify previous professional care for tooth-colored restorations.
3. *Patient Counseling:* Note previous instruction for personal care of restorations; advice given for stain prevention; smoking history past and present and whether smoking cessation was successful.

C. Clinical Examination

1. *Soft Tissue:* Monitor gingiva adjacent to restorative materials.
2. *Periodontal Probing:* Complete probing with an emphasis on gingival margins and probing depths adjacent to restorations.
3. *Dental Examination*
   a. Explore all margins of restorations.
   b. Check documentation of new restorations placed since previous dental hygiene appointment; record dental material(s) used, and determine care needed.

II. PATIENT COUNSELING

Instruct the patient in personal care procedures to preserve the dental material(s) and the teeth. This education must be an integral part of the dental hygiene appointment.

A. Evaluate Patient's Personal Care

1. Use caution when using disclosing agents on tooth-colored restorations because the dye might be absorbed by the tooth-colored dental material.
2. Use minimal disclosing agent in a discreet area to assess the color absorption qualities prior to use of a dye in a large area.
3. May detect soft deposits by running a probe over the surfaces while the patient watches in a mirror.

B. Tobacco Use

1. Prevent health hazards by discussing tobacco cessation.
2. Prevent staining of esthetic restorative materials by discussing tobacco cessation.

C. Dietary Review

1. Prevent dental caries by discussing diet.
2. Discuss relationship of diet and caries/recurrent caries with carbohydrates and sugars on teeth and restorations.
3. Discuss foods as a source of discoloration of esthetic restorations.

III. CLINICAL PROCEDURES

At maintenance appointments the dental hygienist uses instruments and procedures that cannot alter or otherwise harm the surfaces and margins of the dental materials.

REFERENCES

1. **Gilmore**, N. and Sheiham, A.: Overhanging Dental Restorations and Periodontal Disease, *J. Periodontol., 42,* 8, January, 1971.
2. **Highfield**, J.E. and Powell, R.N.: Effects of Removal of Posterior Overhanging Metallic Margins of Restorations Upon the Periodontal Tissues, *J. Clin. Periodontol., 5,* 169, August, 1978.
3. **Pack**, A.R.C., Coxhead, L.J., and McDonald, B.W.: The Prevalence of Overhanging Margins in Posterior Amalgam Restorations and Periodontal Consequences, *J. Clin. Periodontol., 17,* 145, March, 1990.
4. **Jeffcoat**, M.K. and Howell, T.H.: Alveolar Bone Destruction Due to Overhanging Amalgam in Periodontal Disease, *J. Periodontol., 51,* 599, October, 1980.
5. **Rodriguez-Ferrer**, H.J., Strahan, J.D., and Newman, H.N.: Effect on Gingival Health of Removing Overhanging Margins of Interproximal Subgingival Amalgam Restorations, *J. Clin. Periodontol., 7,* 457, December, 1980.
6. **Barnes**, C.M., Covey, D.A., and Walker, M.P.: Maintenance of the Esthetic Integrity of Dental Restorations, *RDH, 23,* 74, March, 2003.
7. **Okuda**, W.H.: Aesthetic Maintenance Protocol in Cosmetic Dentistry, *J. Pract. Hyg., 11,* 31, September/October, 2002.
8. **Hodsdon**, K.A. and Williams III, A.J.: A Comprehensive Approach to Creating and Maintaining Direct Resin Veneers, *J. Pract. Hyg., 9,* 21, September/October, 2000.

SUGGESTED READINGS

Cardoso, M., Baratieri, L.N., and Ritter, A.V.: The Effect of Finishing and Polishing on the Decision to Replace Existing Amalgam Restorations, *Quintessence Int., 30,* 413, June, 1999.

Carr, M.P., Mitchell, J.C., Seghi, R.R., and Vermilyea, S.G.: The Effect of Air Polishing on Contemporary Esthetic Restorative Materials, *Gen. Dent., 50,* 238, May-June, 2002.

Hodsdon, K.A.: Postoperative Care for Aesthetic Restorations: A Challenge to Dental Hygienists, *J. Pract. Hyg., 7,* 19, March/April, 1998.

Hodsdon, K.A.: Polishing to Preserve, *RDH, 22,* 96, August, 2002.

McGuire, M.K. and Miller, L.: Maintaining Esthetic Restorations in the Periodontal Practice, *Int. J. Periodont. Restorative Dent., 16,* 231, June, 1996.

Neme, A.L., Frazier, K.B., Roeder, L.B., and Debner, T.L.: Effect of Prophylactic Polishing Protocols on the Surface Roughness of Esthetic Restorative Materials, *Oper.Dent., 27,* 50, January-February, 2002.

Rogo, E.J.: Overhang Removal: Improving Periodontal Health Adjacent to Class II Amalgam Restorations, *J. Pract. Hyg., 4,* 15, May/June, 1995.

Schatzle, M., Lang, N.P., Anerud, A., Boysen, H., Burgin, W., and Loe, H.: The Influence of Margins of Restorations on the Periodontal Tissues Over 26 Years, *J. Clin. Periodontol., 28,* 57, January, 2001.

Wilder, A.D. Jr., Swift, E.J. Jr., May, K.N. Jr., Thompson, J.Y., and McDougal, R.S.: Effect of Finishing Technique on the Microleakage and Surface Texture of Resin-Modified Glass Ionomer Restorative Materials, *J. Dent., 28,* 367, July, 2000.

Yap, A.U.J., Lye, K.W., and Sau, C.W.: Surface Characteristics of Tooth-Colored Restoratives Polished Utilizing Different Polishing Systems, *Oper. Dent., 22,* 260, November-December, 1997.

Ceramics

Ashe, M.J., Tripp, G.A., Eichmiller, F.C., George, L.A., and Meiers, J.C.: Surface Roughness of Glass-Ceramic Insert-Composite Restorations: Assessing Several Polishing Techniques, *J. Am. Dent. Assoc., 127,* 1495, October, 1996.

Culp, L., McLaren, E.A., Ritter, R.G., Roberts, M., and Trinkner, T.: Selection of Ceramic Materials for Aesthetics and Function, *J. Pract. Hyg., 11,* 13, March/April, 2002.

Goldstein, G.R., Barnhard, B.R., and Penugonda, B.: Profilometer, SEM, and Visual Assessment of Porcelain Polishing Methods, *J. Prosthet., Dent., 65,* 627, May, 1991.

Composites

Harvey, H.L. and Swift, E.J.: Effects of a Calculus Scaling Gel on Microhardness of Composite Resins, *J. Pract. Hyg., 4,* 32, May/June, 1995.

Lopes, G.C., Franke, M., and Maia, H.P.: Effects of Finishing Time and Techniques on Marginal Sealing Ability of Two Composite Restorative Materials, *J. Prosthet, Dent., 88,* 32, July, 2002.

Nash, L.B.: Maximizing Aesthetic Restorations: The Hygienist's Role, *J. Pract. Hyg., 1,* 23, March, 1992.

Settembrini, L., Penugonda, B., Scherer, W., Strassler, H., and Hittleman, E.: Alcohol-Containing Mouthwashes: Effect on Composite Color, *Oper. Dent., 20,* 14, January-February, 1995.

Stoddard, J.W. and Johnson, G.H.: An Evaluation of Polishing Agents for Composite Resins, *J. Prosthet. Dent., 65,* 491, April, 1991.

Strassler, H.E. and Moffitt, W.: The Surface Texture of Composite Resin After Polishing With Commercially Available Toothpastes, *Compend. Cont. Educ. Dent., 8,* 826, November-December, 1987.

Glass Ionomer

El-Badrawy, W.A. and McComb, D.: Effect of Home-Use Fluoride Gels on Resin-Modified Glass-Ionomer Cements, *Oper. Dent., 23,* 2, January-February, 1998.

Momoi, Y., Hirosaki, K., Kohno, A., and McCabe, J.F.: In Vitro Toothbrush-Dentifrice Abrasion of Resin-Modified Glass Ionomers, *Dent. Mater., 13,* 82, March, 1997.

Maintenance for Oral Health: Dental Hygiene Continuing Care

Esther M. Wilkins, BS, RDH, DMD
Anna Matsuishi Pattison, RDH, MS

CHAPTER OUTLINE

The overall purposes of treatment are to arrest disease and provide oral health, function, and comfort for the patient (Table 44-1). After a series of active treatments when evaluation shows that the soft tissue is in optimum health and the dentition has been restored in function, the patient enters a new phase of treatment for continuing supervision and care.

The primary objective of dental hygiene maintenance is to continue the healthy state attained during active therapy. The patient must realize that oral diseases do recur, but *control* is possible by combined personal and professional care. Lifelong preservation of the teeth and their supporting structures is a realistic goal.

Initially the success of the program depends on the understanding by the patient of the maintenance procedure. One way to help the patient become aware is by including the concept of the maintenance phase in the initial care plan. Terms associated with preventive maintenance are defined in Box 44-1.

I. PURPOSES OF THE MAINTENANCE PROGRAM

A. Prevent new disease from starting.
B. Prevent recurrence of previous infections.
C. Monitor educational and behavioral changes.
D. Monitor clinical signs of health and disease.
  1. Periodontal infections.
  2. Dental carious lesions.
  3. Oral mucosal lesions.
E. Provide specialized instruction for new implants, prostheses, and orthodontic appliances.
F. Offer motivational encouragement.

II. APPOINTMENT INTERVALS

A. Frequency Planning

No fixed schedule by which all patients can be maintained in oral health is possible because the frequency depends on the needs of each patient. Appointments may vary from 2 to 6 months. The time interval must be reevaluated periodically and changed in accord with changing needs.

B. Maintenance Frequency: Contributing Factors

1. Risk for periodontal disease activity.
2. Risk for dental carious lesions.
3. Risk for oral cancer: tobacco and alcohol users.
4. Predisposing diseases, conditions, and behaviors for periodontal diseases: diabetes, HIV/AIDS, host genetic factors, smoking, and stress.[1]
5. Compliance: keeping appointments, personal daily biofilm control.

TABLE 44-1 PURPOSES AND OUTCOMES OF DENTAL HYGIENE PERIODONTAL THERAPY

- Resolve inflammation
- Eliminate bleeding on probing
- Restore lost tissues to normal contour and texture
- Create environment for healing
- Arrest disease progression
- Preserve esthetics
- Provide patient comfort
- Encourage patient self-care
- Create environment that deters recurrence of infection
- Motivate patient to cooperate in continuing care

6. Previous treatment: patient who has had previous disease, either dental caries or periodontal infection, is at a greater risk for recurrence.
7. Local factors: rate of calculus formation.
8. Restorative complications: implants, prosthetic replacements.

C. Special Appointment Requirements

Intervals of 2 or 3 months are required for many patients. Examples of patients in this category are described throughout this book. A few are mentioned here.

1. *Patient Undergoing Extensive Dental Care.* The gingival or periodontal treatment may be completed or nearly completed by the time appointments for restorative phases of treatment are under way. The first maintenance appointment should be dated from the completion of the initial gingival and periodontal treatment. When extensive restorative, prosthetic, or other treatment is in progress, frequent tissue maintenance during long-term therapy is essential.
2. *Rampant Dental Caries.* Appointment for continuation of a caries control effort includes topical fluoride applications, dietary supervision, and personal care factors for biofilm control.
3. *Orthodontic Therapy.* Appliances make cleaning and biofilm control difficult; frequent topical

BOX 44-1 KEY WORDS AND ABBREVIATIONS: Maintenance

Compliance: action in accordance with request; extent to which a person's health behaviors coincide with dental/medical health advice. Also called **adherence.**

Consultation: the joint deliberation, usually for diagnostic purposes, between two or more practitioners or between a patient and a practitioner.

Disease activity: ongoing dynamic process that results in loss of clinical attachment and alveolar supporting bone; an area is quiescent when a diseased site becomes inactive or stable without treatment.

End points: criteria for completion of a particular procedure; therapeutic end points generally have been reached when the clinical signs of the treated pathologic condition have been eliminated or reduced.

PMT: periodontal maintenance therapy; also called preventive maintenance, supportive periodontal treatment.

Recall: system of appointments for the long-term maintenance phase of patient care; the system is carried out by computer, telephone, and/or mail.

Refractory: resistant, not responding to routine therapy.

Remission: diminution or abatement of the symptoms of a disease; the period during which the diminution occurs.

Response diagnosis: the diagnosis made at a reevaluation spaced for a period of time after treatment (or a series of treatments); diagnosis that shows the response to prior treatment.

Risk factor: a characteristic, habit, or predisposing condition that makes an individual susceptible to, or in danger of acquiring, a certain disease or disability.

SPT: supportive periodontal therapy; procedures performed at selected intervals as an extension of periodontal therapy to assist the patient in maintaining oral health; includes complete assessment, review of and/or additional instruction in dental biofilm control, and such clinical procedures as scaling and root planing; also called preventive maintenance, periodontal maintenance therapy.

fluoride applications may be indicated; response of gingival tissue to irritants can be marked.

4. *Mentally or Physically Disabled.* Managing the toothbrush may be difficult; when the disability involves the mouth area, opening the mouth may be a problem.

5. *Diabetes.* Diabetes or other disease can predispose patients to lowered resistance to infection; tissues must not be allowed to develop advanced disease.

6. *Cardiovascular Disease or Other Condition.* Brushing is a difficult procedure to carry out and only short appointments at the dental office can be tolerated because of the fatigue factor.

D. Periodontal Maintenance Therapy (PMT)[2]

Any of the types of patients who have been mentioned and any of the "special" patients described in Section VII may have a potentially recurrent periodontal infection or may have had periodontal corrective surgical therapy. Four categories of PMT have been defined:

1. *Preventive PMT:* To prevent the initiation of disease in individuals without periodontal infection.

2. *Trial PMT:* To provide an interim study period for borderline patients with conditions that must be observed and further evaluated before a decision can be made as to whether corrective surgery may be necessary or whether maintenance is possible without further advanced disease therapy.

3. *Compromise PMT:* To slow the progress of disease in patients for whom corrective surgery and other advanced treatment are indicated but cannot be implemented for reasons of health, economics, or other personal factors.

4. *Posttreatment PMT:* To prevent the recurrence of disease and maintain the state of periodontal health attained during periodontal therapy. Such therapy may have been nonsurgical or surgical.

▪ MAINTENANCE APPOINTMENT PROCEDURES

The dental hygiene process of care is described in Chapter 1 and is illustrated in Figure 44-1. As with preparation of the initial dental hygiene care plan (Chapter 22), the steps in the process of care apply for the *maintenance dental hygiene care plan.*

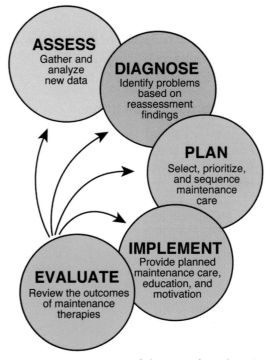

■ **FIGURE 44-1 Components of the Dental Hygiene Process of Care.** Planning for dental hygiene maintenance care unites all of the interrelated components.

I. ASSESSMENT

Preparation of data follows the same plan as that for a new patient. Every patient needs a medical history review; an intraoral and extraoral examination for soft tissue lesions, particularly for cancer; and a blood pressure determination.

At every appointment, whether at 3, 6, or any other number of months, a patient of any age needs a complete probing and special evaluations for the particular problems of previous treatments.

Basic to all examinations are the periodontal examination (pages 103 to 104, 226 to 235) and the dental examination (pages 98 to 102, 269 to 272) with charting.

Steps in preparation of a maintenance appointment work-up include the following:

A. Review of Patient History

Supplementary questions are asked to determine the present state of health, recent illnesses, present medications, and other pertinent data (pages 112 to 121).

B. Blood Pressure Determination (pages 133 to 136)

C. Extraoral and Intraoral Examination

A thorough extraoral and intraoral examination for oral disease, particularly cancer (see pages 176 to 179 and Table 10-1), must be made and recorded.

D. Radiographs

The frequency of radiographic surveys is in accord with the dentist's determination of an individual patient's need (see Table 9-5).[3]

E. Periodontal Examination

1. Observe and record: gingival color, size, shape, position, recession.
2. Complete probing: compare with previous probings.
3. Mucogingival lines; attached gingiva.
4. Occlusion, fremitus, mobility.
5. Calculus: distribution, amount.
6. Biofilm score.

F. Examination of the Teeth

1. Restorations.
2. Sealants.
3. Carious lesions.
4. Sensitivity.

G. Evaluation of Oral Cleanliness and Adequacy of Self-care Measures

Relate biofilm on teeth as observed after applying a disclosing agent to areas of gingival redness, enlargement, and other signs of infection.

H. Examination of Specific Areas

Areas of special problems include endodontically treated teeth, postsurgical areas, implants, occlusal factors, and prosthetic appliances.

I. Microbial Monitoring

Of the more than 400 species of bacteria that reside in the oral cavity, only a few, singly or in clusters, are responsible for periodontal infection leading to tissue destruction. Table 17-3 (page 300) lists major pathogens involved in destructive periodontal diseases. Tests for periodontal pathogens have been developed to aid in the diagnosis and treatment of infections.

1. *Possible Purposes for Testing*
   a. Select treatment procedures: certain bacteria respond to certain treatments.
   b. Monitor treated patients: determine pathogens present before treatment and test again after treatment to determine whether the pathogens have been eradicated.
   c. Screening: to determine sites that are at risk for periodontal infection.

2. *Types of Tests*
   a. Dark-field and phase-contrast microscope: show shifts in size, shape, and motility, but not specific organisms.
   b. Bacterial culture: most accurate method for identifying and quantifying specific organisms.
   c. Immunoassay and nucleic acid probe assay: target certain species by using specific antisera or antibody.
   d. Enzyme assays: test for collagenase, peptidases, and other enzymes specific to certain periodontal pathogens.
   e. DNA probes: identify specific organisms by their DNA.

II. MAINTENANCE CARE PLAN

A care plan is outlined based on the new dental hygiene diagnosis and evaluation of the patient's oral condition. A patient in any of the maintenance categories will require the basic care plan below. Supplemental procedures may be needed.

A. Oral Hygiene Instruction/Motivation

During continuing care, the patient is considered a cotherapist. Compliance in faithful personal daily care is a major feature in the total program if etiologic factors are to be kept under control.

B. Periodontal Scaling and Debridement

C. Dental Caries Control

Prevention with attention to root caries; fluoride applications and diet modifications. Review remineralization protocol (pages 396 to 400).

D. Supplemental Care Procedures

1. Smoking cessation assistance (pages 508 to 515).
2. Desensitization of sensitive areas.
3. Special care for implants or fixed prostheses.
4. Local delivery of antimicrobials for isolated persistent deep pockets (pages 680 to 686).

E. Referral for Retreatment Evaluation

III. CRITERIA FOR REFERRAL DURING MAINTENANCE

There are three points during patient care when the dental hygienist in a general practice must confer with the dentist to determine the need for referral to a periodontist.

The decision can be made initially when the patient is first examined and severe periodontitis is evident, later during the reevaluation of initial scaling, or even later during the maintenance therapy. Criteria for referral during maintenance include:

A. Pocket depth that prohibits access for debridement or maintenance.

B. Furcation involvements and other deep or complex anatomical areas that cannot be instrumented successfully.

C. Mucogingival problems.

■ RECURRENCE OF PERIODONTAL DISEASE

Recurrence of signs and symptoms of periodontal infection indicates recolonization of periodontal pathogens. Recolonization of a pocket can occur within an average of 42 days.[4]

Without daily personal dental biofilm control and regular professional supervision and maintenance procedures, infection can recur. How soon after the completion of treatment it may reappear will vary with each patient depending on a number of contributing factors.

I. CONTRIBUTING FACTORS

A. Inadequate or Insufficient Dental Biofilm Control

B. Lack of Compliance With Maintenance Appointments

1. *Patient Decision:* Misunderstanding of importance; personal reasons.

2. *Professional Laxity:* Insufficient patient counseling; inadequate recall system.

C. Incomplete Professional Treatment

1. *Scaling and Debridement:* Incomplete, especially in areas of difficult access such as furcations and deep proximal pockets.

2. *Biofilm Retention:* Neglect to remove or replace overhanging restorations and other areas that trap biofilm and foster bacterial growth.

D. Tobacco Use[5]

E. Systemic Diseases

Diabetes mellitus,[6] HIV/AIDS, and certain other systemic diseases influence healing and control factors related to bone loss and severity of infections.

Everyday Ethics

(?) There were two full-time dental hygienists in the practice. Jeanette had been there over 15 years, and Wilma less than a year. Wilma had previously practiced with a periodontist in another city for 6 years, and she joined this practice shortly after she moved here. Everything went well. Each hygienist had instruments of their own preference and cared for them relative to sharpening and preparation for the autoclave. Patients usually had appointments with the same dental hygienist. Jeanette usually scheduled a maintenance for 45 minutes, whereas Wilma never felt she had time enough even with an hour.

Occasionally, certain long-standing patients who had been with Jeanette for many years would be scheduled with Wilma when Jeanette could not be in the office.

As Wilma saw more of Jeanette's regular patients, she began to see a pattern of subgingival calculus that could not have formed since the previous 3 or 4 months' maintenance appointment. She had decided to ask the secretary to have Jeanette's patients wait for her return for their appointments.

Mrs. Doubleday had already been scheduled and came for her appointment the next day. After the usual history review, periodontal charting, and treatment started, Wilma had to tell the patient that she needed two appointments and wanted to complete her scaling with local anesthesia. The patient was confused after having only short appointments faithfully and wanted to know whether to reschedule with Jeanette to finish since Jeanette would be back from her vacation soon.

Questions for Consideration

1. Is this an ethical issue or a dilemma? Explain.

2. Using the step procedure of Table 1-2, suggest various possible actions for Wilma.

3. Prepare possible answers Wilma could use for her reply to Mrs. Doubleday's immediate question.

✔ **Factors To Teach The Patient**

- Purposes of follow-up and maintenance appointments.

- Relationship of personal oral care habits to the maintenance of cleanliness provided through professional scaling and debridement.

- Importance of keeping all maintenance appointments.

F. Genetic Factors[7,8]

Risk assessment includes testing for genetic factors.

II. REINFECTION

Transmission of periodontal microorganisms has been shown.[9,10] Colonization in the recipient depends on the number, frequency of exposure, and virulence of the organisms.

■ ADMINISTRATION METHODS

Methods for administration of a maintenance plan vary. For any plan, individual file information includes name, address, telephone numbers, and instructions concerning appointment frequency and available or preferred day and time. The data may be kept on 3 × 5 or 4 × 6-inch file cards or in a computer.

I. PREBOOK METHOD

Make each patient's appointment before the patient leaves the current appointment. An appointment card is given to the patient, who is asked to enter it on the calendar ahead of time. An envelope is prepared for mailing a duplicate card 10 days to 1 week before the scheduled appointment. The card should request the patient to call to confirm. For unconfirmed appointments, a call to the patient the day before must be made.

II. MONTHLY REMINDERS

By this system, individual data are filed alphabetically by the last name of the patient under the month when the patient is due. Each month the cards are pulled and reminders are mailed or telephoned well in advance.

III. COMPUTER ASSISTED

Computers can be helpful in maintaining appointment systems. Either the prebook or the monthly reminders can be used in combination with a computer.

Data stored on a computer can be readily accessible. Computers are capable of printing address labels so that postal cards can be mailed monthly or envelopes containing the prebook appointment card can be sent at the appropriate time.

REFERENCES

1. **Stamm**, J.W.: Periodontal Diseases and Human Health: New Directions in Periodontal Medicine, *Annals Periodontol., 3,* 1, July, 1998.
2. **Schallhorn**, R.G. and Snider, L.E.: Periodontal Maintenance Therapy, *J. Am Dent. Assoc., 103,* 227, August, 1981.
3. **American Dental Association**, Council on Dental Materials, Instruments, and Equipment: Recommendations in Radiographic Practices: An Update, 1988, *J. Am Dent. Assoc., 118,* 115, January, 1989.
4. **Mousqués**, T., Listgarten, M.A., and Phillips, R.W.: Effects of Scaling and Root Planing on the Composition of the Human Subgingival Microbial Flora, *J. Periodont. Res., 15,* 144, March, 1980.
5. **MacFarlane**, G.D., Herzberg, M.C., Wolff, L.F., and Hardie, N.A.: Refractory Periodontitis Associated With Abnormal Polymorphonuclear Leukocyte Phagocytosis and Cigarette Smoking, *J. Periodontol., 63,* 908, November, 1992.
6. **Grossi**, S.G., Skrepcinski, F.B., DeCaro, T., Zambon, J.J., Cummins, D., and Genco, R.J.: Response to Periodontal Therapy in Diabetics and Smokers, *J. Periodontol., 67,* 1094, Supplement, October, 1996.
7. **Hart**, T.C. and Komman, K.S.: Genetic Factors in the Pathogenesis of Periodontitis, *Periodontol. 2000, 14,* 202, 1997.
8. **Kornman**, K.S. and diGiovine, F.S.: Genetic Variations in Cytokine Expression: A Risk Factor for Severity of Adult Periodontitis, *Annals Periodontol., 3,* 327, July, 1998.
9. **Von Troil-Lindén**, B., Torkko, H., Alaluusua, S., Wolf, J., Jousimies-Somer, H., and Asikainen, S.: Periodontal Findings in Spouses: A Clinical, Radiographic and Microbiological Study, *J. Clin. Periodontol., 22,* 93, February, 1995.
10. **Zambon**, J.J.: Periodontal Diseases: Microbial Factors, *Annals Periodontol., 1,* 904, November, 1996.

SUGGESTED READINGS

American Academy of Periodontology, Committee on Research, Science, and Therapy: Position Paper: Supportive Periodontal Therapy (SPT), *J. Periodontol., 69,* 502, April, 1998.

Axelsson, P. and Lindhe, J.: The Significance of Maintenance Care in the Treatment of Periodontal Disease, *J. Clin. Periodontol., 8,* 281, August, 1981.

DeVore, C.H., Hicks, M.J., and Claman, L.: A System for Insuring Success of Long-term Supportive Periodontal Therapy, *J. Dent. Hyg., 63,* 214, June, 1989.

Echeverria, J.J., Manau, G.C., and Guerrero, A.: Supportive Care After Active Periodontal Treatment: A Review, *J. Clin. Periodontol., 23,* 898, October, 1996.

Mann, L.C.: Guidelines for Supportive Periodontal Therapy and When to Refer to a Periodontist, *Can. Dent. Hyg. Assoc. (Probe). 29,* 185, September, 1995.

McCullough, C.: Long-term Maintenance of the Treated Periodontal Patient, *Access, 8,* 45, March, 1994.

Merin, R.L.: Supportive Periodontal Treatment, in Carranza, F.A. and Newman, M.G.: *Clinical Periodontology,* 8th ed. Philadelphia, W.B. Saunders Co., 1996, pp.743–760.

Nevins, M.: Long-term Periodontal Maintenance in Private Practice, *J. Clin. Periodontol., 23,* 273, March, 1996.

Ogilvie, A.L.: Maintenance of the Periodontal Patient, in Schluger, S., Yuodelis, R., Page, R.C., and Johnson, R.H.: *Periodontal Diseases,* 2nd ed. Philadelphia, Lea & Febiger, 1990, pp. 732–746.

Parr, R.W.: *Periodontal Maintenance Therapy.* Berkeley, Calif, Praxis Publishing Co., 1974, 86 pp.

Parr, R.W., Green, E., and Miller, S.R.: *Hygienists in Periodontal Maintenance Therapy.* Berkeley, Calif, Praxis Publishing Co., 1978, 67 pp.

Ramfjord, S.P.: Maintenance Care and Supportive Periodontal Therapy, *Quintessence Int., 24,* 465, July, 1993.

Reiker, J., van der Velden, U., Barendregt, D.S., and Loos, E.G.: A Cross-sectional Study Into the Prevalence of Root Caries in Periodontal Maintenance Patients, *J. Clin. Periodontol., 26,* 26, January, 1999.

Shiloah, J. and Patters, M.R.: Repopulation of Periodontal Pockets by Microbial Pathogens in the Absence of Supportive Therapy, *J. Periodontol., 67,* 130, February, 1996.

Somacarrera, M.L., Lucas, M., Cuervas-Mons, V., and Hernandez, G.: Oral Care Planning and Handling of Immunosuppressed Heart, Liver, and Kidney Transplant Patients, *Spec. Care Dent., 16,* 242, November/December, 1996.

Wang, N.J. and Hoist, D.: Individualizing Recall Intervals in Child Dental Care, *Community Dent. Oral Epidemiol., 23,* 1, February, 1995.

Wang, N.J. and Riordan, P.J.: Recall Intervals, Dental Hygienists and Quality in Child Dental Care, *Community Dent. Oral Epidemiol., 23,* 8, February, 1995.

Wilson, T.G., ed.: Supportive Periodontal Treatment and Retreatment in Periodontics, *Periodontol. 2000, 12,* 1-140 (18 articles), 1996.

Von Troll-Lindén, B., Saarela, M., Matto, J., Alaluusua, S., Jousimies-Somer, H., and Asikainen, S.: Source of Suspected Periodontal Pathogens Re-emerging After Periodontal Treatment, *J. Clin. Periodontol., 23,* 601, June, 1996.

Treatment During Maintenance

Cattabriga, M., Pedrazzoli, V., Cattabriga, A., Pannuti, E., Trapani, M., and Verrocchi, G.C.: Tetracycline Fiber Used Alone or With Scaling and Root Planing in Periodontal Maintenance Patients: Clinical Results, *Quintessence Int., 27,* 395, June, 1996.

Drisko, C.H. and Lewis, L.H.: Ultrasonic Instruments and Antimicrobial Agents in Supportive Periodontal Treatment and Retreatment of Recurrent or Refractory Periodontitis, *Periodontology 2000, 12,* 90, 1996.

Greenstein, G.: Periodontal Response to Mechanical Nonsurgical Therapy: A Review, *J. Periodontol., 63,* 118, February, 1992.

Kaldahl, W.B., Kalkwarf, K.L., Patil, K.D., Molvar, M.P., and Dyer, J.K.: Long-term Evaluation of Periodontal Therapy: I. Response to 4 Therapeutic Modalities, *J. Periodontol., 67,* 93, February, 1996.

Matsuda, S.A.: Instrumentation of Biofilm, *Dimensions D.H., 1,* 26, February/March, 2003.

Pattison, A.M.: The Use of Hand Instruments in Supportive Periodontal Treatment, *Periodontology 2000, 12,* 71, 1996.

Compliance

Novaes, A.B., Novaes, Jr., A.B., Moraes, N., Campos, G.M., and Grisi, M.F.M.: Compliance With Supportive Periodontal Therapy, *J. Periodontol., 67,* 213, March, 1996.

Novaes, Jr., A.B., deLima, F.R., and Novaes, A.B.: Compliance With Supportive Periodontal Therapy and Its Relation to the Bleeding Index, *J. Periodontol., 67,* 976, October, 1996.

Wilson, T.G., Hale, S., and Temple, R.: The Results of Efforts to Improve Compliance With Supportive Periodontal Treatment in a Private Practice, *J. Periodontol., 64,* 311, April, 1993.

Wilson, T.G.: How Patient Compliance to Suggested Oral Hygiene and Maintenance Affect Periodontal Therapy, *Dent. Clin. North Am., 42,* 389, April, 1998.

Patients With Special Needs

INTRODUCTION

An understanding of each patient's general and/or oral health problems requires particular study. Actually, each patient is a "special" patient and must be considered according to individual needs. The patients with special needs who will be considered in the chapters following include patients with oral and general systemic conditions. Variations with respect to age and degree of physical and/or mental disability are considered.

Certain patients, however, have problems related to their age group and/or unusual health factors that may complicate the plan for care generally provided. These special patients require more skillful application of dental hygiene knowledge and ability to accomplish a comparably favorable result than do what might be called "normal" patients.

The dental hygienist's obligation is to see that no patient needs special rehabilitative dental or periodontal services because of any condition that could have been prevented by dental hygiene care.

Consideration of the patient as a whole requires attention to general physical and emotional problems as well as oral problems. Basic psychological needs for affection, belonging, independence, achievement, recognition, and self-esteem frequently influence the outcome of treatment, as does the patient's whole attitude toward dental and dental hygiene care.

Optimum oral health is frequently an important contributing factor in maintaining or restoring the patient's physical, emotional, vocational, economic, and social usefulness to the extent of individual capabilities.

With certain disabilities, oral health has assumed less importance in the mind of the patient because other health problems have demanded so much attention. For some of these patients, neglect has intensified the need for oral care.

▪ SPECIAL ORAL PROBLEMS

In each specialty of dentistry, patients present with problems that can be helped by the services performed by the dental hygienist. Patients with dentofacial handicaps who have missing teeth or congenital malformations, patients requiring surgery, and patients afflicted with habits conducive to the initiation of dental caries are all examples of patients who need special adaptations of the preventive care and instruction the dental hygienist can provide.

▪ PERIODONTAL RISK FACTORS

The new research that ties together periodontal infections with systemic conditions provides the basis for emphasis on periodontal health. Risk factors for peri-odontal infections also may be risk factors for systemic conditions, for example, use of tobacco, certain nutritional deficiencies, and immune dysfunctions.

Periodontal infection is a risk factor for many systemic conditions, including diabetes mellitus, preterm low birth weight, osteoporosis, bacterial pneumonias, and cardiovascular diseases. Certain systemic conditions are risk factors for periodontal conditions, including HIV/AIDS, diabetes mellitus, and medications with side effects of oral manifestations.

▪ ORAL MANIFESTATIONS

The interrelationship between oral conditions and systemic diseases must be revealed through a patient's medical history and identified by clinical changes noted during the extraoral and intraoral examinations.

Oral manifestations may be evident in association with certain acute and chronic systemic diseases, particularly nutritional deficiencies, endocrine disturbances, blood diseases, and many chronic degenerative diseases. When an oral manifestation suggests the possibility of an undiagnosed systemic disease, dental personnel have a responsibility to refer the patient for medical evaluation.

▪ DENTAL HYGIENE CARE

Patients with chronic conditions may or may not be able to go to a dental office or clinic for appointments. Certain conditions, particularly during the advanced stages of a disease, require the patient to remain confined and, in some instances, bedridden. Dental hygienists must understand the special procedures for care in these instances.

The basic approach to oral problems of the patient with a chronic disease or a physical or mental disability is through prevention. Individual initiative is vital if the impact of preventive measures is to be understood and necessary action taken. The public, including dental personnel, must incorporate into daily living fundamental health practices that contribute to optimum health and, hence, to the prevention of chronic disease. Dental hygiene care can improve the general health and influence the resistance to infection of the oral cavity.

A patient may have more than one special need. For example, the patient who requires dental hygiene care prior to oral surgery may have a blood disorder. The pregnant patient may have diabetes. The use of the patient's medical history plays an important role when the total needs of the patient are outlined.

Section VII attempts to integrate learning from other areas of medical and social sciences into the dental and dental hygiene aspects. The dental hygienist is encouraged to supplement knowledge and appreciation of the special needs of patients through the use of additional readings such as those suggested at the end of each chapter. By application of understanding of the patient's needs, clinical techniques and patient counseling may be directed more skillfully to provide *complete dental hygiene care*.

■ ETHICAL APPLICATIONS

The complex medical and dental conditions of certain patients may translate into unique treatment options. Dental hygiene professionals must consider not only the quality of care provided to patients but also their quality of life in general. Increasingly, medically compromised patients are ambulatory and appear in a dental practice or clinic for maintenance and preventive procedures.

The dental hygienist instructs patients about oral hygiene problems and needs related to their systemic disorders and medications. Ethical considerations associated with medically compromised patients center on choosing dental and dental hygiene care that is consistent with physical, mental, and personal capabilities.

Ethically, it is important to understand what the patient values in terms of dental care. If someone other than the patient is responsible for making treatment decisions, the dental team must ensure that those persons are included in all chairside discussions. All information must be carefully documented in the patient's permanent record and reviewed periodically for any updates or changes. Table VII-1 overviews ethical concerns to be considered when presenting treatment options to patients.

■ TABLE VII-1 ETHICAL CONCERNS FOR TREATMENT OPTIONS

QUALITY OF LIFE	DEFINITION	APPLICATIONS
Competency	The patient's ability to make choices about dental and dental hygiene care.	Educates the patient based on intellectual capacity so autonomous consent can be given.
Surrogate	Described as a 'substitute' or proxy with regard to health care decisions.	Acknowledges a 'Durable Power of Attorney' for a patient, where applicable.
Advanced Directives	Individuals may write their choices for limiting health care in the event that they are unable to make choices in the future.	Examples include a 'Living Will', 'Do-Not-Resuscitate (DNR)' order, and 'Patient Values History.'

The Pregnant Patient

Nancy Sisty LePeau, RDH, MS, MA
Esther M. Wilkins, BS, RDH, DMD

CHAPTER OUTLINE

During pregnancy, attention is focused on good health practices for the mother. She is concerned for the health of her baby and for herself. This alertness to total health, of which oral health is an important part, provides an unusual opportunity to help the patient learn principles that may be applied to the future care of the child.

The term *prenatal care* refers to the supervised preparation for childbirth that helps the mother enjoy optimum health during and after pregnancy and that provides the maximum chance for the baby to be born healthy. Such a program involves the combined efforts of the obstetrician and/or midwife, the nurse practitioner, the dentist, the dental hygienist, the dietitian, and the expectant parents. Key words for study with this chapter are defined in Box 45-1.

Obstetricians, family practitioners, and nurses in private and public health settings should recommend dental and periodontal examination early in pregnancy. This brings to the dental office or clinic many women who previously would not have had a regular plan for obtaining professional service. Many of these women have not known the advantages of personal habits of daily care and diet related to the health of the oral tissues. Numerous misconceptions are counteracted when providing up-to-date information about the relationship of pregnancy and oral health.

Women who do not receive routine oral healthcare may appear for emergency dental services and may be receptive to a program of care and instruction to prevent further emergencies. The dental hygienist in public health, especially maternal and child health clinics, participates in community educational programs with public health nurses, whereby some less informed women may learn of the need for professional dental care and advice during pregnancy.

■ FETAL DEVELOPMENT

Pregnancy is arbitrarily divided into three periods of 3 months each called the first, second, and third trimesters. Normal pregnancy, or period of *gestation*, is approximately 40 weeks. *Premature birth* refers to a birth before 37 weeks' gestation.

BOX 45-1 KEY WORDS: Pregnancy

Amniocentesis: a testing procedure on fluid aspirated from the amniotic sac to detect chromosomal abnormalities and metabolic disorders.

Amniotic sac: the innermost of the membranes enveloping the embryo *in utero*; **amniotic fluid** fills the sac in which the embryo is free to move and is protected against mechanical injury.

Anticipatory guidance: the term applied to teaching ahead of time so that untoward, unfavorable conditions can be prevented.

Cesarean section: delivery of a fetus by incision through the abdominal wall and uterus.

Embryo: developing organism from conception to approximately the end of the second month.

Epulis: nonspecific term referring to a growth on the gingiva.

Estradiol: the most potent natural estrogen in humans; the circulating blood level of estradiol rises during the follicular phase of the reproductive cycle and drops when ovulation occurs (see Figure 48-1).

Fetus: developing organism from the second month after conception to birth.

Gestation: the period of pregnancy.

Granuloma: nonspecific term applied to a nodular inflammatory lesion containing macrophages and surrounded by lymphocytes.

    "Pyogenic" granuloma: a misnomer because it does not contain pus, but contains blood vessels and inflammatory cells.

In utero: within the womb; not yet born.

Infant: child younger than 1 year of age.

Intrapartum: occuring during childbirth.

Midwife: a person who attends a woman during delivery.

    Nurse-midwife: a registered nurse specializing in midwifery; requires additional education and special licensure in certain states and countries.

Obstetrics: the branch of medicine that has to do with the care of the pregnant woman during pregnancy and parturition.

    Obstetrician: physician who practices obstetrics.

Parturition: childbirth; labor; giving birth.

Placental abruption: sudden or unexpected breaking off of the connection between uterine and fetal mucous membranes.

Postpartum: pertaining to the period following childbirth or delivery.

Premature birth: birth that occurs before the expected delivery date; denotes an infant born prior to 37 weeks of gestation.

Puerpera: woman who has just given birth to a child.

Pyogenic: producing pus.

Teratogen: nongenetic factors that cause malformations and disease syndromes in utero.

Teratogenic agent: any drug, virus, or irradiation the exposure to which can cause malformation of the fetus.

Trimester: a period of 3 months; one third of a pregnancy.

Physiologic changes in the mother are related to nearly every bodily system. Early development of the embryo is greatly influenced by heredity and the overall health of the mother.

I. FIRST TRIMESTER

During the first trimester, the embryo is highly susceptible to injuries and malformations. Teratogenic effects can be produced by many sources, including maternal poor nutrition, infections, and drug intake.

All organ systems are formed (organogenesis) during the first trimester. By 12 weeks, the fetus moves and swallows. Oral cavity development includes:

A. Teeth

1. Tooth buds develop between the fifth and sixth week.
2. Initial mineralization occurs from the fourth to the fifth month (Table 46-4).

B. Lips and Palate

1. Lips form during the fourth to the seventh week.
2. Palate forms between the eighth and the twelfth week.
3. Cleft lip is apparent by the eighth week; cleft palate, by the twelfth week (page 805).

II. SECOND AND THIRD TRIMESTERS

The organs are completed, and growth and maturation continue. Fetal weight changes from 1 ounce at 3 months to an average of 7.5 pounds at birth.

III. FACTORS THAT CAN HARM THE FETUS

A. Periodontal Infection in the Mother

Severe periodontitis is a significant risk factor for preterm delivery with low birth weight. A pregnant mother with advanced periodontitis has a 7.5- to 7.9-fold increased risk for a preterm low-birth-weight infant.[1,2]

B. Other Infections

Protection from infectious diseases is necessary because damage to and infection of the fetus can result. Women of childbearing age should take advantage of all available vaccines prior to conception.

Defects, deformities, and life-threatening infections in the fetus can result from infection acquired during pregnancy or during delivery and after birth. Rubella (German measles), rubeola, varicella, herpes viruses, hepatitis B (pages 29 to 30), human immunodeficiency virus (HIV) infection (pages 38 and 43), syphilis (congenital syphilis), and gonorrhea all can have serious effects on the fetus.

C. Medications

Ideally, no medications or other drugs should be used during pregnancy. Nearly all drugs can pass across the placenta to enter the circulation of the developing fetus. Many drugs have teratogenic effects. Table 45-1 lists selected drugs with examples of their possible effects on the fetus.

1. *Effect of Tetracycline*. Tetracycline is well known for intrinsic staining of tooth structure. The effect occurs during mineralization of the primary teeth beginning at about 4 months of gestation and of the permanent teeth near and after birth (page 319). When an antibiotic is required during pregnancy, a choice other than tetracycline can be made.
2. *Therapy for HIV Infection*. Prevention of perinatal HIV transmission and health for the fetus and neonate are considered with the plan for optimal healthcare for the mother with HIV/AIDS infection. Some antiretroviral medications are not withheld because of pregnancy.[3] Consideration by the mother can be given to withholding the antiretroviral treatment during the first 14 weeks of pregnancy. That is the period of maximal organogenesis and risk for teratogenicity.

D. Drugs of Abuse

Adverse effects of controlled substances, alcohol, and tobacco products are included in Table 45-1. There are many serious effects from their use. Additional information on the effects of smoking on pregnancy and smoking cessation can be found on page 505.

E. Herbal Dietary Supplements

Herbal dietary supplements are not regulated by the Federal Drug Administration for efficacy. The public is free to purchase them over the counter to self-medicate. Routine medical history taking needs to include questions about the use of herbal supplements, the amount, and the duration. Information about possible problems when taking the supplements is presented to the patient.

1. Common uses are for colds, burns, headaches, allergies, rashes, depression, insomnia, and premenstrual syndrome.
2. Several remedies have implications for dental/dental hygiene treatment, such as:

■ TABLE 45-1 DRUGS CONTRAINDICATED DURING PREGNANCY AND BREAST-FEEDING

CLASSIFICATION	DRUGS PRESCRIBED FOR TREATMENT*	POSSIBLE ADVERSE EFFECTS ON FETUS AND INFANT
Anticoagulant	Warfarin (Coumadin) (D) Dicumarol (D)	Hemorrhagic fetal death Birth malformations
Anticonvulsant	Barbiturates (phenobarbital) (D) Phenytoin sodium (D) Trimethadione (D) Valproate sodium (D)	Congenital malformations Developmental delays Fetal phenobarbital syndrome Fetal hydantoin syndrome Fetal trimethadione syndrome Fetal valproate syndrome
Antimicrobial	Streptomycin (B) Tetracycline (D)	Toxic action on ear: 8th cranial nerve damage Bone growth inhibition; intrinsic dental stain
Antineoplastic	Cyclophosphamide (Cytoxan) (D) Mercaptopurine (D) Methotrexate (D)	Multiple anomalies; fetal death

Hormones	Clomiphene (Clomid) (X)
	Estrogenic substances (X)
	    diethylstilbestrol (X)
	Prednisone (C)
	Progesterone (X)
		Increased anomalies; neural tube defects
		Cancer of the vagina and cervix; genital tract
		    anomalies; congenital heart defects

Psychotrophic	Antianxiety
	    chlordiazepoxide (Librium) (D)
	    diazepam (Valium) (D)
	    meprobamate (Miltown) (D)
	Antimanic
	    lithium carbonate (D)
		Low heart rate, muscle tone, respiration, poor
		    sucking reflex
		Taken near term may cause neonatal withdrawal
		    syndrome or cardiorespiratory instability
		
		Lethargy, cyanosis, teratogenic (dose related)

Drugs of Abuse	Alcohol	Fetal alcohol syndrome (page XX) Spontaneous abortion; low birth rate. Mental retardation

	Cocaine
	    prenatal exposure
	
	    inhale free-base vapors
	    (postpartum)
		Decreased birth weight; prematurity
		Fetal growth retardation; microcephaly
		Teratogenic effects
		Increased rate of seizures

	Narcotics
	    heroin
	    methadone
		Decreased birth weight
		Withdrawal symptoms
		Convulsions; sudden infant death

	Tobacco
	    cigarette smoking
	
	    involuntary smoking
	
	Environmental
		Low birth weight; prematurity; miscarriage;
		    still birth; infant mortality
		Sudden infant death syndrome
		Children: increased respiratory infections and
		    symptoms
		Deficiencies in physical growth, intellectual
		    development
		Higher incidence in mortality rate of infant
		    and child

*United States Food and Drug Administration (FDA) categorizes drugs and their relation to pregnancy as: **A.** No risk demonstrated to fetus in any trimester. **B.** No adverse effects in animals; no human studies available. **C.** Only given after risks to fetus are considered; animal studies have shown no adverse reactions, no human studies available. **D.** Definite fetal risks; may be given in spite of risks if needed in life-threatening conditions. **X.** Absolute fetal abnormalities; not to be used at any time in pregnancy.

a. Echinacea used for colds activates cell-mediated immunity: may cause allergic reactions, decreased effectiveness of immunosuppressants, and immunosuppression with long-term use.

b. Valerian used for insomnia and stress has a sedative effect and may increase the sedative effect of anesthetics and, with long-term use, may increase anesthetic requirements.[4]

■ ORAL FINDINGS DURING PREGNANCY

Gingival inflammatory changes that occur during pregnancy are considered to be an exaggerated response of the tissues to dental biofilm. When the periodontal tissues are in good health and the patient uses adequate personal oral care measures for biofilm control, major adverse gingival changes are not expected.

The gingiva can show a reaction to the physiologic changes of pregnancy, as well as to the influence of the increased circulating levels of female sex hormones. Trauma, poor oral hygiene, and local irritation from calculus or prostheses may be contributory factors.

The gingival reaction in pregnancy is usually seen by the second month. When left untreated, the gingival inflammation continues as the hormones rise to a maximum level by the eighth month.

The symptoms abate after the birth of the child, but a completely healthy condition does not necessarily result. A patient with a gingival disturbance during pregnancy continues to have the disturbance, even if to a somewhat lessened degree, after the birth.

I. GINGIVITIS

A. Clinical Appearance

The appearance varies and shows characteristics of inflamed tissues, including enlargement, redness, smooth, shiny surface, and bleeding on probing.

B. Predisposing Factors

1. Local irritation and infection because of poor oral hygiene leaving dental biofilm on the teeth and gingiva.
2. Hormonal changes during pregnancy that may alter the tissue reaction.[5,6]

C. Microbiology

Increased proportions of *Prevotella intermedia* have been found in gingivitis and elevated serum levels of the hormones of pregnancy (estrogen and progesterone).[7]

II. GINGIVAL ENLARGEMENT

An oral pyogenic granuloma may develop. It is a benign, inflammatory lesion. It has also been called an epulis gravidarum, a pregnancy granuloma, or a pregnancy tumor.[8-10] The use of the word *tumor* is misleading because the lesion is not a tumor but a hyperplasia and also occurs in men and nonpregnant women. When the lesion is removed during pregnancy, there is some tendency for recurrence.

A. Clinical Appearance

The lesion appears as an isolated, discrete, soft, round enlargement near the gingival margin usually associated with an interdental area, as shown in Figure 45-1. It forms in a mushroom-like shape with a smooth, glistening surface. The pressure of the lip or cheek tends to make it flattened.

The color depends on the vascularity and may be purplish-red, magenta, or deep blue, sometimes dotted with red.

B. Symptoms

1. Bleeds readily with slight trauma.
2. Painless unless it becomes large enough to interfere with occlusion and mastication.

C. Significance

1. Interference during mastication: can contribute to inadequate nutritive intake for mother and baby because of discomfort when chewing.
2. Provides a site for bacterial growth: potential development of periodontal attachment loss and eventual bone destruction.

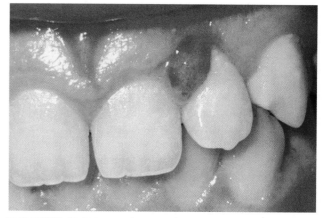

■ **FIGURE 45-1 Pyogenic Granuloma or "Pregnancy Tumor."** Isolated, discrete, round, soft enlargement near the gingival margin; smooth, glistening surface, purplish-red in color.

3. Results in bleeding and pain: may interfere with routine dental biofilm removal using toothbrush and interdental aids.

4. Creates an undesirable esthetic effect.

III. ENAMEL EROSION

Morning sickness with vomiting over an extended period can lead to demineralization and acid erosion primarily of the palatal surfaces. Following are recommendations that can be made to assist patients in dealing with nausea associated with early pregnancy:

- Eat small amounts of nutritious yet noncariogenic foods throughout the day.
- Use a sodium bicarbonate rinse after vomiting to neutralize acid.
- Chew sugarless gum after eating, especially gum containing xylitol.
- Use gentle toothbrushing and low abrasive fluoride toothpaste to prevent damage to demineralized tooth surfaces.

▪ ASPECTS OF PATIENT CARE

I. ASSESSMENT

A. Early Appointment

Dental/dental hygiene appointments are scheduled as early in pregnancy as possible. Anticipatory guidance is mandatory relative to the effects of drugs, tobacco use, and periodontal infection on the development and subsequent health of the infant. However, the first few months may be challenging for the mother-to-be because pregnancy provides an emotional experience with many adjustments.

The second trimester is considered the safest for general dental treatment. However, dental hygiene care should start much earlier to keep the gingival tissues in optimum health and prevent oral infections.

B. Medical History

1. Other health problems: conditions other than pregnancy may be present. For example, diabetes[11] or cardiovascular diseases can involve serious complications. Women with hypertension have greater risk for fetuses with intrauterine growth retardation, *placental abruption*, and a 15% to 20% increase for superimposed preeclampsia later in gestation.

2. Adolescent health: when the expectant mother is an adolescent, her own special needs differ from those of a mature woman. Aspects of adolescent development are described on pages 815 to 817.

C. Consultation

Contact with the patient's physician and/or obstetrician is necessary for integrating general and oral care. All routine treatment is acceptable unless the patient's obstetrician advises otherwise.

When a patient seeks dental and dental hygiene care and is not under the care of a physician, she is urged and assisted to obtain medical supervision for her health and the health of her baby.

II. RADIOGRAPHY

A. Universal Safety Factors

Radiographs are not made for any patient unless necessary. When they are required during pregnancy, the patient is covered with a lead apron, a thyroid collar, and a second apron for the back to prevent secondary radiation from reaching the abdomen. As always, all current methods for radiation safety and protection are applied, including optimum filtration, collimation, use of the fastest film, and extended target film distance.

B. Exposures

Determine the minimum number of film exposures that will produce the required diagnostic information. The use of a paralleling technique does not require angulation directed toward the patient's abdomen. Careful and skillful film placement, angulation, processing, and all phases of technique prevent the need for remaking radiographs that are not acceptable for diagnosis.

III. PERIODONTAL TREATMENT

Areas of food impaction are corrected, and all overhanging restorations are reshaped or replaced. All nonsurgical procedures are carefully and thoroughly completed. Complicated elective surgical periodontal treatment is deferred until after delivery.

IV. OVERALL TREATMENT CONSIDERATIONS

A. Dental Hygiene Care Goal

Optimum periodontal health and hygiene.

B. Dental Care

1. *Elective Treatment*: Postpone until second trimester or early third trimester.

2. *Restorative*: Restorations should be completed with permanent restorative materials. One important contraindication for the use of temporary

restorations is that after the baby is born, the mother may be too busy to attend to appointments because of added family responsibilities and/or a return to career employment.

■ DENTAL HYGIENE CARE

The dental hygienist who is well informed about dental care can motivate the patient and alleviate fears related to certain services. The patient often consults with the dental hygienist for reassurance and interpretation of the dentist's recommendations and procedures.

Gingival disease need not be expected when the patient is motivated to practice conscientious self-care procedures for oral cleanliness and dental biofilm control. This calls for a specific appointment plan for scaling and disease control instruction.

A concentrated plan for dental caries control is indicated. A multiple fluoride program and limitation of cariogenic foods are basic to the preventive efforts.

I. APPOINTMENT PLANNING

A. Frequency

Monthly appointments or appointments three times during the 9-month period may be required. Appointment frequency depends on the patient's needs as well as ability and motivation to maintain a healthy oral environment.

B. Individual Appointments

Patients are more comfortable with short appointments. A series of appointments is indicated when calculus deposits are heavy.

C. Postpartum Maintenance Appointments

For the patient who has not been on a regular maintenance plan prior to pregnancy, emphasis is placed on motivating the patient to continue regular appointments for dental hygiene and dental care after the baby is born.

II. CLINICAL CARE

It is not within the scope of this book to review all the physiologic changes that occur during pregnancy. Common physical changes should be identified because they can affect appointment procedures. Nearly every woman is bothered by one or more minor complaints at some time during her pregnancy.

Attention to details provides the patient with comfort and motivates her to continue oral care. Table 45-2 lists the more common physical changes of pregnancy and suggests a few appointment considerations.

A. Patient Positioning

1. *Effect of Supine Position.* The weight of the developing fetus in the uterus bears down directly on the major vessels, the aorta, and the inferior vena cava. The vessels are pressed between the spinal column and the uterus. During the third trimester, symptoms of circulatory insufficiency can appear when venous return is decreased.
2. *Alternate Positions* (Figure 45-2).[12]
   a. Patient lies on left side.
   b. Elevate the right hip to displace the uterus to the left. Use a pillow or rolled-up blanket.

B. Preventive Measures

When a patient has gingival enlargement and inflammation, a good part of the first appointment is spent on instruction in biofilm control and other preventive measures. At the second appointment, evaluation is made and instruction is continued.

C. Instrumentation

1. Careful instrumentation for calculus removal is indicated. The use of ultrasonic scalers usually is not contraindicated.
2. After consultation with the patient's physician, local anesthetics may be used in moderation. Nitrous oxide–oxygen sedation is contraindicated during the first trimester. If used in the second or third trimester, great precaution is required, including length minimized to 30 minutes with oxygen percentage at 50%.[13]
3. If stain removal is needed, the use of an abrasive cleaning paste is postponed until the tissue has responded to the biofilm control measures.

D. Fluoride Program

1. *Professional Topical Application.* All patients can benefit from a topical application of fluoride solution, gel, or varnish after scaling and root planing. Applications can be indicated, especially for patients with a tendency toward rampant caries and who have numerous restorations. The fluoride agents and techniques are described in Chapter 33.
2. *Self-application.* A fluoride dentifrice is recommended for all patients. Other fluoride recommendations are individualized according to patient need. A daily fluoride, non–alcohol-containing

■ TABLE 45-2 APPOINTMENT ADAPTATIONS FOR THE PRENATAL PATIENT

CHARACTERISTIC	DENTAL HYGIENE IMPLICATION
Fatigues easily, may even fall asleep	Short appointments; several in series, as needed Work with an assistant to accomplish more at each appointment
General awkwardness because of new shape and weight gain	Attend to details, such as gently lowering and straightening chair for patient Make sure rinsing facilities are convenient; or preferably, an assistant attends to evacuation
Frequent urination	Allow sufficient appointment time for interruptions Suggest at beginning of appointment that patient mention need for interruption
Discomfort of remaining in one position too long	Position the patient on her left side and not in supine or Trendelenburg position (Figure 45-2)
Backache	Interrupt in middle of appointment to allow patient to change position Assistance with evacuation during intraoral instrumentation can shorten appointment time
Faintness and dizziness	Be prepared for emergency (Table 66-4, page 1113)
Adverse reaction to strong smells and flavors	Recommend less strong flavored dentifrice
Exaggerated reactions to odors and flavors of medicaments and other office materials	Determine particularly obnoxious odors for an individual patient and remove them; check office ventilation
Unpleasant taste in mouth	Advise: nonalcoholic mouthrinse; use a neutral sodium fluoride rinse Demonstrate tongue cleaning (page 419)
Nausea and vomiting (first trimester)	Explain why not to brush right after vomiting to prevent erosion (page 1006)
Gagging	Recommend a small toothbrush Turn head down over sink while brushing; helps to relax throat and allow saliva to flow out Take care in instrument and radiographic film placement
Physician's recommendation for alleviation of nausea symptoms: frequent eating of small amounts of foods	Encourage use of noncariogenic foods
Unusual food cravings	If cravings are for sweets, clearly define relationship of frequent nibbling of cariogenic foods to dental caries Provide list of nutritious noncariogenic snacks

mouthrinse, gel tray, or other mode of application is essential for some patients. A comprehensive fluoride effort can be particularly helpful for the pregnant adolescent.

■ PATIENT INSTRUCTION

The emphasis on general health during pregnancy provides the ideal setting for instruction relative to many aspects of oral health for the mother, her expected child, and other family members. New developments in disease prevention and control should be explained. Helping the mother learn what to expect before the infant arrives is essential and may be found in Table 46-2, Anticipatory Guidance: Birth to 24 Months.

Printed materials concerning the prevention of periodontal infections and dental caries and the development and care of children's teeth are available from the American Dental Association. (An ADA Product Catalog for the current year may be obtained by writing to the American Dental Association, Catalog Sales, P.O. Box 776, St. Charles, IL 60174, or for ordering the ADA Catalog online, www.adacatalog.org.) Reading material that supplements personal discussions can contribute to patient understanding and cooperation.

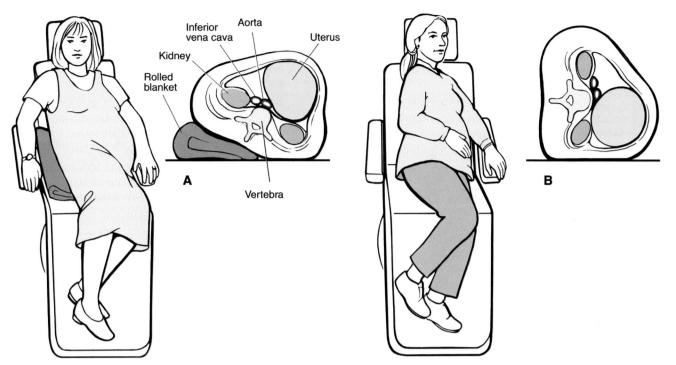

■ **FIGURE 45-2 Positions During Pregnancy.** The supine position allows the weight of the developing fetus to bear down directly on the major vessels. **(A)** Patient lies on left side with a pillow or blanket roll to elevate right hip. **(B)** Patient turned farther to left. Note position of uterus in cross sections of the abdomen.

I. DENTAL BIOFILM CONTROL

A rigid schedule for self-care is demonstrated and supervised. A series of instructional sessions usually is needed.

II. PREVENTION OF PERIODONTAL DISEASE

A. Gingival changes during pregnancy (page 773) require daily attention by the patient and periodic professional appointments.

B. Severity of existing periodontal infection, or potential for the initiation of bone and attachment loss, can have serious effects on both mother and fetus. An example of the effect of periodontal infection of the mother on the fetus is preterm low birth weight.[1,2]

III. SMOKING CESSATION

Use of tobacco, alcohol, and many substances of abuse during pregnancy has moderate to severe influences on the developing fetus as well as on the child after birth. Pregnancy is an ideal time to motivate a patient to quit smoking and use of other harmful substances. The mother's attention is captivated by doing her very best for a healthy child.

A. Explain increased risks for reduced birth weight, spontaneous abortions, perinatal deaths, and sudden infant death syndrome.

B. Explain the effects of secondhand smoke on the fetus and child after birth.

C. Present the steps in a cessation program (pages 513 to 515).

IV. DIET

Instruction is provided in prevention of dental caries and maintenance of the health of the supporting structures of the teeth. The use of a varied diet containing the essential protective food groups, with a minimum of cariogenic foods, is necessary. The food guide pyramid is shown on page 523.

A. Purposes of Adequate Diet During Pregnancy

1. To maintain daily strength and feeling of well-being.
2. To provide the essential building materials for the developing fetus.
3. To protect and promote the health of the oral tissues of the mother.
4. To minimize postpartum problems.

B. Dietary Needs During Pregnancy

The mother's diet must be adequate to maintain her own nutritional status and to meet the needs of the fetus.[14]

The particular needs of the fetus are:
1. Proteins, for general tissue construction.
2. Minerals, especially calcium and phosphorus, for bone and tooth mineralization; iron for blood corpuscles.
3. Vitamins, especially vitamin D for calcium metabolism, folate to prevent neural tube defects and low birth weight, and vitamin A to prevent preterm birth. However, too much vitamin A may cause birth defects.[15]

C. Adolescent Dietary Needs During Pregnancy

Teenagers have higher requirements for calcium, iron, and folic acid. Many young women drink soda instead of milk, eat foods high in sugar and fat, and voluntarily restrict their diet due to concerns about weight gain. Pregnant adolescents often present with these same dietary needs and problems.[14]
1. Diet history taking for oral health focuses on:
    a. Intake from the five food groups.
    b. Number and types of snacks per day.
    c. Frequency of cariogenic foods.
    d. Intake of sweetened beverages, particularly soda.
    e. Use of sugar-containing chewing gum.
2. Dietary recommendations for oral and general health include:
    a. A healthy diet from the five food groups.
    b. 1300 mg of calcium per day or four servings of calcium-rich foods.
    c. Iron and folic acid supplements and iron- and folate-rich foods.
    d. Healthy snacks.
    e. Substitution of water and juice for soda and drinks with caffeine.
    f. Use of sugarless chewing gum with xylitol after eating.

V. DENTAL CARIES CONTROL

A. Incidence During Pregnancy

Some patients believe that they have more dental caries during and because of pregnancy. Research has shown that this is not true and that any relationship is indirect. Factors that result in dental caries formation are the same during pregnancy as at other times (Figure 32-2 and pages 298 to 299).

B. Factors That May Contribute to Apparent Increase in Dental Caries Rate

1. *Previous Neglect.* A patient may not have kept a regular dental appointment plan. The existing dental caries during pregnancy may represent years of accumulation.
2. *Diet During Pregnancy.* Possible increase in intake of cariogenic foods:
    a. Unusual cravings may be for sweet foods.
    b. Frequency of eating: patient may be eating every few hours for prevention of nausea, and these foods may be cariogenic.
3. *Neglect of Personal Oral Care Procedures.* Patient may lack interest in daily dental biofilm removal or be lax about rinsing immediately following intake of a cariogenic food. The smell of toothpaste or the act of brushing may precipitate nausea and reduction in oral care.

C. Calcium and the Mother's Teeth

The misconception concerning the withdrawal of calcium from the mother's teeth and its relationship to dental caries is widespread. It is important to review the known facts because the patient's beliefs may need clarification. In discussing the problem with the patient, a summary of the process of dental caries initiation can be helpful.
1. Minerals contained in the erupted tooth enamel and dentin are not available, and no removal of minerals can occur by way of the pulp.
2. Minerals are removed from the external surface of the enamel and exposed root surface in the process of demineralization. This demineralization is due to incomplete daily dental biofilm removal and overexposure to fermentable carbohydrates rather than the effects of pregnancy.
3. Minerals contained within the alveolar bone are available, as they are from other bones of the body. When the mother's diet does not contain sufficient calcium and phosphorus, her own reserve is utilized. The metabolism of calcium is complex.
4. Most calcium and phosphorus of bones and teeth is added to the fetus during the third trimester. The incidence of dental caries in the mother is not different during that period, although the carious lesions may be larger if the teeth have been neglected throughout the pregnancy.
5. The teeth of the fetus tend to develop and mineralize normally in spite of the diet of the mother because the reserve in her bones is used.

D. Relationship of Fluoride

No direct evidence shows that prenatal fluoride intake influences the rate of dental caries in the child.[16-18]

Everyday Ethics

A 20-year-old single woman, Julie, was referred to the dental practice by a nurse from the Maternal and Child Health Clinic. She is in the first trimester of pregnancy and has not seen a dentist in the past 5 years. She has pain on the left side of her mouth when she eats and states that her gums bleed when she brushes.

Julie's general health history is negative except for smoking. Examination reveals multiple carious lesions, heavy calculus, and 4- to 5-mm proximal probing depths in several molar areas. After initial patient education, follow-up appointments are scheduled with the dental hygienist and with the dentist. The patient does not show up for the appointments.

Questions for Consideration

1. How does the ethical principle of beneficence apply to this situation?

2. What is the role of the dental hygienist, if any, to make further contact with this patient, and why?

3. Describe two courses of action and the possible outcomes of the situation through a dental hygiene care plan.

■ SPECIAL PROBLEMS FOR REFERRAL

I. DEPRESSION DURING PREGNANCY

Childbearing years place women at greatest risk for depression.[19] Oral healthcare professionals can learn to identify signs and symptoms of depression in pregnant patients. Treatment for depression and dental hygiene care for individuals with depression are described on pages 997 to 999 in Chapter 60.

A. Signs of Depression

1. Depressed mood; loss of interest or pleasure in ordinary activities.
2. Disturbed sleep and fatigue.
3. Loss of appetite.
4. Difficulty making decisions.
5. Feelings of worthlessness and suicidal thoughts.[20]

B. Impact on Health of the Fetus

1. Higher tendencies for preeclampsia.
2. Longer labor.
3. Low birth rate.
4. Preterm delivery.

C. What to Do

1. Explain that depression is a biologically based illness caused by a chemical imbalance in the brain.

2. Indicate that depression is treatable, and when treated, can improve the quality of life.
3. Refer the patient to the physician of record or a community mental health resource center.

✔ Factors To Teach The Patient

- The relationship of oral health of the mother to the general health of the fetus and newborn.

- The serious effects of tobacco and other drugs on the health of the fetus, the infant, and the child.

- Reasons for dental hygiene appointments early in the pregnancy, at regular intervals throughout the pregnancy, and after the birth of the baby.

- Reasons for scheduling oral care appointments during the pregnancy in the second trimester or early in the third trimester.

- The rationale for maintaining good personal oral hygiene care to control dental biofilm throughout the pregnancy and after the baby's birth.

- Self-examination of the oral cavity to evaluate the effectiveness of daily dental biofilm removal and the health of the soft tissues.

- Reasons for limiting fermentable carbohydrate intake and maintaining a healthy diet from the five food groups.

II. DOMESTIC VIOLENCE

A. Identification

Identification, assessment, and intervention with victims of domestic violence can be an important part of a dental visit (pages 960 to 964).

B. Most Common Sites of Injury

1. Head
2. Face
3. Neck

C. Obstetrical and Other Manifestations

1. Obstetrical: miscarriages and spontaneous or multiple abortions.
2. Possible substance abuse.
3. Depression.
4. Suicide attempts.[21]

D. What to Do

1. Address the issue with patients.
2. Refer to the Domestic Violence Intervention Program in the community if a case of domestic violence is suspected.[22]

REFERENCES

1. **Offenbacher**, S., Katz, V., Fertik, G., Collins, J., Boyd, D., Maynor, G., McKaig, R., and Beck, J.: Periodontal Infection as a Possible Risk Factor for Preterm Low Birth Weight, *J. Periodontol.*, 67, 1103, October, 1996, Supplement.
2. **Jeffcoat**, M.K., Geurs, N.C., Reddy, M.S., Cliver, S.P., Goldenberg, R.L., and Hauth, J.C.: Periodontal Infection and Preterm Birth: Results of a Prospective Study, *J. Am. Dent. Assoc.*, 132, 875, July, 2001.
3. **Watts**, D.H.: Management of Human Immunodeficiency Virus Infection in Pregnancy, *N. Engl. J. Med.*, 346, 1879, June 13, 2002.
4. **Ang-Lee**, M.K., Moss, J., and Yuan, G.S.: Herbal Medicines and Perioperative Care, *JAMA*, 286, 208, July 11, 2001.
5. **Loe**, H.: Periodontal Changes in Pregnancy, *J. Periodontol.*, 36, 209, May–June, 1965.
6. **Klokkevold**, P.R., Mealey, B.L. and Carranza, F.A.: Influence of Systemic Disease and Disorders on the Periodontium, in Newman, M.G., Takei, H.H., and Carranza, F.A.: *Carranza's Clinical Periodontology*, 9th ed. Philadelphia, W.B. Saunders, 2002, pp. 212–214.
7. **Kornman**, K.S. and Loesche, W.J.: The Subgingival Microbial Flora During Pregnancy, *J. Periodont. Res.*, 15, 111, March, 1980.
8. **Fehrenbach**, M.J., Lemborn, U.E., and Phelan, J.A.: Inflammation and Repair, in Ibsen, O.A.C. and Phelan, J.A.: *Oral Pathology for the Dental Hygienist*, 3rd ed. Philadelphia, W.B. Saunders, 2000, p. 75.
9. **Pindborg**, J.J.: *Atlas of Diseases of the Oral Mucosa*, 5th ed. Philadelphia, W.B. Saunders, 1992, pp. 286–288.
10. **Carranza**, F.A. and Hogan, E.L.: Gingival Enlargement, in Newman, M.G., Takei, H.H., and Carranza, F.A.: *Carranza's Clinical Periodontology*, 9th ed. Philadelphia, W.B. Saunders, 2002, pp. 286–287.
11. **Moore**, P.A., Orchard, T., Guggenheimer, J., and Weyant, R.J.: Diabetes and Oral Health Promotion: A Survey of Disease Preventive Behaviors, *J. Am. Dent. Assoc.*, 131, 1333, September, 2000.
12. **Tarsitano**, B.F. and Rollings, R.E.: The Pregnant Dental Patient: Evaluation and Management, *Gen. Dent.*, 41, 226, May–June, 1993.
13. **Little**, J.W., Falace, D.A., Miller, C., and Rhodus, N.L.: *Dental Management of the Medically Compromised Patient*, 6th ed. St. Louis, Mosby, 2002, p. 310.
14. **Faine**, M.P.: Nutrition in Pregnancy, Infancy, and Childhood, in Palmer, C.A.: *Diet and Nutrition in Oral Health*. New Jersey, Prentice Hall, 2003, pp. 245–250.
15. **Oakley**, G.P. and Erickson, J.D.: Vitamin A and Birth Defects (Editorial). *N Engl. J. Med.*, 333, 1414, November 23, 1995.
16. **Driscoll**, W.S.: A Review of Clinical Research on the Use of Prenatal Fluoride Administration for Prevention of Dental Caries, *ASDC J. Dent. Child.*, 48, 109, March–April, 1981.
17. **Thylstrup**, A.: Is There a Biological Rationale for Prenatal Fluoride Administration? *ASDC J. Dent. Child.*, 48, 103, March–April, 1981.
18. **Bawden**, J.W., ed.: Changing Patterns of Fluoride Intake, Workshop Report Group III, *J. Dent. Res.*, 71, 1224, Special Issue, May, 1992.
19. **Monacs**, R. and Cohen, L.S.: Depression During Pregnancy: Diagnosis and Treatment Options, *J. Clin. Psychiatry*, 63, 24, Supplement 7, 2002.
20. **American Psychiatric Association**: *Diagnostic and Statistical Manual of Mental Disorders, DSM-IV*, 4th ed, Arlington, VA, American Psychiatric Association, 1994, p. 327.
21. **McFarlane**, J., Parker, B., Soeken, K., and Bullock L.: Assessing for Abuse During Pregnancy, *JAMA*, 267, 3176, June 17, 1992.
22. **Love**, C., Gerbert, B., Caspers, N., Bronstone, A., Perry, D., and Bird, W.: Dentists' Attitudes and Behaviors Regarding Domestic Violence, *J. Am. Dent. Assoc.*, 132, 85, January, 2001.

SUGGESTED READINGS

Brown, L.J., Wall, T.P., and Lazar, V.: Trends in Caries Among Adults 18 to 45 Years Old, *J. Am. Dent. Assoc.*, 133, 827, July, 2002.

Casamassimo, P.: *Bright Futures in Practice: Oral Health*. Arlington, VA, National Center for Education in Maternal and Child Health, 1996, pp. 15–18. (Available from: National Maternal and Child Health Clearinghouse, 2070 Chain Bridge Road, Suite 450, Vienna, VA 22182-2536.)

Gibson-Howell, J.C.: Domestic Violence Identification and Referral, *J. Dent. Hyg.*, 70, 74, March–April, 1996.

Goldenberg, R.L., Hauth, J.C., and Andrews, W.W.: Intrauterine Infection and Preterm Delivery, *N. Engl. J. Med.*, 342, 1500, May 18, 2000.

Greenfield, S.F., Reizes, J.M., Magruder, K.M., Muenz, L.R., Kopans, B., and Jacobs, D.G.: Effectiveness of Community-Based Screening for Depression, *Am. J. Psychiatry*, 154, 1391, October, 1997.

Rapaport, M.H., Judd, L.L., Schettler, P.J., Yonkers, K.A., Thase, M.E., Kupfer, D.J., Frank, E., Plewes, J.M., Tollefson, G.D., and Rush, A.J.: A Descriptive Analysis of Minor Depression, *Am. J. Psychiatry*, 159, 637, April, 2002.

Roberts, M.C., Riedy, C.A., Coldwell, S.E., Nagahama, S., Judge, K., Lam, M., Kaakke, T., Castillo, J.L., and Milgrom, P.: How Xylitol-Containing Products Affect Cariogenic Bacteria, *J. Am. Dent. Assoc.*, 133, 435, April, 2002.

Scarr, E.M.: Effective Prenatal Care for Adolescent Girls, *Nurs. Clin. North Am.*, 37, 513, September, 2002.

Pregnancy

Brown, Z.A., Selke, S., Zeh, J., Kopelman, J., Maslow, A., Ashley, R.L., Watts, H., Berry, S., Herd, M., and Corey, L.: The Acquisition of

Herpes Simplex Virus During Pregnancy, *N. Engl. J. Med., 337,* 509, August 21, 1997.

Franko, D.L., Blais, M.A., Becker, A.E., Delinsky, S.S., Greenwood, D.N., Flores, A.T., Ekeblad, E.R., Eddy, K.T., and Herzog, D.B.: Pregnancy Complications and Neonatal Outcomes in Women With Eating Disorders, *Am. J. Psychiatry, 158,* 1461, September, 2001.

Gaffield, M.L., Colley Gilbert, B.J., Malvitz, D.M., and Romaguera, R.: Oral Health During Pregnancy: An Analysis of Information Collected by the Pregnancy Risk Management Monitoring System, *J. Am. Dent. Assoc., 132,* 1009, July, 2001.

Glick, M. and Goldman, H.: Viral Infections in the Dental Setting: Potential Effects on Pregnant HCWs, *J. Am. Dent. Assoc., 124,* 79, June, 1993.

Innes, K.E., Byers, T.E., Marshall, J. A., Baron, A., Orleans, M., and Hamman, R.F.: Association of a Woman's Own Birth Weight With Subsequent Risk for Gestational Diabetes, *JAMA, 287,* 2534, May 15, 2002.

Robert, E.: Treating Depression in Pregnancy (Editorial), *N. Engl. J. Med., 335,* 1056, October 3, 1996.

Wisner, K.L., Zarin, D.A., Holmboe, E.S., Appelbaum, P.S., Gelenberg, A.J., Leonard, H.L., and Frank, E.: Risk-Benefit Decision Making for Treatment of Depression During Pregnancy, *Am. J. Psychiatry, 157,* 1933, December, 2000.

Periodontal Aspects

Krejci, C.B. and Bissada, N.F.: Women's Health Issues and Their Relationship to Periodontitis, *J. Am. Dent. Assoc., 133,* 323, March, 2002.

Lopez, N.J., Smith, P.D., and Gutierrez, J.: Periodontal Therapy May Reduce the Risk of Preterm Low Birth Weight in Women With Periodontal Disease: A Randomized Controlled Trial, *J. Periodontol., 73,* 911, August, 2002.

Machuca, G., Khoshfeiz, O., Lacalle, J.R., Machuca, C., and Bullon, P.: The Influence of General Health and Socio-cultural Variables on the Periodontal Condition of Pregnant Women, *J. Periodontol., 70,* 779, July, 1999.

Silverstein, L.H., Burton, C.H., Garnick, J.J., and Singh, B.B.: The Late Development of Oral Pyogenic Granuloma as a Complication of Pregnancy: A Case Report, *Compend. Cont. Educ. Dent., 17,* 192, February, 1996.

Soorlyamoorthy, M. and Gower, D.B.: Hormonal Influences on Gingival Tissue: Relationship to Periodontal Disease, *J. Clin. Periodontol., 16,* 201, April, 1989.

Yalcin, F., Eskinazi, E., Soydinc, M., Basegmez, C., Issever, H., Isik, G., Berber, L., Has, R., Sabuncu, H., and Onan, U.: The Effect of Sociocultural Status on Periodontal Conditions in Pregnancy, *J. Periodontol., 73,* 178, February, 2002.

Drugs

Gleghorn, T. and Housholder, G.T.: Anti-infective Drug Therapy: Implications for the Lactating Mother and Nursing Infant, *J. Dent. Hyg., 69,* 130, May–June, 1995.

Jacobson, J.L. and Jacobson, S.W.: Intellectual Impairment in Children Exposed to Polychlorinated Biphenyls In Utero, *N. Engl. J. Med., 335,* 783, September 12, 1996.

Rosenberg, N.M., Meert, K.L., Knazik, S.R., Yee, H., and Kauffman, R.E.: Occult Cocaine Exposure in Children, *Am. J. Dis. Child., 145,* 1430, December, 1991.

Singer, L.T., Arendt, R., Minnes, S., Farkas, K., Salvator, A., Kirchner, H.L., and Kliegman, R.: Cognitive and Motor Outcomes of Cocaine-Exposed Infants, *JAMA, 287,* 1952, April 17, 2002.

Tuomala, R.E., Shapiro, E.E., Mofenson, L.M., Bryson, Y., Culnane, M., Hughes, M.D., O'Sullivan, M.J., Scott, G., Stek, A.M., Wara, D., and Bulterys, M.: Antiretroviral Therapy During Pregnancy and the Risk of an Adverse Outcome, *N. Engl. J. Med., 346,* 1863, June 13, 2002.

Tobacco Use

Cunningham, J., Dockery, D.W., and Speizer, F.E.: Maternal Smoking During Pregnancy as a Predictor of Lung Function in Children, *Am. J. Epidemiol., 139,* 1139, June 15, 1994.

DiFranza, J.R. and Lew, R.A.: Effect of Maternal Cigarette Smoking on Pregnancy Complications and Sudden Death Syndrome, *J. Fam. Pract., 40,* 385, April, 1995.

Fried, P.A.: Prenatal Exposure to Tobacco and Marijuana: Effects During Pregnancy, Infancy, and Early Childhood, *Clin. Obstet. Gynec., 36,* 319, June, 1993.

Schoendorf, K.C. and Kiely, J.L.: Relationship of Sudden Infant Death Syndrome to Maternal Smoking During and After Pregnancy, *Pediatrics, 90,* 905, December, 1992.

Waldman, H.B.: Do the Parent(s) of Your Pediatric Patients Smoke? *ASDC J. Dent. Child., 59,* 126, March–April, 1992.

Pediatric Oral Health Care: Infancy Through Age 5

Nancy Sisty LePeau, RDH, MS, MA

Oral health for infants and young children up to the age of 5 years depends primarily on parental interventions. Parents are counseled and given the information needed to assess their child's oral health status. They are taught how to intervene and to anticipate the child's oral health needs at various ages and stages of growth and development. Parents can become well informed through the education they receive from healthcare professionals prior to the birth of their children and at regular intervals thereafter. Box 46-1 defines key words associated with this chapter.

ACCESS TO PARENTS BY HEALTH PROFESSIONALS

Contacts with parents can occur in prenatal and birthing classes, hospitals, and public and private community health centers. Many public and private agencies have begun to send providers into the homes of high-risk families for education and guidance. Daycare and preschool centers and offices of pediatric and family practitioners also present opportunities to educate parents on ways to

---

BOX 46-1 KEY WORDS: Pediatric Oral Health Care: Infants through Age 5

Anticipatory guidance: provide information to parents and caregivers on what to expect in a child's current and next developmental stage so that they can anticipate and provide for their needs.

Dental home: establish a dentist of record in the community early in childhood for continuous and comprehensive preventive interventions, dental hygiene, and dental care.

Grazing: eating or drinking at will throughout the day or evening.

Infant: child younger than 1 year of age.

Neonate: newborn.

Neonatal: refers to the period immediately following birth and continuing through the first month of life.

Nonnutritive sucking: sucking fingers, thumb, pacifiers, or other objects for comfort.

Premature birth: birth that occurs before the expected delivery date; denotes an infant born prior to 37 weeks of gestation.

Sippy cup: a special cup with a lid that may have a straw or a drinking projection to teach a young child to drink.

Toddler: child from age 1 year to approximately 3 years of age.

Wean: to discontinue breast- or bottle-feeding; to nourish the infant with other food.

---

give oral hygiene care, identify problems early, and prevent oral disease. Healthcare personnel in these settings assist parents in establishing a relationship with a dentist in the community by making dental referrals.

▪ FIRST CONTACT WITH PARENT AND CHILD

The American Academy of Pediatric Dentistry recommends that infants be seen by a dentist by 6 months or after the eruption of the first primary tooth and by no later than age 1.[1] More recently, physicians, nurses, dentists, and dental hygienists are educated during their professional programs to identify families at high risk for oral health problems. Emphasis is placed on early intervention before serious oral health problems develop.[2]

Healthcare professionals are taught how to examine the mouths of infants and children for early childhood dental caries, dental biofilm, gingivitis, oral pathologies, and evidence of orofacial trauma and/or possible abuse. Furthermore, they are prepared to guide parents to be aware of and to attend to their infant and children's oral health needs.[3,4] Emphasis on early prevention, identification of problems, and referral for infants and young children should improve oral health status, reduce pain and suffering, and decrease the need for costly treatment.

▪ RISK FACTORS FOR CARIES AND GINGIVITIS

Risk factors[5-7] for early childhood oral disease are identified from the interview with the parents or guardians and are listed in Table 46-1. Parents can be seated in a quiet, private place so that they are able to concentrate and feel comfortable while supplying the information requested. After rapport is established with the parents, an explanation is given as to why the information is needed and the following factors are addressed:

I. FAMILY CONFIGURATION

- Number of people in the household and their relationship to the child.
- Number of family members who work outside the home and their time with the child at home.
- Other caregivers, the time periods, and location.
- Socioeconomic status and educational level of parents or guardians.

II. DENTAL HISTORY OF THE PARENTS AND CHILDREN

- Dentist of record for the family and the frequency of visits for the parents and children.
- Dental caries and periodontal disease experience of parents and children.

▪ TABLE 46-1 EARLY CHILDHOOD RISK FACTORS FOR ORAL DISEASE

Familial Factors	• Low socioeconomic status • Belonging to a minority • Mother and siblings with caries experience • Limited or no oral hygiene provided by parents • Use of nonfluoridated toothpaste • No dentist of record for the family • Infrequent or irregular dental visits • Low dental preventive knowledge of family • No belief in prevention • Fear of dentistry
Health Considerations	• Premature birth • Low birth weight • Severe or chronic illness • Developmental disabilities • Early hospitalization and/or surgery • Developmental dental defects and/or malposed teeth • Frequent use of sweetened medications • Use of antihistamine causing dry mouth • Early childhood caries
Dietary Considerations	• Insufficient fluoride in water supply • Bottles in bed • Sweetened liquids placed in bottle/sippy cup • Prolonged breast/bottle-feeding • Use of bottles/sippy cups at will • Frequent snacking • Diet high in fermentable and retentive carbohydrates

Sources: Casamassimo, P.: *Bright Futures in Practice: Oral Health.* Arlington, VA, National Center for Education in Maternal and Child Health, 1996, pp. 1–41.
Nowak, A. and Crall, J.: Prevention of Dental Disease, in: Pinkham, J.R., ed.: *Pediatric Dentistry: Infancy Through Adolescence,* 3rd ed. Philadelphia, W.B. Saunders Co., 1999, p. 197.

- Tooth eruption patterns of parents and children.
- Parents' personal oral hygiene habits.
- Teething problems exhibited by child.
- Deep pits and fissures in primary molars and no spacing.

III. PRENATAL AND PERINATAL HISTORY

- Physician of record and frequency of visits.
- History of chronic/infectious diseases.
- Prenatal care provided for mother.
- Problems in pregnancy or delivery, including prematurity or low term birth weight.
- Drugs, alcohol consumed during pregnancy.
- Use of tobacco during pregnancy.

IV. MEDICAL HISTORY OF THE CHILD

- Family history of chronic/infectious disease.
- Genetic, developmental, metabolic diseases.
- Hospitalizations/surgeries and reasons.
- Allergies or reactions to medications.
- Frequency of ear infections.

- History of high fevers.
- Current medications.

V. FEEDING PATTERNS

A. Infant (birth to 1 year)

- Breast/bottle fed.
- Formula used and fluoride content of water used for preparation.
- Frequency and method of feeding.
- Problems with feeding.
- Problems with sleeping.
- Pacifier, thumb, or finger use.
- Other liquids besides formula or milk in bottle.
- Age other children in family were weaned.

B. Toddler (1 to 3 years) and Preschool Child (3 to 5 years)

- Number of snacks per day and time period.
- Types of snacks provided.
- Amount of juice or other sweet drinks consumed per day.

- Availability of snacks without supervision.
- Problems with eating, including likes and dislikes.

VI. FLUORIDE EXPOSURE

- History of exposure to fluoride.
- Fluoride level of current water supply, including childcare environments (check public health department records).
- Well water (have water tested for fluoride level).
- Use of nonfluoridated bottled water or water systems using reverse osmosis.
- Type of toothpaste, amount and frequency of use.
- Parental control of fluoride toothpaste.
- Use of fluoride supplementation.

VII. PERSONAL ORAL CARE HABITS

- Parents/caregivers wipe inside mouth daily with wet gauze (infants before teeth erupt).
- Brush teeth with water only until approximately 2 years of age.
- Frequency and time of day oral hygiene care is provided.
- Positioning of child for access to oral cavity.
- Lift lip to brush anterior teeth.
- Child's behavior during oral hygiene care.

VIII. BARRIERS TO DENTAL CARE

- Lack of belief in prevention.
- Language.
- Cost.
- Fear.
- No *dental home.*
- Dentist does not see children under age 3 years.
- Dentist's hours do not fit into parents'/caregivers' schedules.
- Dentist does not accept dental insurance.
- Transportation.

■ ANTICIPATORY GUIDANCE FOR PARENTS, CAREGIVERS, AND PROVIDERS

Anticipatory guidance in oral health counseling assists parents in developing knowledge of what to expect of their children during their current and next developmental stage.[5] Essential information tailored to the child's individual needs is provided to parents verbally and in writing. Parents can learn what constitutes good oral healthcare and how to anticipate the child's future requirements. Proper expectations of what children should be able to do at each age level allows for more positive interactions between parent and child. Aspects addressed when guiding parents are shown in Table 46-2 (Birth to 24 Months) and in Table 46-3 (Age 2 Through 5 Years). Developmental milestones, nutrition and feeding, oral hygiene measures, dental caries prevention, health and safety precautions, and treatment measures are outlined in the tables.[8]

■ ORAL HEALTH CONSIDERATIONS FOR INFANTS

I. NONNUTRITIVE SUCKING

A. Normal Sucking

- Infants engage in nonnutritive sucking patterns during the first year of life and beyond.
- They may suck on their thumb, fingers, or pacifiers for comfort.
- Inform parents that such sucking is normal and acceptable behavior.[9]

B. Characteristics of a Safe Pacifier

- Solid construction so that it cannot be pulled apart. Figure 46-1 shows two types of pacifiers, one has an orthodontic nipple and the other a nonorthodontic. The orthodontic nipple is designed to be more like a mother's breast nipple during nursing.
- Nontoxic material.
- Ventilated shield large enough to prevent swallowing.
- Not tied to the child's clothing, which could lead to strangulation.
- Not cleaned in the parent's/caregiver's mouth since caries-producing bacteria could be transferred to the infant who has teeth.[10]

II. BOTTLE/BREAST-FEEDING

A. Bottle

- Put only formula or milk in the bottle.
- Hold the child during feeding.
- Never place the child in bed with a bottle.
- Do not use the bottle as a pacifier.
- Do not put juice or other sweet liquids in the bottle.

▪ TABLE 46-2 ANTICIPATORY GUIDANCE: BIRTH TO 24 MONTHS

AREA OF CONCERN	BIRTH TO 6 MONTHS	6–12 MONTHS	12–24 MONTHS
Developmental Milestone	• Eruption of first tooth • Pattern of eruption	• Pattern of eruption • Expected new teeth	• Check tooth contacts • Close contacts: teach to floss
Nutrition and Feeding	• Cause of tooth decay by improper bottle/breast-feeding • No propping of bottles in bed • Avoid use of bottle as pacifier • Breast-feeding: passage of alcohol and drugs to infant • Discuss weaning	• Begin weaning • Discontinue bottle feeding by age 1 year • Use small, regular cup • Avoid at-will access to bottle or sippy cup • Discuss sugar use, sugar retention, and caries initiation • Discuss consumption of sugar-sweetened beverages • Snacking safety (aspiration) • Avoid use of food for behavior modification	• Review prior content covered • Nutrition, snacking based on child's diet • Reduce snacking frequency • Review snacking safety • Avoid use of food for behavior modification
Oral Hygiene and Caries Prevention	• Oral health of parents; *Streptococcus mutans* transmission • Clean ridges after each feeding (soft, wet cloth or gauze) • Use of brush (water only) • Position of infant for brushing	• Use of brush • Review position of infant for brushing • Parents look for signs of disease	• Disclose for dental biofilm • Review brushing • Parents are the role models • Parents look for signs of disease
Fluoride Information	• Explain the relation of fluoride to teeth • Anticipate need to supplement • Check water supply for fluoride content at home and daycare	• When water supply is deficient, prescribe supplement (see Table 46-5) • Discuss compliance • Review manner of storage: cool, dry, out of reach	• Update fluoride status • Store fluoride products out of reach of children • Use of small, thin smear of fluoride dentifrice on brush
Trauma Prevention	• Car seat safety	• Discuss highest accident rate is 1 to 2 years • Car seat safety • Trauma-proofing • Confirm emergency access to dental provider	• Car seat safety • Discuss oral electrical burns and child-proofing home • Care of avulsed tooth
Habits/Function Behaviors	• Discuss teething • Discuss nonnutritive sucking	• Discuss oral/head and neck signs of child abuse	• Effects of continued thumb sucking
Environmental (Passive) Smoke	• Detrimental at all ages: smoking parents must start tobacco cessation program	• Provide smoke-free environment	• Children need smoke-free environment
			(continued)

■ TABLE 46-2 ANTICIPATORY GUIDANCE: BIRTH TO 24 MONTHS (Continued)

AREA OF CONCERN	BIRTH TO 6 MONTHS	6–12 MONTHS	12–24 MONTHS
Dental/Dental Hygiene Visit	• Provide rationale for timing of baby's first dental visit • Explain what happens at first dental visit • Encourage parents to make appointments for their own dental care to eliminate *Streptococcus mutans*	• Schedule first dental visit within 6 months of eruption of first tooth • Provide information about how to make the first dental/dental hygiene visit a happy experience • Review need for parents to complete their own dental care	• Home preparation for dental visit • Frequency depends on parent compliance with home preventive measures • Parents emphasize helping/caring nature of dentist/dental hygienist • Toothbrush dental biofilm removal • Discuss findings and recommendations with parents

(Adapted from Nowak A.J. and Casamassimo, P.S.: Using Anticipatory Guidance to Provide Early Dental Intervention, *J. Am. Dent. Assoc., 126,* 1156, August, 1995.)

B. Breast

- Do not allow prolonged, at-will breast-feeding after teeth erupt.
- If the infant sleeps with the mother, do not allow them to suckle at will after the eruption of teeth.
- When the infant falls asleep after sucking, milk collects around teeth and causes demineralization. Dental carious lesions are most often seen first in the maxillary anteriors (Figure 46-2).

III. TEETHING

A. Eruption Patterns

- Tell parents/caregivers when to expect teeth to erupt.
- Provide a table of primary tooth eruption patterns, as shown in Table 46-4.
- Explain that eruption patterns vary widely and are familial in nature.

B. Teething Behaviors

- Excessive chewing and drooling.
- Irritability.
- Change in appetite.
- Interrupted sleep patterns.
- Crying.
- Fever or diarrhea usually are not symptoms and require consultation with a physician to assess the presence of a systemic illness.[4]

C. Palliative Measures

1. Chewing on objects.
   - Cold wash cloth.
   - Hard, solid teething ring.

2. Numbing Solutions.
   - Over-the-counter numbing solutions are not recommended.
   - Products contain a strong anesthetic that is difficult to control.
   - May numb the entire oral cavity and, if swallowed, suppress the gag reflex.[4]

IV. EARLY CHILDHOOD CARIES

Dental disease exhibited in primary teeth of infants and very young children is termed early childhood caries. Baby bottle tooth decay is one form and is usually seen in children who routinely have been given a bottle when going to sleep or who have experienced prolonged at-will breast-feeding. Other names for this condition are nursing caries, baby bottle caries, and rampant caries.[11]

A. Microbiology

1. High levels of *Streptococcus mutans* cultured from the saliva and dental biofilm from the teeth.
2. Transfer of *Streptococcus mutans* from parent's or caregiver's mouth to the infant or young child.[10,12]
3. *Lactobacilli* in large numbers in the dental biofilm.

B. Risk Factors

The risk factors are listed in Table 46-1. Teaching the parents about the cause and effects of early childhood caries is a significant part of anticipatory guidance (Tables 46-2 and 46-3).

■ TABLE 46-3 ANTICIPATORY GUIDANCE: AGE 2 THROUGH 5 YEARS

AREA OF CONCERN	2–3 YEARS	4–5 YEARS
Developmental Milestone	• Primary dentition complete • Evaluate occlusion for possible crowding, overbite, overjet • Bruxing and occlusal wear	• Discuss exfoliation of primary teeth • Eruption patterns and expected new permanent teeth • Discuss sealants for primary molars and first permanent molars
Nutrition and Feeding	• Suggest snacks from fruit, vegetable, milk, and meat groups • Limit juice intake to 4 ounces per day • Avoid use of sweetened beverages • Avoid use of food for behavior modification	• Snacking: suggest healthy snacks • Limit juice and soda • Avoid use of food for behavior modification
Oral Hygiene and Caries Prevention	• Parents continue to assist • Ask about problems • Lift upper lip, brush morning and night • Review signs of disease	• Parents continue to assist • Review signs of disease
Fluoride Information	• Parent controls toothpaste • Evaluate changes in diet and water • Make appropriate fluoride recommendations • Possible fluoride varnish applications	• Parents continue toothpaste control • Check fluoride status • Varnish applications
Trauma Prevention	• Provide trauma management plan at daycare or preschool • Discuss head and neck, oral signs of child abuse • Review safety measures	• Trauma management plan at school • Discuss bike safety • Discuss child abuse • Review safety measures
Habits/Function Behaviors	• Nonnutritive sucking may still be present • Discuss elimination of digit/thumb sucking	• Eliminate digit/thumb sucking
Environmental (Passive) Smoke	• Smoke-free environment required	• Smoke-free environment required
Dental/Dental Hygiene Visit	• Need regular care every 6 months unless need for greater frequency identified • Emphasize helping/caring nature of dentist/dental hygienist • Use disclosing solution to identify dental biofilm • Toothbrush or rubber cup dental biofilm • Radiographic evaluation if indicated • Discuss findings and recommendations with parents	• Need regular care • Radiographic evaluation if indicated • Emphasize helping/caring nature of providers • Use disclosing solution to identify dental biofilm • Assess for calculus requiring scaling • Rubber cup polishing • Discuss findings and recommendations with parents

(Adapted from Nowak, A.J. and Casamassimo, P.S.: Using Anticipatory Guidance to Provide Early Dental Intervention, *J. Am. Dent. Assoc.*, *126*, 1156, August, 1995.)

C. Predisposing Factors

- Placing bottle in bed.
- Bottle contains sweetened milk or other fluid sweetened with sucrose.
- Prolonged at-will breast- or bottle-feeding as a sleep or behavioral control.
- Ineffective or no daily biofilm removal from the teeth.

D. Effects

1. Maxillary anterior teeth and primary molars are the first to be affected, as noted in Figure 46-2.

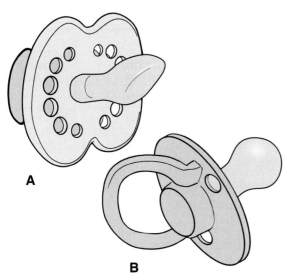

■ **FIGURE 46-1 Criteria for Selecting Pacifiers.** Two styles of pacifier nipples: **(A)** orthodontic and **(B)** nonorthodontic. Criteria for selection of a safe pacifier: size of shield is at least 1 to 1 1/2 inches in diameter; shield has air vents; plastic portion is of sturdy construction to prevent separation and possible choking; nipple is checked frequently for cracking and stickiness, at which time, pacifier is replaced.

2. As the baby falls asleep, pools of sweet liquid can collect around the teeth.
3. While the sucking is active, the liquid passes beyond the teeth.
4. The nipple covers the mandibular anterior teeth; hence, they are rarely affected.

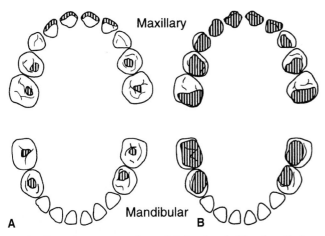

■ **FIGURE 46-2 Progression of Baby Bottle/Nursing Caries.** **(A)** Earliest caries affect the maxillary anterior teeth followed by the molars as they erupt. **(B)** Severe extensive lesions develop in all except the mandibular anterior teeth. Protection for the mandibular incisors and canines is provided by the tongue during the sucking process.

E. Recognition

1. Demineralization or white spot lesions may be noted along the cervical third of the maxillary anterior teeth and proximal surfaces when the upper lip is lifted, as seen in Figure 46-3. These lesions are considered pre-carious.
2. At a later stage the lesions appear dark brown. Eventually, the crowns may be destroyed to the gum line, abscesses may develop, and the child may suffer severe pain and discomfort. An advanced stage of dental caries is shown in Figure 46-4.

V. DAILY DENTAL BIOFILM REMOVAL

A. Gaining Access and Cooperation

1. Infants may cry, fuss, and squirm during oral healthcare.
2. Parents use a knee-to-knee position to control the child's head, arms, and feet as depicted in Figure 46-5. Other positions are shown in Figure 53-13.
3. One parent can cradle the infant's head with one arm and wipe or brush with the opposite hand.
4. Visibility can be improved if the child is placed on a bed, changing table, floor, or lap.
5. Singing, talking, and smiling during this oral cleaning help the child associate the process with a pleasant experience.

B. Wiping Prior to Tooth Eruption

1. Oral health needs prior to tooth eruption include daily, gentle wiping of gum ridges, inside of cheeks, lips, and tongue with a clean, wet cloth or gauze.
2. Infants become used to the oral care routine through this daily activity.
3. Parents often elect to do the wiping at bath time.

C. Tooth Brushing

1. Newly erupted teeth are brushed with a child-sized toothbrush and water only.[13,14]
2. Recommend a good quality toothbrush with soft and end-rounded filaments.
3. Emphasize brushing teeth in the morning and before bed.
4. Replace the brush when filaments are frayed or bent, usually every 3 months.

VI. FLUORIDE SUPPLEMENTATION

A. Discuss fluoride requirements at 6 months according to the guidelines specified in Table 46-5.

■ TABLE 46-4 TOOTH DEVELOPMENT AND ERUPTION: PRIMARY TEETH

		HARD TISSUE FORMATION BEGINS (WEEKS IN UTERO)	ENAMEL COMPLETED (MONTHS AFTER BIRTH)	ERUPTION (MONTHS)	ROOT COMPLETED (YEAR)
Maxillary	Central incisor	14	1½	10 (8–12)	1½
	Lateral incisor	16	2½	11 (9–13)	2
	Canine	17	9	19 (16–22)	3¼
	First molar	15½	6	16 (13–19 boys) (14–18 girls)	2½
	Second molar	19	11	29 (25–33)	3
Mandibular	Central incisor	14	2½	8 (6–10)	1½
	Lateral incisor	16	3	13 (10–16)	1½
	Canine	17	9	20 (17–23)	3¼
	First molar	15½	5½	16 (14–18)	2¼
	Second molar	18	10	27 (23–31 boys) (24–30 girls)	3

From Lunt R.C. and Law, D.B: A Review of the Chronology of Eruption of Deciduous Teeth, *J. Am. Dent. Assoc., 89,* 872, October, 1974.

B. History information regarding fluoride exposure directs decisions regarding fluoride supplementation.

C. Consult with the child's dentist to make this decision.

VII. FEEDING PATTERNS

A. Introducing the Cup

A small, plastic cup is introduced to the child when he or she is ready developmentally, usually 8 to 12 months. The goal is to discontinue use of the bottle by 12 months of age.

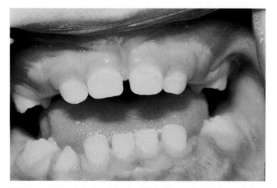

■ **FIGURE 46-3 Risk for Early Childhood Caries.** The upper lip of the child is retracted. White spot lesions are noted along the cervical margins of the maxillary anterior teeth. Slight marginal gingivitis is noted on the maxillary anterior gingival tissues. Parents are instructed to lift the lip of their child's teeth and brush along the cervicals to remove dental biofilm and to examine the teeth visually. Remineralization of lesions may occur through use of fluoride-containing toothpaste and topical fluoride application. Photo: Courtesy of Michael J. Kanellis, DDS, MS.

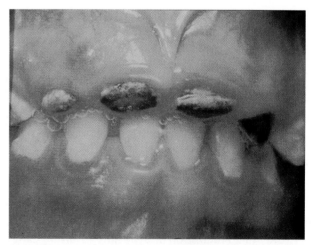

■ **FIGURE 46-4 Severe Baby Bottle/Nursing Caries.** Nearly complete loss of tooth structure of maxillary incisors. Note the abscess on the gingival tissues between the maxillary right central and lateral incisor, and the moderate cervical biofilm on the mandibular incisors.

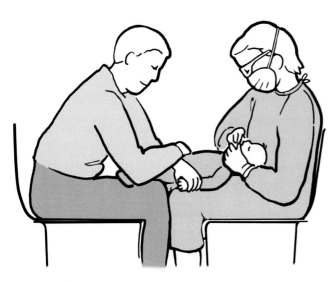

■ **FIGURE 46-5 Infant Dental/Dental Hygiene Visits.** Clinician and parent sit knee-to-knee with the child across their laps. Parent stabilizes the infant's legs and holds the hands in a position that allows a good view of the infant's oral cavity for watching and learning. The clinician does the oral examination, discusses oral findings, and demonstrates proper oral care for the infant. The position of the infant then is reversed so that the parent can position the child and demonstrate proper oral care measures.

B. Diet and Health

1. Teach about the relationship between frequent and large amounts of sweetened beverage intake and dental caries and obesity.[15,16]
2. Provide healthy snacks from the grain, vegetable, fruit, meat, and milk groups between meals.
3. Limit intake of fermentable and retentive carbohydrate foods.

■ **TABLE 46-5 FLUORIDE SUPPLEMENTS DOSAGE SCHEDULE (mg F/day)***

AGE OF CHILD (years)	WATER FLUORIDE CONCENTRATION (PPM)		
	LESS THAN 0.3	BETWEEN 0.3 AND 0.6	GREATER THAN 0.6
Birth–6 mo	0	0	0
6 mo–3 yr	0.25 mg	0†	0†
3–6 yr	0.50 mg	0.25 mg	0
6–16 yr	1.0 mg	0.5 mg	0

*2.2 mg sodium fluoride provides 1 mg fluoride ions.
† Infants receiving their total diet from breast-feeding need a 0.25-mg supplement. (Recommendations from the American Dental Association, Chicago, IL.)

4. Rinse the child's mouth with water immediately following the dispensing of sweetened medications. Medications such as those used for ear infections and nutritional supplementation often are made with a sugar or a syrupy base to disguise medication flavors.

VIII. THE FIRST DENTAL HYGIENE/ DENTAL VISIT

A. Purposes

1. Oral examination by 6 months of age or after the eruption of the first primary tooth.
2. Educate parents.
3. Emphasize prevention of oral disease.

B. Oral Examination: Positioning for Access

1. Seat parent and clinician knee-to-knee.
2. Place child's head on the lap of the examiner, as seen in Figure 46-5.

C. Examination Sequence

1. Look at the child's head and neck, legs, and arms for evidence of abuse. Signs of abuse are described on pages 960 to 963 in Chapter 57.
2. Ask the parent to control the child's extremities while the oral soft tissues are assessed (Tables 46-6 and 46-7).[17,18]
3. If teeth are present, lift the upper lip to observe the condition of the anterior teeth.
4. Examine all teeth for evidence of biofilm, discoloration.
5. Look for malformations (Figure 46-6), and dental caries (Figure 46-4).
6. Show parents the findings and inform them of the significance.
7. Make referrals to the dentist if evidence of pathology is noted (Tables 46-6 and 46-7 and Table 15-4, pages 270 to 271).

D. Homecare Instruction

1. Wiping/brushing is demonstrated by the clinician while the parent/caregiver observes.
2. Move the child's head to the lap of the parent and ask the parent to demonstrate the procedures. Make appropriate suggestions for changes.
3. Provide recommendations orally and in writing based on the information gleaned from the interview and examination.

▪ **TABLE 46-6 ORAL SOFT AND HARD TISSUE CONDITIONS/PATHOLOGY IN INFANTS (1 TO 6 MONTHS)**

CONDITIONS	FINDINGS	SIGNIFICANCE
Soft Tissue		
Pseudomembranous candidiasis (thrush)	Mucosa or tongue; white, curd-like plaques; wipe off leaving red and raw area	Discomfort; antifungal medication
Congenital epulis	Maxillary anterior ridge; pink, smooth pedunculated mass; present at birth	Benign; spontaneous involution or surgical excision
Bohn's nodule	Buccal and lingual aspects of dental ridge; mucous gland remnant; smooth, translucent nodules	No treatment Shed spontaneously
Epstein's pearls	Palate near raphe; smooth, translucent nodules	No treatment
Dental lamina cysts	Crest of maxillary and mandibular ridges; dental lamina origin; smooth, translucent	No treatment
Bifid uvula	Cleft in uvula	Evaluate for possible submucous palatal cleft
Ankyloglossia	Short lingual frenum; may limit tongue mobility	Surgical reduction if interferes with nursing
Teeth		
Natal teeth	85% mandibular primary incisors; present at birth; commonly occur in pairs	Familial tendency; remove if mobile or have sharp edges causing injury
Neonatal teeth	Erupt within 30 days after birth	Same as above

Sources: McDonald, R.E. and Avery, D.R.: *Dentistry for Children and the Adolescent,* 7th ed. St. Louis, Mosby, 2000, pp. 141–144, 155–158, 188–191. Flaitz, C.M.: Oral Pathologic Conditions and Soft Tissue Anomalies, in: Pinkham, J.R., ed.: *Pediatric Dentistry: Infancy Through Adolescence,* 3rd ed. Philadelphia, W. B. Saunders Co, 1999, pp. 12–42.

▪ ORAL HEALTH CONSIDERATIONS FOR TODDLERS AND PRESCHOOLERS

I. ACCIDENT AND INJURY PREVENTION

Toddlers are more active and as a result are subject to injuries. Parents can be taught to protect the child by close supervision, anticipating problems, and making the environment safe by removing dangers. Written information regarding what to do in the event of a traumatic oral injury makes parents feel more prepared. Table 66-5 (page 1119) provides information on a dislocated jaw, facial fracture, and tooth forcibly displaced or avulsed.

II. SUPERVISED BRUSHING AND FLOSSING

A. Establish a Routine

1. Make suggestions as to how to establish and maintain a brushing routine.
2. Recommend brushing in the morning after breakfast and before bedtime.

3. Specify that the most critical time for dental biofilm removal is before bed.

B. Gaining Cooperation

1. At these ages, the child is becoming more independent.
2. Parents can provide a fun activity by making up and singing a brushing song.
3. For 2- to 3-year-olds, teach them to take turns when brushing by using the phrase, "It's your turn to brush," followed by, "It's my turn to brush."
4. To gain better cooperation, connect brushing with a fun activity such as, first we brush teeth and then, we read a story.
5. Provide disclosing solution and 2- or 3-minute timers to be used for motivation during brushing.

C. Parental Supervision

1. Parents keep fluoride toothpaste out of reach of the child and are in charge of placing the proper amount of toothpaste on the toothbrush.

■ TABLE 46-7 ORAL SOFT TISSUE AND HARD TISSUE CONDITIONS/PATHOLOGY IN CHILDREN APPROXIMATELY 6 MONTHS TO 5 YEARS

CONDITIONS	FINDINGS	SIGNIFICANCE
Soft Tissue		
Eruption cysts	Translucent, smooth; may appear blue to blue black if bleeding in cystic space	Usually no treatment
Mucocele	Lower lip, floor of mouth, buccal mucosa most common in order of occurrence; fluid-filled vesicle or blister; trauma, tearing of minor salivary duct	May resolve or require surgical excision
Traumatic ulcer	Reaction to puncture wound	Clean wound; possible suture
Alveolar abscess	Smooth, red or yellowish nodule; tender; primary teeth—more diffuse infections; may be acute or chronic	Radiographic evaluation; drainage and antibiotic may be required
Primary herpetic gingivostomatitis	High fever, 102–104°F; regional lymphadenopathy; diffuse, swollen erythematous gingiva; vesicles form painful ulcers	Resolves in 7–10 days Transmissible
Geographic tongue	Red, smooth areas devoid of filliform papillae on dorsum of tongue; margins well developed, slightly raised; pattern changes	No treatment; brush tongue to reduce bacteria
Verruca vulgaris	Multiple, white, sessile lesions; finger-like projections, rough surface; human papilloma virus in origin	May resolve spontaneously or require excision
Teeth		
Enamel hypoplasia	Disturbance of enamel matrix during tooth development; irregular to round pits of varying size on enamel, usually in a row; multiple causes	Aesthetics
Fluorosis	See enamel hypoplasia; infrequent in primary dentition; usually seen in cervical region of second primary molars	Daily biofilm removal
White spot lesions	Usually cervical and proximal areas of teeth at contacts; first step of caries; loss of hard structure in enamel	Fluoride; daily biofilm removal
Fused teeth	Usually limited to anterior teeth; union of two independently forming primary tooth buds; familial tendency	Possible caries at point of fusion; may be absence of one of corresponding permanent teeth
Gemination	More common in primary teeth; invagination of single tooth germ; bifid crown on single root; crown appears wide	None

Sources: McDonald, R.E. and Avery, D.R.: *Dentistry for Children and the Adolescent,* 7th ed. St. Louis, Mosby, 2000, pp. 141–144, 155–158, 188–191. Flaitz, CM.: Oral Pathologic Conditions and Soft Tissue Anomalies, in: Pinkham, J. R., ed.: *Pediatric Dentistry: Infancy Through Adolescence,* 3rd ed. Philadelphia, W.B. Saunders Co., 1999, pp. 12–42.

2. Until the child develops fine motor coordination, usually about 7 years, the parents/caregivers assist the child to clean the teeth by doing the brushing for them.

3. Parents teach the child to brush and follow up with effective and complete biofilm removal.

4. Parents floss closely approximated primary teeth to remove proximal biofilm.

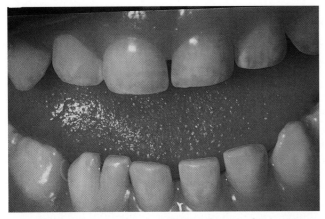

■ **FIGURE 46-6 Developmental Disturbance of Primary Teeth.** Gemination of mandibular right lateral incisor caused by invagination of a single tooth germ and resulting in a notched and grooved crown. Note the presence of six mandibular anterior teeth.

5. Parents are taught how to examine the mouth for signs of gingival inflammation, dental caries, or injury.

III. FLUORIDE

A. Assessments Needed to Recommend Supplements and Topical Applications

- Source and fluoride levels of the child's water supply.
- Type of toothpaste used and frequency of brushing.
- Effectiveness of personal oral healthcare.
- Dietary patterns and caries experience.
- Consultation with the dentist to determine fluoride needs (Table 46-5).

B. Toothpaste

1. Children's toothpastes manufactured in the United States contain the same amount of fluoride as adult toothpastes, whereas manufacturers in several other countries around the world reduce the amount of fluoride in children's toothpastes. Parents/caregivers are informed that they need to prevent problems by controlling the amount of toothpaste used and placing it out of the child's reach.
   a. Young children swallow large amounts of the toothpaste during brushing, which could cause dental fluorosis in developing teeth (Table 33-3).[19]
   b. Children like the taste of toothpaste and may eat a large amount at one time that could result in acute fluoride toxicity.

2. Instructions for parents:
   a. No toothpaste is used for children until age 2.
   b. *At age 2 years,* a tiny touch of fluoride toothpaste is placed on the child's brush by the parent.
   c. For older children, *ages 3 to 5 years,* a small, pea-sized amount of toothpaste is used and spread the length of the brush head, as shown in Figure 46-7.
   d. Spread the toothpaste from the brush on all of the teeth before brushing.
   e. Teach the child to lean over the sink so that collected saliva and fluoride toothpaste can drip in the sink and be spit out.
   f. Continue to control the toothpaste and keep it out of reach.

C. Fluorosis

1. The most critical time for fluorosis to develop in primary teeth as a result of excessive fluoride intake is during the middle of the first year of life.
2. The primary second molar could show evidence of fluorosis along the cervical margin.[20]
3. The most critical time for dental fluorosis of maxillary permanent incisors to occur is when the child is 22 to 26 months of age.[21]

D. Fluoride Varnish Application

1. Fluoride varnish is used on infant and young children's teeth when there is evidence of white spot lesions, indicating demineralization and high risk for early childhood caries.[22,23]

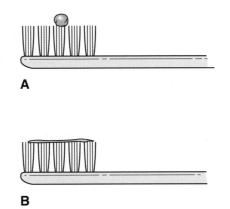

■ **FIGURE 46-7 Dentifrice for a Child 3 to 5 Years of Age.** To prevent ingestion of an excess amount of dentifrice, a parent is instructed to place only a small portion on the brush. **(A)** The appropriate size is that of a small pea. **(B)** The paste is spread in a thin layer over the brush surface and then spread over all of the teeth prior to brushing.

2. Fluoride varnish application is particularly helpful for children identified at high risk for dental caries.
3. Tooth preparation usually requires brushing only unless there is calculus that requires removal.
4. Varnish is easy to apply on infants and young children.
   a. Requires a light source, gauze squares or cotton rolls for drying, and applicators such as cotton swabs or a disposable brush.
   b. Wipe teeth dry with the gauze or cotton roll and apply the varnish to cover the teeth.
   c. Instruct parents to have the child wait for 30 minutes before eating and drinking and avoid brushing the teeth until the next day or at least 4 to 6 hours after application.
   d. Inform parents that the teeth look yellow until the varnish is removed through brushing.
   e. Recommend application at least two times per year and more frequently for children at highest risk for dental caries.

IV. ORAL MALODOR

A. Causes

- Bacteria at the base of the tongue.
- Bacteria between the teeth.
- Postnasal drip.[24]

B. What to Teach Parents

1. Explain bacterial causes.
2. Emphasize thorough dental biofilm removal through daily brushing of the teeth.
3. Teach them to floss their child's teeth.
4. Show them how to gently brush the dorsum of the tongue (page 419).

V. GRAZING ON THE SIPPY CUP

A. Do not allow the child to sip milk or sweet liquids at will, which promotes dental caries.
B. Have the child sit in the chair and complete a drink when they are thirsty.
C. Put any remaining drink away until they are thirsty again.

VI. DIETARY AND FEEDING PATTERN RECOMMENDATIONS

A. Children need a series of small, healthy meals during the day as recommended in the Food Guide Pyramid for Young Children (Figure 46-8).
B. Healthy snacks include foods from the grain, vegetable, fruit, meat, and milk groups that do not promote tooth decay.

C. Sweetened foods and drinks are limited and provided at mealtimes rather than between meals.
D. Juice intake is limited to no more than 4 to 6 ounces per day for children between the ages of 1 and 6 years.[25]
E. Parents or caregivers avoid giving young children carbonated soda drinks that promote caries and may contribute to childhood obesity.[15]
F. Parents or caregivers avoid using food for behavior modification.

VII. PREPARING THE CHILD FOR THE DENTAL VISIT

A. Make the dental office or clinic visit as pleasant as possible for the child.
B. Children are told that the dental hygienist and dentist help them take good care of their teeth.
C. Parents are instructed to avoid using negative words, such as "hurt, pain, do not be scared."
D. When the child is not present, parents are asked if the child has any fears or has had any prior negative experiences.

VIII. REGULAR VISITS TO THE DENTIST

A. Frequency

Visits to the dental hygienist and the dentist are scheduled according to the child's specific needs. The usual appointment plan for children with little or no oral disease is every 6 months.

B. Scheduling

The best time to schedule visits is early in the morning or after naps when the child is not tired and is more apt to listen and cooperate.

C. Purposes

Appointments are planned for assessment, prevention, and introduction to dental hygiene.
1. Develop rapport with the child and the family.
2. Initiate positive preventive measures, such as fluoride usage, feeding practices, and dental biofilm removal.
3. Discover, intercept, and change any parental practices that may be detrimental to the child's oral health.

D. Type of Oral Prophylaxis

The type of oral prophylaxis provided for the child depends on the age and oral findings.

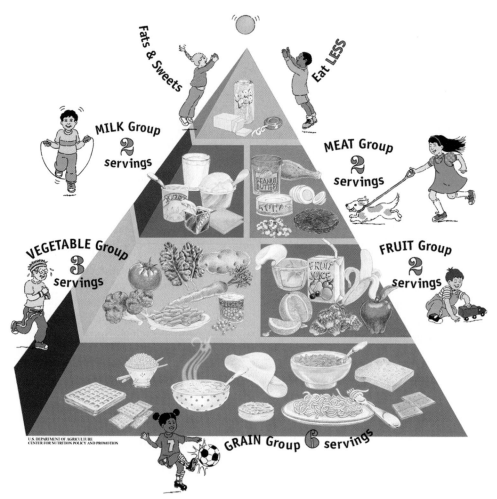

▪ **FIGURE 46-8 The Food Guide Pyramid for Young Children.** Guidelines for 2- to 6-year-old children. Released March 25, 1999 by the United States Department of Agriculture. Emphasizes foods from the five food groups and limiting fats and sweets.

1. Most children under the age of 3 years require only a wet toothbrush for dental biofilm removal.
2. Remove calculus, stain, and heavy dental biofilm not removed during toothbrush instruction.
3. Disclosing solution is extremely helpful for assessment and education.

E. Purpose of the Oral Prophylaxis

1. Provide a positive and enjoyable introductory experience.
2. Remove biofilm, stain, and calculus to facilitate visual examination of the teeth.
3. Educate parents and children regarding proper, daily biofilm control procedures and other preventive measures.
4. Teach parents how to examine their child's mouth for biofilm, gingivitis, dental caries, or injury.

IX. ORAL EXAMINATION

A. Positioning

Older children are able to sit in a dental chair. The size of the chair usually can be modified by removing the headrest and a portion of the backrest.

B. Parental Involvement

1. Plan the assessment and treatment.
    a. Determine the expected developmental milestones of the child according to the chronological age, as outlined in Tables 46-8 and 46-9.[26,27]
    b. Ask parents to identify actual developmental milestones so that proper management can be initiated during the appointment.
    c. Ask parents to provide a general statement regarding the child's temperament and ability to cooperate.

▪ TABLE 46-8 MILESTONES IN CHILD DEVELOPMENT: BIRTH TO AGE 18 MONTHS

AREAS	BIRTH TO 6 MONTHS	6–12 MONTHS	12–18 MONTHS
Language	• 0–2 months quiets to sound • Reflects displeasure at noises • Coos and babbles	• Says dada or mama • Understands name • Pays attention to verbalizations	• Repeats a few words • Says two or more words • Uses expressions "oh, oh" • Points to few body parts • Follows one-step directions
Motor	• 2 months head control • 6 months transfer hand to hand • Grasps with forearm (ulnar grasp)	• 7–9 months sits • 9–10 months plays pat-a-cake • Waves bye, bye	• Pincer grasp • Gives toys on request • 15–18 months good use of cup and spoon
Social/Emotional	• 2 months gaze at human face • Alert to voices	• Inhibited by word "no" • Separation anxiety • Stranger awareness	• Separation anxiety and stranger awareness continue

Sources: Overby, K.J.: Pediatric Health Supervision, in: Rudolph, A.M., Kamei, R.K., and Overby, K.J., eds.: *Rudolph's Fundamentals of Pediatrics,* 3rd ed. New York, McGraw-Hill, 2002, pp. 1–69.
Hangerman, R.J.: Growth and Development, in: Hay, W.W., Hayward, A.R., Levin, M.J., Sondheimer, J.M. eds.: *Current Pediatric Diagnosis and Treatment,* 14th ed. Stamford, CT, Appleton and Lange, 1999, pp. 1–18.

▪ TABLE 46-9 MILESTONES IN CHILD DEVELOPMENT: 18 MONTHS TO 5 YEARS

AREAS	18 MONTHS TO 2 YEARS	2–3 YEARS	3–4 YEARS	5 YEARS
Language	• Has up to 50 words and 2-word sentences • Talks to self • Hums or sings simple songs • Says names of familiar objects • Listens to short rhymes	• Up to 500 words • Converses using simple 2- to 3-word phrases and sentences • Responds to simple directions	• 75%–80% of speech understandable • Knows location words • Likes familiar stories repeated over and over • Knows what, who, why questions	• Five-word sentences • Conversations more mature • Links past and present events
Motor	• Feeds self • Uses straw • Walks well • Helps wash hands • Seats self in chair	• Dresses with supervision • Holds crayon in fist	• Feeds self well • Takes off jacket • Holds crayon with fingers	• Fine motor coordination maturing • Buttons clothing • May be able to tie shoe laces
Social/ Emotional	• Likes to imitate • Independent • Difficulty waiting • Shy with strangers • Likes adult attention • May exhibit anger and temper tantrums	• Likes to see and touch • Attached to parent • Rarely shares • Self-help skills of interest	• Likes to please • Responds to commands	• Distinguishes fantasy from reality • Likes pretend play • Longer attention span • Tolerates parent separation

Sources: Overby, K.J.: Pediatric Health Supervision, in: Rudolph, A.M., Kamei, R.K., and Overby, K.J., eds.: *Rudolph's Fundamentals of Pediatrics,* 3rd ed. New York, McGraw-Hill, 2002, pp. 1–69.
Hangerman, R.J.: Growth and Development, in: Hay, W.W., Hayward, A.R., Levin, M.J., Sondheimer, J.M. eds.: *Current Pediatric Diagnosis and Treatment,* 14th ed. Stamford, CT, Appleton and Lange, 1999, pp. 1–18.

d. Have parents/guardians sign an informed consent prior to treatment (page 369).

2. Evaluate if the parent should accompany the child.

a. At the first visit, a parent often accompanies the child to the treatment room.

b. Advise the parent to let the dental hygienist/dentist explain what they are going to do.

c. Instruct the parent to offer nonverbal reassurance for the child.

d. Ask the parent if they have questions regarding the treatment.

e. If appropriate, explain that the child is ready to go to the treatment room unaccompanied.

e. Inform the parent of your findings and provide verbal and written recommendations and instructions.

f. Have the parent/guardian sign consent for the care plan after the assessment.

X. CHILD MANAGEMENT

A. Establish Rapport

The purpose of the visit is to teach appropriate behaviors and to prevent management problems. Cooperation is usually gained by smiling and talking to establish rapport.

B. Show, Tell, and Do

1. Each piece of equipment and step of the procedure is shown and explained to the child before it is used (*show, tell, and do*).[28]

2. Use fun names for the equipment such as the "elevator chair," "tooth feeler," "tooth mirror," "slurpy straw," and "water fall."

3. Keep explanations brief and do the procedures as quickly as possible.

4. Four- and five-year-olds enjoy holding a hand mirror to watch what you are doing, which often distracts them from possible anxiety and fear of the unknown.

C. Crying

1. Stop the procedure if the child cries.

2. Comfort the child by telling him or her it is all right to cry.

3. The clinician's use of voice is extremely important: use a pleasant and modulated tone.

4. Avoid raising the voice. This frightens the child and indicates that the provider has lost control.

5. Continuous crying after the aversive stimulus is removed means the child is fearful.

6. If crying ceases, ask if they are ready to begin again and then reinitiate the show, tell, and do routine.

D. Positive Reinforcement

1. Use positive verbal reinforcement during the appointment, such as "super," "you are doing great," "what a helper," "great job," "I knew you could do it," "well done."

2. Provide brief breaks in the procedure for compliance and cooperation.

E. Lack of Cooperation

Reschedule the appointment if the child is unable to cooperate.

XI. GINGIVAL EVALUATION

A. **Healthy gingiva** in the primary dentition has the following characteristics:
    - Color is pink or slightly red.
    - Tissue appearance is thick, rounded or rolled, and shiny.
    - Tissue adaptation is not tight to the teeth and less fibrous than in the permanent dentition.
    - Interdental papillae on spaced anterior teeth are flat or saddle-shaped.
    - A col is present between facial and lingual papillae on posterior teeth in contact.

B. **Unhealthy gingiva** exhibits swelling, redness, and bleeding upon brushing or debriding.

XII. DENTAL CARIES EVALUATION

A. Anterior Teeth

1. Retract the lips to expose all of the teeth from the facial aspect.

2. Look for white spot lesions, or demineralization, along the cervical areas and proximal surfaces. Run the side of the tip of the explorer lightly over the area to assess for an intact surface, and, if present, initiate caries control for remineralization (page 399).

3. Observe discolored areas or dental caries interproximally using direct vision or transillumination.

4. Look for the presence of dental caries on smooth surfaces (pages 271 to 272).

B. Posterior Teeth

1. Observe and gently explore the pits and fissures of the primary molars to determine if they are shallow or deep.

2. Look for dark discolorations in the pits and fissures and on interproximal surfaces.
3. Look for open dental carious lesions on occlusal and smooth surfaces.

XIII. RADIOGRAPHIC EVALUATION OF PRIMARY DENTITION

A. Indications for Radiographic Exposures

1. Primary molars are close together and interfere with visualization and exploration.
2. Trauma.
3. Suspected pathology.
4. Problems with growth and development.

B. Use of Leaded Apron and Thyroid Collar

Protection is required because children are more susceptible than adults to low-level radiation.

C. Film Size

Film size is determined by the size of the mouth. Normally, one pediatric-sized film is used on each side to assess the primary molars.

D. Cooperation

Cooperation of the child is required and will depend on age and past experiences.[29]

XIV. OCCLUSION

A. Evaluation

1. Lack of spacing between primary teeth.
2. Malposed, crowded, or congenitally missing teeth.
3. Tooth eruption delays.
4. Discrepancies between the size of the teeth and the size of the mouth.
5. Early loss of primary molars: this condition, if untreated, usually disrupts the eruption and alignment of permanent molars and premolars, as depicted in Figure 46-9.

B. Indications for Referral

1. Severely crowded, malposed, or congenitally missing teeth.
2. Overbite, overjet, or crossbites.
3. Early loss of primary molars requires placement of a space maintainer to preserve arch length and allow for proper eruption of permanent teeth.

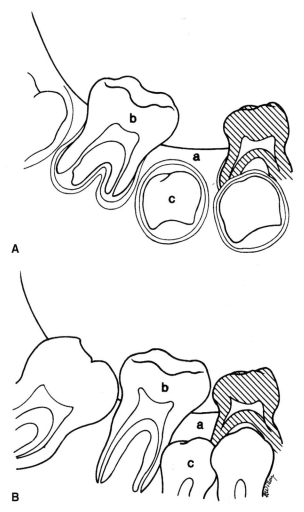

■ **FIGURE 46-9 Premature Loss of Second Primary Molar.**
(A) Developing first permanent molar (*b*) inclines and drifts mesially into the space (*a*) from which the second primary molar was removed. Developing second premolar (*c*) is crowded. **(B)** Space from which molar was removed (*a*) is nearly closed by the mesial drift and eruption of the first permanent molar (*b*). Developing second premolar (*c*) is closed in and prevented from eruption. Note that the second permanent molar has impacted against the first molar.

C. Thumb and Finger Sucking

1. When thumb or finger sucking continues to age 4, parents and clinicians intervene. The intervention is initiated before the time of the eruption of the maxillary anterior permanent teeth to prevent malposition (Figure 46-10).[1]
2. The clinician explains to the child what effects thumb sucking has on the teeth.
3. One approach to use to help the child stop the sucking habit is:
   a. Ask if the child would like to have straight teeth.

Everyday Ethics

? Four-year-old Charlie is accompanied by his mother to the dental office for his first dental visit. As they enter, the mother is overheard saying to her son, "Don't worry, the dentist won't hurt you." The dental hygienist introduces herself to the mother and child, escorts them to the treatment room, and seats Charlie in the dental chair. The mother immediately tells Charlie, "Everything will be all right, so don't be afraid." The dental hygienist talks to Charlie and asks him questions about his family, friends, and favorite games. He does not use eye contact, holds on tightly to the chair arms, and fidgets with his legs. He hesitates to answer, and his mother answers the questions for him.

Questions for Consideration

1. How do the ethical principles of autonomy and nonmaleficence apply in this case?

2. What responsibilities does the dental hygienist have to Charlie and to his mother?

3. Name two choices the dental hygienist can make to manage the situation and how these choices might affect Charlie, his mother, and the dentist.

---

   b. If the child agrees, the clinician asks for help in stopping the digit-sucking habit.
   c. A contract is made between the clinician and child.
   d. A photo is taken to document the current position of the teeth and as a reminder to stop the habit.
   e. A new photograph is taken at a subsequent appointment when changes in tooth positions can be documented.
4. Possible ways for the parents to assist the child in stopping the habit are:
   a. Place a reminder on the thumb or finger at the time the child usually sucks.
   b. The reminder may be a band-aid, glove, or fingernail polish on the nail of the digit.
   c. Provide the child with a small piece of satin ribbon or a soft, stuffed animal to stroke as a substitute for the digit sucking.

   d. Use a chart for daily recording of compliance with stars or stickers.
   e. Agree upon a reward for stopping the habit for 14 continuous days.
   f. Have the child call the clinician to say that the prize has been won.

✔ Factors To Teach The Parents

- How the bacteria that cause dental caries can be transferred to the baby's mouth.

- How fluoride makes enamel stronger and more resistant to the bacteria that cause dental caries.

- Methods to prevent dental caries from developing in a young child's mouth.

- How feeding methods and snacking patterns can contribute to dental caries.

- How the parent can examine the infant's/child's mouth and what to look for during the examination.

- Reasons why the baby's mouth should be examined by an oral health professional at 6 months of age or as soon as the first tooth erupts.

- Ways parents can prepare their young children for visits to the dentist and dental hygienist.

- How parents can prevent accidents and injury in their infants and children.

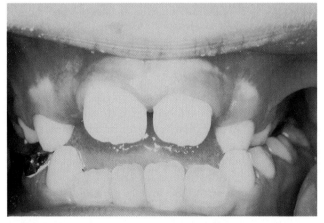

■ **FIGURE 46-10 Effects of Prolonged Thumb Sucking on Teeth.** Anterior openbite with posterior crossbite.

XV. REFERRAL

Appropriate referrals are made when problems are identified that require intervention by other health providers. Conditions that require referral include evidence of systemic illness, pathology, child abuse or neglect, failure to provide safety measures, substance abuse in the family, and evidence of poor parenting skills.[5]

REFERENCES

1. **American Academy of Pediatric Dentistry:** Oral Health Policies, Guidelines, and Quality Assurance Policies, *Pediatr. Dent., 23,* Special Issue, Number 7, Reference Manual, 2001-2002, pp. 16, 31, 39.
2. **Green,** M. and Palfrey, J.S. (eds): *Bright Futures: Guidelines for Health Supervision of Infants, Children, and Adolescents,* 2nd ed. rev. Arlington, VA, National Center for Education in Maternal and Child Health, 2002, pp. 1–15.
3. **McWhorter,** A.G., Seale, N.S., and King, S.A.: Infant Oral Health Education in US Dental School Curricula, *Pediatr. Dent., 23,* 407, September–October, 2001.
4. **Mueller,** W.A. and Abrams, R.B.: Oral Medicine and Dentistry, in: Hay, W.W., Howard, A.R., Levin, M.J., Sondheimer, J.M.: *Current Pediatric Diagnosis and Treatment,* 14th ed. Stamford, CT, Appleton and Lange, 1999, pp. 384–394.
5. **Casamassimo,** P.: *Bright Futures in Practice: Oral Health.* Arlington, VA, National Center for Education in Maternal and Child Health, 1996, pp. 1–41.
6. **Nowak,** A. and Crall, J.: Prevention of Dental Disease, in: Pinkham, J.R., ed.: *Pediatric Dentistry: Infancy Through Adolescence,* 3rd ed. Philadelphia, W.B. Saunders Co., 1999, p. 197.
7. **Albert,** D.A., Findley, S., Mitchell, D.A., Park, K., and McManus, J.M.: Dental Caries Among Disadvantaged 3- to 4-year-old Children in Northern Manhattan, *Pediatr. Dent., 24,* 229, May–June, 2002.
8. **Nowak,** A.J. and Casamassimo, P.S.: Using Anticipatory Guidance to Provide Early Dental Interventions, *J. Amer. Dent. Assoc., 126,* 1156, August, 1995.
9. **Warren,** J.J., Levy, S.M., and Nowak, A.J.: Nonnutritive Sucking Behaviors in Preschool Children: A Longitudinal Study, *Pediatr. Dent., 22,* 187, May–June, 2000.
10. **Kohler,** B. and Andreen, I.: Influence of Caries-Preventive Measures in Mothers on Cariogenic Bacteria and Caries Experience in Their Children, *Arch. Oral Biol., 39,* 907, October, 1994.
11. **Tinanoff,** N. and O'Sullivan, D.M.: Early Childhood Caries: Overview and Recent Findings, *Pediatr. Dent., 19,* 12, January/February, 1997.
12. **Wan,** A.K.L., Seow, W.K. Purdie, D.M., Bird, P.S., Walsh, L.J., and Tudehope, D.I.: Oral Colonization of *Streptococcus mutans* in Six-Month-Old Predentate Infants, *J. Dent. Res., 80,* 2060, December, 2001.
13. **Levy,** S.M., Kiritsy, M.C., Slager, S.L., Warren, J.J., and Kohout, F.J.: Patterns of Fluoride Dentifrice Use Among Infants, *Pediatr. Dent., 19,* 50, January/February,1997.
14. **Pendrys,** D.G.: Risk of Enamel Fluorosis in Nonfluoridated and Optimally Fluoridated Populations: Considerations for the Dental Professional, *J. Amer. Dent. Assoc., 131,* 746, June, 2000.
15. **Harnack,** L., Stang, J., and Story, M.: Soft Drink Consumption Among U.S. Children and Adolescents: Nutritional Consequences, *J. Am. Diet. Assoc., 99,* 436, April, 1999.
16. **Strauss,** R.S. and Pollack, H.A.: Epidemic Increase in Childhood Overweight, 1986-1998, *JAMA, 286,* 2845, December 12, 2001.
17. **McDonald,** R.E. and Avery, D.R.: *Dentistry for Children and the Adolescent,* 7th ed. St. Louis, Mosby, 2000, pp. 141–144, 155–158, 188–191.
18. **Flaitz,** C.M.: Oral Pathologic Conditions and Soft Tissue Anomalies, in: Pinkham, J.R., ed.: *Pediatric Dentistry: Infancy Through Adolescence,* 3rd ed. Philadelphia, W.B. Saunders Co., 1999, pp. 12–42.
19. **Warren,** J.J. and Levy, S.M.: A Review of Fluoride Dentifrice Related to Dental Fluorosis, *Pediatr. Dent., 21,* 265, July/August, 1999.
20. **Levy,** S.M., Hillis, S.L., Warren, J.J., Broffitt, B.A. Islam, M., Wefel, J.S., Kanellis, M.J.: Primary Tooth Fluorosis and Fluoride Intake During the First Year of Life, *Community Dent. Oral Epidemiol., 30,* 286, August, 2002.
21. **Bawden,** J.: Issues Involving Fluoride Supplementation, in: Pinkham, J.R.: *Pediatric Dentistry: Infancy Through Adolescence,* 3rd ed. Philadelphia, W.B. Saunders Co., 1999, p. 203.
22. **Autio-Gold,** J.T. and Courts, F.: Assessing the Effect of Fluoride Varnish on Early Enamel Carious Lesions in the Primary Dentition, *J. Am. Dent. Assoc., 132,* 1247, September, 2001.
23. **Beltran-Aguilar,** E.D., Goldstein, J. W., and Lockwood, S.A.: Fluoride Varnishes: A Review of Their Clinical Use, Cariostatic Mechanism, Efficacy and Safety, *J. Amer. Dent. Assoc., 131,* 589, May, 2000.
24. **Amir,** E., Shimonov, R., and Rosenberg, M.: Halitosis in Children, *J. Pediatr., 134,* 338, March, 1999.
25. **American Academy of Pediatrics,** Committee on Nutrition: The Use and Misuse of Fruit Juice in Pediatrics, *Pediatrics, 107,* 1210, May, 2001.
26. **Overby,** K.J.: Pediatric Health Supervision, in: Rudolph, A.M., Kamei, R.K., and Overby, K.J., eds.: *Rudolph's Fundamentals of Pediatrics,* 3rd ed. New York, McGraw-Hill, 2002, pp. 1–69.
27. **Hangerman,** R.J.: Growth and Development, in: Hay, W.W., Hayward, A.R., Levin, M.J., Sondheimer, J.M. eds.: *Current Pediatric Diagnosis and Treatment,* 14th ed. Stamford, CT, Appleton and Lange, 1999, pp. 1–18.
28. **Pinkham,** J.R.: Patient Management, in: Pinkham, J.R., ed.: *Pediatric Dentistry: Infancy Through Adolescence,* 3rd ed. Philadelphia, W.B. Saunders Co., 1999, pp. 361–362.
29. **Kaakko,** T., Riedy, C.A., Nakai, Y., Domoto, P., Weinstein, P., and Milgrom, P.: Taking Bitewing Radiographs in Preschoolers Using Behavior Management Techniques, *ASDC J. Dent. Child., 66,* 320, September–October, 1999.

SUGGESTED READINGS

Adair, S.M., Milano M., Lorenzo, I., and Russell, C.: Effects of Current and Former Pacifier Use on the Dentition of 24- to 59-month-old Children, *Pediatr. Dent., 17,* 437, November/December, 1995.

Arnrup, K., Broberg, A.G., Berggren, U., and Bodin, L.: Lack of Cooperation in Pediatric Dentistry: The Role of Child Personality Characteristics, *Pediatr. Dent., 24,* 119, March/April, 2002.

Casamassimo, P.S., Christensen, J.R., and Fields, H.W.: Examination, Diagnosis, and Treatment Planning, in: Pinkham, J.R., ed.: *Pediatric Dentistry: Infancy Through Adolescence,* 3rd ed. Philadelphia, W.B. Saunders Co., 1999, pp. 265–286.

Edelstein, B.L., Manski, R.J., and Moeller, J.F.: Pediatric Dental Visits During 1996: An Analysis of the Federal Medical Expenditure Panel Survey, *Pediatr. Dent., 22,* 17, January/February, 2000.

Johnson, E.D. and Larson, B.E.: Thumb-sucking: Literature Review, *ASDC Dent. Child., 60,* 385, November/December, 1993.

King, D.L.: Teething Revisited, *Pediatr. Dent., 16,* 179, May/June, 1994.

Nagahama, S.I., Fuhriman, S.E., Moore, C.S., and Milgrom, P.: Evaluation of a Dental Society-Based ABCD Program in Washington State, *J. Amer. Dent. Assoc., 133,* 1251, September, 2002.

Nowak, A.J.: Rationale for Timing of the First Oral Evaluation, *Pediatr. Dent., 19,* 8, January/February, 1997.

Nowak, A.J. and Casamassimo, P.S.: The Dental Home: A Primary Care Oral Health Concept, *J. Amer. Dent. Assoc., 133,* 93, January, 2002.

Sarnat, H., Arad, P., Hanauer, D., and Shohami, E.: Communication Strategies Used During Pediatric Dental Treatment: A Pilot Study, *Pediatr. Dent., 23,* 337, July/August, 2001.

Warren, J.J., Bishara, S.E., Steinbock, K.L., Yonezu, T, and Nowak, A.J.: Effects of Oral Habits' Duration on Dental Characteristics in the Primary Dentition, *J. Am. Dent. Assoc., 132,* 1685, December, 2001.

Early Childhood Caries

Aaltonen, A.S. and Tenovuo, J.: Association Between Mother-Infant Salivary Contacts and Caries Resistance in Children: A Cohort Study, *Pediatr. Dent., 16,* 110, March/April, 1994.

Berkowitz, R.J. and Jones, P.: Mouth-to-Mouth Transmission of the Bacterium *Streptococcus mutans* between Mother and Child, *Arch. Oral Biol., 30,* 377, Number 4, 1985.

Bowen, W.H., Pearson, S.K., Rosalen, P.L., Miguel, J.C., and Shih, A.Y.: Assessing the Cariogenic Potential of Some Infant Formulas, Milk and Sugar Solutions, *J. Am. Dent. Assoc., 128,* 865, July, 1997.

Febres, C., Echeverri, E.A., and Keene, H.J.: Parental Awareness, Habits, and Social Factors and Their Relationship to Baby Bottle Tooth Decay, *Pediatr. Dent., 19,* 22, January/February, 1997.

Gomez, S.S. Weber, A.A., and Emilson, C.-G.: A Prospective Study of a Caries Prevention Program in Pregnant Women and Their Children Five and Six Years of Age, *J. Dent. Child., 68 ,* 191, May/June, 2001.

Kanellis, M.J.: Caries Risk Assessment and Prevention: Strategies for Head Start, Early Head Start, and WIC, *J. Public Health Dent., 60,* 210, Summer, 2000.

Lai, P.Y., Seow, W.K., Tudehope, D.I., and Rogers, Y.: Enamel Hypoplasia and Dental Caries in Very-Low Birthweight Children: A Case Controlled, Longitudinal Study, *Pediatr. Dent., 19,* 42, January/February, 1997.

Matee, M.I., Mikx, F.H.M., Maselle, S.Y.M., and van Palenstein, W.H.: Mutans streptococci and Lactobacilli in Breast-fed Children With Rampant Caries, *Caries Res., 26,* 183, May/June, 1992.

Muller, M.: Nursing-Bottle Syndrome: Risk Factors, *ASDC J. Dent. Child., 63,* 42, January/February, 1996.

O'Neil, M. and Clarkson, H.: "Reaching Families With Young Children," A Community Health Project for Preventing Early Childhood Caries, *J. Canad. Dent. Hyg. Assoc. (Probe), 36,* 145, July/August, 2002.

O'Sullivan, D.M. and Tinanoff, N.: Social and Biological Factors Contributing to Caries of the Maxillary Anterior Teeth, *Pediatr. Dent., 15,* 41, January/February, 1993.

O'Sullivan, D.M. and Tinanoff, N.: Maxillary Anterior Caries Associated With Increased Caries Risk in Other Primary Teeth, *J. Dent. Res., 72,* 1577, December, 1993.

Peretz, B. and Kafka, I.: Baby Bottle Tooth Decay and Complications During Pregnancy and Delivery, *J. Pediatr. Dent., 19,* 34, January/February, 1997.

Powell, L.V.: Caries Prediction: A Review of the Literature, *Community Dent. Oral Epidemiol., 26,* 361, December, 1998.

Proceedings: Conference on Early Childhood Caries, Bethesda, MD, USA. October, 1997, *Community Dent. Oral Epidemiol., 26 5,* Supplement 1, 1998.

Quinonez, R., Santos, R.G., Wilson, S., and Cross, H.: The Relationship Between Child Temperament and Early Childhood Caries, *Pediatr. Dent., 23,* 5, January/February, 2001.

Ripa, L.W.: Nursing Caries: A Comprehensive Review, *Pediatr. Dent., 10,* 268, December, 1988.

Smith, R.E., Badner, V.M., Morse, D.E., and Freeman, K.: Maternal Risk Indicators for Childhood Caries in an Inner City Population, *Community Dent. Oral Epidemiol., 30,* 176, June, 2002.

Van Houte, J., Gibbs, G., and Butera, C.: Oral Flora of Children With "Nursing Bottle Caries," *J. Dent. Res., 61,* 382, February, 1982.

Fluoride for the Infant and Preschooler

Bentley, E.M., Ellwood, R.P., and Davies, R.M.: Factors Influencing the Amount of Fluoride Toothpaste Applied by the Mothers of Young Children, *Br. Dent. J., 183,* 412, December 13–27, 1997.

Bawden, J.W., ed: Changing Patterns of Fluoride Intake, Workshop Report-Group III, *J. Dent. Res., 71,* 1224, Special Issue, May, 1992.

Levy, S.M., Kiritsy, M.C., and Warren, J.J.: Sources of Fluoride Intake in Children, *J. Public Health Dent., 55,* 39, Winter, 1995.

Mascarenhas, A.K.: Risk Factors for Dental Fluorosis: A Review of the Recent Literature, *Pediatr. Dent., 22,* 269, July/August, 2000.

Naccache, H., Simard, P.L., Trahan, L., Brodeur, J.-M., Demers, M., and Lachapelle, D.: Factors Affecting the Ingestion of Fluoride Dentifrice by Children, *J. Public Health Dent., 52,* 222, Summer, 1992.

Shulman, J.D. and Wells, L.M.: Acute Fluoride Toxicity From Ingesting Home-Use Dental Products in Children, Birth to 6 Years of Age, *J. Public Health Dent., 57,* 150, Summer, 1997.

Slayton, R.L., Kanellis, M.J., Levy, S.M., Warren, J.J., and Islam, M.: Frequency of Reported Dental Visits and Professional Fluoride Applications in a Cohort of Children Followed From Birth to Age 3 Years, *Pediatr. Dent., 24,* 64, January/February, 2002.

The Patient With a Cleft Lip and/or Palate

47

CHAPTER OUTLINE

Cleft lip and/or palate is the most common of the many types of congenital craniofacial anomalies. Cleft lip and/or palate frequently occurs as part of a syndrome with other birth defects.

The person with a cleft lip and/or palate can be dentally dysfunctional unless extensive habilitative care and supervision from birth is available. An interdisciplinary team of medical and dental specialists is required to provide adequate treatment and family counseling as needed. The dental hygienist is an important member of the team with responsibilities to coordinate dental and periodontal care.

Speaking ability and appearance are among the first factors considered when the long-range treatment program is planned because the objective is to help the patient lead a normal life. Dental personnel need to maintain a current list of the health agencies, clinics, and other community resources where the patient and family can obtain assistance for the various phases of treatment and habilitation.

Key words relating to cleft lip and/or palate are defined in Box 47-1.

CLASSIFICATION OF CLEFTS

Classification is based on disturbances in the embryologic formation of the palate as it develops from the premaxillary region toward the uvula in a definite pattern. Interference with normal development of the palate may occur at one stage level of the embryo, and the normal pattern may be re-established at a later stage.

The first six classes are illustrated in Figure 47-1. All degrees are found, from an insignificant notch in the

BOX 47-1 KEY WORDS: Cleft Lip and/or Palate

Autograft: graft transferred from one part of the patient's body to another part.

Bifid uvula: cleft of the uvula of the soft palate that divides the uvula into two parts (Figure 47-1, Class 2).

Cheiloplasty: surgical repair of a lip defect.

Cheilorhinoplasty: plastic surgery of nose and lip.

Cleft lip: a unilateral or bilateral congenital fissure in the upper lip, usually lateral to the midline; can extend into one nostril or both and may involve the alveolar process; caused by defect in the fusion of the maxillary and globular processes.

Cleft palate: a congenital fissure in the palate caused by failure of the palatal shelves to fuse; may extend to connect with unilateral or bilateral cleft lip.

Congenital: present at and existing from the time of birth.

Craniofacial: pertaining to the cranium, the part of the skull that encloses the brain, and the face.

Dentally dysfunctional: abnormal functioning of dental structures.

Graft: tissue that is transplanted and expected to become a part of the host tissue.

Heredity: genetic transmission of traits from parents to offspring; the hereditary material, chromosomes, is contained within the ovum and the sperm (23 chromosomes each), which unite when the sperm penetrates the ovum.

Multifactorial: pertaining to, or arising through the action of, many factors.

Obturator: a prosthesis designed to close a congenital or acquired opening, such as a cleft of the hard palate.

Orthognathic surgery: surgical repositioning of all or parts of the maxilla or mandible.

Orthopedics: branch of surgery dealing with the preservation and restoration of function of the skeletal system, its articulations, and associated structures.

Palatoplasty: plastic reconstruction of the palate.

Premaxilla: anterior part of maxilla that contains the incisor teeth; bilateral cleft lips separate the premaxilla from its normal fusion with the entire maxilla.

Prosthesis: an artificial replacement of an absent part of the human body; a therapeutic device to improve or alter function.

Rehabilitation: the process of restoring a person's ability to live and work as normally as possible after a disabling injury or illness; aims to help the individual to achieve maximum possible physical and psychologic fitness and to regain ability to carry out personal care.

> **Habilitation:** the same goals and objectives as rehabilitation, but for a person with acquired disability for whom the ability to achieve maximum physical and psychologic fitness is acquired for the first time.

Rhinoplasty: plastic surgery of nose.

Speech aid prosthesis: a prosthetic device with a posterior section to assist with palatopharyngeal closure; also called bulb, speech bulb, or prosthetic speech appliance.

> **Pediatric speech aid prosthesis:** a temporary or interim prosthesis used to close a defect in the hard and/or soft palate; may replace tissue lost as a result of developmental or surgical alterations; necessary for intelligible speech.

> **Adult speech aid prosthesis:** a definitive prosthesis to improve speech by obturating (sealing off) a palatal cleft or occasionally assisting an incompetent soft palate.

mucous membrane of the lip or uvula, which produces no functional disability, to the complete cleft defined by Class 6 of this classification.

Class 1. Cleft of the tip of the uvula.

Class 2. Cleft of the uvula (bifid uvula).

Class 3. Cleft of the soft palate.

Class 4. Cleft of the soft and hard palates.

Class 5. Cleft of the soft and hard palates that continues through the alveolar ridge on one side of the premaxilla; usually associated with cleft lip of the same side.

Class 6. Cleft of the soft and hard palates that continues through the alveolar ridge on both sides, leaving a free premaxilla; usually associated with bilateral cleft lip.

Class 7. Submucous cleft in which the muscle union is imperfect across the soft palate. The palate is short, the uvula is often bifid, a groove is situated at the midline of the soft palate, and the closure to the pharynx is incompetent.

■ ETIOLOGY

I.   EMBRYOLOGY[1,2]

Cleft lip and palate represent a failure of normal fusion of embryonic processes during development in the first trimester of pregnancy. Figure 47-2 shows the locations of the globular process and the right and left maxillary processes. With normal fusion, no cleft of the lip results.

Formation of the lip occurs between the fourth and seventh week *in utero*. The development of the palate takes place during the eighth to twelfth week. Fusion begins in the premaxillary region and continues backward toward the uvula.

A cleft lip becomes apparent by the end of the second month *in utero*. A cleft palate is evident by the end of the third month.

II.   RISK FACTORS[3,4]

Genetic and environmental factors can be significant. Rarely a single factor can be found as the specific cause.

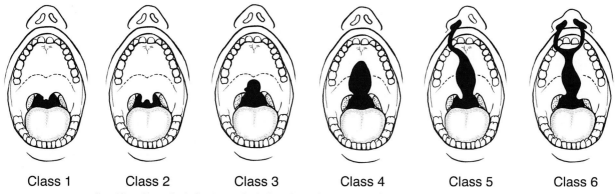

Class 1   Class 2   Class 3   Class 4   Class 5   Class 6

■ **FIGURE 47-1 Classification of Cleft Lip and Cleft Palate.** (Courtesy of O.E. Beder.)

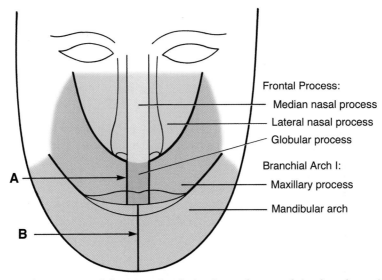

▪ **FIGURE 47-2 Developmental Processes of the Face.** The derivations of parts of the face from the frontal process and the branchial arch. **A.** Location of cleft lip when fusion of the globular process and a maxillary process fails. **B.** Cleft of the mandible can occur at the midline. (Redrawn from Melfi, R.C.: *Permar's Oral Embryology and Microscopic Anatomy,* 8th ed. Philadelphia, Lea & Febiger, 1988.)

They are most often multifactorial. Early in the first trimester is the significant time for influences due to the environmental factors.

A. Genetic

B. Environmental

1. Tobacco smoking.[5,6]
2. Alcohol consumption.[7]
3. Teratogenic agents: phenytoin, vitamin A (isotretinoin), corticosteroids, drugs of abuse (see Table 45-1).
4. Inadequate diet: vitamins, especially folic acid deficiency.
5. Lack of adequate prenatal care and instruction is a risk factor that has influence on all the environmental factors.

▪ ORAL CHARACTERISTICS

I. TOOTH DEVELOPMENT

Disturbances in the normal development of the tooth buds occur more frequently in patients with clefts than in the general population. There is a higher incidence of missing and supernumerary teeth, as well as of abnormalities of tooth form.

II. MALOCCLUSION

A high percentage of patients with cleft lip and palate require orthodontic care.

III. OPEN PALATE

Before surgical correction, an open palate provides direct communication with the nasal cavity.

IV. MUSCLE COORDINATION

A lack of coordinated movements of lips, tongue, cheeks, floor of mouth, and throat may exist and lead to compensatory habits formed in the attempt to produce normal sounds while speaking.

V. PERIODONTAL TISSUES

Dental biofilm accumulation is influenced by the irregularly positioned teeth; inability to keep lips closed; mouth breathing; and the difficulties in accomplishing adequate personal oral care, especially around the cleft areas.

Early periodontal disease with loss of bone and clinical attachment at cleft sites is common in adolescents.[8] Periodontal tissue loss in later years is greatest at the cleft sites.[9]

VI. DENTAL CARIES

The many predisposing factors relating to malpositioned teeth, problems of mastication, diet selection, and dental biofilm retention are intensified for the person with a cleft lip and/or palate.

Feeding difficulties of infants and toddlers have contributed to baby bottle tooth decay. Children with a cleft lip and/or palate are at higher risk for dental caries.[10]

■ GENERAL PHYSICAL CHARACTERISTICS

I. OTHER CONGENITAL ANOMALIES

Incidence is higher than that in noncleft people. In more than 300 disorders, cleft lip, cleft palate, or both represent one feature of a syndrome.[11]

II. FACIAL DEFORMITY

Facial deformities may include depression of the nostril on the side with the cleft lip; deficiency of upper lip, which may be short or retroposed; and overprominent lower lip.

III. INFECTIONS

Predisposition to upper respiratory and middle ear infections is common.

IV. AIRWAY AND BREATHING

The craniofacial anomalies of the nose and throat area predispose the child with a cleft palate to airway obstruction and breathing problems.[12] Early treatment intervention is necessary for the infant to cope with feeding problems. Speech involves breathing and swallowing.

V. SPEECH[13]

Patients with cleft lip and/or cleft palate have difficulty in making certain sounds and may produce nasal tones. Anatomic structure, airway and breathing problems, and hearing difficulties all contribute to speech problems.

VI. HEARING LOSS

The incidence of hearing loss is significantly higher in individuals with cleft palate than in the noncleft population.

■ PERSONAL FACTORS

Most patients with a cleft lip or palate do not have more personality problems than people without clefts. Realization of the social effects of speech and appearance makes it possible to understand why some of these patients exhibit evidences of maladjustment. The ridicule of contemporaries soon leads even young children to think they are "different." Parental acceptance or rejection no doubt can be a strong influence. A few characteristics are suggested here.

I. SELF-CONSCIOUSNESS

Hypersensitivity to taunts or obvious pity.

II. FEELINGS OF INFERIORITY

The result may be a person who is quiet, unresponsive, and withdrawn, or one who is openly brash or rebellious until rapport is established.

■ TREATMENT

Treatment is coordinated by a team of specialists and is based on the patient's progress at each age period. Members of the interdisciplinary team are listed in Box 47-2.

The team is responsible for providing integrated case management. Quality and continuity of care are essential.[14] The need for attention to gingival health throughout the years of treatment cannot be overemphasized.

I. CLEFT LIP

Surgical union of the cleft lip is made before 6 months. The infant's general health is a determining factor.

A. Purposes for Early Treatment

1. Aid in feeding.
2. Encourage development of the premaxilla.
3. Help partial closure of the palatal cleft.
4. Lessen concern of family about appearance of their infant.

B. Orthodontics and Dentofacial Orthopedics[15]

In preparation for cleft closure, orthodontic and orthopedic treatment may be needed to reduce the protrusion and stabilize the premaxilla.

II. CLEFT PALATE

Primary surgery to close the palate should be undertaken by age 18 months or earlier when possible.[14] The combined efforts of many specialists are required (Box 47-2).

A. Goals for Treatment

1. Produce anatomic closure.
2. Maximize maxillary growth and development.
3. Achieve normal function, particularly normal speech.
4. Relieve problems of airway and breathing.
5. Establish good dental aesthetics and functional occlusion.

B. Types of Secondary Surgical Procedures

Secondary surgical care refers to additional surgical procedures after primary closure of the clefts. Secondary surgery may involve the lips, nose, palate, and

---

BOX 47-2 Interdisciplinary Team for Treatment of Patient With Cleft Lip and/or Palate

DENTAL PROFESSION

Dental hygiene

Oral and maxillofacial surgery

Orthodontics

Pediatric dentistry

Prosthodontics

Implantology

Periodontics

MEDICAL PROFESSION

Anesthesiology

Genetics/dysmorphology

Imaging/radiology

Neurology

Neurosurgery

Ophthalmology

Otolaryngology

Pediatrics

Physical anthropology

Plastic surgery

Psychiatry

ALLIED MEDICAL

Nursing

Nutrition

Genetic counseling

Psychology

Social work

Speech-language pathology

Vocational counseling

---

jaws. It may be to improve function, improve appearance, or both.

Treatment plans are individualized to fit the needs of the patient. Team evaluations on a periodic basis determine the effects of treatment to date and outline the next phase. Examples of what may be needed are:

1. Rhinoplasty and nasal septal surgery for an airway problem.
2. Velopharyngeal flap or other pharyngoplasty.
3. Closure of palatal fistulae.
4. Tonsillectomy and/or adenoidectomy.

C. Use of Bone Grafting[16,17]

Bone grafting is used to repair residual alveolar and hard palate clefts.

1. *Alveolar Graft.* Placed before eruption of maxillary teeth at the cleft site, creates a normal architecture through which the teeth can erupt. A need for future prosthetic replacement of missing teeth is reduced. Support is provided for teeth adjacent to the cleft areas.
2. *Hard Palate Graft.* Provides closure of oronasal fistulae and helps to relieve a compromised airway.
3. *Sources for Autogenous Bone for Graft.* Rib, iliac crest, skull, or mandible.

D. Use of Osseointegrated Implant

After bone grafting, implants can be used to replace individual teeth or to support a complete prosthesis.[18,19]

III. PROSTHODONTICS

A. Types of Appliances[20]

A removable prosthesis may be designed to provide closure of the palatal opening (obturator) and/or to complete the palatopharyngeal valving required for speech (speech aid prosthesis).

B. Purposes and Functions of a Prosthesis

The prosthesis may be designed to accomplish one or all of the following:

1. Closure of the palate.
2. Replacement of missing teeth.
3. Scaffolding to fill out the upper lip.
4. Masticatory function.
5. Restoration of vertical dimension.
6. Postorthodontic retainer.

IV. ORTHODONTICS

Treatment may be initiated as early as 3 years of age, depending on the problems of dentofacial development. Each stage of surgery and other treatment may require orthodontic intervention and follow-up.

Final formal orthodontic treatment for realigning the teeth and gaining a functional occlusion may start during the mixed dentition years or later. During that period, an intensive program for dental caries prevention and gingival health must be supervised.

V. SPEECH THERAPY

Training may be started with very young children and is particularly emphasized after the surgical or prosthodontic treatment has been accomplished.

VI. RESTORATIVE DENTISTRY (PEDIATRIC DENTIST OR GENERAL DENTAL PRACTITIONER)

A major problem can be dental caries, leading to tooth loss. With missing teeth, major difficulties arise related to all phases of treatment. Preservation of the primary teeth is very important.

■ DENTAL HYGIENE CARE

Preventive measures for preservation of the teeth and their supporting structures are essential to the success of the special care needed for the habilitation of the patient with a cleft palate.

Each phase of dental hygiene care and instruction, important for all patients, takes on even greater significance in light of the magnified problems of the patient with a cleft lip and/or palate.

Every attempt should be made to avoid the need for removal of teeth, especially around the cleft area. In an area already weakened by lack of bone, the removal of teeth creates further complications. The presence of teeth encourages optimum arch growth.

Understanding by the patient and the parents of the value of preventive procedures is accomplished through explanation and instruction. When the patient has not had specialized care, the dental team has a responsibility to arrange referral to an available agency, clinic, or private practice specialist.

I. PARENTAL COUNSELING: ANTICIPATORY GUIDANCE

Items from Tables 46-2 and 46-3 pertain to the parents and infant with a cleft lip and/or palate. The primary concerns are daily dental biofilm removal and prevention of baby bottle tooth decay.

II. OBJECTIVES FOR APPOINTMENT PLANNING

Frequent appointments, scheduled every 3 or 4 months, are usually needed during the maintenance phase of the patient's care:

- To review biofilm control measures and provide encouragement for the patient to maintain the health of the supporting structures and the cleanliness of the removable prostheses.
- To remove all calculus and smooth the tooth surfaces as a supplement to the patient's personal daily care procedures.
- To supervise a dental caries prevention program for both primary and permanent dentitions with fluorides and sealants.

III. APPOINTMENT CONSIDERATIONS

A. Patient Apprehension

A patient who has been seen often in hospital clinics may become "clinic tired" and be very apprehensive about dental and dental hygiene care.

B. Communication

1. *Speech*. Speech may be almost undiscernible although with repeated contact, understanding can be developed. Referral for speech assessment, if not already done, is recommended.
2. *Hearing*. Depending on the severity of hearing loss, the approach is similar to that for speech difficulties. Suggestions for care of patients with hearing problems are described on pages 954 to 959.

C. Avoid Solicitousness

Approach as a normal patient.

D. Provide Motivations

Quiet, unresponsive, or bold, rebellious patients can be approached in ways that can help them gain an objective attitude toward oral health.

IV. DENTAL HYGIENE INTERVENTIONS

A. Infection Control

Although procedures for infection control should be the same for all patients, one should remember that the open fistulae make the patient with a cleft palate particularly susceptible to infections.

B. Instrumentation

1. Adapt techniques to the oral characteristics. All objectives of scaling and other instrumentation have particular implications for the patient with a cleft palate.
2. Prevent debris or pieces of calculus from passing into or being retained in the clefts.
3. Remove an obturator or prosthesis for cleaning.

Everyday Ethics

? Brian is 6 years old and recently had another surgical procedure completed on his upper lip. He was born with a bilateral clefting of the lip with partial involvement of the palate. There is a university-based dental school and medical center in the city where Brian's family lives, so all treatment has been done locally.

Indent As his dental hygienist, Leona has been delivering dental hygiene care to Brian since he was 3 years old. The status of his oral hygiene continues to decline even though Brian is at a point where he can care for his own teeth. His parents are supportive but want Brian to assume responsibility. Communication is sometimes difficult due to Brian's speech and hearing impairments.

Questions for Consideration

1. What professional role can Leona play as contributor in part of Brian's ongoing treatment plan, which includes surgical procedures related to the clefting?

2. Is Brian competent to act "autonomously" when performing home care procedures? Why or why not?

3. What issues of beneficence, veracity, and justice apply to the medical and dental care Brian receives?

C. Topical Application of Fluoride

Short upper lip may complicate cotton-roll or tray placement.

V. PATIENT INSTRUCTION

A. Personal Oral Care Procedures

The self-conscious patient may actually fear or exhibit rejection toward the oral cavity. With a small child, the parents may be afraid of damaging the deformed areas or hurting the child if cleaning methods are employed. An empathetic approach and plan for continued instruction over a long period of time is needed.

✔ **Factors To Teach The Patient**

- Parental anticipatory guidance (Tables 46-2 and 46-3).

- Biofilm removal methods for cleft areas.

- Prevention of mouth odors by proper cleaning of tongue and removable appliances.

- Necessity for regular dental hygiene appointments to maintain freedom from infection.

- Sources with addresses for team treatment clinics specializing in craniofacial developmental defects.

1. *Teeth and Gingiva.* Select toothbrush, brushing method, and auxiliary aids according to the individual needs. A soft nylon brush with end-rounded filaments is indicated.

2. *Fluoride.* Instigate daily self-application of fluoride by way of mouthrinse, fluoride dentifrice, and diet supplements for a young child in a non-fluoridated community.

3. *Rinsing Instruction.* Young children especially may need instruction in how to rinse when this procedure is new for them (Box 27-5).

4. *Prosthesis or Speech Aid.* Halitosis may be a real problem when the prosthesis forms the soft palate and the floor of the nasal cavity. Mucus secreted in the nasal cavity accumulates on the prosthesis.
   a. Instruct patient in the need for frequent removal of prosthesis for cleaning, particularly following eating.
   b. Method for cleaning the prosthesis is the same as that for a removable partial denture (pages 474 to 475).

B. Diet

1. *Need for a Varied Diet*: Should include adequate proportions of all essential food groups (see Figure 32-1, Adult Food Pyramid; Figure 46-8, Child's Food Pyramid).

2. *Need for Prevention of Dental Caries*: Limitation of cariogenic foods, particularly for between-meal snacks.

C. Smoking Cessation

Patients who smoke or use any form of smokeless tobacco should be informed about the effects of tobacco on all the oral tissues, with emphasis on the potential damage to the periodontal bone. Offer assistance with a smoking cessation program (pages 513 to 515).

VI. DENTAL HYGIENE CARE RELATED TO ORAL SURGERY

A. Presurgery (page 852)

Objectives have particular significance because the patient with a cleft palate is unusually susceptible to infections of the upper respiratory area and middle ear. Every precaution should be taken to prevent complications.

B. Postsurgery Personal Oral Care

In certain of the palate operations, arm restraints are applied to prevent accidental damage to the repaired region. After each feeding (liquid diet for several days, soft diet for the next week), the mouth must be rinsed carefully.

Brushing must be accomplished with great care, usually by the parent or caregiver, to avoid damage to the healing suture lines. In some cases, a toothbrush with suction attachment may be useful (page 916).

Water irrigation using low pressure can also be helpful where jaw repositioning surgery has been completed and wires have been used to stabilize the jaws for a period of time.

REFERENCES

1. **Melfi**, R.C. and Alley, K.E.: *Permar's Oral Embryology and Microscopic Anatomy,*10th ed. Philadelphia, Lippincott Williams & Wilkins, 2000, pp. 25–42.
2. **Ten Cate**, A.R.: *Oral Histology, Development, Structure, and Function*, 5th ed.St. Louis, Mosby, 1998, pp. 46–49.
3. **Slavkin**, H.C.: Meeting the Challenges of Craniofacial-Oral-Dental Birth Defects, *J. Am. Dent. Assoc., 127,* 681, May, 1996.
4. **Berkowitz**, S.: *The Cleft Palate Story.* Chicago, Quintessence, 1994, pp. 45–49.
5. **Shaw**, G.M., Wasserman, C.R., Lammer, E.J., O'Malley, C.D., Murray, J.C., Basart, A.M., and Tolarova, M.M.: Orofacial Clefts, Parental Cigarette Smoking, and Transforming Growth Factor-Alpha Gene Variants, *Am. J. Hum. Genet., 58,*551, March, 1996.
6. **Källen**, K.: Maternal Smoking and Orofacial Clefts, *Cleft Palate Craniofac. J., 34,*11, January, 1997.
7. **Werler**, M.M., Lammer, E.J., Rosenberg, L., and Mitchell, A.A.: Maternal Alcohol Use in Relation to Selected Birth Defects, *Am. J. Epidemiol., 134,*691, October 1, 1991.
8. **Gaggl**, A., Schultes, G., Kärcher, H., and Mossböck, R.: Periodontal Disease in Patients With Cleft Palate and Patients With Unilateral and Bilateral Clefts of Lip, Palate, and Alveolus, *J. Periodontol., 70,* 171, February, 1999.
9. **Brägger**, U., Schürch, E., Salvi, G., von Wyttenbach, T., and Lang, N.P.: Periodontal Conditions in Adult Patients With Cleft Lip, Alveolus, and Palate, *Cleft Palate Craniofac. J., 29,*179, March, 1992.
10. **Bokhout**, B., Hofman, F.X.W.M., van Limbeek, J., Kramer, G.J.C., and Prahl-Andersen, B.: Incidence of Dental Caries in the Primary Dentition in Children With a Cleft Lip and/or Palate, *Caries Res., 31,* 8, January, 1997.
11. **Cohen**, M.M., Jr. and Bankier, A.: Syndrome Delineation Involving Orofacial Clefting, *Cleft Palate Craniofac. J., 28,*119, January, 1991.
12. **Perkins**, J.A., Sie, K.C.Y., Milczuk, H., and Richardson, M.A.: Airway Management in Children With Craniofacial Anomalies, *Cleft Palate Craniofac. J., 34,* 135, March, 1997.
13. **Berkowitz**: op. cit., pp. 113–115.
14. **American Cleft Palate-Craniofacial Association:***Parameters for Evaluation and Treatment of Patients With Cleft Lip/Palate or Other Craniofacial Anomalies*, Revised April, 2000. Official Publication of the American Cleft Palate-Craniofacial Association, 104 South Estes Drive, Suite 204, Chapel Hill, NC 27514.
15. **Figueroa**, A.A., Polley, J.W., and Cohen, M.: Orthodontic Management of the Cleft Lip and Palate Patient, *Clin. Plast. Surg., 20,* 733, October, 1993.
16. **Boyne**, P.J. and Sands, N.R.: Secondary Bone Grafting of Residual Alveolar and Palatal Clefts, *J. Oral Surg., 30,* 87, February, 1972.
17. **Kalaaji**, A., Lilja, J., Friede, H., and Elander, A.: Bone Grafting in the Mixed and Permanent Dentition in Cleft Lip and Palate Patients: Long-term Results and the Role of the Surgeon's Experience, *J. Craniomaxillofac. Surg., 24,* 29, February, 1996.
18. **Jansma**, J., Raghoebar, G.M., Batenburg, R.H.K., Stellingsma, C., and van Oort, R.P.: Bone Grafting of Cleft Lip and Palate Patients for Placement of Endosseous Implants, *Cleft Palate Craniofac. J., 36,* 67, January, 1999.
19. **Lund**, T.W. and Wade, M.: Use of Osseointegrated Implants to Support a Maxillary Denture for a Patient With Repaired Cleft Lip and Palate, *Cleft Palate Craniofac. J., 30,* 418, July, 1993.
20. **Reisberg**, D.J.: State of the Art: Dental and Prosthetic Care for Patients With Cleft or Craniofacial Conditions, *Cleft Palate Maxillofac. J., 37,* 534, November, 2000.

SUGGESTED READINGS

Endriga, M.C. and Kapp-Simon, K.A.: Psychological Issues in Craniofacial Care: State of the Art, *Cleft Palate Craniofac. J., 36,* 3, January, 1999.
Heidbuchel, K.L.W.M., Kuijpers-Jagtman, A.M., Ophof, R., and van Hooft, R.J.M.: Dental Maturity in Children With a Complete Cleft Lip and Palate, *Cleft Palate Craniofac. J., 39,* 509, September, 2002.
Lin, Y.-T.J. and Tsai, C.-L.: Caries Prevalence and Bottle-feeding Practices in 2-Year-Old Children With Cleft Lip, Cleft Palate, or Both in Taiwan, *Cleft Palate Craniofac. J., 36,* 522, November, 1999.
Lucas,V.S., Gupta, R., Ololade, O., Gelbier, M., and Roberts, G.J.: Dental Health Indices and Caries Associated Microflora in Children With Unilateral Cleft Lip and Palate, *Cleft Palate Craniofac. J., 37,* 447, September, 2000.
Quirynen, M., Dewinter, G., Avontroodt, P., Heidbuchel, K., Verdonck, A., and Carels, C.: A Split-Mouth Study on Periodontal and Microbial Parameters in Children With Complete Unilateral Cleft Lip and Palate, *J. Clin. Periodontol., 30,* 49, January, 2003.
Reed, J., Robathan, M., Hockenhull, A., Rostill, H., Perrett, D., and Lees, A.: Children's Attitudes Toward Interacting With Peers With Different Craniofacial Anomalies, *Cleft Palate Craniofac. J., 36,* 441, September, 1999.

Prenatal and Development

Aspinall, C.L.: Dealing With the Prenatal Diagnosis of Clefting: A Parent's Perspective, *Cleft Palate Craniofac. J., 39,* 183, March, 2002.

Jones, M.C.: Prenatal Diagnosis of Cleft Lip and Palate: Detection Rates, Accuracy of Ultrasonography, Associated Anomalies, and Strategies for Counseling, *Cleft Palate Craniofac. J., 39,* 169, March, 2002.

Nuckolls, G.H., Shum, L., and Slavkin, H.C.: Progress Toward Understanding Craniofacial Malformations, *Cleft Palate Craniofac. J., 36,* 12, January, 1999.

Pham, A.N.D., Seow, W.K., and Shusterman, S.: Developmental Dental Changes in Isolated Cleft Lip and Palate, *Pediatr. Dent., 19,* 109, March/April, 1997.

Prescott, N.J. and Malcolm, S.: Folate and the Face: Evaluating the Evidence for the Influence of Folate Genes on Craniofacial Development, *Cleft Palate Craniofac. J., 39,* 327, May, 2002.

Shaw, G.M., Lammer, E.J., Wasserman, C.R., O'Malley, C.D., and Tolarova, M.M.: Risks of Orofacial Clefts in Children Born to Women Using Multivitamins Containing Folic Acid Periconceptionally, *Lancet, 346,* 393, August 12, 1995.

Tolarova, M. and Harris, J.: Reduced Recurrence of Orofacial Clefts After Periconceptional Supplementation With High-Dose Folic Acid and Multivitamins, *Teratology, 51,* 71, February, 1995.

Will, L.A.: Growth and Development in Patients With Untreated Clefts, *Cleft Palate Craniofac. J., 37,* 523, November, 2000.

Wyszynski, D.F. and Wu, T.: Prenatal and Perinatal Factors Associated With Isolated Oral Clefting, *Cleft Palate Craniofac. J., 39,* 370, May, 2002.

Treatment

Anastassov, G.E. and Joos, U.: Comprehensive Management of Cleft Lip and Palate Deformities, *J. Oral Maxillofac. Surg., 59,* 1062, September, 2001.

Eppley, B.L. and Sadove, A.M.: Management of Alveolar Cleft Bone Grafting–State of the Art, *Cleft Palate Craniofac. J., 37,* 229, May, 2000.

Hamamoto, N., Hamamoto, Y., and Kobayashi, T.: Tooth Autotransplantation Into the Bone-Grafted Alveolar Cleft: Report of Two Cases With Histologic Findings, *J. Oral Maxillofac. Surg., 56,* 1451, December, 1998.

LaRossa, D.: The State of the Art in Cleft Palate Surgery, *Cleft Palate Craniofac. J., 37,* 225, May, 2000.

Mehrara, B.J. and Longaker, M.T.: New Developments in Craniofacial Surgery Research, *Cleft Palate Craniofac. J., 36,* 377, September, 1999.

Prahl-Anderson, B.: Dental Treatment of Prenatal and Infant Patients With Clefts and Craniofacial Anomalies, *Cleft Palate Craniofac. J., 37,* 528, November, 2000.

Rivkin, C.J., Keith, O., Crawford, P.J.M., and Hathorn, I.S.: Dental Care for the Patient With a Cleft Lip and Palate. Part 1: From Birth to the Mixed Dentition Stage, *Brit. Dent. J., 188,* 78, January 22, 2000.

Schendel, S.A.: Unilateral Cleft Lip Repair–State of the Art, *Cleft Palate Craniofac. J., 37,* 335, July, 2000.

Preadolescent to Postmenopausal Patients

Patricia A. Cohen, RDH, BS, MS

The endocrine glands are glands of internal secretion. They secrete highly specialized substances—the hormones—that, with the nervous system, maintain body homeostasis.

Hormones are transported by the blood or lymph. They may act directly on body cells or indirectly to control the hormones of other glands. Their complex and unified action augments and regulates many vital functions, including growth and development, energy production, food metabolism, reproductive processes, and the responses of the body to stress.

The major endocrine glands are the pituitary, thyroid, parathyroids, pancreas, adrenals, and gonads. The anterior pituitary is called the master gland because it regulates the output of hormones by other glands. In turn, the pituitary itself is regulated by the hormones of the other glands.

Both hyposecretion and hypersecretion of a hormone can cause physical and mental disturbances. Regulation of hormonal secretion is complex, and the mechanisms are not fully understood. Normally, hormones are secreted when needed. The external temperature, for example, can influence the production of thyroxin by the thyroid gland. The calcium level of the blood affects parathyroid activity.

Hormones of the reproductive system have an effect on the development and function of the individual. Some of the influences on oral health and patient care are described in this chapter. Key words are defined in Box 48-1.

■ ADOLESCENCE AND PUBERTY

I. STAGES OF ADOLESCENCE

The period of life considered adolescence is represented by the years between ages 10 and 21. The adolescent years, which include puberty, are marked by many physical and psychosocial changes.

BOX 48-1 KEY WORDS: Preadolescent to Postmenopausal Patients

Acne vulgaris: a chronic skin disorder with increased production of oil from the sebaceous glands; may be inflammatory or noninflammatory; appears on the face, back, and chest.

Adolescence: the period extending from the time the secondary sex characteristics appear to the end of somatic growth, when the individual is mature.

Amenorrhea: absence of spontaneous menstrual periods in a female of reproductive age.

Circumpubertal: on or around the age of puberty.

Coitus: sexual union; copulation; intercourse.

Dysmenorrhea: difficult and painful menstruation.

Dysphoria: feeling unwell or unhappy, depressed feeling.

Endometrium: the lining of the uterus.

Endometriosis: a condition of the endometrium which causes pelvic pain.

Gynecologist: physician who specializes in conditions specific to women, particularly of the genital tract, female endocrinology, and reproductive physiology.

Homeostasis: the tendency of biologic systems to maintain constant internal stability while continually adjusting to external changes.

Hormone: a chemical product of an organ or of certain cells within the organ that has a specific regulatory effect upon cells elsewhere in the body.

Hormone replacement therapy: prescription of a purified or synthetic hormone to correct or prevent undesirable symptoms of menopause.

Mastalgia: fullness, soreness, or pain in the breast.

Maturity: state of complete growth.

Menarche: onset of menstruation; may occur from ages 9 to 17 years.

Menopause: the time of life when a woman ceases menstruation; defined as a period of 6 to 12 months of amenorrhea in a woman over 45 years of age.

Menses: menstruation.

Oligomenorrhea: menstrual intervals of greater than 45 days.

Premenstrual syndrome: a cluster of behavioral, somatic, affective, and cognitive disorders that appear in the premenstrual (luteal) phase of the menstrual cycle and that resolve rapidly with the onset of menses.

Puberty: period in which the gonads mature and begin to function.

Pubescence: coming to the age of puberty or sexual maturity.

Spermatogenesis: the process of male sperm production.

From a psychosocial aspect, this period can be divided into three overlapping phases:
- Early adolescence, approximately ages 10 to 13.
- Middle adolescence, approximately ages 14 to 17.
- Late adolescence, approximately ages 18 to 21.

II. PUBERTAL CHANGES

Puberty is a dynamic period of development marked by rapid changes in body size, shape, and composition. Puberty is a sign of growing up. Some individuals go through changes earlier and faster than others.

Chronologic age is an unreliable indicator because puberty may begin normally in either sex between 9 and 17 years of age, depending on such factors as race, heredity, and nutritional status. Friends of the same age may look quite different from one another because there is a wide range of normal. Females generally begin puberty before males. The secondary sex characteristics begin to appear between 10 and 13 years of age in females, whereas changes in males start at about 13 or 14 years. The major changes are usually complete in 3 to 4 years.

III. PHYSICAL DEVELOPMENT

A. Hormonal Influences

Pituitary hormones control the hormones produced by the ovaries and the testes. The several hormones produced by the ovaries are known collectively as estrogens, and those produced by the testes are called androgens. They are responsible for the development of the sex organs, the accessory sex organs, and the secondary sex characteristics. They have strong physical, mental, and emotional influences throughout the body.

B. Female Development

1. Accelerated growth spurt.
2. Development of the sex organs: fallopian tubes, uterus, vagina, and breasts.
3. Appearance of secondary sex characteristics:
   * Growth of pubic and axillary hair.
   * Skeletal development, increased height, enlargement of the pelvis.
   * Fat deposition on the hips.
   * Voice drops one or two tones.
4. Beginning of menstruation and ovulation. Menstruation may precede the first ovulation.

C. Male Development

1. Increase in size of testes and scrotum and beginning of spermatogenesis.
2. Development of the sex organs: vas deferens, seminal vesicles, prostate, and penis.
3. Appearance of secondary sex characteristics:
   * Growth of facial, pubic, and axillary hair.
   * Voice deepens.
4. Increased height, increased muscle volume and mass.

D. Growth Spurt

1. Varies in age of occurrence, extent, and duration; usually occurs in females between 11 and 14 years, and in males between 12 and 16 years.

2. Overeating with underexercise, along with psychological problems, makes obesity a difficult and serious problem.
3. Poor coordination and awkwardness in young adolescents may result from irregular, uneven stages of growth.
4. Teens need three health basics: fuel, activity, and rest.

IV. PSYCHOSOCIAL DEVELOPMENT

Psychologically and socially, adolescence is the bridge from childhood to adulthood.

A. Changes

During the stages of development, the changes that take place can be grouped under the following topics, as detailed in Table 48-1.
* Achievement of independence from parents.
* Adoption of peer codes and lifestyles.
* Assignment of increased importance to body image and acceptance of one's own body image.
* Establishment of sexual, ego, vocational, and moral identities.

B. Relevance in Dental Hygiene Care

* Vital for all health professionals to understand the general patterns of growth and development.
* Insight into changes during adolescence can direct patient teaching.

V. NUTRITIONAL REQUIREMENTS

1. Highest of any time in life for males; exceeded only during pregnancy for females.
2. Undernutrition is common.
   * Boys: due to overactivity and poor food selection.
   * Girls: due to voluntary diet restrictions, with poor food selection and fad diets in the attempt to be trim.
   * Teens with a distorted body image may take concern to extremes.
3. Eating disorders
   * Anorexia nervosa and/or bulimia, can lead to severe health complications and even death.
   * Successful treatment usually requires an interdisciplinary team approach involving medical care, psychotherapy, and nutrition and family counseling (pages 1003 to 1006).
4. Iron-deficiency anemia
   * Common among teenage girls, particularly after the onset of menstruation.

■ TABLE 48-1 PSYCHOSOCIAL DEVELOPMENT OF ADOLESCENTS

TASK	EARLY ADOLESCENCE APPROX 10–13 YRS MIDDLE SCHOOL	MIDDLE ADOLESCENCE APPROX 14–17 YRS HIGH SCHOOL	LATE ADOLESCENCE APPROX 17–21 YRS HIGHER EDUCATION OR WORK
Independence	• Less interest in parental activities • Wide mood swings	• Peak of parental conflicts	• Reacceptance of parental values
Body Image	• Preoccupation with self and pubertal changes • Uncertainty about appearance	• General acceptance of body • Concern over making body more attractive	• Acceptance of pubertal changes
Peers	• Intense relationships with same-sex friends	• Peak of peer involvement • Conformity with peer values • Increased sexual activity and experimentation	• Peer group less important • More time spent in sharing intimate relationships
Identity	• Increased cognition • Increased fantasy world • Idealistic vocational goals • Increased need for privacy • Lack of impulse control	• Increased scope of feelings • Increased intellectual ability • Feeling of omnipotence • Risk-taking behavior	• Practical, realistic vocational goals • Refinement of moral religious, and sexual values • Ability to compromise and to set limits

Adapted from Radzik, M., Sherer, S., and Neinstein, L.S.: Psychosocial Development in Normal Adolescents, in Neinstein, L.S.: *Adolescent Health Care: A Practical Guide,* 4th ed. Baltimore, Lippincott Williams & Wilkins, 2002, p. 57. Used with permission.

• Treated with iron supplements, changes in diet, or both (page 1063).

VI. PERSONAL FACTORS

Adolescents are no longer children, yet they have not reached adulthood. They may respond and wish to be treated as adults or as children at different times. They are learning to adapt to body changes, sexual impulses, secondary sex characteristics, and independence. There is no fixed picture. Characteristics listed below are exhibited to one degree or another by many adolescents. Issues can be addressed at the family, school, or individual level.[1]

A. Anxiety

Causes of adolescent anxiety include:
• Health problems. Younger, less healthy teenagers tend to show greater health concerns.
• Violence, substance abuse.
• Sexual issues, peer pressures.
• Family arguments, divorce.
• School performance, concern about the future.

B. Increased Self-interest

• Have a great deal of concern for themselves and respond best to those who show concern for them.

• Want attention and tend to reject those who do not listen.
• Interest in their own health.

C. Growing Independence

• Adolescence is a period of rapidly growing independence of thought and action, with conflicts between feelings of dependence and independence.
• Childhood dependence on parents is gradually given up; the idea of infallibility of parents is lost; teachers and other authority figures are questioned.
• Personal identity is sought; adolescents are uncertain about their place and role in society.
• Independence from parents frequently means increased confidence in and respect for other adults outside the family.
• Teachers, coaches, and health professionals can have a powerful impact at this time.

D. Concern Over Physical Characteristics

• Girls mature earlier than boys; young females are usually taller than their male counterparts. Social problems may result.

- Increased interest in personal appearance; want to dress and be like their peers.
- Issues such as delayed growth and delayed sexual development.
- Obesity may be troublesome. Obesity is a serious health problem and is associated with increased morbidity and mortality.
- Skin disorders may occur. Acne vulgaris commonly results from overactivity of the sebaceous glands. Usually, relief occurs when adolescence is completed, although the condition may persist longer. The impact upon self-esteem can affect social interactions and school performance. Treatment with topical agents or systemic therapy can often be successful.

■ ORAL CONDITIONS

I. DENTAL CARIES

- Incidence higher during adolescence than other age groups, especially in communities without fluoridation.
- Related to eating habits: frequency, demands of rapid growth, emotional issues, peer pressures.
- Cariogenic foods selected: frequent snacks, sweetened carbonated beverages.

II. PERIODONTAL INFECTIONS

Adolescents are subject to all categories of periodontal infections (see Tables 14-2A and 14-2B). Gingival problems are common in this age group. Careful probing and study of radiographs are indicated for each patient. Emphasis must be placed on preventive measures, early assessment, early treatment, and regular maintenance appointments.

A. Biofilm-Induced Gingivitis During Puberty[2]

- Incidence and severity may increase.
- Clinical changes and hormonal changes related to increased dental biofilm.
- Exaggerated response to dental biofilm.

B. Risk Factors for Periodontitis[3]

- Local factors: supragingival and subgingival calculus; dental biofilm accumulations.
- Pathogenic microorganisms, viruses.
- Untreated dental caries and defective restorations.[4]
- Orthodontic appliances.
- Oral hygiene: personal habits of care.

- Infrequent, inadequate dental and dental hygiene care.
- Socioeconomic influences.
- Use of tobacco.
- Systemic diseases such as diabetes and hematological diseases.
- Host immune factors.
- Genetic factors.

C. Destructive Periodontal Diseases

Periodontal diseases in adolescents may be either in the aggressive or chronic classification. Loss of periodontal attachment and supporting bone is evident in 5% to 47% of adolescents around the world.[5]

The two distinct disease categories are localized aggressive periodontitis (LAP) and generalized aggressive periodontitis (GAP). Both types have a familial tendency and may have a neutrophil dysfunction with a compromised immune response.[6]

1. *Localized Aggressive Periodontitis* (LAP)
   - Characterized by severe bone loss involving the first permanent molars and the incisors, with proximal surface attachment loss on at least two permanent teeth.
   - First diagnosed during the circumpubertal years.
   - Pathogenic microorganism of etiologic importance is the *Actinobacillus actinomycetemcomitans,* a powerful microorganism that can invade tissue.
2. *Generalized Aggressive Periodontitis* (GAP)
   - Characterized by generalized proximal surface attachment loss affecting at least three permanent teeth other than the first molars and incisors.
   - Occurs in persons under 30 years of age.
   - Microflora found in pockets of GAP has similarities to the microflora of adult periodontitis.

■ DENTAL HYGIENE CARE

I. IMPACT OF CARE

- Dental hygiene services provided during adolescence can impact oral health throughout the patient's lifetime.
- The concrete information, education, and guidance from interested and caring health professionals will help form the attitudes and health behavior practices developed by adolescents.
- Influences at this time can have wide-reaching significance throughout life.

II. PATIENT APPROACH

- Adolescence is a period of transition and growth spurts. Understanding adolescents, their issues, and their biological changes is critical for promoting health and preventing disease.[7]
- Each situation requires its own approach.
- Health behaviors at this stage of development can have lifelong implications.
- Adolescence is an opportune time to promote health and prevent disease.
- Treat adolescents as adults. Physically, many of them are mature, although their emotional development varies. They are becoming less dependent on the family and paying more attention to the influence of peers.
- Be attentive and show interest in them and their issues. Encourage them to talk, and then listen attentively.
- Avoid lecturing and admonishing. Suggest and advise, but do not become impatient or take offense when they choose to make their own decisions. Adolescents need time to process information about health behavior changes.
- Highlight the positive. Self-concept plays a significant role in mediating changes in dental health behavior. High self-esteem has a strong positive association with oral cleanliness in adolescents.[8,9]
- Question the patient regarding motivations and health behaviors.
- Health, including oral health, may be a real concern.
- Adolescents need information about their oral health; explanations based on science are generally appreciated.

III. PATIENT HISTORY

- *History questions.* Adolescents may provide their own information for the medical and dental histories. Verification by the parent or guardian for additional details is needed, but not in the same interview with the patient and not without the patient's consent.
- *Responsibility for health.* Adolescents need to take increasing responsibility for their own health. Although the initial dental visit may be at the suggestion of a parent or guardian, every effort should be made to focus on the patient.
- *Other health problems.* The patient with diabetes; heart disease; a mental, physical, or sensory disability; or other systemic involvement requires special adaptations of procedures as described in the various chapters of Section VII of this book.

- *Medical clearance.* The parent or legal guardian will need to consent to medical clearance for conditions requiring antibiotic coverage, local anesthesia, or other medication for a patient under legal age.
- *Parental approval.* The dental hygiene care plan requires approval by a parent or legal guardian.

IV. ORAL HEALTH PROBLEMS IN ADOLESCENCE[10]

Dental caries and periodontal infections of the adolescent years have been described. Some examples of other oral problems related to adolescent development and behavior characteristics, including risky health behaviors, are listed here.

- Oral manifestations of sexually transmitted diseases (STDs).
- Effects of tobacco use, such as leukoplakia and periodontal damage.
- Effects of cocaine use and other drugs.
- Potential effects of oral contraceptives on periodontal tissues (page 821).
- Oral findings of anorexia nervosa or bulimia (pages 1004 and 1006).
- Traumatic injury to teeth and oral structures may occur. Contact sports and skateboarding are risky behaviors. Automobile and motorcycle accidents can also cause dental injuries.
- Pregnancy and parenting may be issues for the adolescent. The dental hygienist has the opportunity to use anticipatory guidance in educating the patient on important oral health issues (Tables 46-2 and 46-3).
- Body piercings in the orofacial region are common. Inform patients who are considering a piercing regarding piercing procedures and related health risks. Patients need education regarding daily hygiene of the piercing site to avoid infection.

V. DENTAL BIOFILM CONTROL

1. Educate the patient by explaining the following:
    - Causes and prevention of dental caries and periodontal infections.
    - Effects of dental biofilm accumulation.
    - Purposes of professional calculus removal.
    - Daily self-care and its relation to oral tissue health and halitosis prevention.
2. The total caries-control program

For dental caries prevention, adolescents must appreciate the effects of fluoride and the need to restrict the intake of cariogenic foods. The program is outlined and conducted on the basis of these clear-cut preventive measures.

- Instruction in self-care procedures.
- Continuing reassessment over a series of appointments to develop behavior changes that include daily practices that can be carried over into adult life.

VI. INSTRUMENTATION

- Series of appointments may be required, depending on probing depth and extent of calculus deposits.
- Careful and complete scaling and root planing.
- Removal of all local irregularities, such as inadequate margins of restorations.

VII. FLUORIDE TREATMENT PROGRAM

- A combined fluoride program is indicated for most adolescent patients, particularly for those who have not had the benefit of a fluoridated water supply.
- Topical fluoride applications made in conjunction with dental hygiene appointments; self-administered methods include a fluoride dentifrice and a daily fluoride mouthrinse.
- A daily application of a fluoride gel in a custom-made tray may be necessary in selected cases (page 558).

VIII. DIET CONTROL

A. Dietary Assessment (pages 529 to 531)

A study of the patient's diet and counseling relative to general nutrition and dental caries control can provide important learning experiences for many adolescents. The parent or other person who is responsible for shopping and food preparation is included so that appropriate foods are available. As much responsibility as possible is placed with the adolescent patient.

B. Instruction Suggestions

- *Advise foods from the most recent food guide pyramid* (page 523). Emphasize foods for growth, energy, clear complexion, wellness, and overall good health.
- *Emphasize a nutritious breakfast.* Teenagers tend to omit breakfast, particularly if they have to prepare it for themselves.
- *Snack selection.* Advise selecting nutritious foods, with recognition of cariogenic foods. Suggest snacks such as raw fruits and vegetables, nuts, unsweetened milk, use of sugar-free

foods when possible, and sugarless chewing gum if gum is used.

- *Suggest reading labels.* Recommend that teens learn how to read nutrition labels and become aware of serving size, nutrition information, and total calories.

▪ MENSTRUATION

I. MENSTRUAL CYCLE

The cycle is the period of time from the beginning of one menstrual flow to the beginning of the next menstrual flow.

A. Cyclic Changes in the Uterus.

- Instigated by hormones (Figure 48-1)
- Preparation of the endometrium for pregnancy (Figure 48-1).

B. Conception Does Not Occur

- Fluid discharged during menstruation.
- Composed of blood, mucous, endometrial membrane fragments.
- Length: 3 to 6 days; cycle starts over.

II. CHARACTERISTICS

A. Occurrence

- Cyclic menstruation occurs from puberty to menopause.
- Except during pregnancy and part of breast-feeding.
- Cycle complete in about 28 days, as shown in Figure 48-1 (range, 22 to 35 days).

B. Onset

- Between ages 9 and 19 years.
- May occur before the first ovulation.
- Timing and extent of flow may be irregular for several months or years.

III. IRREGULARITIES

- Variations are common. Many have no problems.
- Factors affecting the cycle: changes in climate, changes in work schedule, emotional trauma, acute or chronic illnesses, weight loss, or excessive exercise.
- Emotional impact: may have a psychological basis.

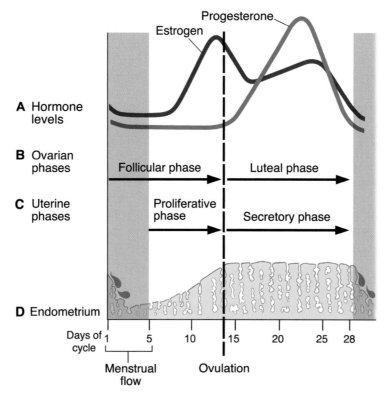

■ FIGURE 48-1 Changes During the Menstrual Cycle. The 28 days of a normal cycle are shown, with ovulation between days 12 and 15 and the menstrual flow between days 1 to 5 and again at day 28. **(A)** Hormonal levels show the estrogen peak shortly before ovulation during the follicular phase of the ovary **(B)** and the proliferative phase of the uterus **(C)**. **(D)** The endometrium builds up at the end of each menstrual flow. This prepares the area for possible implantation of a fertilized ovum.

A. Premenstrual Syndrome

Premenstrual syndrome (PMS) is a distinctive group of physical and emotional changes that may occur 7 to 10 days prior to menstruation.
- *Physical Symptoms.* Fatigue, headache, bloating, mastalgia, skin breakouts, cramps, and food cravings.
- *Affective Symptoms.* Depression, anxiety, irritability, hostility, tearfulness, mood changes, reduced ability to concentrate.
- *Medical Management.* Medical care for severe symptoms, possibly prescription medication.
- *Self-help Methods.* Daily exercise, diet modification to eliminate caffeine, salt, alcohol, and simple carbohydrates, stress reduction, and rest. Over-the-counter (OTC) medications to manage discomfort.[11]

B. Dysmenorrhea

- *Primary or functional dysmenorrhea.* The organs are normal and there are symptoms of hyperactivity and contractions.

- *Secondary or acquired dysmenorrhea.* Associated with abnormal anatomy of the uterus or as the result of an illness such as endometriosis or pelvic inflammatory disease (PID).
- *Physiologic or psychologic factors.* Emotional status, inadequate preparation for the arrival of puberty, poor parental example.

IV. DENTAL HYGIENE CARE

A. Patient History

- Menstruation is normal and healthy; not an illness.
- Terminology for history questions: use "period" or "monthly period."
- Include questions concerning regularity.
- Irregularity: may reflect general health problems.

B. Oral Findings[12]

- No specific gingival changes; occasional problems may occur.
- Exaggerated response to local irritants or unusual gingival bleeding may be noted.

- Prevention through dental biofilm control, self-care measures, and removal of calculus at regular maintenance appointments.

■ HORMONAL CONTRACEPTIVES

Numerous types of hormonal contraceptives are available. Birth control pills, also known as oral contraceptives (OCs) are recognized as a safe and effective method of contraception when they are taken as prescribed. They are used by millions of women throughout the world.

I. TYPES[13]

A. Combination Preparations

1. *Estrogen and Progestin*
   - Combination of synthetic hormones estrogen and progestin is nearly 100% effective in preventing pregnancy when taken appropriately.
   - OCs inhibit the release of gonadotropin-releasing hormone, without which the ovum cannot be released from the ovary.
2. *Schedule of Administration*
   - One pill taken each day for 21 days starting 5 days after the onset of the menstrual flow.
   - For a period of 7 days, a placebo pill is taken.
   - Routine is followed regardless of when menstrual flow starts or stops.

B. Single Preparations: Minipills

- The progestin-only pill has been used when estrogen is contraindicated.
- Pregnancy prevention is slightly less effective with this pill.
- Menstrual cycles tend to be irregular; side effects frequent.

C. Injectible Contraceptive: Depo-Provera™

- Contains synthetic progestin.
- One injection every 12 weeks prevents ovulation.
- Can be helpful for those who have trouble remembering to take daily pill.

D. Subdermal Implant

- Allows for slow release of hormone.
- Provides effective contraception for 5 years.
- Method of action is similar to injectible.

II. CONTRAINDICATIONS[13]

Contraceptives containing hormones should not be used by the patient in the presence of the following:
- Circulatory problems, thromboembolic disorders, cerebrovascular disease, coronary heart disease, severe hypertension.
- Liver disease.
- Cancer of the breast.
- Severe migraine headaches.
- Pregnancy or lactation.

III. SIDE EFFECTS[13]

Side effects may be related to incorrect use of the drug rather than to hormonal effects. Visual problems, mental depression, rashes, and bleeding irregularities occur in some women. The most significant side effects are:
- Cardiovascular (including increased blood pressure).
- Weight gain.
- Decreased effectiveness when certain drugs are used, including antibiotics,[14,15] anticonvulsants, and rifampin.

IV. EFFECT ON THE GINGIVA

An exaggerated response to dental biofilm and other local irritants has been noted. The gingivitis is similar to that described for pregnancy (page 773).

V. APPOINTMENT CONSIDERATIONS

A. Medical History

A record of the use of oral contraceptives should be updated with each history review.

B. Inform the Patient

- Potential oral side effects of hormonal contraceptives.
- The need for exceptional personal oral care and regular professional maintenance appointments to prevent complications.

■ MENOPAUSE

Menopause is the complete and permanent cessation of menstrual flow.
- Menopause generally occurs between the ages of 47 and 55 years.
- The end of fertility due to decreased production of sex hormones by the ovaries.

- Menopause is usually confirmed when a woman has no menstrual period for 12 consecutive months and there is no apparent biologic or physiologic cause.

I. CHARACTERISTICS

Prior to menopause, menstruation changes in frequency, duration, and amount of flow over a period of about 12 to 24 months. Menopause is accompanied by a number of characteristic physiologic changes. Although many women experience minor symptoms, a small percent have problems during menopause.

A. General Symptoms

As ovarian function declines with diminishing estrogen, physiologic changes in body function take place.
1. *Vasomotor Reactions.*
   - Hot flashes, defined as periodic surges of heat involving the whole body; may be accompanied by drenching sweats.
   - Hot flash may begin with a headache; proceed to a flushing of the face, with heart palpitations, and dizziness, followed by a chill.
   - Episodes may last a few minutes or more than 30 minutes.
   - Night sweats can cause sleep disturbances.
2. *Vaginal Changes.*
   - Dryness, irritation, and thinning of tissue may occur.
   - Associated with decreased estrogen levels.
3. *Emotional Disturbances.*
- Alterations in estrogen level may result in mood swings, depression, and difficulty with concentration.
- Some women experience anxiety, tension, and irritability and feel useless.

B. Postmenopausal Effects

1. Reproductive organs atrophy.
2. Bone problems have been associated with the menopausal patient.
3. Skin and mucous membranes decrease in thickness and keratinization, becoming fragile and easily injured.
4. Predisposition to conditions including atherosclerosis, diabetes, and hypothyroidism.

II. ORAL FINDINGS

Oral changes can be related to menopause, but they are not a common feature. Control of local factors through preventive dental hygiene appointments for maintenance will supplement daily personal oral care.

A. Gingiva

- Gingival changes associated with menopause usually represent an exaggerated response to dental biofilm.
- Hormonal changes influence oral tissue response.
- Menopausal gingivostomatitis may develop.[16] It may also occur after removal of, or radiation therapy to, the ovaries.

B. Mucous Membranes and Tongue

- Tissue may appear shiny and may vary in color from abnormal paleness to redness.[16] Dryness with burning sensations may be present.
- Burning mouth syndrome may occur.
- Altered salivary composition in some menopausal women may be due to psychological stress.[17]
- Epithelium may become thin and atrophic with decreased keratinization; tolerance for removable prostheses may lessen, especially with xerostomia.
- Taste perception may be altered, described as salty, peppery, or sour.
- Inadequate diet and eating habits may contribute to the adverse changes of the mucosal tissues. The appearance and symptoms frequently resemble those associated with vitamin deficiencies, particularly B vitamins.

C. Alveolar Bone Loss

As a result of systemic osteoporosis, ridge resorption and loss of teeth can occur.[18] Osteoporotic jaws may be unsuitable for conventional prosthetic devices or dental implants.[19]

III. DENTAL HYGIENE CARE

In the approach to the patient, a specific relationship of oral conditions to menopause need not be emphasized. Emphasize the need for self-care measures. Because of the importance of local factors, attention should be directed to the need for meticulous and daily biofilm control, along with regular and frequent professional care.

A. Appointment Suggestions

The symptoms of physical and emotional changes should be kept in mind when planning and conducting the appointment. In treating women entering menopause, consideration should be given to the stressful phase of life the patient may be experiencing.
- Rapport begins with the clinician's courtesy, personal attention, and friendly, unhurried manner.

Everyday Ethics

? Amy, an 18-year-old female, returns home from her first semester of college and presents with swollen gingiva, weight gain, and stories about considerable amounts of alcoholic beverages being consumed at parties. She also tells Sally, the dental hygienist, that she has just started taking birth control pills. Sally acknowledges Amy's desire to exercise her independence while away at school but also indicates the term "risky behaviors" in the patient's chart.

Questions for Consideration

1. Ethically, what is Sally's role as a primary dental health provider in referring this patient to other professionals for counseling and/or a physical examination?

2. Role play a discussion that might occur between Sally and Amy's parents, who are still financially responsible for the services rendered. Consider what has been entered into the patient's chart—"risky behaviors."

3. Using a decision framework, prioritize the content of the homecare information needed to educate Amy about her oral conditions.

- Give particular attention to details, such as seating the patient promptly, handling materials and instruments efficiently and with calm assurance.
- Consider adjusting the temperature of the room for patient comfort if necessary.

B. Instruction of Patient

- Saliva substitute may be needed to provide relief from xerostomia and aid in the prevention of dental caries.
- Measures for the prevention of periodontal infections can be carefully explained.
- Emphasize reasons for frequent calculus removal as a supplement to meticulous daily self-care.
- Explain the relationship between good general health and oral health.

✔ **Factors To Teach The Patient**

- Self-care procedures that are necessary to maintain good oral health.
- The long-term impact of health behaviors, including lifestyle choices and risk reduction.
- The benefits of fluoride throughout life.
- The importance of nutrition, exercise, and sleep for good health.
- The value of seeking professional help when problems arise.

C. Diet

- Dietary assessment may prove to be a helpful teaching–learning experience by helping the patient identify and correct inadequately balanced food selection (page 529).
- Caries prevention through selection of nutritious and noncariogenic foods is especially important for the patient who tends to indulge in between-meal eating.

D. Fluoride Therapy

A fluoride-containing dentifrice and a brush-on gel applied before bedtime are necessary for nearly all patients in this age group (page 560).

REFERENCES

1. **Resnick**, M.D., Bearman, P.S., Blum, R.W., Bauman, K.E., Harris, K.M., Jones, J., Tabor, J., Beuhring, T., Sieving, R.E., Shew, M., Ireland, M., Bearinger, L.H., and Udry, J.R.: Protecting Adolescents From Harm: Findings From the National Longitudinal Study on Adolescent Health, *JAMA, 278*, 823, September 10, 1997.
2. **Newman**, M.G., Takei, H.H., and Carranza, F.A.: Carranza's *Clinical Periodontology*, 9th ed. Philadelphia, W.B. Saunders, 2002, pp. 212, 287, 311.
3. **Albandar**, J.M. and Rams, T.E.: Risk Factors for Periodontitis in Children and Young Persons, *Periodontol. 2000, 29*, 207, 2002.
4. **Albandar**, J.M., Buischi, Y.A., and Axelsson, P.: Caries Lesions and Dental Restorations as Predisposing Factors in the Progression of Periodontal Diseases in Adolescents: A 3-Year Longitudinal Study, *J. Periodontol., 66*, 249, April, 1995.
5. **Hansen**, B.F., Gjermo, P., Bellini, H.T., Ihanamaki, K., and Saxén, L.: Prevalence of Radiographic Alveolar Bone Loss in Young Adults: A Multinational Study, *Int. Dent. J., 45*, 54, February, 1995.

6. **Armitage**, G.C.: Development of a Classification System for Periodontal Diseases and Conditions, *Ann. Periodontol., 4,* December, 1999.

7. **Susman**, E.J., Reiter, E.O., Ford, C., and Dorn, L.D.: Work Group I: Developing Models of Healthy Adolescent Physical Development, *J. Adolesc. Health, 31,* 171, 2002.

8. **Regis**, D., Macgregor, I.D.M., and Balding, J.W.: Differential Prediction of Dental Health Behaviour by Self-esteem and Health Locus of Control in Young Adolescents, *J. Clin. Periodontol., 21,* 7, January, 1994.

9. **Macgregor**, I.D.M., Regis, D., and Balding, J.: Self-concept and Dental Health Behaviors in Adolescents, *J. Clin. Periodontol., 24,* 335, May, 1997.

10. **American Academy of Pediatric Dentistry**: Oral Health Policies, Statement on Adolescent Oral Health, May, 2001, *Pediatr. Dent., 23,* 7, Special Issue: Reference Manual 2001–2002, November, 2001.

11. **Campbell**, M.A. and McGrath, P.J.: Use of Medication by Adolescents for the Management of Menstrual Discomfort, *Arch. Pediatr. Adolesc. Med., 151,* 905, September, 1997.

12. **Newman**, M.G., Takei, H.H., and Carranza, F.A.: op. cit., p. 212.

13. **Greydanus**, D.E., Patel, D.R., and Rimsza, M.E.: Contraception in the Adolescent: An Update, *Pediatrics, 107,* 562, March, 2001.

14. **American Dental Association**, Council on Scientific Affairs: Antibiotic Interference With Oral Contraceptives, *J. Am. Dent. Assoc., 133,* 880, July, 2002.

15. **American Dental Association**, Health Foundation Research Institute, Department of Toxicology: Antibiotic Interference With Oral Contraceptives, *J. Am. Dent. Assoc., 122,* 79, December, 1991.

16. **Newman**, M.G., Takei, H.H., and Carranza, F.A.: op. cit., p. 214.

17. **Ciberka**, R.M., Nelson, S.K., and Lefebvre, C.A.: Burning Mouth Syndrome: A Review of Etiologies, *J. Prosthet. Dent., 78,* 93, July, 1997.

18. **Jeffcoat**, M.K. and Chesnut, C.H.: Systemic Osteoporosis and Oral Bone Loss: Evidence Shows Increased Factors, *J. Am. Dent. Assoc., 124,* 49, November, 1993.

19. **Friedlander**, A.H.: The Physiology, Medical Management and Oral Implications of Menopause, *J. Am. Dent. Assoc., 133,* 73, January, 2002.

SUGGESTED READINGS

Armitage, G.: Classifying Periodontal Diseases: A Long-standing Dilemma, *Periodontol. 2000, 30,* 9, 2002.

Adolescence

Blum, R.W., Beuhring, T., Shew, M.L., Bearinger, L.H., Sieving, R.E., and Resnick, M.D.: The Effects of Race/Ethnicity, Income, and Family Structure on Adolescent Risk Behaviors, *Am. J. Public Health, 90,* 1879, December, 2000.

Gall, G.B.: Comprehensive Risk Assessment for Adolescents in School-Based Health Centers, *Nurs. Clin. N. Am., 37,* 553, 2002.

Lafferty, W.E., Downey, L., Holan, C.M., Lind, A., Kassler, W., Tao, G., and Irwind, K.: Provision of Sexual Health Services to Adolescent Enrollees in Medicaid Managed Care, *Am. J. Public Health, 92,* 1779, November, 2002.

Martin, H. and Ammerman, S.: Adolescents With Eating Disorders: Primary Care Screening, Identification, and Early Intervention, *Nurs. Clin. N. Am., 37,* 537, 2002.

Sargent, J.D. and DiFranza, J.R.: Tobacco Control for Clinicians Who Treat Adolescents, *CA Cancer J. Clin., 53,* 102, March/April, 2003.

Adolescents' Oral Health Issues

Albandar, J.M. and Tinoco, E.: Global Epidemiology of Periodontal Diseases in Children and Young Persons, *Periodontol. 2000, 29,* 153, 2002.

Berglundh, T., Wellfelt, B., Liljenberg, B., and Lindhe, J.: Some Local and Systemic Immunological Features of Prepubertal Periodontitis, *J. Clin. Periodontol., 28,* 113, February, 2001.

Clerehugh, V., Seymour, G.J., Bird, P.S., Cullinan, M., Drucker, D.B., and Worthington, H.V.: The Detection of *Actinobacillus actinomycetemcomitans, Porphyromonas gingivalis* and *Prevotella intermedia* Using an ELISA in an Adolescent Population With Early Periodontitis, *J. Clin. Periodontol., 24,* 57, January, 1997.

Ellwood, R., Worthington, H.V., Cullinan, M.P., Hamlet, S., Clerehugh, V., and Davies, R.: Prevalence of Suspected Periodontal Pathogens Identified Using ELISA in Adolescents of Differing Ethnic Origins, *J. Clin. Periodontol., 24,* 141, March, 1997.

Machuca, G., Rosales, I., Lacalle, J., Machuca, C., and Bullon, P.: Effect of Cigarette Smoking on Periodontal Status of Healthy Young Adults, *J. Clin. Periodontol., 71,* 73, January, 2000.

Oh, T-J, Eber, R., and Wang, H-L: Periodontal Diseases in the Child and Adolescent, *J. Clin. Periodontol., 29,* 4000, May, 2002.

Women's Health

Danner, V.: The Hormonal Impact, *Access, 16,* 22, March, 2002.

Mosca, L., Collins, P., Herrington, D., Mendelsohn, M., Pasternak, R., Robertson, R., Schenck-Gustafsson, K., Smith, S., Taubert, K., and Wenger, N.: Hormone Replacement Therapy and Cardiovascular Disease: A Statement for Healthcare Professionals From the American Heart Association (AHA Scientific Statement), *Circulation, 104,* 499, July, 2001.

Perno, M.: The Dental Hygienist: Our Role in Women's Health—Management of the Female Client, *Compend. Contin. Ed. Dent., 22,* 39, Special Issue, 2001.

Women's Oral Health Issues

Covington, P.: Women's Oral Health Issues: An Exploration of the Literature, *Can. Dent. Hyg. (Probe), 30,* 173, September/October, 1996.

Fried, J.L.: Women and Tobacco: Oral Health Issues, *J. Dent. Hyg., 74,* 49, Winter, 2000.

Krejci, C.B. and Bissada, N.F.: Womens' Health Issues and Their Relationship to Periodontitis, *J. Am. Dent. Assoc., 133,* 323, March, 2002.

Perno, M.: Burning Mouth Syndrome, *J. Dent. Hyg., 75,* 245, Summer, 2001.

Steinberg, B.J.: Women's Oral Health, *Compend. Contin. Ed. Dent., 22,* 7, Special Issue, 2001.

The Gerodontic Patient

Esther M. Wilkins, BS, RDH, DMD
Janet H. Towle, RN, RDH, BS, MEd

CHAPTER OUTLINE

Preventive measures for the aging population through care and instruction require greater emphasis as the number of people involved in this group increases steadily. Members of the dental team are challenged by the need to help the aging population learn about personal care and seek professional care that will provide continuing oral comfort and function.

As the percentage of people in the older group has increased, the total number of older patients in a general or adult practice has grown. An increasing number of dental hygienists specialize in the care of the elderly and are employed in long-term care and resident facilities for the aged.

Tooth loss increases with age, but not because of age. Dental caries and periodontal diseases are the major causes of tooth loss. Periodontal diseases in the older population represent the cumulative effects of long-standing, undiagnosed, untreated, or neglected chronic infection.

With fluoridation and the application of current knowledge of preventive measures for oral diseases in younger age groups, it is anticipated that future generations of older people will not be subjected to the severe effects of uncontrolled and untreated oral diseases of previous generations. Key words relating to older patients are defined in Box 49-1.

■ AGING

I. BIOLOGIC AND CHRONOLOGIC AGE

When aging is defined from a chronologic viewpoint, the aging population may be recognized as the "older population" (age 55 and over), the "elderly" (age 65 and over), the

---

BOX 49-1 KEY WORDS: Gerodontic Patient

Ageism: discrimination toward/against the aged population.

Aging: the continuous process (biologic, psychologic, social), beginning with conception and ending with death, by which organisms mature and decline.

Alzheimer's disease: a form of irreversible dementia, usually occurring in older adulthood, characterized by gradual deterioration of memory, disorientation, and other features of dementia.

Biologic age: the anatomic or physiologic age of a person as determined by changes in organismic structure and function; takes into account features such as posture, skin texture, strength, speed, and sensory acuity.

Chronologic age: the actual measure of time elapsed since a person's birth.

Dementia: severe mental deterioration involving impairment of mental ability; organic loss of intellectual function.

Dysphagia: difficulty in swallowing.

Emphysema: pathologic accumulation of air in tissues or organs; general use refers to **chronic pulmonary emphysema,** in which terminal bronchioles become plugged with mucus, the lung and tissue lose elasticity, and breathing difficulties ensue.

Geriatric dentistry: the branch of dentistry that deals with the special knowledge, attitudes, and technical skills required in the provision of oral health care for older adults.

Geriatrics: the branch of medicine that deals with the problems and illnesses of aging and their treatment.

Gerontology: study of the aging process; includes the biologic, psychologic, and sociologic sciences.

Hemostasis: arrest of the escape of blood by either natural (clot formation or vessel spasm) or artificial (compression or ligation) means, or by the interruption of blood flow to a part.

Life expectancy: average number of years that a person can be expected to live; expectancy from birth in 1900 averaged 47 years; in 1996 averaged 76.1 years; expectancy for the female population is about 6 years longer than that for the male population.*

Lifestyle: relatively permanent organization of activities, including work, leisure, and associated social activities, characterizing an individual.

Osteoid: young bone that has not undergone calcification.

Osteopenia: decreased calcification or density of bone; inadequate osteoid synthesis.

Osteoporosis: low bone mass resulting from an excess of bone resorption over bone formation, with resultant bone fragility and increased risk of fracture.

Presbyopia: a condition of farsightedness resulting from a loss of elasticity of the lens of the eye due to aging.

Psychologic age: the age of a person as determined by his or her feelings, attitudes, and life perspective.

Senescence: the process of growing old.

Senility: old age; loss of mental, physical, or emotional control; caused by physical and/or mental deterioration.

*Centers for Disease Control and Prevention: Mortality Patterns—Preliminary Data, United States, 1996, *MMWR, 46,* 941, October 10, 1997.

"aged" (75 years and older), and the "very old" (85 years and older).[1] Biologic age is not synonymous with chronologic age, and, hence, signs of aging appear at different chronologic ages in different individuals. In other words, some people are old at 45 years, whereas others are not old at 75 years.

II. CLASSIFICATION BY FUNCTION

The degree of general health and physical activity provides a workable classification not based on age. Relative to the degree of impairment, older persons may be *functionally independent, frail,* or *functionally dependent.*

Another term for the functionally independent is the *well elderly,* a more descriptive term for the many healthy, active, productive people who happen to be older than what is considered to be a reasonable retirement age.[2]

III. AGING AND DISEASE

Normal changes with aging should not be confused with the effects of pathologic influences that accelerate the aging process. Each age level brings changes in body metabolism, activity of the cells, endocrine balance, and mental processes.

An older person's health status is influenced by many factors. Both biologic and environmental factors influence longevity. Genetically, a person may belong to a family of healthy people who have exhibited great resistance to disease factors. Another person may have inherited a specific disease state. Even inherited diseases, for example, diabetes or sickle cell anemia, may be controllable through treatment or genetic counseling.

■ CHANGES WITH AGING

Changes with aging vary among individuals and among organs and tissues of the same individual. In a healthy person, free of chronic diseases and medications with their potential side effects, the tissue changes of aging are more subtle, appear at a later age, and definitely can be influenced by the person's lifestyle.

- Over the years, the risk factors of smoking, poor diet, lack of exercise, and obesity take their toll.
- Helping people to learn early in life the health maintenance procedures that prevent the development of chronic illnesses and disabilities is a responsibility of all health-care personnel.
- During aging, an overall gradual reduction in functional capacities occurs in most organs, with a decrease in cell metabolism and numbers of active cells.
- The tissues may show signs of dehydration, atrophy, fibrosis, reduced elasticity, and diminished reparative ability.
- Many of these characteristics cannot be separated from pathologic changes.

A. Increased Susceptibility to Infection[3]

With aging, an increased susceptibility to infection may be related to one or more of the following:
1. Lowered capacity in cell-mediated and humoral immunity and nonspecific host defenses.
2. Altered skin and mucosal barriers. In the oral cavity, the flora of the mucosa can be changed, especially when systemic conditions or medications lead to xerostomia.

3. Interaction of nutritional factors with underlying chronic conditions.
4. Decreased immunologic functioning of aging is a factor in increased susceptibility of both men and women to HIV infection and AIDS.[4]

B. Response to Disease

1. *Course and Severity:* Although the diseases that affect the elderly person also occur in younger persons, the course and effects of the diseases may differ. In the elderly person, disease may occur with greater severity and have a longer course, with slower recovery.
2. *Pain Sensitivity:* May be lessened.
3. *Temperature Response:* May be altered so that a patient may be very ill without the expected increase in body temperature.
4. *Healing*
   a. Decreased healing capacity.
   b. More prone to secondary infection.

■ SYSTEMS CHANGES AND DISORDERS

A. Cardiovascular System

Effects of aging on the cardiovascular system include the following:
1. Tendency toward increased blood pressure usually secondary to disease.
2. Arteriosclerosis, with decreased circulation to the tissues.
3. Reduced cardiac output; increased heart size.
4. Postural hypotension, with dizziness or weakness when sitting up from recumbent position.

B. Pulmonary Disorders

1. Vital capacity is progressively diminished.
2. Decreased pulmonary efficiency may be related to lifestyle and lack of exercise.
3. Chronic obstructive pulmonary diseases (COPD): chronic bronchitis and emphysema are of particular concern for the longtime smoker.
4. Pneumonia and influenza.
5. Inactive tuberculosis.

C. Musculoskeletal System

1. *Skeletal Integrity:* Significantly influenced by an insufficient intake of calcium, phosphorus, and fluoride.
2. *Bone Volume (Mass):* Decreases gradually after the age of 40, depending on diet, nutrition, and exercise.
3. *Osteoporosis:* Common in individuals older than age 60, and the incidence increases with age.

4. *Loss of Muscle Function:* Development of unsteadiness and tremor, diminishing of muscular strength, and decreased speed of response. Posture may become stooped; joints may stiffen as a result of loss of elasticity in the ligaments.
5. *Osteoarthritis:* A major cause of disability, it affects the weight-bearing joints. Also known as degenerative joint disease.

D. Gastrointestinal System

1. Production of hydrochloric acid and other secretions gradually decreases.
2. Peristalsis is slowed.
3. Evaluation of digestive disorders is complicated by the general indiscriminate use of self-medications.

E. Skin

1. The skin may become thin, wrinkled, and dry, with pigmented spots, loss of tone, and atrophy of the sweat glands.
2. Reduced tolerance to temperature extremes and solar exposure is evident.

F. Special Senses

1. *Vision:* Decline in accommodation and color and depth perception, and difficulty in adapting from light to dark.
2. *Hearing:* Reduced hearing ability, with a loss of sensitivity to high tones.

G. Alcoholism[5,6]

1. *Early-Onset Drinkers:* May have lifetime pattern, with history of trauma, medical problems, hospitalizations, and detoxification.
2. *Late-Onset Drinkers:* Less likely to have chronic illnesses directly related to alcohol abuse; more likely to be living with family than early-onset drinkers.
3. *Related Factors:* Depression, loneliness, lack of social support, and loss of self-image.
4. *Effects of Aging:* Symptoms and effects are similar to younger people; aging people are more vulnerable because of tissue changes and metabolism.

▪ OSTEOPOROSIS

Osteoporosis is a bone disease involving loss of mineral content and bone mass. Although most prominent in postmenopausal women, the condition may also occur at other ages and in men.

I. CAUSES

A. Endocrine: hormonal disturbances; depletion of estrogen after menopause.
B. Calcium deficiency: defective absorption of calcium.

II. RISK FACTORS

Several risk factors have been identified, some of which usually work together. From this list of risk factors, a list of methods for long-term prevention can be derived:
A. Female gender.
B. Caucasian or Asian ethnicity (worldwide, blacks are least affected).
C. Positive family history.
D. Low calcium and vitamin D intake (life-long).
E. Early menopause or early surgical removal of ovaries.
F. Sedentary lifestyle; lack of exercise.
G. Alcohol abuse.
H. Use of corticosteroids.
I. Cigarette smoking.
J. High caffeine intake.

III. RELATION TO PERIODONTAL DISEASE[7,8]

A. Relationship exists between the reduced bone mineral density of osteoporosis and oral bone loss in skeletal and mandibular bone; oral bone loss pertains to periodontal bone destruction and residual ridge loss in the edentulous person.
B. Osteoporosis and periodontal disease have mutual risk factors. Included are smoking, nutritional deficiencies, alcohol use, hormonal status, and others from the above list of risk factors for osteoporosis.
C. Osteoporotic bone is less dense and more readily absorbed; periodontal pathogenic microorganisms can provide the toxic products for increased periodontal breakdown.
D. Osteoporosis can be considered a risk factor for periodontal bone loss.

IV. SYMPTOMS

A. Asymptomatic Period

Osteoporosis develops over many years; therefore, a long asymptomatic period of bone change occurs with no clinical symptoms.

B. Clinical Symptoms

1. Backache: stooping of the posture.
2. Fractures: hip, spine, ends of long bones.

3. Evidence of bone changes in the mandible: residual ridge resorption.

V. TREATMENT

A. Medications[9]

1. Decrease bone resorption: estrogen; calcium and vitamin D.
2. Increase bone formation: sodium fluoride.

B. Activity

1. Activity and exercise require caution and preventive measures to avoid accidental falls.
2. Severe involvement of the spine may require orthopedic support and medication for pain. Questions regarding the patient's medical history can elicit factors of importance.

C. Behavioral

Avoid smoking and excessive alcoholic intake.

■ ALZHEIMER'S DISEASE

Alzheimer's disease is one of the nonreversible types of dementia. Dementia is severe impairment of the intellectual abilities, notably thinking, memory, and personality. At least one half of the patients with dementia have Alzheimer's disease.

I. SYMPTOMS

The common impairments of Alzheimer's disease may be divided into three or four overlapping stages that may extend over many years. In Table 49-1, characteristics are divided into early, middle, advanced, and terminal stages.

II. APPOINTMENT CONSIDERATIONS

During the early stages, perhaps even before a diagnosis of Alzheimer's disease has been made, the patient will be attending routine dental and dental hygiene appointments.

A. Early Stages

An early sign of the disease may be a slow decline of interest in oral hygiene and personal care. Review of the patient's medical and dental history at each maintenance appointment may reveal lapses in memory and other items listed under the "Early Stage" in Table 49-1. An opportunity may be found to help a patient seek professional evaluation and care.

■ TABLE 49-1 COMMON IMPAIRMENTS ASSOCIATED WITH ALZHEIMER'S DISEASE

EARLY STAGE

Forgetfulness
Personality changes
Employment performance difficulty
Social withdrawal
Apathy
Errors in judgment
Inattentiveness
Personal hygiene neglect

MIDDLE STAGE

Disorientation
Loss of coordination
Restlessness/anxiety
Language difficulty
Sleep pattern disturbance
Progressive memory loss
Catastrophic reactions
Pacing

ADVANCED STAGE

Profound comprehension difficulty
Gait disturbances
Bladder and bowel incontinence
Hyperoralia
Inability to recognize family members
Seizures
Aggression
Lack of insight into deficits

TERMINAL STAGE

Physical immobility
Contractures
Dysphagia
Emaciation
Mutism
Pathologic reflexes
Unawareness of environment
Total helplessness

(From Fabiszewski, K.J.: Caring for the Alzheimer's Patient, *Gerodontology,* 6, 53, Summer, 1987, © Beech Hill Enterprises, Inc. Used by permission.)

B. Later Stages

Later stages may require that the patient reside in a long-term care facility. Dental hygienists in specialized facilities develop particular techniques for the variety of patients to be served.

■ ORAL FINDINGS IN AGING

As mentioned earlier in this chapter, changes related to aging must be separated from the long-term effects of chronic diseases.

I. SOFT TISSUES

A. Lips

1. *Tissue Changes.* Dry, purse-string opening results from dehydration and loss of elasticity within the tissues.
2. *Angular Cheilitis.*[10] Angular cheilitis is not specifically an age-related lesion, but it frequently is seen among elderly persons. It appears as skin folds with fissuring at the angles of the mouth and can be related to reduced vertical dimension or inadequate support of the lips. Primary etiologic factors are candidiasis and vitamin B deficiency.

B. Oral Mucosa

Degenerative changes take several forms. The surface texture is affected by changes in lubrication of the tissue with decreased secretion of the salivary and mucous glands. Xerostomia is not a result of aging but is associated with certain diseases and medications.

1. *Atrophic Changes.* The tissue may become thinner and less vascular, with a loss of elasticity. Clinically, the smooth shiny appearance is related to thinning of the epithelium.
2. *Hyperkeratosis.* White, patchy areas may develop as a result of irritation from sharp edges of broken teeth, restorations, or dentures, and from use of tobacco.
3. *Capillary Fragility.* Facial bruises and petechiae of the mucosa are common.

C. Tongue

1. *Atrophic Glossitis (Burning Tongue).* The tongue appears smooth, shiny, and bald, with atrophied papillae. The condition is related to anemia that results from a deficiency of iron or combinations of deficiencies. Elderly people have deficiency anemias more frequently than do those in other age groups because of nutritional factors, but not because of aging specifically.
2. *Taste Sensations.* Taste buds are not reduced in number. Taste may be reduced or abnormal taste reactions may occur, primarily in people with a disease condition, but changes are not routinely observed in the healthy elderly person.
3. *Sublingual Varicosities*
   a. Clinical appearance: Deep, red or bluish nodular dilated vessels on either side of the midline on the ventral surface of the tongue.
   b. Significance: Although frequently occurring, these varicosities do not necessarily have a direct relation to systemic conditions.

D. Xerostomia

Dryness of the mouth is found frequently in older people in conjunction with pathologic states, drug-induced changes, or radiation-induced degeneration of the salivary glands. Healthy people continue to have normal salivary flow.[11]

II. TEETH

A. Color

The teeth may show color changes from long use of tobacco or foods with coloring agents, such as tea or coffee. Dark intrinsic stains from dental restorations may be evident.

B. Attrition

The teeth of elderly people frequently show signs of wear, which may be the long-term effects of diet, occupational factors, or bruxism. Attrition may be accompanied by chipping, and teeth may seem more brittle, particularly compared with teeth of young people.

C. Abrasion

Abrasion at the neck of a tooth may be the result of extended use of a hard toothbrush in a horizontal direction with an abrasive dentifrice. With current preventive measures, use of soft-textured brushes, and attention to abrasiveness of dentifrices, future generations will be less likely to exhibit such tooth alterations.

D. Root Caries

1. *Occurrence.* With roots exposed by periodontal infections, an increase in caries of the cementum can result. An increase in caries with age is the result of root exposure, not of age.
2. *Effect of Fluoride.* Adults with longtime residence in a fluoridated community have substantially fewer root carious lesions than in a nonfluoridated community. This is especially true for lifelong residents where there has been natural fluoride in the water.[12]
3. *Rampant Caries.* Sometimes called "retirement caries." A noticeable increase in dental caries may occur after age 65. Factors influencing the development of dental caries include the following:
   a. Xerostomia. Tooth-protection factors of the saliva are missing.
   b. Masticatory abilities. Oral conditions and, possibly, tooth loss make mastication difficult. This leads to changes in food selections.

c. Lifestyle. After retirement, without a daily work schedule, snacking and irregular meal-times may lead to poor food selections and an excessively cariogenic diet.

E. Dental Pulp[13]

Whether pulpal changes can be considered results of aging is questionable. The pulpal changes develop as reactions to dental caries, restorations, bruxism, and other assaults during the elderly person's long life. The changes noted here may be observed at younger ages but are seen more frequently in older people.

1. Narrowing of pulp chambers and root canals; increased deposition of secondary dentin.
2. Progressive deposition of calcified masses (pulp stones or denticles).

III. PERIODONTIUM

A. Clinical Findings

The periodontal tissues reflect the health and disease of the patient over the years. One of the following may apply to any patient.

1. *The Healthy Periodontium.* Healthy tissues that have been maintained over the years may have had a minimum of disease. The radiographs show little if any bone recession, the gingiva are firm, and the appearance is normal in every way. Probing reveals minimal sulcus depth with no bleeding. The teeth are not mobile.
2. *The Patient With Periodontal Infection.* Neglect or omission of preventive measures and therapy over the years may have resulted in a chronic periodontal infection with extension of tissue destruction into the bone, periodontal ligament, and cementum. Loss of attachment, deep periodontal pockets, tooth mobility, and radiographic signs of periodontitis may be present.
3. *The Treated Patient.* Although the patient was subject to periodontal infection, treatment was completed, and the tissues were maintained in health through personal care and professional supervision. The tissues may show the effects of the treated disease, such as scar tissue. Areas of recession with exposed cementum may also be evident. The teeth are not mobile.

B. Tissue Changes Related to Aging

1. *Bone*
   a. Osteoporosis may be present.[7,8]
   b. Depressed vascularity, a reduction in metabolism, and reduced healing power affect bone.

2. *Cementum.* Increased thickness has been demonstrated. In one series of measurements, the average overall thickness of the cementum at 20 years of age was 0.095 mm, whereas cementum from 60-year-old persons measured 0.215 mm.[14]
3. *Gingiva.* Most gingival changes can be traced to the effects of infection or to anatomic factors. For example, gingival recession is common in older individuals. Predisposing factors may be a lack of sufficient attached gingiva or malposition of the teeth.

■ DENTAL HYGIENE CARE

Certain aging patients have physical and sensory limitations, and for those persons, adaptations are needed. It should be appreciated, however, that many members of the elderly population are independent, agile, and healthy people without systemic disease and who are not dependent on medications.

Care for the older patient should be planned in terms of comprehensive, not palliative, treatment. Long-term maintenance for the prevention of oral disease must be the basic objective.

Many elderly people do not seek dental and dental hygiene care except when an emergency arises. A primary reason for the limited attention to professional care may be a lack of perceived need. Other reasons relate to physical and mental disabilities, chronic disease, and physical barriers such as transportation or accessibility of the dental office. Financial resources may be a reason for some people.

I. OFFICE OR CLINIC FACILITIES

Attention to dental office arrangement that eliminates physical barriers is important. An aged person's impaired vision or limited motor control must be considered.

Hazards, such as small rugs, which can slide on polished floors; loose corners of rugs, which can be tripped over; and irregularities in floor levels, can be eliminated.

II. ASSESSMENT

A. Patient History

Preparation of a careful and detailed medical and dental history takes on particular significance.

Suggestions for good communication include the following:

1. Eliminate distracting background music or sounds.

2. Sit facing the patient because hearing may be a problem.
3. Speak slowly and clearly.
4. Be courteous at all times; show respect for age. Do not call the patient by his/her first name unless the patient suggests doing so.

B. Medications

Older patients use more drugs and have more prescriptions, as well as more over-the-counter drugs, than does any other age group. Many have more than one chronic disease or disability requiring medication.

1. *Obtain the Correct List.* Ask the patient to bring in either the bottles that contain the various medications (over-the-counter as well as prescription items) or a written copy of the labels so that a list may be kept in the patient's record. The patient's physician may be the best source for an accurate list.

   The list of medications must be checked at each maintenance appointment. Changes in health status can mean changes in prescriptions.
2. *References for Checking Drugs.* Each practice center or clinic needs current references, such as the *Physician's Desk Reference (PDR), Merck Manual,* and pharmacology textbooks.
3. Review patient's medication to determine:
   a. Potential adverse side effects.
   b. Possible drug interactions with products recommended or used during the appointment.
   c. A clear understanding of the patient's state of health to assure the clinician that the recommended procedure is best for the patient.

C. Need for Antibiotic Premedication

Many conditions that require prophylactic coverage are found fairly frequently in the elderly person.[15] Those with uncontrolled diabetes or those who receive chemotherapeutic or steroid treatments may have an increased susceptibility to infection. When the patient has a prosthetic joint replacement, pacemaker, or a history of other conditions, consultation with the patient's physician is indicated.

D. Vital Signs

Blood pressure determination is recommended for each visit.

E. Intra-Oral and Extra-Oral Examination

The need for careful, periodic examination of the oral mucosa from lips to throat cannot be over-

stressed at any age, but it is especially crucial for the elderly patient because oral cancer occurs with increasing frequency with advancing years. Many, in fact most, oral lesions exist without the patient being aware of them.

For some early surface lesions, biopsy is definitely indicated. For others, a cytologic smear can be prepared as directed by the dentist.

III. PREVENTIVE CARE PLAN

Older patients need to have frequent appointments to maintain their oral health at a high level through supervision on a regular basis. The content of a care plan resembles that for other age groups, and emphasis on bacterial plaque control dominates.

A. Dental Biofilm Control

Biofilm control is described in detail in a subsequent section. Self-care provides the foundation for all preventive measures.

B. Periodontal Care

Treatment includes complete scaling, root debridement, and follow-up to assess need for additional therapy.

C. Dental Caries Control

1. Diet record covering several days.
2. Diet adjustment to eliminate cariogenic foods and make appropriate substitutions.
3. Emphasis on prevention of root caries.
4. Fluoride therapy by use of daily self-applied preparations of dentifrice, rinse, or brush-on gel as needed.

▪ DENTAL BIOFILM CONTROL

I. OBJECTIVES

Basic objectives do not differ from those for younger people: infection must be eliminated and controlled.

Older individuals need to be as interested in their health and appearance as do people of any age. Esthetic deterioration may create emotional distress, and when aging persons feel insecure or depressed, they may lose their interest in personal oral care and diet. Motivation through expression of sincere interest on the part of dental personnel can be an influencing factor in helping the patient to better health.

Certain people fear dentures because they associate them with "old" people. Patients with partial dentures may already have been impressed with the need for preserving the remaining teeth. Here, in the desire to save the teeth, lies the appeal for preventive measures for both the teeth and their supporting structures, and good use should be made of this very real motivating force.

II. APPROACH TO INSTRUCTION

Self-confidence, which may be diminished because of lowering of physical capabilities and emotional satisfaction, must be built up. Major changes required because previous habits were detrimental must be brought about gradually if cooperation is to be expected. A more optimistic attitude is needed about the degree of oral health the elderly patient can be expected to achieve.

III. DENTAL BIOFILM FORMATION

The incidence and severity of periodontal diseases increase with age as an effect of disease accumulation. The extent of periodontal destruction reflects the length of time the tissues have been exposed to disease-producing factors, primarily biofilm microorganisms.

A. Factors Contributing to Accumulation of Biofilm

1. Gingival recession with wide embrasures that result from periodontal destruction provides a larger surface area for biofilm retention.
2. Exposed cementum with areas of abrasion or dental caries at the neck of a tooth can create undercut areas where special adaptation of plaque removal devices is needed.

B. Biofilm Retention and Removal

1. Exposed untreated cementum may hold biofilm more readily than does enamel. A smooth root surface is less likely to hold biofilm, and biofilm removal efforts are more successful.
2. Decreased saliva production reduces or eliminates the cleansing and lubricating effects of saliva.
3. Restorations and prostheses provide a more complex dentition for personal care. Biofilm removal requires more time, patience, and motivation.
4. Deficient restorations may have overhanging margins that provide areas of biofilm retention.
5. Lack of dexterity related to disabling conditions resulting from chronic diseases, such as arthritis and Parkinsonism, makes biofilm removal more difficult.

IV. SPECIFIC RECOMMENDATIONS

A. Selection of Dental Biofilm Removal Devices

1. Use of a power toothbrush may help certain patients with impaired motor function.
2. Adaptations to alter the handle of a manual brush are described on pages 898 to 899.
3. Methods for the care of fixed and removable prostheses are described on pages 471 to 475.

B. Dentifrice Selection

1. Fluoride ingredient mandatory for root caries prevention.
2. Mild abrasive agent to prevent abrasion of root surfaces.
3. Desensitizing ingredient for exposed dentinal tubules.

C. Relief for Xerostomia

1. Recommendations are described on pages 387 to 388.
2. Provide specific instructions for use of a saliva substitute.

D. Motivation and Instruction

Instruction and motivation techniques are applied gradually and regularly at frequent intervals for best results. Suggestions for adaptations of instruction to the physical and personal characteristics of the patient are listed in Table 49-2.

■ DIET AND NUTRITION

I. DIETARY HABITS

A. Nutritional Deficiencies

Dietary and resulting nutritional deficiencies are common in older people. For example, characteristic changes, such as burning tongue, angular cheilitis, and atrophic glossitis, may be related to vitamin B deficiencies.

B. Factors Contributing to Dietary and Nutritional Deficiencies

1. Limited budget.
2. Living alone or eating alone.
3. Not eating regular meals; frequently using non-nutritious snacks and foods for entertaining.
4. Alcoholism.

■ TABLE 49-2 CHARACTERISTICS AFFECTING INSTRUCTION FOR THE GERODONTIC PATIENT

CHARACTERISTIC OF THE GERODONTIC PATIENT	SUGGESTED RELATION TO PATIENT INSTRUCTION
Tendency for introspection; desire for attention	Patience needed in taking time to listen to complaints and accounts of past experiences
Feelings of insecurity Deprivation of physical capabilities Touchy sensitiveness, exaggerated imaginary or real pains, or attitudes of suspicion	Sympathetic understanding needed Build up self-confidence
Resistance to change; tendency to maintain fixed habits	Should not attempt to change all lifelong habits, only detrimental habits
Vision impaired	For the patient who wears prescription eyeglasses, make sure the glasses are worn while instruction is being given Recommend that eyeglasses be worn at home while performing biofilm control procedures
Hearing impaired; loss of sensitivity to higher tones	Speak distinctly in normal voice Look directly at patient while speaking; many are lip readers
Slowing of voluntary responses Slowing of speed of thought asssociations Difficulty in timing sequential events; skills become separate movements Least comfortable when must respond quickly to demanding sequential stimuli Rate of learning changed, ability to learn not changed Changes in speed of vocalization	Make suggestions gradually, over a series of appointments Do not demand learning a completely new procedure; adapt procedure already used Guide patient's demonstration of toothbrushing to prevent embarassment Do not expect perfection; go slowly, anticipate difficulties, give cues and clues Distinguish between slowness of learning and inability to learn
Memory shortened, mainly the result of lack of attention, lack of interest, or more selection of what patient wants to remember	Use motivating factors carefully. Provide written instruction; spoken instructions may be forgotten or misunderstood
Need for personal achievement	Help patient gain sense of accomplishment; commend for any success however minor Never compare the patient's condition with that of other patients

5. Lacking interest in shopping for or preparing food.

6. Acuteness of senses (taste, smell) lowered; may seek highly seasoned or sweetened foods.

7. Tendency to follow food habits of lifetime; ignorant of newer knowledge of food preparation methods and dietary needs.

8. Inadequate masticatory efficiency because of tooth loss or dentures that no longer fit properly.

9. Adverse food selection may result from social embarrassment over inability to chew.

10. Adaptations in eating habits, made to compensate for deficiency, may interfere with adequate digestion and absorption of nutrients.

11. Following dietary fads that provide only a limited and unbalanced diet.

12. Loss of appetite, which may have physiologic, social, or economic causes.

13. Difficulty in swallowing.

II. DIETARY NEEDS OF THE AGED

The nutritional needs of older persons are not different from those of younger persons, except in quantity. Caloric intake must be decreased to control weight. Protein, vitamins, minerals, and water are particularly important for body function, repair, and resistance to disease.

A necessary objective in geriatric nutrition is to retard the progression of diet-induced chronic diseases. Examples of these are atherosclerosis related to high dietary cholesterol, anemias related to iron and folic

Everyday Ethics

Mr. and Mrs. Bracken were among Doc Roberts' first patients when he began his practice almost 30 years ago. They keep a strict 4-month maintenance plan with the dental hygienist. Rosemary, the new hygienist, is looking forward to meeting and treating the Brackens for the first time as she has heard many wonderful things about this lovely elderly couple.

Upon completion of the oral examination with Mrs. Bracken, Rosemary recorded significant dental biofilm retention and evidence of xerostomia. She immediately begins to give the patient detailed homecare instructions and asks for a complete listing of medications Mrs. Bracken is taking for her arthritis, angina, and diabetes. Mrs. Bracken left the appointment confused and upset.

Questions for Consideration

1. Considering that Mrs. Bracken seemed overwhelmed at the end of her appointment, how may Rosemary have erred in her judgment of the patient and the instruction she gave?

2. To ensure the autonomy of Mr. and Mrs. Bracken while acknowledging their longevity in the practice, how should the medical status of these patients be clarified?

3. With an intent to act beneficently toward Mrs. Bracken and improve her oral health, explain several factors that Rosemary needs to assess in the self-care plan she uses.

---

acid deficiencies, and osteoporosis resulting from calcium and fluoride deficiency.

In addition to a better intake of calcium in the diet, fluoride intake over the years is beneficial in the prevention of osteoporosis and fractures of the bones.

III. INSTRUCTION IN DIET AND ORAL HEALTH

A. Dietary Analysis

A 4- or 5-day record of the patient's diet can provide information to guide recommendations to be made. Difficulties in showing the procedure to the patient and obtaining accurate results may seem insurmountable. Inaccuracy of recent memory is a problem with some elderly people, so that even the 24-hour dietary record prepared during the appointment may not be complete.

The first consideration in making recommendations for aging patients is that a well-balanced diet be used with limited amounts of cariogenic foods for dental caries prevention.

B. Motivation

Appeal to the patient is made through personal concerns for the relationships of dietary deficiencies to appearance, lowered resistance to disease, and premature aging, which may inspire the patient to improve daily habits. Educational materials are available to study with, and to give to, the patient.

Factors To Teach The Patient

- To remember to tell the dentist and dental hygienist all changes in personal health, medical care received since the last appointment, and all changes in prescriptions.

- Importance of drinking the fluoridated water when it is available.

- Good suggestions for little gifts for children that won't harm their teeth.

- How dental caries is a transmissible disease. Therefore, why it is urgent to have all cavities restored and dental biofilm cleaned from the teeth every day.

REFERENCES

1. **World Health Organization:** *Planning and Organization of Geriatric Services.* Geneva, World Health Organization, Technical Report Series, Number 548, 1974, p. 11.
2. **Roddy,** J.A.: Dental Needs: The Well Elderly, *DentalHygienistNews,* 3, 13, Fall, 1990.
3. **Terpenning,** M.S. and Bradley, S.F.: Why Aging Leads to Increased Susceptibility to Infection, *Geriatrics,* 46, 77, February, 1991.
4. **Woolery,** W.A.: Occult HIV Infection: Diagnosis and Treatment of Older Patients, *Geriatrics,* 52, 51, November, 1997.
5. **Wartenberg,** A.A. and Nirenberg, T.D.: Alcohol and Other Drug Abuse in Older Patients, in Reichel, W., ed.: *Care of the Elderly: Clinical Aspects of Aging,* 4th ed. Baltimore, Williams & Wilkins, 1995, pp. 133–141.
6. **Gambert,** S.R.: Alcohol Abuse: Medical Effects of Heavy Drinking in Late Life, *Geriatrics,* 52, 30, June, 1997.

7. von Wowern, N., Klausen, B., and Kollerup, G.: Osteoporosis: A Risk Factor in Periodontal Disease, *J. Periodontol.*, *65*, 1134, December, 1994.

8. Wactawski-Wende, J., Grossi, S.G., Trevisan, M., Genco, R.J., Tezal, M., Dunford, R.G., Ho, A.W., Hausmann, E., and Hreshchyshyn, M.M.: The Role of Osteopenia in Oral Bone Loss and Periodontal Disease, *J. Periodontol.*, *67*, 1076, Supplement, October, 1996.

9. Riggs, B.L. and Melton, L.J.: The Prevention and Treatment of Osteoporosis, *N. Engl. J. Med.*, *327*, 620, August 27, 1992.

10. Robinson, H.B.G. and Miller, A.S.: *Colby, Kerr, and Robinson's Color Atlas of Oral Pathology*, 5th ed. Philadelphia, J.B. Lippincott Co., 1990, p. 141.

11. Baum, B.J.: Salivary Gland Fluid Secretion During Aging, *J. Am. Geriatr. Soc.*, *37*, 453, May, 1989.

12. Stamm, J.W., Banting, D.W., and Imrey, P.B.: Adult Root Caries Survey of Two Similar Communities With Contrasting Natural Water Fluoride Levels, *J. Am. Dent. Assoc.*, *120*, 143, February, 1990.

13. Seltzer, S. and Bender, I.B.: *The Dental Pulp. Biologic Considerations in Dental Procedures*, 3rd ed. St. Louis, Ishiyaku EuroAmerica, 1990, pp. 324–348.

14. Zander, H.A. and Hurzeler, B.: Continuous Cementum Apposition, *J. Dent. Res.*, *37*, 1035, November–December, 1958.

15. Felder, R.S., Nardone, D., and Palac, R.: Prevalence of Predisposing Factors for Endocarditis Among an Elderly Institutionalized Population, *Oral Surg. Oral Med. Oral Pathol.*, *73*, 30, January, 1992.

SUGGESTED READINGS

Berkey, D.B., Berg, R.G., Ettinger, R.L., and Mersel, A.: The Old-Old Dental Patient: The Challenge of Clinical Decision-making, *J. Am. Dent. Assoc.*, *127*, 321, March, 1996.

Bryant, S.R., MacEntee, M.I., and Browne, A.: Ethical Issues Encountered by Dentists in the Care of Institutionalized Elders, *Spec. Care Dent.*, *15*, 79, March/April, 1995.

Friedlander, A.H. and Yoshikawa, T.T.: Pathogenesis, Management, and Prevention of Infective Endocarditis in the Elderly Dental Patient, *Oral Surg. Oral Med. Oral Pathol.*, *69*, 177, February, 1990.

Garcia, R.I.: Geriatric Dentistry, in Reichel, W., ed.: *Care of the Elderly: Clinical Aspects of Aging*, 4th ed. Baltimore, Williams & Wilkins, 1995, pp. 451–459.

Hoad-Reddick, G.: Organization, Appointment Planning, and Surgery Design in the Treatment of the Older Patient, *J. Prosthet. Dent.*, *74*, 364, October, 1995.

Kilmartin, C.M.: Managing the Medically Compromised Geriatric Patient, *J. Prosthet. Dent.*, *72*, 492, November, 1994.

Maddox, M.K. and Burns, T.: Positive Approaches to Dementia Care in the Home, *Geriatrics*, *52*, S54, Supplement 2, September, 1997.

Reichel, W. and Rabins, P.V.: Evaluation and Management of the Confused, Disoriented, or Demented Elderly Patient, in Reichel, W., ed.: *Care of the Elderly: Clinical Aspects of Aging*, 4th ed. Baltimore, Williams & Wilkins, 1995, pp. 142–154.

van der Bijl, P.: Therapeutic Considerations in the Gerodontic Patient, *Compend. Cont. Educ. Dent.*, *15*, 478, April, 1994.

Yellowitz, J.A.: Alzheimer's Disease. An Oral Health Care Provider's Perspective, *DentalHygienistNews*, *7*, 10, Fall, 1994.

Oral Health Problems

Loesche, W.J., Bretz, W.A., Grossman, N.S., and Lopatin, D.E.: Dental Findings in Geriatric Populations With Diverse Medical Backgrounds, *Oral Surg. Oral Med. Oral Pathol. Oral Radiol. Endod.*, *80*, 43, July, 1995.

MacEntee, M.I.: How Severe is the Threat of Caries to Old Teeth? *J. Prosthet. Dent.*, *71*, 473, May, 1991.

Niessen, L.C. and Gibson, G.: Aging and Oral Health: Implications for Women, *Compend. Cont. Educ. Dent.*, *14*, 1542, December, 1993.

Shay, K.: Identifying the Needs of the Elderly Dental Patient: The Geriatric Dental Assessment, *Dent. Clin. North Am.*, *38*, 499, July, 1994.

Soon, J.A.: Effects of Drug Therapy on Oral Health of Older Adults, *Can. Dent. Hyg. J. (Probe)*, *26*, 118, Autumn, 1992.

Vissink, A., Spijkervet, F.K.L., and Amerongen, A.V.N.: Aging and Saliva: A Review of the Literature, *Spec. Care Dent.*, *16*, 95, May/June, 1996.

Youngs, G.: Risk Factors for and the Prevention of Root Caries in Older Adults, *Spec. Care Dent.*, *14*, 68, March/April, 1994.

Periodontal Disease

Baelum, V., Luan, W.-M., Chen, X., and Fejerskov, O.: A 10-Year Study of the Progression of Destructive Periodontal Disease in Adult and Elderly Chinese, *J. Periodontol.*, *68*, 1033, November, 1997.

Burt, B.A.: Periodontitis and Aging: Reviewing Recent Evidence, *J. Am. Dent. Assoc.*, *125*, 273, March, 1994.

Carranza, F.A. and Newman, M.G.: *Clinical Periodontology*, 8th ed. Philadelphia, W.B. Saunders Co., 1996, pp. 51–55, 423–426.

Fransson, C., Berglundh, T., and Lindhe, J.: The Effect of Age on the Development of Gingivitis: Clinical, Microbiological, and Histological Findings, *J. Clin. Periodontol.*, *23*, 379, April, 1996.

Klemetti, E., Collin, H.-L., Forss, H., Markkanen, H., and Lassita, V.: Mineral Status of Skeleton and Advanced Periodontal Disease, *J. Clin. Periodontol.*, *21*, 184, March, 1994.

McArthur, W.P., Bloom, C., Taylor, M., Smith, J., Wheeler, T., and Magnusson, N.I.: Antibody Responses to Suspected Periodontal Pathogens in Elderly Subjects With Periodontal Disease, *J. Clin. Periodontol.*, *22*, 842, November, 1995.

Persson, R.E., Persson, G.R., and Robinovitch, M.: Periodontal Conditions in Medically Compromised Elderly Subjects: Assessments of Treatment Needs, *Spec. Care Dent.*, *14*, 9, January/February, 1994.

Wheeler, T.T., McArthur, W.P., Magnusson, I., Marks, R.G., Smith, J., Sarrett, D.C., Bender, B.S., and Clark, W.B.: Modeling the Relationship Between Clinical, Microbiologic, and Immunologic Parameters and Alveolar Bone Levels in an Elderly Population, *J. Periodontol.*, *65*, 68, January, 1994.

Patient Instruction

Doherty, S.A., Ross, A., and Bennett, C.R.: The Oral Hygiene Performance Test: Development and Validation of Dental Dexterity Scale for the Elderly, *Spec. Care Dentist.*, *14*, 144, July/August, 1994.

Felder, R., James, K., Brown, C., Lemon, S., and Reveal, M.: Dexterity Testing as a Predictor of Oral Care Ability, *J. Am. Geriatr. Soc.*, *42*, 1081, October, 1994.

Felder, R., Reveal, M., Lemon, S., and Brown, C.,: Testing Toothbrushing Ability of Elderly Patients, *Spec. Care Dentist.*, *14*, 153, July/August, 1994.

Garry, P.J. and Vellas, B.J.: Aging and Nutrition, in Ziegler, E.E. and Filer, L.J., eds.: *Present Knowledge in Nutrition*, 7th ed. Washington, D.C., ILSI Press, 1996, pp. 414–419.

Ostuni, E. and Mohl, G.: Communicating More Effectively With the Confused or Demented Patient, *Gen. Dent.*, *43*, 264, May–June, 1995.

Shay, K. and Ship, J.A.: The Importance of Oral Health in the Older Patient, *J. Am. Geriatr. Soc.*, *43*, 1414, December, 1995.

Spencer, P.: The Dental Hygienist and the Senior Client, *Can. Dent. Hyg. J. (Probe)*, *31*, 89, May/June, 1997.

Osteoporosis

Dawson-Hughes, B., Harris, S.S., Krall, E.A., and Dallal, G.E.: Effect of Calcium and Vitamin D Supplementation on Bone Density in Men and Women 65 Years of Age or Older, *N. Eng. J. Med., 337,* 670, September 4, 1997.

Hillier, S., Inskip, H., Coggon, D., and Cooper, C.: Water Fluoridation and Osteoporotic Fracture, *Community Dent. Health, 13,* 63, September, 1996.

Jeffcoat, M.K. and Chesnut, C.H.: Systemic Osteoporosis and Oral Bone Loss: Evidence Shows Increased Risk Factors, *J. Am. Dent. Assoc., 124,* 49, November, 1993.

Kanis, J.A.: Treatment of Symptomatic Osteoporosis With Fluoride, *Am. J., Med., 95,* 53S, November 30, 1993.

Loza, J.C., Carpio, L.C., and Dziak, R.: Osteoporosis and Its Relationship to Oral Bone Loss, *Curr. Opin. Periodontol., 3,* 27, 1996.

Pak, C.Y.C., Sakhaee, K., Rubin, C.D., and Zerwekh, J.E.: Sustained-Release Sodium Fluoride in the Management of Established Postmenopausal Osteoporosis, *Am. J. Med. Sci., 313,* 23, January, 1997.

Talbot, L. and Craig, B.J.: Osteoporosis and Alveolar Bone Loss, *Canad. Dent. Hyg. Assoc. (Probe), 32,* 11, January–February, 1998.

Watson, E.L., Katz, R.V., Adelezzi, R., Gift, H.C., and Dunn, S.M.: The Measurement of Mandibular Cortical Bone Height in Osteoporotic vs. Non-osteoporotic Postmenopausal Women, *Spec. Care Dentist., 15,* 124, May/June, 1995.

The Edentulous Patient

Kathryn Ragalis, RDH, MS, DMD

The completely edentulous patient who wears a removable denture needs an appointment at least annually for careful observation of the oral tissues, as well as for supervision of denture biofilm control for the dentures. The edentulous patient with an implant-supported denture requires more frequent appointments. Since the implants are surrounded and supported by gingival tissue and osseointegrated bone, professional care and supervision is more like that required by natural teeth.

For either type of denture, instruction for the patient who receives new dentures for the first time is a special concern. The patient must learn new personal oral health care and apply new dental biofilm control measures to the new prosthesis. The present chapter is concerned primarily with the traditional type of removable denture. Terminology related to dentures and the edentulous patient is defined in Box 50-1.

Various combinations are found among denture wearers. A patient may have a single complete denture and natural teeth in the opposing dental arch. There may be a complete denture for one arch and natural teeth and a partial fixed or removable denture in the other arch.

Of the completely edentulous population, particularly in the older age groups, some individuals have dentures they do not wear, others have full dentures but wear only one of them, and still others have no dentures. When there is a single denture, more frequently the maxillary denture is worn. It is not unusual to find that the same dentures have been worn for many years without having the dentures or the supporting oral tissues examined.

Dentures occasionally must be constructed to replace primary teeth. The teeth may be congenitally missing (anodontia) or may have required extraction because of rampant caries or trauma. Early childhood

BOX 50-1 KEY WORDS: Edentulous Patient*

Anodontia: congenital absence of all teeth, primary and permanent.

Complete denture prosthodontics: that body of knowledge and skills pertaining to the restoration of the edentulous arch with a removable prosthesis.

Denture: an artificial substitute for missing natural teeth and adjacent tissues.

Complete denture: a removable dental prosthesis that replaces the entire dentition and associated structures of the maxilla or mandible.

Denture adhesive: a material used to adhere a denture to the oral mucosa; over-the-counter product that can be misused without professional instruction.

Denture characterization: modification of the form and color of the denture base and teeth to produce a more lifelike appearance.

Denture placement: the process of directing a prosthesis to a desired oral location; introduction of a prosthesis into a patient's mouth; other terms used are denture delivery or denture insertion.

Immediate denture: a complete denture fabricated for placement immediately following the removal of the natural teeth and/or other surgical preparation of the dental arches.

Implant prosthesis: any prosthesis that utilizes dental implants in part or whole for retention, support, and stability; the prosthesis may be a complete denture.

Overdenture: a removable denture that covers and is partially supported by one or more remaining natural teeth, roots, and/or dental implants and the soft tissue of the residual alveolar ridge; also called overlay denture.

Prosthesis: an artificial replacement of an absent part of the human body.

Dental prosthesis: artificial replacement of one or more teeth and/or associated structures.

Resection: excision of a segment of any part; removal of articular ends of one or both bones forming a joint.

*Definitions are taken from or adapted from and in harmony with the *Glossary of Prosthodontic Terms,* 7th ed., 1999, from the Academy of Prosthodontics Foundation.

dental caries can result in severe breakdown of the teeth soon after eruption.

To provide esthetics and function, dentures can be constructed for the accepting child who is able to cooperate. As the permanent teeth begin to erupt, parts of the denture are cut away (Figure 50-1). A supervised caries prevention program is initiated for protection of the permanent dentition.

■ TYPES OF REMOVABLE COMPLETE DENTURES[1]

A. **Tissue-Supported Complete Denture:** a removable dental prosthesis that replaces the entire dentition and associated structures of the maxilla or the mandible and rests on the mucosal-covered alveolar ridge.

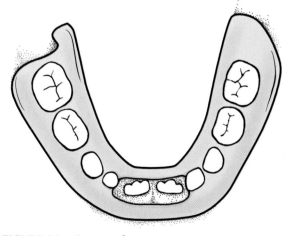

■ **FIGURE 50-1 Denture for a Young Child.** As permanent teeth erupt, parts of the denture are cut away. Shown is the denture alteration for the erupting permanent mandibular incisors.

B. **Implant-Supported Complete Denture:** a dental prosthesis supported by one or more dental implants.

C. **Overdenture:** a prosthesis that covers and is partially supported by remaining natural teeth, tooth roots, and/or dental implants (Figure 29-8, page 482).

D. **Provisional or Interim Prosthesis:** a transitional prosthesis that provides protection, stabilization, and function prior to the fabrication of a definitive prosthesis. It may also be used as a diagnostic device, for function during a healing process, or as a training prosthesis for an apprehensive patient. Originally serving as a transitional partial denture, artificial teeth may be added as natural teeth are removed. The definitive denture can be completed after postextraction tissue changes have occurred.

E. **Immediate Denture:** a denture fabricated for placement immediately following the removal of the natural teeth. An immediate or interim denture tends to loosen after the significant remodeling of bone and soft tissue that follows extractions. Temporarily, the denture may be relined with a soft liner or a tissue conditioning material. The patient may use a denture adhesive until the majority of healing occurs. After approximately 6 months, dentures are remade, relined, or rebased.

▪ THE EDENTULOUS MOUTH

I. BONE

A. Residual Ridges

- After the teeth are removed, the residual ridges enter into a continuing process of remodeling.
- The alveolar bone, which had supported the teeth, undergoes resorption. The rate and amount of bony resorption vary with each individual.
- Major bony changes occur during the first year after the teeth are removed, but changes continue throughout life.
- Mandibular bone loss is generally as much as four times greater than maxillary bone loss.[2]
- Bone remodeling and soft tissue healing usually make it necessary to have dentures rebased, relined, or remade at intervals.

B. Tori

The tori that may interfere with dentures are benign bony outgrowths. Because of the size, shape, or location, a torus often must be removed surgically before a denture can be constructed.

1. *Torus Palatinus.* Bony enlargement located over the midline of the palate.
2. *Torus Mandibularis.* Bony mass(es) generally located on the lingual side in the region of the premolars.

II. MUCOUS MEMBRANE

A. Composition: Mucosa

- Oral mucosa is composed of masticatory, lining, and specialized mucosa.
- *Masticatory* mucosa covers the edentulous ridges and the hard palate. The mucous membrane covering the bony ridges is made up of two layers, the lamina propria and the surface-stratified squamous epithelium, which is keratinized in the healthy mouth.
- *Lining* mucosa covers the floor of the mouth, vestibules, and cheeks.

B. Composition: Submucosa

- Underneath the mucous membrane is the submucosa, which is attached to the underlying bone.
- Composed of connective tissue with vessels, nerves, adipose tissue, and glands.
- The support or cushioning effect for the denture depends on the makeup of the submucosa, which varies in different parts of the mouth.

C. Tension Test

- Examine the edentulous mouth by retracting the lips and cheeks using a tension test technique.
- A line of demarcation similar to the mucogingival junction is apparent, separating the attached tissue over the bony ridge and the loose lining mucosa of the vestibule.
- Frenal attachments can be observed readily.

▪ THE PATIENT WITH NEW DENTURES

I. PATIENT COUNSELING

A. Preparation

- The preparation for denture insertion has to begin well in advance of the day the dentures are delivered.
- Becoming edentulous may be very emotional for a patient and requires great effort to learn to adapt and function with the new prosthesis.

- Anticipatory guidance will help the patient gain a clear idea of what to expect and what procedures to follow.
- Successful after-care and denture satisfaction depend to a large extent on conditioning the patient to the adjustments to be made and to the period of practice and learning with the new dentures that can be expected.

B. Adjuncts

Many dental teams prepare their own printed educational materials, whereas others use those available from outside sources.

II. POSTINSERTION CARE

The preliminary counseling is followed through the initial postinsertion appointments to adjust the prosthesis, teach denture hygiene, and arrange for continuing maintenance appointments.

A. Immediate Denture

- The patient is instructed to leave the immediate denture in place for 24 to 48 hours after extractions to aid in the control of bleeding and swelling.
- When the patient returns and the denture is removed, the mouth is rinsed and appropriate instructions are given.
- After initial healing, the denture care and other instructions are similar to those presented in Table 50-1.

B. New Dentures Over Healed Ridges

1. *Appointments*
   - Following insertion, adjustment appointments are scheduled routinely because adjustments can be expected.
   - The first appointment is made within 48 hours of the time of insertion, and additional appointments are made in accord with individual needs.
2. *Instructions*[3]
   - Too many instructions given on the day of insertion may confuse the patient; limit instruction to basic denture care and other procedures of immediate concern.
   - Slow repetition over several periods helps the patient to develop adequate denture management and hygiene habits.
   - Basic information for the new denture wearer is provided in Table 50-1.

- Denture cleaning methods are described with other biofilm control procedures for the care of dental prostheses on pages 477 to 480.

▪ DENTURE-RELATED ORAL CHANGES

The condition of the mucous membranes, salivary glands, and alveolar bone is influenced by dietary and nutritional deficiencies, age, and various chronic diseases. Tissue alterations for an older patient are described on page 830. Some of the denture-related changes are listed here.

I. BONE CHANGES

A. **Alveolar Ridge Remodeling** may lead to:
   - Loss of denture support.
   - Loss of facial height and lip support.
   - Increased prominence of the chin.
   - Temporomandibular joint manifestations.
   - Occlusal disharmony.
B. **Compensations by the Patient**
   - Patients may adapt to the bone changes by making compensating adjustments in the way they wear and manage the dentures.
   - Other patients may resort to drugstore remedies, such as pads, adhesives, or self-reline materials, which can be detrimental if used improperly.
   - Denture adhesives should never be used to compensate for a poorly designed, poorly constructed, or ill-fitting denture.
C. **Treatment by the Dentist**
   - Dentures need adjusting, repairing, relining, rebasing, or remaking periodically.
   - Patient should be instructed to seek care if any issues relating to denture or oral health arise between scheduled maintenance visits.

II. ORAL MUCOSA

A. Tissue Reaction

- Tissue under a denture varies considerably among individuals.
- One mouth may have thinning of the mucosa, submucosa, and, particularly, the epithelium with an absence of keratinization, and another may have normal keratinization or hyperkeratinization.

▪ TABLE 50-1 PATIENT INSTRUCTION FOR COMPLETE DENTURES

ITEM	FACTORS TO TEACH

Food selection	Use foods from the Food Guide Pyramid (page 523, Figure 32-1)
	Check each day's diet to fulfill needs for a balanced diet
	Older patients: use foods to prevent diet-induced chronic diseases
	New denture wearer:
	  Avoid foods that need incising
	  Avoid raw vegetables, fibrous meats, and sticky foods until experience has been gained
	  Cut food into small pieces
	Practiced denture wearer:
	  Select a variety of foods, but do not expect the same efficiency as with the natural teeth

Incision or biting	Use the canine and premolar area. Insert for biting at the angle of the mouth. Push back as the food is incised; do not pull or tear the food in a forward direction
Chewing	Take small portions Try to chew with some food on each side at the same time to stabilize the denture Be patient and practice
Salivary flow	Anticipate an increased flow of saliva when a new denture is worn
Speaking	Speak slowly and quietly Practice by reading aloud at home, preferably in front of a mirror Repeat and practice words that seem the most difficult
Sneezing, coughing, yawning	Anticipate loss of denture retention Cover mouth with hand and handkerchief
Denture hygiene	Thoroughly clean dentures at least twice each day Immerse dentures in chemical solution and brush for biofilm removal. Rinse thoroughly Complete denture care is described on pages 477 to 480 Devices to aid a disabled person are shown on page 901 and Figure 53-12
Mucosa	Tissues need to rest each day; consult dentist regarding whether it is best to leave the denture out while sleeping Brush and massage the mucosa to clean away biofilm and debris and stimulate circulation
Storage of dentures	After careful cleaning to remove all bacterial biofilm, store the denture in water (or cleaning solution) in a covered container Place in a safe place inaccessible to children or house pets Change water or cleaning solution daily and wash the container
Over-the-counter products	Never attempt to alter the denture for relief of discomfort Do not buy and use self-reline materials, adhesives, or other additives without consulting the dentist. They may be harmful to the dentures and/or the oral tissues Consult the dentist for advice about all denture problems
Maintenance	Understand the importance of the dentist's examination of the denture fit, occlusion, wear, and the condition of the oral mucosa First year: expect reline, rebase, or remake of dentures because bone remodeling is greatest during the first year Subsequent appointments: an examination each year for most patients, provided the denture hygiene is ideal; other patients in the cancer-susceptible category need an examination every 3 months
Seek care	Report any concerns, changes, or problems immediately Dentures may need adjustments to correct occlusion or traumatic sore spots

B. Factors That Influence the Mucosa

- Systemic conditions that alter host response.
- Aging, mucosa tends to become thinner.
- Denture and tissue hygiene.
- Wearing the denture constantly.
- Xerostomia.
- Fit and occlusion of the denture itself.

III. EFFECT OF XEROSTOMIA

The causes of xerostomia are described on page 387. Diminished salivary flow can influence denture retention and tissue lubrication, as well as reduce the resistance of the oral mucosa to trauma and infection.

A. Lubrication

The oral mucosa needs saliva for protection against frictional irritation by the denture.

B. Retention

The film of saliva between the denture and the mucosa contributes to retention and suction of the denture.

IV. SENSORY CHANGES

A. Tactile Sense

- With the dentures in place, sensitivity may be diminished to small objects in the mouth, such as small bones or bits of nut shells.
- Proprioception from the periodontal ligaments that aid, for example, in knowing how hard to chew and when to stop biting, is lost.

B. Taste

- Patients occasionally indicate that since they have been wearing dentures food has a different taste.
- Taste buds that are located in the tongue papillae are not affected by the dentures.
- Taste buds of the palate are covered by the maxillary denture and therefore are ineffective for taste and temperature perception.
- Denture hygiene must be meticulous to ensure that the denture does not develop thick odoriferous biofilm, which may alter food flavors.

▪ DENTURE-INDUCED ORAL LESIONS

When the mouth is examined extraorally and intraorally, the dentures are removed and the mucosa is examined carefully and thoroughly.

- A patient may tell of an area that has been sensitive and thus helpfully call attention to a specific visible lesion.
- A patient may be unaware of chronic mucosal lesions, which are often asymptomatic.
- Because tissue changes can be important indicators of serious disease, such as oral cancer, the intraoral examination must be conducted thoroughly with good illumination.

I. PRINCIPAL CAUSES OF LESIONS UNDER DENTURES

The factors that singly or in combination cause most oral lesions under dentures are ill-fit of the dentures, inadequate oral hygiene, infection, trauma, and wearing the dentures all the time, without relief for the tissues.

A. Ill-Fitting Dentures

- Because tissue changes under dentures occur gradually over a long period, the patient may not be aware of developing disease.
- The patient may not realize or may not have been informed of the importance of having regular professional examinations of the dentures and the oral mucosa.

B. Inadequate Oral Hygiene

- Dentures and the oral mucosa need daily care.
- Neglected dentures can accumulate heavy biofilm and calculus that may irritate the mucosa and cause infection and inflammation.

C. Continuous Wearing of Dentures

- Dentures need to be removed for a part of every 24 hours so that the mucosa can have a rest from the pressure of the hard acrylic during occlusion, bruxism, and clenching.
- A rest period allows the tissue to recover in its natural environment, where the tongue and saliva provide a cleansing effect.

II. INFLAMMATORY LESIONS

A. Contributing Factors

The following may occur singly or in combination.
- Denture trauma from the fit, occlusion, or parafunctional habits.
- Inadequate denture hygiene and care of the mucosa.
- Chemotoxic effect from residual cleansing paste or solution not thoroughly rinsed from the denture.

- Allergy to the denture base (rare).
- Continuous denture wearing without relief for the tissues.
- Patient self-treatment with over-the-counter products for relining.
- Systemic influence on the tolerance of the tissues to trauma and lowered resistance to infection; for example, vitamin and other nutritional deficiencies and immunosuppressant therapy, such as chemotherapy.

B. Localized Inflammation (Sore Spots)

1. *Appearance.* Isolated, red, inflamed area, sometimes ulcerated.
2. *Contributing Factors.* Trauma from an ill-fitting denture, a rough spot on a denture surface, a tongue bite, or a foreign object caught under the denture.

C. Generalized Inflammation

1. *Other Names.* "Denture sore mouth," "denture stomatitis."
2. *Appearance.* Generalized redness over the tissues that support the denture. The patient may have pain and a burning sensation; occurs more frequently in the maxilla.

D. Candida albicans Infection[4]

C. albicans is a customary member of the oral flora of people with or without teeth. In denture stomatitis, or in recognizable candidiasis, the numbers of the yeast-like fungus increase. Conditions that promote *C. albicans* overgrowth include:
- Depression of immune system by disease or medications.
- Radiation therapy.
- Prolonged antibiotic therapy.

III. ULCERATIVE LESIONS

- Localized ulcer-shaped lesions usually are related to an overextended denture border.
- The ulcer may resemble a cancerous lesion and should be biopsied if it persists longer than expected of a healing traumatic ulcer (7–14 days).

IV. PAPILLARY HYPERPLASIA[5]

A. Appearance

Papillary hyperplasia is located on the palate, rarely outside the confines of the bony ridges (Figure 50-2). The overall lesion appears as a group of closely arranged, pebble-shaped, red, edematous projections.

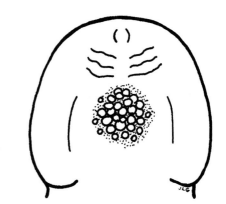

■ **FIGURE 50-2 Papillary Hyperplasia.** Outline of an edentulous palate shows the characteristic location of papillary hyperplasia within the bony ridges.

B. Contributing Factors

The cause is unknown but it is associated with poor denture hygiene, ill-fitting dentures, and possible *Candida albicans* infection.

V. DENTURE IRRITATION HYPERPLASIA (EPULIS FISSURATUM)[5]

Long-standing chronic inflammatory tissue appears in single or multiple elongated folds related to the border of an ill-fitting denture.

VI. ANGULAR CHEILITIS[6]

A. Appearance

- Fissuring at the angles of the mouth, with cracks, ulcerations, and erythema.
- Moist with saliva or sometimes dry with a crust.

B. Contributing Factors

- Lack of support of the commissure because of overclosure from loss of vertical dimension of occlusion and by moistness from drooling.
- Secondarily, a riboflavin deficiency or an infection by *Candida albicans* or other organisms may be involved.
- Prescription antifungal medication may be indicated.

▪ PREVENTION

I. DENTURE HYGIENE

- Dentures must be cleaned after each meal.
- Cleansing solutions must be changed daily.

II. ORAL MUCOSA

- Brush to clean and massage.
- Perform digital massage.

III. REST FOR THE TISSUES

- Having the dentures out while sleeping may be the best procedure to provide rest for the oral tissues for many patients. However, the potential for damage to the temporomandibular joint from lack of support needs checking.
- Daytime for as long as a period as possible, such as while bathing.
- Place dentures in a container with cleaning solution when out of the mouth.
- Clean and massage the underlying mucosa.

IV. DIET AND NUTRITION

- Teaching of food selection cannot be overemphasized.
- Emphasis on foods from the basic food groups as shown in the pyramid (Figure 32-1) is necessary.
- Control of weight and avoidance of foods that are related to specific chronic conditions are important.
- A dietary analysis can provide a foundation for making specific recommendations.
- Diet problems of the elderly patient have been described on pages 833 to 835. Factors that contribute to dietary deficiencies in patients of any age are magnified when dentures are ill-fitting or painful and masticatory efficiency is decreased. The patient tends to overlook food value and to select foods that are within the limits of chewing ability or that can be swallowed without chewing.
- Learning to adapt to an initial denture may affect nutrition. Patient should be instructed to attempt small amounts of a soft diet to relearn to chew.

V. RELIEF FROM XEROSTOMIA

The use of a saliva substitute may be recommended.

VI. DENTAL CARIES CONTROL FOR OVERDENTURE WEARERS

- Meticulous denture hygiene and dental biofilm control for the natural teeth are mandatory.
- Care of the overdenture is described on pages 481 to 482.
- Fluoride dentifrice is used while brushing the teeth. Daily fluoride application is made by placing gel drops inside the overdenture.

■ MAINTENANCE

I. APPOINTMENT FREQUENCY

A. First Year

After the initial adjustments, the patient can expect the dentures to need reline, rebase, or remake in 6 months to 1 year.

B. Subsequent Maintenance Period

1. For most patients, one appointment each year may be adequate.
2. For patients who are careless with denture and tissue care, at least two appointments each year are recommended.
3. For patients who are at high cancer risk because of age, tobacco use, and alcohol-drinking habits or who have a previous history of cancer, examination three to four times per year should be scheduled.
4. Patients should be informed to seek an appointment at any time if discomfort or concerns arise with the denture or any tissue area.

II. MAINTENANCE APPOINTMENT

Maintenance procedures are followed with necessary adaptations for the edentulous patient.

A. Procedures

1. Review patient history; make necessary additions to the record.
2. Determine blood pressure.
3. Perform an extraoral and intraoral examination.
4. Examine dentures for cleanliness and evidence of patient care.
5. Ask patient to demonstrate the personal hygiene care procedures used routinely.
6. Supplement with additional demonstration and instruction when the care is less than adequate.
7. Clean the dentures to remove calculus and stain.

B. Procedures for the Dentist

- Review the complete assessment.
- Examine the oral tissues and the fit and occlusion of the dentures.
- Treat as needed.

C. Subsequent Appointment

- Make necessary appointments for continuing current treatment and for maintenance.

- All tissues must be examined at least annually for oral cancer screening and any other changes indicative of oral or systemic disease.

▪ DENTURE MARKING FOR IDENTIFICATION[7]

The need for denture marking is apparent in a variety of situations. A universal system for marking would be ideal. Marking is required by law in some countries and in most states of the United States. In forensic dentistry, or for identification of victims of war, such disasters as flood or fire, or transportation catastrophes, the dentition has been used increasingly as a means of identification.

Dentures provide a method for immediate identification. Prompt identification can be urgent when an individual is found unconscious from illness or injury or is suffering from amnesia as a result of psychiatric or traumatic causes, as well as from Alzheimer's disease.

The dentures of people in long-term residence or care facilities must be marked. Mislaid dentures can be returned, and mix-ups by the direct care staff can be prevented. An important contribution to an oral health program is to introduce a plan for denture marking.

I. CRITERIA FOR AN ADEQUATE MARKING SYSTEM

Information on the denture must be specific so that rapid identification is possible.

A. Relative to the Denture

1. Must have no adverse effects on denture material.
2. Must not change the strength, surface texture, or fit of the denture.
3. Must be cosmetically acceptable; the label must be placed in an unobtrusive position.

B. Relative to the Procedure

1. Readily learned and simple to carry out.
2. Inexpensive.
3. Durable result. When the information is incorporated during denture processing, indefinite durability can be expected. A surface marker for a denture already in use should be able to withstand denture cleaning methods for a reasonable period of time.

C. Characteristics of the Material Used

1. *Fire and Humidity Resistant.* When the label is placed inside the posterior section of a denture, the surrounding tongue and maxillofacial parts offer protection except in the most severe conflagration.
2. *Radiopaque.* A metal marker can be of use as a means of identification by radiographic examination in the event the radiolucent acrylic denture is accidentally swallowed.

II. INCLUSION METHODS FOR MARKING

A. New Dentures

- A typewritten or printed enclosure is inserted as a denture is being processed.
- Labels are positioned on the impression surfaces of the maxillary and mandibular dentures (Figure 50-3).
- Cover label, just before the final closure of the flask, with a clear acrylic material.
- A label may be typewritten on onionskin paper or the tissue paper that separates sheets of packaged baseplate wax.[7,8]
- Another system uses a thin metal strip for the insert. Stainless steel matrix bands, orthodontic bands, and thin metal strips (shim stock) have been used.[9]
- *Microchip* can be incorporated for denture marking because of the small size, aesthetic acceptability, forensic identification qualities, and information they can contain. They have a higher cost than other methods.[10]
- *Copper vapour laser* has been used to mark dentures with metal frameworks, removable partial dentures, and other metallic restorations.[11]

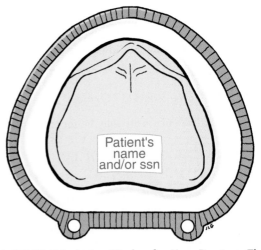

▪ **FIGURE 50-3 Inclusion Marker for New Denture.** The label is inserted on the impression surface as the denture is being processed. In the flasked maxillary denture shown, the marker is positioned near the posterior border.

Everyday Ethics

Mr. Ryan presents for his yearly denture examination and oral cancer screening. He faithfully keeps his appointment every year because the cigarette stains build up on his full upper and lower dentures and he likes the way his dental hygienist, Kaitlin, gets them very clean.

During this visit, Kaitlin notices a small area on the alveolar ridge under the denture near the area of tooth #29. Mr. Ryan is aware of the lesion and sometimes doesn't wear his lower denture, but he indicates that it doesn't really bother him. Kaitlin informs Mr. Ryan that she will get the dentist to check the area. Mr. Ryan becomes annoyed at her concern. He just wants to have his denture cleaned and to leave.

Questions for Consideration

1. Since Mr. Ryan has been a heavy smoker for over 40 years, what actions are indicated to document and evaluate the lesion?

2. What are Kaitlin's 'obligations' to the patient in communicating the possible serious nature of her findings?

3. What can be done if Mr. Ryan leaves the office without having the lesion evaluated?

B. Existing Dentures[12]

1. Clean the dentures thoroughly.
2. Use a No. 6 or 8 round bur and an inverted cone to cut small, shallow, box-like preparations in the posterior buccal flange of the maxillary denture and the lingual posterior flange of the mandibular denture (Figure 50-4). Do not go through to the impression surface.
3. Typewrite two copies of the patient's name (or other choice of identification) on onionskin paper, and trim the papers to fit the box-like preparations.

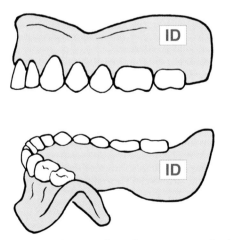

■ **FIGURE 50-4 Surface Markers for Dentures.** The labels are placed on the external denture surfaces for existing dentures. As shown, the markers are on the maxillary buccal flange and the mandibular lingual flange.

4. Cover the paper with cold-cure clear acrylic and fill to a slight excess; after the acrylic has cured, polish to a smooth finish.

III. SURFACE MARKERS

Surface markers are not as durable, but instruction can be provided for persons not trained in dental laboratory methods. In a skilled nursing facility or other long-term institution that has no resident dentist or dental hygienist, it may be possible to teach a nurse or other staff member to mark dentures of residents as they are admitted. The methods described as follows have been used for this purpose.

A. Indelible Pen or Ballpoint

• After cleaning and drying the denture, a small area near the posterior of the outer or polished denture surface is rubbed with an emery board until it is rough (Figure 50-4).
• Name, initials, or other identification is printed on the roughened area with an indelible pen and dried.
• Two or three coats of a fingernail acrylic (heavy nail protector) are painted over the area; each layer is dried before applying the next.
• Surface markings have been found to last at least 6 months.[13]
• Light-cured materials may also be used.[14,15]

B. Engraving Tool

An engraving tool is used to enter the name on the denture, and the grooves created are darkened with a special pencil before a sealing liquid is applied. Materials are available in a commercial kit.[16]

✔️ **Factors To Teach The Patient**

- Dentures are not permanent prostheses.

- Dentures and tissues must be examined at least once a year for care of the tissue-supported removable prosthesis; for the implant-supported prosthesis, more frequently. Teach frequency of maintenance appointments for the individual, depending in part on that individual's ability to clean the dentures and maintain them free of biofilm, stain, and calculus.

- Dentures may need replacement periodically. Tissues under the denture change.

- Avoid use of drugstore remedies, reliners, and other home-applied materials unless the dentist has provided specific instruction.

- Specific methods of care for dentures.

- Leaving the dentures out of the mouth overnight in accord with the dentist's directions.

- Where to obtain and how to use a saliva substitute.

IV. INFORMATION TO INCLUDE ON A MARKER

- For residents of a home or institution, using only the person's name and initials should suffice for temporary surface marking.
- In a community, country, or international situation, the name alone would not provide enough identification, and the social security number, armed services serial number, or the equivalent in other countries should be included.
- Other identification, such as blood type and vital drug or disease condition, has been suggested.
- In certain countries, the dentist's registration or hospital number has been used. In Sweden, the patient's date of birth and national registration number have been marked on the dentures.
- Markings that can provide *immediate* identification are the most significant.

REFERENCES

1. **Academy of Prosthodontics Foundation:** The Glossary of Prosthodontic Terms, 7th ed, *J. Prosthet. Dent., 81,* 39, January, 1999.
2. **Tallgren,** A.: The Continuing Reduction of the Residual Alveolar Ridges in Complete Denture Wearers: A Mixed-Longitudinal Study Covering 25 Years, *J. Prosthet. Dent., 27,* 120, February, 1972.

3. **Gallagher,** J.B.: Insertion and Postinsertion Care, in Clark, J.W., ed.: *Clinical Dentistry,* Volume 5, Revised Edition—1984. Philadelphia, J.B. Lippincott Co., Chapter 14, pp. 1–27.
4. **Iacopino,** A.M. and Wathen, W.F.: Oral Candidal Infection and Denture Stomatitis: A Comprehensive Review, *J. Am. Dent. Assoc., 123,* 46, January, 1992.
5. **Robinson,** H.B.G. and Miller, A.S.: *Color Atlas of Oral Pathology,* 5th ed. Philadelphia, J.B. Lippincott, 1990, pp. 94–95.
6. **Robinson** and Miller: op. cit., p. 141.
7. **American Dental Association,** Council on Prosthetic Services and Dental Laboratory Relations: *Techniques for Denture Identification.* Chicago, American Dental Association, 1984, 12 pp.
8. **Dentsply International, Inc.:** *Method for Placing Permanent Record Data in Denture Base Without Affecting Tissue Adaptation,* Technical Bulletin, Dentsply International, Inc., York, PA 17404.
9. **Turner,** C.H., Fletcher, A.M., and Ritchie, G.M.: Denture Marking and Human Identification, *Br. Dent. J., 141,* 114, August 17, 1976.
10. **Rajan,** M. and Julian, R.: A New Method of Marking Dentures Using Microchips, *J. Forensic Odontostomatol., 20,* 1, June, 2002.
11. **Ling,** B.C., Nambiar, P., Low, K.S., and Lee, C.K.: Copper Vapour Laser ID Labelling on Metal Dentures and Restorations, *J. Forensic Odontostomatol., 21,* 17, June, 2003.
12. **Bauer,** T.L.: Technique for Denture Identification, *J. Indiana Dent. Assoc., 58,* 28, Number 6, 1979.
13. **Deb,** A.K. and Heath, M.R.: Marking Dentures in Geriatric Institutions. The Relevance and Appropriate Methods, *Br. Dent. J., 146,* 282, May 1, 1979.
14. **Richards,** E.E., Williams, J.E., and Gauthier, G.: A Modified Light-Cured Denture Identification Technique, *Spec. Care Dentist., 12,* 81, March/April, 1992.
15. **Lamb,** D.J.: A Simple Method for Permanent Identification of Dentures, *J. Prosthet. Dent., 67,* 894, June, 1992.
16. **Identure,** Geri, Inc., P.O. Box 9086, North St. Paul, MN 55109.

SUGGESTED READINGS

Anttila, S.S., Knuuttila, M.L., and Sakki, T.K.: Relationship of Depressive Symptoms to Edentulousness, Dental Health, and Dental Health Behavior, *Acta. Odontol. Scand., 59,* 406, December, 2001.
Cordioli, G., Majzoub, Z., and Castagna, S.: Mandibular Overdentures Anchored to Single Implants: A Five-year Prospective Study, *J. Prosthet. Dent., 78,* 159, August, 1997.
Douglass, C.W., Shih, A., and Ostry, L.: Will There Be a Need for Complete Dentures in the United States in 2020?, *J. Prosthet. Dent., 87,* 5, January, 2002.
Fiske, J., Davis, D.M., and Horrocks, P.: A Self-help Group for Complete Denture Wearers, *Br. Dent. J., 178,* 18, January 7, 1995.
Jones, J.A., Orner, M.B., Spiro, A., 3rd, and Dressin, N.R.: Tooth Loss and Dentures: Patients' Perspectives, *Int. Dent. J., 53,* 327, Supplement 5, 2003.
Joshipura, K.J., Willett, W.C., and Douglass, C.W.: The Impact of Edentulousness on Food and Nutrient Intake, *J. Am. Dent. Assoc., 127,* 459, April, 1996.
Kulak, Y., Arikan, A., and Delibalta, N.: Comparison of Three Different Treatment Methods for Generalized Denture Stomatitis, *J. Prosthet. Dent., 72,* 283, September, 1994.
Ramos, V., Giebink, D.L., Fisher, J.G., and Christensen, L.C.: Complete Dentures for a Child With Hypohidrotic Ectodermal Dysplasia: A Clinical Report, *J. Prosthet. Dent., 74,* 329, October, 1995.
Sebring, N.G., Guckes, A.D., Li, S.-H., and McCarthy, G.R.: Nutritional Adequacy of Reported Intake of Edentulous Subjects Treated With New Conventional or Implant-Supported Mandibular Dentures, *J. Prosthet. Dent., 74,* 358, October, 1995.

Assessment

Allen, C.M.: Diagnosing and Managing Oral Candidiasis, *J. Am. Dent. Assoc., 123,* 77, January, 1992.

Ansari, I.H.: Panoramic Radiographic Examination of Edentulous Jaws, *Quintessence Int., 28,* 23, January, 1997.

Guggenheimer, J. and Hoffman, R.D.: The Importance of Screening Edentulous Patients for Oral Cancer, *J. Prosthet. Dent., 72,* 141, August, 1994.

Kogon, S.L., Stephens, R.G., and Bohay, R.N.: An Analysis of the Scientific Basis for the Radiographic Guideline for New Edentulous Patients, *Oral Surg. Oral Med. Oral Pathol. Oral Radiol. Endod., 83,* 619, May, 1997.

Moltzer, G., van der Meulen, M.J., and Verheij, H.: Psychological Characteristics of Dissatisfied Denture Patients, *Community Dent. Oral Epidemiol., 24,* 52, February, 1996.

Denture Hygiene and Microbiology

Blair, Y., Bagg, J., MacFarlane, T.W., and Chestnutt, I.: Microbiological Assessment of Denture Hygiene Among Patients in Longstay and Daycare Community Places, *Community Dent. Oral Epidemiol., 23,* 100, April, 1995.

Danser, M.M., van Winkelhoff, A.J., and van der Velden, U.: Periodontal Bacteria Colonizing Oral Mucous Membranes in Edentulous Patients Wearing Dental Implants, *J. Periodontol., 68,* 209, March, 1997.

Danser, M.M., Van Winkelhoff, A.J., De Graaff, J., and van der Velden, U.: Putative Periodontal Pathogens Colonizing Oral Mucous Membranes in Denture-Wearing Subjects With a Past History of Periodontitis, *J. Clin. Periodontol., 22,* 854, November, 1995.

Kulak, Y., Arikan, A., and Kazazoglu, E.: Existence of *Candida albicans* and Microorganisms in Denture Stomatitis Patients, *J. Oral Rehabil., 24,* 788, October, 1997.

Marsh, P.D., Percival, R.S., and Challacombe, S.J.: The Influence of Denture-Wearing and Age on the Oral Microflora, *J. Dent. Res., 71,* 1374, July, 1992.

Radford, D.R. and Radford, J.R.: A SEM Study of Denture Plaque and Oral Mucosa of Denture-Related Stomatitis, *J. Dent., 21,* 87, April, 1993.

Adhesives, Materials

Granström, G.: Upper Airway Obstruction Caused by a Do-It-Yourself Denture Reliner, *J. Prosthet. Dent., 63,* 495, May, 1990.

Grasso, J.E.: Denture Adhesives: Changing Attitudes, *J. Am. Dent. Assoc., 127,* 90, January, 1996.

Jagger, D.C. and Harrison, A.: Denture Fixatives—An Update for General Dental Practice, *Br. Dent. J., 180,* 311, April 20, 1996.

Jagger, D.C. and Harrison, A.: Complete Dentures—The Soft Option: An Update for General Dental Practice, *Br. Dent. J., 182,* 313, April 26, 1997.

Kelsey, C.C., Lang, B.R., and Wang, R.-F.: Examining Patients' Responses About the Effectiveness of Five Denture Adhesive Pastes, *J. Am. Dent. Assoc., 128,* 1532, November, 1997.

Shay, K.: Denture Adhesives: Choosing the Right Powders and Pastes, *J. Am. Dent. Assoc., 122,* 70, January, 1991.

Tassarotti, B.: A Clinical and Histologic Evaluation of a Conditioning Material, *J. Prosthet. Dent., 28,* 13, July, 1972.

Waters, M.G.J., Williams, D.W., Jagger, R.G., and Lewis, M.A.O.: Adherence of *Candida albicans* to Experimental Denture Soft Lining Materials, *J. Prosthet. Dent., 77,* 306, March, 1997.

Denture Identification

Berry, F.A., Logan, G.I., Plata, R., and Riegel, R.: A Postfabrication Technique for Identification of Prosthetic Devices, *J. Prosthet. Dent., 73,* 341, April, 1995.

Borrman, H.I., DiZinno, J.A., Wasen, J., and Rene, N.: On Denture Marking, *J. Forensic Odontostomatol., 17,* 20, June, 2002.

Coss, P. and Wolfaardt, J.F.: Denture Identification System, *J. Prosthet. Dent., 74,* 551, November, 1995.

Cunningham, M. and Hoad-Reddick, G.: Attitudes to Identification of Dentures: The Patients' Perspective, *Quintessence Int., 24,* 267, April, 1993.

Goshima, T., Gettleman, L., Goshima, Y., and Yamamoto, A.: Evaluation of Radiopaque Denture Liner, *Oral Surg. Oral Med. Oral Pathol., 74,* 379, September, 1992.

Milward, P.J., Shepherd, J.P., and Brickley, M.R.: Automatic Identification of Dental Appliances, *Br. Dent. J., 182,* 171, March 8, 1997.

The Oral and Maxillofacial Surgery Patient

Oral and maxillofacial surgery is the specialty of dentistry that includes the diagnostic, surgical, and adjunctive treatment of diseases, injuries, and defects involving both the functional and the aesthetic aspects of the hard and soft tissues of the oral and maxillofacial regions.[1] Box 51-1 lists types of treatment included in this specialty, with examples.

The practice of an oral surgeon may be primarily in a group clinical setting, in a hospital, or in a private office with outpatient hospital facilities available. With the oral surgeon is a team of specially trained individuals that might include surgical assistants, anesthetists, registered nurses, and dental hygienists. Terminology that relates to maxillofacial surgery is defined in Box 51-2.

The surgeon is involved with various dental practitioners, including general dentists and specialists. Maxillofacial surgery can be programmed, for example, with prosthodontists, orthodontists, implantologists, and specialists caring for any of the patients suggested by the list in Box 51-1.

Surgery for treatment of diseases and correction of defects of the periodontal tissues is categorized specifically as *periodontal surgery*. Within the scope of periodontal surgery are procedures for pocket elimination, gingivoplasty, treatment of furcation involvements, correction of mucogingival defects, treatment for bony defects about the teeth, and placing implants. Preparation for periodontal surgery is not specifically described in this chapter.

BOX 51-1 Categories of Oral and Maxillofacial Treatments

DENTOALVEOLAR SURGERY

Exodontics

Impacted tooth removal

Alveolar bone surgery: alveoloplasty

INFECTION

Abscesses

Osteomyelitis

TRAUMATIC INJURY

Fractures of jaws, zygoma

Fracture of teeth, alveolar bone

NEOPLASM

Cysts

Tumors

DENTAL IMPLANT PLACEMENT

PREPROSTHETIC RECONSTRUCTION

Maxillofacial prosthetics

Immediate denture

ORTHOGNATHIC SURGERY

Prognathism correction

Facial aesthetics

CLEFT LIP/PALATE

TEMPOROMANDIBULAR DISORDERS (TMD)

SALIVARY GLAND OBSTRUCTION

■ PATIENT PREPARATION

I. OBJECTIVES

Dental hygiene care and instruction prior to oral and maxillofacial surgery may contribute to the patient's health and well-being by one or more of the following:

A. Reduce Oral Bacterial Count

1. Aid in the preparation of an aseptic field for the surgery.
2. Make postsurgical infection less likely or less severe.

B. Reduce Inflammation of the Gingiva and Improve Tissue Tone

1. Lessen local bleeding at the time of the surgery.
2. Promote postsurgical healing.

C. Remove Calculus Deposits

1. Remove a source of dental biofilm retention and thus improve gingival tissue tone.
2. Prevent interference with placement of surgical instruments.
3. Prevent pieces of calculus from breaking away.
   a. Danger of inhalation, particularly when a general anesthetic is used.
   b. Possibility of calculus falling into a socket or other surgical area and acting as a foreign body to inhibit healing.

D. Instruct in Presurgical Personal Oral Care Procedures

Such instruction contributes to reducing inflammation and thus improves tissue tone and helps to prepare the patient for postsurgical care.

E. Instruct in the Use of Foods

The patient should be instructed about foods that provide the elements essential to tissue building and repair during pre- and postsurgical periods.

For the patient who will have teeth removed and immediate complete or partial dentures inserted, the importance of a diet containing all essential food groups should be emphasized.

F. Interpret the Dentist's Directions

Explanation should be given for the immediate presurgical preparation with respect to rest and dietary limitations, particularly when a general anesthetic is to be administered.

G. Motivate the Patient Who Will Have Teeth Remaining

The patient who will have teeth remaining after surgery should be motivated to prevent further tooth loss through routine dental and dental hygiene professional care and personal oral care procedures.

II. PERSONAL FACTORS

The extent of the surgery to be performed and previous experiences affect the patient's attitude. Many patients who are in the greatest need of presurgical dental hygiene care and instruction may be people who have neglected their mouths for many years. They have been indifferent to or unaware of the importance of obtaining adequate care. Their only visits to a dentist may have been to have a toothache relieved. Their knowledge of preventive measures may be limited. A few possible characteristics are suggested here.

BOX 51-2 KEY WORDS: Oral and Maxillofacial Surgery

Comminution: act of breaking or condition of being broken into small fragments.

Ecchymosis: a hemorrhagic spot, larger than a petechia, in the skin or mucous membrane caused by extravasation of blood; forms a nonelevated, rounded, or irregular purplish patch.

Exodontics: branch of dentistry dealing with the surgical removal of teeth.

Exostosis: benign new growth projecting from the surface of bone.

Intermaxillary fixation: fixation of the maxilla in occlusion with the mandible held in place by means of wires and elastic bands; the healing parts are stabilized following fracture or surgery.

Maxillofacial: pertaining to the jaws and the face.

Maxillofacial prosthetics: the branch of prosthodontics concerned with the restoration of the mouth and jaws and associated facial structures that have been affected by disease, injury, surgery, or a congenital defect.

Orthognathic surgery: surgery to alter relationships of the dental arches and/or supporting bone; usually coordinated with orthodontic therapy.

Orthognathics: science dealing with the causes and treatment of malposition of the bones of the jaws.

Osteosynthesis: internal fixation of a fracture by mechanical means, such as metal plates, pins, or screws.

> **Miniplate osteosynthesis:** a method of internal fixation of mandibular fractures utilizing miniaturized metal plates and screws formerly made of titanium or stainless steel and currently made primarily of biodegradable or resorbable synthetic materials.

Trismus: motor disturbance of the trigeminal nerve with spasm of masticatory muscles and difficulty in opening the mouth (lockjaw).

A. Apprehensive and Fearful

1. Apprehensive and indifferent toward need for personal care of teeth.
2. Fearful of all dental procedures, particularly oral surgery and anesthesia.
3. Fearful of cancer or other disease.
4. Fearful of personal appearance after surgery.

B. Impatient

When teeth have caused discomfort and pain, the patient may have difficulty understanding the need for delay while oral hygiene procedures are accomplished.

C. Resigned

Feeling of inevitableness of the situation; lack of appreciation for natural teeth.

D. Discouraged

Over tooth loss or development of soft tissue lesions.

E. Resentful

1. Toward time lost from work.
2. Toward the financial aspects of dental care.
3. Toward inconvenience and discomfort.

▪ DENTAL HYGIENE CARE

A review of the patient's record shows preliminary procedures that need to be completed. For example, a thorough intraoral and extraoral examination, a recording of vital signs, photographs, and additional radiographs may be required. The patient's medical and dental history reveals essential information relative to the need for prophylactic antibiotics or other precautions.

I. PRESURGERY TREATMENT PLANNING

The pending date for the surgery and the patient's attitude may limit the time to be spent.

A. First Appointment

1. Develop rapport; explain purposes of presurgical appointments.

2. Explain and demonstrate dental biofilm control principles. Demonstrate appropriate technique using new soft toothbrush.
3. Present initial dietary information (pages 522 to 524).
4. Perform scaling to prepare for tissue healing.
5. Give postappointment instruction for rinsing with basic saline or with chlorhexidine 0.12% for tissue conditioning.

B. Second Appointment

1. Observe gingival tissue response; apply disclosing agent. Review disease control procedures. Introduce the use of dental floss or other interdental aids when applicable.
2. Continue the dietary instruction. Present diet recommendations (pages 528 to 535).
3. Complete or continue the scaling. More than two appointments may be needed for patients who will have surgery for oral cancer or who have a cardiovascular or other condition for which all periodontal and dental treatment must be completed before surgery. When radiation or chemotherapy will be used following surgery for oral cancer, or when a prosthetic heart valve or total joint replacement will be involved, complete oral care is described on page 869.

II. PATIENT INSTRUCTION

A. Dental Biofilm Control

1. *Brush.* Soft.
2. *Technique.* For a patient who may not have practiced careful brushing on a regular plan, a simple brushing technique is preferred. Time for establishing habits may be limited until postsurgical healing is complete. Use of disclosing agent for the patient's own evaluation can be motivating.

B. Auxiliary Procedures

Removal of dental biofilm from proximal tooth surfaces and care of fixed and removable prostheses are included in instruction. The patient who is to have multiple extractions for the placement of an immediate denture or other prosthesis, such as an obturator following cleft palate, tumor, or other surgery, needs postsurgical instruction for the specific care of the prosthesis.

III. INSTRUMENTATION

A. Scaling

1. *Problems*
   a. Teeth with large carious lesions.
   b. Mobile teeth.

c. Edentulous areas.
d. Sensitive, enlarged gingival tissue that bleeds readily.
2. *Suggestions for Procedure*
   a. Provide preprocedural antimicrobial rinse to lessen bacteremia and aerosol contamination.
   b. Use local anesthetic.
   c. Maintain a clear field, using evacuation techniques.
   d. Use alternate finger rests to adapt to mobile teeth or edentulous areas; stabilize mobile teeth during scaling strokes.
   e. Ultrasonic scaling may be the technique of choice; high-power evacuation is essential.

B. Stain Removal

1. *Contraindications*
   a. Enlarged, inflamed, sensitive gingiva.
   b. Deep pockets.
   c. Profuse hemorrhage.
2. *Effects*
   a. Irritation to tissue by polishing abrasive and action of rubber polishing cup.
   b. Abrasive particles forced into the gingival tissues by movement of rubber cup.

C. Rinsing Instruction

1. *Objectives.* To promote tissue healing following scaling and to remove debris; to initiate the habit of rinsing for postsurgical care later.
2. *Rinsing Solution.* Warm, mild, hypertonic salt solution.
3. *Frequency.* Recommended for several times each day after the surgical procedure.

D. Follow-up Evaluation

Scaling and planing should be planned for a few weeks after oral surgery. Emphasis must be placed on review and redemonstration of personal daily care.

IV. PATIENT INSTRUCTION: DIET SELECTION

The nutritional state can influence the resistance to infection and wound healing, as well as general recovery powers. Nutritional deficiencies can occur because of the inability to ingest adequate nutrients orally.

Specific recommendations of what to include and not to include in the diet should be given to the patient. Postsurgical suggestions may differ from presurgical; for example, when difficulty in chewing is a postsurgical problem, a liquid or soft diet may be required. When major oral surgery requires hospitalization, tube feeding may be used during the initial healing period. Tube feeding is described on page 861.

A. Nutritional and Dietary Needs

Diets outlined are designed to include the essential foods from the Food Guide Pyramid (Figure 32-1).

1. *Essential for Promotion of Healing.* Protein and vitamins, particularly vitamin A, vitamin C, and riboflavin.

2. *Essential for Building Gingival Tissue Resistance.* A varied diet that includes adequate portions of all essential food groups.

3. *Essential for Dental Caries Prevention.* Noncariogenic foods. When a patient has not been able to masticate properly, the diet employed frequently may have included many soft and cariogenic foods.

B. Suggestions for Instruction

1. Provide instruction sheets that show specific pre- and postsurgery meal plans. Foods for liquid and soft diets are listed on page 861.

2. Express nutritional needs in terms of quantity or servings of foods so that the patient clearly understands.

3. For the patient who will receive dentures, careful instruction must be provided over a period of time. Information for the patient with new dentures is described on page 840 and in Table 50-1.

   When the patient loses the teeth because of dental caries, the diet has likely been highly cariogenic. Emphasis should be placed on helping the patient include nutritious foods for the general health of the body and, more specifically, the health of the alveolar processes, which will support the dentures.

V. PRESURGICAL INSTRUCTIONS[2]

At the appointment just prior to the oral surgery appointment, instructions relative to the surgical procedure should be discussed with the patient. The objective is to let the patient know what to expect so that full cooperation is possible. The patient may have concerns about the anesthesia, the surgical procedure, and the outcome.

A. Explain the general procedures for anesthesia and surgery.

B. Provide printed instructions concerning the following:

   1. *Food and Liquid Intake.* Specify the number of hours before the time of the surgery when the patient stops further intake of food and fluids.

   2. *Alcohol and Medication Restrictions.* Certain medications, supplements, and alcohol are not compatible with the anesthetic and drugs to be used during and following the surgical procedure. The patient is instructed to discontinue use.

   3. *Transport to and From the Appointment.* When a general anesthetic or light sedation is used, the patient must not drive. Plans for someone to accompany and assist the patient should be made.

   4. *The Night Before the Appointment.* In addition to food and alcohol restrictions, a good night's rest is advocated.

   5. *Personal Items*
      a. Clothing. The clothing worn should be loose and comfortable. The sleeves should be easily drawn up over the elbows for taking blood pressure.
      b. Care of contact lenses and prostheses. The patient will be asked to remove prostheses, and may be asked to remove contact lenses, so needs to bring containers for their safe keeping.

VI. POSTSURGICAL CARE

A. Immediate Instructions

Printed postsurgical instructions are provided following all oral procedures. The prepared material is reviewed with the patient after surgery. Specific details vary, but basic information for postsurgical instruction sheets includes the following:

1. *Control Bleeding.* Keep the sponge in the mouth over the surgical area for 1/2 hour; then discard it. When bleeding persists at home, place a gauze pad or cold wet teabag over the area and bite firmly for 30 minutes.

2. *Rinsing.* Do not rinse for 24 hours after the surgical appointment. Then use warm salt water (1/2 teaspoonful salt in 1/2 cup [4 ounces] of warm water) after toothbrushing and every 2 hours.

3. *Dental Biofilm Control.* Brush the teeth and floss more than usual. Avoid the surgery site.

4. *Rest.* Get plenty of rest; at least 8 to 10 hours of sleep each night. Avoid strenuous exercise during the first 24 hours, and keep the mouth from excessive movement.

5. *Diet.* Use a liquid or soft diet high in protein. Drink water and fruit juices freely. Avoid foods that require excessive chewing or are acidic.

6. *Pain.* If needed, use a pain-relieving preparation prescribed by the dentist. Adhere to directions.

7. *Icepack.* Following a flap procedure or when swelling is likely to occur, apply icepack (ice cubes in a plastic bag) for 15 minutes followed by 15 minutes off, or apply for 15 minutes after 30 minutes off, as directed by the dentist. Heat is not used for swelling.

8. *Complications.* Include the telephone number to call after office hours, should complications arise; complications may include uncontrollable pain, marked bleeding, temperature rise, difficulty in opening the mouth, or unusual swelling a few days after the surgery.

B. Follow-up Care

The dental hygienist may participate in suture removal, irrigation of sockets, and other postsurgical procedures when the patient returns. Appropriately, instruction concerning biofilm control, rinsing, oral irrigation, and other personal care, as well as diet supervision, can be continued.

■ PATIENT WITH INTERMAXILLARY FIXATION

The limited access for personal oral care procedures and the effect of the liquid diet required for most cases define the need for special dental hygiene care for the patient with intermaxillary fixation. Attention to rehabilitation of the oral tissues during the period following the removal of appliances takes on particular significance lest permanent tissue damage result or inadequate oral care habits be continued indefinitely.

Descriptions in this section are related to a fractured jaw, but intermaxillary fixation is required for a variety of corrective surgeries and other conditions, including temporomandibular joint treatment and reconstructive and orthognathic surgeries. Regardless of the reason for intermaxillary fixation, instructions for dental hygiene care (pages 860 to 862) are similar, and the patient's problems are much the same.

■ FRACTURED JAW

The patient with a fractured jaw may be hospitalized. A dental hygienist employed in a hospital would be called upon to assume a part of the responsibility for patient care or to give oral hygiene instruction to direct-care personnel. After dismissal from the hospital, the patient may require special attention in the private dental office for a long period of time.

Treatment of a fractured jaw may be complex, and the patient may suffer considerably, both physically and mentally. Some basic knowledge of the nature of fractures and their treatment is helpful in understanding the patient's needs.

I. CAUSES OF FRACTURED JAWS

A. Traumatic

Interpersonal violence, sporting injuries, falls, road traffic accidents (including bicycles), and industrial accidents.

B. Predisposing

Pathologic conditions, such as tumors, cysts, osteoporosis, or osteomyelitis, weaken the bone; thus, slight trauma or even tooth removal can cause fracture.

II. EMERGENCY CARE

- Immediate attention must be paid to measures for care of the patient's general condition.
- Emergency care is given for airway, breathing, and circulation ("A-B-C-D," Figure 66-4, page 1100).
- Hemorrhage, shock, and skull or internal head injuries are next in the sequence of concern.
- Almost any category of emergency care may be required (Tables 66-4 and 66-5).
- Although treatment for the fractured jaw must not be postponed for any great length of time, its immediate care takes second place to the vital aspects of patient care.
- Tetanus prophylaxis may be indicated as soon as medical treatment is available.

III. RECOGNITION

A. History

Except for a pathologic fracture, a history of trauma should be available.

B. Clinical Signs

- Pain, especially on movement, and tenderness on slight pressure over the area of the fracture.
- Teeth may be displaced, fractured, or mobile. Because of muscle pull or contraction, segments of the bones may be displaced, and the occlusion of the teeth may be irregular.
- Muscle spasm is a common finding, particularly when the fracture is at the angle or ramus of the mandible.
- Crepitation can be heard if the parts of bone are moved.
- Soft tissue in the area of the fracture may show laceration and bleeding, discoloration (ecchymosis), and enlargement.

IV. TYPES OF FRACTURES

A fracture is classified by using a combination of descriptive words for its *location, direction, nature,* and *severity.* Fractures may be single or multiple, bilateral or unilateral, complete or incomplete.

A. Classification by Nature of the Fracture (Figure 51-1)

1. *Simple.* Has no communication with outside.
2. *Compound.* Has communication with outside.
3. *Comminuted.* Shattered.
4. *Incomplete.* "Greenstick" fracture has one side of a bone broken and the other side bent. It occurs in incompletely calcified bones (young children, usually). The fibers tend to bend rather than break.

B. Mandibular (described by location)

1. Alveolar process.
2. Condyle.
3. Angle.
4. Body.
5. Symphysis.

C. Midfacial

1. *Alveolar Process.* The alveolar process fracture does not extend to the midline of the palate.
2. *Le Fort.*[3] The Le Fort classification is used widely to identify the three general levels of maxillary fractures, as shown in Figure 51-2.

- Le Fort I is a horizontal fracture line above the roots of the teeth, above the palate, across the maxillary sinus, below the zygomatic process, and across the pterygoid plates.
- *Le Fort II.* The midface fracture extends over the middle of the nose, down the medial wall of the orbits, across the infraorbital rims, and posteriorly, across the pterygoid plates.
- *Le Fort III.* The high-level craniofacial fracture extends transversely across the bridge of the nose, across the orbits and the zygomatic arches, and across the pterygoid plates.

V. TREATMENT OF FRACTURES[4,5]

Each fracture differs from the next, and the methods used in treatment vary with the individual case.

A. Treatment Planning

Many factors are involved when the oral surgeon selects the methods to be used, particularly the location of the fracture or fractures, the presence or absence of teeth, existing injuries to the teeth, other head injuries, and the general health and condition of the patient. All fractures do not require active intervention. Examples are fractures of the condylar and coronoid processes, nondisplaced fractures of an edentulous mandible, and greenstick fractures of children.

Basic treatment consists of *reduction* (open or closed) of the fracture, *fixation* of the fragments, and *immobi-*

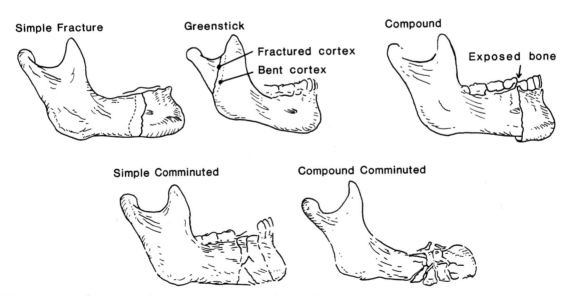

■ **FIGURE 51-1 Types of Fractures.** (From Kruger, G.O.: *Textbook of Oral and Maxillofacial Surgery,* 6th ed. St. Louis, Mosby, 1984.)

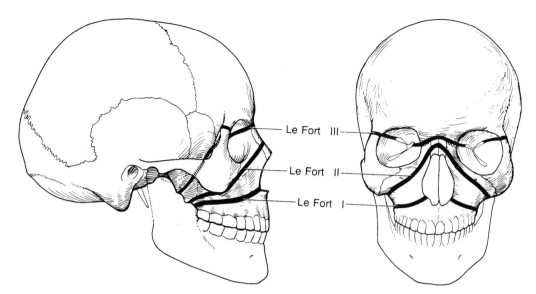

■ **FIGURE 51-2 Le Fort Classification of Facial Fractures.** *Le Fort I,* horizontal fracture above the roots of the teeth, below the zygomatic process, and across the pterygoid plates. *Le Fort II,* midface fracture over the middle of the nose and across the intraorbital rims. *Le Fort III,* transversely across the bridge of the nose, across the orbits and the zygomatic bone. (From Archer, W.H.: *Oral and Maxillofacial Surgery,* 5th ed. Philadelphia, W.B. Saunders Co., 1975; from Committee on Trauma, American College of Surgeons: *Early Care of the Injured Patient.* Philadelphia, W.B. Saunders Co., 1972.)

lization for healing. Control of complications of treatment centers around prevention of infections, malunion of the parts, and malocclusion of the dentition.

B. Healing

Union is affected by the location and character of the fracture. Much depends on the patient's general health and resistance, as well as on cooperation. Six weeks is considered the average for the uncomplicated mandibular fracture, and 4 to 6 weeks for the maxillary. The major cause of complication is infection.

■ MANDIBULAR FRACTURES

Reduction means the positioning of the parts on either side of the fracture so they are in apposition for healing and restoration of function.

- *Open reduction* refers to the use of a surgical flap procedure to expose the fracture ends and bring them together for healing.
- *Closed reduction* is accomplished by manipulation of the parts without surgery.

I. CLOSED REDUCTION

- The closure of the teeth in normal occlusion for the individual is the usual guide for position of the fracture parts in the dentulous patient.

- To identify the customary relation of the teeth can be difficult, especially in the partially edentulous mouth.

II. INTERMAXILLARY FIXATION (IMF)

After reduction, a method of fixation and then immobilization that has been used for many years is *intermaxillary fixation*. It still is indicated under certain circumstances and in certain parts of the world.

A. Description

- Intermaxillary fixation is accomplished by applying wires and/or elastic bands between the maxillary and mandibular arches (Figure 51-3).
- *Arch bars.* Ready-made, contoured arch bars are adapted to fit accurately to each tooth and provide hooks for connecting the arches (Figure 51-3C). A small horizontal elastic may be positioned across the fracture to reduce the lateral displacement (Figure 51-3D).

B. Evaluation: Advantages

- Relative simplicity without surgical requirement: noninvasive.
- Lower cost; shorter hospital stay (depending on other injuries).

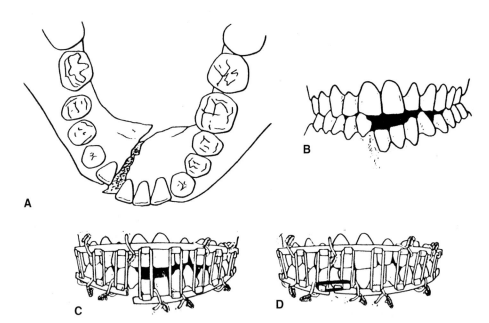

■ **FIGURE 51-3 Intermaxillary Fixation. (A)** Location of fracture of the mandible. **(B)** Segments of bone on either side of the fracture are displaced by muscle pull or contraction. **(C)** Arch bars with hooks for metal wires or rubber bands positioned to provide a steady pull for fracture reduction. **(D)** Note small horizontal rubber band extending from the hook at the mandibular right central incisor to the mandibular right canine to reduce the lateral displacement. (From Archer, W.H.: *Oral and Maxillofacial Surgery,* 5th ed. Philadelphia, W.B. Saunders Co., 1975.)

- In less developed countries, resources and trained surgeons may be limited.
- Person can return to activity and work sooner; can use outpatient facility for follow-up.

C. Evaluation: Contraindications and Disadvantages

- Patients with chronic airway diseases who cough and expectorate: Asthma, chronic obstructive pulmonary diseases.
- Patients who vomit regularly, notably, during pregnancy.
- Patients with a mental illness.
- Dietary problems: patients lose weight with liquid, monotonous diet, often with cariogenic content.
- Oral hygiene and dietary limitations lead to increased dental caries and periodontal infection.

III. EXTERNAL SKELETAL FIXATION (EXTERNAL PIN FIXATION)

A. Description

Two special bone screws are placed via skin incisions on either side of the fracture (Figure 51-4A). An acrylic bar is molded and, while still pliable, is pressed over the threads of the bone screws and locked into position with the screw nuts (Figure 51-4B).

B. Indications

Management of a fracture cannot always be accomplished satisfactorily by intermaxillary wiring alone. The following are indications for external fixation:

1. Insufficient number of teeth in good condition for intermaxillary fixation.
2. As a supplement to intermaxillary fixation when no teeth are present in the fractured portion of the mandible.
3. Loss of bone substance.
   - When bone substance is lost because of an accident, a gunshot wound, or a pathologic condition, a bone graft may be indicated.[6]
   - The extraoral fixation is used first to hold the fractured parts in a normal relationship, and then to immobilize the area during healing following the bone graft surgery.
4. Certain patients may be unable to have the jaws closed for a long period. Examples of these are:
   - Patient with a vomiting problem, such as during pregnancy.
   - Patient with a mental or physical disability, such as cerebral palsy, epilepsy, or mental retardation.
5. Edentulous mandible when the fracture fragments are greatly displaced, when the fracture is at the angle of the mandible, or when the mandible is atrophic or thinned.

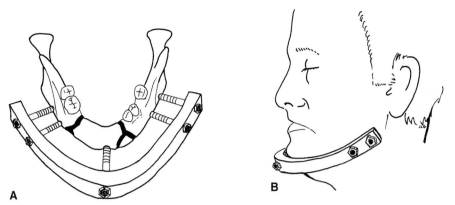

■ **FIGURE 51-4 External Skeletal Fixation. (A)** Precision bone screws placed on either side of the fractures shown by heavy black lines. **(B)** Molded acrylic bar positioned over the bone screws and locked into position with nuts.

IV. OPEN REDUCTION

A. Principles for Treating Skeletal Fractures

- Anatomic reduction.
- Functionally stable fixation.
- Atraumatic surgical technique.
- Active function.
- Prevention of infection.

B. Description

- Surgical approach to bring the fracture parts together.
- Anesthesia: anesthesia selected in accord with patient history.
- Types of systems used or immobilization include:
  - Transosseous wiring (osteosynthesis)
  - Plates of various sizes
  - Titanium mesh
  - Bone clamps, staples, screws
  - Materials: Miniplates, screws and other parts made of biodegradable or resorbable synthetic materials

C. Clinical Example

- Figure 51-5 illustrates various positions for miniplates to provide stability for the reduced fracture parts.
- Care is needed so that the screws are not placed over a fracture line or over the roots of teeth and so that they do not infringe on the mandibular canal.

■ MIDFACIAL FRACTURE

I. PRINCIPLES

- Maxillary fractures are more difficult to manage because of the number of bones, the associated

anatomy, and the complications of basal skull fractures.
- Not all midface fractures need fixation following reduction.
- Both function and cosmetics are involved.

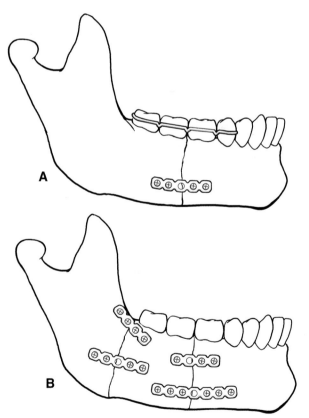

■ **FIGURE 51-5 Miniplates for Immobilization of Fracture. (A)** Tension band on the teeth to aid in maintaining correct occlusion while miniplate holds fracture ends in apposition. **(B)** Examples of possible positions for miniplates.

II. DESCRIPTION

A. Older Methods

- Internal wire suspension.
- External cranial suspension to a stable bone such as uninvolved zygoma.
- Headcaps.

B. Current Therapeutic Interventions

- Open reduction with internal fixation.
- Use of bone plates of various sizes.
- Grafts for reconstruction of midface defects.
- Early reconstruction before scarring and soft tissue contracture deform the surrounding area.

■ ALVEOLAR PROCESS FRACTURE

The most common fracture is of the alveolar process, maxillary or mandibular.

I. CLINICAL FINDINGS

- Face: bruising, areas of swelling.
- Teeth: fractures, mobility, avulsion, displacement.
- Lips and Gingiva: bruising, bleeding lacerations from contact with teeth at time of impact.
- Bone fracture: most frequently in anterior.

II. TREATMENT

1. Replantation of displaced teeth.
2. Immobilization with interdental wiring. A temporary fixed splint of acrylic may be placed over the wires. The teeth must be tested periodically for vitality.
3. Endodontic therapy may be required later.

■ DENTAL HYGIENE CARE

I. PROBLEMS

Fixation apparatus, however carefully placed to prevent tissue irritation, interferes with normal function. Identification of possible effects of treatment provides the basis for planning dental hygiene care.

A. Development of Gingivitis or Periodontal Complications

1. Thick biofilm formation and food debris accumulation provide sources of irritation to the gingiva.

2. Gingivitis can develop in 9 to 19 days.[7]
3. Lack of normal stimulation to the circulation of the periodontium and of cleansing effects usually provided by the action of the tongue, lips, and facial muscles contributes to stagnation of saliva and accumulation of debris and bacteria.
4. Tender, sensitive gingiva make biofilm control more difficult, even on available surfaces.

B. Initiation of Demineralization

An appetizing soft or liquid diet is difficult to plan using limited cariogenic foods for dental caries prevention.

C. Loss of Appetite

Loss of appetite related to monotonous liquid or soft diet may lead to weight loss and lowered physical resistance. Secondary infections, including those of the oral tissues, may result.

D. Difficulty in Opening the Mouth

1. When the temporomandibular joint has been injured, the patient wearing fixation appliances that involve only the mandible has difficulty in applying a toothbrush to the lingual surfaces of teeth.
2. After removal of appliances, all patients have a degree of muscular trismus that limits personal oral care and mastication.

II. INSTRUMENTATION

A. Presurgical

Gross calculus is removed, insofar as possible, before open reduction procedures. Trauma to surrounding soft tissues of lip, tongue, and cheeks limits accessibility.

B. During Treatment

Periodic scaling contributes to oral health. Although access is only from the facial aspect for a patient with intermaxillary wiring, some benefit can be obtained. An assistant must provide continual suction during treatment.

C. After Removal of Appliances

A few weeks after removal of appliances, when the patient can open the mouth normally and personal daily oral care has been initiated, complete scaling and planing can be performed.

III. DIET

Many patients with fractured jaws tend to lose weight, which is generally related to an inadequate nutrient and caloric intake. Objectives in planning the diet are:

- To help the patient maintain an adequate nutritional state.
- To promote healing.
- To increase resistance to infection.
- To prevent new carious lesions.

Attention must be given to the patient's willingness and ability to follow the recommendations made. The patient may be in the hospital for a few days to a few weeks, depending on the severity of other injuries. A greater length of time is spent as an outpatient, when the diet is much more difficult to supervise. The patient's understanding of dietary instructions and what is expected may appear more significant than the specific components of the diet recommended.

A. Nutritional Needs

After a surgical fixation procedure, the diet must be planned to promote tissue building and repair.

1. All essential food elements.
2. Emphasis on protein, vitamins, particularly A and C, and minerals, particularly calcium and phosphorus.
3. Usual caloric requirements for patient's age, taking into consideration lack of physical exercise and loss of appetite while ill.

B. Methods of Feeding

1. *Plastic Straw.* Liquid is sucked through the teeth or through an edentulous area. Straw can be bent to accommodate a patient who cannot sit up.
2. *Spoon Feeding.* When a patient's arms are not functional, direct assistance is needed. The mouth may have injuries that prevent sucking food through a straw.
3. *Tube Feeding.* Tube feeding may be indicated following various types of extensive oral surgery, facial trauma, burns, immobilized fractured jaw, and other conditions that prevent ingesting sufficient calories and nutritional foods by way of the mouth.

   A nasogastric tube is used. Blenderized food can be prepared, or special tube formulas are available commercially. When commercial preparations are used, contents can be selected to meet the specific nutritional and caloric requirements of an individual patient.

C. Liquid Diet

A *clear liquid* diet to help prevent dehydration may be prescribed initially, but it can be nutritionally inadequate. A *full liquid* diet to provide high protein and other healing elements is of a consistency to be taken by a cup. A *blenderized liquid* diet can be passed through a straw.

1. *Indications*
   a. All patients with jaws wired together.
   b. All patients with no appliance or single-jaw appliance who have difficulty in opening the mouth because of a condition, such as temporomandibular joint involvement or tongue or lip injury, that hinders insertion of food or manipulation of food in the mouth.
2. *Examples of Foods.* Fruit juices, milk, eggnog, meat juices and soups, cooked thin cereals, and canned baby foods. Strained vegetables and meats (baby foods) may be added to meat juices and soups.
3. *Use of a Blender.* Regular table foods can be mixed in a food blender. With liquid, such as clear soup or milk, added, a fluid consistency can be obtained that will pass through a straw (Figure 51-6).

D. Soft Diet

1. *Indications*
   a. Patient with no appliance or with single-jaw appliance without complications in opening the mouth or in movement of the lips and tongue.

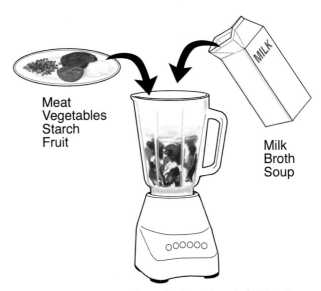

■ FIGURE 51-6 Preparation of a Liquid or Soft Diet. Regular table foods can be blended with milk or other nutritious liquid.

b. Patient who has been maintained on liquid diet throughout treatment period. After appliances are removed, the soft diet is recommended for several days to 1 week to provide the stomach with foods that are readily digestible rather than making a drastic change to a regular diet. A soft diet can also aid by protecting tender oral tissues from the rough textures of a regular diet until the tissues have had a chance to respond to softer foods.

2. *Examples of Foods.* Soft-poached, scrambled, or boiled eggs; cooked cereals; mashed soft-cooked vegetables, including potato; mashed fresh or canned fruits; soft, finely divided meats; custards; plain ice cream.

E. Hints for Diet Planning With the Nonhospitalized Patient

1. Provide instruction sheets that show specific meal plans.
2. Express nutritional needs in quantities or servings of foods.
3. Show methods of varying the diet. A liquid or soft diet is at best monotonous because of the sameness of texture.
4. Encourage limitation of cariogenic foods as an aid to prevention of dental caries.

IV. PERSONAL ORAL CARE PROCEDURES

Every attempt to keep the patient's mouth as clean as possible for comfort and sanitation, and as free of dental biofilm as possible for disease prevention, should be made. The extent of possible care depends on the appliances; the condition of the lips, tongue, and other oral tissues; and the cooperation of the patient.

Encouragement must be given to the patient to begin toothbrushing as soon as possible after the surgical procedure, but until the patient is able, a plan for care is outlined for a caregiver.

A. Irrigation

1. *Indications.* During the first few days after the surgical procedure, while the mouth may be too tender for brushing, frequent irrigations are required; irrigation also serves as an adjunct to toothbrushing.
2. *Method.* In a hospital, irrigations with suction are possible. At home, the patient irrigates with the head lowered over a sink (page 447).
3. *Mouthrinse Selection.* The oral surgeon should be consulted for specific instructions.

a. Physiologic saline.
b. Chlorhexidine gluconate (page 445).
c. Fluoride rinse after toothbrushing, after each meal, and before going to sleep (page 558).

B. Early Mouth Cleansing

While the patient is in the hospital, a soft toothbrush with suction can be used. The toothbrush with suction is described on pages 916 to 917.

C. Personal Care by the Patient

- As soon as possible, the patient is instructed in personal care.
- A toothbrushing method and other aids, such as those used for orthodontic appliances, are recommended and demonstrated (pages 457 and 459).
- Because interdental and proximal tooth-surface care is limited to access only from the facial approach, the choice of devices is limited.[8] Some spaces permit insertion of an interdental brush. With instruction, most patients can use a toothpick in a holder (page 436).
- When the tongue is not injured, the patient can be instructed to use the tongue as an aid in cleaning the lingual surfaces of the teeth and massaging the gingiva.
- The ambulatory patient can use a water irrigator. A low-pressure setting is used, and the spray is directed carefully to prevent tissue injury (pages 445 to 447).

D. After Appliances Are Removed

Except for the patient who had practiced good personal oral care before the accident, a step-by-step series of lessons is usually necessary.

A method for daily self-applied fluoride, such as a mouthrinse, brush-on gel, or customized fluoride trays, should be introduced along with the use of a fluoride dentifrice. Demineralization and dental caries can result from biofilm retention about the appliances.

▪ DENTAL HYGIENE CARE PRIOR TO GENERAL SURGERY

Completing dental and dental hygiene treatment and bringing the oral cavity to a state of health have special significance for certain patients who will have surgical procedures other than oral. When emergency surgery is performed, preparation of the mouth is not possible, and

Everyday Ethics

(?) Mrs. Squires was involved in a severe automobile accident that fractured her mandible and required fixation. Fortunately, Mrs. Squires had some presurgical debridement prior to placement of the intermaxillary wiring. This is her first appointment with William, the dental hygienist, since the accident 10 months ago. He documents the moderate amounts of calculus and heavy dental biofilm throughout the mouth. Mrs. Squires also demonstrates difficulty opening her mouth completely and seems apprehensive when William continually asks her to "open wide."

Questions for Consideration

1. How can William demonstrate "empathy" toward Mrs. Squires?

2. What steps in the decision model (page 10) should be exercised to deliver optimal oral health services to benefit this patient?

3. What is the role of the dental hygienist in coordinating preventive care with the posttreatment examinations Mrs. Squires has with the oral maxillofacial surgeon?

---

postsurgical examination and care may be complicated by various limitations.

When surgery is elective, or planned well in advance, the patient can be encouraged to have complete dental and periodontal treatment. Protection against complications related to broken appliances or restorations can be very meaningful to the hospitalized patient. Types of patients are described briefly here. Other examples are found in the various special patient chapters throughout this section of the book.

✔ Factors To Teach The Patient

Accident Prevention

- Always use seat belts in automobiles and other vehicles.

- Use mouthguards and all safety devices during contact sports.

- Wear motorcycle and bicycle helmets.

For the Patient Who Will Have General Surgery

- Why it is necessary to have dental and dental hygiene care completed before the surgery.

- Significance of a clean mouth during general anesthesia.

- Postsurgery oral problems related to specific diseases.

I. PATIENTS IN WHOM SURGICAL PROCEDURES AFFECT THEIR RISK STATUS

Susceptibility to infection is greatly increased in certain patients, for example, those with prosthetic heart valves, prostheses for joint replacement, and transplanted organs. Patients who receive chemotherapeutic agents as partial treatment after surgery for various types of cancer, and others who use immunosuppressant drugs, require special management to prevent complications during dental and dental hygiene appointments. Antibiotic premedication to prevent infective endocarditis and other infections is mandatory for certain patients (pages 122 to 125).

Prior to surgery for prostheses, transplants, cancer, and other serious conditions, patients can be informed of the need for completing oral care treatments and practicing preventive daily personal care.

II. PREPARATION OF THE MOUTH PRIOR TO GENERAL INHALATION ANESTHESIA

Because the mouth is an entrance to the respiratory chamber, the possibility always exists that bacteria, debris, and fluids may be inhaled from the mouth. Inhalation could occur during the administration of an anesthetic or when the patient coughs.

III. PATIENT WITH A LONG CONVALESCENCE

Patients whose surgery requires a long convalescence are unable to keep a regular maintenance appointment. When the patient has a healthy mouth before the hospitalization and convalescence, the problems of postsurgical oral care are lessened but not eliminated.

Instruction for the caregiver may be needed. A home visit by the dental hygienist may be possible.

REFERENCES

1. **American Dental Association**, Council on Dental Education, Chicago, 1990.
2. **Chuong**, R.: Perioperative Management of the Surgical Patient, in Peterson, L.J., ed.: *Oral and Maxillofacial Surgery.* Philadelphia, J.B. Lippincott Co., 1992, pp. 63–85.
3. **Haskell**, R.: Applied Surgical Anatomy, in Rowe, N.L. and Williams, J.L.: *Maxillofacial Injuries.* London, Churchill Livingstone, 1985, pp. 21–24.
4. **Luyk**, N.H.: Principles of Management of Fractures of the Mandible, in Peterson, L.J., ed.: *Oral and Maxillofacial Surgery.* Philadelphia, J.B. Lippincott Co., 1992, pp. 407–434.
5. **Banks**, P. and Brown, A.: *Fractures of the Facial Skeleton.* Oxford, Wright, 2001, pp. 81-106.
6. **Boyne** , P.J.: *Osseous Reconstruction of the Maxilla and the Mandible.* Chicago, Quintessence, 1997, pp. 64–74.
7. **Löe**, H., Theilade, E., and Jensen, S.B.: Experimental Gingivitis in Man, *J. Periodontol., 36,* 177, May–June, 1965.
8. **Phelps-Sandall**, B.A. and Oxford, S.J.: Effectiveness of Oral Hygiene Techniques on Plaque and Gingivitis in Patients Placed in Intermaxillary Fixation, *Oral Surg., 56,* 487, November, 1983.

SUGGESTED READINGS

Acton, C.H., Nixon, J.W., and Clark, R.C.: Bicycle Riding and Oral/Maxillofacial Trauma in Young Children, *Med. J. Aust., 165* , 249, September 2, 1996.

Alexander, R.E.: Patient Understanding of Postsurgical Instruction Forms, *Oral Surg., Oral Med., Oral Pathol., Oral Radiol., and Endod., 87,* 153, February, 1999.

Bunn-Minsky, K.C., Hunt, V., Mona, R.A., and Tal, K.: Nutrition of the Hospitalized Patient, in Zambito, R.F., Black, H.A., and Tesch, L.B., eds.: *Hospital Dentistry: Practice and Education.* St. Louis, Mosby, 1997, pp. 243–282.

Fun-Chee, L. and Shanmuhasuntharam, P.: A Simple Method to Enable Feeding During Maxillomandibular Fixation of the Jaws, *Oral Surg. Oral Med. Oral Pathol., 75,* 549, May, 1993.

Holman, A.R., Brumer, S., Ware, W.H., and Pasta, D.J.: The Impact of Interpersonal Support on Patient Satisfaction With Orthognathic Surgery, *J. Oral Maxillofac. Surg., 53,* 1289, November, 1995.

Kaban, L.B.: Diagnosis and Treatment of Fractures of the Facial Bones in Children 1943–1993, *J. Oral Maxillofac. Surg., 51,* 722, July, 1993.

Schmidt, B., Kearns, G., Perrott, D., and Kaban, L.B.: Infection Following Treatment of Mandibular Fractures in Human Immunodeficiency Virus Seropositive Patients, *J. Oral Maxillofac. Surg., 53,* 1134, October, 1995.

Seyer, B.A., Grist, W., and Muller, S.: Aggressive Destructive Midfacial Lesion From Cocaine Abuse, *Oral Surg., Oral Med., Oral Pathol., Oral Radiol., Endod., 94,* 465, October, 2002.

Torres, H.O., Ehrlich, A., Bird, D., and Dietz, E.: *Modern Dental Assisting,* 5th ed. Philadelphia, W.B. Saunders, 1995, pp. 579–597.

Mandibular Fracture

Bavitz, J.B. and Collicott, P.E.: Bilateral Mandibular Subcondylar Fractures Contributing to Airway Obstruction, *Int. J. Oral Maxillofac. Surg., 24,* 273, August, 1995.

Ellis, E.: Treatment Methods for Fractures of the Mandibular Angle, *Int. J. Oral Maxillofac. Surg., 28,* 243, August, 1999.

Eyrich, G.K.H., Grätz, K.W., and Sailer, H.F.: Surgical Treatment of Fractures of the Edentulous Mandible, *J. Oral Maxillofac. Surg., 55,* 1081, October, 1997.

Shonberg, D.C., Stith, H.D., Jameson, L.M., and Chai, J.Y.: Mandibular Fracture Through an Endosseous Implant, *Int. J. Oral Maxillofac. Implants, 7,* 401, Fall, 1992.

Tolman, D.E. and Keller, E.E.: Management of Mandibular Fractures in Patients With Endosseous Implants, *Int. J. Oral Maxillofac. Implants, 6,* 427, Winter, 1991.

Tuovinen, V., van Steenis, K., and Sindet-Pedersen, S.: Internal Fixation of a Mandibular Fracture in a 6-month-old Girl—A Case Report, *Int. J. Oral Maxillofac. Surg., 24,* 210, June, 1995.

The Patient With Cancer

Care of the patient with cancer before, during, and after therapy has as its main purposes attaining and maintaining oral health at the highest possible level and contributing to the patient's general and mental health. The patient may be under the care of a team of specialists, including the dentist, oral surgeon, dental hygienist, oncologist, nurse, dietitian, and pharmacist. Special rehabilitation personnel, such as a plastic surgeon, psychiatrist, speech therapist, physical therapist, maxillofacial prosthodontist, and social worker are frequently involved.

Oral cancers and leukemias are forms of cancer that have particular relevance because the cancers themselves and their treatment modalities (radiation, chemotherapy, surgery, and transplantation) have significant effects on the oral tissues. In Box 52-1, terminology relating to cancer is defined.

BOX 52-1 KEY WORDS: Cancer

Alopecia: a loss of hair.

Anaplasia: an irreversible alteration in adult cells toward more primitive (embryonic) cell types; characteristic of tumor cells.

Benign: not malignant; not recurrent; remains localized; favorable for recovery (Table 52-1).

Carcinogen: an agent that may cause cancer; may be chemical, physical (ionizing radiation), or biologic; biologic carcinogens may be external (for example, viruses) or internal (genetic defects).

Carcinoma: a malignant tumor of epithelial origin.

Chemotherapy: treatment of illness by chemical means, that is, by medication or drugs.

Dysgeusia: distortion of the sense of taste.

Dysplasia: an abnormality of development; in pathology, alteration in size, shape, and organization of adult cells.

Endoscopy: visual examination of interior structures of the body with an endoscope.

Hematologic profile: an analysis of the blood and blood-forming tissues.

Hematopoiesis: formation and development of blood cells.

Hyperbaric oxygen: the patient is placed in a sealed chamber and given pure oxygen through a face mask. At the same time, compressed air is introduced into the chamber to raise the atmospheric pressure to several times normal. This equalizes the pressure inside and outside of the body, thereby flooding the tissues with oxygen. An increase in oxygen to the irradiated tissues can temporarily compensate for the reduction in circulation.

Imaging: the production of diagnostic images, including radiography, ultrasonography, or scintigraphy.

Infiltration: the diffusion or accumulation in a tissue of cells or substances not normal to it or in amounts in excess of normal; in leukemia, for example, white blood cells infiltrate body tissues.

Infusion: slow therapeutic introduction of fluid other than blood into a vein; infusion flows by gravity.

In situ: in its normal place; confined to the site of origin.

Interstitial: pertaining to, or situated in, the interstices (small spaces) of a tissue.

Intrathecal: within a sheath; through the theca of the spinal cord into the subarachnoid space; in leukemia, for example, the location for the delivery of various chemotherapeutic drugs.

Isogenic: having the same genetic constitution; syngeneic.

Leukemia: an acute or chronic progressive malignant neoplasm of the blood-forming organs, marked by diffuse proliferation of immature white blood cells (leukocytes); subsequent reduction in erythrocytes and platelets results.

Lymphadenectomy: excision of one or more lymph nodes.

Malignant: tending to become progressively worse and to result in death; having the properties of anaplasia, invasiveness, and metastasis; said of tumors (Table 52-1).

Metastasis: transfer of disease from one organ or part to another not directly connected with it; for example, regional or distant spread of cancer cells from the site primarily involved.

Neoplasm: any new and abnormal growth, specifically one in which cell multiplication is controlled and progressive; may be benign or malignant.

Oncology: the sum of knowledge regarding tumors: the study of tumors.

Palliative: affording relief, but does not cure.

Pancytopenia: abnormal depression of all cellular elements of the blood.

KEY WORDS: Cancer, continued

Pleomorphism: occurrence in more than one form; the assumption of various distinct morphologic types by a single organism or cell.

Radiotherapy: the treatment of disease by ionizing radiation; may be external megavoltage or internal by use of interstitial implantation of an isotope (radium).

Radium: a highly radioactive chemical element found in uranium minerals; used in the treatment of malignant tumors in the form of needles or pellets for interstitial implantation.

Radon: radioactive element produced by the disintegration of radium and is used in radiotherapy; referred to as **radium emanation.**

Relapse: the return of a disease weeks or months after its apparent cessation.

Remission: diminution or abatement of the symptoms of a disease; the period during which such diminution occurs.

Sarcoma: a tumor, often highly malignant, composed of cells derived from connective tissue such as bone and cartilage, muscle, blood vessel, or lymphoid tissue.

Staging: the succinct, standardized description of a tumor with regard to origin and spread. This clinical classification is based on physical assessments, biopsy, imaging, endoscopy. Each stage (I–IV) consists of three components: T (size of tumor); N (lymph node involvement); and M (presence or absence of distant metastasis).

Trismus: limitations of opening because of spasm and/or fibrosis of the muscles of mastication and/or temporomandibular joint located in the field of radiation.

■ DESCRIPTION

Cancer refers to a group of neoplastic diseases in which there is transformation of normal body cells into malignant ones. As cancer cells proliferate, the mass of abnormal tissue that is formed enlarges and sheds cells that spread the disease locally or to distant sites (metastasis). Characteristics of benign and malignant neoplasms are compared in Table 52-1.

There are numerous types of cancers. They are classified on the basis of the (1) origin of the tissue involved, that is, carcinomas from epithelial tissue, and sarcomas from connective tissue; and (2) type of cell from which they arise, namely, an epithelial or connective tissue cell.[1]

I. INCIDENCE

Cancer is the second leading cause of death in the United States. The three most commonly diagnosed cancers among women involve the breast, colon and rectum. Among men, the most common cancers are of the prostate, lung and bronchus, and colon and rectum.[2]

A. Survival Rates

A cured patient is one that shows no evidence of disease and has the same life expectancy as a person who has never had cancer. Most forms of cancer are considered cured after survival for 5 years without symptoms following treatment.

B. Oral Cancer

Oral/pharyngeal cancers annually account for 3.3% of cancers in men and 1.6% in females.[2] The incidence rate for oral/pharyngeal cancer is about 1.5 times higher in African Americans than in whites. The overall mortality rate has declined slightly over the past 15 years. The 5-year survival rate for posterior oral structures such as the pharynx is lower than that for anterior oral structures, namely the lip.[3] Approximately 90% of all oral carcinomas are of the squamous cell type. They spread by local extension and the lymphatic system.

C. Leukemia

Many new cases of leukemia occur annually. Slightly more than half of the cases occur in males. An equal number of leukemia cases are chronic as are acute in type. Cancer is the leading cause of death in children aged 1 to 14; approximately one third of the deaths occur from leukemia.[3]

II. ETIOLOGY AND PREDISPOSING FACTORS

Although the etiologic factors of cancer are not known, extensive research is being conducted. Several factors predispose an individual to cancer formation. Implicated

▪ TABLE 52-1 CHARACTERISTICS OF BENIGN AND MALIGNANT NEOPLASMS

CHARACTERISTIC	BENIGN	MALIGNANT
Cell Characteristics	Cells resemble normal cells of the tissue from which the tumor originated	Cells often bear little resemblance to the normal cells of the tissue from which they arose; there is both anaplasia and pleomorphism
Mode of Growth	Tumor grows by expansion and does not infiltrate the surrounding tissues; encapsulated	Tumor grows at the periphery and sends out processes that infiltrate and destroy the surrounding tissues
Rate of Growth	Rate of growth is usually slow	Rate of growth is usually relatively rapid and is dependent on level of differentiation; the more anaplastic the tumor, the more rapid the rate of growth
Metastasis	Does not spread by metastasis	Gains access to the blood and lymph channels and metastasizes to other areas of the body
Recurrence	Does not recur when removed	Tends to recur when removed
General Effects	Is usually a localized phenomenon that does not cause generalized effects unless by location it interferes with vital functions	Often causes generalized effects, such as anemia, weakness, and weight loss
Destruction of Tissue	Does not usually cause tissue damage unless location interferes with blood flow	Often causes extensive tissue damage as the tumor outgrows its blood supply or encroaches on blood flow to the area; may also produce substances that cause cell damage
Ability to Cause Death	Does not usually cause death unless its location interferes with vital functions	Usually causes death unless growth can be controlled

(From Porth, C., *Pathophysiology: Concepts of Altered Health States,* 2nd ed. Philadelphia, J. B. Lippincott Co., 1986.)

have been weakened immunity, a history of syphilis and other infections, diet, and tobacco. Table 52-2 lists the sites of cancer and their risk factors.

A. Risk Factors for Oral Cancer[3]

1. Excessive use of alcohol and tobacco in combination. Chronic alcoholic persons have more lesions of the tongue and floor of the mouth than of other locations of the oral cavity.
2. Long-term exposure to the chemical carcinogens of tobacco (smoking or smokeless).
3. Poor oral hygiene, particularly in chronic alcohol and tobacco users.
4. Overexposure to sunlight. Persons with occupations requiring outdoor activity in the sun and weather have a higher risk for developing lip cancer.

B. Risk Factors for Leukemia[3]

1. Radiation.
2. Toxic exposure to chemicals, namely, benzene.
3. Previous bone marrow disorders.
4. Congenital disorders such as Down's syndrome.

▪ PREPARATION FOR TREATMENT

Time may be a factor for the patient with advanced malignancy. Once the extent and severity of the cancer has been ascertained, or staging has been completed, as is the case with tumors of the head and neck, the type and length of therapy can be determined and initiated. Basic preparation follows the same general outline for a patient undergoing oral surgery.

I. OBJECTIVES

The aim in preparation of a patient for the treatment of cancer is to restore the mouth to optimal health prior to radiation, chemotherapy, surgery, or bone marrow transplantation. The objectives of preparing a patient for treatment include steps to:
A. Assess the oral cavity.
B. Eliminate sources of infection.
C. Motivate the patient in preventive oral care measures.
D. Reduce the oral microbial count.

■ TABLE 52-2 RISK FACTORS FOR CANCER

AGENT	SITES OF CANCER
Tobacco related	Lung, bladder, kidney, renal pelvis, pancreas, cervix
Tobacco and alcohol related	Oral cavity, esophagus
Diet related	High fat, low fiber, low in vegetables & fruits—large bowel, breast, pancreas, prostate, ovary, endometrium Pickled, salted foods, low in vegetables & fruits—stomach Alcohol, certain mushrooms—liver, esophagus
Bacterial	*Helicobacter pylori*—stomach
Sunlight	Skin (melanoma)
Occupational	Various carcinogens—bladder, liver, other organs
Lifestyle and Occupation	Tobacco and asbestos; tobacco and mining; tobacco and uranium and radium—lung, respiratory tract
Iatrogenic	Radiation, drugs—diverse organs, leukemia
Genetic	Retinoblastoma, soft-tissue sarcomas
Viral	Human T-cell lymphotropic virus type 1 (HTLV-1); adult T-cell lymphoma; human papillomavirus—cervix, penis, anus
Origin Uncertain	Lymphomas, leukemias, sarcomas, cervical cancer

(Adapted from the *American Cancer Society Cancer Statistics,* 1988[2], and the *Textbook of Clinical Oncology,* 1995, p. 18.[3])

E. Provide a better environment for therapeutic procedures.

F. Improve the conditions for healing.

II. ORAL FINDINGS

The extent and severity of the oral side effects of cancer therapy are related to the condition of the teeth and soft tissues before therapy and the patient's hematologic profile. If some or all of the following oral findings are encountered they must be corrected prior to therapy:

A. Extensive carious lesions.

B. Retained root tips.

C. Periodontal involvement.

D. Ill-fitting prostheses (partial or complete dentures).

E. Orthodontic appliances that cause excessive irritation may require removal or wax coverage to protect soft tissues.

F. Poor oral hygiene.

■ DENTAL/DENTAL HYGIENE TREATMENT PLAN[4,5]

Dental procedures, such as tooth removal, periodontal surgery, and endodontic treatment, that could open a channel for infection to reach the bone or systemic circulation are contraindicated during cancer therapy and, in the case of radiation, after therapy as well. When con-

sideration is given to proper preparation of the oral cavity prior to cancer therapy and supervision of preventive measures continues during and after therapy, the incidence of harmful effects can be minimized.

The patient's total treatment plan prior to the initiation of therapy should include at least the following:

I. ASSESSMENT

A complete oral and dental assessment must be performed to establish a baseline for measuring changes and evaluating the effectiveness of oral care. Areas of assessment should include:

A. Oral–facial soft tissue.

B. Hard tissues for dental caries, impacted teeth, ill-fitting prostheses.

C. Periodontium for presence of deposits on the teeth, probing depths, bone loss.

D. Amount and consistency of saliva.

E. Previous history of oral complications associated with cancer therapy.

F. Cultures performed before and throughout treatment when it is suspected that a patient is exhibiting an oral mucosal infection, such as *Candidiasis.*

II. PREVENTION PROGRAM

A. Dental Biofilm Control

1. Start oral hygiene instruction at first appointment.

2. Emphasize preventive infection control procedures and potential oral side effects associated with cancer therapy.

B. Daily Fluoride Therapy

1. Indicated for patients about to undergo head and neck radiation therapy, if the salivary glands are in the field of radiation.
2. Make impressions and fabricate custom fluoride trays.
3. Advise patient to apply custom trays lined with 1.1% neutral sodium fluoride gel to the teeth for 4 minutes once daily or use brush-on method, if trays are not feasible.
4. Advise patient to refrain from eating, drinking, or rinsing for 30 minutes following tray removal.

C. Dietary Instructions

1. Instruct patient or caregiver in the preparation of foods in a blender.
2. Avoid highly cariogenic or spicy foods.

D. Avoid Alcohol and Smoking

III. PERIODONTAL THERAPY

A. Complete scaling and root debridement.
B. Perform surgical procedures when time permits follow-up for healing.
C. Adjust occlusion when necessary.

IV. RESTORATION OF CARIOUS LESIONS

A. Restore all clinically and radiographically detected caries.
B. Remove all overhanging margins.
C. Finish and polish all restorations.
D. Seal newly erupted teeth.

V. PROSTHODONTIC THERAPY

A. Correct ill-fitting prostheses.
B. Instruct patient to leave prostheses out of the mouth as much as possible once therapy has begun.
C. Fabricate new prostheses 3 to 6 months after radiation.
D. Motivate patient to maintain meticulous denture hygiene.[6]
   1. Dentures should be cleansed and soaked in an antimicrobial solution overnight.
   2. Disposable cups should be used to soak the denture. Change solution daily.
   3. Denture adhesives should be avoided.

VI. REMOVAL OF NONRESTORABLE TEETH

A. Indications

Extensively involved teeth may need extraction because of severe bone loss, mobility, and other signs of advanced periodontal infection, large carious lesions with pulpal exposures not conducive to endodontic therapy, or periapical radiographic findings.

B. Rationale

In the past, treatment frequently called for complete extraction of all teeth that would be in the pathway of radiation whether or not they were broken down or diseased. Now, only teeth that are definitely beyond saving or loose primary teeth are removed.

C. Healing

Alveoloplasty to remove bone spicules is necessary. A healing period of at least 10 to 14 days should be allowed before starting radiation therapy because when bone is irradiated, healing and remodeling cease.

VII. SURGICAL PROCEDURES

Removal of residual root tips, gingival opercula, which have the potential to trap food debris and become infected, and other subsurface pathologic areas that are found in radiographs of edentulous areas is advised.

VIII. ENDODONTIC THERAPY

Endodontic therapy for essential abutment teeth may be necessary. Treatment planning for prosthetic replacements must be done in advance so that abutment teeth can receive proper treatment before radiation therapy.

▪ RADIATION THERAPY[7,8]

Therapeutic radiation may be the only treatment for oral cancer or it may be used in conjunction with surgery.

I. OBJECTIVES

A. As a Total Treatment

Exposures are usually given as daily doses, made in fractions of the total dose.

B. In Conjunction With Surgery

1. *Preoperatively.* To reduce the size of the neoplasm as an aid to surgery by limiting the surgical area.
2. *Postoperatively.* To control residual disease.

II. TYPES

A. External Beam

1. *Orthovoltage.* Low-yield radiation may be used for superficial lesions, such as lip lesions or small lesions in the oral cavity, where radiation is applied by an intraoral cone.

2. *Megavoltage or Supervoltage.* High-yield radiation includes cobalt-60 and the linear accelerator. It has a spraying effect on skull and bone and less scatter radiation to surrounding tissues than does orthovoltage. Divided doses are given over 6 to 8 weeks on an outpatient appointment plan.

3. *Field of Radiation.* Areas of application. Figure 52-1 illustrates exposure areas for external irradiation. The neoplasms and regional lymph nodes cannot be exposed without radiation also going to the oral cavity, salivary glands, maxilla, and mandible. The side effects to the exposed normal tissues are induced by the unwanted radiation.

B. Internal: Interstitial Implant

The source of radiation is placed within the body. Less radiation is delivered to surrounding tissues than when an external source is utilized. Radium needles and radioactive radon and gold seeds are used.

III. DOSAGE AND DURATION

A. Dosage

The dosage of radiation therapy may range from 3,000 to > 7,000 centigray (cGy) for a 3- to 8-week period.

B. Factors Affecting Duration

1. Tumor type and location.
2. Single or combination therapy.
3. Patient's ability to tolerate therapy.
4. Infiltration of cancer cells into CNS.

■ ORAL EFFECTS OF RADIATION THERAPY AND MANAGEMENT[4,9-14]

Irradiation is the exposure of tissues to electromagnetic radiation (e.g., heat, light, x rays). The purpose is to destroy cancerous cells. Damage to surrounding normal

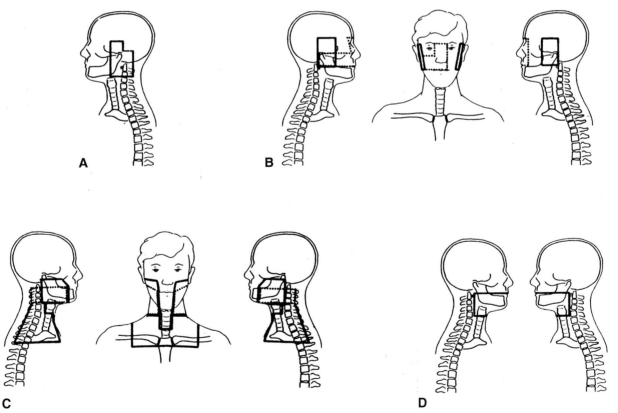

■ **FIGURE 52-1 Common Fields of Radiation for Head and Neck Tumors.** Dark lines show fields when increased dosages are needed. **(A)** Parotid field. **(B)** Antrum field. **(C)** Oropharynx field. **(D)** Floor of mouth field. (From Jansma, J.: *Oral Sequelae Resulting From Head and Neck Radiotherapy.* Groningen, Drukkerij van Denderen B.V., 1991.)

tissue cannot be avoided, but the severity of damage can be minimized.

I. TISSUE CHANGES

Ionizing radiation induces tissue changes, some of which are apparent during the treatment period and may continue for a few weeks or months after cessation of irradiation. Other changes may not be evident until after treatment and may have long-term significance. Therefore, the patient should be seen often during therapy (at least once weekly), and indefinitely following therapy.

A. Onset: Early Changes (damage to exposed tissues in the field of radiation with rapid cell turnover rates)

1. Dermatitis.
2. Mucositis.
3. Alopecia.
4. Reduced salivary flow.

B. Late Changes (damage to exposed tissues in the field of radiation with slow turnover rates)

1. Xerostomia.
2. "Radiation Caries."
3. Osteoradionecrosis.
4. Trismus.

II. MUCOSA

A. Inflammatory Changes

1. *Time Sequence.* Inflammation of the mucosa usually occurs 1 to 2 weeks after the onset of radiation therapy.
2. *Severity.* Effects of radiation are more severe in patients with susceptible oral tissues secondary to alcoholism and/or heavy smoking.

B. Cellular Changes

1. *Initial Inflammatory Response.* Edema of the tissues is noted first, followed by ulcerations and necrosis with sloughing.
2. *Latent Response.* Fibrosis develops as a result of chronic inflammation.

C. Clinical Signs

1. Sensitivity to pressure and temperature extremes.
2. Unpleasant odor from necrotic tissue.
3. Bleeding.
4. Tenderness.

5. Dental biofilm accumulation.
6. Inability to tolerate prostheses over thin, fragile epithelium.

D. Recovery

1. *Immediate.* Severe signs heal and disappear within a few weeks after radiation is completed.
2. *Long Range.* Thin, fragile mucosa with compromised blood supply never completely recovers, and healing remains difficult in response to exposure to future infections.

III. ORAL MANAGEMENT

Personal care may be neglected because of preoccupation with medical concerns or sensitivity of the oral tissues, but the patient must be urged to be compliant with biofilm control and daily fluoride application.

A. Toothbrushing

1. Use of a super-soft toothbrush to remove biofilm is highly recommended.
2. Lemon-glycerine swabs are ineffective in the removal of biofilm and may further dry the oral mucosa.
3. A flavored dentifrice may not be tolerated, but a dentifrice containing fluoride is essential.

B. Mouthrinses

1. Rinsing with a baking soda/saline solution throughout the day followed by a plain water rinse is suggested. Salt may be eliminated.
2. Chlorhexidine rinsing may also be recommended to reduce inflammation, particularly when mechanical biofilm control methods are compromised owing to mucositis pain.
3. Commercial mouthwashes with high alcohol content should be avoided owing to their drying and irritating effects.
4. Hydrogen peroxide should be diluted with water to a 1:4 concentration. Use of hydrogen peroxide 3% should be limited to short-term use to prevent disruption of the normal oral flora.
5. Gauze or a tooth sponge may be employed as a vehicle for applying rinsing agents to the teeth and sensitive oral soft tissues.

C. Diet

1. Topical anesthetic or anti-inflammatory rinses, ointments, or gels may be applied as needed or before eating to alleviate mucositis pain.

2. Liquids are needed with meals to moisten food for swallowing.
3. A soft, bland, noncariogenic diet eaten at a low temperature is recommended.

D. Habits

Alcoholic beverages and tobacco products must be avoided.[15]

IV. SALIVARY GLANDS

Radiation to the salivary glands may be unavoidable, depending on the location of the tumor. The radiation primarily affects the serous gland cells, causing a reduction in secretion.

A. Xerostomia

A reduced quantity of saliva may be noticed as early as the third or fourth day after the beginning of radiation, thus decreasing the self-cleansing ability of the oral cavity. Subsequent candidiasis or periodontal infections may develop.

1. *Changes in Saliva.* Saliva is more acidic and viscous, thus increasing the risk for enamel demineralization. Mastication and swallowing become impaired by the combination of xerostomia and mucositis, making nutritional intake difficult.
2. *Changes in Mucosa.* Dry friable mucosa may be prone to cracks and bleeding, creating a portal of entry for infection. The patient who wears a denture may be unable to tolerate it because of a reduced surface tension between the dry mucosa and the prosthesis.

B. Management

1. *Pilocarpine Therapy.* This parasympathomimetic drug has been shown to be effective in relieving symptoms of xerostomia and improving salivary flow when given in a dosage of 5–10 mg 3 to 4 times daily.[16-19]
2. *Saliva Substitutes.* Adjunctive artificial salivas with fluoride may be used as often as needed to provide temporary relief from xerostomia. The only contraindication is if the patient is on a low-sodium diet. The patient should be instructed to spray directly on the tissues, or if in gel form, place a drop or two in the mouth and spread around with the tongue.
3. *Water and Ice Chips.* Frequent sips of water or sucking on ice chips help to alleviate xerostomia on a short-term basis.

4. *Diet.* The patient is advised to eat moist foods, chew sugarless gum, and avoid sucking on lozenges or candy with sugar to moisten the mouth.
5. *Humidify Air.* Humidifiers can be used to manage dry air at home, particularly during the winter months when the house is heated.

V. TEETH

A. Radiation Caries

1. *Description.* Teeth with exposed root surfaces are especially susceptible. The lesions develop in the gingival third and gradually encircle the necks of the teeth (Figure 15-3, page 266). The carious lesions appear black or dark brown.
2. *Predisposing Factors.* Xerostomia, neglect of biofilm control measures, soft cariogenic diet, sore mouth, and changes in oral flora are responsible, not radiation directly.
3. *Prevention.* Intensified preventive measures involving daily fluoride application, dental biofilm control, and noncariogenic diet are warranted. The use of a saliva substitute containing fluoride is also indicated.

B. Tooth Development

Radiation in children can affect the odontogenic cells. A tooth bud may be completely destroyed if irradiated before mineralization has started.[20]

C. Sensitivity of Teeth

Teeth with dental caries are particularly sensitive, but all teeth may react to temperature extremes. Daily fluoride therapy and tooth sensitivity dentifrices with fluoride will also lessen tooth sensitivity. Extreme hot or cold foods should be avoided.

VI. INFECTIONS

A. Fungal

Candidiasis is the most common oral infection during or after radiation therapy. The increase in *Candida* infection is related to hyposalivation and the changed composition of the saliva. Fungal infections should be treated with an antifungal agent, ideally one that does not contain sugar.

B. Bacterial

Radiation leaves the patient with susceptible oral tissues. Gram-negative bacilli increase and are often related to the secondary infections occurring in the later stages of ulcerative mucositis.

VII. BONE: OSTEORADIONECROSIS

Radiation damages bone cells and blood vessels within the bone. Changes in the endothelial cells lead to sclerosis of the vessels. The result is change in the growth potential of the bone and lowered resistance to infection.

A. Portals of Entry for Infection

1. Mucosal ulceration.
2. Dental biofilm.
3. Deep periodontal pockets.
4. Periapical lesion.
5. Open socket from tooth extraction.

B. Signs

1. Pain.
2. Trismus.
3. Exposed bone, sequestration, pathologic fracture.
4. Suppuration.
5. Halitosis.

C. Management

Administration of a series of hyperbaric oxygen treatments to facilitate healing of the compromised bone is the treatment for osteoradionecrosis. Advanced cases may involve extended antibiotic therapy and surgery for the removal of the sequestra, or even part of the mandible.[21-24]

D. Prevention

Correct preradiation and postradiation procedures have had a definite effect on lowering the incidence of osteoradionecrosis. Maintenance of oral cleanliness and health are contributing preventive factors.

E. Development

Children who receive radiation to the developing facial bones may experience altered craniofacial growth.[20]

VIII. DYSGEUSIA

A. Changes

Taste can be altered or lost by degeneration of taste buds or by changes in the quantity of saliva.

B. Duration

Altered taste may begin as early as the first 200–400 cGy. Taste acuity is usually regained in 2 to 4 months after therapy, if saliva flow is adequate.

C. Management

Taste aversions should be considered if a person other than the patient is responsible for preparing meals. Meats, for example, may elicit a metallic taste. Dietary supplements of zinc have been recommended to alleviate taste disturbances.[21]

IX. LOSS OF APPETITE

A. Factors

1. Sore mouth; alteration in taste.
2. Diminished saliva; inability to wear prostheses.
3. Depression.

B. Sequelae

1. Dehydration; weight loss.
2. Impaired healing.
3. Fatigue.

X. TRISMUS

A. Duration

Trismus may occur 3 to 6 months after therapy has stopped. Opening of the mouth is difficult and often painful. Oral care, eating, and speaking may be adversely affected.

B. Management

Exercises and stretching appliances have been used for treatment.

▪ POSTRADIATION THERAPY[4,5,13]

When radiation therapy has been completed and the acute oral side effects have resolved, dental hygiene care must continue on a routine basis to eliminate the risk of infection. The risk of osteoradionecrosis in the patient who has undergone radiation therapy persists throughout life. The dental hygienist's contribution to the oral health success after radiation therapy is as significant as the care and supervision required before and during therapy.

I. DENTAL HYGIENE ASSESSMENT AND CARE PLAN

A. Evaluate Periodontal Health

1. Complete periodontal examination with charting.
2. Assess dental biofilm control and provide additional motivation and instruction.
3. Perform scaling and root debridement.

B. Examine and Chart Dental Caries

1. Review home fluoride program.
2. Administer topical application.

C. Assess Salivary Flow

Review care plan for xerostomia.

D. Counsel in Dietary Practices

E. Manage Additional Effects of the Radiation Therapy

F. Make Referrals for Dental Treatment

G. Arrange Frequent Maintenance Appointments

II. DENTAL TREATMENT FOLLOW-UP

A. New or Routine Adjustment of Prostheses

B. Restoration of Carious Lesions

C. Extractions

If extraction is the only option to manage extensive dental or periodontal disease, hyperbaric oxygen therapy before and after tooth removal, antibiotic prophylaxis, and meticulous surgical technique are warranted.

D. Extraction Alternative: Endodontic therapy

E. Implants Preceded by Hyperbaric Oxygen Therapy[25,26]

■ CHEMOTHERAPY[13,14,27-30]

Chemotherapeutic agents destroy or deactivate rapidly dividing cancer cells with as little destruction of normal cells as possible. Side effects from the drugs are significant and frequently involve the oral tissues.

I. OBJECTIVES

A. Control widely scattered neoplasms.
B. Supplement surgery and/or radiation.
C. Palliative care for patients with advanced squamous cell carcinomas of the head and neck.[21]

II. TYPES OF CHEMOTHERAPEUTIC AGENTS[31]

A. Categories (Table 52-3)

B. Use: Single or combination therapy

■ TABLE 52-3 CATEGORIES OF CANCER CHEMOTHERAPY DRUGS
Alkylating Agents
Antibiotics
Antimetabolites
Plant Alkaloids
Steroids/Hormones
Miscellaneous

III. SYSTEMIC SIDE EFFECTS OF CHEMOTHERAPY

Rapidly proliferating normal cells are susceptible to the suppression action of chemotherapeutic agents. The most common side effects include:

A. Alopecia.
B. Myelosuppression (bone marrow suppression causing a reduction in blood counts leading to anemia, leukopenia, and thrombocytopenia).
C. Immunosuppression (inhibition of antibody responses resultant from leukopenia).
D. Nausea and vomiting, diarrhea.
E. Loss of appetite.

IV. ORAL EFFECTS OF CHEMOTHERAPY AND MANAGEMENT[32]

For chemotherapy-induced oral complications identical to those encountered in the patient undergoing head and neck radiation, follow the management recommendations outlined in Table 52-4.

A. Factors Affecting Severity of Oral Effects

1. Dosage and duration of drugs administered.
2. Patient's age.
3. Patient's oral health status and dietary habits.
4. Patient's systemic condition/hematologic profile.

B. Direct Cytotoxic Effects

Chemotherapy drugs act on the oral structures.
1. Ulcerative mucositis.
2. Transient xerostomia.
3. Jaw pain.
4. Abnormal enamel and root development.[20]
5. Delayed eruption.[20]

C. Indirect Cytotoxic Effects

Chemotherapy drugs act indirectly on the oral tissues; caused by myelosuppression.
1. Hemorrhage
   a. Gingival bleeding.
   b. Oral petechiae and ecchymoses.

■ TABLE 52-4 ORAL COMPLICATIONS OF CANCER THERAPY AND THEIR MANAGEMENT

ORAL COMPLICATION	DENTAL MANAGEMENT	PATIENT SELF MANAGEMENT
Infection: • Fungal • Viral • Bacterial	Appropriate prescription for: • Antifungal medication • Antiviral medication • Antibiotic medication Prescription chlorhexidine gluconate rinses	Daily oral hygiene practices: • Thorough, complete biofilm removal • Gentle technique Use daily fluoride to help prevent caries Use saliva substitute if needed
Mucositis	Saliva substitutes Topical anesthetics	Frequent water drinking and rinses
Salivary gland dysfunction Xerostomia	Saliva substitutes Fluoride treatments Prescription pilocarpine	Avoid irritants: • Alcohol • Acidic and spicy foods • All tobacco
Functional Impairments: • Eating • Swallowing • Talking • Alterations in taste • Trismus; muscle dysfunction	Physical therapy, stretching Nutritional counseling	Stress management Report any problems immediately Maintain optimum general health and nutrition
Pain	Prescription systemic analgesic Topical analgesics Palliative rinses	Seek frequent maintenance appointments

2. Infection
   a. Bacterial (gram-negative, *Pseudomonas*, *Klebsiella*, *Proteus*, *E. coli*, *Serratia*, or *Enterobacter*).
   b. Viral (herpes simplex).
   c. Fungal (*Candida*).

V. ORAL CARE

A. Scheduling

Appoint patient and determine need for antibiotic prophylaxis in consultation with the oncologist. The best time to schedule treatment is after the patient's blood counts have recovered, usually just prior to the next course of chemotherapy.

B. Blood Counts

Request blood values the day before or the day of the dental appointment to confirm that the patient can be treated.

C. Platelet Transfusions[4]

Platelet replacement may be necessary prior to any dental procedures if the platelet count is less than 40,000/mm^3.

D. Antibiotic Prophylaxis

The granulocyte count and the presence of an indwelling catheter may suggest the need for antibiotic coverage prior to dental procedures.

VI. PREVENTION

A. Recommend use of super-soft toothbrush and frequent rinsing.
B. Disinfect brush with chlorhexidine; change toothbrush often.
C. Prevent mucosal lacerations with subsequent bacteremia during periods of profound neutrope-

nia and thrombocytopenia: avoid using tooth-picks, irrigating devices, and floss and eating crunchy or sharp foods.

VII. REMISSION

A. Characteristics of Remission

1. Neoplastic cells diminish.
2. Blood counts return to normal.
3. Oral complications subside.

B. Place on Routine Dental Hygiene Maintenance

C. Relapse

The cycle of therapy begins again, and the need for bone marrow transplantation is evaluated.

■ SURGICAL TREATMENT

Surgery may be required to remove a tumor located in the head and neck area.

I. INDICATIONS FOR SURGERY[7]

A. Neoplasms that are not radiosensitive and could not be treated by radiotherapy alone.
B. Neoplasms recurring in an area that had already undergone radiotherapy.
C. Situations where side effects of radiation could be more severe than healed surgical defects.
D. Neoplasms involving bone, lymph nodes, and salivary glands.

II. TYPES OF SURGERY

A. Primary Lesion

Surgical treatment is to remove the primary lesion and the regional lymph nodes. Some small lesions are totally removed when a biopsy is used for diagnosis.

B. Cervical Lymphadenectomy ("Neck Dissection")

1. *Area.* The neck dissection includes wide removal of tissues around a tumor.
2. *Purposes.* To ensure removal of as many neoplastic cells as possible from the oropharynx and neck and to prevent the spread of the cancer to the lymph nodes.

■ BONE MARROW TRANSPLANTATION (BMT)[33,34]

Bone marrow transplantation is used to treat a variety of neoplasms and blood diseases. The purpose is to substitute bone marrow from a healthy, compatible donor to restore or reconstitute the blood cell–producing capacity of the bone marrow of the patient.

I. TYPES OF TRANSPLANTS

The five basic types of transplants are shown in Table 52-5.

II. STAGES OF THE TRANSPLANTATION PROCESS[33]

A. Patient Selection

1. Indications: patient not responsive to chemotherapy alone; relapse occurs after one or more remissions.
2. Evaluation: medical and dental assessments are completed to ensure patient is free of infection and physically stable to undergo preparative regimen.

B. Donor Regimen

1. Histocompatibility matching.
2. Bone marrow aspirated from iliac crest, ribs, or sternum.

■ TABLE 52-5 TYPES OF BONE MARROW TRANSPLANTS

TYPE OF TRANSPLANT	DONOR SOURCE	FREQUENCY
Autologous	Self	30–50%
Unrelated	Any matched donor (complete or partial)	25–30%
Allogeneic	Sibling	15–25%
Haploidentical	Parent	<5%
Syngeneic	Identical twin	<5%

(Adapted from Rhodus, N.L. and Little, J.W.: Dental Management of the Bone Marrow Transplant Patient, *Compend. Cont. Educ. Dent.,* 13, 1040, November, 1992.)

C. Conditioning of Patient to Receive Bone Marrow Graft

1. Preparative high-dose immunosuppressive regimen: chemotherapy alone or with total-body irradiation.
2. Purposes
   a. Kill malignant cells.
   b. Suppress immune system so new marrow can engraft.

D. Transplantation

Intravenous infusion of donor's marrow.

E. Pancytopenic Period

All cellular elements of the blood are depressed.
1. Protective isolation for patient is required; patient highly susceptible to infection.
2. Function of new marrow (to produce peripheral blood elements) begins after 10 to 20 days.

F. Recovery

Immune recovery 3 to 12 months; long-term recovery 1 to 3 years.

III. PRIMARY COMPLICATIONS

A. Oral Effects

1. Mucositis, candidiasis, and xerostomia are similar in signs and symptoms to those resulting from chemotherapy and radiotherapy.
2. Daily oral care supervision is similar to management for chemotherapy- and radiotherapy-induced oral effects.
3. Team supervision is essential.

B. Opportunistic Infection

Interstitial pneumonia.

C. Graft Versus Host Disease[33,35]

1. *Description.* Bone marrow recipient adversely reacts to the donated marrow and rejects it, or when the donor's immunologically competent cells react against the host.
2. *Symptoms*
   a. Acute. Skin rash on palms and soles; persistent anorexia and/or diarrhea; liver disease during first 3 months after transplant.
   b. Chronic. Facial rash, arthritis, and obstructive lung and liver disease occur or persist beyond 3 months after the transplantation.

3. *Prevention and Treatment*
   a. Antirejection drugs.
   b. Steroids.
4. *Oral Care*
   a. Meticulous oral hygiene.
   b. Only consider emergency dental needs for treatment.
   c. Consult physician regarding blood counts and need for antibiotic prophylaxis.

▪ PERSONAL FACTORS[36]

Patient attitudes and feelings may be similar to those of any patient with a major chronic disease or disability. As with other diseases with limited hope for cure, strong feelings of hopelessness and despair predominate.

The very word *cancer* brings fear and anxiety to the patient. The concerns of a patient may differ at different stages of treatment.

I. PATIENT PROBLEMS

A. Early Fears and Anxieties

1. Outcome.
2. Imminent surgery, radiation, chemotherapy, or other treatment.
3. Disfigurement, changes in appearance, and pain.
4. Extended hospitalization.
5. Financial stress.

B. During and Following Therapy

1. Preoccupation with details of examinations, treatments, symptoms, or medications.
2. Depression and grief, which may lead to withdrawal and isolation.
3. Major concerns may include obvious facial deformity, speech difficulty, swallowing difficulty, drooling, hair loss, weight loss, nausea, and odors from debris collection and tissue changes.

II. SUGGESTIONS FOR APPROACH TO PATIENT

A. Provide explanations before and after therapy to prevent misconceptions and apprehensions and to attempt to allay fears.
B. Provide paper and pencil for patient with a speech difficulty to write questions and requests.
C. Show acceptance. Acknowledge the appropriateness of the patient's concerns.
D. Express empathy, but avoid oversolicitousness.

Everyday Ethics

All of the patients, staff, and dentist had left the office. Ashley, the dental hygienist, was reviewing patient records at the front desk, glad to enjoy the quiet time after hours to complete her work.

The telephone rang and Ashley answered it. It was Gina, the daughter of a longtime patient, Mr. Prisby. Gina lives out of state but is visiting her 70-year-old father who is undergoing radiation and chemotherapy treatments for throat cancer. When she arrived, she was shocked to find her father unable to open his mouth completely and a white coating on the inside of his cheeks. He is unable to eat anything but the softest of foods due to the discomfort and dryness. Gina is concerned that her father cannot eat enough to be healthy. She asks what can be done.

Ashley puts Gina on hold and pulls Mr. Prisby's record. She sees that he had a complete examination and all treatment performed that left him in good dental health 3 months ago, just before he started his cancer treatment. The white coating that Gina describes may be candidiasis and require medication. Ashley considers phoning in the prescription in the dentist's name to save time.

Questions for Consideration

1. What advice can Ashley give to Gina, considering the stipulations of patient confidentiality?

2. Describe the ethical and legal consequences of Ashley phoning in a prescription for Mr. Prisby.

3. What decisions and/or actions are appropriate for Ashley to pursue within the scope of her duties at this time?

E. Help to direct thoughts and efforts toward restoration of functional activity.

F. Instill trust and security by demonstrating genuine interest.

G. Assist the patient who is alcoholic, uses tobacco products excessively, or has other habits that have to be eliminated. The patient may need the help of psychiatry, Alcoholics Anonymous, counseling for a tobacco cessation program, or other type of support.

H. When a patient is referred to a specialist or specialty clinic, a check must be made to ascertain that the patient arrives for the appointment. Frightened patients may become confused or may postpone the visit if they do not realize the urgency of the condition.

 Factors To Teach The Patient

- The importance of oral soft tissue screening and complete oral examination at regular frequent intervals.

- Dental biofilm control methods, gel-tray application, use of saliva substitute, and all other details of personal care to reduce oral side effects induced by the disease and/or therapy.

- Encourage adherence to daily oral care regimen.

- Why use of alcohol and tobacco must be stopped.

- Instruction for family members in oral health care for the sick and dependent patient.

REFERENCES

1. **Miller**, B.F. and Keane, C.B.: *Encyclopedia and Dictionary of Medicine, Nursing, and Allied Health*, 6th ed. Philadelphia, W.B. Saunders Co., 1997.

2. **Cancer Statistics**, 2004, *CA.*, *54*, 8 January/February, 2004.

3. **Murphy**, G.P., Lawrence, W., and Lenhard, R.E., eds.: *Clinical Oncology*, 2nd ed. Atlanta, GA, American Cancer Society, 1995, pp. 1–39.

4. **Little**, J.W., Falace, D.A., Miller, C.S., and Rhodus, N.L.: *Dental Management of the Medically Compromised Patient*, 5th ed. St. Louis, Mosby–Year Book, 1997, pp. 532–542.

5. **Stevenson-Moore**, P.: Essential Aspects of Pretreatment Oral Examination, *NCI Monogr., 9,* 33, 1990.

6. **DePaola**, L.G. and Minah, G.E.: Isolation of Pathogenic Microorganisms From Dentures and Denture Soaking Containers of Myelosuppressed Cancer Patients, *J. Prosthet. Dent., 49,* 20, January, 1983.

7. **Kraus**, D.H. and Pfister, D.G.: Head and Neck Oncology, in Noble, J., ed.: *Textbook of Primary Care Medicine*, 2nd ed. St. Louis, Mosby, 1996, pp. 467–475.

8. **Harrison**, L.B. and Fass, D.E.: Radiation Therapy for Oral Cavity Cancer, *Dent. Clin. North Am., 34,* 205, April, 1990.

9. **Whitmyer**, C.C., Waskowski, J.C., and Iffland, H.A.: Radiotherapy and Oral Sequelae: Preventive and Management Protocols, *J. Dent. Hyg., 71,* 23, January–February, 1997.

10. **Semba**, S.E., Mealey, B.L., and Hallmon, W.W.: The Head and Neck Radiotherapy Patient: Part I—Oral Manifestations of Radiation Therapy, *Compend. Cont. Educ. Dent.,* 15, 250, February, 1994.

11. **Madeya**, M.L.: Oral Complications From Cancer Therapy: Part 1—Pathophysiology and Secondary Complications, *Oncol. Nurs. Forum,* 23, 801, June, 1996.

12. **Madeya**, M.L.: Oral Complications From Cancer Therapy: Part 2—Nursing Implications for Assessment and Treatment, *Oncol. Nurs. Forum,* 23, 808, June, 1996.

13. **Barker**, G.J., Barker, B.F., and Gier, R.E.: *Oral Management of the Cancer Patient. A Guide for the Health Care Professional,* 5th ed. Kansas City, MO, Biomedical Communications, University of Missouri-Kansas City, School of Dentistry, January, 1996, 19 pp.

14. **American Academy of Periodontology**, Committee on Research, Science, and Therapy: Position Paper: Periodontal Considerations in the Management of the Cancer Patient, *J. Periodontol.,* 68, 791, August, 1997.

15. **Browman**, G.P., Wong, G., Hodson, I., Sathya, J., Russell, R., McAlpine, L., Skingley, P., and Levine, M.N.: Influence of Cigarette Smoking on the Efficacy of Radiation Therapy in Head and Neck Cancer, *N. Engl. J. Med.,* 328, 159, January 21, 1993.

16. **Wiseman**, L.R. and Faulds, D.: Oral Pilocarpine: A Review of Its Pharmacological Properties and Clinical Potential in Xerostomia, *Drugs,* 49, 143, January, 1995.

17. **Zimmerman**, R.P., Mark, R.J., Tran, L.M., and Juillard, G.F.: Concomitant Pilocarpine During Head and Neck Irradiation Is Associated With Decreased Posttreatment Xerostomia, *Int. J. Radiat. Oncol. Biol. Phys.,* 37, 571, February 1, 1997.

18. **Garg**, A.K. and Malo, M.: Manifestations and Treatment of Xerostomia and Associated Oral Effects Secondary to Head and Neck Radiation Therapy, *J. Am. Dent. Assoc.,* 128, 1128, August, 1997.

19. **Guchelaar**, H.J., Vermes, A., and Meerwaldt, J.H.: Radiation-Induced Xerostomia: Pathophysiology, Clinical Course and Supportive Treatment, *Support Care Cancer,* 5, 281, July, 1997.

20. **Ried**, H., Zietz, H., and Jaffe, N.: Late Effects of Cancer Treatment in Children, *Pediatr. Dent.,* 17, 273, July/August, 1995.

21. **Peterson**, D.E. and D'Ambrosio, J.A.: Nonsurgical Management of Head and Neck Cancer Patients, *Dent. Clin. North Am.,* 38, 425, July, 1994.

22. **Ashamalia**, H.L., Thom, S.R., and Goldwein, J.W.: Hyperbaric Oxygen Therapy for the Treatment of Radiation-Induced Sequelae in Children: The University of Pennsylvania Experience, *Cancer,* 77, 2407, June 1, 1996.

23. **Neovius**, E.B., Lind, M.G., and Lind, F.G.: Hyperbaric Oxygen Therapy for Wound Complications After Surgery in the Irradiated Head and Neck: A Review of the Literature and a Report of 15 Consecutive Patients, *Head Neck,* 19, 315, July, 1997.

24. **Wong**, J.K., Wood, R.E., and McLean, M.: Conservative Management of Osteoradionecrosis, *Oral Surg., Oral Med., Oral Pathol., Oral Radiol., Endod.,* 84, 16, July, 1997.

25. **Granström**, G., Jacobsson, M., and Tjellström, A.: Titanium Implants in Irradiated Tissue: Benefits From Hyperbaric Oxygen, *Int. J. Oral Maxillofac. Implants,* 7, 15, Spring, 1992.

26. **Esser**, E. and Wagner, W.: Dental Implants Following Radical Oral Cancer Surgery and Adjuvant Radiotherapy, *Int. J. Oral Maxillofac. Implants,* 12, 552, July, 1997.

27. **Savarese**, D.: Principles of Cancer Therapy, in Noble, J., ed.: *Textbook of Primary Care Medicine,* 2nd ed. St. Louis, Mosby, 1996, pp. 777–788.

28. **NIH Consensus Development Conference Statements**: Oral Complications of Cancer Therapies: Diagnosis, Prevention, and Treatment, *NCI Monogr., 9,* 3, 1990.

29. **DeBiase**, C.B.: *Dental Health Education: Theory and Practice,* Philadelphia, Lea & Febiger, 1991, pp. 228–239.

30. **Krywulak**, M.L., Hsu, E., Vietti, T., and DeBiase, C.B.: Mouth and Dental Care, in Ritchey, K., ed.: *Pediatric Oncology Group Supportive Care Manual.* Smith Kline Beecham, 1996, pp. 1–14.

31. **Terezhalmy**, G.T., Whitmyer, C.C., and Markman, M.: Cancer Chemotherapeutic Agents, *Dent. Clin. North Am.,* 40, 709, July, 1996.

32. **Little**, Falace, Miller, and Rhodus: op. cit., pp. 543–544.

33. **Rhodus**, N.L. and Little, J.W.: Dental Management of the Bone Marrow Transplant Patient, *Compend. Cont. Educ. Dent.,* 13, 1040, November, 1992.

34. **DeBiase**, C.B.: Oral Care for the Bone Marrow Transplant Patient, *Case Stud. Periodont. Mgmt.,* 2, 1, November, 1996.

35. **Appelbaum**, F.R.: The Use of Bone Marrow and Peripheral Blood Stem Cell Transplantation in the Treatment of Cancer, *CA,* 46, 142, May/June, 1996.

36. **Allen**, J.: The Psychosocial Effects of Cancer and Its Treatment in the Elderly, *Spec. Care Dentist.,* 4, 13, January/February, 1984.

SUGGESTED READINGS

Barasch, A. and Safford, M.M.: Management of Oral Pain in Patients With Malignant Diseases, *Compend. Cont. Educ. Dent., 14,* 1376, November, 1993.

Joyston-Bechal, S: Prevention of Dental Diseases Following Radiotherapy and Chemotherapy, *Int. Dent. J., 42,* 47, February, 1992.

Lunn, R.: Oral Management of the Cancer Patient. Part I: Overview of Cancer and Oral Cancer, *Can. Dent. Hyg. Assoc.* (PROBE), *31,* 137, July/August, 1997.

Schein, J.: The Many Faces of Cancer: Sifting Through the Facts, *RDH, 15,* 24, October, 1995.

Souliman, S.K. and Christie, J.: Pacemaker Failure Induced by Radiotherapy, *PACE, 17,* 270, March, 1994, Part I.

Toth, B.B., Martin, J.W., and Fleming, T.J.: Oral Complications Associated With Cancer Therapy: An M.D. Anderson Cancer Center Experience, *J. Clin. Periodontol., 17,* 508, August, 1990 (Part II).

Yellowitz, J.A., Goodman, H.S., and Farooq, N.S.: Knowledge, Opinions, and Practices Related to Oral Cancer: Results of Three Elderly Racial Groups, *Spec. Care Dentist., 17,* 100, May/June, 1997.

Children

Berg, J. and Bleyer, A.: Pediatric Dentistry in Care of the Cancer Patient, *Pediatr. Dent., 17,* 257, July/August, 1995.

Chan, K.W.: Pediatric Bone Marrow Transplantation, *Pediatr. Dent., 17,* 291, July/August, 1995.

Kennedy, L. and Diamond, J.: Assessment and Management of Chemotherapy-Induced Mucositis in Children, *J. Pediatr. Oncol. Nurs., 14,* 164, July, 1997.

Chemotherapy

Peterson, D.E. and Sonis, S.T., eds.: *Oral Complications of Cancer Chemotherapy.* The Hague/Boston/London, Martinus Nijhoff Publishers, 1983, pp. 1–12.

Rosenberg, S.W.: Oral Care of Chemotherapy Patients, *Dent. Clin. North Am., 34,* 239, April, 1990.

Semba, S.E., Mealey, B.L., and Hallmon, W.W.: Dentistry and the Cancer Patient: Part 2—Oral Health Management of the Chemotherapy Patient, *Compend. Cont. Educ. Dent., 15,* 1378, November, 1994.

Radiation

Epstein, J.B. and van der Meij, E.H.: Complicating Mucosal Reactions in Patients Receiving Radiation Therapy for Head and Neck Cancer, *Spec. Care Dentist., 17,* 88, May/June, 1997.

Epstein, J.B., Corbett, T., Galler, C., and Stevenson-Moore, P.: Surgical Periodontal Treatment in the Radiotherapy-Treated Head and Neck Cancer Patient, *Spec. Care Dent., 14*, 182, September/October, 1994.

Meraw, S.J. and Reeve, C.M.: Dental Considerations and Treatment of the Oncology Patient Receiving Radiation Therapy, *J. Am. Dent. Assoc., 129*, 201, February, 1998.

Wang, R.R., Pillai, K., and Jones, P.K.: In vitro Backscattering From Implant Materials During Radiotherapy, *J. Prosthet. Dent., 75*, 626, June, 1996.

Whitmeyer, C.C., Esposito, S.J., and Terezhalmy, G.T.: Radiotherapy for Head and Neck Neoplasms, *Gen. Dent., 45*, 363, July/August, 1997.

Patient Health and Oral Hygiene

Addems, A., Epstein, J.B., Damji, S., and Spinelli, J.: The Lack of Efficacy of a Foam Brush in Maintaining Gingival Health: A Controlled Study, *Spec. Care Dentist., 12*, 103, May/June, 1992.

American Cancer Society 1996 Advisory Committee on Diet, Nutrition, and Cancer Prevention: Guidelines on Diet, Nutrition, and Cancer Prevention: Reducing the Risk of Cancer With Healthy Food Choices and Physical Activity, *CA, 46*, 325, November/December, 1996.

Bland, K.I.: Quality-of-Life Management for Cancer Patients, *CA, 47*, 194, July/August, 1997.

Epstein, J.B., van der Meij, E.H., Lunn, R., Le, N.D., and Stevenson-Moore, P.: Effects of Compliance With Fluoride Gel Application on Caries and Caries Risk in Patients After Radiation Therapy for Head and Neck Cancer, *Oral Surg. Oral Med. Oral Pathol. Oral Radiol. Endod., 82*, 268, September, 1996.

Ghalichebaf, M., DeBiase, C.B., and Stookey, G.K.: A New Technique for the Fabrication of Fluoride Carriers in Patients Receiving Radiotherapy to the Head and Neck, *Compend. Cont. Educ. Dent., 15*, 470, April, 1994.

Care of Patients With Disabilities

Kathryn Ragalis, RDH, MS, DMD

Many types of disabilities require special attention and adaptations during dental and dental hygiene appointments, and others have no effect on dental care. Some disabilities severely impact the daily activities and function of an individual and can lead to poor oral hygiene, rampant dental disease, and dental neglect.

The general term *disability* refers to any reduction of a person's activity that has resulted from an acute or chronic health condition and affects motor, sensory, or mental functions. A disability may be permanent or temporary. A temporary impairment may be physical, such as a fracture of a leg, or physiologic with physical limitations, such as during pregnancy. Chronic systemic diseases may result in crippling disabilities. The causes of disabilities may be factors of heredity, systemic disease, trauma, or combinations of these.

Oral health for the individual with a disability takes on more than usual significance and presents a challenge to dental personnel. For the patient, the disability provides enough of a burden without additional oral problems, which can reduce an already lowered potential for normal living. Preventive measures must be encouraged and promoted to minimize oral problems.

Imagination, ingenuity, flexibility, and persistence are necessary for those involved in treating people with disabilities. Individualization and modification of usual procedures may be necessary. Patience, calmness, and kindness are keys to approaching the special patient. Box 53-1 supplies key words and definitions pertaining to impairments, disabilities, and handicaps.

■ DISABILITIES

I. DEFINITIONS

    A. The *United States Americans With Disabilities Act (ADA)* defines an individual with a disability as a person who *"has a physical or mental impairment that substantially limits one or more major life activities, has a record of such impairment, or is regarded as having such impairment."*[1]

    B. The *International Classification of the World Health Organization* clarifies the meaning of impairment, disability, and handicap.[2]

       • An *impairment* is an abnormality of structure or function of a limb or body organ, whereas the *disability* is the inability to perform a task or activity as a result of the impairment.

       • The *handicap* is the disadvantage or limitation that an individual has when compared with others of the same age, sex, and background that has resulted from the impairment and the disability.

       • Table 53-1 lists categories and examples of each.

II. OCCURRENCE

    • Approximately 1 of 5 persons is affected by a disability.

    • Progress in medical care has increased initial survival of those born with a disability and increased the survival rate of those experiencing a disabling condition.

    • As life expectancy increases, so does the likelihood of acquiring a disability.

III. REHABILITATION TRENDS

    • Trends toward deinstitutionalization have brought alternative living, educational, and work arrangements to many individuals with physical and mental disabilities.

    • Children taken out of institutional life and trained for community living in transitional homes are integrated or "mainstreamed" into regular school and health programs.

    • Persons with disabilities may receive vocational and educational counseling, medical and dental services, and work placement.

    • Specially staffed community housing for group living has been made available.

IV. TYPES OF CONDITIONS

    • A variety of impairments are found among persons with disabilities, and an individual may have more than one type of disability.

    • The lists in Table 53-1 are representative.

    • Many of the diseases and syndromes with symptoms of impairments are described in the various chapters throughout Part VII of this book.

V. BARRIERS TO DENTAL CARE

    • People with disabilities must overcome many barriers to live as independently as possible.

    • Dental professionals need to be familiar with the barriers so progress can be made to ensure accessibility to the same level of dental care as the general population.

    • Barriers involve the patient, the family, caregivers, guardians, and dental professional, as described in Table 53-2.

■ DENTAL AND DENTAL HYGIENE CARE

I. OBJECTIVES

The dental team can make a significant contribution to the well-being, independence, and sense of personal value of a

BOX 53-1 KEY WORDS: Impairment, Disability, Handicap

Accessibility standards: the ADA prohibits discrimination on the basis of a disability and requires places of public accommodation and commercial facilities to meet requirements of accessibility by removing architectural, transportation, and communication barriers.

AwDA: Americans with Disabilities Act; abbreviation sometimes used to prevent confusion with the ADA (American Dental Association).

Barrier-free: area that is freely accessible to all without discrimination on the basis of a disability; obstacles to passage or communication have been removed.

Behavior modification: an approach to correction of undesirable conduct that focuses on changing observable actions; modification of behavior is accomplished through systematic manipulation of the environmental and behavioral variables related to the specific behavior to be changed.

Behavior therapy: an approach in which the focus is on the patient's observable behavior rather than on conflicts and unconscious processes presumed to underlie the maladaptive behavior; accomplished through systematic manipulation of the environmental and behavioral variables related to specific behavior to be modified.

Deinstitutionalization: returning patients to home and community as quickly as possible after treatment rather than housing them permanently or for long periods in custodial institutions; the elimination of mental health institutions, for example, has been made possible by (1) the use of new medications that control the symptoms of illness and (2) community health centers that serve as support.

Desensitization: the treatment of phobias and related disorders by intentionally exposing the patient, in imagination or real life, to emotionally distressing stimuli; desensitization of a fearful patient to accept dental treatment might consist, for example, of short exposures to the dental chair, instruments, air syringe, and the sound of a handpiece along with building trust in the dental team members.

Developmental disability: a substantial handicap of indefinite duration with onset before the age of 18 years, attributable to mental retardation, autism, cerebral palsy, epilepsy, or other incurable neuropathy.

Disability: any restriction or lack of ability (resulting from an impairment) to perform an activity in the manner or within the range considered normal for a human being of the same age, sex, and background.

Handicap: a disadvantage for an individual, resulting from an impairment or a disability, that limits or prevents fulfillment of a role that is within the normal range for a human of the same age, sex, and social and cultural factors as the affected individual.

Impairment: any loss or abnormality of psychologic, physiologic, or anatomic structure or function.

Mainstreaming: integration of people with disabilities into their community through programs of rehabilitation; process by which persons with special needs (educational, physical, psychologic) are included within the mainstream of society rather than segregated.

Normalization: making available to all individuals patterns and conditions of everyday life that are as close as possible to the norms and patterns of the mainstream of society.

patient with a disability. Whether employed in private practice, working in an institutional or community clinical and educational setting, or contributing on a volunteer basis, the dental team must have as its objectives to:

- Motivate the patient and the caregiver. Personal oral care practices conducive to maintaining healthy oral tissue with freedom from infection must be developed.

- Contribute to the patient's general health, of which oral health is an integral part. Prevention of tooth loss increases the ability to masticate food, which is essential to prevent malnutrition and to increase resistance to infection. Identify any signs and symptoms of systemic problems and make appropriate referral.

■ TABLE 53-1 IMPAIRMENTS, DISABILITIES, AND HANDICAPS

IMPAIRMENTS	DISABILITIES	HANDICAPS
Intellectual impairments	Behavior disabilities	Orientation handicap
Mental retardation	Awareness	To surroundings
Memory, thinking	Motivation	Relates to behavior and
Psychologic impairments	Communication disabilities	communication disability
Consciousness	Speaking	Physical independence handicap
Perception	Listening	Dependence on others
Language impairments	Personal care disabilities	Mobility handicap
Communication	Personal hygiene	Reduced mobility
Voice function	Dressing	Dwelling restriction
Aural impairments	Locomotor disabilities	Occupation handicap
Hearing impairment	Ambulation	Adjusted occupation
Auditory sensitivity	Transport	Restricted because of disability
Ocular impairments	Body disposition disabilities	Social integration handicap
Visual acuity	Subsistence	Restricted participation
Blindness	Dexterity disabilities	Socially isolated
Visceral impairments	Daily activity	Economic self-sufficiency handicap
Internal organs	Grasping	Fully self-sufficient
Impaired mastication, swallowing	Situational disabilities	Impoverished
Skeletal impairments	Environmental temperature	
Mechanical and motor	Dependence	
Deficiency of parts	Endurance	
Paralysis	Particular skill disability	
Disfiguring impairments	Task fulfillment	
Structural deformity	Learning ability	
Generalized, sensory impairment	Dexterity	
Susceptible to trauma		

(From World Health Organization: *International Classification of Impairments, Disabilities and Handicaps,* Geneva, 1980.)

- Prevent the need for extensive dental and periodontal treatment that the patient may not be able to undergo because of lowered physical stamina or the inability to cooperate. Dentures or other removable prostheses can be hazardous for certain patients or impossible for others.
- Aid in the improvement of appearance, thereby contributing to social acceptance. A person without halitosis and with clean teeth is more socially accepted.
- Make appointments pleasant and comfortable experiences.

■ TABLE 53-2 EXAMPLES OF BARRIERS TO DENTAL CARE

	PATIENT	FAMILY, CAREGIVER, GUARDIAN	DENTAL PROFESSIONAL
Attitude Barriers	May not comprehend importance of dental health or want to or be able to cooperate.	May not care for own dental health, may be overstressed with other patient health issues.	May not feel adequately trained to safely treat medically compromised patient.
Physical Barriers	Fear of not being able to cope with architectural barriers, fear of falling, or fear of attracting attention in an embarrassing way; all can be hindrances to seeking oral care.	May not be able to transport patient and wheel chair to appointment, may be unable to lift patient into car or dental chair.	Office may not be wheelchair accessible or operatory may be too small to comfortably accommodate wheelchair; rest room may not be accessible; no parking spaces available.
Financial Barriers	May have limited income because disability affects employability.	May be unable to take time off from work to accompany patient to appointment.	May need construction to build handicapped-accessible features or buy specialized equipment. Longer appointment time may be needed for same fee.

II. PRETREATMENT PLANNING

Most patients with disabilities can be treated in the private dental office setting. Only a relatively small number need hospitalization due to difficulties in management or a systemic condition that requires special medical supervision.

A. Preliminary Contact

- Information may be obtained from the patient, guardian, parent, relative, advocate, or other person responsible for the patient.
- The essential information can be obtained in advance by telephone interview, or medical forms can be mailed to the home for completion.
- Advance information permits the dental team to be prepared to make the appointment successful

and a positive experience for the patient and dental professionals.

B. Guardian

- If a person is declared incapacitated in a legal process, a guardian is appointed.
- The guardian must give consent for any treatment, including signatures on consent forms.
- Written proof of guardianship should be obtained and kept in the patient record.

C. Information to Obtain

- In addition to the usual topics covered by the questions in Table 7-3, basic information, medical and dental history, and supplemental questions should be asked and are listed in Box 53-2.

BOX 53-2 Information to Obtain About the Patient Before the Appointment

BASIC INFORMATION

Has a guardian been legally appointed? Obtain written documentation.

Is there a caregiver, case worker, or counselor that works with the patient?

Will someone accompany the patient to appointments?

Does the patient give consent to discuss care with other individuals?

Degree of independence, self-care, and way to communication with the patient.

MEDICAL HISTORY

Specific list of disabilities or disabling conditions.

When diagnosed.

History of treatments, hospitalizations, or institutionalization.

Current medications and other therapy.

Names and addresses of specialists.

Any restrictions, such as dietary or for safety (leg braces, helmet).

DENTAL HISTORY

Previous dental experiences and patient's attitude.

Difficulties in obtaining appointments, barriers to dental care experienced.

Most recent care: procedures, setting, success.

History of oral infections and oral habits.

Fluoride history, including self- or professionally applied topical methods.

Current home care methods: aids and special devices, frequency, degree of self-care.

Concepts of perceived needs, attitudes, and apparent emphasis on dental care.

Modifications and successful techniques used before and during appointments.

SUPPLEMENTAL INFORMATION

Are any of the following affected by disability:

- Muscular coordination, mobility, walking
- Sitting tolerance
- Sitting position
- Ability to cooperate/involuntary movements
- Communication: speech, hearing, vision
- Breathing, including when reclined
- Swallowing, control of saliva
- Bowel or bladder control
- Mental capacities
- Dexterity, ability to brush and floss teeth
- Ability to chew or eat

OPEN-ENDED OTHER INFORMATION

Does patient require any additional assistance or have any other issues of concern?

- To avoid unpleasant situations, do not make assumptions but ask direct questions about a patient's disability.

C. Consultations With Physicians, Other Specialists, and Sources

- Management of a patient with disabilities can be very complex because the patient is medically compromised.
- Consultation with the other professionals involved may be required to help determine a plan for patient treatment and continued care.
- Pertinent information may be obtained from other medical specialists and the social worker.
- Extra time may be required to access information about the conditions and medications prior to appointment.

D. Interaction With Caregiver

- A patient with a disability may depend on a caregiver for daily life activities.
- May or may not be legal guardian of patient and contact person to plan appointments.
- Caregivers are an excellent source of information, help, and suggestions for gaining cooperation from the patient, and dental personnel must make every effort to work with them.
- Special help may be needed during the appointment and for supervision of oral care on a daily basis in the total preventive care program.
- Solicit help in preparing the patient for the appointments; ask that procedures and facilities be described in advance in a pleasant and positive manner to reassure the patient.
- Invite to the office before the appointment to see the facility and become familiar with the surroundings and staff.
- List special aids the patient must bring to the appointment, such as a transfer board for transfer into the dental chair, hearing aid, dental prostheses, and biofilm control devices currently in use.

■ APPOINTMENT SCHEDULING

I. DETERMINE SPECIAL REQUIREMENTS

Determine what preparation needs to be taken prior to appointment to allow time in the schedule, for example, to move furniture, retrieve and set up special equipment, or premedicate the patient.

II. TRANSPORTATION REQUIREMENTS

- Wheelchair patient may need to reserve a public wheelchair transport vehicle and be limited by the time schedule.
- Patient may arrange a ride transportation service that must be contacted when the patient has completed the appointment; forms may need to be completed.

III. TIME OF APPOINTMENT

A. Patient

Determine whether the patient's daily schedule influences time selection. The cooperation of the patient may be decreased if basic routines are disturbed, for example:

- Appointment for the patient with diabetes must not interfere with medication, meal, or between-meal eating schedules.
- The elderly person who rises early may feel better during a morning appointment.
- Patients with arthritis may have greater mobility late in the morning or in the afternoon.
- Child's nap schedule should be respected.
- Early morning appointment may be difficult for a patient who requires a long time for morning preparation, such as a patient with a spinal cord injury or colostomy.

B. Caregiver

The schedule of the caregiver who accompanies the patient must be considered.

C. Dental Facility

- Arrange a time when the patient will not have to wait a long time after arrival.
- Schedule a challenging patient when the clinician is at optimum energy and patience.
- Allow sufficient time so that the patient does not feel rushed; many persons with disabilities cannot hurry.
- Consider incontinence issues and the difficulties and time needed for rest room visits; encourage emptying bladder before being seated in dental operatory.

IV. FOLLOW-UP

The frequency of maintenance appointments for all patients must be individualized. Frequent appointments are encouraged for the following reasons:

- To decrease length of single appointment by keeping the oral tissues at an optimum level of health.

- To assist the patient whose disability limits the ability to perform personal oral hygiene adequately.
- To provide motivation through monitoring of biofilm and review of procedures for the patient and the parent or other caregiver involved.

▪ BARRIER-FREE ENVIRONMENT

- In general, a facility that is barrier-free for a patient in a wheelchair is accessible to all other individuals. The patient in a wheelchair requires more space for turning and positioning.
- Additional features are needed for other specific disabilities, for example, braille floor indicators can be installed beside the numbers on elevators; doorways, steps, and stairways can be outlined with bright colors that contrast with the background for people with limited vision.
- Guidelines and specifications for a barrier-free environment are available. The descriptions that follow represent general features based on governmental regulations for accessibility standards, along with suggested applications for a dental clinic or office.[3]

I. EXTERNAL FEATURES

A. Parking

A reserved area, clearly marked, should be close to the building entrance and 13 feet wide (8-foot car space with 5-foot access aisle) to permit a person with a disability to open car doors for exiting and reboarding.

B. Walkways

- A 3-foot-wide walkway is needed for wheelchair accommodation.
- The surface must be solid and nonslip, without irregularities.
- Curb ramps (cuts) from the street and from the parking area are necessary.

C. Entrance

- At least one entrance to the building should be on ground level or be accessible by a gently sloping ramp (rise of 1 inch for every 12 inches).
- An easily grasped handrail (height 30 to 34 inches) is needed on at least one side, and preferably both sides, to accommodate left- and right-handed cane and one-crutch users.

D. Door

The lightweight door with a lever type of handle must open at least 32 inches for a wheelchair and a person using a tall crutch, as shown in Figure 53-1.

II. INTERNAL FEATURES

Official regulations specify dimensions for accessibility of all aspects, including passageways, floors, drinking fountains, and restrooms. A few are described here.

A. Passageways

- The passageways should be at least 3 feet wide, with handrails along the sides.
- They should be free from obstructions, such as hanging signs with which a tall blind person could collide.

B. Floors

- Level floors with nonslip surfaces are important.

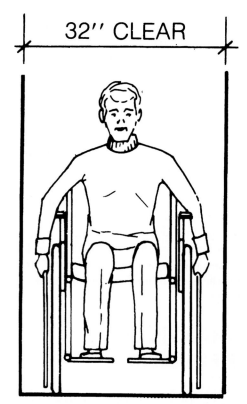

▪ **FIGURE 53-1 Wheelchair Accessibility.** Wheelchairs designed for adults vary in width from 2 feet 3 inches to 2 feet 8 inches. A clear door width of 32 inches to accommodate these wheelchairs has been accepted as the official regulation.

- Thick or small unattached movable rugs or carpets present obstacles for wheelchairs or walkers and hazards for a patient with crutches, cane, or leg brace.

C. Reception Area

- At least part of the furniture should permit easy access during seating and rising.
- Preferred are chairs with 18-inch-high, flat, firm seats and arms for support when pushing oneself up by the arms.
- Chairs must not slide or tip as the person rises.

III. THE TREATMENT ROOM

In a group of several treatment rooms, only one room needs to be made accessible. Dental personnel should be versatile in exchanging rooms to serve special patients.

A. Dimensions

- Space is needed for the dental chair, related dental equipment, and the wheelchair.
- The doorway must be at least 32 inches wide.
- The wheelchair is placed beside and parallel to the dental chair for patient transfer. In a small facility, the dental chair can be rotated to allow for turning the wheelchair.
- The dental chair selected should be able to be lowered to 19 inches from the floor and should be accessible from both sides for wheelchair transfer.
- An x-ray machine in the same treatment room can simplify the problems of moving the patient into a separate radiography room.

B. Wheelchair Used During Treatment

When the patient is in a total support wheelchair, transfer to the dental chair may not be advisable. The wheelchair of a patient who is unable to transfer can be positioned for direct utilization; some wheelchairs are self-reclining and have headrests.
- *Portable Headrest.* A portable headrest may be attached to the wheelchair handles, as shown in Figure 53-2.
- *Position of Dental Chair.* The dental chair can be swiveled to permit the wheelchair to be backed up to place the patient's head in a usual treatment position. The dental light can then be directed into the patient's oral cavity and the equipment adjusted for easy access.

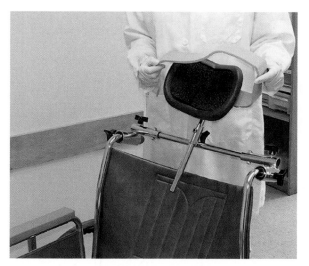

■ **FIGURE 53-2 Portable Headrest Attached to Wheelchair.**

- *Wheelchair Lift.* An automatic wheelchair lift that tilts the chair back to a usual working position can be obtained for a clinical facility where wheelchair patients are treated frequently.

IV. PATIENT INSTRUCTION

When a teaching area is planned for patient instruction, attention must be given to ensure accessibility for a patient in a wheelchair. The same facility can be used by all patients.

A. Dimensions

The tabletop and washbasin built at a height of 32 to 34 inches permit clearance underneath for knees and wheelchair arms, as shown in Figure 53-3.

B. Washbasin

- Lever- or blade-type handles on faucets are usable by patients who have difficulty gripping handles or have no hands; prevent burning the patient who cannot sense temperature.
- Hot pipes under the sink must be covered or insulated because patients who have no sensation in their legs could be burned.

C. Mirror

- Mirrors and dispensers are positioned low, a tilt mirror could provide better viewing of the teeth during instruction for most patients.
- An unattached hand mirror, preferably on a pedestal that tilts, supplements the wall mirror.
- A magnifying mirror can provide an excellent aid for viewing the disclosed biofilm and the devices for biofilm removal.

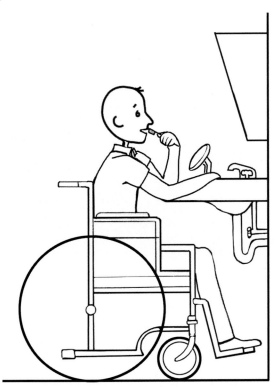

▪ **FIGURE 53-3 Biofilm Control Facility.** The tabletop and washbasin in a patient instruction area or lavatory should be built at a height of 32 to 34 inches to provide clearance underneath for knees of the patient and arms of the wheelchair. Hot pipes under a sink must be covered or insulated because patients with no sensation could be burned.

▪ PATIENT RECEPTION: THE INITIAL APPOINTMENT

The orientation of a patient with a disability paves the way for long-term success of dental and dental hygiene supervision and care.

I. ORIENTATION

- The first appointment includes and, when necessary, may be devoted entirely to a basic orientation to the facilities, the dental chair, and the personnel.
- The examination of the oral cavity is started, and dependent on the degree of patient cooperation, various steps in the assessment may be completed.
- Preventive personal care instructions are initiated, and participation of the caregiver is solicited.

- Several orientation visits may be necessary to acclimate the patient to surroundings and to desensitize.

II. COMMUNICATION

- Each patient is different, and members of the dental team must watch, listen, and learn procedures that will develop the patient's trust.
- Parents and other caregivers can explain how best to communicate, if appropriate.
- The caregiver can help interpret the changing moods of the patient, identify problems, and note changes in behavior that may indicate a dental problem.
- Even for the patient who cannot or will not speak or may appear withdrawn, the ability to understand what is being said should not be underestimated. The patient should always be addressed with instructions and respect.
- Nonverbal communication using facial expressions, pointing, body language, and demonstration helps certain patients to respond. Other patients write messages on a pad of paper or use sign language, a language board, or other devices the dental personnel can learn to use. Suggested procedures for the hearing-impaired patient are described on page 954.

III. PREVENTIVE CARE INTRODUCTION

- Whether or not the assessment and treatment plan are completed at the initial visit, the personal oral daily care program should be introduced. After finding out what the current daily care has been, instruction for the parent or other caregiver is presented along with that for the patient.
- The first step in treatment is the control of gingival infection by daily biofilm removal instruction and diet evaluation.
- The complete instruction and prevention program is described on page 897.

▪ WHEELCHAIR TRANSFERS[4,5]

Three basic transfer techniques are described, and selection is influenced by the size, weight, and mobility of the patient, along with any special physical conditions. The patient may prefer to transfer from the left or the right side of the dental chair, depending on which side of the body is stronger. Transfer from the wheelchair can be a frightening experience to the patient owing to fear of falling and injury. Always inform the patient of your intended actions before starting.

I. PREPARATION FOR WHEELCHAIR TRANSFER

A. Clear the Area

- Before starting a transfer, clear the area: move the clinician's stool, bracket tray, portable unit, and dental light.
- After the transfer, release the wheelchair brake to move it aside.
- In a small treatment room, the wheelchair may be folded and set aside.

B. Special Needs of Patient

- *Chair Padding.* Special padding used in a wheelchair as protection from pressure sores. Depending on the length of the appointment, the patient will decide whether the padding should be moved to the dental chair. Pressure sores are described on page 925.
- *Bags and Catheters.* Patients who do not have control of urine discharge, such as those with paraplegia or quadriplegia, have a bag with tubing for collection. The bag may be attached to the leg of the patient or to the wheelchair. After transfer, the tubing must be checked to be sure it is not bent or twisted.
- *Spasms.* Ask the patient about susceptibility to spasms and about procedures to follow for prevention.
- *Advice Concerning Transfer.* Ask the patient, family member, or caregiver how best the clinician can help during the transfer. The patient must be allowed to do as much as possible.

II. MOBILE PATIENT TRANSFER

When a patient can support his or her own weight, the "stand and pivot" technique can be used, as shown in Figure 53-4.

A. Position the Wheelchair

Face the wheelchair in the same direction as the dental chair at approximately an angle of 30°; set brakes; remove footrests and wheelchair armrests. The patient will adjust a power-driven chair and set the brakes before turning it off.

B. Prepare Dental Chair

Adjust the dental chair to the same height as or lower than the wheelchair; clear a path for transfer by uplifting the dental chair arm.

C. Approach to Patient

- Detach patient's safety belt.
- Face the patient and place feet outside the patient's feet for pivoting. Clinician's knees should be close to or against the patient's knees to prevent buckling.
- Place hands under the patient's arms and grasp the waist belt in back. Patient places arms around clinician's neck or places hands on wheelchair arms to push up. Clinician lifts patient to standing position, as in Figure 53-4B.

D. Pivot to Dental Chair

- Pivot together slowly until the patient is backed up to the side of the dental chair, with the backs

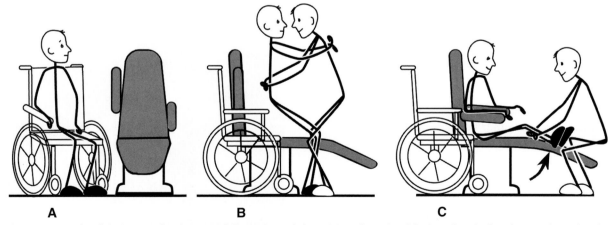

| A | B | C |

■ **FIGURE 53-4 Wheelchair Transfer for a Mobile Patient. (A)** Position the wheelchair at level of or lower than the dental chair; set wheel locks, remove footrests and arm rests, and raise the dental chair arm. **(B)** Clinician places feet outside of the patient, grasps the patient around the waist under the arms, locks hands or grasps belt in back; patient holds clinician around shoulders or neck; patient is lifted up and pivoted to dental chair side. **(C)** Patient is gently lowered to sitting position; dental chair arm is lowered; clinician grasps legs together to lift onto dental chair.

of the legs touching. The patient is gently lowered to a sitting position. Reposition the arm of the dental chair.

- Grasp the patient's legs together between the ankles and knees, and lift them onto the dental chair, as shown in Figure 53-4C.

E. Repeat in Reverse

After the appointment, return the patient to the wheelchair in the reverse order of procedure.

III. IMMOBILE PATIENT TRANSFER

When the patient is unable to support his or her own weight, two aides are required. The parent or other caregiver may serve as the second person.

A. Position the Wheelchair

1. Position the wheelchair in the same direction and parallel with the dental chair; set brakes; remove footrests.
2. Adjust the dental chair to the same height as or lower than the seat of the wheelchair.
3. Move the arm of the dental chair out of the transfer area, and remove the arm of the wheelchair.

B. First Aide

1. Aide I is positioned behind the wheelchair.
2. Place feet, one on either side of the rear wheel nearest the dental chair; place hands under the patient's arms below the elbows, pressing forearms against the patient's lower thorax area.
3. Clasp hands or wrists under the patient's rib cage.

C. Second Aide

Aide II may do either of the following, depending on the size and weight of the patient.
- Face patient and grasp hands under the patient's knees.
- Face dental chair; place one arm under the thighs and the other under the calves of the lower legs.

D. Transfer

On a prearranged signal and a steady motion, lift and gently transfer the patient to the dental chair.

E. Repeat in Reverse

After the appointment, the patient is returned to the wheelchair in the reverse order of procedure.

IV. SLIDING BOARD TRANSFER

A patient may bring a sliding board or one may be kept in the office or clinic. A transfer board is shown in Figure 53-5.

A. Position the Wheelchair

1. Position the wheelchair in the same direction as and parallel with the dental chair; set the brakes; remove the footrests, as show in Figure 53-5.
2. Adjust the seat of the dental chair to slightly lower than the wheelchair seat.
3. Move the arm of the dental chair out of the transfer area, and remove the arm of the wheelchair.

B. Adjust the Sliding Board

- Patient or clinician places the sliding board well under the hip of the patient.
- The board is extended across the dental chair.

C. Transfer

1. Patient shifts weight, balances on hands, and walks the buttocks across the board. The clinician can assist or do the transfer by holding the patient under the axillae. Two persons are needed when the patient is heavy or less mobile.
2. Board is removed and replaced after the appointment.

D. Repeat in Reverse

Dental chair is positioned slightly higher than the wheelchair seat for the return transfer.

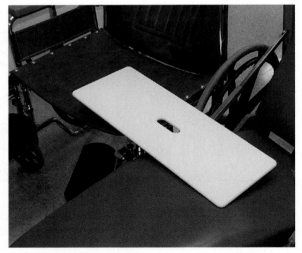

▪ **FIGURE 53-5 Transfer Board.** Transfer board placement between wheelchair and dental chair.

V. WALKING FRAME, CRUTCHES, CANE

The clinician asks the patient for instructions in how to assist.

A. Walking Frame to the Dental Chair

1. Adjust the dental chair upright, with arm out of the way and seat to level of back of patient's knees.
2. Patient backs up to dental chair until back of legs touch, then lowers into the chair. Clinician stabilizes the walking frame.
3. Clinician takes patient by the ankles to lift legs and turn patient onto the dental chair.
4. Remove walker to a place out of the way of dental personnel.

B. Walking Frame From the Dental Chair

1. Raise the dental chair to upright and ask the patient to wait while the walker is positioned. Allow ample time for the patient to adjust to the upright position to prevent effects of postural hypotension.
2. Move the arm of the dental chair; position the chair to the approximate height of the patient's knees.
3. Grasp ankles, gently turn patient, and swing legs down.
4. Reposition the walker.
5. The patient uses one hand to push up and the other to grasp the walker. When the walker is used for balance, one hand must be in the middle to prevent tipping.
6. If the patient wants assistance when rising, the clinician can hook an arm under the patient's arm on left side if the patient is right-handed. The patient's dominant hand is used to grasp the walker.

C. Crutches

1. The dental chair is positioned upright at a level with the patient's knees. Some patients need the chair higher so seating does not require knees to be bent.
2. The clinician assists, as directed by the patient, while the patient lowers into the chair; the legs are lifted onto the dental chair.
3. After the appointment, with the patient seated on the side of the dental chair, pass the crutches together to one hand. The patient usually uses the other hand to push up. If assistance in rising is requested, the clinician can hook an arm under the patient's arm as directed.

D. Cane

1. The dental chair is positioned at the level of the patient's knees or higher if the patient may have difficulty in bending the knees.
2. The patient may need assistance in lifting the legs onto the dental chair.
3. After the appointment, when the patient is seated on the side of the dental chair, the clinician passes the cane to the patient and assists the patient to rise only as directed.

■ PATIENT POSITION AND STABILIZATION

- The objectives in patient positioning and stabilization are to let the patient feel comfortable and secure while the professional person performs in a position that provides adequate illumination, visibility, and accessibility.
- A hyperactive patient or a patient with involuntary muscle movements can wear a special stabilizing device to enable the clinician to work and to prevent damage to the oral tissues by accidental movement of instruments.
- Extreme care must be given to placement of any patient with a swallowing defect; the patient is unable to prevent aspiration of fluids or any object placed in the mouth.

I. CHAIR POSITION
A. Tip Chair Back Slowly

Start to tip the chair back feet up first to provide balance so that the patient cannot fall. While tipping back the chair, place one hand on the patient's shoulder to offer assurance and support. Never place the chair back quickly. Advance in steps to allow the patient to adjust.

B. Chair Up

A patient with a respiratory complication must have the chair back up. A patient with a cardiac disease or a patient wearing a pacemaker should be asked, "How many pillows do you use at night?" The chair can be adjusted accordingly.

II. BODY ADJUSTMENTS

During the appointment, patients with a spinal cord injury must do a "push up" and patients with quadriplegia must shift their weight every 20 minutes for 10 to 15 seconds. By doing so, the patient can maintain good circulation and healthy tissue of the buttocks, where there is no sensation. The procedure is a preventive measure for decubitus ulcers and should be a consideration during long dental procedures, as on page 925.

III. BODY STABILIZATION

Body movement can be limited by providing support. When a support of any type is to be used, it should be explained to the patient that the devices are used to help the clinician and to make the patient more comfortable and are by no means a form of punishment. Body stabilization is used to help prevent injury to the patient and the dental practitioner, but any use of restraint has the risk of causing injury. Advanced training in the use of body stabilization is required. Written consent should be obtained for any use of restraint or stabilization, and the least restrictive method should be used.

A. Body Enclosure

Although a small patient may be held by a parent, such positioning can be tiring and insecure and is not recommended. Better cooperation is usually obtained by the use of aids, such as commercial wraps, which are available, or improvised wraps.

- *Pediwrap.* The *Pediwrap* is made of nylon mesh and encloses the patient from neck to ankles. It is available in three sizes to fit infants and children through 10 years of age. It is frequently used with support straps about the patient's legs and arms.
- *Papoose Board.* A *papoose board* is a board with padded wraps to enclose a patient, as in Figure 53-6. It is available in three sizes, from a small child size to an adult size.
- *Bed Sheet or Blanket.* The parent can bring from home a blanket or sheet that is familiar to the patient. The sheet or blanket is folded firmly around the patient twice and is held securely by a Velcro strap around the body. Support straps about the legs and body provide the patient with additional control.

B. Support Straps

Adhesive tape (2 or 3 inches wide), canvas, or Velcro straps may be used with or without a body enclosure. A soft strap may be made from a soft material, such as flannel, with a padded section to place over the wrists, ankles, or where needed. Ties 4 to 6 inches wide may be passed around the dental chair or may be tied to the arms of the chair.

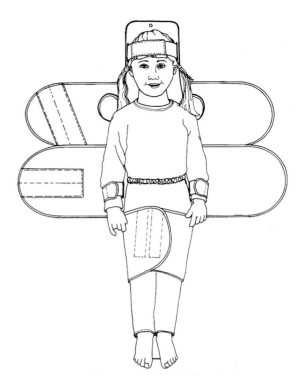

▪ **FIGURE 53-6 Papoose Board.** Stabilization is accomplished by three body wraps and a head restrainer. The arms are secured at the wrists, as shown, before the large center wrap is closed. (From King, E.M., Wieck, L., and Dyer, M.: *Illustrated Manual of Nursing Techniques.* Philadelphia, J.B. Lippincott Co., 1977, p. 311.)

C. Head Stabilization

1. *Arm of Clinician.* From a working position at 12 o'clock (top of the patient's head), the nondominant arm is placed around the patient's head to hold it in position.
2. *Mouth Prop,* as described on page 908.

▪ ORAL MANIFESTATIONS

Oral diseases of individuals with disabilities are not different from those of nondisabled persons. The two principal diseases found are dental caries and periodontal infections. Other oral findings include congenital malformations, oral injuries, and malocclusions. In the chapters devoted to describing specific individuals with disabilities, oral characteristics of each are included.

For a majority of patients with disabilities, dental and dental hygiene treatment is not different once the patient is in the dental chair, sedated if needed, and stabilized physically. For a few other patients, an oral manifestation can be caused by, or be a result of, the patient's disabling condition or the treatment for it. Examples are included here.

I. CONGENITAL MALFORMATIONS

A. **Cleft Lip or Palate** as discussed on page 805.
B. **Other Craniofacial Anomalies**
C. **Tooth Defects**

An increased incidence of malformations has been observed with developmental disabilities, for example:

1. Variations in number and structure of teeth.
2. Dentinogenesis imperfecta, amelogenesis imperfecta, enamel hyperplasia, and other abnormalities of tooth structure.

II. ORAL INJURIES

A. Attrition

Attrition caused by bruxism is particularly common among individuals with cerebral palsy and mental retardation.

B. Trauma to Teeth and Soft Tissues

*   Trauma to teeth and soft tissues may result from accidents (instability, falling), self-abuse, or seizures.
*   The individual with epilepsy is particularly susceptible to accidents. Chipped and fractured teeth, as well as residual scars in the tongue and lips, may be seen frequently.

III. FACIAL WEAKNESS OR PARALYSIS

When a patient has muscle weakness or paralysis of one side of the face, bilateral mastication is not possible. Biofilm usually collects more heavily, and food debris is retained on the involved side. Certain patients may have bilateral weakness.

IV. MALOCCLUSION

Malocclusion is frequently found among persons with developmental disabilities. Factors contributing to problems of occlusion include skeletal and muscular deformities, macroglossia, congenitally missing teeth, and such oral habits as tongue thrust and mouth breathing.

V. THERAPY-RELATED ORAL FINDINGS

A. Phenytoin-Induced Gingival Overgrowth

Patients whose treatment for seizures requires phenytoin (Dilantin) or other antiseizure medication may be susceptible to a slight to severe gingival enlargement. The severity of the enlargement usually depends on the maintenance of healthy gingival tissue associated with adequate daily biofilm control. A description of phenytoin-induced gingival overgrowth is included on pages 973 to 975.

B. Chemotherapy

Oral ulcerations, mucositis, and susceptibility to infection are frequent manifestations following cancer chemotherapy. Patients with leukemia have a high incidence of oral manifestations, including lymphadenopathy, gingival changes with bleeding, and petechiae, which are more severe following chemotherapy.

C. Radiation Therapy

When radiation therapy of the head and neck area involves the cells of the salivary glands, xerostomia can result and can contribute to an increased incidence of dental caries. The symptoms and treatment aspects of radiation therapy are described on pages 873 to 875.

D. Other Medications

Patients with disabilities tend to be treated with medications. All side effects of medications, particularly xerostomia, must be addressed.

■ DENTAL HYGIENE CARE PLAN

I. PREVENTIVE THERAPY

A. Biofilm Control

B. Fluoride Program

1. Supervision of self-applied daily fluoride.
2. Periodic professionally applied topical fluoride.

C. Pit and Fissure Sealants

II. EDUCATIONAL

A. Orientation

Patient orientation to each dental hygiene and dental procedure.

B. Counseling

Parental counseling starting as early as possible after an infant is known to have a disability.

C. Instruction in Disease Control

1. Biofilm control for natural teeth and prostheses.
2. Daily fluoride, systemic and/or topical.
3. Dietary and nutritional effects.

III. THERAPEUTIC

A. Patient's biofilm control for therapeutic purposes until tissue health is attained, followed by planned maintenance.

B. Complete scaling and root debridement.

C. Removal of overhanging fillings.

D. Reevaluation for additional periodontal therapy.

E. Restorative phase; finishing restorations.

▪ DISEASE PREVENTION AND CONTROL

I. PREVENTIVE PROGRAM COMPONENTS

A. Dental biofilm control.

B. Fluorides.

C. Pit and fissure sealants.

D. Diet counseling.

E. Smoking cessation.

F. Regular professional examinations and treatment at intervals as recommended by the dentist and dental hygienist.

II. FUNCTIONING LEVELS

For a patient who does not have a mental or physical disability, neglect of personal oral hygiene usually can be explained by either a lack of knowledge and understanding about the need for biofilm removal and how it is accomplished or a lack of motivation to carry out the necessary daily routines. For certain patients with disabilities, the problem of disease control becomes greatly magnified because of a lack of the necessary mental and/or physical coordination to carry out the simplest of oral hygiene measures.

Depending on the severity of the disability, many patients need either complete or partial assistance. Assistance must be provided by parents and other family members when living at home, or by an aide or other caregiver responsible for the patient's care in a residence or long-term care setting. There is a twofold responsibility to teach and supervise the patient and the patient's caregivers. Suggestions for in-service education are on pages 905 to 907.

A *high, moderate,* or *low* functioning level refers to the daily living skills (bathing, toothbrushing, dressing, for example) an individual can do alone, what range or degree of assistance is needed, or whether the person depends on others for complete care. The functioning levels have also been called *self-care, partial care,* or *total care.* In another concept, the terms *supervised, supervised/assistance,* and *maintenance (by others)* have been used.[6]

A. High Functioning Level

The high-functioning, self-care group includes those capable of flossing and brushing their own teeth. Many patients, particularly children and those of all ages who are mentally retarded, need varying degrees of encouragement, motivation, and supervision.

B. Moderate Functioning Level

The moderate-functioning, partial-care group includes those capable of carrying out at least part of their oral hygiene needs but who require considerable training, assistance, and direct supervision. The assistance may be verbal, gestural, or hand-over-hand.

C. Low Functioning Level

The low-functioning, total-care group includes those who are unable to attend to their own care and are therefore dependent. Patients in this group may be bedridden and nonambulatory, although others may be confined to wheelchairs. With training, some may be able to attempt a part of their own care.

III. PREPARATION FOR INSTRUCTION

A. Basic Planning Questions

1. What is the patient's functioning level?
2. Will the patient do all or part of the biofilm removal personally or require partial or total care?
3. Is the patient involved in any community dental health programs (home, school, or day activity), and can the dentist and/or dental hygienist in such a program be contacted to coordinate the instruction given?
4. Will the parent or caregiver do part or all of the oral care?
5. What disabilities have the greatest influence on the extent of self-care possible and the anticipated success of the overall preventive program? Mental? Physical? Sensory? Learning? Oral?
6. Which techniques and procedures will best fit the situation of the particular patient and the parent or caregiver?
7. How can the patient be helped to be as independent as possible?

B. Introduction

For the answers to these questions, an initial plan is made, with the realization that the system is on a trial-and-error basis. As the skills of the patient and parent improve and less biofilm is observed and recorded on succeeding appointments, adaptations can be made. In the meantime, communication improves and the patient's trust develops as the sincere concern of the dental team is realized.

For all patients, with or without a disability, the aim is complete daily biofilm control. Such an ideal result may seem far from reality with a moderate- or low-functioning person, but with continuing reinforcement and inspiration, progress can be made. Patient and parental attitudes, willingness to participate, and acceptance of the recommended procedures must be taken into consideration.

▪ DENTAL BIOFILM REMOVAL

I. COMPONENTS

General procedures for instruction and methods for toothbrushing, interdental biofilm removal, and care of fixed and removable prostheses are described in Chapters 23 through 26. Individualization for each patient's needs and abilities is necessary for all patients. Each step must be explained carefully.

A. Provide Basic Information

Biofilm formation and disease development are described on a level at which the patient and parent can learn and be motivated.

B. Disclose and Show Biofilm

An ongoing record of the extent of biofilm in graphic form by which the patient and caregiver can watch progress may help to motivate many patients.

C. Toothbrushing

1. Provide a soft toothbrush and ask the patient to remove the disclosed biofilm from the teeth. For the completely dependent patient, the parent will demonstrate. Alternative positions for the parent are described on page 903 and in Figure 53-13.
2. Biofilm removal is more important than the specific technique used, as long as damage is not done to the gingiva or teeth. A scrub-brush or circular Fones method may be appropriate and within the capability of certain patients, as described on page 414.
3. Explain each step and demonstrate slowly.
4. Adaptations for brush handles and other devices to promote or make possible a patient's independent performance are described on pages 898 to 901.

D. Dentifrice

A dentifrice containing fluoride is recommended for patients who can use a dentifrice. An ingestible dentifrice may prove useful. The factors to consider when deciding whether a standard noningestible dentifrice should be used include the following:

1. When a patient cannot control saliva, rinse or expectorate, a dentifrice should not be used. The person who is severely disabled may be treated with a suction brush, as described on pages 916 to 917 to help prevent aspiration.
2. When a parent or other caregiver is performing the brushing, the paste may limit visibility for thorough biofilm removal. When a paste is used, only a small amount should be placed on the brush (pea size, Figure 46-7).
3. Dentifrice may increase a gag reflex for certain patients.
4. For the patient whose problem is brush manipulation, and for whom special adaptations of the brush are recommended, management of the dentifrice may be awkward and messy.
5. Dentifrice is not essential to biofilm removal, and other means of daily fluoride application may prove easier for certain patients. A brush-on gel may be recommended.

E. Dental Floss

With time and repeated instruction, many patients with disabilities can learn to use dental floss, and some can learn to use other interdental aids. The use of a floss holder can make flossing possible for certain patients, such as those with limited digital dexterity or the use of only one hand, as shown in Figures 53-10 and 53-11. The holder may also be useful for the parent or other caregiver. Methods for increasing the size of a toothbrush handle may be adapted for the handle of a floss holder.

II. EVALUATION

Many patients, parents, and other caregivers can learn with demonstration and practice how to examine the teeth and gingiva. The signs of healthy gingiva, especially color and absence of bleeding on brushing, can be noted.

For selected patients, the thoroughness of brushing can be improved if a disclosing agent is used at the start. The visible objective then is to remove all the color. Another system is to apply a disclosing agent after brushing to determine completion of biofilm removal. Then, any additional biofilm noted is brushed and removed.

When a patient brushes first, followed by the caregiver, the disclosing agent might be applied by the caregiver so the task of removal can be completed. Because the patient is encouraged to do as much as possible and is praised for whatever successes are accomplished, the biofilm disclosed for the caregiver to remove may be a factor of discouragement to the patient who really had done the very best to the extent of individual capability. A better plan could be for the patient to do all the brushing and flossing once a day, and for the caregiver to do all the brushing and flossing at a different time.

▪ SELF-CARE AIDS

Although a caregiver may be willing to brush the patient's teeth, as much as possible should be carried out by the patient. Psychological benefits to the patient result in feelings of self-esteem and accomplishment when able to manage the important and worthwhile task of brushing, particularly with patients who have physical but no cognitive disability.

For patients of all ages whose main deterrent to personal self-care is related to grasp, manipulation, or control of a toothbrush, adaptations of the brush have been devised.[7–9] Modifications to accommodate specific needs include enlarged handles, hand attachments, and elongated handles.

I. GENERAL PREREQUISITES FOR A SELF-CARE AID

A. Cleanable.
B. Durable. Can withstand exposure to water and saliva.
C. Resistant to absorption of oral fluids.
D. Replaceable.
E. Inexpensive.

II. TOOTHBRUSHING

A. For Patient With Fingers Permanently Fixed in a Fist

Insert the brush handle into the grasp.

B. For Patient Who Cannot Grasp and Hold

1. *Objective.* To fasten the brush handle to the open hand.
2. *Methods*
   a. Velcro strap around hand has a slit on the palm side into which the brush handle can be inserted. A vinyl pocket with an adjustable Velcro strap is commercially available. The toothbrush handle fits into the pocket, as shown in Figure 53-7A. The

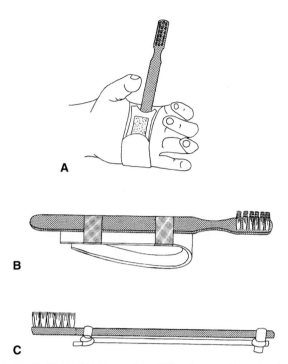

▪ **FIGURE 53-7 Aids for Patient Who Cannot Grasp and Hold. (A)** Adjustable Velcro strap around hand has a pocket designed to hold the toothbrush handle. **(B)** Handle of a fingernail brush attached to toothbrush by adhesive tape. **(C)** Rubber tubing attached firmly to toothbrush handle enables patient to hold brush across the palm of the hand. A floss holder also may be held by these methods.

device can be used to hold other objects for the patient, such as eating utensils.
   b. Handle of fingernail brush attached to toothbrush by adhesive water-resistant tape, as shown in Figure 53-7B.
   c. Wide rubber strap or a length of small-diameter rubber tubing attached through the hole in the toothbrush handle and tied adjacent to the brush head so the patient's hand can be slipped under the rubber and the brush can be held firmly, as shown in Figure 53-7C.

C. For Patient With Limited Hand Closure (unable to manipulate usual toothbrush handle or floss holder)

1. *Objective.* Enlarge the diameter of the handle.
2. *Methods*
   a. Bicycle handle grip. Insert toothbrush handle, as shown in Figure 53-8A.
   b. Soft rubber ball or a styrofoam ball. Push brush handle, as in Figure 53-8B. Styrofoam balls are available in various sizes from craft shops.

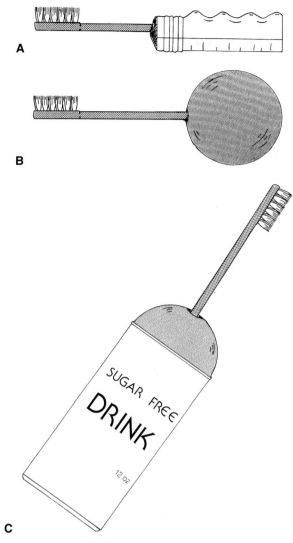

A

B

C

■ **FIGURE 53-8 Aids for Patient With Limited Grasp. (A)**
Toothbrush inserted into a bicycle handle grip. **(B)** Toothbrush inserted into a soft rubber ball. **(C)** Toothbrush in
soft rubber ball inserted into a juice or soda pop can may
provide a handle of appropriate diameter for patients
with limited hand closure.

   c. Juice or soda pop can. Place the rubber ball
      with toothbrush inside the can, as shown in
      Figure 53-8C.
   d. Foam rubber hair roller. Insert brush han-
      dle.
   e. Quick-cure acrylic. Obtain an impression of
      the hand grasp by having the patient grasp a
      cylinder of base plate wax. Then, fill the
      wax cylinder with quick-cure acrylic. Insert
      the toothbrush handle before the acrylic
      sets. The angle may be adjusted to set the
      brush head for the patient's convenient use.
      Polish the acrylic.

D. For Patient Unable to Lift Hand or Arm (with limited shoulder or elbow movement)

1. *Objective.* Lengthen the handle of the brush.
2. *Prerequisite.* The material must be strong or
   rigid enough to maintain the brush contact with
   sufficient lateral pressure to remove biofilm from
   the tooth surfaces.
3. *Methods*
   a. Cylinder of wood with brush handle
       cemented inside.[7]
   b. Two brushes. Cut the head from an old
       brush and fasten the handle to the end of
       the new brush handle (glue, tape, heat).
   c. Tongue depressors taped to the brush
       handle, then one or two other tongue
       depressors taped to overlap and provide an
       extension.
   d. Bicycle spoke, coat hanger, or other means
       for elongation fixed with a handle of acrylic
       resin. The metal tip may be heated and
       pushed into the toothbrush handle.[10,11] Use
       double or triple thickness to avoid flexibility.

E. For Patient Who Can Hold and Position the Toothbrush But Cannot Manipulate to Make Strokes for Biofilm Removal

1. *Specially Designed Toothbrush*
   • A manual brush that brushes exposed tooth
     surfaces simultaneously, as shown in Figure
     53-9.

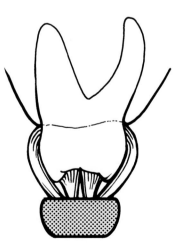

■ **FIGURE 53-9 Aid for Patient With a Brushing Problem.**
A specially designed toothbrush is shown on the mesial of
a maxillary second primary molar. Used with a back-and-
forth motion, the filaments remove debris and dental
biofilm simultaneously from the facial, lingual (palatal),
and occlusal tooth surfaces.

- The brush with curved outer filaments and a short stiff center row of filaments.
- Research showed a similar reduction in debris and biofilm with this brush compared with such reduction with a conventional brush.[12]
- This type of brush can also aid those with hand tremors, such as with Parkinson's disease, by stabilizing brush placement in position.

2. *Patient Moves Head Instead of Hand* . Guide patient to learn to move the head up and down and from side to side while a conventional soft brush is held against the teeth.[11]

F. Use of a Power Toothbrush

A power toothbrush can be a beneficial adjunct for many patients with disabilities and can motivate selected patients. This type of appliance can provide independence and improve quality of life for certain patients.

However, a power toothbrush can cause significant trauma if used incorrectly by, for example, a patient unable to hold the heavier weight of the power toothbrush or one lacking the comprehension for proper use.

1. *Advantages and Disadvantages*[13]
   - The extra size and weight of the handle may be advantageous for some patients or difficult for others with limited strength.
   - The on/off mechanism may be difficult to use for those lacking finger strength and coordination.
   - The larger handle can aid those who have difficulty grasping objects.
   - The vibrations created during use cannot be tolerated by certain patients.
   - Cost is higher than conventional brushes.

2. *Suggestions for Use*
   - Patients are instructed to follow manufacturers' instructions for proper use as indicated on each package.
   - Patients are instructed to bring their toothbrushes to dental appointments to demonstrate proper use.
   - Care for a power toothbrush should be reviewed with the patient including periodic replacement of the brush tip.
   - A patient with limited grasp can adapt a Velcro cuff around the handle to aid in holding the brush, similar to those shown in Figure 53-7.
   - Cross contamination can be a problem, particularly in group living situations. Ensure

each patient has a separate marked toothbrush and is kept apart from others.

3. *Other Power Oral Care Devices*

Power devices are continually developed and modified. Power-assisted flossers are available and may be an appropriate recommendation for use by certain patients. Dental professionals must evaluate new products available and make appropriate suggestions for use with each individual patient.

III. USE OF FLOSS HOLDER

A. Types

Several types of plastic floss holders are available, as shown in Figure 53-10.

B. Use

Careful instruction should be provided and supervision given periodically to prevent tissue damage. As threaded into a holder, the floss is in a straight line, as shown in Figure 53-11A.

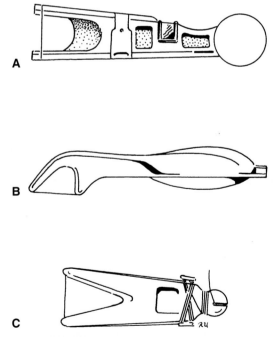

▪ **FIGURE 53-10 Floss Holders.** A variety of floss holders are available. **(A)** A holder with a replaceable floss container. **(B)** A holder with a replaceable floss cartridge and a thin edge for cleaning the tongue. **(C)** A holder with a threading mechanism for a 24-inch length of floss applied at each use. A fourth type, shown in Figure 53-11, is operated in a manner similar to that shown in C.

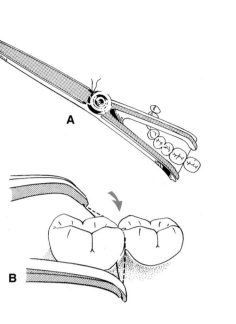

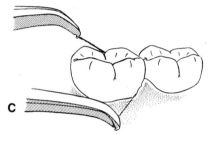

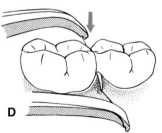

■ **FIGURE 53-11 Use of a Floss Holder. (A)** The floss is held over the proximal contact for insertion. A hand rest should be applied on the chin to prevent excess pressure. **(B)** As the floss is lowered gently and drawn through the contact area, the holder should be pulled mesially when the floss is applied to the distal surface and pushed distally when the floss is applied to the mesial surface. **(C)** Floss is lowered slightly below the gingival margin. **(D)** Floss cut in the papilla when used incorrectly.

To avoid cutting the papilla when applied interproximally:
- Use a rest or fulcrum to prevent snapping through the contact.
- Pull the floss mesially (to clean the distal surface of a tooth) or push distally (to clean the mesial surface) to allow floss to be positioned on the side of the papilla, as shown in Figure 53-11C.

IV. CLEANING REMOVABLE DENTAL PROSTHESES[7,14]

The details for cleaning removable prostheses are described on pages 474 to 475. The same materials and procedures are recommended for the patient with a disability or for another person who cares for the prosthesis.

Management of both the prosthesis and the brush requires attention and skill, and instruction in methods that prevent accidents is necessary. In all procedures, the sink must be partially filled with water and/or a face cloth or small towel should be placed in the sink to serve as a cushion should the denture be dropped.

A. Grasp Problem

For the patient with difficulty grasping or holding the brush, a denture brush handle may be adapted by any of the methods described for the regular toothbrush, as shown in Figure 53-8. A fingernail brush may be used instead of a standard denture brush provided all denture surfaces can be reached for biofilm removal.

B. One Hand

For the patient handicapped by hemiplegia or for the patient with use of two hands but who needs to grasp the denture with two hands to prevent accidents, the following are recommended:
1. Fingernail brush with suction cups.
2. Denture brush in mounting that has suction cups. These are available commercially, as shown in Figure 53-12A.
3. Denture brush with suction cups to attach low inside the sink bowl, as shown in Figure 53-12B.

■ INSTRUCTION FOR CAREGIVER

Individuals who need partial or total care present with varying degrees of ability to cooperate, depending on the nature of the disability. The size of the patient and whether the patient is ambulatory, bedridden, or in a wheelchair are among the factors that influence the technique for management.

The instruction for the parents or the other caregiver should be given where the specific techniques can actually be demonstrated as they will be done at home. When the patient lies down with the head in the parent's lap, for example, a suitable couch should be used, or chairs can be placed together. Time and repeated practice sessions are needed for successful biofilm removal for a difficult patient.

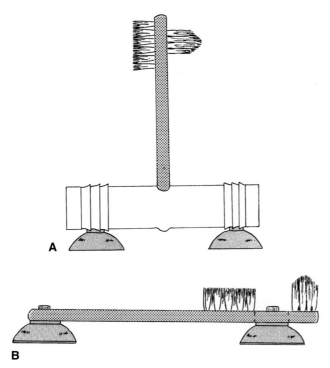

■ **FIGURE 53-12 Denture Brushes With Suction Cups. (A)** Denture brush in a commercially available mounting. **(B)** Suction cups attached directly to a denture brush. Either brush may be positioned in a sink to aid the person who has one hand or who needs to grasp the denture with two hands to prevent accidental dropping and breakage.

I. SELF-CARE AND ATTITUDE

Whenever possible, instruction for the parents, family members, or other caregivers begins with their own personal oral care. The most success comes when those who care for the patient have knowledge and understanding of the purposes and techniques and can demonstrate their own biofilm removal.

An appreciation for the need for preventive care and for why the health of the teeth and gingiva are of great importance to the well-being and overall health of the patient can help those responsible to develop the patience and take the necessary time from their own busy schedules.

II. GENERAL SUGGESTIONS

A. Place

The biofilm removal procedures must be performed where both the patient and the caregiver can be comfortable and relaxed. A small bathroom may be the least desirable place because positioning the patient may be awkward, except when a standing position can be used.

Good light, easy visibility of the teeth, and control of the head of the person with the disability are prerequisites.

B. Teaching Techniques for Biofilm Removal

1. *Use of Finger and Hand Rests.* The person performing the biofilm removal must learn how to balance the toothbrush, dental floss, floss aid, or any other implement with a finger or hand rest on the side of the patient's face or chin. Such contact contributes to total patient control and to effective use of the biofilm removal device.
2. *Use of a Mouth Prop.* For certain patients, biofilm removal is impossible without a mouth prop, and demonstration for insertion on both sides is needed. For home use, a washable rubber prop is practical.

III. POSITIONS

General positions that involve one or two people are suggested here.[15] When the patient is young, hyperactive, and unable to cooperate, and the assistance of a second person is not available, the use of a blanket or sheet wrap may be necessary (page 894).

In the following description, the term "parent" is used to mean the family member or other caregiver who may be performing the biofilm removal.

A. Parent Standing

With the parent standing from behind, the arm is brought around the patient's head and the chin is cupped while using the thumb and index finger to retract the lips and cheeks. The other hand applies the toothbrush, floss aid, or other device. This technique requires that the patient be able to bend the head back far enough for the parent to see the maxillary teeth. The procedure may be applicable for the following.

1. Short patient standing in front of and backed up to the parent.
2. Tall patient seated in a chair with the head tipped back to lean against the parent, or seated in a large chair or sofa with the head stabilized against the top of chair back.
3. Patient in a wheelchair leaning back against the parent. Wheelchair brakes are set.

B. Parent Seated

1. Patient seated on pillow on floor in front of parent, with back close to the chair and head turned back into parent's lap, as shown in Figure 53-13A. The parent may place his/her legs over the shoulders of the patient to restrain arms and body movements, as shown in Figure 53-13B.

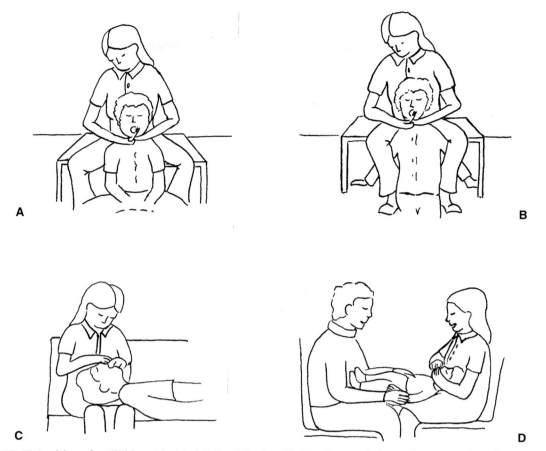

■ **FIGURE 53-13 Positions for Child or Disabled Patient During Biofilm Removal. (A)** Patient seated on floor with head turned back into the lap of the caregiver. **(B)** Patient's arms restrained by legs of caregiver. **(C)** Patient reclining on couch with head in lap of caregiver. **(D)** Two people participating with small child between. One holds patient for stabilization while the other holds the head for toothbrushing and flossing.

2. Parent is seated at the end of a sofa or couch, and patient is lying down with the head in parent's lap, as shown in Figure 53-13C.

3. For a bedridden patient, the parent may sit at the patient's head and place the head in the lap. When body and arm movements must be controlled, the parent can sit beside the patient, lean across the patient's chest, and hold the patient's arm against the body with the elbow. The hand of the restraining arm can hold the mouth prop, retract, or do whatever is necessary. If the patient is particularly difficult, a sheet or blanket wrap is indicated.

C. Two People

In any of the positions previously mentioned, the parent may need the assistance of a second person to hold the hands and arms or otherwise restrain the patient.

A small child may be placed across the laps of two persons seated facing each other. One stabilizes the head and brushes and flosses while the other person holds hands, arms, and legs as needed, as shown in Figure 53-13D.

■ FLUORIDES

Selection of a multiple fluoride program for an individual patient depends on the age, the caries status, and the concentration of fluoride in the water supply. In addition, for a patient with a disability, the abilities to cooperate, to accept the vehicle and mode of application, and to master the technique required for a self-administered preparation dictate the final recommendation.

I. FLUORIDATION

A. Community Water Fluoridation

As more communities begin to fluoridate the water supplies, more of the total population, including persons with disabilities, will benefit.

B. Institutional Water Fluoridation

Research has shown the benefits derived from fluoridation of a school water supply when the community in which the school was located could not or did not have fluoridation. These programs are summarized on page 550.

Institutions where individuals with disabilities reside may have a water supply that could be fluoridated. Installation is a relatively inexpensive procedure when the health benefits and the decreased need for professional care are realized.

II. DIETARY SUPPLEMENTS

When the community water supply is deficient in fluoride content, the fluoride level is below optimum, or the water intake by a child is low, a supplement is recommended, as shown in Table 33-1. Depending on the masticatory function of the child, that is, whether chewing or rinsing is possible, the fluoride can be prescribed in the form of a chewable tablet, lozenge, drops, or mouthwash to swallow after swishing.

III. PROFESSIONALLY APPLIED TOPICAL FLUORIDE

When water fluoridation is not available or when the benefits of water fluoridation must be supplemented, at least two topical applications per year are indicated, and more frequently if the dental caries rate is high. The method for application and the system for isolation of the teeth depend on the patient's ability to cooperate.

IV. SELF-APPLIED PROCEDURES

- Whether the individual with a disability is a child or an adult, a home fluoride program is indicated.
- After disease control techniques for flossing and toothbrushing have been completed before the patient retires, a mouthrinse, for the patient who can rinse; a gel applied by tray or toothbrush; or a chewable tablet, for the patient who can chew and who needs a fluoride supplement, may be advised.
- For a young, dependent, low-functioning person, brushing with a gel or swabbing with a fluoride rinse might be most applicable.
- Caregiver supervision and cooperation are essential. Motivation of the parent or caregiver needs regular reinforcement by the dental team.

▪ PIT AND FISSURE SEALANTS

Pit and fissure sealants have been used for children with developmental disabilities with satisfactory results.[16,17] The principles for application are the same as those described for all patients, as described on page XX. The use of a rubber dam is especially important for patients with excess saliva, hyperactivity of the tongue, or other management difficulties.

When a severely disabled patient will be administered general anesthesia for restorative procedures, pit and fissure sealants should be placed in all noncarious occlusal surfaces while the patient is under control. For all young patients, the sealant can be placed as soon after eruption as the tooth will hold a rubber dam.[15]

▪ DIET INSTRUCTION

Efforts to help adults who are disabled and the parents, family members, advocates, and other caregivers responsible to understand the general dietary requirements for oral health and how to put the principles into daily practice are a distinct part of the total preventive program. Information from Chapter 32 is applicable to patients with special needs as well as to all patients.

A careful assessment of current eating habits, extent of knowledge, family customs, and economic factors as they relate to a patient's condition is necessary before specific recommendations can be made. In an institutional setting, efforts can be directed to contact and work with the administrative personnel, teachers, dietitians, and aides. Coordination of biofilm control, snack selection, and snack availability, together with the fluoride program, opens the way to caries control.

I. FACTORS THAT INFLUENCE DIET HABITS

For certain patients, diet selection and utilization center on problems of mastication, whereas for others, the transport of food to the mouth is a major undertaking. The problems of the elderly patient are described on pages 833 to 835.

The following partial list of problems is suggested to help during dietary analysis and counseling. Many of the problems are directly related to increases in biofilm accumulation and resultant dental caries and periodontal infections.

A. Masticatory or Feeding Problems

Problems in eating can lead to the use of a soft diet, often composed mainly of carbohydrates.

B. Overindulgence in Sucrose-Containing Foods

- Sweets are sometimes used as rewards or bribes by unsuspecting family members or teachers involved in behavior modification procedures in training programs.

- Nonambulatory or otherwise confined patients may have less access to between-meal foods and, therefore, may eat more regularly, as served.
- The confined person may have snacks and sweets readily available, which can lead to dental destruction.

C. Inability to Accomplish Personal Biofilm Control Measures

Problems of daily biofilm removal can be related to a physical disability or lack of assistance from a parent or aide, combined with a diet high in cariogenic foods, which leads to dental caries development.

D. Lack of Professional Care and Instruction

Many patients do not receive adequate professional care because of unavailability, inability to obtain care because of physical barriers, inadequate financial support, lack of knowledge of the importance of oral health, or preoccupation with other major health problems.

E. Medications

- Medications with a side effect of xerostomia contribute to dental caries.
- Medications that diminish appetite as a side effect influence diet habits.
- Medications contained within a sucrose base designed to mask the flavor of the agent or to pacify the patient contribute to dental caries incidence.[18]

F. Obesity

Obesity is a problem with certain patients who suffer from inactivity, overeating, boredom, or lack of knowledge of proper food selection.

G. Food Preparation

Difficulty of food preparation can be a major limitation to diet selection for adults with neuromuscular disorders. Wheelchair confinement, lack of muscular coordination, hemiplegia or paraplegia, and dependence on others for grocery shopping are examples of problems encountered.

II. DIET ASSESSMENT AND COUNSELING

A. Food Record

- A high-functioning patient may be able to keep a food diary, and participation should be encouraged.

- The parent, advocate, or other caregiver can assist or, in the case of a low- or moderate-functioning person, may complete the entire diary.
- With the aid of the record and the information from the medical and dental histories, items for counseling can be selected.

B. Recommendations

General procedures for assessment and counseling are described on page 529. Adaptations involve long-range planning for gradual modification of each patient's diet.

The person who selects and prepares the food must be involved in the planning. Sugarless snacks and sugarless rewards during behavior modification training are especially important to control.

Parents need instruction as early as possible after a newborn is known to be developmentally disabled so that fluoride, diet, early personal hygiene, and the prevention of baby bottle caries can be coordinated into the daily program. The infant's early care should include an oral examination by the dentist and dental hygienist within 6 months of the eruption of the first tooth and no later than 12 months of age, as described on page 791.

■ GROUP IN-SERVICE EDUCATION

In-service programs may be provided for teachers, registered nurses, other health professionals, parents, and volunteers in school and community preventive programs. For example, all persons mentioned could be involved in the preparation of a program about classroom weekly rinsing with a fluoride mouthrinse. When a program is citywide and many dental hygienists are involved, in-service preparation for the dental hygienists themselves is necessary.

A special need exists for in-service instruction in oral health measures for caregivers in extended care institutions. Many patients in such facilities are unable to care for their own needs and may require total care, partial assistance, supervision, or regular reminders. The dental hygienist is able to work with the caregivers to teach them appropriate techniques and to motivate them to incorporate oral care into the daily routine for each resident or patient.

The general suggestions outlined in the following sections pertain to preparation and content for in-service workshops for the oral care of long-term patients.

I. PREPARATION FOR AN IN-SERVICE PROGRAM

A. Planning

- An in-service program needs careful planning. For many groups, time for an in-service is taken from an already busy work schedule. Nonmotivated participants require special considerations. A leading factor contributing to the success of a program is the genuine concern and enthusiasm of the program leader in motivating the participants.

- The material must be clear and to the point, interestingly presented with appropriate visual aids, and stimulating for learning. Objectives should be defined in writing and serve as a guide to preparation and evaluation.

- Problems of the staff must be recognized. Some members may have negative oral health attitudes, minimal educational background, and poor personal oral health.

- Initially, basic preparation includes learning about the functioning levels of the clients and assessing the procedures used for their oral care. A survey of the biofilm control materials and devices available and in current use, methods for labeling or storing individual brushes, and the frequency of use is important.

B. Use of Clinic Records

- Clinic records for each patient should be examined for information relative to the dental status and to those who wear dentures.

- Medical histories must be reviewed so that special general or oral health problems can be considered and necessary precautions can be taken.

- When a dental hygienist is employed regularly within an institution, a much more complete assessment can be made.

- The dental hygienist invited to the institution for the specific purpose of presenting the workshop must arrange a preworkshop visit for observing the caregivers and the clients.

C. Gingival/Biofilm Index

- The use of a gingival or biofilm index can provide a baseline of information from which progress can be evaluated.

- The caregivers could carry out the daily biofilm program and see the changes that take place by comparing survey results at a later date.

- Such continuing participation could provide real motivation to the group.

II. PROGRAM CONTENT

A. The Participants' Own Biofilm Control

- Based on the premise that persons who are motivated to care for their own mouths have a clearer understanding of the effects and importance of oral care and give a higher priority to the time spent daily, an in-service education group needs to participate in a personal biofilm control program.

- A biofilm-free score, as described on page 330, or another evaluation device can be used.

- A group may be willing to work in pairs and learn to evaluate and score each other, thereby learning the techniques to be applied to their clients.

B. Facts About Cause and Prevention

Basic information about biofilm, its formation, and how gingivitis and dental caries develop are important to most groups. The progress of disease from reversible gingivitis to severe periodontitis can be explained, as can the process of dental caries, which begins with a small white spot of demineralization and progresses to a diseased pulp. Prevention through biofilm control, fluoride, dietary controls, sealants, and early treatment for restorations must be carefully presented. Handout materials and colorful visual aids promote learning.

C. Oral Examination

1. *Oral Mucosa.* Techniques demonstrated and practiced by the participants on each other should include the use of a tongue depressor to retract, a disposable mouth mirror, and a light source to see the oral mucosa.

2. *Tongue.* How to hold the tongue, using a sponge to lift and inspect all parts, can be shown.

3. *Gingiva.* Color, size, and bleeding that occurs spontaneously or while brushing can be explained and demonstrated. When projection is possible, slides can be included for all aspects of the instructional material. When a camera is available for intraoral photography, "before" and "after" pictures of the patients can be shown. Changes effected by the biofilm control supervised by the caregivers are more meaningful than are pictures of strangers.

4. *Biofilm.* Inspection for biofilm can be demonstrated when the disclosing agent is used prior to biofilm scoring and removal.

5. *Denture-Supporting Mucosa.* Patients with dentures need the supporting tissues examined

periodically by the dentist, but caregivers can notice changes that should be called to the dentist's attention as a result of their daily cleaning and massaging of the mucosa while the denture is out of the mouth for cleaning.

6. *Dentures.* Sample dentures may be used to help the participants learn to examine each denture for cracks or sharp edges. Examination for deposits can be made by the patient and the caregivers and compared with the denture after it has been cleaned.

D. Techniques of Mouth Care and Disease Control

Staff members can be trained to work in pairs.[19] Working in pairs is more efficient, particularly in the care of difficult patients.

A plan for each patient can be worked out with the caregivers so that individual problems relative to dental caries prevention, gingival disease control, or complete or partial denture care can be solved. Teaching some or all of the following may be included, depending on the needs of the clients.

1. *Biofilm Control.* Instruction includes positioning of the patient (Figure 53-13), application of disclosing agent, examination for biofilm on the teeth, toothbrush selection and technique, use of a mouth prop, and flossing with or without a floss aid. The use of a portable or bedside suction unit for removing debris from a patient's mouth can be practiced by a paired team.[19]
2. *Fluoride Application.* The objectives and techniques for brushing with a gel, swabbing with a mouthrinse, assisting the patient with a chewable tablet, or applying a gel tray can be included.
3. *Denture Care.* Procedures for care of dentures and of the mucosa under the denture are shown.
4. *Saliva Substitute.* Use of saliva substitute for dry mouth is demonstrated; instruction includes how to use a swab with saliva substitute to provide relief for certain patients (page 388).

E. Denture Marking Procedure

- All dentures should be marked for patient identification.
- Most dentures are marked during processing.
- The techniques for denture marking are outlined on page 846.

III. RECORDS

- A record form to be completed for each patient is essential to follow-up and evaluation.

- During the instruction periods, the staff can learn how to complete the record and where to file the copies.
- The form can be designed with spaces to record information obtained during the oral examination, the functioning level and degree of cooperation, the procedures needed for dental caries control, periodontal health, and/or denture care.
- In addition, the instruction provided, the implements and materials used, the planned future instruction, the prognosis, and any other notes can be included. Successful techniques should be described, and suggestions for future appointments can be made.

IV. FOLLOW-UP

- After caregivers have tried their newly learned procedures, an opportunity to have questions answered should be provided.
- Direct observation by the dental hygienist of techniques performed with and for the patients, advice concerning oral problems of particular patients, and corrections when necessary can motivate and encourage both patient and caregiver.
- Disclosing and recording the biofilm for comparison of scores before and after the program can show the progress being made.

V. CONTINUING EDUCATION

- Individual instruction must be provided for each new employee during the orientation period for that employee.
- Periodic updating for all employees can be accomplished at regular intervals. Questions and problems can be discussed, and plans can be introduced for changing a certain procedure based on new research evidence.
- A specific plan for scheduled oral health programs may be a requirement for licensure of a health-care facility.
- Advanced education programs are available for extensive training in care of the disabled patient.

■ INSTRUMENTATION

Customary procedures must be adapted. With basic knowledge of methods for maintaining patient stability, adequate visibility of working area, secure instrument grasps and finger rests, and well-controlled strokes, instrumentation for calculus removal and root planing can be effectively accomplished.

Patients who are hyperactive, lack muscular control, or have a mental impairment provide many challenges. With some patients, the tasks of keeping the head and mouth positioned, the profuse saliva controlled, and the oversized or hyperactive tongue held back may seem insurmountable. Patience, a gentle but firm touch, and continuing experience are essential.

I. PREPARATION FOR INSTRUMENTATION

A. Premedication

- Antibiotic coverage as indicated for susceptible patients, as discussed on pages 122 to 124.
- Sedative for control of selected patients.

B. Biofilm Control Instruction Precedes Scaling

- Provide a clean mouth for professional instrumentation (conditioning).
- Disclose and present or review information on biofilm.
- Continue practice on biofilm removal methods selected for the particular patient.
- The patient and caregiver demonstrate.

II. STABILIZATION

For certain patients, opening the mouth is difficult, and maintaining the mouth in an open position is impossible. A mouth prop can be used to assist the patient. Verbal encouragement of the patient must continue throughout the appointment.

A. Ratchet Type (Molt's Mouth Gag)

The most stable mouth prop is a sterilized prop that can be nearly closed for insertion between the teeth. It can be opened gradually to hold the jaws to the necessary position. The tips are covered with rubber tubing and are positioned over the maxillary and mandibular teeth on one side while the clinician treats the opposite side.

B. Bite Blocks

Rubber: Different types of rubber bite blocks are available, for example, Figure 53-14 shows one that allows for placement of a suction tip. A long piece of dental floss should be tied through the holes in a commercially available rubber mouth prop so that, in case of a sudden respiratory change, the prop can be quickly pulled out and breathing normalized.

C. Tongue Depressors

A practical, disposable mouth prop can be made from three to six tongue depressors taped together. A folded

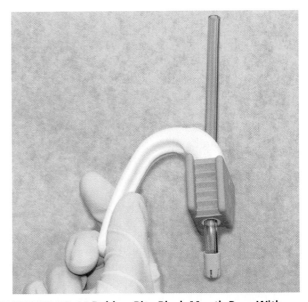

■ **FIGURE 53-14 Rubber Bite Block Mouth Prop With Saliva Ejector.**

sponge should be placed under the tape to provide a cushion, as shown in Figure 53-15 along with an example of a prefabricated bite stick.

D. Precautions for the Use of a Mouth Prop

- Mobile teeth could be knocked out and aspirated.
- Loose primary teeth in young patient.

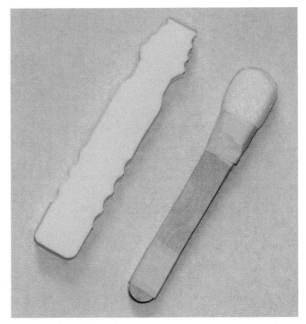

■ **FIGURE 53-15 Examples of Bite Sticks.** Left, a prefabricated model. Right, a self-made example made from bite sticks taped together with a gauze pad for a comfortable biting surface.

- Mobile teeth in advanced periodontal infection.
- Fatigue of the patient's facial and masticatory muscles and temporomandibular joint.
- Patient must know that all stabilization devices are for comfort and to make the work easier and that they are in no way meant to hurt or punish.

III. TREATMENT BY QUADRANTS

For many patients, particularly those with generalized heavy supragingival and subgingival calculus, treatment by quadrants under local anesthesia is the procedure of choice. Removal of calculus and overhanging fillings can be completed more efficiently.

A. Scaling Requirements

- The occurrence of generalized heavy calculus deposits in disabled patients is not unusual. The reason may be inadequate personal and professional care or factors related to the disabling condition.
- The objective of the clinical procedures is the complete removal of calculus and periodontal pocket debridement. The compromising or rationalization of complete treatment neglects the patient's needs and permits advanced periodontal disease to develop.

B. Need for Assistance

Four-handed dental hygiene procedures (page 926) are needed while treating many types of patients with disabilities. Many patients have excess saliva, whereas others have uncontrollable tongue and general body movements, all of which can hinder instrumentation.

1. *Stabilization and Visibility.* With assistance for stabilization, visibility, and maintenance of a clear field, the procedure is less traumatic for the patient and less time-consuming for all.
2. *Precaution During Evacuation.* Patients with chronic lung disorders, asthma, or cystic fibrosis and patients with cerebral palsy are considered "aspiration risks." For example, a sudden spasm in the facial, neck, or throat areas could cause a patient with cerebral palsy to aspirate foreign matter from the mouth into the airway.

C. Instruments

- Unbreakable mirrors are recommended for use with a patient subject to spasm or sudden closure.
- Use single-end sharp instruments to prevent accidents. When an unrestrained patient moves involuntarily, the nonworking end of an instrument can be a hazard.
- Use of an ultrasonic scaler is contraindicated for an aspiration-risk patient. It also should not be used for patients who overreact to sensory stimuli, such as a patient with autism (pages 987 to 990).

D. Technique Suggestions

- *Introduce Each Procedure and Sound to Prevent Startling a Patient.* Follow the basic instruction rule to "show, tell, then do." When a patient is blind or deaf, the rule has double significance.
- *Finger Rests.* Firm, dependable finger rests are needed. Supplemental or reinforced rests can contribute to instrument stability. With certain patients, external finger and hand rests may be safer for the clinician.[20]

Everyday Ethics

When Mrs. Becker has her dental appointment, Lauren the dental hygienist must rush to finish the previous patient so she can have time to go to the storage closet in the basement and get the transfer board so Mrs. Becker can slide over to the dental chair from her wheelchair. Mrs. Becker has numerous medical and dental problems that she tends to complain about. She has been very difficult to motivate to perform daily biofilm control. Her current dental status indicates that she should be placed on more frequent 2- to 3-month maintenance appointments. Lauren feels overstressed to prepare for and treat Mrs. Becker in the time she is allowed for appointments. Lauren is considering ignoring the plan for more frequent maintenance visits and scheduling Mrs. Becker in 6 months to avoid another unpleasant experience for both of them.

Questions for Consideration

1. What issues could Lauren discuss with her employer to defend her request for a longer appointment time?

2. What efforts could Lauren make to improve biofilm control with Mrs. Becker?

3. What might Mrs. Becker feel about her dental experiences, including with Lauren?

REFERENCES

1. **United States Equal Employment Opportunity Commission and the U.S. Department of Justice:** *Americans With Disabilities Act Handbook.* EEOC-BK-19, October, 1991, Appendix N. Title II Highlights.
2. **World Health Organization:** *International Classification of Impairments, Disabilities, and Handicaps.* Geneva, World Health Organization, 1980.
3. **United States Equal Employment Opportunity Commission and the U.S. Department of Justice:** *Americans With Disabilities Act Handbook.* EEOC-BK-19, October, 1991, Appendix B. ADA Accessibility Guidelines.
4. **Posnick, W.R. and Martin, H.H.:** Wheel Chair Transfer Techniques for the Dental Office, *J. Am. Dent. Assoc., 94,* 719, April, 1977.
5. **Felder, R.S., Gillette, V.M. and Leseberg, K.:** Wheelchair Transfer Techniques for the Dental Office, *Spec. Care Dentist., 8,* 256, November–December, 1988.
6. **Meador, H.G.:** Toothbrushing: A Sensible Approach for the Mentally Retarded, *Dent. Hyg., 53,* 462, October, 1979.
7. **Duncan, J.L.:** Incorporating Oral Hygiene Procedures in Geriatric Nursing Homes, *Dent. Hyg., 53,* 519, November, 1979.
8. **Price, V.E.:** Toothbrush Modifications for the Handicapped, *Dent. Hyg., 54,* 467, October, 1980.
9. **Sroda**, R. and Plezia, R.A.: Oral Hygiene Devices for Special Patients, *Spec. Care Dentist., 4,* 264, November–December, 1984.
10. **Albertson, D.:** Prevention and the Handicapped Child, *Dent. Clin. North Am., 18,* 595, July, 1974.
11. **Ettinger, R.L. and Pinkham, J.R.:** Oral Hygiene and the Handicapped Child, *J. Int. Assoc. Dent. Child., 9,* 3, July, 1978.
12. **Williams, N.J. and Schuman, N.J.:** The Curved-Bristle Toothbrush: An Aid for the Handicapped Population, *ASDC J. Dent. Child., 55,* 291, July–August, 1988.
13. **Mulligan, R.A.:** Design Characteristics of Electric Toothbrushes Important to Physically Compromised Patients, *J. Dent. Res., 59,* 450, Abstract 731, Special Issue A, March, 1980.
14. **Ettinger, R.L. and Pinkham, J.R.:** Dental Care for the Homebound—Assessment and Hygiene, *Aust. Dent. J., 22,* 77, April, 1977.
15. **Nowak, A.J.:** *Dentistry for the Handicapped Patient.* St. Louis, Mosby, 1976, pp. 167–192.
16. **Ripa, L.W. and Cole, W.W.:** Occlusal Sealing and Caries Prevention: Results 12 Months After a Single Application of Adhesive Resin, *J. Dent. Res., 49,* 171, January, 1970.
17. **Richardson, B.A., Smith, D.C., and Hargreaves, J.A.:** A 5-Year Clinical Evaluation of the Effectiveness of a Fissure Sealant in Mentally Retarded Canadian Children, *Community Dent. Oral Epidemiol., 9,* 170, August, 1981.
18. **Feigal, R.J. and Jensen, M.E.:** The Cariogenic Potential of Liquid Medications: A Concern for the Handicapped Patient, *Spec. Care Dentist., 2,* 20, January–February, 1982.
19. **Gertenrich, R.L. and Hart, R.W.:** Utilization of the Oral Hygiene Team in a Mental Health Institution, *ASDC J. Dent. Child., 39,* 174, May–June, 1972.
20. **Pattison, A.M. and Pattison, G.L.:** *Periodontal Instrumentation,* 2nd ed. Norwalk, CT, Appleton & Lange, 1992, pp. 355–408.

SUGGESTED READINGS

Alty, C.T.: Finding a Place in Your Heart for Special Smiles, *RDH, 16,* 19, February, 1996.

Belles, M.T.: Long-Term Care Facilities: An In-service Education Program, *DentalHygienistNews, 6,* 14, Spring, 1993.

Boj, J.R. and Davila, J.M.: Differences Between Normal and Developmentally Disabled Children in a First Dental Visit, *ASDC J. Dent. Child., 62,* 52, January–February, 1995.

Brandes, D.A., Wilson, S., Preisch, J.W., and Cassamassimo, P.S.: A Comparison of Opinions From Parents of Disabled and Non-disabled Children on Behavior Management Techniques Used in Dentistry, *Spec. Care Dentist., 15,* 119, May–June, 1995.

Carr, M.P.: Ensuring Treatment for the Special Needs Population, *Access, 8,* 33, February, 1994.

Finger, S.T. and Jedrychowski, J.R.: Parents' Perception of Access to Dental Care for Children With Handicapping Conditions, *Spec. Care Dentist., 9,* 195, November–December, 1989.

Glassman, P., Miller, C., Wozniak, T., and Jones, C.: A Preventive Dentistry Training Program for Caretakers of Persons With Disabilities Residing in Community Residential Facilities, *Spec. Care Dentist., 14,* 137, July/August, 1994.

Lange, B.M., Entwistle, B.M., and Lipson, L.F.: *Dental Management of the Handicapped: Approaches for Dental Auxiliaries.* Philadelphia, Lea & Febiger, 1983, 169 pp.

Lawton, L.: Providing Dental Care for Special Patients: Tips for the General Dentist, *J. Am. Dent. Assoc., 133,* 1666, December, 2002.

Ogasawara, T., Watanabe, T., Hosaka, K., and Kasahara, H.: Hypoxemia Due to Inserting a Bite Block in Severely Handicapped Patients, *Spec. Care Dentist., 15,* 70, March/April, 1995.

Perlman, S.P. and Miller, C.: Preventive Oral Health Care for Patients With Disabilities, *Compend. Cont. Educ. Oral Hyg., 4,* 3, Number 2, 1997.

Ramsey, W.O.: Valved Feeding Devices: Adjuncts in Rehabilitation of the Oral Phase of Swallowing, *Int. J. Periodontics Restorative Dent., 10,* 321, Number 4, 1990.

Raynak, S.: Dental Hygiene Care for Individuals With Special Needs, *Can. Dent. Hyg. Assoc./Probe, 29,* 184, September, 1995.

Saunders, R.H., Davila, C.E., Hayes, A.L., Fu, J., and Zero, D.T.: The Effectiveness of Sponge-Type Intraoral Applicators for Applying Topical Fluorides in Institutionalized Older Adults, *Spec. Care Dentist., 14,* 224, November/December, 1994.

Sfikas, P.M.: What's a "Disability" Under the Americans With Disabilities Act? *J. Am. Dent. Assoc., 127,* 1406, September, 1996.

Tesini, D.A. and Fenton, S.J.: Oral Health Needs of Persons With Physical or Mental Disabilities, *Dent. Clin. North Am., 38,* 483, July, 1994.

Waldman, H.B.: Respite Care: A New Social Program for Children at Risk, *ASDC J. Dent. Child., 58,* 241, May–June, 1991.

Wyatt, C.C.L. and MacEntee, M.I.: Dental Caries in Chronically Disabled Elders, *Spec. Care Dentist., 17,* 196, November/December, 1997.

Patient Management

American Academy of Pediatric Dentistry: Oral Health Policies: Guidelines for Behavior Management, *Pediatr. Dent., 18,* 40, Number 6, Special Issue, December, 1996.

Burtner, A.P. and Dieks, J.L.: Providing Oral Health Care to Individuals With Severe Disabilities Residing in the Community: Alternative Care Delivery Systems, *Spec. Care Dentist., 14,* 188, September/October, 1994.

Carroll, B.: Dental Hygiene and Preventive Care for People With Disabilities, *Access, 11,* 35, April, 1997.

Casamassimo, P.S.: A Primer in Management of Movement in the Patient With a Handicapping Condition, *J. Mass. Dent. Soc., 40,* 23, Winter, 1991.

Chalmers, J.M., Levy, S.M., Buckwalter, K.C., Ettinger, R.L., and Kambhu, P.P.: Factors Influencing Nurses' Aides' Provision of Oral Care for Nursing Facility Residents, *Spec. Care Dentist., 16,* 71, March/April, 1996.

Frankel, R.I.: The Papoose Board® and Mothers' Attitudes Following Its Use, *Pediatr. Dent., 13,* 284, September/October, 1991.

Gordon, S.M., Dionne, R.A., and Snyder, J.: Dental Fear and Anxiety as a Barrier to Accessing Oral Health Care Among Patients With Special Health Care Needs, *Spec. Care Dentist., 18,* 88, March/April, 1998.

Kayser-Jones, J., Bird, W.F., Redford, M., Schell, E.S., and Einhorn, S.H.: Strategies for Conducting Dental Examinations Among

Cognitively Impaired Nursing Home Residents, *Spec. Care Dentist.,* *16,* 46, March/April, 1996.

Malamed, S.F., Gottschalk, H.W., Mulligan, R., and Quinn, C.L.: Intravenous Sedation for Conservative Dentistry for Disabled Patients, *Anesth. Prog., 36,* 140, July–October, 1989.

Nunn, J.H., Davidson, G., Gordon, P.H., and Storrs, J.: A Retrospective Review of a Service to Provide Comprehensive Dental Care Under General Anesthesia, *Spec. Care Dentist., 15,* 97, May/June, 1995.

Williams, E.O. and Seals, R.R.: Treating Patients in Wheelchairs, *J. Prosthet. Dent., 67,* 431, March, 1992.

Dental Biofilm Control

Brownstone, E.: Handicapped Dental Patients: Mechanical Methods and Modifications for Oral Hygiene Care, *Can. Dent. Hyg./Probe, 24,* 32, Spring, 1990.

Carr, M.P., Sterling, E.S., and Bauchmoyer, S.M.: Comparison of the Interplak® and Manual Toothbrushes in a Population With Mental Retardation/Developmental Disabilities (MR/DD), *Spec. Care Dentist., 17,* 133, July/August, 1997.

Finizio, J.M., Fox, D.W., and Yasser, D.S.: Power-Assisted Toothbrushes Simplify Hygiene for Those Who Need Extra Help, *RDH, 16,* 42, January, 1996.

Stiefel, D.J., Truelove, E.L., Chin, M.M., and Mandel, L.S.: Efficacy of Chlorhexidine Swabbing in Oral Health Care for People With Severe Disabilities, *Spec. Care Dentist., 12,* 57, March/April, 1992.

Stiefel, D.J., Truelove, E.L., Chin, M.M., Zhu, X.C., and Leroux, B.G.: Chlorhexidine Swabbing Applications Under Various Conditions of Use in Preventive Oral Care for Persons With Disabilities, *Spec. Care Dentist., 15,* 159, July/August, 1995.

The Patient Who Is Homebound or Bedridden

Esther M. Wilkins, RDH, DMD
Charlotte J. Wyche, RDH, MS

■ HOMEBOUND PATIENTS

Within recent years, efforts have been made through research and organized programming to devote more attention to the oral health needs of people with a chronic illness and a disability. Patients of all age groups who are confined to hospitals, hospices, institutions, nursing homes, skilled nursing facilities, or private homes need special adaptations for oral care. Portable equipment is available, and special training for dental personnel is encouraged.

Dental care for the chronically ill must be completed in a variety of surroundings. For the hospitalized person, dental clinics may be available to provide care for in-patients. Those who are not hospitalized may be confined to their homes or may be able to be transported to the dental office or clinic in a wheelchair, depending on the severity and extent of disability.

Private practice clinicians have occasion to attend to patients confined to their homes. Dental hygiene procedures lend themselves to care for the homebound because nearly the entire treatment can be completed with manual instruments. Instruction in personal oral

preventive procedures has particular significance for the comfort, as well as the health, of the patient. Suggestions relative to planning and conducting a home visit are included in this chapter. Key words and definitions are included in Box 54-1.

I. OBJECTIVES OF CARE

- Provide routine screening to detect lesions that may be pathologic, particularly those that may be early cancer.
- Aid in preventing dental caries and periodontal infections that require extensive treatment.
- Assist in preventing further complication of the patient's state of health by lessening oral care problems.
- Contribute to the patient's comfort, mental ease, general well-being, and quality of life.
- Encourage adequate personal care procedures, whether performed by the patient or a caregiver.
- Contribute to general rehabilitation or habilitation of the patient.
- Provide palliative care for the individual with a shortened life span.

BOX 54-1 KEY WORDS: Homebound and Bedridden Patients

Coma: state of unconsciousness from which the patient cannot be aroused.

> **Irreversible coma:** brain death.

Comatose: pertaining to or affected with a coma.

Hospice: a medically directed, nurse-coordinated program providing a continuum of home and inpatient care for the terminally ill patient and family; employs an interdisciplinary team acting under the direction of an autonomous hospice administration; the program provides palliative and supportive care to meet the special needs arising out of the physical, emotional, spiritual, social, and economic stresses that are experienced during the final stages of illness and during dying and bereavement.[1]

Interdisciplinary team: consists of specialists from many fields; combines expertise and resources to provide insight into all aspects of a given special area.

Palliative: affording relief but not cure.

Sordes: foul matter that collects on the lips, teeth, and oral mucosa in low fevers; consists of debris, microorganisms, epithelial elements, and food particles; forms a crust.

Terminally ill patient: a person who is experiencing the end stages of a life-threatening disease, for whom there is no longer hope of a cure.

II. PREPARATION FOR THE HOME VISIT

A. Understanding the Patient

1. Consider the characteristics associated with the particular chronic illness or disease and the effect oral infection may have on the severity of the illness.
2. Consider special problems related to age. (For example, for the gerodontic patient, see Chapter 49.)
3. Review patient's medical history.
   - Mail form to complete and send back.
   - Telephone to ask questions.
4. Determine precautions that must be taken.
5. Arrange with dentist and physician when premedication or other prescription is required.

B. Instruments and Equipment

1. *Protective Barriers.* Mask, protective eyewear, gloves, and gown.
2. *Instruction Materials.* Toothbrush, interdental aids (several types, until needs of patient are known).
3. *Sterile Equipment.* Sterile instruments and other items are transported in the sealed packages in which they were sterilized.
4. *Disposable Items.* Napkins, gauze sponges, cotton rolls and pellets, fluoride application trays, and other essential disposable items are prepared in packages that are convenient to open and use at the bedside.
5. *Pharmaceuticals.* Pretreatment mouthrinse, disclosing agent, and topical fluoride preparation (fluoride varnish is particularly easy to apply in this setting).
6. *Coverall.* A large plastic drape can be helpful because in certain types of illness the patient's coordination during rinsing may be limited.
7. *Emesis Basin for Patient Rinsing.* Although a small basin would be available at the home, the kidney-shaped emesis basin facilitates the rinsing process.
8. *Lighting.* Adaptation of available possibilities.
   - Headlight or reflector. Dentist may have as part of the office equipment; with practice, the dental hygienist can learn to use with ease.
   - Photography spotlight. Might be available either from the dentist or from the patient's home; need a type with a narrow, concentrated beam.
   - Gooseneck lamp. Might be available in patient's home; need bulb of adequate wattage.
9. *Miscellaneous Items Usually Available at the Home.* Arrangements must be made (by telephone) in advance of appointment.
   - Large towels. For covering pillows.
   - Pillows. Types of pillows available that may be

firm enough to assist in maintaining patient's head in reasonably stationary position.
- Hospital bed. Can be adjusted most effectively for patient's position.
- Container for prosthesis.
- Hand mirror for patient instruction.
- Power toothbrush.

C. Appointment Time

Arrange during the patient's usual waking hours at as convenient a time as possible in relation to nursing care and mealtime schedule.

III. APPROACH TO PATIENT

Because a majority of patients who come to the dental office are active people with good general health, the adjustment to the relatively helpless, chronically ill person is sometimes difficult. One may tend to be oversolicitous, an attitude that may not contribute to the development of a cooperative patient.

Usually, a direct approach with gentle firmness is most successful. Establishment of rapport with the patient may depend in part on whether the patient has requested and anticipated the appointment or whether those caring for the patient have insisted on and arranged for the visit.

A. Personal Factors

- The well-adjusted chronically ill person may show more appreciation for the care provided than does the healthy patient who comes to the dental office.
- An ill patient may be well aware of the difficulties under which the clinician is working.
- Cooperation obtained may depend on the patient's attitude toward the illness or disability.

B. Effects of Inactivity

A prolonged illness that may have been accompanied by suffering is not conducive to a healthy outlook on life. Monotonous confinement contributes to the development of characteristics such as those that follow.
- Unable to maintain a cheerful attitude.
- Bored or dissatisfied with sameness of daily routine.
- Easily depressed.
- Discouraged about recovery; leads to mental state that may retard recovery.
- Sensitive and easily offended.
- Demanding; enjoys being waited on if used to having prompt attention to each request.
- Indifferent to personal appearance and general rules of personal hygiene.

- Preoccupied with details of medical examinations, tests, treatment, medications, and symptoms.

C. Suggestions for General Procedure

1. Request the caregiver to be present to assist as needed and to learn method for care of the patient's mouth on a daily basis. Other visitors should be asked to remain out of the room during the appointment to prevent distraction of patient.
2. Introduce each step slowly to be sure patient knows what is being done.
3. Do not make the patient feel rushed. Listen attentively: socializing is one of the best ways to establish rapport.
4. Regardless of inconvenience of arrangements, plan two or more appointments when extensive scaling is required.
   - Need to avoid tiring the patient.
   - Need for observing tissue response.
   - Need to give encouragement in biofilm control procedures.

▪ DENTAL HYGIENE CARE AND INSTRUCTION

I. WORKING SITUATION

Because many patients can sit up in a chair or wheelchair for at least 1 or 2 hours each day, only rarely must procedures be performed while the patient is in bed. For the patient in a chair, a kitchen or large bathroom may be most satisfactory for working. In either situation, ingenuity is needed to arrange patient position, head stabilization, and proper lighting to maintain patient comfort and yet provide access for the clinician.

A. Patient in Bed

1. Hospital bed. Adjust to lift patient's head to desirable height.
2. Ordinary bed. Use firm pillows to support patient.

B. Patient in Wheelchair

1. Portable headrest may be attached to back of plain chair or wheelchair (Figure 53-2, page 889).
2. Although the chair can be backed against a wall and a pillow inserted for the head, the patient preferably should be moved to a davenport or chair where a more stable headrest could be provided.

C. Small Patient

Positions for biofilm control described on page 902 and shown in Figure 53-12 may be applicable during treatment.

D. Suggestions for Lighting

- Overhead lighting. Turn off to reduce shadows in the mouth.
- Headlight. Usually the most convenient and efficient form of lighting because of concentrated beam.
- Head reflector. Reflect light from bed lamp attached to bed behind patient's head.
- Gooseneck or photographer's light. Care must be taken not to direct the light into patient's eyes.

E. Instrument Arrangement

Use instruments directly from a sterile package or cassette.

II. ASSESSMENT TREATMENT PLAN

   A. Vital signs.
   B. Extraoral/intraoral examination.
   C. Periodontal assessment.
   D. Dental examination.

III. PERSONAL ORAL CARE

   A. Provide specific instruction for caregiver of help-less or uncoordinated patient.
   - Demonstrate in patient's mouth.
   - A power-assisted toothbrush may prove valuable for certain patients.
   B. Specific instruction for cleaning and care of prostheses is needed.
   C. Xerostomia can be a serious problem with patients using certain medications.
   - Avoiding cariogenic candies and beverages is mandatory.
   - Instruction for use of a saliva substitute.

IV. INSTRUMENTATION

- Anesthesia when indicated.
- Scaling is complicated by instability of the head.

V. FLUORIDE APPLICATION

Selection of method for fluoride application varies with the patient and the home situation.
- Professional: fluoride varnish lends itself to easy application.
- Self-care: depends on the patient's disability and the cooperation of the caregiver. The greatest benefit will be from daily toothpaste (at least twice daily), mouthrinse with alcohol-free fluoride rinse, chewable tablet (to swallow when nonfluoridated water is used), or gel applied in tray or brush-on.

VI. DIETARY SUGGESTIONS

- Consultation with physician concerning a prescribed diet is necessary. When significant relationships of diet to oral health are suspected, they should be reported to the physician. The patient's problem then can be discussed with the physician and dietary adjustments made.
- Dietary assessment instigated and follow-up recommendations made (pages 528 to 535).
- When significant relationships of current dietary habits detrimental to oral health exist, they can be discussed with physician.
- Cariogenic foods should be avoided as snacks. The patient and those who provide the patient's food need specific suggestions for food substitutes that are noncariogenic.
- Factors influencing suggestions for diet:
  - Patient's appetite may be poor, particularly if the patient is discouraged about the state of health.
  - The patient who is finicky in food selection may have affected the general nutritional state or may have used cariogenic foods in excess.
  - Monotony of meals may have lessened the desire to eat.

VII. APPOINTMENT PLAN FOR MAINTENANCE

- Determine frequency: 2 to 3 months depending on patient and caregiver cooperation on daily care.
- For caries-susceptible patient, fluoride varnish application every 2 to 3 months can be beneficial.

■ THE UNCONSCIOUS PATIENT

Personal oral care procedures for the unconscious patient are accomplished by the caregiver. Planning and conducting an oral health in-service program for a nursing staff and other caregivers are described on pages 905 to 907.

Understanding the possible procedures for oral care of hospitalized patients is important to all dental hygienists, whether or not they are employed in a hospital. Dental hygienists can appreciate ramifications of dental hygiene care for the many types of patients with special needs.

Skill is required to carry out routine methods of tooth-brushing, rinsing, and cleaning of removable dentures for the conscious patient who is able to cooperate. Methods must be adapted when the patient's head cannot be elevated. When the patient's illness or injury involves the oral cavity, the advice and recommendations of the attending oral surgeon are followed.

Maintenance of oral cleanliness for the acutely ill or unconscious patient requires special procedures because of the complete helplessness of the patient. Objectives and methods described in the following sections have application for patients with other special needs, for example, the patient with a fractured jaw (pages 860 to 862) or severe mental retardation (page 985).

I. OBJECTIVES OF CARE

- Observe the overall health of the oral tissues and provide routine screening to detect lesions that may be pathologic, particularly those that may be early cancer.
- Prevent debris and microorganisms in the mouth from being aspirated.
- Minimize the possibility of oral infection.
- Clean the mouth and provide comfort for the patient.
- Relieve mouth dryness.

II. CARE OF REMOVABLE DENTURES

A. Remove dentures from the patient's mouth. Usual hospital policy requires removal of dentures when a patient is unconscious. When already removed, locate them.
B. Procedure for removal is described on pages 474 and 476.
C. Clean the dentures (page 474) and store in water in a covered container by the patient's bedside. Instruct caregiver to change the water or denture cleanser daily to prevent bacterial growth.[2]

III. GENERAL MOUTH CLEANING: INSTRUCTION FOR CAREGIVER

A. Edentulous and Dentulous

- Clean the mouth at least three times each day to prevent dryness and sordes.
- Sordes is a crust-like material that collects on the lips, teeth, and gingiva of a patient with a fever or dehydration in a chronic debilitating disease.
- A soft toothbrush and other devices such as swabs and gauze sponges can be used to wipe the oral mucosa. Swabs and sponges are less effective and more time consuming than a toothbrush for the removal of dental biofilm.[3]

B. Brush

A power toothbrush may be more efficient and thorough than a manual brush when a caregiver must brush a helpless patient's teeth. A mouth prop can be placed in one side while the other side is retracted.

IV. TOOTHBRUSH WITH SUCTION ATTACHMENT

The toothbrush with attached suction provides an efficient and safe method for patient care.

A. Description of Brush[4,5]

1. Soft-textured nylon brush with the hole drilled between the filaments in the middle of the head of the brush.
2. Small plastic tubing inserted into hole; end adjusted slightly below level of brushing plane.
3. Other end of tubing passed across back of brush handle and attached to handle by small rubber bands (Figure 54-1).

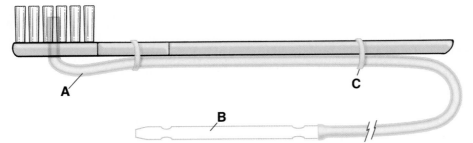

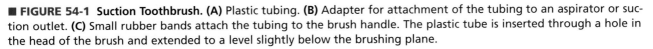

▪ **FIGURE 54-1 Suction Toothbrush. (A)** Plastic tubing. **(B)** Adapter for attachment of the tubing to an aspirator or suction outlet. **(C)** Small rubber bands attach the tubing to the brush handle. The plastic tube is inserted through a hole in the head of the brush and extended to a level slightly below the brushing plane.

4. Tubing is connected by an adapter to aspirator or suction outlet.
5. Suction brushes are also manufactured commercially.[6]

B. Procedure for Use of Brush

The detailed procedure should be outlined for hospital personnel and included in the nursing procedures manual. An abbreviated outline of the basic steps is included here.

1. Prepare patient.
   a. Although not able to respond in a usual manner, the patient may be aware of what is going on.
   b. Tell patient that the teeth are going to be brushed, and thereafter maintain a one-way conversation despite patient's inability to respond verbally.
   c. Turn patient on a side and place a pillow at the back for support.
   d. Place a face towel under patient's chin and over bedding.
2. Attach toothbrush to suction outlet and lay brush on towel near patient's mouth.
3. Place a rubber bite block on one side of the patient's mouth between the teeth. Floss tied to bite block is fastened to the patient's gown with a safety pin.
4. Dip brush in fluoride mouthrinse; turn on suction.
5. Gently retract lip and carefully apply the appropriate toothbrushing procedures; apply suction over each tooth surface with particular care at each interproximal area. Moisten brush frequently.
6. Move bite block to opposite side of mouth and continue brushing procedure.
7. Place brush in cup of clear water to allow water to be sucked through to clear the tubing during the procedure if there is clogging and to clean the tube after brushing.
8. Remove bite block; wipe patient's lips with paper wipe and apply a water-based lubricant, such as plain hydrous lanolin.
9. Wash brush and bite block; prepare materials for next use.

V. RELIEF FOR XEROSTOMIA

A. Use Saliva Substitute

- Swab the oral mucosa using a saliva substitute containing fluoride.[7]
- Lemon and glycerin swabs formerly were used by hospital personnel, but the acidic effect of the lemon led to demineralization of enamel, and the drying effect of the glycerin was contradictory to the intended outcome.[8,9]
- Swabs prepared with saliva substitute are available to relieve xerostomia and can be used as frequently as needed throughout the day and night.[10]

B. Composition of Saliva Substitutes

- *Remineralizing Effect.* Products containing fluoride (F), calcium (Ca), and phosphorus (P) ions have remineralizing capacity.
- *Alcohol and Glycerin.* Avoid products that contain alcohol or glycerin, which are drying to the oral tissues.

Everyday Ethics

Elena is 55 years old and is dying of esophageal cancer. She has been involved in an outpatient hospice program and receives all medical services in her home. Elena's daughter contacts the dental office of Dr. Gray and asks if someone can please come to the house and check her mother's teeth.

Sandy, the dental hygienist in the practice, offers to go and provide whatever "comfort care" she can for Elena.

Questions for Consideration

1. What legal and ethical concerns need to be addressed before going to Elena's home since care will be limited?

2. Reviewing the principle of justice, if Elena's homebound status prevents her from accessing dental care, what options can the dental team offer to her at this time?

3. Describe several "virtues" that can be exhibited by the dental team to benefit this patient.

▪ THE TERMINALLY ILL PATIENT

The role of the dental hygienist in the care of the terminally ill patient is to provide comfort care. The emphasis is on symptom relief and a clean environment, which may enhance the patient's sense of dignity and improve quality of life, no matter how brief the life is to be.

Although complicated dental procedures are not usually indicated for terminally ill patients, there is no excuse for neglect of oral cleanliness. Daily oral hygiene must be provided.

While hospice program caregivers are becoming more aware of the oral care needs of their patients, standardized oral health protocols are not followed in many programs.[11] The major difference in caring for a terminally ill patient is that the focus is on short-term palliative care rather than long-term preventive care.

I. OBJECTIVES OF CARE

- Provide oral care that emphasizes patient comfort rather than only preventive or restorative aspects of care.
- Provide relief of painful or aggravating symptoms of oral disease or lesions.
- Provide a "clean mouth" environment to reduce malodor and improve appearance, which may enhance personal interaction with caregivers and family members.

II. GENERAL MOUTHCARE CONSIDERATIONS

A. Cleanliness

Gentle but thorough daily cleaning of teeth, tongue, and oral mucosa is necessary. It is important to provide cleansing in any way the patient will allow. Dentifrice or other oral products are not necessary, but they can add a refreshing flavor that the patient may like.

B. Visual Inspection

Frequent visual inspection of the patient's mouth is necessary to identify oral lesions that can cause discomfort or lead to serious infection.

C. Oral Lesions

Mucosal soreness and ulceration, candidiasis, glossitis, and xerostomia are frequently found on clinical examination.

✔ **Factors To Teach The Patient**

- The contribution of good oral health to general health.

- How a clean mouth can contribute to wellness and quality of life factors.

- Need for prevention of dental caries by not using sugary snacks and sugar-sweetened beverages, especially between meals.

---

1. *Candidiasis Infection.* Oral cultures of *Candida albicans* have been found in as many as 79% of terminally ill patients.[12] The infection may become life threatening in immunocompromised individuals. It is easily treated with antifungal medication.

2. *Xerostomia.* Xerostomia is common among terminally ill individuals owing to medications, dehydration, or mouthbreathing.[11,12] Intraoral tissues and lips should be moistened constantly using water, ice chips, or appropriate over-the-counter products as mentioned earlier in this chapter.

3. *Oral Mucosa.* Approximately 75% of hospice patients in one study had evidence of pathologic changes in the oral mucosa, and 42% reported soreness of the oral mucosa.[12] Active oral lesions in the terminally ill may cause extreme discomfort when eating or talking as well as present an opportunity for development of secondary infec-

---

✔ **Factors To Teach The Caregiver**

- How to care for the patient's natural teeth: toothbrushing, flossing, rinsing, and other personal needs.

- Removable denture care: cleaning daily; storage in a safe covered container when not in the mouth; changing solution for denture care daily.

- Selecting foods and snacks that are not cariogenic.

- How to use a suction toothbrush, power brush, or other device that can mean better oral care for the patient.

tions. Daily examination of tissues and immediate care of developing lesions is recommended.

4. *Denture Problems.* Because of severe weight loss, many terminally ill patients find that dentures no longer fit. More than 70% of hospice patients who wore dentures reported having some kind of difficulty wearing their dentures.[12]

Individuals who continue to wear ill-fitting prostheses may find chewing and talking difficult. A more serious concern would be development of active intraoral lesions secondary to denture movement along with the collection of denture biofilm microorganisms due to lack of daily cleaning of the denture. Denture-induced lesions are described in Chapter 50, pages 843 to 844. Several soft reline materials are available that may solve the problem for the duration of the patient's life.

REFERENCES

1. **National Hospice Organization** (NHO), 1978, in Zimmerman, J.M.: *Hospice Complete Care for the Terminally Ill,* 2nd ed. Baltimore-Munich, Urban & Schwarzenberg, 1986, p. 17.

2. **DePaola**, L.G. and Minah, G.E.: Isolation of Pathogenic Microorganisms From Dentures and Denture-Soaking Containers of Myelosuppressed Cancer Patients, *J. Prosthet. Dent., 49,* 20, January, 1983.

3. **Seto**, B.G., Wolinsky, L.E., Tsutsui, P., and Avera, C.: Comparison of the Plaque-Removing Efficacy of Four Nonbrushing Oral Hygiene Devices, *Clin. Prev. Dent., 9,* 9, March–April, 1987.

4. **Capps**, J.S.: New Device for Oral Hygiene, *Am. J. Nurs., 58,* 1532, November, 1958.

5. **Tronquet**, A.A.: Oral Hygiene for Hospital Patients, *J. Am. Dent. Assoc., 63,* 215, August, 1961.

6. **Trademark Medical Corporation,** 1053 Headquarters Park, Fenton, Missouri, 63026. *www.trademarkmedical.com.*

7. **American Dental Association:** *ADA Guide to Dental Therapeutics,* latest edition. ADA Publishing, 211 East Chicago Ave., Chicago, IL 60611.

8. **Daeffler**, R.J.: Oral Care, *Hospice J., 2,* 81, Spring, 1986.

9. **Poland**, J.M.: Xerostomia in the Oncologic Patient: Combating Complications of Treatment, *Am. J. Hospice Care, 4,* 31, May/June, 1987.

10. **Moi-stir Oral Swabsticks,** Kingswood Laboratories, Inc., 10375 Hague Road, Indianapolis, IN 46256.

11. **Wyche**, C.J. and Kerschbaum, W.E.: Michigan Hospice Oral Healthcare Needs Survey, *J. Dent. Hyg., 68,* 35, January/February, 1994.

12. **Aldred**, M.J., Addy, M., Bagg, J., and Finlay, I.: Oral Health in the Terminally Ill: A Cross-sectional Pilot Survey, *Spec. Care Dentist., 11,* 59, March/April, 1991.

SUGGESTED READINGS

Bowes, D. and Murray, K.: The Palliative Care Team and the Dental Hygienist, *Can. Dent. Hyg. Assoc./Probe, 31,* 127, July/August, 1997.

Crosson, B.: Mobile Oral Hygiene Services, *Can. Dent. Hyg. Assoc./Probe, 30,* 72, March/April, 1996.

Epstein, J., Ransier, A., Lunn, R., and Spinelli, J.: Enhancing the Effect of Oral Hygiene With the Use of a Foam Brush With Chlorhexidine, *Oral Surg. Oral Med. Oral Pathol., 77,* 242, March, 1994.

Fiske, J.: The Delivery of Oral Care Service to Elderly People Living in a Noninstitutionalized Setting, *J. Public Health Dent., 60,* 321, Fall, 2000.

Kambhu, P.P. and Levy, S.M.: An Evaluation of the Effectiveness of Four Mechanical Plaque-Removal Devices When Used by a Trained Care-Provider, *Spec. Care Dentist., 13,* 9, January/February, 1993.

Lugo, R.I., Braun, R.J., and Gray, S.A.: Homebound Dental Care of the HIV+ Individual, *J. Dent. Educ., 60,* 189, Abstract no. 58, February, 1996.

Paunovich, E.: Assessment of the Oral Health Status of the Medically Compromised Homebound Geriatric Patient: A Descriptive Pilot Study, *Spec. Care Dentist., 14,* 80, March/April, 1994.

Practice Profile: Bruce Coyle: Dental Hygienist Provides Mobile Dental Hygiene Services, *Can. Dent. Hyg. Assoc./Probe, 32,* 15, January/February, 1998.

Simons, D.: Who Will Provide Dental Care for Housebound People With Oral Problems? *Brit. Dent. J., 194,* 137, February 8, 2003.

Strayer, M.S.: Perceived Barriers to Oral Health Care Among the Homebound, *Spec. Care Dentist., 15,* 113, May/June, 1995.

Sweeney, M.P. and Baggs, J.: The Mouth and Palliative Care, *Am. J. Hosp. Palliat. Care, 17,* 118, March-April, 2000.

Wiseman, M.A.: Palliative Care Dentistry, *Gerodontology, 17,* 49, July, 2000.

Terminally Ill

Bennett, L.: Hospice Care, *Can. Dent. Hyg. Assoc./Probe, 31,* 92, May/June, 1997.

Brown, J.O. and Hoffman, L.A.: The Dental Hygienist as a Hospice Care Provider, *Am. J. Hosp. Palliat. Care, 7,* 31, March–April, 1990.

Brown, J.: Community Hospices: Their Role in Palliative Care, *Can. Dent. Hyg. Assoc./Probe, 31,* 50, March/April, 1997.

Cassel, C.K. and Vladeck, B.C.: ICD-9 Code for Palliative or Terminal Care, *N. Engl. J. Med., 335,* 1232, October 17, 1996.

Chiodo, G.T., Tolle, S.W., and Madden, T.: The Dentist's Role in End-of-Life Care, *Gen. Dent., 46,* 560, November–December, 1998.

Jobbins, J., Bagg, J., Finlay, I.G., Addy, M., and Newcombe, R.G.: Oral and Dental Disease in Terminally Ill Cancer Patients, *Br. Med. J., 304,* 1612, June 20, 1992.

Kutscher, A.H., Schoenberg, B., and Carr, A.C.: *The Terminal Patient: Oral Care.* New York, Foundation of Thanology, 1973, 273 pp.

Kutscher, A.H., Schoenberg, B., Carr, A.C., Rappaport, S., DeBellis, R., and Blitzner, A.: *Oral Care: The Mouth in Critical and Terminal Illness.* New York, Arno Press, 1980, 216 pp.

Nursing Homes and Hospitals

Anderson, J.L.: Dental Treatment for Homebound and Institutionalized Patients, in Nowak, A.J.: *Dentistry for the Handicapped Patient.* St. Louis, Mosby, 1976, pp. 211–224.

Hardy, D.L., Brangan, P.P., Darby, M.L., Leinbach, R.M., and Welliver, M.R.: Self-Report of Oral Health Services Provided by Nurses' Aides in Nursing Homes, *J. Dent. Hyg., 69,* 75, March–April, 1995.

Helgeson, M.J. and Smith, B.J.: Dental Care in Nursing Homes: Guidelines for Mobile and On-site Care, *Spec. Care Dentist., 16,* 153, July/August, 1996.

Henry, R.G. and Ceridan, B.: Delivering Dental Care to Nursing Home and Homebound Patients, *Dent. Clin. North Am., 38,* 537, July, 1994.

Kambhu, P.P., Warren, J.J., Hand, J.S., Levy, S.M., and Cowen, H.J.: Medical and Functional Changes Among Nursing Facility Residents: Implications for Dentistry, *Spec. Care Dentist., 16,* 22, January/February, 1996.

Meurman, J.H., Sorvari, R., Peittari, A., Rytömaa, I., Franssila, S., and Kroon, L.: Hospital Mouth-Cleaning Aids May Cause Dental Erosion, *Spec. Care Dentist., 16*, 247, November/December, 1996.

Pellegrini, J.M., Fitch, J.A., Munro, C.L., and Glass, C.A.: Oral Hygiene in the Intensive Care Unit: An Interdisciplinary Approach to Oral Health, *J. Pract. Hyg., 6*, 15, July/August, 1997.

Thai, P.H., Shuman, S.K., and Davidson, G.B.: Nurses' Dental Assessments and Subsequent Care in Minnesota Nursing Homes, *Spec. Care Dentist., 17*, 13, January/February, 1997.

Warren, J.J., Kambhu, P.P., and Hand, J.S.: Factors Related to Acceptance of Dental Treatment Services in a Nursing Home Population, *Spec. Care Dentist., 14*, 15, January/February, 1994.

The Patient With a Physical Impairment

Kathryn Ragalis, RDH, MS, DMD and
Esther M. Wilkins, RDH, BS, DMD

Many diseases of the locomotor system and nervous system have as a symptom or leave as a chronic aftereffect loss of function in the form of a physical impairment. Many patients who experience physical impairments are unable to perform daily life activities and are dependent on others. Most patients with a physical impairment do not have any mental impairment.

This chapter contains brief descriptions of selected diseases or conditions to illustrate the types of care necessary and the adaptations that must be made by the patient, as well as by the professional person, during treatment appointments. Box 55-1 lists key words and their definitions relating to physical impairments and disabilities.

General suggestions that may be adapted to a variety of patients with disabilities are described in Chapter 53. From those descriptions, methods and materials can be selected as they apply in the situations created by the different disorders included in this chapter and encountered in practice.

▪ SPINAL CORD DYSFUNCTIONS

The oral cavity has great added significance for those who have lost sensation in other areas of the body. There is added functional importance to increase independence when the patient is fitted with a mouth-held implement used to control an electric wheelchair and operate a computer.

There are many causes of disruption of spinal cord function. Major causes are listed here, with examples provided in parentheses.
- Trauma (spinal cord injury).
- Neoplasms (within the cord or extradural).
- Viral or bacterial infections (poliomyelitis).
- Progressive degenerative disorders (multiple sclerosis).
- Vascular accidents (hemorrhage, thrombus, embolus, hematoma).
- Compression from an arthritic spur (spondylitic osteoarthritis).
- Congenital anomalies or deformities (myelomeningocele, meningocele, spina bifida).

▪ SPINAL CORD INJURY

Spinal cord injury is the impairment of spinal cord function resulting from the application of an external traumatic force. The effect is partial or complete paralysis to a degree related to the spinal cord level and the extent of the injury.

I. OCCURRENCE

At least one half of the trauma cases result from motor vehicle accidents; other causes are falls, diving accidents, and violence, such as from gunshot or stabbing wounds. The vast majority of patients are teenage or young adult men.

II. THE INITIAL INJURY

Total or partial loss of sensory, motor, and autonomic function occurs below the level of injury. The injury may be diagonal and leave one side with better function than the other at that particular level.

A. Types of Injury

Damage to the spinal cord may result from one or more of the following:
- Fracture, dislocation, or both, of one or more vertebrae.
- Compression, stretching, bending, or severing of the spinal cord.

B. Emergency Patient Care[1,2]

At the scene of an accident, severe damage can be done by inexpert care. The patient should be immobilized in a supine position. Any twisting motion may produce irreversible injury to the spinal cord by bony fragments cutting into or severing the cord. When transfer is made, the patient must be moved by at least four persons and placed on a board for transport.

C. Spinal Shock

Immediately after the injury, spinal shock causes a complete loss of reflex activity. The result is a flaccid paralysis below the level of injury that may last from several hours to 3 months.

III. CHARACTERISTICS OF SPINAL CORD INJURY

The pattern of signs and symptoms depends on the nature and level of injury to the spinal cord. There are 7 cervical (C), 12 thoracic (T), and 5 lumbar (L) vertebrae, with paired spinal nerves extending from each.

The areas of the body that are controlled at the different levels are illustrated in Figure 55-1. The patient's condition is referred to by the letter C, T, or L, followed by the specific vertebra number where the injury occurred. The most severely disabled patients have a lesion level above C6, which refers to the sixth cervical vertebral level.

BOX 55-1 KEY WORDS: Physical Impairments

Akinesia: absence or loss of power of voluntary motion.

Ankylosis: immobility due to direct union between parts.

> **Bony ankylosis:** union of bone with bone or bone with tooth resulting in complete immobility; the periodontal ligament of an ankylosed tooth is completely obliterated.

Aphasia: defect in, or loss of power of, expression by speech, writing, or signs, or of comprehension of spoken or written language.

Ataxia: failure of muscular coordination; irregularity of muscle action.

Atrophy: wasting; decrease in size; occurs when muscle fibers are not used or are deprived of their blood supply, or when the nerve connection is interrupted.

Bradykinesia: abnormal slowness of movements.

Cerebrovascular accident (CVA): a focal neurologic disorder caused by destruction of brain substance as a result of intracerebral hemorrhage, thrombosis, embolism, or vascular insufficiency; also called stroke.

Decubitus ulcer: ulcer that usually occurs over a bony prominence as a result of prolonged, excessive pressure from body weight; also called pressure sore or bed sore.

Demyelinate: destruction/removal of the myelin sheath of a nerve.

Dialysate: a mixture that passes through the dialyzing membrane during dialysis.

Dialysis: an artificial means to filter the blood.

Diplopia: double vision; perception of two images of a single object.

Dysphagia: difficulty in swallowing.

Hypercholesterolemia: excess of cholesterol in the blood.

Ischemia: deficiency of blood caused by functional constriction or actual obstruction of a blood vessel.

Kyphosis: abnormally increased convexity in the curvature of the thoracic spine (viewed from the side).

Microcephaly: head that is small in relation to the rest of the body; contrast with macrocephaly, head that is large in relation to the rest of the body.

Myopathy: any disease of muscle.

Orthosis: orthopedic appliance or apparatus used to support, align, prevent, or correct deformities or to improve the function of a movable part of the body.

Pallidotomy: surgical excision or destruction of part of the globus pallidus in the basal ganglia to prevent symptoms of Parkinsonism, including tremor, muscular rigidity, and bradykinesia.

Paralysis: a symptom of the loss or impairment of motor function in a body part caused by a lesion of the neural or muscular mechanism.

> **Diplegia:** paralysis of like parts on either side of the body.

> **Hemiplegia:** paralysis of one side of the body; usually caused by CVA or a brain lesion.

> **Paraplegia:** paralysis of the legs and in some cases the lower part of the body.

> **Quadriplegia:** paralysis of all four limbs from neck down; tetraplegia.

> **Triplegia:** paralysis of three limbs; hemiplegia with additional paralysis of one limb on the opposite side.

Paresis: slight or incomplete paralysis.

Paresthesia: abnormal sensation, such as burning, prickling, tingling.

Parkinsonism: a symptom complex comprising any combination of tremor, akinesia or bradykinesia, rigidity, loss of postural reflexes, and flexed posture. There are many causes of parkinsonism, one of which is Parkinson's disease.

KEY WORDS: Physical Impairments, continued

Sclerosis: induration or hardening; especially hardening from inflammation and in disease of the interstitial substance.

Shunt: passage between two natural channels; to bypass or drain an area.

Ventriculoatrial shunt: surgical creation of a communication between a cerebral ventricle and a cardiac atrium by means of a plastic tube; for relief of hydrocephalus.

Ventriculoperitoneal shunt: communication between a cerebral ventricle and the peritoneum by means of a plastic tube; for relief of hydrocephalus.

TIA: transient ischemic attack; brief episode of cerebral ischemia that results in no permanent neurologic damage; symptoms are warning signals of impending CVA (stroke).

Visceral: pertaining to internal organs (digestive, respiratory, urogenital, endocrine, spleen, heart, and great vessels).

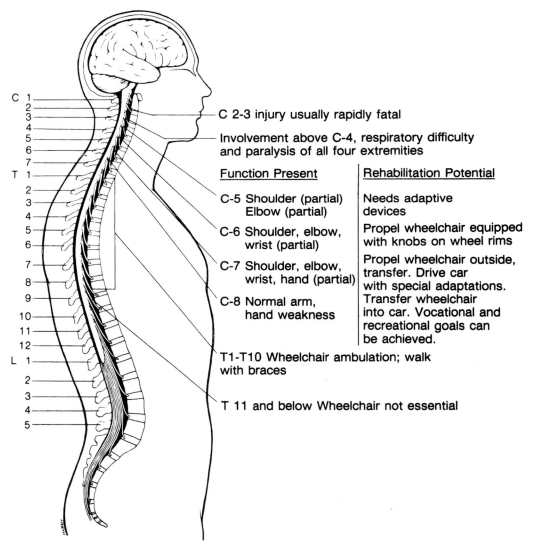

■ **FIGURE 55-1 Levels of Spinal Cord Injury.** On the left, the vertebrae are designated as C (cervical), T (thoracic), and L (lumbar). The effects of spinal cord injury depend on the level of injury, as shown by the information under Function Present at the specific level. The most severely disabled patient has a lesion above level C6. (From Smeltzer, S.C. and Bare, B.G.: *Brunner and Suddarth's Textbook of Medical-Surgical Nursing,* 7th ed. Philadelphia, J.B. Lippincott Co., 1992, p. 1739.)

A. Sensorimotor Effects

- *Complete Lesion.* A complete transection or compression of the spinal cord leaves no sensation or motor function below the level of the lesion.
- *Incomplete Lesion.* Partial transection or injury of the spinal cord leaves some evidence of sensation or motor function below the level of the lesion. The sensation and motor function may return within a few hours after injury, and maximum return may occur in 6 months to 1 year.

B. Other Possible Effects

- Impairment of voluntary bladder and bowel control.
- Impairment of sexual function.
- Impairment of vasomotor and body temperature regulatory mechanisms.

IV. SECONDARY COMPLICATIONS THAT MAY OCCUR[3,4]

Most of the complications described here do not occur in patients with lesions below the T6 level.

A. Respiratory Function

- Respiratory difficulties may occur.
- Attention to patient position and continuous suction to keep passageways clear are vital.
- Any patient with impaired respiratory function or gag reflex is at risk for aspiration.
- Some quadriplegic patients are unable to elicit a functional cough and need assistance. By placing manual pressure over the abdomen, below the diaphragm, after the patient has inhaled, the patient may be assisted while an attempt to cough is made.[3]

B. Tendency for Pressure Sores

- A pressure sore (*decubitus ulcer*) is caused by pressure exerted on the skin and subcutaneous tissues by bony prominences and the object on which they rest, such as a mattress. The result is tissue anoxia or ischemia.
- The cutaneous tissue becomes broken or destroyed, thereby leading to destruction in the subcutaneous tissue. The ulcer that forms may become infected by secondary bacterial invasion and be slow to heal; anemia and poor nutrition may also contribute.
- Prevention of pressure can be accomplished by the use of padding and by regular turning of the patient.

- The dental chair can be positioned to prevent pressure, padding can be used during the appointment, and the patient should be asked to provide instruction for the dental personnel so correct procedures can be followed.

C. Spasticity

- As spinal shock subsides, muscle-reflex spasticity develops from a slight to a severe degree.
- Stimuli, such as pressure sores, infections, and sensory irritation, may bring on a spasm.
- Before dental hygiene treatment, the patient should be asked about susceptibility to spasms and to describe the procedure to follow should one occur.

D. Body Temperature

- High-level quadriplegic patients are unable to regulate body temperature; a blanket may be needed in colder weather and air cooling during summer.
- When air conditioning is not available, the patient's temperature should be monitored. In the event of a rise in temperature, treatment should be postponed.

E. Vulnerability to Infection

Complications related to elimination (urinary tract infections, renal stones), decubitus ulcer, and respiratory problems are the most common.

F. Autonomic Dysreflexia

1. *Definition.* Autonomic dysreflexia, or hyperreflexia, is a life-threatening *emergency* condition in which the blood pressure increases sharply. It may occur in patients with lesions at T6 or above, but not below that level. A variety of stimuli may precipitate dysreflexia, especially an irritation to the bowel or bladder.
2. *Symptoms*
   - Increased blood pressure with slowed pulse rate. The blood pressure may rise to 300/160 mmHg.
   - Pounding headache.
   - Flushing, chills, perspiration, stuffy nose.
   - Restlessness; increased spasticity.
3. *Emergency Care*[3]
   - Position chair upright gradually. Do NOT recline the chair because increased blood pressure in the brain could result.
   - Monitor the blood pressure.
   - Call for medical aid.
   - Check bladder distention and unclamp catheter.

V. PERSONAL FACTORS

- The typical patient is a young man, possibly a former athlete. Depression and discouragement along with the pain and pressure of treatment and rehabilitation make psychiatric therapy necessary for many patients.
- Physical and occupational therapists provide self-care training and preparation for discharge from the rehabilitation hospital. As much responsibility as possible is given to the patient for personal care.
- Daily oral care, which at first may be carried out by others, should gradually become a part of the daily hygiene routine accomplished by the patient, depending on the cord level of injury.

VI. DENTAL HYGIENE CARE

- Emergency dental care may be needed during the patient's hospital period of recovery and treatment. Routine care should be delayed until the condition is stabilized.
- By the time the patient is able to be transported to a dental office or clinic, physical and psychological preparation for daily living is at a stage where the patient has developed a stable routine.
- Most of the information necessary for patient management and instruction is presented in Chapter 53. A few special considerations are described here.

A. Dental Chair

1. Wheelchair transfers (page 891) into the dental chair.
2. Chair angle[3]
   - For the patient with a gravity-drained urinary appliance, the chair may be adjusted to accommodate the drainage, or the patient should be uprighted at intervals to allow drainage to take place. The bag may require emptying during the appointment.
   - The chair angle should not be changed abruptly because of the patient's susceptibility to postural hypotension.
3. Allow frequent changes of the patient's body position in the chair by lifting and turning at intervals to prevent pressure sores and pain in muscles and joints.
4. Padding that the patient brings to the appointment or obtained by the dental facility can be used under areas of the patient to relieve pressure and help prevent sores.

B. Four-Handed Dental Hygiene

Precautions for the patient with spinal cord injury relate to the problems of respiration, aspiration, pressure sores, spasms, autonomic dysreflexia, temperature control, wheelchair transfers, and other factors described earlier. It is necessary to:
1. Monitor vital signs.
2. Watch the patient for signs of body needs, emergencies.
3. Assist with rubber dam. A rubber dam should always be used for appropriate procedures, such as application of topical fluorides, sealants, and polishing of restorations, because of danger of a respiratory complication should materials be inhaled.
4. Suction
   - Prevent aspiration of any material, such as calculus.
   - Use ultrasonic instruments with great caution, if at all. When use of such instruments is unavoidable, care must be taken to prevent aspiration of water, to avoid spraying the throat and stimulating a gag reflex or cough, and to watch for patient sensitivity.
5. Assist with all procedures to make the total treatment time as brief and efficiently used as possible without sacrificing patient comfort.

C. Disease Control

- A complete preventive program with biofilm control, fluorides, and diet counseling is essential.
- Frequent appointments usually are necessary to motivate, follow up with additional instruction, and assist the patient in carrying out the recommended procedures.
- Instruction for the caregiver must be provided.
- Care of removable appliances includes cleaning of mouth-held implements.

VII. MOUTH-HELD IMPLEMENTS

The patient without hands or without the use of hands may utilize the mouth for performing many tasks and the teeth for holding objects. The maintenance of optimum oral health has special significance for these individuals because many functions could not be accomplished in an edentulous mouth.

A. Uses

Mouth-held appliances have been fabricated that are effective in carrying out a variety of basic procedures and that contribute to increased independence for a person without the use of hands. A device makes possible such activities as pressing light switches, writing, typing on a computer, pressing telephone buttons, pushing an elevator button, or turning the pages of a book.

B. Criteria

The formerly used plain mouthsticks required gripping the stick with the teeth, which could cause chipping, uneven pressures led to periodontal trauma, and tipping and extrusion of teeth. Criteria for an adequate oral orthosis include the following[5]

1. Does not harm the oral tissues.
   - Stabilization of occlusion with contact for all fully erupted teeth and the biting forces distributed to as many teeth as possible.
   - Is not traumatic to the periodontal supporting structures.
   - Does not prevent eruption of teeth.
2. Is comfortable and does not cause fatigue.
   - Patient can talk, swallow, and moisten the lips.
   - Orthosis can be inserted and removed by the patient.
   - Orthosis is adaptable for the various needs of the quadriplegic patient.
3. Can be cleaned and cared for easily.
4. Is relatively easy to construct; inexpensive.

C. Oral Care

- Before making impressions for constructing a mouthpiece, periodontal and restorative therapy should be completed and the occlusion adjusted.
- Biofilm control procedures must be effective, and the patient must be instructed carefully in the importance and methods of oral hygiene and appliance care.

▪ MYELOMENINGOCELE[6]

- *Spina bifida* is a congenital defect or opening in the spinal column. A portion of the spinal membranes may protrude through the opening with or without spinal cord tissue. When the spinal cord protrudes through the spina bifida, the condition is called *myelomeningocele*.
- Anticipatory guidance prior to conception must include the use of multivitamins containing *folic acid*. A reduced risk of offspring with spina bifida and other neural tube defects has been shown when mothers received folic acid.[7]

I. DESCRIPTION

- Embryologically, a neural tube forms during the first month of pregnancy.

- From the neural tube, the brain, brain stem, and spinal cord arise, and, eventually, the vertebrae form and enclose the spinal cord.
- When a place in the spinal column fails to close, the result is an open defect in the spinal canal, which is called a spina bifida.

II. TYPES OF DEFORMITIES

A. Myelomeningocele

A myelomeningocele is a protrusion or outpouching of the spinal cord and its covering (meninges) through an opening in the bony spinal column. Because part of the spinal cord and nerve roots protrude, flaccid paralysis of the legs and part of the trunk results, depending on the level of the protrusion (herniation).

B. Meningocele

A meningocele is a protrusion of the meninges through a defect in the skull or spinal column. Because no neural elements are contained in the protrusion, paralysis is uncommon.

C. Spina Bifida

Spina bifida is a congenital cleft in the bony encasement of the spinal cord. When no outpouching of the meninges or spinal cord exists, the condition is called *spina bifida occulta*. Usually, spina bifida occulta has no symptoms.

III. PHYSICAL CHARACTERISTICS

Depending on the level of the myelomeningocele, some or all of the signs and physical characteristics listed here may be found.

A. Bony Deformities

Muscle imbalance from paralysis can cause dislocation of the hip, club foot, and spinal curvatures, such as humpback (kyphosis), curvature (scoliosis), or swayback (lordosis).

B. Loss of Sensation

Lack of skin sensitivity to pain, temperature, and other sensations can lead to problems of inadvertent burn or trauma unrecognized by the patient or caregiver or to pressure sores, described on page 925. Frequent position changes are necessary.

C. Bladder and Bowel Paralysis

The nerve supplies to the bladder and bowel are usually affected. Lack of bowel and bladder control requires continual attention. Kidney infection with loss of kidney function is one cause of shorter life expectancy.

D. Hydrocephalus

- A high percentage of children with myelomeningocele have hydrocephalus. Hydrocephalus is a condition characterized by an excessive accumulation of fluid in the brain. The fluid dilates the cerebral ventricles, causes compression of brain tissues, and separates the cranial bones as the head enlarges (Figure 55-2).
- Development is slowed, and mental retardation is present.
- Many of these patients have seizures.

IV. MEDICAL TREATMENT

Surgical, orthopedic, medical, urologic as well as physical and occupational therapy may constitute a minimum of specialties involved in the care of a patient with myelomeningocele.

A. Neurosurgery

- *Closure of the Myelomeningocele*. Surgical closure helps to prevent infections that may otherwise enter into the spinal cord. Paralysis is not lessened by the surgery.
- *Treatment of the Hydrocephalus*. Permanent drainage systems may be accomplished in the form of a ventriculoatrial shunt between the cerebral ventricle and the atrium of the heart (Figure 55-3). Sometimes, drainage by way of

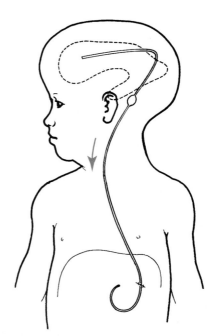

■ **FIGURE 55-3 Shunt for Hydrocephalus Treatment.** Fluid is drained by way of a ventriculoatrial or ventriculoperitoneal shunt. (Adapted from Bleck, E.E. and Nagel, D.A.: *Physically Handicapped Children: A Medical Atlas for Teachers*. New York, Grune & Stratton, 1975.)

the abdomen in the form of a ventriculoperitoneal shunt is used.

B. Orthopedic Surgery

- Orthopedic surgical procedures can assist by reducing or correcting deformities.
- Bracing to support the trunk and lower limbs is used in accord with the extent of the individual's paralysis.
- Ambulation varies from dependency on a wheelchair, walker, crutches, or cane to near normal with only foot problems.

V. DENTAL HYGIENE CARE

A. General Management

- Management for the physical impairments of the patient with myelomeningocele can be adapted from the information in Chapter 53.
- Wheelchair transfers and assistance for patients with crutches are described on pages 892 to 893.

B. Need for Premedication

Ventriculoatrial shunts, but not ventriculoperitoneal shunts, need antibiotic premedication for dental and dental hygiene instrumentation.[8]

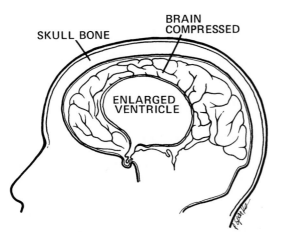

■ **FIGURE 55-2 Hydrocephalus.** The ventricle is enlarged because of the accumulation of fluid. Brain tissues are compressed. (From Bleck, E.E. and Nagel, D.A.: *Physically Handicapped Children: A Medical Atlas for Teachers*. New York, Grune & Stratton, 1975.)

C. Latex Allergy

- Patients with spina bifida appear to be specifically at risk for latex allergy.[9,10]
- Proper precautions must be taken (page 60).

D. Gingival Care

- Special adaptations for biofilm control techniques are needed when the cervical or thoracic body level is involved, and the assistance of an attendant may be required.
- Patients with seizures treated with antiepileptic medication such as phenytoin may need gingival treatment for phenytoin-induced gingival overgrowth. The condition is described on pages 973 ot 975.

▪ CEREBROVASCULAR ACCIDENT (STROKE)

- Cerebrovascular accident (CVA) or stroke is a sudden loss of brain function resulting from interference of the blood supply to a part of the brain.
- CVA is the clinical manifestation of cerebrovascular disease.
- The patient is frequently disabled by changes in motor, communication, and perception. Hemiplegia or hemiparesis is common.
- Stroke is the third leading cause of death, following heart disease and cancer, in the United States.

I. ETIOLOGIC FACTORS[11]

The stroke may be severe and followed by death within minutes. The less severe attack leaves the patient with the symptoms and signs described below. Strokes are usually brought on by one of the following:

A. Thrombosis

- A clot within a blood vessel of the brain or neck closes or occludes the vessel and shuts off the oxygen supply to the portion of the brain supplied by that vessel, resulting in cerebral infarction.
- Cerebral thrombosis is the most common cause of stroke.

B. Intracerebral Embolism

- A blood vessel is blocked by a clot or other material carried through the circulation from another part of the body.

- Atherosclerotic plaque build-up in a blood vessel (atheroma) can become an embolism and increases the risk of stroke. Calcifications in the carotid artery may be observable in a panoramic radiograph and indicate an increased risk of CVA.

C. Ischemia

The blood flow decreases to an area of the brain, usually as a result of an atheromatous constriction of the arteries supplying the area.

D. Cerebral Hemorrhage

A cerebral blood vessel may rupture and bleed into the brain tissues.

E. Predisposing Factors

Patients with certain conditions may be considered "risk" patients, or persons more susceptible to having strokes. Early diagnosis and treatment for control of the following predisposing factors are necessary in the prevention of stroke and its devastating effects.

- Atherosclerosis (page 1046)
- Hypertension, the greatest risk factor that leads to stroke (page 1043).
- Hypercholesterolemia, hypertriglyceridemia.
- Cigarette smoking.
- Cardiovascular disease (rheumatic heart disease, congestive heart failure, history of TIAs).
- Diabetes mellitus.
- Use of oral contraceptives (enhanced by hypertension, cigarette smoking, age over 35, and high estrogen levels).
- Drug abuse (especially in adolescents and young adults).

II. SIGNS AND SYMPTOMS

The effects of a stroke depend on the location of the damage to the brain, as well as on the degree or extent of involvement.

A. Transient Ischemic Attack (TIA)

- A brief event where the blood supply to a localized area of the brain is interrupted and the patient may have transient signs or symptoms of a stroke.
- These "little strokes" may last a few minutes to an hour and may leave no permanent damage.
- A history of transient attacks is a possible risk factor or warning for a stroke.

B. Acute Symptoms of a Stroke

Acute symptoms and emergency procedures are included in Table 66-4 (page 1114).

C. Residual or Chronic Effects

Approximately two thirds of those who survive have some degree of permanent disability. Temporary or permanent loss of thought, memory, speech, sensation, or motion results. The side of the brain affected influences the symptoms.

The side of the face and body affected is opposite that of the brain injury (Figure 55-4). Persons with right hemiplegia have more difficulty with verbal communication and are more apt to be cautious, anxious, and disorganized. Patients with left hemiplegia have difficulty with action requiring physical coordination and may respond impulsively with overconfidence.

Common signs and symptoms are described briefly here for application during clinical patient care.

- *Paralysis.* Hemiplegia (one side of the body) or portions, such as an arm, leg, or the face.
- *Articulation.* Difficulty of speech, which may be caused by involvement of the tongue, mouth, or throat, as well as aphasia by brain damage related to the speech centers, and the patient may have difficulty finding the right word.
- *Salivation.* Difficulty in control of saliva complicated by difficulty in swallowing; aspiration.
- *Sensory.* Loss in affected parts may result in superficial anesthesia, or the opposite may occur

with resultant increased sensitivity to pain and touch.

- *Visual Impairment.* Blurred vision, or diminished visual acuity.
- *Mental Function.* May be unaffected, but slowness, poor memory, and loss of initiative are common. Brain deterioration may occur over a period of time.
- *Personal Factors.* Personality changes relate to emotional trauma, fear, discouragement, and dependency. Anxiety neuroses and periods of depression, which are common, may require assistance from a psychiatrist, psychologist, or social worker.

III. MEDICAL TREATMENT

A. Surgical

Treatment may include surgical correction of aneurysms, clots, or malformations. Newer developments include surgery in the intracranial arteries using an operating microscope to remove very small clots or to perform minute grafting to bypass blocked vessels and provide collateral circulation.

B. Physical and Occupational Therapy

Rehabilitation techniques are vital to the patient's functioning.

C. Drugs

Careful recording of the medical history includes the listing of medications. The patient may be taking a variety of drugs for some or all of the following purposes:

1. Anticoagulant (to thin the blood).
2. Antihypertensive (to lower the blood pressure).
3. Thrombolytic (to dissolve clots).
4. Vasodilator (to relax the blood vessels of the brain).
5. Steroid (to control brain swelling).
6. Antiepileptic (to help to control seizures).

IV. DENTAL HYGIENE CARE

A. Timing

- Elective dental treatment is not usually advisable until 6 months or more after a stroke, but, when possible, preventive measures and biofilm control procedures should be introduced or reinstated early.
- Regular appointments for preventive care should be initiated as soon as a release can be obtained from the physician.

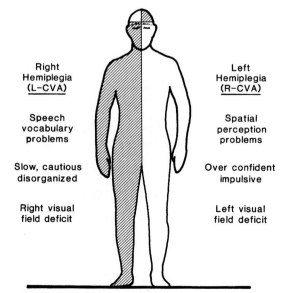

■ FIGURE 55-4 Cerebrovascular Accident (Stroke). Right hemiplegia is the result of left-sided brain damage; left hemiplegia results from right-sided brain damage.

B. Appointment Procedures

*   Patients may be homebound or brought to the clinic or office by wheelchair or walker. Factors described in Chapter 53 apply to the patient who has had a stroke.
*   Because of weakness, treatment may best be accomplished in shorter appointments and small increments of instrumentation.
*   The application of four-handed dental hygiene during instrumentation is necessary for all the same reasons described on page 926 for the patient with a spinal cord injury.
*   Effects of medications must be considered, particularly if the patient is on anticoagulation.

C. Disease Control

*   Every attempt should be made to provide complete care because temporary care may increase the severity of needs at a later time. Complete scaling and root planing to control the periodontal status are especially important and may need special adaptation techniques.
*   When the right-handed person is paralyzed on the right side (or the left-handed on the left), development of dexterity for the manipulation of biofilm removal implements with the nondominant hand takes time and patience. The patient must be as self-sufficient as possible but should be encouraged to have the paralyzed side cleaned daily (brush, floss, and supplementary aids) by a family member or other caregiver for whom instruction has been provided.
*   The paralyzed side of the face tends to sag or droop, and, because of inactivity of the tongue on the same side, self-cleansing is ineffective. Lack of sensation hinders the patient from realizing that collection of food debris and tooth deposits may be extensive.
*   Rinsing is difficult or impossible. Daily fluoride application can be the use of a gel tray by the caregiver or the brushing of the teeth with a fluoride gel. When xerostomia is present, substitute saliva can be recommended (page 388).
*   Modified handles for toothbrushes and floss holders are shown on pages 898 to 901. The patient who wears dentures requires a suction cup brush to clean the denture with one hand (Figure 53-12).

D. Disease Risk Detection

*   All panoramic radiographs should be evaluated for the evidence of calcifications in the carotid artery. If present, and because of the increased risk of stroke, the patient needs referral for immediate medical evaluation.
*   Calcifications in the carotid artery are observable inferior and posterior to the inferior border of the mandible on a panoramic radiograph.
*   Radiation therapy is associated with an accelerated form of atherosclerosis formation and risk of stroke.[12]

■ MUSCULAR DYSTROPHIES[13]

The muscular dystrophies are genetic myopathies characterized by progressive severe weakness and loss of use of groups of muscles. The term *dystrophy* means degeneration and is associated with atrophy and dysfunction.

The syndromes of muscular dystrophy have been separated by clinical and genetic means and range from mild types (Becker) with a later onset to more severe types (Duchenne, facioscapulohumeral). The cause of each type is not known, but the underlying pathologic processes do not differ. Generally, the diseases are limited to skeletal muscles, with cardiac muscle only rarely involved.

All muscular dystrophies are rare. The two types described are the more common.

I. DUCHENNE MUSCULAR DYSTROPHY (PSEUDOHYPERTROPHIC)

A. Occurrence

The Duchenne type is primarily limited to males and transmitted by female carriers.

B. Age of Onset

The condition is present at birth and becomes apparent during early childhood, usually between 2 and 5 years, but before 10 years.

C. Characteristics

1. *Musculature*. Enlargement (pseudohypertrophy) of certain muscles, particularly the calves, is present in early years.
2. *Weakness of Hips*. Child falls frequently, has increasing difficulty in standing erect.
3. *Lordosis*. With an abdominal protuberance.
4. *Gait*
    *   Waddling. Either walks on toes or flatfoot as a result of muscle contracture.
    *   Balance. Precarious; patient arches back in attempt to find center of gravity; gait is slow because balance must be attained with each step.

5. *Progressive Muscular Wasting.* Eventual involvement of thighs, shoulders, trunk; weakness of respiratory muscles; inactivity is detrimental and increases the individual's helplessness and dependency.

6. *Intellectual Impairment.* Average IQ in the range of 80 to 90; some patients have normal intelligence and others have a moderate to severe level of retardation.

D. Prognosis

Disablement severe by puberty; child is confined to a wheelchair. Patients rarely live to reach their third decade.

II. FACIOSCAPULOHUMERAL MUSCULAR DYSTROPHY

A. Occurrence

Males and females are equally affected.

B. Age of Onset

Between 10 and 18 years, with an average at 13 years, after puberty. Mild symptoms may appear at later ages.

C. Characteristics

- Facial muscles involved, particularly the obicularis oris.
- Scapulae prominent; shoulder muscles weak; difficulty in raising the arms.
- Difficulty in closing eyes completely.

D. Prognosis

- Progression is slower than that of the Duchenne type.
- Most patients live a normal life span and become incapacitated late in life.

III. MEDICAL TREATMENT

- A specific treatment is not known. Symptoms may be relieved. The patient is encouraged to lead as full a life as possible and to keep active.
- Preventive treatment consists of prenatal diagnosis, carrier detection, and genetic counseling.

IV. DENTAL HYGIENE CARE

Adaptations depend on the patient's disability. Patients may have slight muscular involvement, may be ambulatory but have balancing difficulties, may be in a wheelchair, or may be bedridden. Factors described for general consideration of patients with disabilities have application (Chapter 53). Suggestions that follow are useful for certain patients.

A. Patient Reception and Seating

1. *Assistance for the Walking Patient*
   - Certain patients do better without assistance because they have developed their own method of balancing and the slightest touch may upset them.
   - Many patients gain balance by holding both hands on the partially flexed forearm of a person walking beside them.

2. *Seating Preparation.* Raise chair and chair arm. Allow patient to sit directly. Lift patient's legs onto dental chair if such assistance is needed.

3. *Seated Patient.* Tilt chair back gently; balance is precarious while sitting as well as standing; patient may fall forward.

4. *Assistance for Patient While Rising From Chair*
   - Stand directly in front of patient. Lock arms around lower back and pull forward near hips.
   - Allow patient to sway upper trunk back while rising to standing position.
   - Provide support until balance is obtained for walking.

B. Patient Instruction

1. *Problems of Oral Cleanliness*
   - Facial muscle weakness may interfere with self-cleansing mechanisms and prevent adequate rinsing by the patient with facioscapulohumeral dystrophy.
   - Effect of gaping lips on oral tissues is similar to that of mouth breathing.
   - Weakness of arm and shoulder causes difficulty in applying toothbrush. A power-assisted brush under supervision or an adapted handle for a regular brush (page 898) may have advantages.

2. *Oral Disease Control*
   - Instruct parent or other caregiver.
   - When patient is receiving therapy, solicit assistance and advice from the occupational and physical therapists.

▪ MYASTHENIA GRAVIS

Myasthenia gravis is an autoimmune neuromuscular disease characterized by weakness and fatigability of symmetrical voluntary muscles. It is caused by an autoimmune process that results in a defect in nerve impulse transmission at the neuromuscular junctions. In myasthenia gravis, the numbers of acetylcholine receptors in each neuromuscular junction are reduced markedly compared with the normal number of receptors.[14]

The patient with myasthenia gravis has a special significance for dental professionals because the facial and oral parts served by certain cranial nerves are involved early. Muscles of the eyes, facial expression, mastication, and swallowing are affected. In advanced severe forms of the disease, muscle involvement may be extensive and result in total paralysis.

I. OCCURRENCE

The onset of myasthenia gravis may occur at any age. The early peak at about age 20 affects women twice as frequently as men. In late adult life, more men than women are affected.

II. SIGNS AND SYMPTOMS

A. Early Signs

- Weakness of eye movements with double vision (diplopia) and drooping eyelids (ptosis) may be the initial indicators.
- In certain patients, the disease may not progress further.

B. Oral and Facial Problems

- Involvement of muscles of the face, mastication, and tongue lead to swallowing difficulties (dysphagia) and a lack of facial expression.
- Disturbed speech and expression, with a weak voice that sounds tired and muffled, are typical.
- A patient may support the chin with one hand to help during talking.

C. Progressive Involvement

- When the muscles that are used during breathing become involved, serious respiratory complications can result.
- Because of the lack of facial expression, distress may be difficult for the patient to convey.
- Generalized fatigue is usually not so evident in the morning or immediately after rest. Weakness may increase as the day goes by, a factor pertinent to the time selected for dental and dental hygiene appointments.

D. Precipitating Factors

- Individual reactions vary, but the more common predisposing, aggravating factors affecting the severity of muscular involvement include emotional excitement, surgical procedures, loss of sleep, alcoholic intake, and, especially, infections.
- Prevention of oral infections and of the need for dental or periodontal surgery contributes to patient stability.
- Myasthenic crisis is best avoided by elimination and prevention of infection and all precipitating factors.

E. Types of Crises

1. *Myasthenic Crisis*[15]
   a. Cause. A myasthenic crisis may result from undermedication or increased severity of the disease, or it may be precipitated by one of the aggravating factors previously mentioned. The relative deficiency of acetylcholine, which leads to the crisis symptoms, can usually be corrected by the administration of anticholinesterase by the physician.
   b. Symptoms and signs. The inability to swallow, speak, or maintain a patent airway is sudden. Marked weakness of respiratory and pharyngeal muscles leads to depression of respiration and obstruction. The patient may also have double vision and drooping eyelids.
   c. Emergency care.
      - Suction.
      - Provide a patent airway.
      - Obtain medical assistance; transport to hospital emergency facility.
2. *Cholinergic Crisis*
   a. Cause. The cholinergic crisis results from overmedication with anticholinesterase.
   b. Symptoms and signs. Increased muscle weakness occurs within 30 to 60 minutes of taking the medication. Excessive pulmonary secretion, cramps, and diarrhea also are characteristic.
   c. Treatment. No further medication should be taken at that time. Medical assistance is needed promptly. When respiratory symptoms develop, ventilation is urgent (page 1112).

III. MEDICAL TREATMENT[14]

- Medical treatment may have two purposes: to influence the course of the disease and to induce disease remission.
- Anticholinesterase agents are used for most patients at intervals during the day. A sustained-release preparation may be used at bedtime, particularly for the patient who awakens with severe weakness.

- Current therapy for attempting to induce remission includes surgical removal of the thymus gland, particularly if a tumor of the gland develops, and drug therapy. Immunosuppressive medications include corticosteroids, azathioprine (when corticosteroids are contraindicated), and cyclosporin. Among the side effects of cyclosporin is gingival enlargement (page 257).

IV. DENTAL HYGIENE CARE

Dental hygiene care takes on special significance because the presence of infection can worsen the myasthenic weakness. Treatment with immunosuppressive drugs makes the patient vulnerable to infection. The health of the oral cavity with minimal inflammation of the periodontal tissues contributes to the overall health of the patient.

A. Appointment Factors

1. *Time and Length*. Short appointments planned early in the day and in conjunction with the patient's medication schedule. Weakness worsens with activity.
2. *Maintenance*. Frequent appointments to aid the patient in obtaining and maintaining freedom from oral infection.
3. *Preparation for the Appointment*.
   - Office emergency equipment for a possible respiratory emergency must be checked and in order.
   - Stress-reduction procedures should be followed.
   - At the outset, the patient should be asked about medication and whether it has been taken on schedule prior to the appointment.

B. Four-Handed Dental Hygiene

For any patient who is a potential respiratory risk, an assistant is needed to aid in observing the patient and to monitor vital signs. Because the patient with myasthenia gravis may have difficulty in providing a warning of distress, the need for supervision is indicated.

1. *Suction*. An assistant is needed to maintain the airway, to ensure no problem of aspiration, and to provide a clean field for efficient instrumentation to minimize appointment time. A side effect of the anticholinesterase medication is increased salivation.
2. *Rubber Dam*. Apply for appropriate procedures to prevent aspiration of harmful substances.

C. Patient Instruction for Disease Control

1. *Diet Evaluation*. A dietary survey and instruction are recommended. The patient with myasthenia gravis may have difficulty in masticating and swallowing, and adequate food selection for oral health and dental caries prevention may be difficult.
2. *Biofilm Control*. Weakness and fatigue may have discouraged the patient's routine daily biofilm control efforts. A power-assisted brush or other aids can be recommended. Instruction for a family member or other caregiver may be needed to provide the severely disabled patient with assistance.

▪ MULTIPLE SCLEROSIS[16,17]

Multiple sclerosis is a chronic demyelinating disease of the central nervous system characterized by progressive disability. It is a genetically linked disease of adults with motor, sensory, cognitive, and emotional (depression, mania) changes. Women are affected twice as frequently as men.

Pathologically, the myelin sheath is destroyed within the white matter of the central nervous system. The sheath degenerates in patches called *MS plaques* and is replaced by sclerotic tissue. There is interference with the transmission of nerve impulses and frequent involvement of the spinal cord and optic nerves.

I. OCCURRENCE

- Usually, the onset is between 20 and 40 years of age, rarely before 15 or after 55 years.
- The disease is more prevalent in temperate climates.

II. CHARACTERISTICS

A. Initial Symptoms

1. May be visual impairment, diplopia, difficulty in coordination, tremor, fatigue, or weakness.
2. Transient tingling paresthesia of the hands or feet.
3. May have a sudden onset of severe illness with paralysis or marked weakness.

B. Course of Disease

1. *Relapses and Remissions*. An attack may last several days or weeks and be followed by a symptom-free period. Physical impairment varies, but the condition worsens with each attack.

2. *Risk Factors for Exacerbations*
   a. Infection.
       •   Various types of infection, systemic or local, can stimulate a relapse.
       •   Oral infections are no exception.
   b. Pregnancy.
       •   For certain patients, pregnancy may appear to increase the risk and bring on an attack. Because the effect is more likely to be noticed during the first several months after delivery, fatigue and stress may be the direct precipitating effects.
       •   Effects of multiple sclerosis on the pregnancy should also be recognized. Possible side effects of medications on the developing fetus should be considered because certain medications used may have to be discontinued if they are teratogenic.
3. *Longevity.* People with multiple sclerosis may live many years. Fewer than half of those afflicted may eventually become nonambulatory.

C. Physical Symptoms

A wide distribution of areas is affected. Symptoms fluctuate, and several years may elapse between attacks. With extended rest, symptoms usually subside.
1. Fatigue.
2. Involuntary motion of eyes (nystagmus); may later become partially or completely blind.
3. Speech disorders; possible loss of speech in advanced stages.
4. Changes in muscular coordination and gait; loss of balance; spasms.
5. Paralysis of one or more extremities; occasionally, facial paralysis.
6. Autonomic derangements, such as urinary frequency and urgency; later urinary incontinence.
7. Susceptibility to infection, particularly upper respiratory.

III. CATEGORIES

A. **Relapsing-Remitting:** acute episodes worsening with recovery and a stable course between relapses.
B. **Secondary Progressive:** gradual neurologic deterioration with or without superimposed acute relapses in a patient who previously had relapsing-remitting multiple sclerosis.
C. **Primary Progressive:** gradual, nearly continuous neurologic deterioration from the onset of symptoms.
D. **Progressive Relapsing:** gradual neurologic deterioration from the onset of symptoms but with subsequent superimposed relapses (very uncommon).

IV. TREATMENT

A. Objectives of Treatment

Since the direct cause of multiple sclerosis is not known, the first objective is to prevent relapses and progressive worsening of the disease. Prompt diagnosis and early treatment by 6 months is crucial to prevent neurological damage. Treatments are based on the following:
1. *Psychological Support.* The ramifications of having an incurable disease can be devastating. Understanding dental personnel can contribute in this area.
2. *Disease Course Modification.* Patients with relapsing-remitting multiple sclerosis have the best responses to treatment.
3. *Symptom Relief;* palliative treatment.

B. General Treatment Procedures

•   General hygienic care; adequate nutrition, rest, avoidance of strain, prevention of infections, and prevention of injury.
•   Physical and occupational therapy; exercise, but not strenuous exertion, is important.
•   Patient should continue in a usual occupation as long as possible; activity should be encouraged.
•   Psychotherapy for personality problems and morale building is frequently necessary.

C. Medications

•   *Corticosteroids.* Anti-inflammatory and immunomodulatory effects.
•   *Interferon Beta (1a and 1b).* Reduce or prevent severity and frequency of future exacerbations.
•   *Glatiramer Acetate.* Reduce or prevent relapse. Useful for patients who become resistant to interferon-beta.
•   *Methotrexate.* Used for progressive multiple sclerosis to slow the disease process.

V. DENTAL HYGIENE CARE

Because relapses may be precipitated by infections, dental hygiene care for the prevention of periodontal infection assumes particular significance.

Many factors described in Chapter 53 have direct application for the patient with a disability associated with multiple sclerosis. For the patient with paraplegia or quadriplegia, items from the section on patients with spinal cord injuries can be used (page 926).

A. Appointment Considerations

1. Provide a warm, quiet, comfortable atmosphere. The patient needs to remain relaxed mentally and physically; people nearby cannot be tense, restless, or noisy.
2. Frequent short appointments contribute to the prevention of fatigue, emotional stress, and advanced dental or periodontal conditions.

B. Patient Instruction

1. *Problems of Personal Oral Care*
   - Involvements of the tongue and facial muscles interfere with the self-cleansing mechanisms.
   - Paralysis may make grasping and manipulating a toothbrush difficult or impossible. Adaptive aids are described on page 898.
2. *Factors Affecting Teaching*
   - Slow response of patient; give instruction slowly and simply.
   - Visual disturbances (pages 951 to 952).

▪ CEREBRAL PALSY

Palsy means impairment of the ability to control movement, and *cerebral palsy* means a condition in which injury to parts of the brain has occurred prenatally, natally, or postnatally and has resulted in paralysis or disruption of motor parts. Such a condition can occur at any age as a result of brain injury from a variety of causes.

Cerebral palsy can be caused by anoxia during pregnancy or delivery, maternal infection during pregnancy (for example, rubella), blood type incompatibility, severe nutritional lack during pregnancy, or maternal diabetes endocrine imbalance. Later in infancy, infectious diseases, such as meningitis or encephalitis, lead poisoning, direct trauma from accidents, or battering (nonaccidental injury) may be implicated.

Symptoms usually can be observed during the first year after birth but may not appear for several years. General symptoms that may occur are tense, contracted muscles; uncontrolled movements of limbs, eyes, or head; poor coordination; muscle spasms; problems with hearing and/or seeing; and a lack of manual dexterity.

I. TYPES OF CHARACTERISTICS[18,19]

Classified by motor activity, six types have been named. In each type, different parts of the brain are damaged, and the symptoms vary respectively. More than 50% of those with cerebral palsy are in the spasticity group, 15% to 20% are athetoid, and the remainder are divided among the other four types or have mixed types.

A. Spasticity

- Muscles have increased tone, tension, and activity.
- Condition characterized by spasms, which are sudden, involuntary contractions of single muscles or groups of muscles.
- Patient has complete or partial loss of ability to control muscular movement; therefore, movements are awkward and stiff.
- Lack of control causes patient to fall easily; patient tends to avoid activity and thus may gain weight, particularly during teenage years; caloric requirement is therefore low.
- Brain damage to motor area of cerebral cortex (Figure 55-5).

B. Athetosis

1. Condition characterized by constant, involuntary, unorganized muscular movement.
2. Patient lacks ability to direct muscles in the motions desired; probably the most difficult dental patient.
3. Grimacing, drooling, and speech defects are common.
4. Factors influencing movements
   - Effort by patient to control muscle activity results in exaggerated muscle movement.
   - May be initiated and aggravated by stimuli outside body, such as sudden noises, bright lights, or quick movements by people or things in the area.
   - Intensity influenced by emotional factors. Patient is least in control in an emotionally charged environment, such as the dental office.
5. Patient constantly in motion; burns up energy; usually very thin; caloric requirement of diet is therefore high.
6. Brain damage to basal ganglia (Figure 55-5).

C. Ataxia

1. Loss of equilibrium; balance and orientation difficult; walk uncertain; has difficulty in sitting straight.
2. Lack of coordination; needs time to execute changes.
3. Patient inactive because of balance disturbance; tends to put on weight; caloric requirement in diet is therefore low.
4. Brain damage to cerebellum (Figure 55-5).

D. Rigidity

1. Muscles may be rigid and stiff, with resistance to movement and hypertonicity.
2. Tendency to lack of activity.

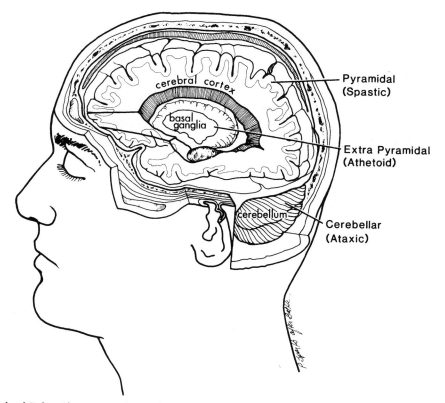

■ **FIGURE 55-5 Cerebral Palsy.** Shown are the major parts of the brain involved in each of the three major types of cerebral palsy—spastic, athetoid, and ataxic. (From Bleck, E.E. and Nagel, D.A.: *Physically Handicapped Children: A Medical Atlas for Teachers.* New York, Grune & Stratton, 1975.)

E. Tremor

Involuntary muscle quivering may affect part or all of the body.

F. Flaccidity

1. Hypotonia or atonia of muscles that are flabby and weak.
2. Unable to stand or raise head.
3. Drooling; difficulty in swallowing and chewing; speech problems.

G. Mixed

Various combinations of the six types occur.

II. CONDITIONS ACCOMPANYING MOTOR ACTIVITY

In addition to impaired movement, weakness, and lack of coordination, the following disabling conditions may also occur.

A. Mental Retardation

Fewer than 50% of individuals with cerebral palsy also have mental retardation.

B. Learning Disabilities

Of the 50% who are not mentally retarded, many have problems of learning because of sensory defects, especially hearing and seeing, and perceptive-cognitive deficiencies. Speech difficulties and inability to move about freely can also contribute to learning problems.

C. Seizures

Between 25% and 30% have seizures and undergo related drug therapy.

D. Sensory Disorders

Seeing and hearing problems are common.

III. MEDICAL TREATMENT

- Surgical, orthopedic, and medical care, as well as speech, physical, and occupational therapy, may constitute a minimum of specialties involved in the care of a patient with cerebral palsy.
- Bracing to support the lower limbs and the use of canes, crutches, walkers, or wheelchairs help to increase function.
- Surgery may be needed for orthopedic deformities or for correcting eye or ear difficulties.

- Patients may use tranquilizers to reduce tension or aid in limiting problems associated with nerve damage. Other medication may include drugs for seizure control. Cerebral palsy has no cure.

IV. ORAL CHARACTERISTICS

A. Disturbances of Musculature

Facial grimacing, abnormal muscle function, facial asymmetry, and problems of mastication and swallowing are common. Opening of the mouth may present problems during dental and dental hygiene therapy, as well as during biofilm control at home.

B. Malocclusion

The incidence of malocclusion is high. Oral habits of mouth breathing, tongue thrusting, and faulty swallowing contribute to orthodontic needs.

C. Attrition

Severe, constant, involuntary grinding of teeth wears down tooth structure and restorations. Bruxism is most extensive in the athetoid group.

D. Fractured Teeth

Patients fall frequently; accidents to anterior teeth result.

E. Dental Caries

The rate of dental caries may be slightly higher, but the factors that operate for the patient with cerebral palsy are the same as those for the physically normal population. Difficulties in maintaining biofilm control and problems of mastication, which lead to the use of a soft diet, may predispose to an environment for biofilm formation.

F. Periodontal Infections

Periodontal or gingival infections are found in a high percentage of patients with cerebral palsy.
- *Phenytoin-Induced Gingival Overgrowth.* When phenytoin is used for the prevention of seizures, the patient is susceptible to gingival enlargement. The condition and its prevention are described on page 973.
- *Predisposing Factors to Periodontal Involvement.* Mechanical difficulties related to biofilm control, mouth breathing, and increased food retention because of ineffective self-cleansing all lead to increased periodontal involvement and biofilm collection. Many patients with cerebral palsy have heavy calculus deposits.

V. DENTAL HYGIENE CARE

- Procedures described in Chapter 53 apply in the management of the patient with cerebral palsy. Many special adaptations are needed, and experience contributes to developing the necessary patience and confidence.
- Dental hygiene care is complicated by the difficulties the patient has in cooperating and by the oral manifestations previously listed. Understanding the physical characteristics is particularly necessary to the success of the appointments. Athetoid movements should not be interpreted as lack of cooperation, and a patient's inability to communicate does not mean lack of comprehension. Address patient directly, not only through caregiver.
- Dentists occasionally must use general anesthesia in a hospital situation for the patient who is unmanageable.
- Dangers for both the patient and dental personnel may result from the uncontrolled movement of the patient, eg, the sudden forceful closure of the mouth on the finger of the clinician or on a mouth mirror. Consider use of a mouth prop (page 908) during dental appointments and for caregiver in home setting.
- Assistance throughout appointments is important. Suggestions for management should be solicited from family or caregivers. Sedation through premedication may be possible, and various stabilizing procedures may be used (page 894).
- Selected patients with cerebral palsy may use a mouth-held instrument, as described on page 926. Oral care and preventive measures are vital to this group of patients.

▪ BELL'S PALSY

Bell's palsy is paralysis of the facial muscles innervated by the facial or seventh cranial nerve. Although the cause is not known, various possible agents have been implicated, including bacterial and viral infections, particularly herpes simplex, trauma from tooth removal, or surgery of the parotid gland area, such as the removal of a tumor.

I. OCCURRENCE

- Although relatively rare, the incidence increases with each decade of life.
- Women are more frequently affected than men in younger age groups, but after age 50, the disorder is more common in men.

II. CHARACTERISTICS[20]

A. Signs and Symptoms

Abrupt weakness or paralysis of facial muscles, usually without preceding pain, occurs on one side of the face.
- *Mouth*. The corner of the mouth droops, and salivation with drooling is uncontrollable.
- *Eye*. Eyelids cannot be closed. Watering and drooping of the lower lid invite infection.

B. Functional Problems

Speech and mastication are difficult.

C. Prognosis

A majority of patients experience a return to normal within a month; many have a spontaneous recovery. Others may have lasting residual effects or permanent paralysis.

III. MEDICAL TREATMENT

Without knowledge of the specific cause, treatment has not been definitive. Temporary palliative measures, such as protecting the eye during sleep and massaging the involved muscles, provide some relief.

A. Drugs

Steroids have been used to improve the prognosis.

B. Surgical

The objectives for surgical procedures have been to improve the appearance, provide facial symmetry with voluntary motion, and provide control of the eye and the mouth. Surgery has included repair of the facial nerve, nerve transplantation and grafting, crossover nerve grafts from the uninvolved side of the face, muscle transfers, and free muscle grafts. Prosthetic rehabilitation has been combined with surgical treatment.

IV. DENTAL HYGIENE CARE

- Instruction and frequent appointments to supplement the patient's efforts usually are needed. A removable prosthesis needs daily care because debris and biofilm collect readily. The involved side needs meticulous biofilm removal because self-cleansing ability has been lost.
- When only the seventh nerve is affected, sensory responses are still intact. When anesthesia is used on the opposite side, special precautions should be provided for posttreatment care until the anesthesia has worn off.
- Protective eyewear should be worn by all patients. Care is necessary to ensure that calculus, polishing paste, or other foreign material does not enter the eye because the eyelid lacks its natural ability to close for protection.

■ PARKINSON'S DISEASE

Parkinson's disease is a progressive disorder of the central nervous system characterized by loss of postural stability, slowness of spontaneous movement, resting tremor, and muscular rigidity. It is also known as *paralysis agitans* and *Parkinson's syndrome*.

Although the cause is not known, the basis for the specific group of symptoms is degeneration of certain neurons in the substantia nigra of the basal ganglia, where posture, support, and voluntary motion are controlled. In addition, a severe deficiency of dopamine, one of the substances that participates in nerve transmission, occurs.

I. OCCURRENCE

Parkinson's disease affects middle-aged and older persons primarily, with a higher incidence in men than in women.

II. CHARACTERISTICS

The signs and symptoms center around tremor, rigidity, and loss or impairment of motor function (akinesia). These three factors also occur in other conditions, which must be differentiated by a physician when a diagnosis is made.

A. General Manifestations

- Body posture bent, with bent head and general stiffness.
- Motion and responses slowed; difficulty in keeping balance.
- Gait slow and shuffling.
- Speech monotonous and slow.
- Tremor of one or both hands; the fingers may be involved in a pill-rolling motion in which the thumb and index finger are rubbed together in a circular movement. The tremor can be reduced or stopped when the person engages in purposeful action.
- Intellect is seldom affected except in the advanced stages.
- Eventually, after 10 to 20 years, the person may become incapacitated and may require complete care.

B. Face and Oral Cavity

- Expression is fixed and masklike, with diminished eye blinking.
- Tremor in lips, tongue, and neck, and difficulty in swallowing.
- Excess salivation and drooling.

III. TREATMENT

- Maintenance of good general health, with plenty of rest and nutritious meals, is encouraged. Professional physical therapy and occupational therapy have particular significance for a patient's well-being.
- Although no known cure exists for Parkinson's disease, symptomatic control can be accomplished, at least in part, by replenishing the dopamine shortage with levodopa. Side effects are common, and may indicate an overdose. Orthostatic hypotension and dizziness may be expected and should be considered when adjusting the dental chair.
- Surgical relief for symptoms has been accomplished using pallidotomy. The surgery alters the globus pallidus in the basal ganglia. The location of the basal ganglia in the brain is shown in Figure 55-5.

IV. DENTAL HYGIENE CARE

- Various adaptations of procedures can be anticipated from knowledge of the physical characteristics previously noted. Personal interest, attention, and encouragement contribute to help the patient bear the stresses of the disability.
- General suggestions for the gerodontic patient in Chapter 49 may prove useful, as well as suggestions related to physical disabilities in Chapter 53. Special adaptations for biofilm control may be needed.

▪ ARTHRITIS

Diseases of the joints, including arthritis, are among the most common causes of chronic illness in the United States. In addition to arthritis as a disease entity, arthritic manifestations are produced as part of various other chronic diseases. The disability may be temporary or permanent, partial or complete. A person may suffer from more than one type at a time.

Arthritis means inflammation in a joint. It may occur in an acute or chronic form and may be localized or generalized. When many joints are involved, the term *polyarthritis* may be applied.

Factors that have been implicated in the cause of rheumatic and arthritic diseases include infectious agents, traumatic disorders, endocrine abnormalities, tumors, allergy and drug reactions, and inherited or congenital conditions. When the cause is known, specific medical, physical, and surgical therapies may be available to alleviate pain and disability.

I. RHEUMATOID ARTHRITIS

Rheumatoid arthritis is a chronic, immunologic systemic disease in which inflammation of the joints occurs in exacerbations and remissions. The cause is unknown, and the means by which the inflammation in the joints is initiated remains a question.

A. Occurrence

- The onset usually occurs between ages 20 and 40, although it may occur at any age.
- More women than men are affected.
- It is rare in tropical countries.

B. Signs and Symptoms

- Joint pain and swelling. Rheumatoid arthritis is a polyarthritis with migratory pain, swelling, tenderness, and warmth in symmetrical joints. Fingers, hands, and knees are usually affected first.
- Morning stiffness and stiffness after periods of inactivity.
- Weakness, fatigue, loss of appetite and weight, anemia, low-grade fever.
- Subcutaneous nodules in elbows, wrists, or fingers in approximately 20% of the patients; nodules may appear in other body organs.
- Possible temporomandibular joint involvement. There may be pain with jaw movements and difficulty in chewing. Ankylosis may develop but is not a common finding.
- Progressive deformity, with limited motion in the more severely involved joints and muscle atrophy adjacent to the joints.

C. Medical Treatment

- Without a specifically known cause, therapy is limited to an individualized program involving pain relief, physical and occupational therapy, and overall health maintenance with adequate nutrition.
- Drugs used in treatment include nonsteroidal anti-inflammatory drugs (NSAIDs), and drugs to aid in controlling the disease including methotrexate, gold compounds, azathioprine, and cyclosporin.[21]

- Selected patients have been treated by joint replacement surgery.

D. Relationship to Periodontal Disease[22]

Rheumatoid arthritis and periodontitis are both chronic inflammatory diseases. The pathogenesis of both is very similar, although etiology differs.
- Indications are that the extent and severity of periodontal disease and rheumatoid arthritis are related.
- Medications used to manage one of these conditions may have implications for treatment of both.

II. JUVENILE RHEUMATOID ARTHRITIS

- Rheumatoid arthritis occurring in children under 16 years of age differs from the disease in adults. The onset is usually more acute, with prolonged fever and enlargement of the spleen and lymph nodes.
- The inflammation of many joints, particularly knees, wrists, and spine, may appear after a few weeks. Figure 55-6 shows the shape of affected fingers. The temporomandibular joint may be involved, with pain and limited oral opening.
- Many patients have complete remissions, some have increasing disability, and others may have mild arthritic symptoms that continue for years. Children are encouraged to lead as normal a life as possible.
- The long-term treatment program includes activity to maintain function and drugs to relieve pain.

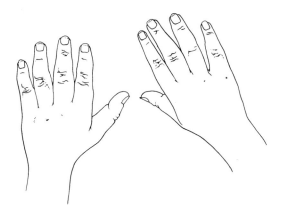

■ **FIGURE 55-6 Child With Rheumatoid Arthritis.** The fingers are tapered from fat central areas. The joint nearest the tip of the finger is the least involved. (From Bleck, E.E. and Nagel, D.A.: *Physically Handicapped Children: A Medical Atlas for Teachers.* New York, Grune & Stratton, 1975.)

III. DEGENERATIVE JOINT DISEASE[23]

- Degenerative joint disease (DJD), or osteoarthritis as it is frequently called, affects the weight-bearing joints particularly. Because inflammation is not the basic joint problem, degenerative joint disease is a more accurate term.
- No specific cause is known, but predisposing factors may include repeated trauma, obesity, age-related changes in the joint tissues, mechanical stresses to the weight-bearing joints, and genetic predisposition.

A. Occurrence

The onset occurs between 50 and 70 years of age, with the average onset 20 years later than that of rheumatoid arthritis. As many as 85% of people over age 70 have evidence of degenerative joint disease.

B. Symptoms

At first insidious, with slight stiffness of a single joint, the eventual condition leads to much pain, deformity, and limitation of movement.
- Hips, knees, fingers, and vertebrae affected most frequently.
- Swelling rare; ankylosis does not occur.
- Stiffness in the morning on rising and after periods of inactivity; diminishes with exercise.
- Pain aggravated by temperature changes and bearing body weight.
- Temporomandibular joint usually without pain or other clinical symptoms, although crepitation, clicking, or snapping may occur when the joints are exercised.

C. Medical Treatment

- Moderate exercise, pain-relieving drug therapy, weight reduction for obese patients, physical therapy, and selected orthopedic surgical procedures comprise the general treatments available.
- Total hip or knee joint replacement has proved satisfactory for many patients and has been used more widely for DJD than for rheumatoid arthritis.

IV. PERSONAL FACTORS

With long-term illnesses, patients are frequently discouraged or apprehensive. Certain patients may be worried, pessimistic, or resigned. Some may be impatient and tend to harm themselves by overexercise. A few are irritable, a characteristic related to the pain that has been suffered.

V. DENTAL HYGIENE CARE

A high standard of general health contributes to the well-being of the patient with arthritis. Maintenance of oral health contributes to general health.

Adjustments for physical disabilities of the patient with arthritis are given in Chapter 53. Assistance with ambulation, chair positioning, and other special adaptations are needed.

A. Patient History

*   Questions to determine whether the patient has a joint prosthesis should be included in the patient history. Because of the susceptibility to infection at the interface of the bone and the prosthesis, prophylactic antibiotic premedication to prevent bacteremia is recommended for certain patients and procedures, as described on pages 122 to 125.[24]
*   A patient who is anticipating surgery for a joint replacement should be counseled to complete all needed periodontal and restorative therapy before the surgery to prevent the need for repeated antibiotic premedication.

B. Instrumentation

*   For the patient with arthritis of the temporomandibular joint, instrumentation may need adaptations to accommodate a minimal opening of the mouth. Fatigue in the joint may be reduced by rest periods, by minimizing the pressure on the mandible, and by overall efficiency to shorten the necessary appointment time.
*   More frequent appointments can contribute to keeping the oral health at a maximum and thus preventing long, difficult scaling sessions.

C. Dental Biofilm Control

*   Because of hand and arm involvement, a patient may have difficulty grasping a toothbrush or lifting the arm for sufficient periods to clean the mouth completely.
*   Adapted brushing procedures may be applied (page 898).

D. Diet and Nutrition

*   No special nutritional factors are known to be associated with the course or treatment of arthritis.
*   Physicians generally recommend a normal, well-balanced diet with a controlled caloric intake for weight control.

*   Encouragement of restriction of sweets and selection of noncariogenic between-meal snacks can help improve oral health.
*   Obtaining a food diary for several days to a week can be important for dietary analysis and counseling, especially for the gerodontic arthritic patient.

■ SCLERODERMA (PROGRESSIVE SYSTEMIC SCLEROSIS)

Scleroderma is an autoimmune disease of connective tissue characterized by an overproduction of collagen. The most striking physical symptom is the immobility and rigidity of the skin, but inflammation and sclerosis occur throughout the body. Thus, the disease has the full title of *progressive systemic sclerosis*.

The cause is not known, but collagen synthesis irregularities, associated immunologic disorders, and microvascular abnormalities have been implicated. Hereditary factors are not involved.

I. OCCURRENCE

*   Scleroderma usually has its onset between ages 30 and 50, but it may affect persons of any age, even infants.
*   It may develop over months or years and is 2 to 5 times more common in females.

II. CHARACTERISTICS

Scleroderma may be localized and involve only the skin, or it may be generalized and involve all body organs. The most notable changes are in the skin, gastrointestinal tract, kidneys, heart, muscles, and lungs. Eventual death results from renal failure, cardiac failure, pulmonary insufficiency, or intestinal malabsorption. Symptoms vary, and all individuals do not have all the symptoms and signs that follow.

A. General Manifestations

*   *Joints*. Pain, swelling, and stiffness of the fingers and knee joints.
*   *Polyarthritis*. Symmetrical polyarthritis, similar to rheumatoid arthritis.
*   *Skin*. Hard and fixed; ivory-white, yellow, or gray, sometimes with brown pigmentation in the late stages.
*   *Face*. When affected, the face becomes mask-like and expressionless.

B. Oral Characteristics

- *Lips*. Thin, rigid, with oral stricture and difficulty in opening and closing.
- *Mucosa*. Thin, pale, tender, rigid, with poor healing capacity.
- *Gingiva*. Pale and unusually firm.
- *Teeth*. Mobility is common.
- *Radiographic Findings*. Marked widening of the periodontal ligament spaces. This finding is sometimes considered pathognomonic for scleroderma.
- *Mastication*. Difficult; temporomandibular joint movement is limited.
- *Tongue*. May be immobile; speech difficult.

III. MEDICAL TREATMENT

Specific therapy is not known. Medications that retard collagen deposition have not yet been effective for scleroderma. Treatment, therefore, has been directed at specific system complications, physical therapy, and attempts to maintain normal activities.

IV. DENTAL HYGIENE CARE

- The tightening of the skin and lips limits opening of the mouth and complicates all dental and dental hygiene procedures, as well as daily self-care by the patient.
- Every effort for preservation of the teeth and gingiva in health should be made to prevent the need for extensive treatment.
- With oral stricture, the preparation and wearing of dentures are difficult or impossible as the disease becomes more severe.
- Patients with scleroderma are sensitive to cold and dampness, stress, undue emotional tension, and fatigue. All these factors can be considered for the dental hygiene appointment.

■ KIDNEY DISEASE[25]

- Kidney disease is a major health care problem. Impaired renal function may be congenital or caused by disease or injury.
- Dental and dental hygiene care is affected for those with impaired renal function, undergoing dialysis, or have renal transplantation.
- Antibiotic premedication may be required; medication choices may be limited.
- No oral treatment should occur until kidney function is evaluated.
- A healthy individual may have a kidney removed for donation to another.

I. KIDNEY FUNCTIONS

- Composed of nephrons, each kidney filters fluids, excretes waste, and produces urine.
- Controls electrolyte balance in the body, including sodium, bicarbonate, potassium, and calcium.
- Produces erythropoietin, which stimulates the bone marrow to produce red blood cells.
- Regulates serum pH.

II. IMPAIRED KIDNEY FUNCTION

Effects of decreased kidney function include:
- Anemia, lowered hematocrit.
- Hypertension.
- Bone changes.
- Increased bleeding, bruising, petechiae.
- Vascular disease.
- Peripheral edema, inflammation.
- Hyperpigmentation.

III. LABORATORY TESTS

- *Urinalysis:* Presence of protein and abnormal specific gravity reveal kidney disease when urine is tested.
- *Blood Tests:* Elevated creatinine and blood urea nitrogen (BUN) levels indicate renal dysfunction.

IV. TREATMENT OF END-STAGE RENAL DISEASE

When kidney function is reduced to a very low level, a patient requires an alternative method to perform functions of the kidney. Patients may need antibiotic premedication prior to dental procedures.

A. Peritoneal Dialysis

- A plastic catheter tube is placed into abdomen (peritoneum).
- The catheter is filled with a dialysate, and fluids and waste are drawn out of blood.
- Performed daily at home, work, or other setting several times throughout the day or overnight.

B. Hemodialysis

An artificial kidney (hemodialyzer) removes waste and other materials from the blood.
1. Procedure
   - Blood is transported out of the body via an arteriovenous shunt, located in the arm or leg, to the hemodialyzer.
   - Usually performed 3 times per week at a health care facility.

Everyday Ethics

? John had an accident when diving into surf at the beach 2 years ago at age 18. He is now quadriplegic. At his biannual dental maintenance visit, Amy, the dental hygienist, was assisting in the wheelchair transfer into the dental chair. During the transfer, John's t-shirt was inadvertently lifted slightly, and Amy noticed obvious decubitus ulcers. Amy continues to safely transfer him into the dental chair and then stops to quickly consider what to do next. Dramatic images from a lecture in dental hygiene school flash through her mind. She will never forget those photographs of patients suffering from neglect.

Questions for Consideration

1 If John is unaware of the sores, and they are not being treated, what actions should Amy take and what issues need to be addressed before the appointment can occur? Serious infections need to be resolved prior to elective treatment.

2. John came to the appointment with his mother, who is his primary caregiver. What options should Amy consider if the mother denies the existence of the problem?

3. Is the possibility that John is a victim of neglect an ethical issue or ethical dilemma? What responsibility does Amy have to inform the patient or others?

---

2. Relation to dental and dental hygiene appointments
   * Heparin usually is used to prevent coagulation of blood during the hemodialysis treatment, therefore, dental or dental hygiene procedures that cause bleeding should not be performed on the day of dialysis.

✓ Factors To Teach The Patient

* The need to communicate is key to successful dental treatment and oral health and is achieved by speaking openly about medical history and limitations.

* Daily, thorough biofilm removal is particularly necessary to reduce the occurrence of oral disease.

* Regular maintenance appointments are important to promote oral health.

* Why maintaining periodontal health has added value for teeth used as abutments for a mouth-held implement.

* How to clean and maintain the mouth-held implement.

* The need to maintain teeth in order to tolerate a mouth-held aid.

* Because of the risks associated with the shunt, antibiotic premedication is recommended for invasive dental treatment.[26]

C. Kidney Transplant

* Kidney transplantation can be a successful treatment for end-stage renal disease.
* Patients are treated with immunosuppressive therapy after transplantation.
* Cyclosporin may be used; side effects include gingival enlargement.

V. ORAL FINDINGS

Impaired renal function may produce the following oral changes:
* Petechiae.
* Ammonia in saliva with urine-like smell and taste changes.
* Stomatitis, erythema, edema, candidiasis.
* Dimineralization of bone in radiograph.

VI. MEDICATIONS

Medications or their metabolites are cleared in urine through the kidneys. If kidney function is decreased, toxic levels may accumulate. Some common drugs that use the kidney as a major pathway of elimination are contraindicated or should be used with caution. Included are:
* Lidocaine/Xylocaine local anesthetic.
* Aspirin and nonsteroidal anti-inflammatory drugs (NSAIDs).
* Acetaminophen.

- Penicillin.
- Clarithromycin.

VII. DENTAL HYGIENE CARE

- Primary objective: to obtain and maintain the highest level of oral health to eliminate possible sources of infection.
- Complete medical history must be taken to establish extent of kidney function; may require consultation with physician.
- Screen patient for bleeding or other hematologic disorder. Obtain bleeding time, prothrombin time (PT), international normalized ratio (INR), partial thromboplastin time (PTT), hematocrit, hemoglobin, complete blood cell count (CBC).
- Take blood pressure of all patients; follow recommendations for referral to physician as described on page 1043.
- Patient needs antibiotic premedication prior to dental and dental hygiene treatment if hemodialysis shunt is present, if recommended by consultation with physician, or if patient has a history of another condition that necessitates coverage.
- Consider schedule of dialysis, appoint patient on day other than that of hemodialysis.
- Systemic medications prescribed may be cleared with dialysis.
- Perform thorough diet evaluation; patient may be on a special diet that may impact oral health.

REFERENCES

1. **Smeltzer**, S.C. and Bare, B.G.: *Brunner and Suddarth's Textbook of Medical-Surgical Nursing*, 7th ed. Philadelphia, J.B. Lippincott Co., 1992, pp. 1737–1744.
2. **Chiles**, B.W. and Cooper, P.R.: Acute Spinal Injury, *N. Engl. J. Med., 334,* 514, February 22, 1996.
3. **Schubert**, M.M., Snow, M., and Stiefel, D.J.: *Dental Treatment of the Spinal Cord Injured Patient*. Disability Dental Instruction, 4919 NE 86th Street, Seattle, WA 98115, 34 pp.
4. **Thornton**, J.B., Sneed, R.C., Tomaselli, C.E., and Boraz, R.A.: Dental Management of Patients With Spinal Cord Injury, *Compend. Cont. Educ. Dent., 13,* 122, February, 1992.
5. **Ruff**, J.C.: Selection Criteria for Static and Dynamic Mouthsticks, *Gen. Dent., 38,* 414, November–December, 1990.
6. **Akar**, Z.: Myelomeningocele, *Surg. Neurol., 43,* 113, February, 1995.
7. **Green**, N.S.: Folic Acid Supplementation and Prevention of Birth Defects, *J. Nutr., 132,* 2356S, Supplement 8, 2002.
8. **Little**, J.W., Falace, D.A., Miller, C.S., and Rhodus, N.L.: *Dental Management of the Medically Compromised Patient*, 6th ed. St. Louis, Mosby, 2002, pp. DM55, 435.
9. **Engibous**, P.J., Kittle, P.E., Jones, H.L., and Vance, B.J.: Latex Allergy in Patients With Spina Bifida, *Pediatr. Dent., 15,* 364, September/October, 1993.
10. **Nelson**, L.P., Soporowski, N.J., and Shusterman, S.: Latex Allergies in Children With Spina Bifida: Relevance for the Pediatric Dentist, *Pediatr. Dent., 16,* 18, January/February, 1994.
11. **Malamed**, S.F.: *Medical Emergencies in the Dental Office,* 5th ed. St. Louis, Mosby, 2000, pp. 287–301.
12. **Friedlander**, A.H. and Freymiller, E.G.: Detection of Radiation-Accelerated Atherosclerosis of the Carotid Artery by Panoramic Radiography: A New Opportunity for Dentists, *J. Am. Dent. Assoc., 134,* 1361, October, 2003.
13. **Bennett**, J.C. and Plum, F., eds.: *Cecil Textbook of Medicine,* 20th ed. Philadelphia, W.B. Saunders Co., 1996, p. 2161.
14. **Drachman**, D.B.: Myasthenia Gravis, *N. Engl. J. Med., 330,* 1797, June 23, 1994.
15. **Appel**, S.H.: Myasthenia Gravis, in Rakel, R.E., ed.: *Conn's Current Therapy, 1998.* Philadelphia, W.B. Saunders Co., 1998, p. 929.
16. **Silberberg**, D.H.: Multiple Sclerosis, in Rakel, R.E., ed.: *Conn's Current Therapy, 1998.* Philadelphia, W.B. Saunders Co., 1998, p. 922.
17. **Rudick**, R.A., Cohen, J.A., Weinstock-Guttman, B., Kinkel, R.P., and Ransohoff, R.M.: Management of Multiple Sclerosis, *N. Engl. J. Med., 337,* 1604, November 27, 1997.
18. **Sorenson**, H.W.: Physically Handicapped, in Nowak, A.J.: *Dentistry for the Handicapped Patient.* St. Louis, Mosby, 1976, pp. 23–38.
19. **Danforth**, H.A., Snow, M., and Stiefel, D.J.: *Dental Management of the Cerebral Palsied Patient.* Disability Dental Instruction, 4919 NE 86th Street, Seattle, WA 98115, 30 pp.
20. **Dawidjan**, B.: Idiopathic Facial Paralysis: A Review and Case Study, *J. Dent. Hyg., 75,* 316, Fall, 2001.
21. **Cash**, J.M. and Klippel, J.H.: Second-Line Drug Therapy for Rheumatoid Arthritis, *N. Engl. J. Med., 330,* 1368, May 12, 1994.
22. **Mercado**, F.B., Marshall, R.I., and Bartold, P.M.: Inter-Relationship Between Rheumatoid Arthritis and Periodontal Disease, *J. Clin. Periodontol., 30,* 761, September, 2003.
23. **Neustadt**, D.H.: Osteoarthritis, in Rakel, R.E., ed.: *Conn's Current Therapy, 1998.* Philadelphia, W.B. Saunders Co., 1998, p. 995.
24. **American Dental Association; American Academy of Orthopaedic Surgeons:** Antibiotic Prophylaxis for Dental Patients With Total Joint Replacements, *J. Am. Dent. Assoc., 134,* 895, July, 2003.
25. **Little**, Falace, Miller, Rhodus: Op. Cit., pp. 147–159.
26. **Werner**, C.W. and Saad, T.F: Prophylactic Antibiotic Therapy Prior to Dental Treatment for Patients With End-Stage Renal Disease, *Spec. Care. Dentist., 19,* 106, May/June, 1999.

SUGGESTED READINGS

Anderson, R.A. and Ewell-Jackson, T.: Scleroderma in Pediatric Patients, *ASDC J. Dent. Child., 57,* 462, November–December, 1990.
Frey, L. and Hauser, W.A.: Epidemiology of Neural Tube Defects, *Epilepsia, 44,* 4, Supplement 3, 2003.
Hughes, G.B.: Acute Peripheral Facial Paralysis (Bell's Palsy), in Rakel, R.E., ed.: *Conn's Current Therapy, 1998.* Philadelphia, W.B. Saunders Co., 1998, p. 943.
Kellman, R.: The Cervical Spine in Maxillofacial Trauma: Assessment and Airway Management, *Otolaryngol. Clin. North Am., 24,* 1, February, 1991.
Rosenberg, D. and Fetter, C.: Product Guide, *Spec. Care Dentist., 21,* 232, November/December, 2001.
Sonies, B.C. and Dalakas, M.C.: Dysphagia in Patients With Post-polio Syndrome, *N. Engl. J. Med., 324,* 1162, April 25, 1991.
Spackman, G.K.: Scleroderma: What the General Dentist Should Know, *Gen. Dent., 47,* 576, November-December, 1999.
Waldman, H.B., Perlman, S.P., and Swerdloff, M.: Periodontics and Patients With Special Needs, *J. Periodontol., 71,* 330, February, 2000.
Zuckerman, J.D.: Hip Fracture, *N. Engl. J. Med., 334,* 1519, June 6, 1996.

Arthritis

Akerman, S., Jonsson, K., Kopp, S., Petersson, A., and Rohlin, M.: Radiologic Changes in Temporomandibular, Hand, and Foot Joints of Patients With Rheumatoid Arthritis, *Oral Surg. Oral Med. Oral Pathol., 72,* 245, August, 1991.

Carpenter, E.H., Plant, M.J., Hassell, A.B., Shadforth, M.F., Fisher, J., Clarke, S., Hothersall, T.E., and Dawes, P.T.: Management of Oral Complications of Disease-Modifying Drugs in Rheumatoid Arthritis, *Br. J. Rheumatol., 36,* 473, April, 1997.

Gynther, G.W., Holmlund, A.B., Reinholt, F.P., and Lindblad, S.: Temporomandibular Joint Involvement in Generalized Osteoarthritis and Rheumatoid Arthritis: A Clinical Arthroscopic, Histologic, and Immunohistochemical Study, *Int. J. Oral Maxillofac. Surg., 26,* 10, February, 1997.

Harris, E.D: Rheumatoid Arthritis: Pathophysiology and Implications for Treatment, *N. Engl. J. Med., 322,* 1277, May 3, 1990.

Haas, S.E.: Implant-Supported, Long-Span Fixed Partial Denture for a Scleroderma Patient: A Clinical Report, *J. Prosthet. Dent., 87,* 136, February, 2002.

Liang, M.H. and Fortin, P.: Management of Osteoarthritis of the Hip and Knee, *N. Engl. J. Med., 325,* 125, July 11, 1991.

Risheim, H., Kjaerheim, V., and Arneberg, P.: Improvement of Oral Hygiene in Patients With Rheumatoid Arthritis, *Scand. J. Dent. Res., 100,* 172, June, 1992.

Russell, S.L. and Reisine, S.: Investigation of Xerostomia in Patients With Rheumatoid Arthritis, *J. Am. Dent. Assoc., 129,* 733, June, 1998.

Tanchyk, A.P.: Dental Considerations for the Patient With Juvenile Rheumatoid Arthritis, *Gent. Dent., 39,* 330, September–October, 1991.

Wright, E.F., DesRosier, K.F., Clark, M.K., and Bifano, S.L.: Identifying Undiagnosed Rheumatic Disorders Among Patients With TMD, *J. Am. Dent. Assoc., 128,* 738, June, 1997.

Zifer, S.A., Sams, D.R., Potter, B.J., and Jerath, R.: Clinical and Radiographic Evaluation of Juvenile Rheumatoid Arthritis: Report of a Case, *Spec. Care Dentist., 14,* 208, September/October, 1994.

Spinal Cord Injury

Ditunno, J.F. and Formal, C.S.: Chronic Spinal Cord Injury, *N. Engl. J. Med., 330,* 550, February 24, 1994.

Lancashire, P., Janzen, J., Zach, G.A., and Addy, M.: The Oral Hygiene and Gingival Health of Paraplegic Inpatients—A Cross-sectional Survey, *J. Clin. Periodontol., 24,* 198, March, 1997.

Shute, N.: A Super Feeling: Are There Signs of Hope in Christopher Reeve's Modest Recovery?, *US News World Rep., 133,* 58, September 23, 2002.

Stiefel, D.J., Truelove, E.L., Persson, R.S., Chin, M.M., and Mandel, L.S.: A Comparison of Oral Health in Spinal Cord Injury and Other Disability Groups, *Spec. Care Dentist., 13,* 229, November/December, 1993.

Taniguchi, M.H. and Schlosser, G.A.: Adolescent Spinal Cord Injury: Considerations for Post-acute Management, *Adolesc. Med., 5,* 327, June, 1994.

Mouth-Held Orthosis

Blaine, H.H. and Nelson, E.P.: A Mouthstick for Quadriplegic Patients, *J. Prosthet. Dent., 29,* 317, March, 1973.

Budning, B.C. and Hall, M.: A Practical Mouthstick for Early Intervention With Quadriparetic Patients, *J. Can. Dent. Assoc., 56,* 243, March, 1990.

DiPietro, G.J., Warfield, D.K., and Bradshaw, A.J.: A Jaw-Operated Proximity Switch for a Paraplegic Patient, *J. Prosthet. Dent., 56,* 711, December, 1986.

Drago, C.J.: Design Considerations for Construction of a Mouthstick Prosthesis, *Quintessence Dent. Technol., 10,* 451, July–August, 1986.

Hock, D.A.: The Use of the Maxillary Interocclusal Splint as a Mouthpiece for the Mouthstick Prosthesis, *J. Prosthet. Dent., 62,* 56, July, 1989.

Nunn, J.H. and Wood, I.: The Use of a Vacuum-Molded Polyvinyl Acetate-Polyethylene Copolymer (PVAC.PE) for a Handicapped Patient, *Spec. Care Dentist., 12,* 122, May/June, 1992.

Rodeghero, P., Claman, L., Cellier, S., and Lotz, J.W.: The Long-term Effect of Mouthsticks on Periodontal Support, *Spec. Care Dentist., 5,* 251, November/December, 1985.

Stroke

Bronner, L.L., Kanter, D.S., and Manson, J.E.: Primary Prevention of Stroke, *N. Engl. J. Med., 333,* 1392, November 23, 1995.

Carter, L.C., Haller, A.D., Nadarajah, V., Calamel, A.D., and Aguirre, A.: Use of Panoramic Radiography Among an Ambulatory Dental Population to Detect Patients at Risk of Stroke, *J. Am. Dent. Assoc., 128,* 977, July, 1997.

Ostuni, E.: Stroke and the Dental Patient, *J. Am. Dent. Assoc., 125,* 721, June, 1994.

Reddy, M.P. and Reddy, V.: After a Stroke: Strategies to Restore Function and Prevent Complications, *Geriatrics, 52,* 59, September, 1997.

Roth, E.J.: Rehabilitation of the Stroke Patient, in Rakel, R.E., ed.: *Conn's Current Therapy, 1998.* Philadelphia, W.B. Saunders, 1998, p. 868.

Wright, S.M.: Denture Treatment for the Stroke Patient, *Br. Dent. J., 183,* 179, September 13, 1997.

Muscular Dystrophy

Darras, B.T., Harper, J.F., and Francke, U.: Prenatal Diagnosis and Detection of Carriers With DNA Probes in Duchenne's Muscular Dystrophy, *N. Engl. J. Med., 316,* 985, April 16, 1987.

Eckhardt, L. and Harzer, W.: Facial Structure and Functional Findings in Patients With Progressive Muscular Dystrophy, *Am. J. Orthod. Dentofacial Orthop., 110,* 185, August, 1996.

Myasthenia Gravis

Nicolle, M.W.: Myasthenia Gravis, *Neurolog., 8,* 2, January, 2002.

Patton, L.L. and Howard, J.F.: Myasthenia Gravis: Dental Treatment Considerations, *Spec. Care. Dentist., 17,* 25, January/February, 1997.

Weijnen, F.G., van der Bilt, A., Kuks, J.B., van der Glas, H.W., Oudenaarde, I., and Bosman, F.: Masticatory Performance in Patients With Myasthenia Gravis, *Arch. Oral Biol., 47,* 393, May, 2002.

Multiple Sclerosis

Dyment, D.A. and Ebers, G.C.: An Array of Sunshine in Multiple Sclerosis, *N. Engl. J. Med., 347,* 1445, October 31, 2002.

Fiske, J., Griffiths, J., and Thompson, S.: Multiple Sclerosis and Oral Care, *Dent. Update, 29,* 273, July–August, 2002.

Robinson-Akande, D.A.: Trigeminal Neuralgia as a Complication of Multiple Sclerosis, *Gen. Dent., 43,* 436, September–October, 1995.

Symons, A.L., Bortolanza, M., Godden, S., and Seymour, G.: A Preliminary Study Into the Dental Health Status of Multiple Sclerosis Patients, *Spec. Care Dentist., 13,* 96, May/June, 1993.

Trapp, B.D., Peterson, J., Ransohoff, R.M., Rudick, R., Mörk, S., and Bö, L.: Axonal Transection in the Lesions of Multiple Sclerosis, *N. Engl. J. Med., 338,* 278, January 29, 1998.

Cerebral Palsy

Bhat, M., Nelson, K.B., Cummins, S.K., and Grether, J.K.: Prevalence of Developmental Enamel Defects in Children With Cerebral Palsy, *J. Oral Pathol. Med., 21,* 241, July, 1992.

Croft, R.D.: What Consistency of Food Is Best for Children With Cerebral Palsy Who Cannot Chew? *Arch. Dis. Child., 67,* 269, March, 1992.

Hallet, K.B., Lucas, J.O., Johnston, T., Reddihough, D.S., and Hall, R.K.: Dental Health of Children With Cerebral Palsy Following Sialodochoplasty, *Spec. Care Dentist., 15,* 234, November/December, 1995.

Kaufman, E., Meyer, S., Wolnerman, J.S., and Gilai, A.N.: Transient Suppression of Involuntary Movements in Cerebral Palsy Patients During Dental Treatment, *Anesth. Prog., 38,* 200, November–December, 1991.

Kuban, K.C.K. and Leviton, A.: Cerebral Palsy, *N. Engl. J. Med., 330,* 188, January 20, 1994.

Loiacono, C.: Dental Hygiene Care for the Patient With Cerebral Palsy, *Access, 10,* 34, July, 1995.

MacDonald, D.: Cerebral Palsy and Intrapartum Fetal Monitoring (Editorial), *N. Engl. J. Med., 334,* 659, March 7, 1996.

Nelson, K.B., Dambrosia, J.M., Ting, T.Y., and Grether, J.K.: Uncertain Value of Electronic Fetal Monitoring in Predicting Cerebral Palsy, *N. Engl. J. Med., 334,* 613, March 7, 1996.

Nielsen, L.A.: Caries Among Children With Cerebral Palsy: Relation to CP-Diagnosis, Mental and Motor Handicap, *ASDC J. Dent. Child., 57,* 267, July–August, 1990.

Parkinson's Disease

Agid, Y.: Parkinson's Disease: Pathophysiology, *Lancet, 337,* 1321, June, 1, 1991.

Clough, C.G.: Parkinson's Disease: Management, *Lancet, 337,* 1324, June 1, 1991.

Grandinetti, A., Morens, D.M., Reed, D., and MacEachern, D.: Prospective Study of Cigarette Smoking and the Risk of Developing Idiopathic Parkinson's Disease, *Am. J. Epidemiol., 139,* 1129, June 15, 1994.

Kennedy, M.A., Rosen, S., Paulson, G.W., Jolly, D.E., and Beck, F.M.: Relationship of Oral Microflora With Oral Health Status in Parkinson's Disease, *Spec. Care Dentist., 14,* 164, July/August, 1994.

Persson, M., Osterberg, T., Granérus, A.-K., and Karlsson, S.: Influence of Parkinson's Disease on Oral Health, *Acta Odontol. Scand., 50,* 37, February, 1992.

Salzman, E.W.: Living With Parkinson's Disease (Editorial), *N. Engl. J. Med., 334,* 114, January 11, 1996.

The Patient With a Sensory Disability

Successful management and treatment of any patient depend to a large extent on the interpersonal communication between the patient and the clinician. When a patient has a vision or hearing impairment, communication assumes a different dimension. Suggestions for adaptations for patients with hearing or visual problems are described in this chapter. Box 56-1 contains key words and definitions pertaining to sensory impairments.

The Americans With Disabilities Act defines an individual with a disability as a person who has a physical or mental impairment that substantially limits a major life activity. The examples of physical and mental impairments provided with the Act include visual and hearing impairments. For the visually impaired, certain qualifications related to physical facilities are specified, such as the removal of physical barriers and the use of braille markers for elevators.

In the section on communications, the Act specifies that communications with individuals with hearing and vision impairments must be as effective as communications with nondisabled people, and appropriate auxiliary aids must be provided. Examples of auxiliary aids are such services and devices as qualified interpreters, assistive listening headsets, text telephone devices for deaf persons (TTYs), readers, taped texts, brailled materials, and large-print materials.

Special skills used to counsel, motivate, and educate a patient with a sensory disability must be developed and

practiced. Although visual channels provide a primary method of communication with the deaf person, audible and "touch" channels are essential for the person with visual disability.

■ VISUAL IMPAIRMENT

Limitations of sight cover a broad spectrum from the slightly affected to the completely blind with no perception of light. Loss of sight is a major physical deprivation. In many persons, blindness is secondary to a primary condition that may have been the cause of the blindness and in itself may be disabling.

In the United States, "legal blindness" is defined as follows: having central vision (or acuity) of not more than 20/200 in the better eye with correction (glasses), or having peripheral fields (side vision) of no more than 20° diameter or 10° radius. Only approximately 3% of legally blind persons are totally blind. The term "legal blindness" is a legal term, not a medical one, but certification of the degree of severity of blindness is obtained from an ophthalmologist.

I. CAUSES OF BLINDNESS

The leading causes of blindness are diabetic retinopathy, age-related macular degeneration, senile cataracts, glaucoma, vascular disease, trauma, and infections. At least

BOX 56-1 KEY WORDS AND ABBREVIATIONS: Sensory Disabilities

VISION

Astigmatism: impaired vision caused by irregularities in the curvature of the cornea or lens.

Blind spot: the area on the retina that marks the site of entrance of the optic nerve.

Blindness: no perception of visual stimuli; lack or loss of ability to see.

Legal blindness: less than 20/200 vision with corrective eyeglasses (see text).

Braille: a system of writing and printing by means of raised points representing letters; enables people with a visual disability to read by touch.

Cataract: clouding or opacity of the lens of an eye.

Color blindness: inability to distinguish between certain colors; most common is red/green confusion; color vision is a function of the cones of the retina.

Diplopia: double vision; perception of two images of a single object.

Glaucoma: group of diseases of the eye characterized by intraocular pressure from pathologic changes in the optic disc; person has visual-field defects.

Hyperopia: farsightedness; eyeball is shorter behind the retina; vision is better for distant objects than for near objects.

Myopia: nearsightedness; longer eyeball from front to back so the image is focused in front of the retina.

Nyctalopia: night blindness; may be hereditary or related to vitamin deficiency.

Ocular: pertaining to the eye.

Ophthalmologist: physician who specializes in diagnosing and prescribing treatment for defects, injuries, and diseases of the eye (obsolete term: oculist).

Ophthalmology: the branch of medicine that deals with the anatomy, diagnosis, pathology, and treatment of the eye.

Optician: technician who prepares and adapts lenses; fills prescriptions from an ophthalmologist.

Optometrist: a specialist in optometry, the measurement of visual acuity and the adaptation of lenses for correction of visual defects.

Retinitis: inflammation of the retina.

Retinopathy: noninflammatory disease of the retina; identified by the chronic disease of which it is a symptom; for example, diabetic retinopathy reflects the retinal manifestations of diabetes mellitus, including microaneurysms.

Retinopathy of prematurity: a condition peculiar to premature infants; characterized by opaque tissue behind the lens resulting from a high concentration of oxygen, which causes spasm of the retinal vessels, leads to retinal detachment, and arrests eye growth and development; prevented by keeping oxygen administration as low as possible and discontinuing the oxygen as soon as possible.

HEARING

Audiogram: graphic record of the findings of an audiometer.

Audiologist: certified allied health worker, often with advanced degrees; trained in the identification, diagnosis, measurement, and rehabilitation of hearing impairment.

Audiometer: instrument used to determine degree and type of hearing ability.

Aural: pertaining to the ear.

Decibel: unit for expressing the relative loudness of a sound; abbreviation, dB.

KEY WORDS AND ABBREVIATIONS: Sensory Disabilities, continued

Hearing: the sense by which sounds are perceived; conversion of sound waves into nerve impulses, which are then interpreted by the brain.

Otitis: inflammation of the ear.

Otitis media: inflammation of the middle ear.

Otologist: physician specialist in otology, the branch of medicine dealing with the anatomy, physiology, pathology, and treatment of the ear.

Speechreading: recognizing spoken words by watching the speaker's lips, face, and gestures.

TDD: Telecommunication Device for the Deaf.

Tinnitus: noise in the ears, as ringing, buzzing, or roaring.

TTY: Text telephone device.

Tuning fork: instrument used to test for hearing loss; vibrations of the fork produce sound waves that can be heard in both ears by a person with normal hearing when the stem is placed on top of the head; sound is heard louder in an ear affected by conductive loss and softer in an ear affected by sensorineural loss.

Tympanic membrane: ear drum; vibrates when sound waves strike; transmits waves to nerve endings by way of ossicles in the middle ear and to cochlea in the inner ear.

Vertigo: sensation of rotation or movement of one's self (subjective vertigo) or of one's surroundings (objective vertigo); a subtype of dizziness, but not a synonym.

one half of the blindness in children is of prenatal origin, particularly resulting from maternal infections (rubella, syphilis, toxoplasmosis). Other causes are injuries, neoplasms, and retinopathy of prematurity (formerly called retrolental fibroplasia). The incidence of retinopathy of prematurity has increased as more premature babies survive.

II. PERSONAL FACTORS

- Consider each patient in relation to individual aptitudes, interests, abilities, and potentialities, with sight as one factor involved.
- No pattern of patient attitudes and personality characteristics can be described.
- The only common characteristic this group of patients has is difficulty in seeing. A few suggestions of factors involved are mentioned here.

A. Patient History

- Assistance in completing the personal questionnaire may be needed.
- Specific details of the patient's limitations must be recorded so that adaptations can be made during the appointment.

B. Child

1. *Learning Ability*
   - Sensory defects often mask a child's intellectual capacity because responses cannot be the same as in other children.
   - Blind children may learn to speak later than sighted children and may start school when they are a year or two older.
   - A blind child takes longer than does the sighted child to cover the same amount of material; therefore, the educational level for the blind child may be different from that for the sighted child of the same chronologic age.
   - Blind children are deprived of the opportunity to learn by imitation.

2. *Personal Factors*
   - Environment influences the child's adjustment, and parental attitude affects the blind child as it does the sighted child.
   - When the parent is overindulgent and protective, the child may be self-centered, dependent, and emotionally less stable.

C. Adult

- The adult who has always been blind or has been so since childhood has made adjustments and may be employed in a limited but useful occupation.

- The greater number of those who become blind after adulthood experience an immediate natural reaction of depression and feeling of helplessness.
- When loss of vision is incipient, the reactions of shock and upheaval usually are less, but dread, worry, and anxiety may be experienced for years in anticipation.
- When the patient begins to accept the disability, efforts for rehabilitation are made easier.
- Independence and self-confidence are needed. The patient must be helped to avoid helplessness.

III. DENTAL HYGIENE CARE: TOTALLY BLIND

A. Factors in Patient Care

1. A blind person can perceive a new experience readily if told about it in detail.
2. Because of the visual disability, the patient must rely more on other senses and cultivate them.
3. A blind person must be neat and orderly. If something is put down, it must be located readily again.
4. A blind person does things deliberately and slowly to gain perception and prevent accidents.
5. A blind person learns to interpret and rely on tone of voice more than do persons with sight who can watch facial expressions.

B. Patient Reception and Seating

1. Lower dental chair prior to receiving patient; move other dental equipment, such as the bracket tray and clinician's stool, from pathway.
2. Guide to dental chair. Patient holds arm and is led without being pushed or pulled (Figure 56-1).
3. Provide forewarnings of potential hazards in the pathway.
4. The patient who has become familiar with office arrangement from previous appointments needs to be informed of changes to prevent embarrassment.
5. Protective eyewear. The patient usually will prefer to wear the personal glasses regularly worn. Many wear dark glasses.
6. When leaving the treatment room during the appointment, explain absence; prevent embarrassment of patient speaking to someone who is not there; speak when re-entering the room.

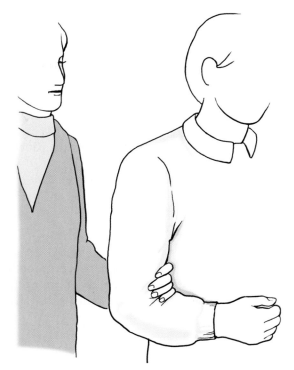

■ **FIGURE 56-1 Escorting a Blind Person.** The blind person holds the arm of the guide just above the elbow and walks beside and slightly behind. The guide verbally gives advance notice of approaching changes. The blind person can sense the body motion of the guide and anticipate changes.

C. The Dog Guide

- Do not distract a dog guide on duty by speaking to or touching it.
- Ask the patient where the best place would be for the dog to stay during the appointment. The dogs are gentle, carefully trained animals, and may lie quietly in a corner of the treatment room as directed by the patient.

D. Introduce Clinical Procedures

1. Describe each step in detail before proceeding. Explain instruments and materials, and how each will be applied. Mention flavors.
2. Permit patient to handle dull instruments, such as a mouth mirror. This applies particularly to a child patient who is not familiar with dental procedures.
3. Use other instruments of a similar size and shape when describing scalers or explorers because handling sharp instruments would be dangerous for the patient.
4. Prepare patient for power-driven instruments.
   a. Avoid surprise applications of compressed air, water from syringe, or power-driven instruments.
   b. Apply moving rubber cup to child's finger.

5. Speak before touching the patient. By maintaining contact of a finger on a tooth or through retraction while changing instruments, repeated orientation can be avoided.
6. Rinsing
   a. Use evacuator when possible.
   b. Without evacuation, explain the water syringe and place rinsing cup in the patient's hand each time. Do not expect the patient to pick it up from unit.
   c. Help the patient avoid embarrassment if water is spilled.

E. Instructions for Patient

1. Give instructions clearly and concisely.
2. Demonstrate toothbrushing in patient's mouth. Help learning by the feeling of the filament tips on and under the gingival margin and the feeling of clean teeth.

IV. DENTAL HYGIENE CARE: PARTIALLY SIGHTED

Persons with sight often underestimate how useful a little vision can be. Patience is needed to help a patient make full use of available vision, without oversolicitousness. Although many of the procedures described for the totally blind person can be applied to the partially sighted person, a few additional hints are suggested here.

Elderly patients with failing sight rarely admit such an impairment. Sight failure in the older individual or lowered vision in a person of any age may be suspected from the patient's unusual squinting, blinking, or lack of continued attention. Procedures can be adapted without mention of sight to the patient.

A. Patient Position

Adjust for patient comfort. Tilting back a patient with glaucoma may increase pain and pressure in the eyes.

B. Light

Avoid glare of the dental light in the patient's eyes. Sensitivity to light is characteristic of many eye conditions.

C. Patient Instruction

1. Position patient for best vision. For example, a patient with glaucoma has no peripheral vision; thus, instruction should be given directly from the front.
2. Do not expect a patient to see fine detail, such as that in a radiograph or on a small model.

3. Work patiently and give instruction slowly. Patient may have slow visual accommodation.

▪ HEARING IMPAIRMENT

When hearing is impaired to the extent that it has no practical value for the purpose of spoken communication, a person is considered deaf. When hearing is defective but functional with or without a hearing aid, the terms "a person who is hard of hearing" or "a person with hearing loss" are used. Terminology is changing and reflects the ways in which people prefer to identify themselves.

I. CAUSES OF HEARING IMPAIRMENT

The auditory system includes the anatomic parts from the outer ear to the termination of the auditory nerve in the brain. The cause of hearing loss may be associated with the outer, middle, or inner ear mechanisms, singly or in combinations.

Many factors may contribute to deafness. Heredity, prenatal infection in the mother, especially rubella, and birth trauma are significant in the earliest years. Chronic inner ear infections, infectious diseases (meningitis), trauma, and toxic effects of drugs have all been implicated.

II. TYPES OF HEARING LOSS

A. Conductive Hearing Loss

Outer or middle ear involvement of the conduction pathways to the inner ear.

B. Sensorineural Hearing Loss

Damage to the sensory hair cells of the inner ear or the nerves that supply the inner ear.

C. Mixed Hearing Loss

Combination of conductive and sensorineural.

D. Central Hearing Loss

Damage of the nerves or nuclei of the central nervous system in the brain or the pathways to the brain.

III. CHARACTERISTICS SUGGESTING HEARING LOSS

Partial deafness may not have been diagnosed, or certain patients, particularly an elderly person, may not admit hearing limitation. Clues to the identification of a hearing problem are listed as follows.

A. Lack of attention; fails to respond to conversation.
B. Intentness; strained facial expression; stares at others.
C. Turns head to one side; hearing may be good on one side only.
D. Gives unexpected answer unrelated to question; does one thing when told to do another.
E. Frequently asks others to repeat what was said.
F. Unusual speech quality.

IV. HEARING AIDS

A hearing aid is an electronic device that amplifies and shapes sound waves that enter the external auditory canal. Current hearing aids are more technically advanced, more esthetic in their invisibility, and more commonly used. Standards for the manufacture and distribution of hearing aids are set by the United States Food and Drug Administration. A medical evaluation is required along with extensive audiologic testing.

Figure 56-2 shows five types of hearing aids. The body aid and the eyeglass models are used less frequently as the newer types are more electronically sophisticated and powerful. The small units may be difficult to operate for people without finger dexterity. The aids are delicate and require special instruction for care.

A. Body Aid Model

The unit is in a case for carrying in a pocket or attaching to clothing.

B. Eyeglass Model

A thickened temple bar of the eyeglasses holds the essential parts, and the earmold is connected by a small tube.

C. Behind-the-Ear Model

The device hooks over the ear and contains tone controls.

D. In-the-Ear Model

Because the unit is practically invisible and lightweight, the in-the-ear model has been a frequent choice.

E. Canal Aid

This model fits entirely within the canal and is the most cosmetically acceptable of all types. It may take extra skill to adjust and remove.

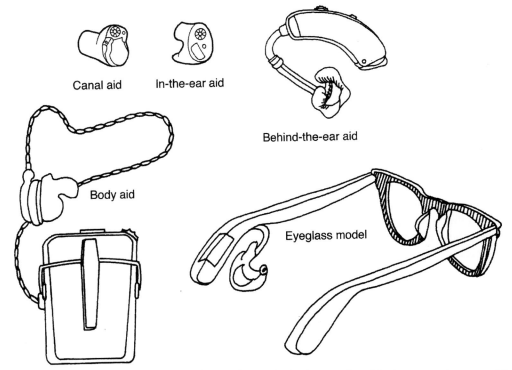

Canal aid   In-the-ear aid

Behind-the-ear aid

Body aid

Eyeglass model

■ **FIGURE 56-2 Types of Hearing Aids.** Hearing aids are electronic devices made with tiny controls to amplify sounds. The hearing aids may be able to fit over or inside the ear, connect to eyeglasses, or be fastened to clothing. None of the illustrations are drawn to scale. (From Series 2: *The Ear and Hearing.* Gallaudet University, 1986. Used with permission.)

V. MODES OF COMMUNICATION

A person with a hearing loss may learn a particular way of personal communication. Choices include speaking, speechreading, writing, manual, or a combination. Manual communication includes using sign language or "signing" and fingerspelling. *Always ask your patient which means of communication is preferred and how you can improve communication.*

A. American Sign Language (ASL)

The American manual alphabet is shown in Figure 56-3.[1] A few examples of signs are shown in Figure 56-4.

American Sign Language is a visual/gestural language with a unique grammar and syntax. Many deaf people who prefer this mode of communication grew up using ASL and consider themselves part of a cultural group. Other individuals who have become deaf in later years may learn sign language and use the signs in English word order.

Some deaf people prefer to communicate using ASL in medical or dental situations. They can request the services of an ASL interpreter.

Although a universal sign language has not been recognized, many countries have their own.

B. Fingerspelling

Spelling "in the air" is often combined with sign language. When making an introduction, for example, the name may be fingerspelled. New words that enter the scientific language often do not have signs and are fingerspelled.

C. Oral Communication

Oral communication by a deaf person means a combination of some speech, residual hearing, and speechreading.

D. Speechreading

- Speechreading consists of recognizing spoken words by watching the lips, face, and gestures.
- Many of the mouth movements for spoken words have the same appearance as one or more other words, so speechreading may need to be combined with another method of communication.
- Speechreading is not a reliable means of communication for extended, complex discussions for most people with hearing loss.

E. Writing

Writing may be an alternative when other methods are not satisfactory.

VI. DENTAL HYGIENE CARE

Patients with hearing problems are of all ages; some have been deaf all their lives, and others lost their hearing later in life. Each has special problems. Determination of the mode of communication is an important step at the outset. Always ask the patient.

When the patient's preferred mode of communication is sign language and the clinician does not know sign language, or when the patient lip reads but cannot read the clinician's lips because the clinician is wearing a mask, writing on a pad of paper may be the first choice. Some deaf individuals may not be fluent in the English language and will need the services of an interpreter for extensive communication such as review of an involved treatment plan.

A. Patient With Hearing Aid

1. Be careful not to touch a hearing aid when it is turned on.
2. Ask the patient to turn off or remove a hearing aid when a power-driven dental instrument, particularly a power-driven scaler, will be used. The noise can be amplified many times, much to the discomfort of the patient.

B. Patient With Partial Hearing Ability

1. Speak clearly and distinctly. When it is necessary to talk, be sure the patient can see your face. With the dental light directed toward the patient's mouth, the clinician's face may be in the background.
2. Eliminate interfering noises from the street outside or from saliva ejector suction.

C. Speechreader

1. Be sure patient is looking; do not turn to side; speak directly.
2. Speaker's face must be clearly visible so patient can read lips easily; difficult when dental light is directed to patient's face or the clinician has back to window.
3. Speak in normal tone; do not exaggerate words; slow the pace of speech; pause more frequently than usual.
4. Do not raise voice; raising voice can distort lip movements and make lip reading more difficult.
5. When the patient cannot understand, use alternate words to express the same thought; many letters and combinations of letters look the same on the lips; others are not visible at all.

(*continued on page –958*)

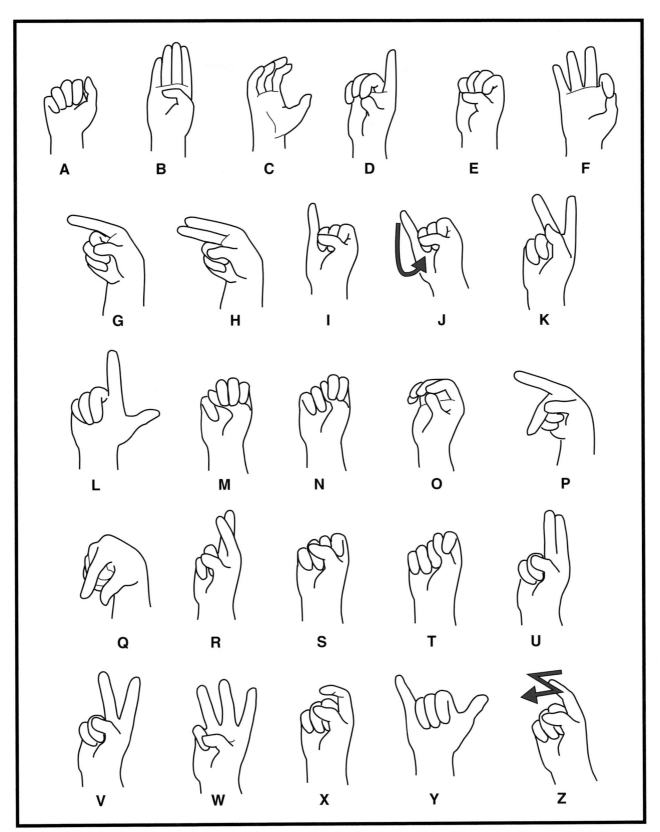

▪ **FIGURE 56-3 American Manual Alphabet.** Fingerspelling is used in combination with signs and lip reading. (From Lane, L.G.: *The Gallaudet Survival Guide to Signing*. Washington, D.C., Gallaudet University Press, 1990. Reproduced by permission.)

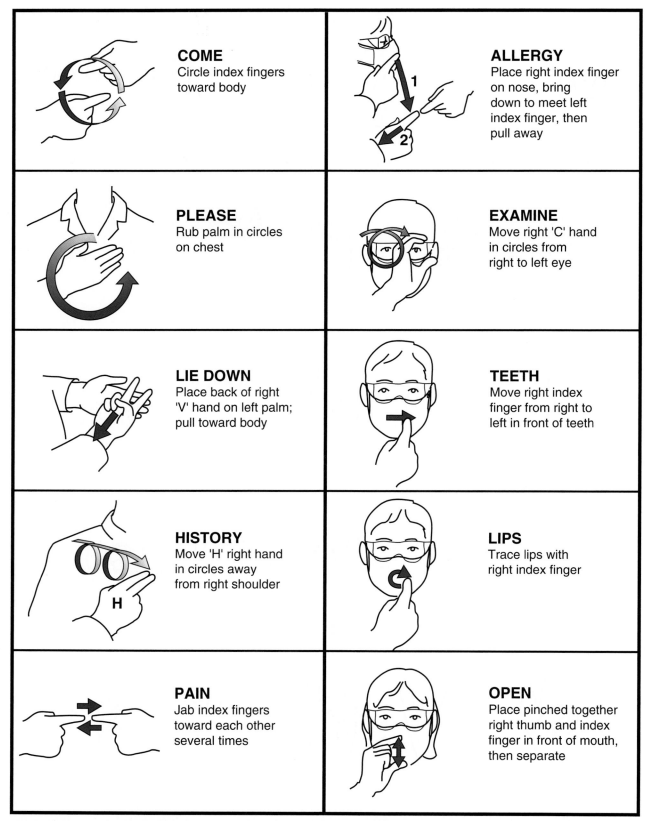

COME
Circle index fingers toward body

ALLERGY
Place right index finger on nose, bring down to meet left index finger, then pull away

PLEASE
Rub palm in circles on chest

EXAMINE
Move right 'C' hand in circles from right to left eye

LIE DOWN
Place back of right 'V' hand on left palm; pull toward body

TEETH
Move right index finger from right to left in front of teeth

HISTORY
Move 'H' right hand in circles away from right shoulder

LIPS
Trace lips with right index finger

PAIN
Jab index fingers toward each other several times

OPEN
Place pinched together right thumb and index finger in front of mouth, then separate

▪ **FIGURE 56-4 Examples of Signing.** Selected words that may be used during a patient's dental appointment. (Adapted from Lane, L.G.: *The Gallaudet Survival Guide to Signing.* Washington, D.C., Gallaudet University Press, 1990.)

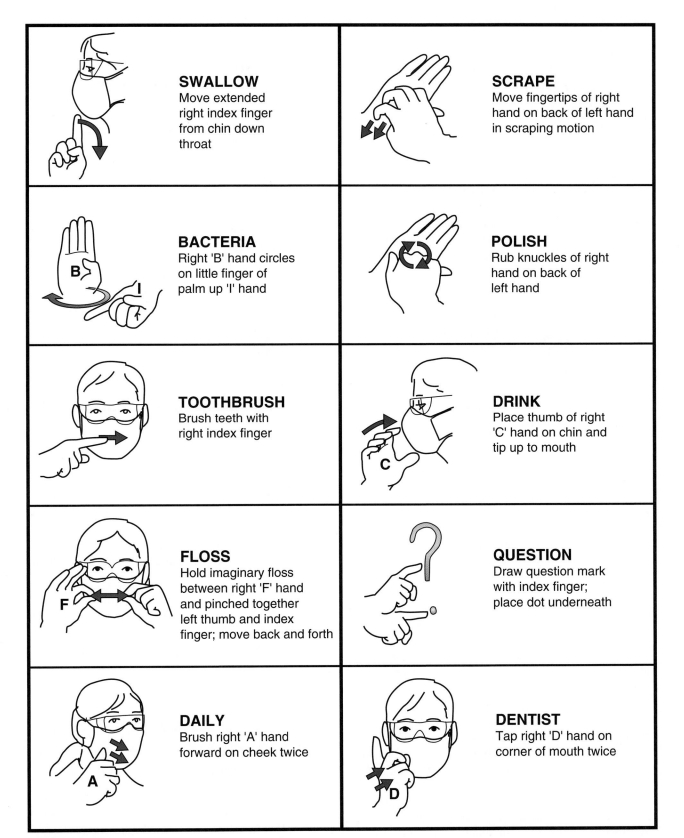

SWALLOW
Move extended right index finger from chin down throat

SCRAPE
Move fingertips of right hand on back of left hand in scraping motion

BACTERIA
Right 'B' hand circles on little finger of palm up 'I' hand

POLISH
Rub knuckles of right hand on back of left hand

TOOTHBRUSH
Brush teeth with right index finger

DRINK
Place thumb of right 'C' hand on chin and tip up to mouth

FLOSS
Hold imaginary floss between right 'F' hand and pinched together left thumb and index finger; move back and forth

QUESTION
Draw question mark with index finger; place dot underneath

DAILY
Brush right 'A' hand forward on cheek twice

DENTIST
Tap right 'D' hand on corner of mouth twice

■ **FIGURE 56-4 Continued.**

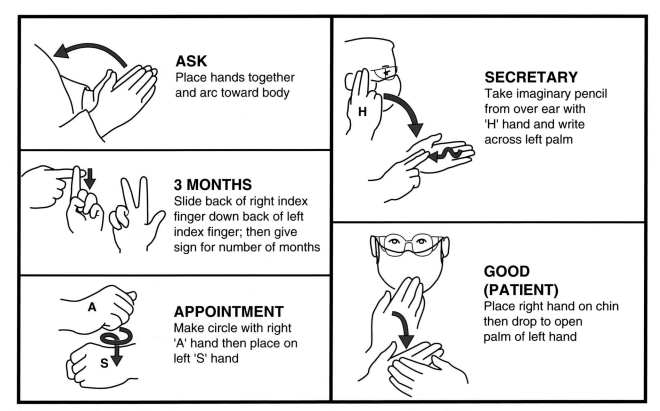

ASK
Place hands together and arc toward body

3 MONTHS
Slide back of right index finger down back of left index finger; then give sign for number of months

APPOINTMENT
Make circle with right 'A' hand then place on left 'S' hand

SECRETARY
Take imaginary pencil from over ear with 'H' hand and write across left palm

GOOD (PATIENT)
Place right hand on chin then drop to open palm of left hand

▪ **FIGURE 56-4 Continued.**

6. Keep calm; display of irritation or annoyance over difficulties in conversing can discourage or upset the patient.
7. Write proper names or unusual words the patient fails to understand.
8. When wearing a mask, certain gestures may be agreed upon in advance.

D. Sign Language

- All the points previously mentioned for the speechreader apply to patients who use sign language because lips are read along with signs.
- When a dental hygienist knows a few signs to use, a deaf patient will greatly appreciate them.

Everyday Ethics

? Mr. Dolson was scheduled for 11:00 AM with Regan, the newest dental hygienist in the practice. He arrived about 15 minutes late, so Regan was ready and waiting to begin the maintenance appointment. She quickly escorted Mr. Dolson to the chair and began the oral examination without much talking. Mr. Dolson sensed that Regan was in a hurry but was uncertain of what to say. He wore a hearing aid but didn't always turn it on. He had been known to "blurt out" his thoughts rather loudly at times not realizing the volume or tone of his voice. "Tell me if I'm doing a good job with my brushing," began Mr. Dolson. Rather startled, Regan said "You're really not brushing well at all!" Mr. Dolson grew very quiet.

Questions for Consideration

1. Professionally and ethically, how would you describe the provider-patient relationship in this scenario?

2. Was Regan's response to Mr. Dolson justified? Why or why not? Explain your rationale.

3. How should virtue ethics apply to a patient with special needs such as a hearing impairment or other loss of sensory functions?

Factors To Teach The Patient

- Why it is important to always provide complete information when the medical history is reviewed.

- New ways for better biofilm control.

- For the person with limited sight: why to avoid using toothpicks or other sharp objects to clean the teeth.

- Ways to prevent dental caries, especially for children and teenagers with limited sight.

- The importance of oral care for the dog guide.

- Learning basic sign language and fingerspelling can provide health-care workers with added skills and reduce stress for the deaf patient.

E. General Suggestions

1. For written messages, use a clipboard with a marker-type pen attached and large paper, at least 8 1/2 x 11 inches. Write clearly.

2. Ask the patient if a gentle tap on the hand or arm is an appropriate way to get attention.

3. Plan in advance for a signal the patient can give to show reaction or discomfort.

4. Teach by demonstration
   a. Use mirror and show dental biofilm removal methods directly on teeth.
   b. Younger child may be taught to rinse by watching and imitating.
   c. Provide reassurance and approval by maintaining eye contact and smiling.

5. Person with hearing loss should always have a written appointment card to ensure complete understanding.

6. Use the state Telecommunication Relay Service (TRS) to call a deaf patient directly with appointment reminders.

7. Use judgment in prolonging conversation with a deaf person. Certain patients are under tension and tire easily, whereas others enjoy the opportunity to communicate.

REFERENCE

1. **Lane**, L.G.: *The Gallaudet Survival Guide to Signing.* Washington, DC, Gallaudet University Press, 1990.

SUGGESTED READINGS

Brock, A.M.: Communicating With the Elderly Patient, *Spec. Care Dentist., 5,* 157, July–August, 1985.

Dahle, A.J., Wesson, M.D., and Thornton, J.B.: Dentistry and the Patient with Sensory Impairment, in Thornton, J.B. and Wright, J.T., eds.: *Special and Medically Compromised Patients in Dentistry.* Littleton, MA, PSG Publishing Co., 1989, pp. 63–72.

Engar, R.C. and Stiefel, D.J.: *Dental Treatment of the Sensory Impaired Patient.* Disability Dental Instruction, 4919 Northeast 86th Street, Seattle, WA 98115, 65 pp.

Lange, B.M., Entwistle, B.M., and Lipson, L.F.: *Dental Management of the Handicapped: Approaches for Dental Auxiliaries.* Philadelphia, Lea & Febiger, 1983, pp. 11–38.

Visual Impairment

Cohen, S., Sarnat, H., and Shalgi, G.: The Role of Instruction and a Brushing Device on the Oral Hygiene of Blind Children, *Clin. Prev. Dent., 13,* 8, July–August, 1991.

Geurink, K.M.: The Visually Impaired: Creating a Comfortable Dental Environment, *DentalHygienistNews, 7,* 15, Fall, 1994.

Hunter, L.H.: "The Way We See It"—Dental Health for the Visually Handicapped, *Dental Health* (London), 27, 3, June/July, 1988.

O'Donnell, D.: The Prevalence of Nonrepaired Fractured Incisors in Visually Impaired Chinese Children and Young Adults in Hong Kong, *Quintessence Int., 23,* 363, May, 1992.

O'Donnell, D. and Crosswaite, M.A.: Dental Health Education for the Visually Impaired Child, *Dent. Health* (London), 30, 8, February/March, 1991.

Schein, J.: Keeping an Eye on Your Vision, *RDH, 9,* 28, August, 1989.

Hearing Impairment

Arnos, K.S.: Hereditary Hearing Loss (Editorial), *N. Engl. J. Med., 331,* 469, August 18, 1994.

Busch, L.: Communication: The Key to Treatment of the Hearing Impaired, *Spec. Care Dentist., 2,* 150, July–August, 1982.

Clark, C.A., Cangelosi-Williams, P., Lee, M.A., and Morgan, L.: Dental Treatment for Deaf Patients, *Spec. Care Dentist., 6,* 102, May–June, 1986.

Glicken, S.R.: Health Care for Deaf Adolescents, *Adolesc. Med., 5,* 345, June, 1994.

Graves, C.E. and Portnoy, E.J.: Identifying Hearing Impairment Among Older Adults, *J. Dent. Hyg., 65,* 138, March–April, 1991.

Hollingsworth, R.A.: Sign for the Times, *RDH, 12,* 40, June, 1992.

Merrell, H.B. and Claggett, K.: Noise Pollution and Hearing Loss in the Dental Office, *Dent. Assist., 61,* 6, Third Quarter, 1992.

Nadol, J.B.: Hearing Loss, *N. Engl. J. Med., 329,* 1092, October 7, 1993.

O'Brien, S.: A Special Challenge, *RDH, 9,* 18, March, 1989.

Smela, D.-M.: Interacting With the Hearing Impaired, *DentalHygienistNews, 7,* 11, Summer, 1994.

Zazove, P. and Kileny, P.R.: Devices for the Hearing Impaired, *Am. Fam. Physician, 46,* 851, September, 1992.

Family Abuse and Neglect

Kathleen M. Nace, RDH, AA

The entire dental team needs to be aware of the problem of family abuse and neglect and identify and report suspected cases to authorities. Those most at risk for family abuse are children, the elderly, people with disabilities, and women. Family abuse may be categorized as physical, emotional, or sexual abuse; neglect; or financial exploitation. Abuse of women can include spouse abuse and dating violence. Table 57-1 summarizes the major types of family maltreatment.

Recognition of abuse can be detected during the initial assessment of a patient, particularly during the extraoral and intraoral examination. Head and facial injuries, oral trauma, lesions, and abnormal pathology can lead to a suspicion of abuse and neglect. Patients may be seen in the dental office or clinic, whereas others may be taken to a hospital emergency department because serious bodily injuries have been inflicted. Key words associated with family abuse and neglect are defined in Box 57-1.

Professional skill in the recognition and management of abused or neglected patients can be developed through experience and special education. Many governing boards require completion of continuing education courses before licensure and relicensure to practice dental hygiene.

One such program for proper training of dental personnel is the coalition "Prevent Abuse and Neglect through Dental Awareness" (P.A.N.D.A.).[1] The coalition is a public-private partnership committed to the education of all dental personnel in the recognition and reporting of suspected cases of abuse.

The P.A.N.D.A. coalition was created by Dr. Lynn Mouden of the Missouri Department of Health in conjunction with Delta Dental Plan and the Missouri Dental Association. P.A.N.D.A. offers dental professionals referral sources for families concerned with child abuse. The free seminars include child abuse and neglect indicators, legal ramifications, and dealing with sensitive issues.

CHILD MALTREATMENT

Child maltreatment can be categorized as abuse and neglect. It involves children ranging from infants through teenagers. Special needs children are more likely to be victims of abuse and neglect. Several thousands a year die as a result of severe physical damage, and others suffer

■ TABLE 57-1 MAJOR TYPES OF FAMILY MALTREATMENT

CATEGORY	DESCRIPTION
Physical abuse	Nonaccidental injuries on family members by parents, caregivers, spouses, or siblings
Psychological abuse	Mental anguish and despair caused by ridicule, intimidation, humiliation, name calling, harassment, threats, and controlling behavior
Sexual abuse	Nonconsensual or exploitive sexual contact, including sexual intercourse, oral sex, fondling, or pornographic activities on one family member by another
Neglect	Willful or unwillful failure of the caregiver or parents to provide the basic necessities to individuals in their care

permanent brain damage or physical deformities as well as emotional trauma. As much as 50% to 65% of child physical abuse involves injuries to the head, neck, or mouth.[2] Maltreatment should be considered in the differential diagnosis for any injury involving a child.

I. DEFINITIONS

A. *Abuse.* The nonaccidental physical, emotional, or sexual acts against a child under the age of 18 by a person who is responsible for the child's welfare.

B. *Neglect.* The intentional or unintentional failure to provide what is necessary for physical, intellec-

tual, and emotional development of a child by a person who is responsible for the child's welfare.

C. *Dental Neglect.* The willful failure of a parent or guardian to seek and follow through with treatment necessary to ensure a level of oral health essential for adequate function and freedom from pain and infection.[3]

II. GENERAL SIGNS OF ABUSE AND NEGLECT

Recognition of signs of suspected abuse is the first step toward protection of the child. As the child enters the treatment room, identifiable characteristics may be displayed that are suggestive of abuse or neglect.

BOX 57-1 KEY WORDS: Family Abuse and Neglect

Acute primary herpetic gingivostomatitis: clinical presentation of an initial HSV infection from HSV-1 (oral) or HSV-2 (genital) that can appear as multiple ulcerations on both keratinizing and gland-bearing mucosa.

Alopecia: baldness.

Traumatic alopecia: an area of baldness on the head caused by pulling out the hair at the roots.

Battle sign: postauricular bruising caused by basilar skull fracture.

Cachexia: ill health, malnutrition, wasting (emaciating).

Condyloma acuminatum: multiple papillary or focal sessile-based lesions caused by the human papilloma virus (HPV-6 or HPV-11).

Differential diagnosis: identifying a disease by comparing the symptoms of two or more diseases that are similar.

Ecchymosis: discoloration on the skin that is blue-black, irregularly formed hemorrhagic areas. Color changes with time to yellow or greenish-brown.

Edema: swelling.

Forensic: pertaining to or used in legal proceedings.

Idiopathic thrombocytopenia purpura: hemorrhages on the skin caused by abnormal decrease in the number of blood platelets with unknown etiology.

Lichenification: area of skin that has thickened and hardened from continuous irritation.

Raccoon sign: bilateral periorbital ecchymosis, which can occur as a result of a basilar skull fracture.

A. Overall Appearance

1. Clothing with long sleeves and long pants, even in warm weather, may suggest that bruises and lacerations are being covered.
2. Uncleanliness and other signs of lack of care.
3. Failure to thrive; malnutrition.
4. Infestation of lice.
   - Live bugs on the scalp.
   - Bug bite marks on the scalp.
   - Nits or lice eggs on the shaft of the hair; appear as tiny silvery tear.
   - Drops that can be attached anywhere along the hair shaft from the scalp to the ends and that do not move or fall off.

B. Behavioral

In Table 57-2, behavioral indicators are separated into categories of abuse and neglect.
- May be very fearful and cry excessively or will show no fear at all.
- May appear unhappy and withdrawn.
- May not exhibit normal behavior consistent with the present age of the child.

■ TABLE 57-2 BEHAVIORAL INDICATORS OF CHILD ABUSE OR NEGLECT

TYPE OF ABUSE OR NEGLECT	BEHAVIORAL INDICATORS
Physical abuse	• Behavioral extremes: aggressive/withdrawn • Frightened of caregiver • Cautious of adult contacts • Uneasy when others cry • Reports abuse by parent or caregiver • Frightened to return home
Physical neglect	• Begging or stealing food/drinks • Arrives early to school and stays late • Constantly tired/fatigued • Alcohol/drug abuse • States there is no caregiver
Sexual abuse	• Will not change in front of peers • Fantasy or immature behavior • Mature sexual awareness • Reports sexual abuse
Emotional abuse	• Habits, including sucking, rocking • Antisocial, destructive • Sleep disorders • Phobias, obsessions, compulsions • Behavior extremes • Developmental lags • Suicide attempts

■ TABLE 57-3 CONDITIONS THAT CAN MIMIC ABUSE

APPEARANCE	POSSIBLE CONDITIONS
Bruising	Accidental injuries Idiopathic thrombocytopenia purpura Hemophilia
Burns/red lesions	Port-wine stain Accidental burns
Skin lesions	Bullous impetigo Birthmarks

- May act differently when the parent is present than when alone, which may provide clues to the type of relationship that exists.
- May be evidence of developmental delays, including those of language or motor skills.

III. EXTRAORAL WOUNDS AND SIGNS OF TRAUMA

Abrasions and lacerations may be present at varying degrees of healing inconsistent with explanations given by the caregiver. Recognizing injuries to the head and neck and connecting them to suspected child abuse can save the lives of the children involved. Table 57-3 lists possible conditions that can mimic lesions from abuse.
- Skull injuries; edema, combined with ecchymosis of varying stages.
- Bald spots (traumatic alopecia); caused by pulling the hair out by the roots.
- Battle sign; postauricular (behind the ears) bruising, which indicates fracture of the basilar area of the skull.
- Raccoon sign: bilateral periorbital ecchymosis.
- Nose fractures or displacements.
- Lip bruises and lacerations; angular bruising, lichenification, or scarring, which can be caused from gags applied to the mouth.
- Marks on the skin that form a pattern of an object like a belt buckle or handprint.
- Human bite marks.

IV. INTRAORAL SIGNS OF ABUSE

Care must be given to the assessment of intraoral traumatic injuries. Many injuries of the mouth in children can also be caused by accidental means.
- Lacerations of the tongue, buccal mucosa, or palate.
- Lingual and labial frenal tears.
- Teeth that are fractured, displaced, avulsed, or nonvital.
- Radiographic evidence of fractures in different degrees of healing.

V. SIGNS OF SEXUAL ABUSE

A. Bruising or petechiae of the palate can indicate forced oral sex.

B. Sexually transmitted genital lesions found intra-orally.
1. Condyloma acuminatum presents as focal sessile-based lesions and also as a multiple papillary lesion. When present, it is necessary to look for other signs of oral sexual abuse because condyloma acuminatum can also occur with contact to verruca vulgaris or from self-inoculation.
2. Primary herpetic gingivostomatitis can occur as a primary infection of herpes simplex virus type 2 (HSV-2), which is a genital infection transmitted through oral sex.

C. Exhibits difficulty in walking or sitting.

D. Extreme fear of the oral examination.

E. Pregnancy, especially in the early adolescent years.

VI. INTRAORAL SIGNS OF NEGLECT

Failure of the caregiver who is responsible for the child to seek dental care for the child can be considered intentional or unintentional neglect. Neglect becomes intentional when the caregiver is negligent in following through with the recommended treatment.

A. Signs of Dental Neglect

- Signs of lack of personal daily care.
- Untreated disease, including rampant dental caries, pain, gingival inflammation, and bleeding.
- Lack of regularity of dental care: appointments may have been made primarily for tooth or mouth pain.

B. Responsibilities of Dentist and Dental Hygienist

- Provide education to the caregivers and age-appropriate children in the required personal care and disease prevention procedures.
- Inform the caregiver of the total treatment plan necessary to control oral diseases.
- Provide information about access to care, financial aid, and transportation, when needed.

VII. PARENTAL ATTITUDE

A. Reasons for Dental Neglect: Parental Factors Involved

- Oral healthcare considered a low priority.
- Lack of education concerning the significance of oral healthcare and the relation to general health.

- Limited finances.
- Family isolation: access to care.
- Religious beliefs.

B. General Attitudes of Abusers

- Disinterest or denial in relationship to the child; may be critical, scolding, or belittling in front of others, including dental personnel.
- Lack of interest in proposed dental and dental hygiene treatment plan, with a tendency to want only pain relief for the child. Such an attitude may not be shown toward other children in the family.
- Unavailable for consultation. Does not usually accompany the child for dental appointments, but sends the child with another sibling.
- Provides inconsistent information about the sources and causes of damaged teeth, bruises, or other signs of trauma.

C. Contributing Factors to Abusive Parents

- Immature and unprepared for accepting the responsibilities of parenthood.
- May have been abused by their own parents.
- Unable to handle daily stresses of financial difficulties, work stress, job loss, marital conflicts.
- Drug use and alcoholism are sometimes involved.

■ ELDER MALTREATMENT

I. GENERAL CONSIDERATIONS

- Elder abuse is much more than physical pain inflicted at the hands of a caretaker.
- Mistreatment occurs in institutional settings as well as in family home environments.
- Harm to the elder can occur through intentional infliction or by unintentional neglect.
- It is consistently reported that family members are the primary elder abusers.[4]
- The dental team, as in child abuse, can be a key source for the gathering of information to prove or disprove abuse of the elder patient.

II. DEFINITIONS

A. *Physical abuse.* The intentional use of force that results in bodily injury, pain, or anguish.

B. *Physical neglect.* The failure to provide basic necessities such as food, clothing, water, shelter, medicine, dental care, personal hygiene. This type of neglect can be intentional or unintentional due to the caregiver's lack of ability to provide such care.

C. *Psychological abuse.* Mental anguish and despair caused by ridicule, name calling, humiliation, harassment, threats, and controlling behavior.

D. *Psychological neglect.* Nonverbal anguish caused by the lack of communication and isolation.

E. *Financial/material abuse.* Improper, illegal, or unethical use of funds or assets.

F. *Sexual abuse.* Sexual contact with an elder who is unable to consent or otherwise nonconsensual sexual contact or exploitation.

G. *Self-neglect.* This can occur owing to depression from a loss of a loved one. The elder may feel unable to continue living.

III. GENERAL SIGNS OF ABUSE AND NEGLECT

When assessing for the possibility of abuse it is necessary to have a working knowledge of lesions that are related to aging, health problems, or medications. Taking a thorough history and comparing it with lesions present will help determine an appropriate differential diagnosis.

- Appears withdrawn, anxious, and shy and has low self-esteem.
- Gives an illogical explanation of how an injury occurred.
- Depression and hostility may be evident.
- May seem to dodge a motion of another person as if expecting to be hit.
- Overly eager to please and to be compliant.

IV. PHYSICAL SIGNS OF ABUSE AND NEGLECT

- Bruises in various degrees of healing or in areas of restraint like the legs or wrists.
- Traumatic alopecia.
- Human bite marks.
- Dislocations or sprains accompanied by fingertip pattern.
- Poor personal hygiene.
- Inadequate clothing for the season.
- Scratches or burns.
- Patterned marks and bruising indicating object used to inflict injury such as belt buckle, ropes, or a hand.
- Cachexia

V. EXTRAORAL SIGNS OF ABUSE AND NEGLECT

- Lip trauma.
- Bruising of facial tissues.
- Eye injuries.
- Fractured or bruised mandible.
- Temporomandiblar joint pain.

VI. INTRAORAL SIGNS OF ABUSE AND NEGLECT

- Fractured, displaced, or avulsed teeth.
- Bruising of the edentulous ridge. May indicate forced oral sex.
- Sexually transmitted disease lesions: condyloma acuminatum, primary herpetic gingivostomatitis.
- Lesions or sore areas in the mouth from ill-fitting dentures: epulis fissuratum, atrophic candidiasis. (Lesions that occur under dentures are described on page 843.)
- Fractured denture.
- Poor oral hygiene.
- Rampant caries.
- Untreated periodontal disease.

▪ PARTNER ABUSE

Spouse or partner abuse is another type of abuse that can be detected in the dental setting. The dental team is in a good position to examine and evaluate the oral areas of injury to a battered partner.

I. SIGNS AND ATTITUDES OF THE ABUSED

- Many of the same injuries listed for the elder person are also evident with partner abuse. They involve most frequently the face, eyes, and neck.
- The battered partner may be very reluctant to admit abuse because of threats of more serious harm.
- The abused may deny the abuse, defend the abuser, or provide excuses.

II. DENTAL HYGIENIST'S APPROACH

- Provide support; encourage open communication; be a source of reassurance.
- Discuss clinical findings in a nonjudgmental manner.
- Maintain patient confidentiality; talk in a private setting (door closed to treatment room).
- Provide references for counseling; telephone numbers.
- Prepare to share your findings with authorities when called to provide evidence.
- When it is known that the interview will be used in a legal setting, a witness needs to be present.

■ DOCUMENTATION

I. PURPOSES OF THOROUGH AND ACCURATE DOCUMENTATION

- For future reference and comparison.
- To provide authorities meticulous information to support an investigation.
- To protect the abused patient from harmful circumstances or even death. A second person should be present to witness the examination and interview.

II. CONTENT OF THE RECORD

- Obtain thorough histories of the injury from both the caregiver and the patient. Identify inconsistencies.
- Document the date, time, and place of the examination.
- Record all observable facts.
- Record questions asked to the abused patient and document all answers in the patient's exact words.
- Document all lesions, giving descriptive location, size, shape, and color. Pay close attention to ecchymoses of varying colors and injuries that appear bilaterally.
- Use diagrams showing the location, size, and description.

- Photographs and radiographs can also be used to supplement findings. Photographs must have patient consent and could be released only with consent. There may be special provisions by law that allow the taking and releasing of photographs without consent if the healthcare provider is required by law to report suspected abuse.
- Scale photography would be necessary for bite marks so further analysis can be done.
- Use the words *suspected abuse* if the patient denies abuse.

The decision must be made by the dental team whether or not to discuss the suspicion of abuse with the caregiver. If the decision is made to confront the parent or caregiver, the professional must never accuse anyone and must refrain from being judgmental. The legal obligation to report a suspected case of abuse can be explained.

■ REPORTING ABUSE AND NEGLECT

Each state has laws regarding the reporting of abuse and neglect to the proper authorities. It is imperative to research the laws for the state and have them available for reference in the office. Each office needs a written protocol for the documentation and reporting of abuse and neglect. If necessary, training in the recognition and

---

Everyday Ethics

Sarah, a young, usually vivacious patient in Dr. Stuart's practice for about 2 years, presents for a maintenance appointment with Amy, the dental hygienist. Since her previous appointment, Sarah had had a big wedding. Amy was expecting to hear about it and maybe even see pictures.

When Sarah came into the treatment room, she seemed very quiet and avoided eye contact with Amy. Upon completion of Sarah's oral assessment, the following was noted: Class II mobility on #6, #7, and #8; disto-incisal edge fractures on #7 and #8; a 4-mm scar on the vermillion border of the upper lip. Sarah explained that she slipped and fell on a wet kitchen floor. She could not remember how she got the scar, which was not present 6 months ago. Amy is not sure that Sarah is telling the truth. She sus-

pects Sarah may be in an abusive relationship with her new husband. There is not enough time to have a long discussion with Sarah or with Dr. Stuart, who is in the middle of a crown prep.

Questions for Consideration

1. Legally, what is Amy's role as a healthcare professional to obtain more details from the patient? Explain what documentation should be included in the patient's chart.
2. Would discussion of the oral assessment with Dr. Stuart be a breach of confidentiality? Why or why not?
3. How would Amy incorporate her suspicions about Sarah into the home care recommendations without violating the patient's rights?

reporting of abuse and neglect should be implemented in every dental office. Abusers may avoid the same medical doctor but frequently return to the same dentist.

All 50 states in the United States mandate reporting child abuse. When reporting suspected child abuse it is necessary to have the following information available:

- Name and address of the child and parents or other persons having custody of the child.
- Child's age.
- Names of siblings if there are any.
- Nature of the child's condition, including evidence of previous injuries.
- Any information that might be helpful in establishing the cause of abuse or neglect and the identity of the person believed to have caused such abuse or neglect.

■ FORENSIC DENTISTRY

Forensic dentistry is that aspect of dental science that relates and applies dental facts to legal problems. Forensic dentistry encompasses dental identification, malpractice litigation, legislation, peer review, and dental licensure.

There are instances when it becomes necessary to request the aid of a forensic odontologist to determine if a particular injury, usually a bite mark, is a result of abuse by a particular suspect.

- Many times the abuser will state that the bite mark occurred from a sibling squabble, an animal bite, or the child biting him/herself.
- When photographs have been obtained and the history of the injury does not match the location of the marks, a bite mark analysis can be requested of the forensic odontologist.
- Impressions and a bite registration are taken from the suspect/caregiver. A careful analysis will determine if the bite came from that suspect.
- The information can then be taken into the legal process involved with prosecuting a child abuser.

Dental forensics are not used only to determine cases of abuse. Forensic procedures are utilized in the identification of victims of a disaster. Forensic teams include dentists, dental hygienists, and assistants with special training in the process of identifying remains by comparing the dentition of the remains with dental records. Each member of the team is assigned a task, and the team works together to check and double check results so the families of the victims can have closure regarding the loss of a loved one. Dental hygienists were an integral part of the identification teams after the September 11, 2001, disaster in New York, New York.[5]

✔ Factors To Teach The Patient

Factors to Teach the Abused or Neglected Child

- The value of oral hygiene with age-appropriate materials.
- What the dental biofilm is on teeth, using disclosing agent.
- How to use the new toothbrush the child just received from the dental hygienist.
- Why it is especially important to brush the teeth and tongue just before going to sleep.

Factors to Teach the Abused Elder or Battered Spouse

- Where help can be obtained: emergency assistance including phone numbers and referrals.
- The tendency for the maltreatment to increase in severity and frequency over time.

REFERENCES

1. **Prevent Abuse and Neglect Through Dental Awareness (P.A.N.D.A.):** Lynn Douglas Mouden, DDS, MPH, Director, Office of Oral Health, 4815 W. Markham St, Slot 41, Little Rock, Arkansas 72205, (501) 661-2595; fax (501) 661-2055, Lmouden@healthyarkansas.com.
2. Senn, D.R., McDowell, J.D., and Alder, M.E.: Dentistry's Role in the Recognition and Reporting of Domestic Violence, Abuse, and Neglect, *Dent. Clin. North Am.*, 45, 343, April, 2001.
3. **American Academy of Pediatric Dentistry:** Reference Manual 2001-2002, Clinical Guideline on Oral and Dental Aspects of Child Abuse and Neglect, *Pediatr. Dent.*, 23, 33, Number 7, Special Issue, 2001.
4. Cowen, H.J. and Cowen, P.S.: Elder Mistreatment: Dental Assessment and Intervention, *Spec. Care Dentist.*, 22, 23, January/February, 2002.
5. Kim, J.: Responding to Disaster. The Story of a Hygienist in New York, *Contemp. Oral Hyg.*, 1, 8, November/December, 2001.

SUGGESTED READINGS

Cammer Paris, B.E., Meier, D.E., Goldstein, T., Weiss, M., and Fein, E.D.: Elder Abuse and Neglect: How to Recognize Warning Signs and Intervene, *Geriatrics*, 50, 47, April, 1995.

Chiocca, E.M.: Documenting Suspected Child Abuse, Part I, *Nursing*, 28, 17, August, 1998.

Chiocca, E.M.: Documenting Suspected Child Abuse, Part II, *Nursing*, 28, 25, September, 1998.

Dym, H.: The Abused Patient, *Dent. Clin. North Am.*, 39, 621, July, 1995.

Gibson-Howell, J.C.: Domestic Violence Identification and Referral, *J. Dent. Hyg., 70,* 74, March–April, 1996.

Gray-Vickery, P.: Protecting the Older Adult, *Nursing Management, 32,* 36, October, 2001.

Johnson, T.E., Boccia, A.D., and Strayer, M.S.: Elder Abuse and Neglect: Detection, Reporting, and Intervention, *Spec. Care Dentist., 21,* 141, July/August, 2001.

Kairys, S.W., Alexander, R.C., Block, R.W., and Everett, V.D.: When Inflicted Skin Injuries Constitute Child Abuse, *Pediatrics, 110,* 644, September 2002.

Kempe, C.H., Silverman, F.N., Steele, B.F., Droegemueller, W., and Silver, H.K.: The Battered Child Syndrome, *JAMA, 181,* 17, July 7, 1962.

McDowell, J.D., Kassebaum, D.K., and Stromboe, S.E.: Recognizing and Reporting Victims of Domestic Violence, *J. Am Dent. Assoc., 123,* 44, September 1992.

Mouden, L.D. and Bross, D.G.: Legal Issues Affecting Dentistry's Role in Preventing Child Abuse and Neglect, *J. Am Dent Assoc., 126,* 1173, August, 1995.

Mouden, L.D.: The Role for Dental Professionals in Preventing Child Abuse and Neglect, *J. Calif. Dent. Assoc., 26,* 737, October, 1998.

The Patient With a Seizure Disorder

Kathryn Ragalis, RDH, MS, DMD

A seizure is a paroxysmal event that results from abnormal brain activity. A seizure may involve loss of consciousness or awareness with or without convulsive movements or spasms. About 10% of the population will have one or more seizures at some point in life. About 1% to 3% of the population has a chronic seizure disorder called *epilepsy*. Epilepsy is a term to describe a group of functional disorders of the brain that are characterized by recurrent seizures. Seizures are a symptom of epilepsy.

The patient's medical history may reveal a susceptibility to seizures. A complete evaluation is required in all cases. Treatment modalities of epilepsy and a seizure itself may affect the oral cavity and dental treatment. Dental personnel must be aware of the issues associated with seizures to evaluate the patient and know how to apply emergency measures in and out of the dental office.

Care of the oral cavity is important for its relationship both to general health and to oral accidents that may occur during a seizure. All patients are advised by their

physicians to live a moderate lifestyle and to pay strict attention to general health.

Occupation and lifestyle may be limited for patients who have recurrent seizures. A person with epilepsy cannot participate in activities that may precipitate a seizure or that provide hazards in the event of a seizure. Such limitations may lead to loss of driving privileges or loss of work and may lead to depression. Box 58-1 contains key words used in this chapter.

■ EPILEPTIC SYNDROMES

I. SEIZURE DEFINITION

- A sudden paroxysmal electrical discharge of neurons in the brain.
- Results from a transient, uncontrolled alteration in brain function.

BOX 58-1 KEY WORDS: Seizures

Absence: a generalized seizure of sudden onset characterized by a brief period of unconsciousness. Formerly called **petit mal.**

Anticonvulsant: a drug that inhibits or suppresses convulsions.

Antiepileptic: a remedy for epilepsy.

Ataxia: failure of muscular coordination; irregularity of muscular action.

Atonic: relaxed; without normal tone or tension.

Aura: warning sensation felt by some people immediately preceding a seizure; may be flashes of light, dizziness, peculiar taste, or a sensation of prickling or tingling.

Automatism: involuntary motor activity, such as lip smacking or repeated swallowing.

Autonomic symptoms: pallor, flushing, sweating, pupillary dilation, cardiac arrhythmia, incontinence.

Clonic: alternate contraction and relaxation of muscle; **clonic phase** is the convulsion phase of a seizure.

Consciousness: degree of awareness and/or responsiveness of a person to externally applied stimuli.

Convulsion: violent spasm.

Cryptogenic: a disorder for which the cause is hidden or occult.

Diplopia: perception of two images of a single object; double vision.

Dyspepsia: impairment of the power or function of digestion.

Electroencephalography: the recording of changes in electric potentials in various areas of the brain by means of electrodes placed on the scalp or on/in the brain itself and connected to a vacuum-tube radio amplifier that amplifies the impulses more than a million times; the impulses move an electromagnetic pen that records the brain waves; a clinical test used for partial diagnosis of epilepsy.

Facies: expression or appearance of the face.

Grand mal: former name for a generalized or major seizure as contrasted with **petit mal,** a minor or relatively mild seizure.

Hirsutism: abnormal hairiness; **Hypertrichosis:** excessive growth of hair.

Ictal: pertaining to or resulting from a stroke or a seizure.

Myoclonus: isolated or repetitive shock-like contractions of a muscle or group of muscles; adj., myoclonic.

Paresthesia: an abnormal sensation, such as burning, prickling, or tingling.

Paroxysm: sharp spasm or convulsion; sudden recurrence or intensification of symptoms.

Petit mal: attack or brief impairment of consciousness often associated with flickering of the eyelids and mild twitching of the mouth.

Prodrome: a premonitory symptom; a symptom indicating the onset of a disease or condition; adj., prodromal.

Psychic: pertaining to the mind or psyche.

Refractory epilepsy: not readily yielding to basic treatment; usually with a single antiepileptic drug.

Seizure: paroxysmal spell of transitory alteration in consciousness, motor activity, or sensory phenomenon; convulsion.

Spasm: sudden involuntary contraction of a muscle or group of muscles; may be tonic or clonic; may vary from small twitches to severe convulsions.

Status epilepticus: rapid succession of epileptic spasms without intervals of consciousness; life threatening; emergency care urgent.

Teratogenesis: production of deformity in the developing embryo.

Tonic: state of continuous, unremitting action of muscular contraction; patient appears stiff.

Tonic-clonic: in a seizure, a sudden sharp tonic contraction of muscles followed by clonic convulsive movements.

- Seizures are usually unprovoked, unpredictable, and involuntary.
- A seizure begins with an abrupt onset of symptoms that may be of a motor, sensory, cognitive, or emotional nature, depending on which brain cells are involved.
- As a seizure progresses, it may or may not cause loss of consciousness or awareness, tonic and/or clonic movements, incontinence, or tongue biting.
- Length of seizure is uncontrollable.
- Other terms: convulsion, fit, spell, ictus.

II. CLASSIFICATION

The epileptic syndromes are complex. Diagnosis is made from:
- Clinical signs and symptoms.
- History.
- Electroencephalography (EEG).
- Functional neuroimaging.

The syndromes have been classified by the following:
- Age-related onset.
- Symptoms (particularly the type of seizure).
- Anatomic localization in the brain (temporal, frontal, parietal, or occipital lobes).

III. TYPES OF SEIZURES[1,2]

- The two basic types of seizures are *generalized* and *partial*.
- The international classification of seizures is outlined in Box 58-2.
- A seizure of focal origin that involves only a part of the brain is called a partial seizure.
- A generalized seizure affects the entire brain at the same time.

IV. ETIOLOGY

In addition to epilepsy, seizures can be a symptom of many different conditions. The causes can be divided into primary and secondary.

A. Primary (Idiopathic)

Genetic predisposition to seizures or to other neurologic abnormalities for which seizure may be a symptom.

B. Secondary (Symptomatic)

Seizures can arise during many neurologic and non-neurologic medical conditions, such as:
- Congenital conditions, such as maternal infection (rubella); toxemia of pregnancy.
- Perinatal injuries.
- Brain tumor.

BOX 58-2 INTERNATIONAL CLASSIFICATION OF SEIZURES

Partial Seizures (Seizures Beginning Locally)
Simple Partial Seizures (without loss of consciousness)

- With motor signs
- With somatosensory or special sensory symptoms
- With autonomic symptoms
- With psychic symptoms

Complex Partial Seizures

- Simple partial onset followed by impairment of consciousness
- With impairment of consciousness at onset

Partial Seizures Evolving to Generalized Tonic-Clonic Convulsions (secondarily generalized)

Generalized Seizures (bilaterally symmetrical, without local onset)

Nonconvulsive Seizures

- Absence seizures
- Atypical absence seizures
- Myoclonic seizures
- Atonic seizures

Convulsive Seizures

- Tonic-clonic seizures
- Tonic seizures
- Clonic seizures

Unclassified Epileptic Seizures

(From International League Against Epilepsy, Commission on Classification and Terminology: Proposal for Revised Clinical and Electroencephalographic Classification of Epileptic Seizures, *Epilepsia, 22,* 489, August, 1981.)

- Cerebrovascular disease (stroke).
- Trauma (head injury).
- Infection (meningitis, encephalitis, opportunistic infections of AIDS).
- Degenerative brain disease.
- Metabolic and toxic disorders, including alcoholism and drug abuse; seizures are common during drug withdrawal.
- Complication of cancer.

V. PROGNOSIS[3]

Prognosis for seizure control is good. Approximately 75% of patients become seizure-free. Seizure disorders tend to be stable, and do not worsen over time.

VI. IMPLICATIONS

Owing to the possibility of severe injury, accidents, or embarrassment, patients who experience recurrent seizures may choose to avoid or be legally restricted from participating in certain activities. These may include:

- *Vocation:* occupations that involve use of machinery or physical coordination may not be an option.
- *Licenses:* certain licenses, such as driver's license, may be restricted until the patient is deemed to be seizure-free.
- *Independent living:* ability to live alone may not be advised due to health risks.

■ CLINICAL MANIFESTATIONS[4]

I. PRECIPITATING FACTORS

A patient may have factors that precipitate a seizure. The patient or a caregiver may provide helpful information to prepare health care workers to handle an emergency. Possible precipitating factors include:

- Psychological stress; apprehension.
- Fatigue; sleep deprivation.
- Sensory stimuli, such as flashing lights, noises, peculiar odors.
- Alcohol use or withdrawal or other substances.

II. AURA

- Not all patients have a warning, or aura, before a seizure.
- A patient with a warning may seek a safe place to sit or lie down in privacy.
- In the dental environment, the patient can inform the personnel so that procedures can be terminated and brief preparations can be made.
- The aura may be a special sensory stimulus, a sensation of numbness, tingling, or a twitching or stiffness of certain muscles.

III. THE SEIZURE

The following are some of the clinical manifestations that may or may not occur during several types of seizures. Patients may experience only one type of seizure or differing types.

A. Partial (more common in adults)

1. *Simple*
   - Cessation of ongoing activity.
   - Staring spell; dizziness.
   - Jerking of muscles around the mouth.
   - No loss of consciousness.
2. *Complex*
   - Trance-like state with confusion lasts usually for a few minutes to hours.
   - Consciousness is impaired to varying degrees.
   - Patient may manifest purposeless movements or actions followed by confusion, incoherent speech, ill humor, unpleasant temper; does not remember what happened during the attack.

B. Generalized

1. *Absence (Petite Mal) Seizure*
   - Loss of consciousness begins and ends abruptly in about 5 to 30 seconds.
   - Most common in children, and might lead to learning difficulties if not identified.
   - Patient has blank stare, usually does not fall, posture becomes fixed, may drop whatever is being held.
   - May become pale.
   - May have rhythmic twitching of eyelids, eyebrows, head, or chewing movements.
   - Attack ends as abruptly as it begins. Patient quickly returns to full awareness, resumes activities, unaware of what occurred.
2. *Tonic Clonic (Grand Mal) Seizure*
   - Muscles of the chest and pharynx may contract at the same time, forcing air out and a sound known as the "epileptic cry."
   - Loss of consciousness is sudden and complete, the patient becomes stiff and falls or may slide out of the dental chair.
   - Musculature contraction: tonic phase tension with rigidity, clonic movements follow with intermittent muscular contraction and relaxation.
   - Skin color turns pale to bluish, breathing is shallow or stops briefly.
   - Possible loss of bladder and rarely bowel control. Tongue may be bitten.
   - Incident usually lasts 1 to 3 minutes.
   - Respiration returns.
   - Saliva, which previously could not be swallowed, may become mixed with air and appear as foam.
   - Patient begins to recover, may be confused, tired, complain of muscle soreness or injury; falls into a deep sleep.

- Phases of seizure may be called preictal, ictal, and postictal.
- Grand mal seizure may continue without recovery and progress to *status epilepticus*.

▪ TREATMENT

I. MEDICATIONS

Antiepileptic drug therapy is one method used to control seizures.

A. Choices

- Patients may be on one antiepileptic drug or a combination of several.
- Choice of therapy is related to type of seizure disorder and possibly to desired side effect or elimination of an undesirable side effect.
- Frequently prescribed medications are listed in Table 58-1.

B. Side Effects

1. *Each* medication has side effects that patients experience to varying degrees and should be investigated for their use, side effects, and mode of action.

▪ TABLE 58-1 ANTIEPILEPTIC MEDICATIONS	
GENERIC NAME	**BRAND NAME**
Older Medications	
Carbamazepine	Tegretol, Carbatrol
Phenytoin	Dilantin
Valproic acid/valproate	Depakote
Phenobarbitol	Luminal
Primidone	Mysoline
Ethosuximide	Zarontin
Clonazepam	Klonipin
Clorazepate	Tranxene
Newer Medications	
Felbamate	Felbatol
Gabapentin	Neurontin
Lamotrigine	Lamictal
Topiramate	Topamax
Tiagabine	Gabitril
Levetiracetam	Keppra
Oxcarbazepine	Trileptal
Zonisamide	Zonegran

2. *Side Effects Include:*
   - Allergic reaction, rash.
   - Fatigue, drowsiness, weakness, ataxia, headache, slurred speech.
   - Nausea, vomiting.
   - Memory loss, behavioral and cognitive deficits.
   - Damage to liver, interactions of medications processed in liver.
   - Leukopenia: delayed healing and infection.
   - Thrombocytopenia or decreased platelet aggregation: increased bleeding, petechiae.
   - Osteoporosis.
   - Increased or unknown risk of birth defects.
   - Hirsutism; hypertrichosis.
   - Oral change of *gingival enlargement* most common with phenytoin.
   - Numerous drug interactions, including other antiepileptic drugs, acetaminophen, non-steroidal anti-inflammatory drugs, erythromycins, and reduction in efficacy of *oral contraceptives.*
3. Elderly and children
   - Are more sensitive to side effects of weakness, unsteadiness, cognitive alterations.
   - Elderly more likely to be on other medications with possible drug interactions and more likely to forget to take medications.

C. Herbal Supplements

- Some over-the-counter herbal supplements are reported to help prevent seizures. These supplements may interfere with the prescribed antiepileptic drug and cause serious complications.
- Patients must inform their physician and dental team when using.
- Herbal supplements may also affect dental treatment, for example, with the common side effect of increased bleeding.

II. SURGERY[5]

A variety of surgical interventions are available and indicated when epilepsy is refractory to traditional antiepileptic drug therapy. Treatments have been made possible through the advances in identifying the epileptogenic area with magnetic resonance imaging, electroencephalographic studies, tomography, neuropsychological testing, and other analyses. Surgical options include:

- *Resection* of the epileptogenic area in the brain.
- *Multiple subpial transections,* which are a series of small parallel slices, which are removed, if total resection may lead to unacceptable deficits.

- *Gamma-knife radiosurgery* involves delivery of a focused dose of radiation to the epileptogenic area in the brain. This technique reduces: risk of infection, bleeding, and hospitalization.

III. VAGUS NERVE STIMULATION[6]

- Some patients are treated with an implantable vagus nerve stimulator.
- This pacemaker-like device is implanted in the upper left chest and delivers an intermittent signal to the vagus nerve.
- It causes voice alteration, swallowing difficulty, and neck and throat pain during stimulation.
- Some dental devices, such as the diathermy devices for electrosurgery and electric pulp testing, may interfere with implantable devices and must not be used.

IV. KETOGENIC DIET

- The goal of the ketogenic diet is to induce fat metabolism and maintain ketosis.
- It is initiated by a starvation period, which induces fat metabolism and the production of ketones.
- When food is reintroduced, it is mainly fat and low proteins with nearly no carbohydrates.
- This diet has been shown to be an effective treatment for patients with epilepsy, particularly children.

■ ORAL FINDINGS

Epilepsy in itself produces no oral changes. Specific changes relate to side effects of antiepileptic drugs or other therapy, results of oral accidents during a seizure, or side effects of the epilepsy, such as depression leading to poor oral hygiene and neglect.

I. EFFECTS OF ACCIDENTS DURING SEIZURES

A. Scars of Lips and Tongue

- Oral tissues, particularly tongue, cheek, or lip, may be bitten.
- Scars may be observed during the extraoral/intraoral examination, and the cause may be differentiated from other types of healed wounds.

B. Fractured Teeth

- Teeth may be clamped and bruxing may be forceful enough to fracture teeth.
- Fractured teeth may be sharp and lacerate tissue and should be smoothed or restored.

- Fractures may extend into pulp of tooth, allowing bacterial infection, which requires treatment with root canal therapy or extraction.

II. GINGIVAL OVERGROWTH/GINGIVAL HYPERPLASIA

- Gingival overgrowth occurs in 25% to 50% of persons using phenytoin for treatment.[7]
- Other antiepileptic drugs also induce gingival overgrowth less frequently.[8]
- Phenytoin and the other antiepileptic drugs have been used in the treatment of many conditions other than epilepsy, including stuttering, headaches, neuromuscular disturbances, and cardiac conditions, and therefore should not lead to the assumption that the patient has epilepsy.
- When related to phenytoin use, gingival enlargement is also called Dilantin hyperplasia, diphenylhydantoin-induced hyperplasia, diphenylhydantoin gingival hyperplasia, Dilantin-induced gingival fibrosis, and phenytoin-induced hyperplasia.

A. Mechanism

- Phenytoin may cause fibroblasts and osteoblasts to deposit excessive extracellular matrix, causing gingival overgrowth.
- Tissue color and texture are generally within normal limits with lobular shape.
- Local irritants such as biofilm or ill-fitting appliances make response more excessive.
- Meticulous oral hygiene has been found to reduce the occurrence and severity of gingival overgrowth.

B. Occurrence[9]

- Incidence is greater in younger patients than in older patients just beginning therapy.
- The gingiva may start to enlarge within a few weeks or even after a few years following the initial administration of the drug.
- The size of the dose and the length of treatment are not necessarily factors in the incidence or nature of the gingival enlargement.
- The anterior gingiva are usually more affected than are the posterior, and the maxillary more than the mandibular.
- Facial and proximal areas are usually more affected than lingual and palatal areas.
- Although rare, an overgrowth of tissue may occur in an edentulous area and is usually associated with trauma, irritation from a denture, the presence of retained roots, or unerupted teeth.[10,11]

- Overgrowth of tissue surrounding dental implants can occur.[12]

C. Effects[13]

- Poses dental biofilm control problem.
- May affect mastication.
- May alter tooth eruption.
- May interfere with speech.
- May cause serious aesthetic concerns.

D. Tissue Characteristics

- **Early Clinical Features:** The overgrowth appears as a painless enlargement of interdental papillae with signs of inflammation. Eventually, the tissue becomes fibrotic, pink, and stippled, with a mulberry- or cauliflower-like appearance, as in Figure 58-1B.
- **Advanced Lesion:** The tissue increases in size, extends to include the marginal gingiva, and

covers a large portion of the anatomic crown. Often, cleft-like grooves occur between the lobules, as shown in Figure 58-1A.
- **Severe Lesion:** Large, bulbous gingiva may cover the enamel, tend to wedge the teeth apart, and interfere with mastication. Note the severe growth about the mandibular left canine to lateral incisor area in Figure 58-2.
- **Microscopic Appearance:** During therapy, phenytoin is present in the saliva, blood, gingival sulcus fluid, and dental biofilm. The number of fibroblasts and the amount of collagen in the connective tissue increases. The stratified squamous epithelium is thick, with long rete ridges. Inflammatory cells are in greatest abundance near the base of the pockets.

E. Complicating Factors

1. **Dental Biofilm and Gingivitis**
   - Biofilm appears to be the most important determinant of the severity of phenytoin-induced gingival enlargement.[14]
   - Adequate biofilm control, particularly if started before the administration of phenytoin, helps control the extent of gingival overgrowth.
2. **Contributing Factors**
   - Mouth breathing.
   - Overhanging and other defective restorations.
   - Large carious lesions.
   - Calculus and other biofilm-retaining factors encourage gingival overgrowth.

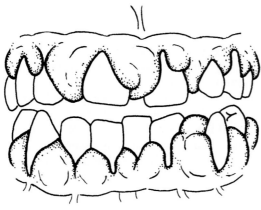

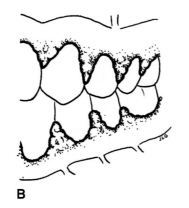

A

B

■ **FIGURE 58-1 Phenytoin-Induced Gingival Enlargement. (A)** Papillary enlargement with cleft-like grooves. Note the effect of the pressure of the fibrotic tissue on the position of teeth. Maxillary incisors and the mandibular left canine have been wedged away from normal positions. **(B)** Mulberry-like shape of interdental papillae.

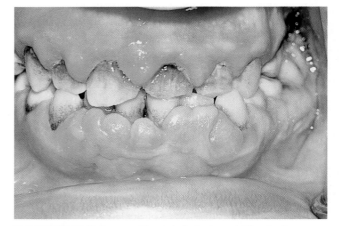

■ **FIGURE 58-2 Severe Phenytoin-Induced Gingival Enlargement.** Note extent of gingival overgrowth on lower left between canine and lateral incisor and presence of local irritants of biofilm, calculus, and stain. Used by permission from Langlais, R.P. and Miller, C.S.: *Color Atlas of Common Oral Diseases,* 3rd ed. Lippincott Williams & Wilkins, 2003, p. 81.

- Treatment must include removal of these factors by polishing overhangs, placing or replacing restorations, and removing calculus.

F. Treatment[15]

There are varying modes to treat gingival enlargement based on the medication used and the clinical presentation of the lesion. Figure 58-3 is a decision tree to help determine the type of treatment indicated.

1. **Change in Drug Prescription**
   - Since the medication is the cause, the physician could be approached concerning the possibility of changing the prescription to a different drug with a lower chance of causing gingival enlargement.
   - If possible, such a change should be made just prior to a surgical removal procedure that may be planned.
2. **Nonsurgical Treatment**
   - Scaling with a concentrated program of biofilm control may help early lesions regress.
   - Once the tissue has become fibrotic, however, shrinkage cannot be expected.
   - A program of prevention and control should be started prior to, or simultaneously with, the initial administration of the medication.
   - Chlorhexidine gluconate rinses have been used with some success to prevent return of gingival enlargement caused by another medication.[16,17]
   - A positive pressure appliance has been used with some success to reduce gingival enlargement.[18]
3. **Surgical Removal**
   - If a sufficient band of attached gingiva exists, one surgical procedure that has been used for tissue removal has been *gingivectomy*.
   - A *periodontal flap* procedure may be the choice for healing and esthetics.
   - Prior to surgery, a regulated program of biofilm control should be introduced and continued after surgical dressings have been removed.
   - For the patient with epilepsy, general health has special significance, and oral health contributes to general health.
   - For the patient with drug-induced gingival enlargement, emphasis in appointments is on a rigid oral hygiene program if the gingival overgrowth is to be kept to a minimum.

G. Differential Diagnosis of Medications Causing Gingival Enlargement[19]

Numerous medications may cause gingival enlargement. These medications include:

- Antiepileptic medications, especially phenytoin and to a lesser extent ethosuximide, valproic acid, and primidone.
- Calcium channel blocking agents used for the treatment of hypertension and other diseases.
- Immunosuppressant cyclosporin used frequently with organ transplant patients. Tacrolimus may be able to be substituted with less occurrence of gingival overgrowth.

■ DENTAL HYGIENE CARE PLAN

The majority of patients with epilepsy or a history of seizure can and should receive the same level of dental care as the general population.

I. PATIENT HISTORY

- Most patients with epilepsy have regular, thorough medical examinations.
- The physician must be contacted if the patient is unable to provide needed information or is noncompliant, if seizure activity has increased or changed, and if treatment for epilepsy is impacting dental treatment, such as gingival overgrowth.
- A well-controlled patient with epilepsy may still have a seizure.
- When seizure prone, a person should wear the Medical Alert jewelry (page 1092).

II. INFORMATION TO OBTAIN

Information to obtain from a patient with a history of seizures is in Box 58-3.

III. PATIENT APPROACH

- Provide a calm, reassuring atmosphere and treat with patience and empathy.
- Encourage self-expression, particularly if the patient tends to be quiet and withdrawn and has narrowed interests.
- Recognize possible impairment of memory when reviewing personal oral care procedures.
- Help the patient develop an interest in caring for the mouth; commend all little successes.
- Drugs used in treatment tend to make the patient drowsy, and chronic illness sufferers tend to have more frequent health issues that interfere with appointments.
- Be understanding when the patient is late or misses an appointment; plan telephone reminder at opportune time; do not mistake drowsiness (effect of drugs) for inattentiveness.

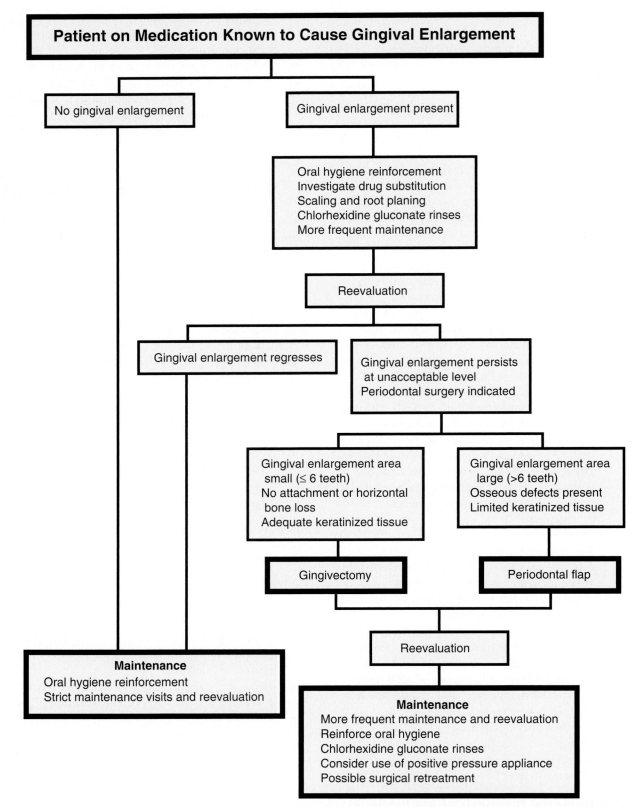

▪ **FIGURE 58-3 Decision Tree of Treatment for Gingival Enlargement.** Adapted from Camargo, P.M., Melnick, P.R., Pirih, F.Q.M., Lagos, R., and Takei, H.H.: Treatment of Drug-Induced Gingival Enlargement: Aesthetic and Functional Considerations, *Periodontology 2000,* 27, 131, 2001.

BOX 58-3 INFORMATION TO OBTAIN FROM PATIENT

Basic Information

- Thorough medical history review, including date of last physical exam, other medical conditions or risk factors present.

- Physician name and phone number.

- Emergency contact person and phone number.

Additional Factors

- Inquire about recent illness, stress, alcohol use, menstrual cycle, fatigue, or pain as factors that may provoke a seizure.

- General well-being, refer for evaluation for any signs or symptoms of other conditions such as depression.

Treatment

- Medications, surgery, or diet.

- Effectiveness of seizure control treatment.

- Investigate each medication for possible interaction with proposed dental treatment and side effects.

- Nonprescription, herbal supplement use.

- Adherence to prescribed treatment; medications taken on schedule.

About the Seizures

- Type of seizure(s) experienced, severity, and duration of episodes.

- Age at onset.

- The precipitating factors or cause of seizure if known.

- Frequency of seizures.

- Description of prodrome, aura if known.

- Experience alteration or loss of consciousness.

- Characteristic motor movements.

- Urinary/fecal incontinence.

- History of injuries, including oral injuries, broken teeth, tongue lacerations.

- Postictal symptoms such as confusion.

Suggestions

- Any other helpful information that may be provided by patient for comfort and management.

IV. CARE PLAN: INSTRUMENTATION

All patients should be instructed and motivated to comply with an effective biofilm control program, complete removal of all deposits on teeth, and any needed root planing. This is particularly important to patients who plan to or are taking an antiepileptic medication, particularly phenytoin. Options for treatment of gingival enlargement are found in Figure 58-3.

A. Prior to and at the Start of Phenytoin Therapy

A rigorous biofilm control program and complete scaling are introduced in preparation for phenytoin therapy. The patient (and caregivers) must understand that, with controlled oral hygiene and emphasis on all phases of prevention, gingival overgrowth can be prevented to a large degree.

B. Initial Appointment Series for the Patient Treated With Phenytoin

Weekly appointments for complete biofilm control instruction and scaling are planned with the following objectives:

1. *Slight or Mild Gingival Overgrowth.*
   - Nonsurgical treatment, including frequent thorough scalings, can be expected to lead to tissue reduction, provided the patient cooperates in daily biofilm control.
   - Frequent maintenance appointments can contribute to function and comfort with minimum periodontal involvement.

2. *Moderate Gingival Overgrowth.*
   - After the initial series of weekly biofilm instruction and scalings, reevaluation of the tissue can determine whether further procedures are needed.
   - An optimum level of oral health may be attained by changing the medication to another antiepileptic drug, using surgical pocket removal, and continuing frequent maintenance appointments.

3. *Severe Fibrotic Overgrowth.*
   - Initial scaling and biofilm control are carried out to prepare the mouth for surgical pocket removal.
   - Plans for changing the drug or altering the dose should be discussed with the patient's physician.

C. Maintenance Appointment Intervals

Frequent appointments on a 1-, 2-, or 3-month plan are indicated, depending on the severity of the gingival enlargement and the ability and motivation of the patient to maintain the oral health. Most patients need continuing assistance and supervision, and their response is influenced by the instruction and devotion of the dental personnel.

V. CARE PLAN: PREVENTION

- Daily biofilm removal and fluoride therapy, the use of pit and fissure sealants, and dietary control all have a vital part in the care of the patient with a seizure disorder.
- Initiation of preventive measures as soon as possible after the disorder has been diagnosed can contribute to the total health and well-being of the patient.

▪ EMERGENCY CARE

I. OBJECTIVES

To prevent body injury and accidents related to the oral structures, such as:
- Tongue bite.
- Broken or dislocated teeth.
- Dislocated or fractured jaw.
- Broken fixed or removable dentures.
- To ensure adequate ventilation.

II. DIFFERENTIAL DIAGNOSIS OF SEIZURE[20]

- Syncope.
- Migraine headache.
- Transient ischemic attack.
- Cerebrovascular accident, stroke.
- Sleep disorder such as narcolepsy.
- Movement disorders such as dyskinesia, common, for example, in patients with cerebral palsy or multiple sclerosis.
- Overdose of local anesthetic.
- Hypoglycemia or insulin overdose in a patient with diabetes.
- Hyperventilation.

III. PREPARATION FOR APPOINTMENT

When the patient's medical history indicates epilepsy, precautions may prevent complications should a seizure occur.
- Emergency materials should be in a convenient place.
- Have patient remove dentures for duration of appointment.
- Provide a calm and reassuring atmosphere.
- Have other dental personnel available in case of an emergency.

IV. EMERGENCY PROCEDURE

The dental clinic or office team has assigned responsibilities during any emergency. Initiation of procedures for seizure emergency follows the usual practice. When a seizure occurs, no attempt should be made to stop the convulsion or to restrain the patient.
- Terminate procedure; call for assistance.

Everyday Ethics

Lillian, the dental hygienist, just finished treating her last patient of the day. Diana is a very pleasant woman with excellent oral health and a history of a car accident with concussion over a month ago. She has no other medical findings. While passing the window, Lillian notices that Diana has collapsed in the parking lot and is convulsing. She calls for assistance from the dentist and assistant, and they rush out. By the time they reach Diana, she is getting to her feet and says she just tripped and fell.

Individuals with seizures may have their driver's license revoked because of the potential for serious automobile accidents that may occur during a seizure. Diana is about to get into her car to drive home.

Questions for Consideration

1. What actions of beneficence should the dentist and/or hygienist take toward Diana?

2. Given the patient's medical history, what condition could Diana be experiencing? How should this information be documented, remain confidential, or be shared with the patient's family, authorities, license bureau, and others?

3. Describe the rights of the patient and the professional duties of the dental hygienist having witnessed the incident. Explain your answer using the principles of autonomy and paternalism.

Factors To Teach The Patient

- Relationship of systemic health to oral health.
- Importance of careful daily care of mouth.
- Need for providing complete medical history information for dental appointments.
- Antiepileptic medication side effects, including gingival enlargement and how to minimize its growth.
- Seek immediate care if any oral change or injury is suspected.

- Protect the patient from injury. Position patient; lower chair and tilt to supine; raise feet. Keep from falling out of dental chair.
- Push aside sharp objects, movable equipment, and instrument trays.
- Loosen tight belt, collar, necktie.
- Do NOT place (or force) anything between the teeth.
- Establish airway; check for breathing obstruction; provide basic life support when indicated. Place on side recovery position. Use high-speed suction with wide tip to remove any vomit.
- Monitor vital signs.
- Stay beside the patient to prevent personal injury and reassure.
- Check for level of consciousness and determine if emergency medical assistance is required.
- If seizure in still occurring or has recurred within 5 minutes, activate emergency medical system.

V. POSTICTAL PHASE

- Complete the record of emergency, as described in Figure 66-1 (page 1097).
- Allow the patient to rest.
- Talk to the patient in a low, reassuring tone. Ask onlookers to leave the patient in privacy.
- Check oral cavity for trauma to teeth or tissues. Palliative care can be administered. When a tooth is broken, the piece must be located so that aspiration can be prevented.
- Contact the patient's family/friend to accompany the patient if requested.

VI. STATUS EPILEPTICUS

- Status epilepticus is defined as one or more seizures that lasts longer than 30 minutes.

- This prolonged seizure may not end spontaneously; brain injury may occur and result in long-term morbidity or death.
- Generally, a seizure lasting more than 5 minutes should be considered to progress to status epilepticus unless emergency intervention is taken.
- Emergency medical assistance must be sought immediately, and the patient must be transported to the emergency department.
- Basic life support and intravenous lorazepam or diazepam are given.

REFERENCES

1. **International League Against Epilepsy**, Commission on Classification and Terminology: Proposal for Revised Clinical and Electroencephalographic Classification of Epileptic Seizures, *Epilepsia, 22,* 489, August, 1981.
2. **International League Against Epilepsy**, Commission on Classification and Terminology: Proposal for Revised Classification of Epilepsies and Epileptic Syndromes, *Epilepsia, 30,* 389, July/August, 1989.
3. **Brodie**, M., de Boer, H.M., and Johannessen, S.I.: Epidemiology, *Epilepsia, 44,* Supplement 6, 17, 2003.
4. **Malamed**, S.F. and Robbins, K.S.: *Handbook of Medical Emergencies in the Dental Office,* 4th ed. St. Louis, Mosby, pp. 279–297.
5. **Nguyen**, D.K. and Spencer, S.S.: Recent Advances in the Treatment of Epilepsy, *Arch. Neurol., 60,* 929, July, 2003.
6. **Roberts**, H.W.: The Effect of Electrical Dental Equipment on a Vagus Nerve Stimulator's Function, *J. Am. Dent. Assoc.,133,* 1657, December, 2002.
7. **Angelopolous**, A.P. and Goaz, P.W.: Incidence of Diphenylhydantoin Gingival Hyperplasia, *Oral Surg, Oral Med. Oral Pathol., 34,* 898, December, 1972.
8. **Rees**, T.D. and Levine, R.A.: Systemic Drugs as a Risk Factor for Periodontal Disease Initiation and Progression, *Compend. Cont. Educ. Dent., 16,* 20, January, 1995.
9. **Hassell**, T.M.: *Epilepsy and the Oral Manifestations of Phenytoin Therapy.* Monographs in Oral Science, Volume 9. London, S. Karger, 1981, pp. 116–127.
10. **Bredfeldt**, G.W.: Phenytoin-Induced Hyperplasia Found in Edentulous Patients, *J. Am. Dent. Assoc., 123,* 61, June, 1992.
11. **McCord**, J.F., Sloan, P., and Hussey, D.J.: Phenytoin Hyperplasia Occurring Under Complete Dentures: A Clinical Report, *J. Prosthet. Dent., 68,* 569, October, 1992.
12. **Chee**, W.W.L. and Jansen, C.E.: Phenytoin Hyperplasia Occurring in Relation to Titanium Implants: A Clinical Report, *Int. J. Oral Maxillofac. Implants, 9,* 107, No. 1, 1994.
13. **Camargo**, P.M., Melnick, P.R., Pirih, F.Q.M., Lagos, R., and Takei, H.H.: Treatment of Drug-Induced Gingival Enlargement: Aesthetic and Functional Considerations, *Periodontology 2000, 27,* 131, 2001.
14. **Majola**, M.P., McFadyen, M.L., Connolly, C., Nair, Y.P., Govender, M., and Laher, M.H.: Factors Influencing Phenytoin-Induced Gingival Enlargement, *J. Clin. Periodontol., 27,* 506, July, 2000.
15. **Camargo**, P.M. and Carranza, F.A.: Treatment Options, in Newman, M.G., Takei, H.H., and Carranza, F.A.: Carranza's *Clinical Periodontology,* 9th ed. Philadelphia, W.B. Saunders Co., 2002, pp. 756–759.
16. **Saravia**, M.E., Svirsky, J.A., and Friedman, R.: Chlorhexidine as an Oral Hygiene Adjunct for Cyclosporine-Induced Gingival Hyperplasia, *J. Dent. Child., 57,* 366, September–October, 1990.

17. **Pilatti**, G.L. and Sampaio, J.E.: The Influence of Chlorhexidine on the Severity of Cyclosporin A–Induced Gingival Overgrowth, *J. Periodontol.*, *68,* 900, September, 1997.

18. **Aiman**, R.: The Use of Positive Pressure Mouthpiece as a New Therapy for Dilantin Gingival Hyperplasia, *Chron. Omaha Dent. Soc.*, *131,* 244, 1968.

19. **Jaiarj**, N.: Drug-Induced Gingival Overgrowth, *J. Mass. Dent. Soc.*, *52,* 16, Fall, 2003.

20. **Shneker**, B. F. and Fountain, N.B.: Epilepsy, *Dis. Mon.*, *49,* 426, July, 2003.

SUGGESTED READINGS

Asconape, J.J.: Some Common Issues in the Use of Antiepileptic Drugs, *Semin. Neurol.*, *22,* 27, March, 2002.

Fiske, J. and Boyle, C.: Epilepsy and Oral Care, *Dent. Update*, *29,* 180, May 2002.

Hupp, W.S.: Seizure Disorders, *Oral Surg. Oral Med. Oral Pathol. Oral Radiol. Endod.*, *92,* 593, December, 2001.

Kanner, A.M.: The Complex Epilepsy Patient: Intricacies of Assessment and Treatment, *Epilepsia*, *44,* 3, Supplement 5, 2003.

Karolyhazy, K., Kovacs, E., Kivovics, P., Fejerdy, P., and Aranyi, Z.: Dental Status and Oral Health of Patients With Epilepsy: An Epidemiologic Study, *Epilepsia*, *44,* 1103, August, 2003.

Koutroumanidis, M., Pearce, R., Sadoh, D.R., and Panayiotopoulos, C.P.: Tooth Brushing–Induced Seizures: A Case Report, *Epilepsia*, *42,* 686, May, 2001.

Liporace, J. and D'Abreu, A.: Epilepsy and Women's Health: Family Planning, Bone Health, Menopause, and Menstrual-Related Seizures, *Mayo Clin. Proc.*, *78,* 497, April, 2003.

Manno, E.M.: New Management Strategies in the Treatment of Status Epilepticus, *Mayo Clin. Proc.*, *78,* 508, April, 2003.

Oh, D., Siddarth, P., Gurbani, S., Koh, S., Tournay, A., Shields, W.D., and Caplan, R.: Behavioral Disorders in Pediatric Epilepsy: Unmet Psychiatric Need, *Epilepsia*, *44,* 591, April, 2003.

Patsalos, P.N. and Perucca, E.: Clinically Important Drug Interactions in Epilepsy: Interactions Between Antiepileptic Drugs and Other Drugs, *Lancet Neurol.*, *2,* 473, August, 2003.

Patsalos, P.N. and Perucca, E.: Clinically Important Drug Interactions in Epilepsy: General Features and Interactions Between Antiepileptic Drugs, *Lancet Neurol.*, *2,* 347, June, 2003.

Ryvlin, P.: Beyond Pharmacotherapy: Surgical Management, *Epilepsia*, *44,* 23, Supplement 5, 2003.

Sirven, J.I.: The Current Treatment of Epilepsy: A Challenge of Choices, *Curr. Neurol. Neurosci. Rep.*, *3,* 349, July, 2003.

Thiele, E.A.: Assessing the Efficacy of Antiepileptic Treatments: The Ketogenic Diet, *Epilepsia*, *44,* 26, September, 2003.

Tyagi, A. and Delanty, N.: Herbal Remedies, Dietary Supplements, and Seizures, *Epilepsia*, *44,* 228, February, 2003.

Wyllie, E.: *The Treatment of Epilepsy: Principles and Practice*, 3rd ed. Baltimore, Lippincott Williams & Wilkins, 2001.

Drug-Induced Gingival Overgrowth

Abdollah, M. and Radfar, M.: A Review of Drug-Induced Oral Reactions, *J. Contemp. Dent. Pract.*, *4,* 10, February 15, 2003.

Guggenheimer, J.: Oral Manifestations of Drug Therapy, *Dent. Clin. North Am.*, *46,* 857, October, 2002.

Kamali, F., McLaughlin, W.S., Ball, D.E., and Seymour, R.A.: The Effect of Multiple Anticonvulsant Therapy on the Expression of Phenytoin-Induced Gingival Overgrowth, *J. Clin. Periodontol.*, *26,* 802, December, 1999.

Majola, M.P., McFadyen, M.L., Connolly, C., Nair, Y.P, Govender, M., and Laher, M.H.: Factors Influencing Phenytoin-Induced Gingival Enlargement, *J. Clin. Periodontol.*, *27,* 506, July, 2000.

Seymour, R.A., Ellis, J.S., and Thomason, J.M.: Risk Factors for Drug-Induced Gingival Overgrowth, *J. Clin. Periodontol.*, *27,* 217, April, 2000.

Silverstein, L.H., Garnick, J.J., Szikman, M., and Singh, B.: Medication-Induced Gingival Enlargement: A Clinical Review, *Gen. Dent.*, *45,* 371, July–August, 1997.

Spolarich, A.E.: Managing the Side Effects of Medications, *J. Dent. Hyg.*, *74,* 57, Winter, 2000.

The Patient With Mental Retardation

Ann Overton Dickinson, RDH, MS

With trends toward deinstitutionalization and emphasis on special training and education in local agencies and schools, more people with mild and moderate mental retardation have appeared in private dental offices and clinics, as well as in school and community dental facilities. Opportunities are available in all settings to contribute to the health and well-being of this special group.

■ MENTAL RETARDATION

Mental retardation refers to significantly reduced general intellectual functioning with onset before 18 years that exists concurrently with deficits in adaptive behavior. Mental retardation is one of several developmental disorders that usually are first diagnosed in infancy, childhood, or adolescence. Box 59-1 lists the major categories of developmental disorders, and Box 59-2 provides descriptive terminology and other key words.

The levels of intellectual functioning are designated *mild, moderate, severe,* and *profound.* Standardized intelligence tests are used to determine individual levels. The Intelligence Quotient (IQ) expresses the test results. A category of *Unspecified Mental Retardation* is used when standard tests cannot be performed because of lack of cooperation, severe impairment, or infancy.

Adaptive functioning refers to the person's effectiveness in social skills, communication, and daily living skills, as well as to how standards of personal independence and social responsibility characteristic of the age and cultural group are met. Adaptive functioning is influenced by such factors as motivation, education, and social and vocational opportunities and has more chance for improvement by remedial efforts than does IQ, which tends to be more fixed.[1]

Adaptive functioning is described briefly for each of the categories listed in the following sections. An understanding of expected capabilities can help to provide

---

BOX 59-1 Disorders Usually First Diagnosed in Infancy, Childhood, or Adolescence

MENTAL RETARDATION

Mild, moderate, severe, profound

LEARNING DISORDERS

Reading

Mathematics

Written expression

MOTOR SKILLS DISORDERS

Coordination

PERVASIVE DEVELOPMENTAL DISORDER

Autistic disorder

DISRUPTIVE BEHAVIOR DISORDERS

Overaggressiveness, hostility, hyperactivity, inattention, impulsiveness

Poor attention span

Conduct disorder; delinquency

Use of alcohol; stealing; destructive acts

ANXIETY DISORDERS

Unrealistic fears of the unfamiliar

Fear of separation

FEEDING DISORDERS

Failure to eat adequately

Pica

Rumination disorder

TIC DISORDERS

Tourette's syndrome

Chronic motor or vocal tic disorder

COMMUNICATION DISORDERS

Expressive language

Stuttering

(Adapted from American Psychiatric Association: *DSM-IV,* 1994, pp. 37–38.)

---

necessary background information for teaching basic oral care procedures.

I. MILD RETARDATION

A. IQ

50–55 to approximately 70.

B. Adaptive Functioning

1. *Child.* In special classes for the educable, the child advances to a level of third to sixth grade. Practical skills can be learned.
2. *Adult.* At adult level, the individual cares for personal hygiene and other necessities, with reminders. Communication is good, although the attention span and memory are less than average. Activities that do not require involved planning or rapid implementation can be carried out satisfactorily. Most educable individuals can engage in semiskilled or simple skilled work with guidance, and so maintain themselves.

II. MODERATE RETARDATION

A. IQ

35–40 to 50–55.

B. Adaptive Functioning

1. *Child.* A marked developmental lag occurs in the early years, but the child can be trained in personal care and hygiene with help. These children attend classes and learn simple habits and skills, but they do not learn to read and write. They speak in short sentences and understand best when single-thought, short sentences are used. They participate well in group activities.
2. *Adult.* As adults, these individuals attend to personal care, with reminders, and have a relatively short attention span and memory. Although they may have problems of coordination, they perform simple tasks and are conscientious about taking responsibility for errands and helpful duties. Although not completely capable of self-maintenance, many do unskilled work with direct supervision.

III. SEVERE RETARDATION

A. IQ

20–25 to 35–40.

BOX 59-2 KEY WORDS: Mental Retardation

Autism: a developmental disability, generally evident before age three (3), affecting verbal and nonverbal communications and social interaction.

Brachycephalic: having a short, wide head.

Coprolalia: involuntary utterance of vulgar or obscene words.

Dysmorphism: abnormality in morphologic development.

Echolalia: echo reaction; the involuntary repetition of a word or sentence just spoken by another person.

Epicanthus: a vertical fold of skin on either side of the nose, sometimes covering the inner canthus; a normal characteristic in persons of certain races.

Hyperactivity: abnormally increased activity.

> **Development hyperactivity (hyperkinesis):** characterized by constant motion, fidgetiness, excitability, impulsiveness, and a short attention span.

Intelligence quotient (IQ): numeric rating determined through psychologic testing that indicates the approximate relationship of a person's mental age (MA) to chronologic age (CA).

Macroglossia: very large tongue.

Microcephaly: small size of head in relation to the rest of the body.

Mutism: inability or refusal to speak; deafness may prevent learning to speak.

> **Elective mutism:** persistent refusal to talk in children with demonstrated ability to speak.

Pathognomonic: characteristic or indicative of a particular disease or syndrome; especially one or more typical symptoms.

Pervasive: throughout entire individual, entire development is severely and markedly impaired, as in autism.

Pica: persistent craving/eating of nonnutritive substances or unnatural articles of food.

Rumination: repeated regurgitation of food in the absence of any associated gastrointestinal illness.

Self-injury: act of deliberate harm to one's own body. Also called self-abuse, self-directed aggression, self-harm, self-inflicted injury, self-mutilation.

Tic: an involuntary, sudden, rapid, recurrent, nonrhythmic, stereotyped motor movement or vocal sound.

> **Tourette's syndrome:** multiple motor and one or more vocal tics; may involve squatting, twirling, grunts, barks, sniffs, and coprolalia.

Ultrasonography: the location, measurement, or delineation of deep structures by measuring the reflection or transmission of ultrasonic waves. Used in examination of fetus to determine birth defects.

B. Adaptive Functioning

1. *Child.* Children at this level can benefit from systematic habit training and may make attempts at personal care and dressing with assistance. They usually walk, use some speech, and respond to directions.
2. *Adult.* Adults conform to a daily routine and may help with household and other small tasks, in spite of a limited attention span. Many adapt to life in the community in group homes or with their families.

IV. PROFOUND RETARDATION

A. IQ

Below 20 or 25.

B. Adaptive Functioning

1. *Child.* Delays occur in all phases of development, and close supervision and care are necessary.
2. *Adult.* Many remain inert and placid throughout the early years and never learn to sit up. In a highly structured setting and with constant supervision, self-care and communication skills may improve. Some perform simple tasks in a sheltered, supervised setting.

■ ETIOLOGY OF MENTAL RETARDATION

Mental retardation represents a more or less important symptom in well over 200 different conditions. Many of these are rare. A variety of means of classification is found in the literature. It has been convenient to divide the causes into factors occurring before birth, at birth, and after birth.

A majority of cases of mental retardation results from prenatal influences; a small number is effected as injuries at birth. Diagnosis may be complicated and difficult, and many cases can only be classified as of unknown origin.

I. PREDISPOSING FACTORS[1]

A. Heredity.
B. Early alterations of embryonic development.
C. Pregnancy and perinatal problems.
D. General medical disorders acquired in childhood.
E. Environmental influences.
F. Unknown.

II. EXAMPLES DURING PRENATAL PERIOD

A. Infections

Brain damage can result from maternal infection during pregnancy. Serious infections during the first trimester are most likely to cause physical malformations.

1. *Congenital Rubella Syndrome.* German measles virus infection during the first trimester may cause abnormalities, including mental retardation. The rubella syndrome also may include cataracts, cardiac anomalies, deafness, and microcephaly.

   Immunization with rubella vaccine has reduced the incidence of the disease, and retardation related to the virus infection has been reduced.
2. *Congenital Syphilis.* Transfer of syphilis from the mother leads to numerous symptoms. When the central nervous system is involved, hydrocephalus, convulsions, and mental retardation can result. Hutchinson's triad, which is associated with the late stage of congenital syphilis, includes deafness, interstitial keratitis, and dental defects. Hutchinsonian incisors, which are notched and tapered, mulberry molars, and microdontia are typical (Figure 15-5, page 268).
3. *Neonatal Congenital Toxoplasmosis.* Infection of the fetus transplacentally may lead to miscarriage, stillbirth, or a living baby with severe clinical disease. The effects may include hydrocephalus or microcephalus, blindness, and mental retardation.

B. Drugs Used During Pregnancy

1. *Contraindicated Drugs.* Table 45-1 (page 772) lists drugs contraindicated during pregnancy and the possible adverse effects the drugs can have on the fetus. Malformations and syndromes that include mental retardation are identified.
2. *Fetal Alcohol Syndrome (FAS).* The signs and symptoms of FAS are described on page 1014, and the facial features are shown in Figure 61-1.

C. Metabolic Disorders

1. *Phenylketonuria (PKU).* Phenylketonuria results from an error of metabolism in which the enzyme necessary for digestion of the amino acid phenylalanine is missing. Severe mental retardation is a consequence. Early recognition of the missing enzyme with early dietary control lessens the severity of retardation. Many states require blood and urine screening tests soon after an infant is born. A diet free of animal and vegetable protein is necessary.
2. *Congenital Hypothyroidism.* Cretinism results from partial or complete absence of the thyroid gland at birth. Symptoms of defective development include mental retardation.

D. Chromosomal Abnormality

Down syndrome is described in a separate section on page 986.

III. EXAMPLES DURING BIRTH

A. Mechanical Injury at Birth

Damage leading to mental retardation may have a variety of causes, including complications of labor and delivery.

B. Hypoxia

Asphyxiation from prolonged oxygen deficiency may result from labor complications.

IV. EXAMPLES DURING POSTNATAL PERIOD

A. Infections

Cerebral infection may be caused by a wide variety of diseases, including encephalitis and meningitis.

B. Postnatal Trauma

Accidents may result in a fractured skull or prolonged unconsciousness.

■ GENERAL CHARACTERISTICS

I. PHYSICAL FEATURES

Because most individuals with mental retardation are in the borderline and mild categories, no unusual physical characteristics should be expected. There may be delayed growth and development.

Facial or other characteristics may be pathognomonic for a particular condition or syndrome; for example, Down syndrome, described later in this chapter.

Skull anomalies include microcephaly (smaller), hydrocephalus (larger, contains fluid), spherical, conical, or otherwise asymmetrical shapes. Other dysmorphic features, such as asymmetries of the face, malformations of the outer ear, anomalies of the eyes, or unusual shape of the nose, may become apparent as the child develops.

II. ORAL FINDINGS

A higher incidence of oral developmental malformations has been observed, some specifically associated with particular syndromes or conditions. Oral findings that have been observed to occur more frequently in individuals with mental retardation than in those with normal intelligence include the following:

A. Lips

Increased thickness of the lips is common. Lip biting is one of the self-injurious habits.

B. Tooth Anomalies

Teeth may be imperfectly formed; eruption patterns may be delayed or irregular.

C. Periodontal Conditions

Gingivitis and periodontitis are common in individuals with mental retardation. Patients with Down syndrome have more severe disease than do those from other groups with mental retardation. The incidence is greater among the institutionalized patients when compared with those living in the community.[2]

D. Habits

Incidence of clenching, bruxing, mouthbreathing, and tongue thrusting is increased.

E. Dental Caries[2]

The factors that are effective in the control of dental caries in the special group are the same as those in the general population. These factors include exposure to fluoridation and other forms of fluoride, form and frequency of cariogenic foods in the diet, and the control of dental biofilm.

When all degrees of retardation are grouped together, dental caries incidence is generally higher for noninstitutionalized than for institutionalized patients, particularly among the profoundly retarded group. Institutionalized individuals have a controlled diet with less food available between meals. They also may have less accessibility to snacks containing refined carbohydrates, except those brought by visitors.

When located in nonfluoridated areas, some institutions have chosen to fluoridate their private water supplies. Noninstitutionalized individuals may also reside in areas with community water fluoridation.

When the figures for dental caries incidence are separated according to degree of retardation, the severely and profoundly retarded patients have been shown to have significantly more dental caries.[2] Patients with mild and moderate retardation can be trained in self-care.

■ DENTAL AND DENTAL HYGIENE CARE AND INSTRUCTION

Procedures for management and care of a patient with a disability are described in Chapter 53, with suggestions for various types of adaptations. The patient with mental retardation may have physical and sensory disabilities or systemic disease problems; therefore, information from various chapters can be applied during treatment. Patients with any type of mental retardation need basic periodontal therapy consisting of intensive daily biofilm control, scaling, and frequent maintenance supervision. Patience and repetition are needed to learn and develop motor skills.

In the following pages, the special characteristics and problems of patients with Down syndrome and autistic disorder are described.

▪ DOWN SYNDROME

A special and unique group of individuals with mental retardation has a chromosomal abnormality manifested in Down syndrome or trisomy 21 syndrome. Prenatal serum testing and genetic counseling have contributed to lowering the incidence of Down syndrome.

Formerly, the incidence of births of babies with Down syndrome increased with advancing maternal age. In recent years, however, the average age of mothers of infants with Down syndrome has decreased.[3] Also, statistical evidence shows that the father can be the source of the chromosomal abnormality.[4]

Patients with Down syndrome have a combination of characteristic abnormalities that is relatively constant. They tend to resemble one another.

I. PHYSICAL CHARACTERISTICS

A. Stature

Small, with a short neck; awkward, waddling gait; general growth retardation.

B. Head

Microcephaly; flat on facial and occipital sides; short, underdeveloped nose with depressed bridge; scanty hair.

C. Eyes

Oblique slant laterally with narrow opening between eyelids; fold of skin continues from upper eyelid over the inner angle of the eye (epicanthic fold) (Figure 59-1). Nearsightedness, eyes crossing inward, and cataracts are common.

D. Hands

Broad, with short stubby fingers. The little fingers are curved inward. A single transverse palmar crease may also be present (Figure 59-2).

II. LEVEL OF MENTAL RETARDATION

Generally, the IQ of patients with Down syndrome is under 70. Those who have been institutionalized for a long period of time may show lower IQ scores. Socially, many of the children are more advanced and may appear to have more intelligence than actually exists. The characteristics of friendliness and personal interaction are described later.

Many people with Down syndrome are fond of music and have a good sense of rhythm. They enjoy singing, playing an instrument, and listening to music. Background music in the dental office or clinic may be helpful in gaining rapport with these special patients.

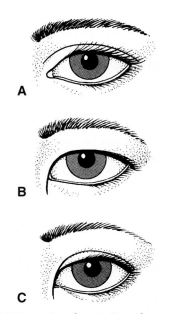

▪ **FIGURE 59-1 Down Syndrome: Eye Characteristics. (A)** Absence of an epicanthic fold. **(B)** Epicanthic fold in Oriental populations. **(C)** Epicanthic fold of person with Down syndrome. (Redrawn from Smith, G.F. and Berg, J.M.: *Down's Anomaly,* 2nd ed. Edinburgh, Churchill Livingstone, 1976.)

III. PERSONAL CHARACTERISTICS

The newborn baby with Down syndrome is considered a "good" baby by the parents. Later, many of the small children are cheerful, happy, and responsive to learning. Individual differences can be noted, and personality disturbances may occur.

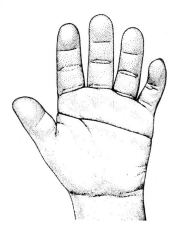

▪ **FIGURE 59-2 Down Syndrome: Hand.** Short, stubby fingers with little finger curved inward are characteristic. An identifying feature is the single transverse palmar crease. (From Smith, G.F. and Berg, J.M.: *Down's Anomaly,* 2nd ed. Edinburgh, Churchill Livingstone, 1976.)

Typical characteristics listed here may suggest management approaches for dental and dental hygiene appointments.

- Like attention; require affection for feeling of security.
- Cheerful disposition; rarely irritable; easily amused.
- Sociable, observant; take initiative.
- Tendency to imitate; mischievous.
- Periods of stubbornness; obstinate and determined to have their own way. Parental discipline is necessary. In the dental hygiene appointment, the initial approach can be important to continued control and cooperation.

IV. ORAL FINDINGS

A. Lips

Habitually, the young person with Down syndrome holds the mouth open with the tongue protruded. The lips are often thickened, cracked, and dry, a result of excessive bathing in saliva while the mouth is open.

Mouth breathing is common. Because respiratory infections frequently exist, and the tonsils and adenoids are often enlarged, breathing through the nose may not be easy.

B. Tongue and Palate

The tongue is generally deeply fissured and appears large. The narrow jaws and short, narrow palate tend to force the tongue into protrusion. It appears larger than it actually may be.

The incidence of cleft lip, cleft palate, or cleft uvula is greater than that in the general population.[5]

C. Teeth

Eruption is delayed and irregular in sequence. There may be microdontia and congenitally missing teeth. Such anomalies as fused teeth and peg lateral incisors occur frequently.

D. Occlusion

Angle's Class III and posterior crossbite are common and relate to the flat face and underdevelopment of the midfacial region. Frequently, the teeth are spaced because certain anomalous teeth are narrow and require less space.

E. Periodontal Disease[6,7]

Periodontal conditions are more severe in people with Down syndrome. Even at early ages, bone loss and other effects of periodontal infection are present. Leukocyte function is altered by impaired chemotaxis and phagocytosis, and the altered immune system contributes to the increased severity of periodontal infection.

Necrotizing ulcerative gingivitis (NUG), superimposed over gingivitis or periodontitis, has been found more in patients with Down syndrome than in those with other types of mental retardation.

V. HEALTH PROBLEMS SIGNIFICANT TO DENTAL HYGIENE CARE

The mortality rate has been high during the early years because of high susceptibility to respiratory infections, leukemia, and congenital heart lesions. More recent improvements in child healthcare and immunizations have brought a longer life expectancy.

A. Susceptibility to Infection

Defects in the body's immune defense mechanisms lead to greater susceptibility to various infections.

B. Obstructive Airway Problems[8]

1. Contributing factors: macroglossia, increased secretions, frequent respiratory infections, obesity, enlarged tonsils and adenoids.
2. Dental hygiene adaptations: chair position, fluid suctioning, gag reflex.

C. Congenital Heart Lesions

Antibiotic premedication will be needed for many patients. There is a high incidence of mitral valve prolapse in this population.[9]

D. Relation to Alzheimer's Disease

Adults with Down syndrome age prematurely. Many over the age of 40 develop an Alzheimer's-like dementia with pathologic brain changes similar to those of Alzheimer's disease.[10] Changes occur in memory, speech, gait, personality, and other characteristics. Alzheimer's disease is described on page 829.

■ AUTISTIC DISORDER

Autism is a developmental disability marked by limitations in the ability to understand and communicate. In autism, brain function is severely disordered, and the way the brain uses or transmits information is affected. Autism usually appears during early childhood and persists throughout life.[11]

Autistic disorder is manifested by a range of impairments rather than by the presence or absence of a certain behavior or symptom. Variations of autistic behavior have been grouped by the American Psychiatric Association as related disorders under the broad heading *Pervasive Development Disorder (PDD)*, a general category of disorders marked by severe and pervasive impairment in several areas of development.

The *DSM-IV* uses the terms PDD and ASD (Autism Spectrum Disorder) to describe five variations of autistic behavior. Major points that distinguish the differences between the categories are outlined in Table 59-1.[12]

I. CHARACTERISTICS

Autistic disorder has a spectrum of symptoms that range from mild to severe. The social, communication, and behavioral features of autism are shown in Box 59-3. Not all individuals have the same degree of impairment; *any combination* of symptoms and behaviors *in any degree of severity* can be exhibited.

Characteristic features include:
- Problems with social interactions.
- Problems with verbal and nonverbal communication.
- Ritualistic or compulsive behaviors.
- Atypical responses to the environment.

II. PREVALENCE

Once thought rare, prevalence rates for autism are not consistent with rates for a rare disease. Statistics from the 1960s indicated a prevalence rate of 4 to 5 cases in 10,000; current estimates range from 1 in 500 to 1 in 1,000 cases in the United States.[13] Some of the increased prevalence could be attributed to recent changes in diagnostic criteria and in the conditions categorized under the PDD and ASD umbrella terms. Autism occurs in all racial, ethnic, and social groups worldwide. It occurs four times more frequently in boys (usually the firstborn) than in girls.

III. ETIOLOGY

The exact cause of autism is uncertain. A variety of factors have been identified and related, including genetics, viruses, chemicals, and a lack of oxygen at birth. Studies suggest a strong genetic basis, leading researchers to theorize that faulty genes might make a person vulnerable to develop autism in the presence of such factors. Outdated theories of poor-quality parenting as a cause of or contributing factor for autism have been proven false.

IV. INTERVENTIONS

There is no "cure," in the medical sense, for autism. Interventions based on the management of autism as a brain-based disorder have changed treatments dramatically since it was first described by Dr. Leo Kanner.[14]

A. Pharmacological Treatments

- Purpose: relief of negative behavioral symptoms (such as aggression, self-injury, and other more difficult behaviors).

▪ TABLE 59-1 PERVASIVE DEVELOPMENTAL DISORDER AND AUTISM SPECTRUM DISORDER	
Autistic Disorder (aka: classic autism)	• Impairments in verbal and nonverbal communication and social interaction, and restrictive or repetitive patterns of behavior, interests, and activities • Symptoms are usually measurable by 18 months of age; formal diagnosis is usually made between ages 2 to 3 years, when delays in language development are apparent
Asperger's Disorder	• Characterized by impairments in social interactions and restricted interests and activities, without clinically significant delays in language, cognitive ability, or developmental age-appropriate skills
Pervasive Developmental Disorder—Not Otherwise Specified (aka: atypical autism)	• Severe and pervasive impairment in specified behaviors, without meeting all of the criteria for a specific diagnosis
Rett's Disorder (aka: Rett syndrome)	• Occurs only in girls, causing the development of autism-like symptoms after a period of seemingly normal development • Purposeful use of hands is lost and replaced by repetitive hand movements beginning between ages 1 to 4 years • In 1999, researchers identified a gene responsible for Rett syndrome
Childhood Disintegrative Disorder	• Characterized by normal development for at least the first 2 years followed by a significant loss of previously acquired skills
Adapted from Rapin, I.: Perspective: The Autistic-Spectrum Disorders. *N. Engl. J. Med., 347*, 302, August 1, 2002.	

BOX 59-3 Characteristics of Autism

A. Impairment in Social Interaction

1. Impairment in use of nonverbal behaviors (e.g., eye-to-eye gaze, facial expression, gestures)

2. Failure to develop peer relationships appropriate to developmental level

3. Lack of spontaneous seeking to share enjoyment, interests, or achievements with others

4. Lack of social or emotional reciprocity

B. Impairment in Communication

1. Delay or total lack of spoken language

2. Individuals with adequate speech: impairment in conversational abilities

3. Repetitive use of language

4. Lack of spontaneous make-believe play

C. Restricted Repetitive and Stereotyped Patterns of Behavior

1. Preoccupation with stereotyped and restricted patterns of interest

2. Inflexible adherence to routines or rituals

3. Repetitive body movements and mannerisms

4. Persistent preoccupation with parts of objects

D. Delays or Abnormal Functioning Prior to Age 3 Years

1. Social interaction

2. Language as used in social communication

3. Symbolic or imaginative play

Adapted from American Psychiatric Association, *DSM-IV*, 1994, pp. 70–71.

- Types of drugs: stimulants (such as methylphenidate *Ritalin*), antidepressants, opiate blockers, and tranquilizers.
- *Risperidone*, an atypical antipsychotic medication, has been shown to be significantly more effective than placebo in improving behavior, representing the largest positive effect by a medication ever observed in children with autism.[15]
- Identification and medical management of comorbid, potentially treatable conditions such as epilepsy seizures, allergies, gastrointestinal problems, or sleep disorders can lead to quality-of-life improvements.

B. Behavioral Therapy Treatments

- Purpose: help people with autism lead more normal lives by decreasing symptoms and increasing their ability to respond.[16]

- Examples: special teachers in intensive structured programs directed toward individual instruction, applied behavior analysis, sensory integration, music therapy, occupational therapy, speech and language therapy, and auditory integration training. No one behaviorally based or educational approach is effective in alleviating symptoms in all cases of autism because of the spectrum nature of the condition and the many behavior combinations that can occur.[16]

C. Prognosis

- Life expectancy: normal.
- Social and communication deficits continue in some form throughout life; some of the negative behaviors may change or diminish over time with appropriate treatment.[13,16]

■ DENTAL HYGIENE CARE

Appointments for medical or dental health care may be frightening, difficult experiences for some patients with autism. Dental care may have been neglected due to problems with social interactions, language and communication problems, or difficult behaviors.

Severity of symptoms dictates the appropriate setting for the delivery of dental care services for the patient with autism. With some modifications to the treatment plan, patients with mild manifestations of the condition may often be treated successfully in the general dental setting. Patients with more severe symptoms may require major treatment plan modifications, such as sedation, general anesthesia, or immobilization, in a specialized setting.

I. ORAL HEALTH PROBLEMS

Except when autism is combined with a developmental disability of a different nature, no specific oral manifestation exists. Several factors can contribute to poor oral health.

A. Previous Dental Care

* Dental care may have low priority.
* Caregivers may not seek dental services for the individual owing to fear of embarrassment over difficult behaviors or fear of discomfort or injury.
* Satisfactory quality of previous services may not have been achievable.

B. Dental Caries

* Feeding problems can lead to offering foods the child accepts, without regard for nutritive content or dental caries prevention.
* Dietary selection may have been limited by needs for sameness, with the possibility of serving excess cariogenic foods.
* Sweet food rewards for behavior modification, repeated frequently over time, promote dental caries development.

C. Oral Hygiene

* Daily oral care procedures may be inadequate for the uncooperative autistic individual, even when delivered by an informed caregiver.

II. DENTAL STAFF PREPARATION

A. Learn how to work with the patient
* Review medical, dental, and personal histories in advance.
* Discuss information with physician, psychiatrist, teacher, or other persons associated with the patient.

B. Plan several short orientation appointments initially.

C. Involve the same members of the dental team at each appointment to avoid distressing the patient and losing time for reorientation.

Everyday Ethics

? At the Caring Community Dental Health Clinic, the first and third Mondays of every month are reserved for special needs patients who have been referred by health professionals in the local area. Mentally retarded adults, adults and children with Down syndrome, and adults and children with autism are frequently scheduled for dental hygiene appointments on those days. With only one full-time and one part-time dental hygienist, more hygiene appointment time has been needed; dental hygiene students from a nearby dental hygiene program have recently begun to rotate through the clinic for community practicum experience.

Questions for Consideration

1. Two days before a scheduled assignment, Ellie, a student, confides to her classmate, Julie, that she cannot participate in this field experience because she is too afraid of people with mental disabilities. What are the ethical issues in this situation?

2. When arriving at the assignment, the students are greeted and oriented by the part-time hygienist, Ms. Gray. She advises the students, "Just get 'em in and get 'em out. They don't understand anything anyway and it's a waste of your time to try to talk to them for patient instruction." What are the ethical principles applicable to this situation?

3. How might the students handle the ethical dilemmas being faced using a formal decision model to determine an acceptable course of action?

✔ Factors To Teach The Patient

- Encourage oral self-care to the extent possible for each patient.

- Instruction of caregivers in oral health care principles and procedures. Promote assistance as needed for patients with limited abilities.

- Encourage caregivers to include oral care procedures in patient behavior modification.

- Emphasize the significance of a total preventive program.

- Explain the importance of complete oral examinations and oral hygiene care services at regular frequent intervals.

III. DENTAL HYGIENE CARE PLAN

A. Plan four-handed dental hygiene for the difficult patient.

B. Frequent appointments to include all phases of prevention:
- Dental biofilm control for the patient and the caregiver.
- Scaling.
- Fluoride therapy, including the use of fluoride varnish that can be especially helpful for patients unable to cooperate with biofilm control. Varnish application is an easy and simple procedure (page 555).
- Sealants.

IV. APPOINTMENT INTERVENTION

A. Provide a predictable and consistent experience.

B. Create a quiet environment free from sensory stimuli.
- Avoid loud, inconsistent background music, noisy dental apparatus, and irrelevant conversations.
- Avoid touching, as this may be disturbing to the patient.

C. Desensitization
- Begin with orientation to the setting and each part of the equipment.
- If patient is not ready, instrumentation may not be included at the first appointment.
- Instruction takes the form of "show-tell-do" repeated many times. Patience and firmness are necessary elements.

- Have caregiver help condition the patient by giving a plastic mouth mirror and a few dental films to take home for practice in the mouth each day.
- Use behavior modification procedures when the patient is familiar with that method. Involve caregiver(s) while presenting preventive measures in a simple step-by-step manner. Provide reinforcing rewards immediately following each success. Model the use of nonedible items and explain rationale against cariogenic food rewards.

D. Physical immobilization
- Various procedures were described in Chapter 53.
- A papoose board (Figure 53-6, page 894) may provide a safe environment for a severely autistic child unable to respond to desensitization.

REFERENCES

1. **American Psychiatric Association:** *Diagnostic and Statistical Manual of Mental Disorders* (DSM-IV). Washington, DC, American Psychiatric Association, 1994, pp. 37–43.

2. **Tesini,** D.A.: An Annotated Review of the Literature of Dental Caries and Periodontal Disease in Mentally Retarded Individuals, *Spec. Care Dentist., 1,* 75, March/April, 1981.

3. **Holmes,** L.B.: Decreasing Age of Mothers of Infants With the Down's syndrome, *N. Engl. J. Med., 298,* 1419, June 22, 1978.

4. **Cohen,** F.L.: Paternal Contributions to Birth Defects, *Nurs. Clin. North Am., 21,* 49, March, 1986.

5. **Schendel,** S.A. and Gorlin, R.J.: Frequency of Cleft Uvula and Submucous Cleft Palate in Patients With Down's Syndrome, *J. Dent. Res., 53,* 840, July–August, 1974.

6. **Izumi,** Y., Sugiyama, S., Shinozuka, O., Yamazaki, T., Ohyama, T., and Ishikawa, I.: Defective Neutrophil Chemotaxis in Down's Syndrome Patients and Its Relationship to Periodontal Destruction, *J. Periodontol., 60,* 238, May, 1989.

7. **Modéer,** T., Barr, M., and Dahllöf, G.: Periodontal Disease in Children With Down's Syndrome, *Scand. J. Dent. Res., 98,* 228, June, 1990.

8. **Jacobs,** I.N., Gray, R.F., and Todd, N.W.: Upper Airway Obstruction in Children With Down syndrome, *Arch. Otolaryngol. Head Neck Surg., 122,* 945, September, 1996.

9. **Barnett,** M.L., Friedman, D., and Kastner, T.: The Prevalence of Mitral Valve Prolapse in Patients With Down's Syndrome: Implications for Dental Management, *Oral Surg., Oral Med., Oral Pathol., 66,* 445, October, 1988.

10. **Sigal,** M.J. and Levine, N.: Down's Syndrome and Alzheimer's Disease, *J. Can. Dent. Assoc., 59,* 823, October, 1993.

11. **American Psychiatric Association:** op. cit., pp. 66–71.

12. **Rapin,** I.: Perspective: The Autistic-Spectrum Disorders. *N. Engl. J. Med., 347,* 302, August 1, 2002.

13. **United States, National Institute of Child and Maternal Health:** *Autism Questions and Answers for Health Care Professionals.* Bethesda MD, National Institute of Child Health and Human Development, Publication #0186, 2001.

14. **Kanner,** L.: Early Infantile Autism, *J. Pediatr., 25,* 211, September, 1944.

15. **Pediatric Psychopharmacology Autism Network,** Risperidone in Children With Autism and Serious Behavioral Problems, *N. Engl. J. Med., 347,* 314, August 1, 2002.

16. **Longe**, J.L.: *The GALE Encyclopedia of Medicine*, 2nd ed, Vol. 1 A-B. Detroit, Thomson Learning, 2002, pp. 417–421.

SUGGESTED READINGS

Brooks, C., Miller, L.C., Dane, J., Perkins, D., Bullock, L., Libbus, M.K., Johnson, P., and Van Stone, J.: Program Evaluation of Mobile Dental Services for Children With Special Health Care Needs, *Spec. Care Dentist., 22,* 156, July/August, 2002.

Dicks, J.L. and Banning, J.S.: Evaluation of Calculus Accumulation in Tube-Fed, Mentally Handicapped Patients: The Effects of Oral Hygiene Status, *Spec. Care Dentist., 11,* 104, May/June, 1991.

Drews, C.D., Yeargin-Allsopp, M., Decoufle, P., and Murphy, C.C.: Variation in the Influence of Selected Sociodemographic Risk Factors for Mental Retardation, *Am. J. Public Health, 85,* 329, March, 1995.

Figueiredo, L.C., Toledo, B.E.C., and Salvador, S.L.: The Relationship Between Place BANA Reactivity and Clinical Parameters in Subjects With Mental Disabilities, *Spec. Care Dentist., 20,* 195, September/October, 2000.

Lange, B., Cook, C., Dunning, O., Froeschle, M.L., and Kent, D.: Improving the Oral Hygiene of Institutionalized Mentally Retarded Clients, *J. Dent. Hyg., 74,* 205, Summer, 2000.

Loiacono, C., Jenkins, J., and Campbell, P.R.: Management of the Patient With Mental Retardation: A Case Report, *Can. Dent. Hyg. Assoc.(PROBE), 32,* 18, January/February, 1998.

Magalhaes, M.H.C.G., Kawamura, J.Y., and Araujo, L.C.A.: General and Oral Characteristics in Rett Syndrome, *Spec. Care Dentist., 22,* 147, July/August, 2002.

Messini, M., Skourti, I., Markopulos, E., Koutsia-Carouzou, C., Kyriakopoulou, E., Kostaki, S., Lambraki, D., and Georgopoulos, A.: Bacteremia After Dental Treatment in Mentally Handicapped People, *J. Clin. Periodontol., 26,* 469, July, 1999.

Shapira, J., Efrat, J., Berkey, D., and Mann, J.: Dental Health Profile of a Population With Mental Retardation in Israel, *Spec. Care Dentist., 18,* 149, July/August, 1998.

Waldman, H.B. and Perlman, S.P.: What About Dental Care for People With Mental Retardation? A Commentary, *J. Am. Coll. Dent., 69,* 35, Spring, 2002.

Down Syndrome

Acerbi, A.G., deFreitas, G., and deMagalhaes, M.H.C.G.: Prevalence of Numeric Anomalies in the Permanent Dentition of Patients With Down Syndrome, *Spec. Care Dentist., 21,* 75, March/April, 2001.

Buxton, R. and Hunter, J.: Understanding Down's Syndrome: A Review, *J. Dent. Hyg., 73,* 99, Spring, 1999.

Chaushu, S., Becker, A., Chaushu, G., and Shapira, J.: Stimulated Parotid Salivary Flow Rate in Patients With Down Syndrome, *Spec. Care Dentist., 22,* 41, January/February, 2002.

Cooley, W.C. and Graham, J.M.: Common Syndromes and Management Issues for Primary Care Physicians: Down Syndrome—An Update and Review for the Primary Pediatrician, *Clin. Pediatr., 30,* 233, April, 1991.

Desai, S.S.: Down Syndrome: A Review of the Literature, *Oral Surg. Oral Med. Oral Pathol. Oral Radiol. Endod., 84,* 279, September, 1997.

Hunt, N.: *The World of Nigel Hunt: The Diary of a Mongoloid Youth.* New York, Garrett, 1967, 126 pp.

Morinushi, T., Lopatin, D.E., and Tanaka, H.: The Relationship Between Dental Caries in the Primary Dentition and Anti *S. mutans* Serum Antibodies in Children With Down's Syndrome, *J. Clin. Pediatr. Dent., 19,* 279, Summer, 1993.

Shapira, J. and Stabholz, A.: A Comprehensive 30-Month Preventive Dental Health Program in a Pre-adolescent Population With Down's Syndrome: A Longitudinal Study, *Spec. Care Dentist.,16,* 33, January/February, 1996.

United States Center for Disease Control and Prevention: Racial Disparities in Median Age at Death of Persons With Down Syndrome—United States, 1968-1997, *MMWR, 50,* 463, June 8, 2001.

Down Syndrome: Periodontal

Amano, A., Kishima, T., Kimura, S., Takiguchi, M., Ooshima, T., Hamada, S., and Morisaki, I.: Periodontopathic Bacteria in Children With Down Syndrome, *J. Periodontol., 71,* 249, February, 2000.

Amano, A., Kishima, T., Akiyama, S., Nakagawa, I., Hamada, S., and Morisaki, I.: Relationship of Periodontopathic Bacteria With Early-Onset Periodontitis in Down's Syndrome, *J. Periodontol., 72,* 368, March, 2001.

Barr-Agholme, M., Dahllof, G., Modéer, T., Engstrom, P.-E., and Engstrom, G.N.: Periodontal Conditions and Salivary Immunoglobulins in Individuals With Down Syndrome, *J. Periodontol., 69,* 1119, October, 1998.

Hanookai, D., Nowzari, H., Contreras, A., Morrison, J.L., and Slots, J.: Herpesviruses and Periodontopathic Bacteria in Trisomy 21 Periodontitis, *J. Periodontol., 71,* 376, March, 2000.

Autism

Armstrong, D. and Matt, M.: Autoextraction in an Autistic Dental Patient: A Case Report, *Spec. Care Dentist., 19,* 72, March/April, 1999.

Barton, M. and Volkmar, F.R.: How Commonly Are Known Medical Conditions Associated With Autism? *J. Autism Develop. Disorders, 28,* 273, August, 1998.

Bryson, S.E. and Smith, I.M.: Epidemiology of Autism: Prevalence, Associated Disorders, and Implications for Service Delivery, *Ment. Retard. Develop. Disabil. Res. Rev., 4,* 97, December,1998.

Faulks, D. and Hennequin, M.: Evaluation of a Long-term Oral Health Program by Carers of Children and Adults With Intellectual Disabilities, *Spec. Care Dentist., 20,* 199, September/October, 2000.

Filipek, P.A., Accardo, P.J., Baranek, G.T., Cook, E.H. Jr., Dawson, G., Gordon, G., Gravel, J.S., Johnson, C.P., Kallen, R.J., Levy, S.E., Minshew, N.J., Prizant, B.M., Rapin, I., Rogers, S.J., Stone, W.L., Teplin, S., Tuchman, R.F., and Volkmar, F.R.: The Screening and Diagnosis of Autistic Spectrum Disorders, *J. Autism Develop. Disorders, 29,* 439, December, 1999.

Folstein, S.E.: Autism, *Int. Rev. Psychiatry, 11,* 269, November, 1999.

Johnson, C.D., Matt, M.K., Dennison, D., Brown, R.S., and Koh, S.: A Case Report Preventing Factitious Gingival Injury in an Autistic Patient, *J. Am. Dent. Assoc., 127,* 244, February, 1996.

Klein, U. and Nowak, A.J.: Autistic Disorder: A Review for the Pediatric Dentist. *Pediatr. Dent., 20,* 312, September–October, 1998.

Regn, J.M., Mauriello, S.M., and Kulinski, R.F.: Management of the Autistic Patient by the Dental Hygienist, *J. Pract. Hyg., 8,* 19, January/February, 1999.

The Patient With a Mental Disorder

Esther M. Wilkins, BS, RDH, DMD
Janet H. Towle, RN, RDH, BS, MEd

CHAPTER OUTLINE

A mental disorder is a complex, clinically significant behavioral or psychological syndrome or pattern that is associated with present distress or disability. The causes may be related to behavioral, psychologic, or biologic dysfunction in the individual.[1]

A classification of mental disorders does not classify people, but rather it is the disorders that people have that are classified. For example, the patient should be referred to as "an individual with schizophrenia," not as "a schizophrenic."[1]

With the discovery and official approval of new psychotropic drugs for more effective therapy, and with the current policies of deinstitutionalization, more individuals with mental disorders are seeking dental and dental hygiene care in dental offices and clinics. Care for a person with a psychiatric illness, or for one who may be undergoing an emotional crisis, presents increased challenges for health professionals.

The American Psychiatric Association has classified more than 200 types of mental disorders in the document *Diagnostic and Statistical Manual of Mental Disorders (DSM-IV)*. The *DSM* is in accord with the *International Classification of Diseases (ICD)* published by the World Health Organization.[2] Each disorder has characteristic signs and symptoms. Terminology related to the disorders is listed and defined in Box 60-1.

This chapter includes descriptions of frequently encountered psychiatric disorders, namely, schizophrenia, mood disorders, anxiety disorders, and eating disorders. Other disorders are described elsewhere in the text,

BOX 60-1 KEY WORDS: Mental Disorders

Affect: emotion or feeling; tone of reaction to persons and events.

Agitation: excessive motor activity, usually nonpurposeful and associated with internal tension.

Anxiolytic medication: ability to relieve anxiety or emotional tension, also called antianxiety agent.

Bradykinesia: abnormal slowness of movement; sluggish physical and mental responses.

Catatonia: no voluntary movement; physical rigidity; fixed position may be maintained for hours.

Cognitive: mental process of comprehension, judgment, memory.

Decompensate: appearance or exacerbation of a mental disorder.

Delusion: false belief firmly held though contradicted by social reality.

Dementia: loss of cognitive and intellectual functions sufficiently severe to interfere with social and occupational functioning.

Electroconvulsive therapy (ECT): electroshock therapy; a form of somatic therapy in which an electric current is used to produce convulsions; primarily used to treat depression.

Euphoria: feeling of well-being; in psychiatry, abnormal or exaggerated sense of well-being.

Hallucination: false sensory perception in the absence of an actual external stimulus.

Illusion: a mental impression derived from misinterpretation of an actual sensory stimulus; a false perception.

Insomnia: wakefulness; inability to sleep in the absence of noise or other disturbance.

Neurosis: a mental disorder that usually involves the use of unconscious defense mechanisms as a means of coping; individual is not out of touch with reality.

Noncompliance: failure to carry out prescribed healthcare plan, for example, failure to take medications as prescribed.

Paranoia: mental disorder characterized by delusions of persecution, illusions of grandeur, or combination of both.

Perimylolysis: erosion of enamel and dentin as a result of chemical and mechanical effects.

Phobia: persistent, unrealistic pathologic fear or dread out of proportion to the stimulus from a particular object or situation.

Prodrome: a premonitory symptom; a symptom indicating the onset of disease.

Psychosis: a significant major mental disorder that so greatly impairs perception, thinking, emotional response, and/or personal orientation that the individual loses touch with reality.

Psychotherapy: treatment of emotional, behavioral, personality, and psychiatric disorders by means of individual or group verbal or nonverbal communication with the patient.

Psychotropic medication: a medication that alters the mind; the major categories are antipsychotic, antianxiety, antidepressant, an antimanic agents.

Tardive dyskinesia: involuntary movements of the mouth, lips, tongue, and jaws, usually associated with long-term use of antipsychotic medication.

for example, alcoholism (Chapter 61), Alzheimer's disease (Chapter 49), and dementia due to Parkinson's disease (Chapter 55).

Knowledge of the types of mental disorders and their signs and symptoms can help the clinician to recognize a patient's needs and to understand a patient's behaviors. Confidence and trust by the patient are essential for communication and the patient's acceptance of clinical care.

Principles of informed consent are applied for patients of all ages with mental disorders. Many patients with mental disorders are capable of signing their own consent form. Information for obtaining informed consent is described on page 369.

■ SCHIZOPHRENIA

Schizophrenia is a complex, chronic mental disorder. Disturbances in feeling, thinking, and behavior significantly impair function to a level below normal for the individual. Schizophrenia is a major psychotic illness in which the individual may be out of touch with reality. Symptoms include delusions, hallucinations, disorganized thinking, and incoherence.

The onset is usually between the ages of 17 and 25 in females, slightly older than for males. Although the cause is not fully understood, genetic factors can make an individual more vulnerable. Periods of remission and recurrence may occur.

I. SYMPTOMS OF SCHIZOPHRENIA

The disturbance progresses from subchronic to remission with acute exacerbations of varying frequencies. Symptoms may be triggered by social, psychologic, or environmental stresses.

The three phases are described as *prodromal, active,* and *residual*. Prodromal symptoms may appear as signs of deterioration for as long as 1 year before the active phase. Box 60-2 shows the symptoms of each phase.

Active-phase symptoms are *positive,* those that reflect unusual, profound behavior, or *negative,* those that show the absence of behavior that might be expected normally.

Rates of alcohol and drug abuse are high among patients with schizophrenia. Many patients diagnosed with schizophrenia also qualify for a diagnosis of alcohol abuse. Drug and alcohol abuse can aggravate psychiatric symptoms and lead to poor treatment compliance, increased hospitalization, homelessness, and suicide.[3]

II. TREATMENT OF SCHIZOPHRENIA

The response to initial treatment is a critical predictor of the long-term prognosis. The prognosis has generally been considered guarded to poor. Evidence shows that although deterioration may occur during the early years, the condition may stabilize with treatment during middle age.

A. Pharmacotherapy[4]

The objectives of treatment are to reduce or alleviate the delusions, hallucinations, and other positive symptoms (Box 60-2) and to enable the patient to function in daily living. The use of antipsychotic medications has improved the outcomes of treatment and led to the process of deinstitutionalization.

Schizophrenia is associated with an excess of dopamine at specific synapses in the brain. Medications are used to block dopamine receptors.

1. **Typical Antipsychotic Drugs**[4,5]
a. Phenothiazines (chlorpromazine [Thorazine™])
b. Butyrophenones (haloperidol [Haldol™])
c. Thioxanthenes (thiothixene [Navane™])

BOX 60-2 Symptoms of Schizophrenia

Prodromal and Residual Symptoms	**Active-Phase Symptoms**
Marked social isolation or withdrawal	Positive Symptoms
Marked impairment in role functioning (as wage earner, student, homemaker)	Delusions
Markedly peculiar behavior	Hallucinations
Marked impairment in personal hygiene	Disorganized speech
Blunted or inappropriate affect	Catatonia
Digressive, vague speech or lack of speech	Disorganized or bizarre behavior
Odd beliefs or magical thinking	Negative Symptoms
Unusual perceptual experiences	Flat affect
Marked lack of initiative, interests, or energy	Lack of voluntary action
	Speechlessness
	No pleasure from events that usually give pleasure

Adapted from American Psychiatric Association: *DSM-IV,* 1994, pp. 285, 290.

2. **Atypical Drugs**
a. Dibenzodiazepines (clozapine [Clozaril™])
b. Benzisoxazoles (risperidone [Risperdal™])
c. Other drugs

B. Adverse Effects of Medications

Careful monitoring is essential because side effects can be severe. For example, weekly white blood cell counts are needed during clozapine therapy because of the high risk of agranulocytosis.[5] Table 60-1 lists a few of the many side effects of antipsychotic medications, with suggestions for appointment adaptations.

C. Maintenance

After an acute episode, the dosage is adjusted for the remission period. A minimal effective dose is important because of the risk of tardive dyskinesia. Non-compliance in continuing medication is a common cause of psychotic relapse and rehospitalization.[4]

D. Psychosocial Therapy

Psychosocial therapy is integrated with pharmacotherapy. Objectives include to ensure compliance with the use of prescribed medications and to give support in the effort to cope with stress.

Long-term treatment for psychosocial and vocational recovery after an acute psychotic episode must include family and all those close to the patient. Psychotherapy may include a variety of vocational rehabilitation efforts and training in social skills.

III. DENTAL HYGIENE CARE

A. Oral Implications[6,7]

1. Overall degeneration of health factors may have occurred because of neglect of diet, exercise,

▪ TABLE 60-1 EFFECTS OF ANTIPSYCHOTIC MEDICATION

SIDE EFFECTS	IMPLICATIONS FOR APPOINTMENT
Dystonia Muscle contractions	Laryngeal spasm; coughing Unable to turn head
Dysarthria Difficult speech	Communication problem
Parkinson-like syndrome Shuffling gait Muscular rigidity Resting tremor (pill rolling) Facial grimacing Bradykinesia	Difficult to gain cooperation Patient positioning Instrument positioning; retraction
Akathisia Restlessness Pacing	Plan short appointments
Akinesia Loss of voluntary movement Lethargy, fatigue feelings	Adjust patient position
Tardive dyskinesia Involuntary mouth and jaw movements	Difficulty in instrumentation Wearing dentures difficult or impossible Muscle fatigue; may need mouth prop
Anticholinergic effects Xerostomia Blurred vision	Dental caries prevention Fluoride dentifrice; saliva substitute Seeing visual aids
Cardiovascular Postural hypotension Tachycardia, palpitations	Have patient sit up slowly and wait before standing Monitor vital signs
Sedation Drowsiness	Interfere with patient's daily routine Patient may be late; needs reminders
Blood Reduced leukocytes Agranulocytosis	Increased susceptibility to infection Oral candidiasis may be present

sleep, general cleanliness, personal grooming, and oral care.

2. Concurrent alcohol and/or drug abuse, as well as smoking, can influence dental and periodontal health.

3. Xerostomia leads to an increase in rampant dental caries. Candy used for stimulating saliva can have devastating effects.

B. Appointment Planning

Elective dental and dental hygiene treatment is not carried out during an acute exacerbation. Treatment is undertaken when the patient's symptoms are reasonably controlled by medications.

If the patient decompensates during a dental or dental hygiene appointment, immediate referral is needed. Because schizophrenia is most often a lifelong disorder, planning for future oral health is essential.

C. Appointment Interventions

1. Review medical and medications history; study possible drug side effects for necessary appointment modifications (Table 60-1).

2. Review consultation notes from mental health physician (psychiatrist) relative to medications, alcohol or other substance use, and medical-legal competence for informed consent.

3. Plan a simple routine. For a series of appointments and maintenance, use a familiar, organized routine that is comfortable for the patient.

4. Decrease stimulation; create a restful atmosphere; if background music is present, keep it low and soft.

5. Provide instruction in oral care.
   a. Help the patient to improve the level of personal oral care on a daily basis.
   b. When applicable, evaluate the patient's personal caregiver for attitude and knowledge and provide information and instruction.

6. Use a mouth prop to assist the patient with tardive dyskinesia. Remember the patient does not have control of mouth movements and can appreciate stability.

■ MOOD DISORDERS

The primary mood disorders are *major depressive disorder* and *bipolar disorder.* A major depressive disorder is unipolar, whereas a bipolar disorder is marked by severe mood swings from depression to elation (mania). Both unipolar and bipolar disorders are characterized by periods of remission and recurrence.

BOX 60-3 Risk Factors for Depression

Prior episodes of depression

Family history of depression

Prior suicide attempts

Female gender

Age at onset <40 years

Postpartum period

Lack of social support

Stressful life events

Personal history of sexual abuse

Current substance abuse

Adapted from Stuart, G.W. and Sundeen, S.J.: *Principles & Practice of Psychiatric Nursing,* 5th ed. St. Louis, Mosby, 1995, p. 431.

Depression is among the most common of the many psychiatric illnesses, yet it may not always be recognized and treated. Bipolar disorder may begin by ages 25 to 30, whereas major depression is more often first evident in middle age. All ages may be affected, but middle-aged women and elderly persons of both sexes are particularly vulnerable to severe depression. Risk factors for depression are listed in Box 60-3.

Transient depressed moods occur in the lives of most people. Sadness over unforeseen tragic events, illnesses, death, or disappointments in career or other life plans causes depressed feelings.

Depression is a disturbance marked by apathy, fear, sadness, and loss of mobility and energy. Transient depressed moods usually can be overcome in time and need to be differentiated from depression as a major depressive illness.

■ MAJOR DEPRESSIVE DISORDER

I. CHARACTERISTICS OF A MAJOR DEPRESSIVE EPISODE

Characteristics of a major depressive episode are listed in Box 60-4. Both thought disorders and physical signs are involved. Depression increases the risk of suicide.

The manifestations of depression can vary considerably among patients and between age groups. Some

BOX 60-4 Characteristics of a Major Depressive Episode

- Depressed mood
- Markedly diminished interest or pleasure in all or almost all activities
- Significant weight loss or gain
- Insomnia or hypersomnia
- Psychomotor agitation or retardation
- Fatigue or loss of energy
- Feelings of worthlessness or excessive guilt
- Diminished ability to concentrate; indecisiveness
- Recurrent thoughts of death or suicide
- Feelings of hopelessness

Adapted from American Psychiatric Association: *DSM-IV*, 1994, p. 327.

individuals experience only one episode of major depression in their entire lives.

For children, depression interferes with interrelations with other children and with motivations to learn and play. The adolescent may demonstrate with substance abuse, antisocial behavior, school difficulties, and/or poor hygiene.[8]

Depressed adults may lack motivation and initiative and may find interactions with people at work or in social settings difficult. Elderly depressed individuals can feel isolated because of the many losses in their lives. In addition, their lives may be influenced by physical and mental changes associated with aging.

II. TREATMENT OF DEPRESSION

Antidepression medications are the primary treatment for individuals with depression. In addition, treatment may include lifestyle changes, correction of sleep disorders, new diet and eating patterns, and exercise, along with counseling and practical psychotherapy.

Hospitalization may be indicated when potential danger of suicide or harm to others exists. Severe health problems can be related to self-neglect with excessive weight loss.

A. Psychopharmacotherapy[9,10]

Antidepressive medications are indicated for major depression and the depressive stage of bipolar disorder. For a patient with a substance-induced mood disorder, antidepressant or mood-stabilizing therapy is withheld for at least 30 days to confirm medical diagnosis of primary mood disorder.

Each drug has characteristic adverse reactions. Xerostomia is the major oral problem.
1. SSRIs (Selective Serotonin Re-uptake Inhibitors)
    a. Often the initial therapy for depressive illness.
    b. Advantages: tolerability better than earlier drugs; better compliance; safety in overdose.
    c. Specific products: fluoxetine (Prozac™); sertraline (Zoloft™); paroxetine (Paxil™); fluvoxamine (Luvox™).
2. Tricyclic Antidepressants
    a. Less used than in past: risk of overdose.
    b. Xerostomia often a serious side effect.
3. MAOIs (monoamine oxidase inhibitors): certain foods and other drugs must be avoided to prevent hypertensive crisis.
4. Number of atypical antidepressant medications is increasing.

B. Psychotherapy

Patients with lesser degrees of depression may benefit from psychotherapy alone. Psychotherapy and pharmacotherapy lend support to each other. Improvement in work performance and social adjustment with increased compliance in carrying out basic personal health needs, including oral hygiene, can be noted.

C. Electroconvulsive Therapy: Indications

1. Patient for whom antidepressant medications are contraindicated.
2. Patient who is nonresponsive to optimal pharmacotherapy.
3. Patient with major depression who also has delusions.
4. Patient with overwhelming suicidal preoccupation or substantially diminished food intake.
5. The need for an immediate response (such as for a catatonic patient).

III. DENTAL HYGIENE CARE

The patient with a major depressive disorder and the patient with the depressive phase of bipolar disorder have the same general characteristics as those described in this section.

A. Personal Factors

The symptoms of the depressed individual not controlled by medication are listed in Box 60-4 and can be considered in preparation for dental hygiene care. By appearance and facial expression, the patient may appear to be pessimistic and show feelings of sadness and gloom. Inattentiveness, memory impairment, and diminished motivation are typical. On the other hand, the medicated patient may demonstrate symptoms of the side effects of medication.

When food and alcoholic beverages are used as coping mechanisms, weight gain may be considerable. Food choices frequently include many sweets, which contribute to dental and periodontal breakdown. Oral problems related to alcohol abuse are described on page 1018.

B. Oral Health Implications[11]

1. Side effects of medications: xerostomia, which leads to high risk of enamel and root caries and to problems of denture retention.
2. Omission of general health habits and neglect of oral care make the person susceptible to various infections and illnesses.
3. Loss of taste perception can contribute to a diet high in cariogenic foods with high levels of sucrose.

C. Appointment Interventions[11,12]

1. Assessment
   a. Monitor the medical and medications histories closely; note side effects and contraindications for new drug therapies.
   b. Review consultations with medical/psychiatric specialists caring for the patient.
   c. Intraoral/extraoral examination: check for signs of xerostomia.
2. Approach
   a. Provide positive reinforcement and reassurance. Avoid negative guilt-inducing words. Depressed patients already blame themselves for all bad things.
   b. Show genuine interest, but avoid attempts to cheer the patient by joking or laughing or making such remarks as, "Let's see you smile now."
3. Preventive Instruction
   a. Dental biofilm control: Teach patient and caregivers the need for daily measures to preserve the teeth and periodontal tissues.
   b. Xerostomia
      i. Home fluoride custom tray daily
      ii. Saliva substitute containing fluoride
      iii. Alcohol-free, over-the-counter fluoride rinse or brush-on gel
4. Scaling and Debridement
   a. Adjust dental light carefully and provide tinted protective eyewear for the patient with photosensitivity, a side effect of certain medications.

   b. Use local anesthesia. Anxious and depressed patients can be sensitive and may need profound anesthesia.
   c. Provide fluoride treatment after scaling.
   d. Use care to prevent postural hypotension. Sit the patient up slowly from a reclined position and have the patient remain seated a few moments before standing.

▪ BIPOLAR DISORDER

Bipolar disorder is the major mood disorder in which episodes of mania (elation) and depression occur. It was formerly called "manic-depressive" disorder. When untreated, periods of elation can average 6 months in duration, whereas periods of depression may last longer. A return to normal behavior between episodes is usual.

I. PHASES AND SYMPTOMS

A. Depressive Phase

The characteristics for a major depressive episode (Box 60-4) and for a depressed episode of bipolar disorder are similar.

B. Manic Phase

Mania is characterized by excessive elation, hyperactivity, and accelerated thinking and speaking. A severe manic episode causes marked impairment in occupational and social functioning. Characteristics of a manic episode are listed in Box 60-5.

BOX 60-5 Characteristics of Manic Episode

- Inflated self-esteem or grandiosity
- Decreased need for sleep
- More talkative than usual or pressure to keep talking
- Flight of ideas
- Distractibility (that is, attention easily drawn to unimportant or irrelevant external stimuli)
- Increase in goal-directed activity (socially, at work or school, or sexually) or psychomotor agitation
- Excessive involvement in pleasurable activities that have a high potential for painful consequences (for example, engages in unrestrained buying sprees, sexual indiscretions, or foolish business investments)

Adapted from American Psychiatric Association: *DSM-IV,* 1994, p. 332.

II. TREATMENT OF BIPOLAR DEPRESSION

Three distinct treatment strategies apply, one for the manic phase, one for the depressive phase, and one for the normal phase, which requires maintenance therapy. Treatment for the depressive phase is described under major depression on page 998.

Both pharmacotherapy and psychotherapy are used for the manic phase. Initially, hospitalization may be needed to protect the individual from harm to self or others.

A. Pharmacotherapy[9,13,14]

Treatment requires a three-pronged approach.
1. Sedation is often needed for the acute stage of mania.
2. Antidepressant therapy may be needed for the patient with moderate to severe depression.
3. Maintenance therapy: lithium carbonate.[9,13]
   - Prevents recurrence of bipolar disorder when given on a maintenance drug level.
   - Possible side effects include gastrointestinal irritation, fine hand tremor, thirst, polyuria, and muscular weakness. Prolonged use may lead to renal tube damage and hypothyroidism.
   - Frequent monitoring is important to guard against lithium toxicity, which can occur with long-term drug use.
   - Antiepileptic drugs are used as an alternative to lithium in selected cases.

B. Psychotherapy

Psychotherapy can help to lower stress factors and uncover early warning signs of an approaching high or low mood. Psychosocial support is important to prevent relapse.

III. DENTAL HYGIENE CARE

A. Personal Factors

Characteristics of an individual during a manic episode can be studied in Box 60-5. During the manic phase, the patient is overactive, restless, and in constant motion, and may behave in an aggressive, fearless manner.

Many patients talk quickly, jump from thought to thought, and have a short attention span. A tendency to argue and become irritable may be apparent if pressured in any way.

B. Oral Health Implications

1. Oral hygiene needs are often unmet.

2. Patient unlikely to report injury or illness; a complete oral assessment can be especially significant.
3. Gingival tissues may appear abraded and lacerated because of overeager grandiose brushing motions.
4. Xerostomia from long-term use of medications will require use of a saliva substitute. A complete preventive program with daily fluoride therapy and an anticariogenic diet is important.
5. Lithium may impart a metallic taste in the mouth.

C. Appointment Interventions

Lithium medication and other treatments usually provide control for the nonhospitalized patient. The need for protecting the patient and others from overactive behavior may not be experienced in the private clinical setting because elective dental and dental hygiene appointments usually are postponed until the patient is under medical control.
1. Simplify the surroundings; provide a comfortable uncluttered environment.
2. Do not rush the patient, as doing so can lead to anger and hostility.
3. Use quiet persuasion; keep the voice firm and low-pitched with a coaxing quality.
4. When applicable, help the patient's caregiver to learn procedures for dental caries prevention and periodontal health.
5. Patient instruction is difficult because the patient has a short attention span and may not like fine detail. Avoid long descriptions.

▪ POSTPARTUM MOOD DISTURBANCES[15]

The puerperium is the 6-week period after childbirth when the body undergoes physical and physiologic changes. During the entire postpartum period, many physiologic and psychologic stresses are related to the changes taking place in the mother's life. Degrees of emotional reactions are evident and range from postpartum blues to psychosis. Postpartum psychosis is considered a major psychiatric emergency.

I. POSTPARTUM BLUES

A period of nonpsychotic depression for a few days after giving birth is not uncommon. There may be crying, irritability, and mood shifts.

II. POSTPARTUM DEPRESSION

A moderate to severe depression may begin by the second to third week postpartum. Symptoms include excessive fatigue, insomnia, loss of appetite, and loss of interest and enthusiasm.

III. POSTPARTUM PSYCHOSIS

Postpartum or puerperal psychosis is a mood disorder. It may be of a depressive or manic type.

A. Underlying Causes

1. Secondary to preexisting mental illness, such as bipolar disorder or schizophrenia.
2. Stress.
3. Conflicts about motherhood, such as unwanted pregnancy, fears about mothering, and marital problems.

B. Symptoms

1. *Early*. Complaints of insomnia, restlessness, tearfulness, fatigue, and emotional unsteadiness.
2. *Progressive*. Confusion, irrationality, delirium, and obsessive concerns about the baby. Thoughts of bringing harm to the baby or oneself are not unusual.

C. Treatment

Without treatment, risk of suicide, infanticide, or both exists. A favorable outcome can be expected with appropriate treatment, family support, and no preexisting illness.
1. *Medical Care*. Treat for other (organic) illnesses.
2. *Suicidal Precautions*. Baby should not be left alone with mother.
3. *Pharmacotherapy*. In accord with symptoms of depression.
4. *Psychotherapy*. Individual and marital. Arrangements for assistance at home must be made before hospital release.
5. *Extended Treatment*. Counseling in infant care with observation for emergence of major mood disorder.

■ ANXIETY DISORDERS

Anxiety is experienced as apprehension, tension, or dread that results from the anticipation of danger, the source of which is unknown or unrecognized. Anxiety is the result of feeling a threat to the person's being, self-esteem, or identity. Fear, on the other hand, is an emotional or physiologic response to a recognized source of danger.

In normal life, some mild anxiety provides an effective stimulus to improved performance. As a psychiatric symptom, anxiety can be excessive, irrational, and beyond the control of the individual.

I. TYPES AND SYMPTOMS OF ANXIETY DISORDERS[16]

The most common anxiety disorders are described in this section. The disorders have symptoms of fear, excess worry, and avoidance behavior that are revealed in a variety of ways and degrees of severity. The anxiety disorders also can produce varying degrees of occupational and social dysfunction. Certain patients may have secondary problems of alcohol and other substance abuse. The abuse may be the result of an attempt at self-medication.

A. Panic Attack

The symptoms that may occur in a panic attack are listed in Box 60-6. The panic attack itself is a symptom in several of the anxiety disorders. *An overwhelming sense of impending doom is the cardinal symptom of the attack.*

A panic attack may be unexpected (uncued) or "situationally bound" (cued). A situationally bound panic attack invariably results from exposure to a specific trigger. Such triggers are characteristic of social and specific phobias that are described in this section.

BOX 60-6 Symptoms of Panic Attack

- Shortness of breath
- Dizziness, unsteady feelings, or faintness
- Palpitations or accelerated heart rate
- Trembling or shaking
- Sweating (clammy hands)
- Choking
- Nausea or abdominal stress
- Numbness or tingling sensations
- Flushes (hot flashes) or chills
- Chest pain or discomfort
- Fear of dying
- Fear of going crazy or losing control

Adapted from American Psychiatric Association: *DSM-IV,* 1994, p. 395.

B. Panic Disorder

Panic disorder is characterized by recurrent panic attacks that are usually unexpected. Panic disorder may occur alone or with agoraphobia.

Agoraphobia is the fear of being in places or situations from which escape might be difficult or embarrassing or in which help might not be available in the event of a panic attack. The fear is of open spaces, of crowds, or of going outside the home alone and away from a safe place.

C. Posttraumatic Stress Disorder

An initiating traumatic event has occurred outside the range of usual human experience. It may be destruction to the home or family or may result from a man-made disaster, such as war, imprisonment, torture, rape, or other exposure associated with intense horror, fear, or serious threat to life. A child may have stress disorder brought on by physical or sexual abuse.

Flashbacks of the traumatic experience and the attendant terror may be precipitated by a stimulus that can be readily associated with the original event. Through dreams or recollections, the patient may have the feeling of reliving the event. Symptoms of depression or panic attacks may be evident in an acute episode.

D. Generalized Anxiety Disorder

There is persistent, pervasive anxiety and excessive worry but not associated with life-threatening fears or "attacks." It may be complicated by depression, alcohol abuse, or anxiety related to a general medical condition.

II. TREATMENT OF ANXIETY DISORDERS[17]

A. Basic Therapeutic Approach

1. Eliminate the intake of caffeine, alcohol, and drugs of abuse. Anxiety disorders are frequently complicated by alcohol abuse.
2. Diagnose and treat other medical and psychiatric problems. Anxiety disorders may emerge with depression, which should be treated first or at least simultaneously.
3. Exercise. Participation in vigorous aerobics or an active sport helps to eliminate physical and psychologic symptoms and enhances the patient's sense of control. Working and keeping busy are important.

B. Cognitive-Behavioral Therapy

A skilled behavioral therapist is needed. Relaxation, biofeedback, and other behavioral therapies have shown selective successes. The support of family and friends can be significant.

C. Pharmacotherapy

As few medications as possible should be used. Treatment can best be focused on the patient's sleeping habits, physical activity, and attainment of personal control in general. Determination of a patient's specific problem is essential because treatment for each disorder is different. When treatment is indicated, antianxiety and antidepressant medications are the drugs of choice.

1. *Antianxiety Medications.* Benzodiazepines.
   a. Objectives: Reduce tension and relieve anxiety; induce sleep.
   b. Prescription: Short-term basis for immediate need only; gradual discontinuance to prevent withdrawal symptoms.
   c. Possible side effects: Confusion, dizziness, muscle weakness, difficulty in speaking, skin rash.
   d. Adverse effects: Potential for addiction, withdrawal symptoms, diminished alertness (drowsiness), impaired eye-hand coordination, xerostomia.
2. *Antidepressant Medication.* Antidepressants may be used in the treatment of panic attack (page 998).

III. DENTAL HYGIENE CARE

A. Personal Factors

Each anxiety disorder has its own specific characteristics. Individuals suffering from an anxiety disorder maintain contact with reality and may be aware of the type of their disorder. Relationships with other people are often strained.

Physical complaints, such as rapid heartbeat, hyperventilation, tightness in the throat, and constant fatigue, are common. Such symptoms may lead to an anxiety about the anxiety.

B. Oral Implications

1. Hypersensitivity of the teeth, related to patient's general tenseness and irritability, may be present.
2. Xerostomia related to medications can cause severe problems for dental caries. Candy or cariogenic beverages used to allay dry mouth lead to enamel and root caries.
3. Oral cleanliness may not be present, even in a patient with an obsession for cleanliness. The opposite may be true, however, and a patient may perform such excessive, vigorous toothbrushing that gingival and dental abrasion result.

Clark, D.B.: Dental Care for the Patient With Bipolar Disorder, *J. Can. Dent. Assoc., 69,* 20, January, 2003.

Elter, J.R., White, B.A., Gaynes, B.N., and Bader, J.D.: Relationship of Clinical Depression to Periodontal Treatment Outcome, *J. Periodontol., 73,* 441, April, 2002.

Friedlander, A.H., Friedlander, I.K., and Marder, S.R.: Bipolar I Disorder: Psychopathology, Medical Management and Dental Implications, *J. Am. Dent. Assoc., 133,* 1209, September, 2002.

Friedlander, A.H. and Norman, D.C.: Late-Life Depression: Psychopathology, Medical Interventions, and Dental Implications, *Oral Surg. Oral Med. Oral Pathol. Oral Radiol. Endod., 94,* 404, October, 2002.

Rigolizzo, D. and Gurenlian, J.R.: Depression, *Access, 16,* 40, April, 2002.

Robert, E.: Treating Depression in Pregnancy (Editorial), *N. Engl. J. Med., 335,* 1056, October 3, 1996.

Spolarich, A.E.: Treating Clients Who Take Antidepressants, *Access, 14,* 32, July, 2000.

Anxiety

Coyle, J.T.: Drug Treatment of Anxiety Disorders in Children, *N. Engl. J. Med., 344,* 1326, April 26, 2001.

Friedlander, A.H., Freymiller, E.G., Yagiela, J.A., and Eth, S.: Dental Management of the Adolescent With Panic Disorder, *ASDC J. Dent. Child., 60,* 365, November–December, 1993.

Friedlander, A.H. and Eth, S.: Dental Management Considerations in Children With Obsessive-Compulsive Disorder, *ASDC J. Dent. Child., 58,* 217, May–June, 1991.

Schmaling, K.B. and Bell, J.: Asthma and Panic Disorder, *Arch. Fam. Med., 6,* 20, January/February, 1997.

Ursano, R.J.: Post-traumatic Stress Disorder (Editorial), *N. Engl. J. Med., 346,* 130, January 10, 2002.

Yehuda, R.: Post-traumatic Stress Disorder, *N. Engl. J. Med., 346,* 108, January 10, 2002.

Eating Disorders

Austin, L.D. and Crafton, B.: The Bulimic Patient: Confrontation, Intervention, Referral, *Access, 14,* 35, December, 2000.

Becker, A.E., Grinspoon, S.K., Klibanski, A., and Herzog, D.B.: Eating Disorders, *N. Engl. J. Med., 340,* 1092, April 8, 1999.

Ediger, M.: Do the Eating Habits of Anorexics and Bulimics Have an Effect on Their Oral Health? *J. Canad. Dent. Hyg. Assoc./ Probe, 28,* 139, July/August, 1994.

Gurenlian, J.R.: Eating Disorders, *J. Dent. Hyg., 76,* 219, Summer, 2002.

Kneisl, C.R., ed.: Eating Disorders (12 articles), *Nurs. Clin. North Am., 26,* 665–800, September, 1991.

Robb, N.D., Smith, B.G., and Geidrys-Leeper, E.: The Distribution of Erosion in the Dentitions of Patients With Eating Disorders, *Br. Dent. J., 178,* 171, March 11, 1995.

The Patient With an Alcohol-Related Disorder

The use of alcohol is common in a large percentage of the population of all ages from teenage through the elderly. Some people are considered light drinkers, some moderate, and others heavy or problem drinkers. A small percent are dependent on alcohol and suffer from *alcoholism*. Alcohol dependence is a chronic, progressive disease that is treatable and can be arrested. Treatment for this illness implies control, not complete cure. The *recovering alcoholic* must be dedicated to lifelong abstinence.

People from each category of alcohol use appear as patients needing dental and dental hygiene care. Knowledge of their social and physical health histories and of the effect alcohol use may have on oral health is essential to dental hygiene care planning.

■ DESCRIPTION

Key words and terminology to describe the use and abuse of alcohol are defined in Box 61-1. Alcohol used for drinking purposes is ethyl alcohol or ethanol. Other alcohols are methyl, an industrial solvent, and isopropyl, used for rubbing alcohol.

I. CLINICAL PATTERN OF ALCOHOL USE

Alcohol dependency develops after periods of use of alcohol followed by pathologic abuse. In the early period, the person functions appropriately in work, family, and social situations.

BOX 61-1 KEY WORDS AND ABBREVIATIONS: Alcoholism

Abstinence: refrain from use; complete abstinence from alcohol is the objective of a recovering alcoholic.

Abuse: substance abuse with respect to alcohol abuse involves persistent patterns of heavy alcohol intake associated with health consequences and/or impairment in social functioning.

Acne rosacea: facial skin condition usually characterized by a flushed appearance; often accompanied by puffiness and a "spider-web" effect of broken capillaries.

Addiction: physiologic and/or psychologic dependence.

> **Drug addiction:** state of periodic or chronic intoxication produced by repeated consumption of a drug; characterized by an overwhelming desire to continue the use of the drug and a tendency to increase the dosage.

Alcoholism: alcohol dependence; progressive chronic disease with physiologic, psychologic, and behavioral implications.

Amnesia: impairment of long- and/or short-term memory.

Analgesia: loss of sensibility to pain without loss of consciousness.

Antabuse: brand name of the generic drug **disulfiram;** used to deter consumption of alcohol by persons being treated for alcohol dependency by inducing vomiting.

Blackout: temporary amnesia occurring during periods of intensive drinking; person is not unconscious.

Chemical dependence: a primary chronic disease with genetic, psychosocial, and environmental factors influencing its development and manifestations.

Delirium: extreme mental and usually motor excitement marked by a rapid succession of confused and unconnected ideas; often with illusions and hallucinations; may be accompanied by tremors.

Delirium tremens: "DTs"; a serious, acute condition associated with the last stages of alcohol withdrawal.

Dementia: condition of deteriorated mentality characterized by a marked decline of intellectual functioning.

Dependence: drug or substance dependence; with respect to alcohol refers to a physical and psychologic dependence on alcohol that results in impaired ability to control drinking behavior; dependence is differentiated from abuse by manifestations of craving, tolerance, and physical dependence, as well as by an inability to exercise restraint over drinking.

Detoxification: treatment designed to assist in recovery from the toxic effects of a drug; involves withdrawal and may include pharmacologic and/or nonpharmacologic treatment with psychotherapy and counseling.

DSM-IV: *Diagnostic and Statistical Manual of Mental Disorders,* 4th ed., published by the American Psychiatric Association.

Euphoria: feeling of well-being, elation; without fear or worry.

Fetal alcohol effects (FAE): offspring of alcoholic mother who does not have all of the criteria of FAS.

Fetal alcohol syndrome (FAS): an abnormal pattern of growth and development in some children born to chronically alcoholic mothers.

Hallucination: a sensory impression (sight, touch, sound, smell, or taste) that has no basis in external stimulation; may have psychologic causes, or may result from use of drugs (including alcohol), brain tumor, senility, or exhaustion.

Hyperthermia: greatly increased temperature.

Illicit: illegal; not authorized; not sanctioned by law.

Micrognathia: abnormal smallness of the jaws, especially of the mandible.

Nystagmus: involuntary, rapid, rhythmic movement of the eyeball.

Polysubstance dependence: addiction to at least three categories of psychoactive substances (not including nicotine or caffeine) but in which no single psychoactive substance predominates.

KEY WORDS AND ABBREVIATIONS: Alcoholism, continued

Psychotropic drug: a drug capable of modifying mental activity; used in the treatment of mental illness.

Recovering alcoholic: a person afflicted with the disease of alcoholism who is abstaining from the use of alcohol; recovering alcoholics prefer the term "recovering" to reformed, cured, "ex," or recovered because recovering implies an ongoing process.

Tolerance: ability to endure without effect or injury.

Drug tolerance: the need for higher and higher doses of a drug to achieve the same effects.

As drinking continues in the alcoholic person, episodes may occur of alcohol intoxication with amnesia and blackouts. Early evidences of withdrawal symptoms require more alcohol for self-treatment, thus creating a vicious circle leading to dependency.

A. Signs of Alcohol Abuse[1]

1. *Adult*
   a. Health problems.
   b. Arrest, accident involvement.
   c. Impairment of job performance.
   d. Difficulties in personal relationships.
2. *Adolescent*
   a. Poor school performance.
   b. Trouble with parents.
   c. Involvement with law enforcement personnel.

B. Signs of Alcohol Intoxication[1]

Intoxication results from recent ingestion of excessive amounts of alcohol. It is characterized by behavioral changes that tend to alter the usual behavior of the individual.

1. *Behavioral Changes.* Aggressiveness, mood instability, impaired judgment, impaired social or occupational functioning, and impaired attention and memory.
2. *Physical Characteristics.* Slurred speech, incoordination, unsteady gait, nystagmus, and flushed face.
3. *Complications*
   a. Irresponsible actions in work and family settings.
   b. Accidents with resultant bruises, fractures, or brain trauma.
   c. Suicide.

C. Signs of Alcohol Dependence

1. Impaired control: inability to stop drinking before intoxication occurs; inability to cut down or limit drinking in spite of repeated attempts; binge drinking.

2. Amnesia for events happening during a period of intoxication.
3. Continuation of drinking in spite of other serious physical or mental disorder that is aggravated by alcohol use.
4. Tolerance; increased amount of alcohol needed to achieve intoxication.
5. Preoccupation with drinking: spending excess time on activities related to drinking.
6. Withdrawal leads to withdrawal symptoms, such as morning-after "shakes"; relief obtained by use of more alcohol.

II. ETIOLOGY[2]

Genetic, psychosocial, and environmental factors influence the development of alcoholism. Children of alcohol-dependent parents have a significantly higher incidence of alcoholism than do children of nonalcoholics.

Various precipitating factors may be involved when considering environmental influences. Included are psychologic stress, social contacts, being raised in a setting where heavy drinking is encouraged or tolerated as acceptable, and current lifestyle.

▪ METABOLISM OF ALCOHOL[3]

I. INGESTION AND ABSORPTION

A. Upon intake, alcohol is promptly absorbed from the stomach and small intestine; less rapidly in the presence of food.
B. Transported to liver for metabolism; it is also partly metabolized in the stomach.

II. LIVER METABOLISM

More than 90% of ingested alcohol is converted into acetaldehyde, then into acetone, and finally into carbon dioxide and water, by action of various liver enzymes. High acetaldehyde levels and chronic alcohol consumption impair liver function and lead to liver damage.

III. DIFFUSION

A. Alcohol is quickly diffused into all cells and intercellular fluid of the body.

B. Less than 10% is excreted directly through the lungs, skin, and kidney (breath, sweat, and urine).

IV. BLOOD ALCOHOL CONCENTRATION (BAC)[4]

A. Within 5 minutes after ingestion, alcohol can be detected in the blood. BAC is measured in milligrams per deciliter (mg/dL).

B. BAC is used in the legal testing of automobile drivers. In most states in the United States, 100 mg/dL (0.1%) or less is the maximum legal driving level. The blood level usually is not measured; it is estimated from the amount present in the expired air and is expressed as a percentage.

C. Effects of BAC at Various Levels

1. The tolerance level varies among individuals. Whereas the inexperienced drinker may lose self-control and become nauseated with low levels of alcohol, the experienced drinker tolerates a higher level of alcohol without nausea.

2. Ethanol is a powerful depressant of the central nervous system. In low doses, alcohol can act as a disinhibitor and as a relaxant. Euphoria may be produced. In high doses, alcohol can produce analgesic effects, with reduction of anxiety generally accompanied by reduced alertness and reduced judgment.

3. BACs at various levels produce the following characteristic effects.

    50 mg/dL
      sedation, tranquility
      fine motor coordination reduced
      unsteadiness on standing
    50–100 mg/dL
      reduced anxiety
      enhanced self-esteem
      reduced critical judgment
      reduced alertness; slowed reaction time
      impulsive risk-taking behavior
    100–200 mg/dL
      slowed reaction time
      slurred speech
      staggering
      mood swings
      memory deficits (blackouts)
      increased aggressive behavior

    300–400 mg/dL
      labored breathing
      nystagmus
      lowered blood pressure
      lowered body temperature
      loss of consciousness
    400–500 mg/dL
      depressed respiration
      alcoholic coma
      possibly fatal

▪ HEALTH HAZARDS

Prolonged alcohol use causes many serious medical disorders. The alcohol-dependent person is most seriously afflicted, but even less heavy drinkers may have complications. Alcohol-related illnesses may involve any body system. A few are mentioned here.

I. LIVER DISEASE

A. Of all the body organs, the liver is the most severely affected. Chronic alcohol abuse is the most outstanding cause of morbidity and mortality from liver diseases.

B. Injurious effects of alcohol lead to fatty liver, early fibrosis, alcoholic hepatitis, and cirrhosis.

II. IMMUNITY AND INFECTION

A. Alcoholic persons have diminished immune response: suppression of immune system defense and disturbed function of neutrophils.

B. Risk for many bacterial infections is increased, particularly pulmonary diseases (pneumonia, tuberculosis) and viral infections (hepatitis B).

III. DIGESTIVE SYSTEM

A. Alcohol ingestion alters the stomach mucosa, stimulates gastric acid secretion, and affects gastric function.

B. Bleeding lesions may develop with desquamation of the stomach lining (acute gastritis).

C. Injury to small intestines can lead to diarrhea, weight loss, and vitamin deficiencies.

IV. NUTRITIONAL DEFICIENCIES

A. The diet of a person who consumes large quantities of alcohol regularly may be limited because the person loses interest in food. The alcohol provides an excess of caloric intake.

B. Marked deficiencies can result from malabsorption of vitamins and other essential nutrients.

C. Secondary malnutrition develops because of the direct effects of alcohol on the gastrointestinal tract. Malabsorption and maldigestion occur following cellular changes in the intestinal wall.

V. CARDIOVASCULAR DISEASES

A. Risk for cardiomyopathy, hypertension, sudden death, and hemorrhagic stroke is greater for chronic alcohol abusers; decreased risk for heart attack and stroke is associated with light to moderate alcohol use.[5]

B. Heavy alcohol consumption increases the death rate from cardiovascular disease.

VI. NEOPLASMS

A. Alcohol use increases the risk for many types of cancers, notably of the alimentary and respiratory tracts.[6]

B. Alcohol combined with tobacco use has long been associated with increased neoplasms of the oral cavity, pharynx, and larynx.

VII. NERVOUS SYSTEM

A. Central and Peripheral

Long-term alcohol abuse combined with malnutrition can lead to damage of both central and peripheral nervous systems. Other factors may be involved, including alcohol-related head injuries and psychiatric status.

Early changes affect intellectual actions, such as judgment and learning ability. With prolonged and heavy alcohol consumption, chronic brain damage results.

B. Wernicke-Korsakoff's Syndrome[7]

This disorder involves ocular and gait disturbances, confusion, and psychosis. It is a result of nutritional deficiency, specifically thiamine deficiency, in conjunction with chronic alcoholism and liver damage.

VIII. REPRODUCTIVE SYSTEM

Alcohol affects every branch of the endocrine system, directly and indirectly, through the body's organization of the endocrine hormones. Possible effects of chronic alcohol abuse are listed here.

A. Female

Menstrual disturbances, failure to ovulate, and early menopause. Fetal alcohol syndrome is described in the next section.

B. Male

Testicular atrophy, suppression of testosterone, loss of mature sperm cells, feminization, and failure of gonadal function.

▪ FETAL ALCOHOL SYNDROME (FAS)

I. ALCOHOL USE DURING PREGNANCY

A. No Safe Amount

The use of alcohol during the prenatal period can be seriously threatening to the health of the baby. Even children born to mothers who have been occasional drinkers, but not alcoholics, may have alcohol-related developmental or behavioral problems. The amount of alcohol, if any, that might be considered "safe" to consume during pregnancy has not been established. Complete abstinence is safest.

B. Other Factors

Many women who abuse alcohol have poor health habits and inadequate nutritional intake, use tobacco regularly, and abuse other substances. These other factors also may influence the health of the baby.

C. No Placental Barrier

Alcohol passes freely across the placenta. Increased incidence of spontaneous abortions and stillbirths has been related to alcohol intake. The most severe effects result in fetal alcohol syndrome (FAS).

D. Fetal Growth Pattern

A characteristically abnormal pattern of growth and development can be found in children with fetal alcohol syndrome. Individually, the signs or symptoms of alcohol-related birth defects cannot be considered specific for alcohol because they appear in other conditions; however, grouped together, they form the syndrome.

II. CHARACTERISTICS OF FETAL ALCOHOL SYNDROME

The minimal criteria for describing FAS include prenatal and postnatal growth deficiencies, central nervous system impairment, and facial dysmorphology.[8] For individuals with only some of the criteria, the designation is either "fetal alcohol effects" (FAE) or "alcohol-related birth defects" (ARBD).

A. Prenatal and Postnatal Growth Retardation

1. Microcephaly.
2. Abnormalities in length and weight.

B. Central Nervous System (CNS) Involvement

1. Mental retardation; learning disabilities.
2. Behavioral dysfunction.
3. Poor motor coordination; abnormal gait.
4. Hyperactivity; irritability.

C. Facial Dysmorphology (Figure 61-1)

1. Eyes: short palpebral fissure (eye openings); epicanthal folds.
2. Thin upper lip, smooth philtrum.
3. Midface: flattened, depressed; underdeveloped maxilla.
4. Nose: short, upturned, with sunken nasal bridge.
5. Micrognathia.
6. Ears: anomalies of shape and position.

D. Other Characteristics

A variety of other health problems may result from major organ malformations, including cardiac, hepatic, muscular, skeletal, and renal. There may be hearing and vision defects. Immune system function may be compromised, leading to susceptibility to infections.

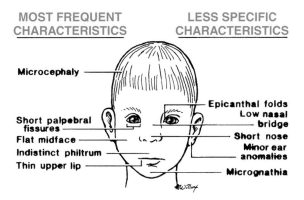

MOST FREQUENT CHARACTERISTICS

LESS SPECIFIC CHARACTERISTICS

Microcephaly

Short palpebral fissures
Flat midface
Indistinct philtrum
Thin upper lip

Epicanthal folds
Low nasal bridge
Short nose
Minor ear anomalies
Micrognathia

▪ **FIGURE 61-1 Fetal Alcohol Syndrome.** The characteristic abnormal facial features of a child born to a mother who is alcohol dependent. Growth deficiency is also a recognized feature, as are many other signs of developmental and behavioral problems. (Adapted from Little, R.E. and Streissguth, A.P.: *Alcohol, Pregnancy and the Fetal Alcohol Syndrome Unit in Alcohol Use and Its Medical Consequences: A Comprehensive Teaching Program for Biomedical Education. Project Cork of Dartmouth Medical School.* Milner-Fenwick, Inc., 2125 Greenspring Drive, Timonium, MD 21093.)

▪ ALCOHOL WITHDRAWAL SYNDROME[1]

Withdrawal consists of the disturbances that occur after abrupt cessation of alcohol intake in the alcohol-dependent person. Withdrawal signs appear within a few hours after drinking has stopped. Even a relative decline in blood concentration can precipitate the syndrome.

I. PREDISPOSING FACTORS

Malnutrition, fatigue, depression, and physical illnesses aggravate withdrawal symptoms.

II. FEATURES

A. Tremor of hands, tongue, eyelids.
B. Nervousness and irritation; anxiety.
C. Malaise, weakness, headache.
D. Dry mouth.
E. Autonomic hyperactivity; sweating, rapid pulse rate, elevated blood pressure.
F. Transient visual, tactile, or auditory hallucinations.
G. Insomnia.
H. Grand mal seizures.
I. Nausea or vomiting.

III. COMPLICATIONS

A. Alcohol Withdrawal Delirium (Delirium Tremens, "DTs")

1. May occur within 1 week of cessation of heavy alcohol intake.
2. Features
   a. Marked autonomic hyperactivity: rapid heart beat, sweating.
   b. Vivid hallucinations (visual, auditory, tactile).
   c. Delusions and agitated behavior; tremor.
   d. Confusion and disorientation.

B. Alcohol Hallucinosis

1. Auditory and visual hallucinations develop within 48 hours after abruptly stopping or reducing heavy alcohol intake of long-standing dependency.
2. Features
   a. May last weeks or months.
   b. Impairment is severe, with schizophrenic symptoms, although schizophrenia is not a predisposing factor.
   c. Delirium is not present.

▪ TREATMENT

The overall objective of treatment is to help the person achieve and maintain total abstinence. An alcohol-dependent person probably can never drink even small amounts of alcohol without eventually resuming dependency.

Treatment includes a combination of medical and psychiatric therapy with self-help. Patients are encouraged not to take other psychoactive drugs, including minor tranquilizers and caffeine.

I. EARLY INTERVENTION

When problem drinkers who are not yet dependent can be identified, counseling may help to reduce and perhaps eliminate the use of alcohol.

II. DETOXIFICATION

The term detoxification applies to the management of acute intoxication and the withdrawal syndrome. A variety of treatments may be involved.

A. Treatment for Immediate Emergencies

An alcoholic may have been in an accident or have a medical emergency other than that of the alcohol withdrawal syndrome. Fractures, head injury, internal bleeding, or other problems may require initial attention. In fact, alcohol dependency may be revealed after a patient is admitted for other reasons and withdrawal symptoms appear within a few hours or days.

B. Removal From Source of Alcohol: Abstinence

One of the advantages of hospitalization is that supervision is available. The patient does not have access to usual sources of alcohol.

C. Rest, Sleep, Exercise, and Proper Diet

One goal of therapy is to restore general physical health by treating nutritional deficiencies and encouraging a normal daily pattern of sleep and meals.

D. Treatment for Medical Complications

Possible medical complications were described with their systemic effects earlier in this chapter. Most alcoholics have additional illnesses.

E. Relief From Acute Withdrawal Signs

Tranquilizers may be prescribed for short-term use. Vitamins, particularly thiamine, are usually administered.

III. PHARMACOTHERAPY[9,10]

A. Medications Used in Alcoholism Treatment

Agents for withdrawal management include:
1. Alcohol-sensitizing agents (cause aversive reactions in combination with alcohol).
2. Anticraving agents (decrease desire for and consumption of alcohol).
3. Amethystic agents (reverse the acute intoxicating and depressant effects of alcohol).
4. Medications for treatment of coexisting psychiatric disorders, such as depression and anxiety.

B. Disulfiram (Antabuse): Alcohol-Sensitizing Agent

The drug disulfiram interferes with the metabolism of alcohol by acting on the enzyme that converts acetaldehyde to acetone in the liver. As a result, acetaldehyde accumulates in the tissues. When both alcohol and disulfiram are taken at the same time, nausea and vomiting with hypotension result, and the patient becomes very ill. The drug acts as a deterrent to provide an adjunct to comprehensive therapy in selected patients.

C. Naltrexone (Trexan): Anticraving Agent

The drug naltrexone produces an aversive reaction. It can help decrease craving and consumption by the alcohol-dependent person. Although there are some side effects, it has been shown to be efficacious as an adjunct to psychosocial treatment.

IV. REHABILITATION

A. Counseling and Education

The patient must recognize that alcoholism is a serious disease and must be willing to be helped. Family and work associates may be recruited to cooperate with the program. Behavior therapy and psychotherapy have been used.

B. Group Therapy

Alcoholics Anonymous (AA) is one source of possible help for motivated individuals. Other people prefer special clinics and centers for treatment.

AA is a fellowship of men and women who help themselves and others to recover from alcoholism. Al-Anon is a separate program for parents, adult children, siblings, and spouses, as well as other persons concerned with the recovering alcoholic. Alateen is a program for teenage children.

C. Psychiatry

Treatment is needed for patients with psychiatric disorders. An increased frequency of schizophrenia, psychoneurosis, sociopathy, and manic-depressive diseases is being recognized among alcohol-dependent people.

D. Aftercare Services

Because recovery takes a long time, an extended period of aftercare is needed. Early relapse is more likely when a recovering alcoholic leaves a treatment system too early. A typical follow-up includes weekly aftercare group meetings for 9 to 12 months.

■ DENTAL HYGIENE CARE

Only a small percentage of individuals with an alcohol-use problem are incapacitated, homeless, shabbily dressed, or socially disoriented. Most alcohol-dependent people continue to maintain home, work, and social relationships, at least initially, and many for a span of years.

In dental and dental hygiene practice, patients who consume alcohol include the occasional social drinker, the light to moderate drinker, the problem drinker, the alcohol abuser, and the alcohol-dependent person. The abstainer or "teetotaler" is particularly important to identify because that patient may be a recovering alcoholic.

Many patients with an alcohol use disorder are polysubstance abusers. They may use other psychoactive drugs, such as cocaine, heroin, amphetamines, marijuana, and assorted sedatives or hypnotics.

I. PATIENT ASSESSMENT

The quality of the content and the frequent updating of the medical history are essential to patient care because of the many general health-related problems of alcohol ingestion that can influence oral health and treatment procedures.

A. Obtain Patient Confidence

Information about substance use and abuse must be obtained from patients of all age levels. Adolescents of all socioeconomic groups may be involved. The number of elderly alcohol consumers is ever increasing; some of these are alcoholics.[11]

Unfortunately, people are hesitant to reveal personal information about alcohol use because of the social stigma attached to alcoholism. A patient first needs to understand the reasons for obtaining the information as a health-safety measure. More than that, the patient must know that personal information will remain confidential.

B. Present Questions Carefully

Questions must be asked privately and without sign of disapproval or judgment. A patient's family members may provide an alert to the patient's problem.

The basic questionnaire or interview format must have a few leading questions to provide basic facts. Care must be taken not to place the patient on the defensive.

1. *Suggested Content for Routine Questions*
   a. Pattern of alcohol consumption, frequency, amount on an average day.
   b. Systemic conditions suggestive of alcohol-related diseases.
   c. Hospitalizations suggestive of alcohol-related accidents or detoxification program.
   d. Information about medications; self-prescribed, over-the-counter, and prescribed drugs. A relationship to polydrug abuse or treatment for alcoholism may be evident.
   e. History of drinking problem.
2. *Screening for Alcohol Abuse or Dependency.* Various questionnaires have been used in the attempt to detect alcoholism. One of these, the **CAGE**, has four selected questions. Although these questions may not provide a positive diagnosis, research has shown that they can alert the interviewer and provide a high index of suspicion. One positive reply can lead to further inquiry. The four questions are as follows[12]:
   a. Have you ever felt you ought to Cut down on your drinking?
   b. Have people Annoyed you by criticizing your drinking?
   c. Have you ever felt bad or Guilty about your drinking?
   d. Have you ever had a drink first thing in the morning to steady your nerves or to get rid of a hangover (Eye-opener)?

II. PATIENT EXAMINATION[13]

Except for the increased risk of oral cancer in persons who use alcohol heavily, no specific oral finding can be attributed directly to alcohol as the etiologic agent. The characteristics listed here have been observed frequently. When present, they assist in patient evaluation and dental hygiene care planning.

A. Extraoral Examination

1. *Breath and Body Odor of Alcohol and of Tobacco.* Many alcohol users are also heavy tobacco users.
2. *Tremor of Hands, Tongue, Eyelids.* Signs of withdrawal.

3. *Skin.* Redness of forehead, cheeks, nose; acne rosacea; dilated blood vessels that produce spider petechiae on the nose.
4. *Face Color.* Light yellowish brown may indicate jaundice from liver disease.
5. *Eyes.* Red, baggy eyes or puffy facial features; bloated appearance.
6. *Evidences of Trauma.* Facial injuries related to falls when intoxicated. Alcohol abusers are especially prone to traumatic accidents.
7. *Lips.* Angular cheilitis related to poor nutrition.
8. *Parotid Glands.* Swelling.

B. Intraoral Examination

1. *Mucosa, Lips, Tongue.* Dry; xerostomia.
2. *Tongue.* Coated; glossitis related to nutritional deficiencies.
3. *Periodontal Infection*
   a. Generalized poor oral hygiene; heavy biofilm not unusual.
   b. Calculus deposits may be generalized, depending on patient neglect.
   c. Gingiva that bleeds spontaneously or on probing.
4. *Teeth*
   a. Chipped and fractured from falls and injuries; stained from tobacco use.
   b. Attrition secondary to bruxism.
   c. Erosion secondary to frequent vomiting.
   d. Dental caries. Except for neglect of dental care, dental caries incidence may be no different from that for the usual population of the age level. An alcoholic who uses primarily wine or sweetened cocktails and frequently snacks on cariogenic foods is likely to have more carious lesions, particularly if gingival recession and root exposures have occurred. Lack of dental biofilm removal also favors increased incidence of dental caries.
5. *Evidence of Minimal Dental Care.* Although subject to great variation, the overall tendency is for the alcoholic patient to put off dental and dental hygiene care, sometimes in the interest of money needed to purchase alcohol or, for the polysubstance abuser, additional drugs.

   The alcohol-dependent person also may tend to use dental care primarily for emergency purposes for pain relief. The evidence may be noted in a patient who has more missing teeth than treated teeth. The indication can be that dental caries was neglected to the point where extraction was requested.

6. *Dentures.* Chipped, missing; may require frequent repairs.

III. CONSULTATION

Information in the patient history may not reveal accurately the extent of a patient's alcohol use, but clinical observations along with the medical history may provide a high degree of suspicion. From that, further inquiry and consultation with the patient's physician may help to confirm precautions needed during clinical procedures.

When a patient does not have a regular physician and has not had a recent medical evaluation, referral to a physician should be made.

IV. VITAL SIGNS

Routine recording of vital signs is indicated. Blood pressure is frequently increased. Fluctuations can be particularly significant.

V. CLINICAL TREATMENT PROCEDURES

The clinical procedures for dental hygiene care are greatly influenced by the many health problems that can result from chronic ingestion of alcohol. Some of the effects were described earlier in this chapter.

A. Nonalcoholic Rinses

Preprocedural rinse, antibacterial agents, or any oral hygiene product that contains alcohol must be avoided for all patients suffering from an alcohol use problem. This is absolutely necessary for the recovering alcoholic because recovery depends on a medication-free lifestyle. The most minute amount of alcohol ingested by a patient being treated with disulfiram can cause an emergency.

B. Scaling and Debridement

The usual oral tissue response expected following periodontal instrumentation may be limited by the changes in the patient's tissues. These can be summarized as follows:

1. Decreased overall reserve that has resulted from degeneration of multiple organ systems.
2. Impaired healing
   a. Prolonged bleeding time; impaired clotting mechanism from chronic liver disease.
   b. Interference with collagen formation and deposition.
   c. Decreased immune system function.
3. Increased susceptibility to infection.

Everyday Ethics

Naka hurried back from lunch to promptly greet her 1:00 patient, Mr. Lumot. He was a salesman that juggled many appointments throughout the day. As he was seated in the treatment room, he stated he had just come from a luncheon meeting where an important contract was signed. Before beginning the examination, Naka measured Mr. Lumot's blood pressure, which was elevated from the recording made at his last visit.

She noticed an odor of alcohol on his breath and became concerned because she remembered a positive response on his medical history regarding his daily alcoholic beverage consumption.

Questions for Consideration

1. In the process of care, what steps should Naka pursue to find out more about Mr. Lumot's drinking habits without seeming judgmental?

2. Ensuring the patient's autonomy, what specific questions need to be asked about his daily alcohol use that have bearing on the current appointment procedures?

3. In addition to the dental hygiene therapy, how should the observations from today's appointment be recorded in the patient's record?

C. Power-Driven Instruments

The patient with chronic alcohol abuse or dependency, particularly one who also inhales tobacco smoke, most likely has pulmonary complications. Lung infections are common. Lung abscesses can be caused by bacteria taken into the lungs from the oral cavity or by abnormal breathing during intoxication.

Power-driven instruments, particularly ultrasonic scalers and air-powder stain-removal devices, must be used with caution to prevent inhalation of oral microorganisms by the patient. High-powered suction applied by an assistant is essential.

■ PATIENT INSTRUCTION

I. DENTAL BIOFILM CONTROL

Teaching oral health and cleanliness can be especially important. Motivation may be difficult because many patients with alcohol or polysubstance dependency are preoccupied with alcohol or drugs and place less priority on personal hygiene.

A preventive care program for a recovering alcoholic should become part of the total rehabilitation process.

II. DIET AND NUTRITION

A. Relation of Diet to Alcoholism

1. Alcoholic beverages contain calories; a day's allotment of calories may be ingested when alcohol is used in excess.
2. The calories of alcohol are "empty" calories without nutritional elements, and the balance of the diet can be very limited.

3. Alcohol unfavorably affects the absorption and digestion of many nutrients by the changes it produces in the mucosa of the gastrointestinal tract.

✔ Factors To Teach The Patient

- Alcohol abuse is a great risk to overall health.

- Incidence of oral cancer is increased by the use of alcohol and tobacco.

- Mixing alcohol with other drugs (prescription or over-the-counter) can lead to medical emergencies. Always check each drug and its actions before using it in combination with alcohol.

- Alcoholism is a disease with serious implications. Advise young people of the dangers involved and discourage them from drinking alcohol.

- Commercial antibacterial and fluoride mouthrinses may contain up to 30% alcohol. Labels must be read carefully. Keep mouthrinse bottles out of reach of children.

- Use of alcohol during pregnancy must be avoided because of possible devastating effects on the baby. Be alert to the alcohol content of certain foods and drugs.

- Alcohol readily enters breast milk and is transmitted to the infant during nursing.

4. Liver damage has a major detrimental influence on the metabolism of nutrients.

B. Dietary Deficiencies

Malnutrition is clearly associated with alcohol abuse. The severe malnutrition that has been described applies primarily to the derelict or "skid row" alcoholic who has limited resources for proper food.

Many middle and upper class alcohol dependents do not consume an acceptable "balanced" diet, but they cannot be considered with the severely malnourished group.

C. Instruction

After a dietary assessment is reviewed with the patient, help can be provided by reviewing the basic dietary needs and encouraging the use of foods from the food guide pyramid (page 523).

III. CONTINUING CARE

Compliance with self-care measures and keeping scheduled appointments for dental hygiene care are major problems. A special effort must be made to provide the patient with the supervision and periodic treatment needed. The moderate and excess user of alcohol, especially when tobacco is also used, is at risk for oral cancer and periodontal bone and attachment loss. Regular screening is necessary.

REFERENCES

1. **American Psychiatric Association:** *Diagnostic and Statistical Manual of Mental Disorders* (DSM-IV). Washington, DC, American Psychiatric Association, 1994, pp. 195–199.
2. **United States Department of Health and Human Services,** Secretary of Health and Human Services: *Eighth Special Report to the U.S. Congress on Alcohol and Health.* Rockville, MD, National Institute on Alcohol Abuse and Alcoholism, September, 1993, pp. 61–77.
3. **United States Department of Health and Human Services:** op. cit., pp. 147–149.
4. **United States Department of Health and Human Services:** op. cit., p. 89.
5. **United States Department of Health and Human Services:** op. cit., p. 175.
6. **Lieber,** C.S.: Medical Disorders of Alcoholism, *N. Engl. J. Med., 333,* 1058, October 19, 1995.
7. **United States Department of Health and Human Services:** op. cit., pp. 180–181.
8. **Sokol,** R.J. and Clarren, S.K.: Guidelines for Use of Terminology Describing the Impact of Prenatal Alcohol on the Offspring, *Alcohol. Clin. Exp. Res., 13,* 597, August, 1989.
9. **Kranzler,** H.R.: Alcoholism, in Rakel, R.E., ed.: *Conn's Current Therapy, 1997.* Philadelphia, W.B. Saunders, 1997, p. 1139.
10. **United States Department of Health and Human Services:** op. cit., pp. 332–335.
11. **Friedlander,** A.H. and Solomon, D.H.: Dental Management of the Geriatric Alcoholic Patient, *Gerodontics, 4,* 23, February, 1988.
12. **Ewing,** J.A.: Detecting Alcoholism: The CAGE Questionnaire, *JAMA, 252,* 1905, October 12, 1984.
13. **Friedlander,** A.H., Mills, M.J., and Gorelick, D.A.: Alcoholism and Dental Management, *Oral Surg., Oral Med., Oral Pathol., 63,* 42, January, 1987.

SUGGESTED READINGS

Biron, C.R.: Help Patients Before They Hit Rock Bottom, *RDH, 15,* 20, August, 1995.
Boffetta, P., Mashberg, A., Winkelmann, R., and Garfinkel, L.: Carcinogenic Effect of Tobacco Smoking and Alcohol Drinking on Anatomic Sites of the Oral Cavity and Oropharynx, *Int. J. Cancer, 52,* 530, October 21, 1992.
Brickley, M.R. and Shepherd, J.P.: Alcohol Abuse in Dental Patients, *Br. Dent. J., 169,* 329, November 24, 1990.
Dobkin, P.L., Tremblay, R.E., Desmarais-Gervais, L., and Depelteau, L.: Is Having an Alcoholic Father Hazardous for Children's Physical Health? *Addiction, 89,* 1619, December, 1994.
Glick, M.: Medical Considerations for Dental Care of Patients With Alcohol-Related Liver Disease, *J. Am. Dent. Assoc., 128,* 61, January, 1997.
Halsted, C.H.: Alcohol: Medical and Nutritional Effects, in Ziegler, E.E. and Filer, L.J., eds.: *Present Knowledge in Nutrition,* 7th ed. Washington, DC, ILSI Press, 1996, pp. 547–556.
Harris, C.K., Warnakulasuriya, K.A.A.S, Johnson, N.W., Gelbier, S., and Peters, T.J.: Oral Health in Alcohol Misusers, *Community Dent. Health, 13,* 199, December, 1996.
Leonard, R.H.: Alcohol, Alcoholism, and Dental Treatment, *Compend. Cont. Educ. Dent., 12,* 274, April, 1991.
McDiarmid, M.: Dental Treatment and the Alcoholic, *N. Z. Dent. J., 92,* 83, September, 1996.
Michels, R. and Marzuk, P.-M.: Progress in Psychiatry (Second of Two Parts), *N. Engl. J. Med., 329,* 628, August 26, 1993.
Robb, N.D. and Smith, B.G.N.: Chronic Alcoholism: An Important Condition in the Dentist-Patient Relationship, *J. Dent., 24,* 17, January/March, 1996.
Talamini, R., Franceschi, S., Barra, S., and La Vecchia, C.: The Role of Alcohol in Oral and Pharyngeal Cancer in Non-smokers, and of Tobacco in Non-drinkers, *Int. J. Cancer, 46,* 391, September 15, 1990.

Fetal Alcohol Syndrome

Coles, C.D.: Impact of Prenatal Alcohol Exposure on the Newborn and the Child, *Clin. Obstet. Gynecol., 36,* 255, June, 1993.
Haney, K. and Bothwell, E.: Fetal Alcohol Syndrome. Implications for Dental Health Professionals, *DentalHygienistNews, 7,* 8, Summer, 1994.
Lewis, D.D. and Woods, S.E: Fetal Alcohol Syndrome, *Am. Family Physician, 50,* 1025, October, 1994.
Seo, P.: Treating the Patient With Fetal Alcohol Syndrome, *Access, 11,* 60, May–June, 1997.
Spohr, H.-L., Willms, J., and Steinhausen, H.-C.: Prenatal Alcohol Exposure and Long-term Developmental Consequences, *Lancet, 341,* 907, April 10, 1993.

The Patient With a Respiratory Disease

Janet B. Selwitz-Segal, RDH, CDA, MS

Patients with respiratory diseases have increased risks for complications due to decreased breathing function, medications used, and drug interactions. By understanding the cause and symptoms of the respiratory condition and the need to modify dental hygiene services, the prevention of an acute episode and a safe dental hygiene appointment can be facilitated.

Many respiratory diseases are caused or aggravated by tobacco use. Dental hygienists have a unique opportunity to educate their patients about this health hazard. Patients with respiratory distress may need emergency treatment for which dental hygienists are prepared to prevent or treat if necessary. The signs and symptoms and medical emergency procedures for respiratory failure, airway obstruction, hyperventilation, allergic reactions, and local anesthesia reactions are found in Table 66-4.

A significant relationship between oral infections, particularly periodontal disease, and several respiratory conditions has been recognized. The periodontal status of the patient may serve as an indicator of risk.[1] Dedication of the dental hygienist to the prevention and control of periodontal infections will have a major influence on the overall health of the patient. Box 62-1 defines key words related to respiration and respiratory diseases.

BOX 62-1 KEY WORDS: Respiration and Respiratory Diseases

Acute: (of a disease or disease symptom) beginning abruptly with marked intensity or sharpness, then subsiding after a relatively short time, opposite of chronic.

Analgesic: relieving pain.

Anaphylaxis: an exaggerated life-threatening hypersensitivity reaction to a previously encountered allergen.

Antigen: any environmental substance that produces inflammation. When used to describe an allergic response, these antigens are called **allergens.**

Antipyretic: pertaining to a substance or procedure that reduces fever.

Atopy: (Atopic) hereditary tendency to experience immediate allergic reactions (allergic asthma).

Bronchodilator: a drug that relaxes contractions of the smooth muscle of the bronchioles to improve ventilation of the lungs.

Chronic: (of a disease or disorder) developing slowly and persisting for a long period, often for the remainder of a person's lifetime, opposite of acute.

Communicable disease: (contagious) any disease transmitted from one person or animal to another. *Direct:* from excreta or other bodily discharges. *Indirect:* from substances or inanimate objects (contaminated drinking glasses, water, insects, or toys).

Coryza: profuse discharge from mucous membrane of the nose.

Dyspnea: labored or difficult breathing.

Edema: abnormal accumulation of fluids in the connective and supporting spaces of tissues causing swelling.

Gastroesophageal reflux: backflow of stomach contents into the esophagus where gastric juices produce a burning sensation.

Goblet cell: specialized epithelial cell that secretes mucus.

Hemoptysis: spitting of blood from lesion in the larynx, trachea, or lower respiratory tract.

Hyperventilation: greater rate and volume of breathing than metabolically necessary for pulmonary gas exchange, which may lead to dizziness and possible syncope.

Hypoxia: inadequate oxygen at the cellular level characterized by tachycardia, hypertension, peripheral vasoconstriction, mental confusion.

Malaise: a vague uneasy feeling of body weakness, often marking the onset and persisting throughout a disease.

Mast cell: constituent of connective tissue; releases substances in response to injury or infection.

Mediator: intermediary substance that effects a change.

Mucus: (n.) viscous, slippery secretion of mucous membranes and glands. Contains mucin, white blood cells, inorganic salts and exfoliated cells. **Mucous (adj.)**

Myalgia: muscle pain accompanied with malaise.

Nosocomial: pertaining to a hospital.

　　　Nosocomial pneumonia: pneumonia contracted during confinement in a hospital or nursing home.

Orthopenia: an abnormal condition in which a person must sit or stand to breathe deeply or comfortably.

Otalgia: pain in the ears.

Pleura: delicate membrane enclosing the lungs.

KEY WORDS: Respiration and Respiratory Diseases, continued

Pleuritic: pertaining to inflammation of the lungs; dyspnea, stabbing pain, restriction of normal breathing, symptoms of pneumonia and tuberculosis.

Pneumothorax: collection of air or gas causing the lungs to collapse.

Pulmonary hypertension: condition of abnormally high pressure within the pulmonary circulation.

Tachypnea: abnormally rapid rate of breathing (more than 20 breaths per minute).

Tracheostomy: direct opening into the trachea through the neck to facilitate breathing or removal of secretions.

■ THE RESPIRATORY SYSTEM

I. ANATOMY[2]

Structures: Sinuses, nasal cavity, larynx, pharynx, trachea, bronchi, lungs, and pleura (Figure 62-1A).

II. PHYSIOLOGY

The respiratory tract from nasal cavity to lungs serves as a passageway for air exchange (Figure 62-1A).
- *Inhaled fresh air:* warmed and filtered in the nasal cavity, enters the lungs.
- *Exhaled air:* with carbon dioxide, leaves the body.
- *Gas exchange:* at the cellular level, occurs in the alveoli at the ends of the bronchioles, as shown in Figure 62-1B.
- *Cardiovascular system:* functions with the respiratory system to pump oxygenated blood from the lungs to every cell in the body and deoxygenated blood back to the lungs.

III. FUNCTION OF THE RESPIRATORY MUCOSA

Figure 62-2 shows ciliated epithelial cells and mucous-secreting goblet cells that line the respiratory tract to make up the respiratory mucosa.
- **Mucus** secreted from goblet cells moistens inspired air, prevents delicate alveolar walls from becoming dry, and traps dust and other airborne particles.
- **Cilia** assist in removing foreign material and contaminated mucus by a constant beating and wavelike motion that propels this material back into the larger bronchi and trachea where it can be expectorated (coughed up) or swallowed.

- **Lack of function** results when the inflammatory process (of asthma and chronic bronchitis) initiates an overabundance of mucus. Congestion is created, preventing the cilia from assisting with normal breathing.

IV. ROLE OF BIOFILM[3]

A. Definition

Biofilms are structured communities of bacteria bound together by a carbohydrate matrix and surrounded by water channels that deliver nutrients and remove waste.

B. Characteristics

- Adheres to inanimate objects (contact lenses, mechanical heart valves, catheters) or living surfaces (oral mucosa and gingiva).
- Bacteria in biofilm are more difficult to kill with antibiotics than their "planktonic" (free-floating) counterparts.
- Dental biofilm is complex and may serve as a reservoir of infection, especially in hospital patients.
- Examples of diseases and devices involving biofilm are shown in Box 62-2.

V. CLASSIFICATION OF RESPIRATORY DISEASES (BOX 62-3)

A. Upper Respiratory Tract Diseases

Diseases of the nose, sinuses, pharynx, and larynx.

B. Lower Respiratory Tract Diseases

Diseases of the trachea, lungs, and bronchi and bronchioles.

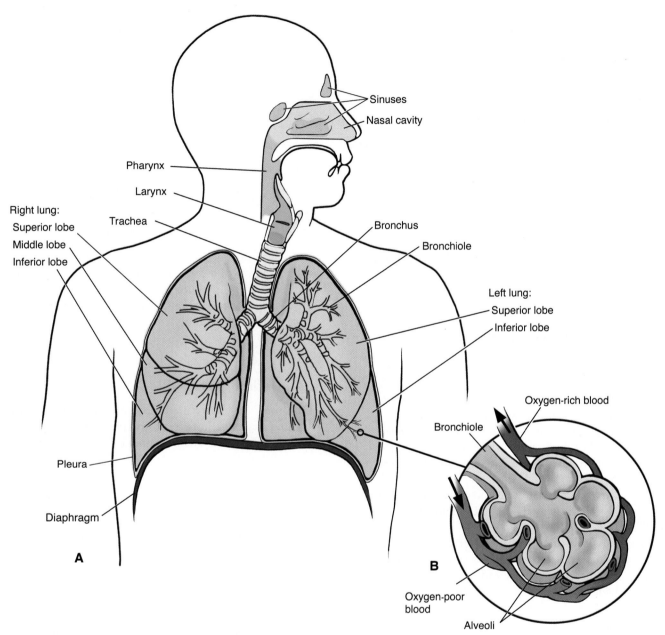

■ FIGURE 62-1 Structures of the Respiratory System. (A) Structures. The major anatomic structures of the respiratory system are shown. Each bronchus branches out to the bronchioles. **(B)** Gas exchange. Exchange of oxygen and carbon dioxide occurs in the alveoli of the bronchioles.

■ UPPER RESPIRATORY TRACT DISEASES

The more common disorders of the upper respiratory tract are caused by infections or allergic reactions that result in inflammation. Signs and symptoms, etiology, medical treatment, and oral findings are summarized in Table 62-1.[4,5]

I. MODE OF TRANSMISSION[6]

- Direct oral contact.

- Inhalation of airborne droplets.
- Indirectly by hands or articles freshly soiled with discharge of nose and throat of infected person.

II. DENTAL HYGIENE CARE

A. Disease Prevention

Observe standard precautions to prevent transmission of pathogens from patient to clinician and to prevent healthcare-associated infections for the patient.

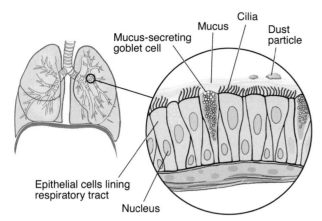

■ FIGURE 62-2 Lining of the Respiratory Mucosa.
Ciliated epithelial cells and mucus secreted by goblet
cells help to remove foreign objects (dust particles). The
material is either expectorated (coughed up) or
swallowed.

B. Appointment Management[7]

- Delay dental and dental hygiene treatment until
  patient is well or is no longer infectious.
- Noninfectivity can be determined by temperature return to normal and regression of oral
  lesions such as erythematous lesions of the soft
  palate and erythema multiforme.

BOX 62-2 Examples of Diseases/Devices Involving Biofilms

Dental caries

Periodontitis

Otitis media

Cystic fibrosis pneumonia

Nosocomial infections

      Intensive care unit (ICU) pneumonia

      Contact lens

      Intrauterine device (IUD)

      Endotracheal tubes

      Mechanical heart valves

Unit water lines

Adapted from Costerton, J.W., Stewart, P.S., and Greenberg,
E.P.: Bacterial Biofilms: A Common Cause of Persistent Infections, *Science, 284,* 1318, May 21, 1999.

■ LOWER RESPIRATORY TRACT DISEASES

Disorders of the lower respiratory tract requiring adaptation during dental hygiene care are listed in Box 62-3.

I. ACUTE DISEASES

Pneumonia.

II. CHRONIC DISEASES

Tuberculosis, asthma, chronic obstructive pulmonary
disease (COPD), and cystic fibrosis.

■ PNEUMONIA

Pneumonia, an inflammation of the lungs, may be caused
by viruses, bacteria, and, rarely, fungi. Normally, host
defense mechanisms eliminate these pathogens. If the
body fails to clear the contamination, pneumonia may
result. Viral and bacterial pneumonias are compared in
Table 62-2.

BOX 62-3 Classification of Respiratory Diseases

Upper Respiratory Tract Diseases

      Upper respiratory infection (common cold)

      Allergic rhinitis (hay fever)

      Otitis media (earache)

      Sinusitis

      Pharyngitis/tonsilitis

      Influenza (flu)

Lower Respiratory Tract Diseases

      Pneumonia

      Tuberculosis

      Asthma

      Chronic obstructive pulmonary disease (COPD)

         Chronic bronchitis

         Emphysema

      Cystic fibrosis

■ **TABLE 62-1 UPPER RESPIRATORY DISEASES: SIGNS/SYMPTOMS, ETIOLOGY, MEDICAL TREATMENT AND ORAL FINDINGS**

SIGNS/SYMPTOMS	ETIOLOGY	MEDICAL TREATMENT	ORAL FINDINGS
Upper Respiratory Infections—Infectious Rhinitis (Common Cold)			
• Sneezing • Nasal obstruction • Nasal discharge (Coryza) • Headache • Watering of the eyes	• Viral	• Analgesic for sore throat, muscle ache • Anticholinergic agent to decrease nasal discharge • Oral decongestant to decrease nasal congestion • Antihistamine for itching, sneezing, "runny nose"	• May observe small round erythematous lesions on soft palate, enlarged tonsils, erythema multiforme, acute ulcerative gingivitis • Decongestants and mouth breathing may cause dry mouth
Allergic Rhinitis (Hay Fever)			
• Watering, burning eyes • Sneezing • Nasal congestion	• Seasonal triggers: grass, trees, pollen, mold spores • Perennial triggers: dust mites, animal dander	• Avoidance of the allergen • Pharmacotherapy medication: antihistamines, decongestants • Immunotherapy: allergy injections	• Dry mouth • Oral candidiasis from long-term use of topical corticosteroids
Otitis Media (Earache)			
• Otalgia • Fever	• Viral/bacterial	• Antibiotics for bacterial infections	• Oral candidiasis from long-term use of antibiotics
Sinusitis			
• Nasal obstruction • Fever, chills • Constant mid-face head pain, more severe when lying down • Palpation over sinus area: tenderness, swelling	• Bacterial infection of the epithelial lining of the sinus • Triggers include upper respiratory infections, dental infections, direct trauma	• Antibiotics • Decongestants	• Dry mouth • Sinus congestion creates pressure on nearby maxillary molar roots and may cause symptoms of toothache; *important to determine if pain originates from tooth or sinus infection*
Pharyngitis/Tonsillitis			
• Sore throat	• Mostly viral • Rarely bacterial: Group A beta-hemolytic streptococcus infection	• Viral: treat symptoms • Bacterial: antibiotics • Patient is no longer infective after 1 day on antibiotics	• Enlarged tonsils • Erythematous tissues
Influenza (Flu)			
• Chills, fever • Headache • Coryza • Malaise • Myalgia	• Viral	• Bed rest • Analgesics • Fluids • Monitor for secondary bacterial infection	• Dry mouth

Adapted from Lepore, M., Anolik, R., and Glick, M.: Diseases of the Respiratory Tract, in Greenberg, M.S. and Glick, M., eds: *Burket's Oral Medicine,* 10th ed. Hamilton, BC Decker Inc., 2002, pp. 341–348; and Bricker, S.L., Langlais, R.P., and Miller, C.S.: *Oral Diagnosis, Oral Medicine, and Treatment Planning,* 2nd ed. Hamilton, BC Decker Inc., 2001, pp. 165–170.

■ TABLE 62-2 COMPARISON OF VIRAL AND BACTERIAL PNEUMONIA

ITEM	VIRAL	BACTERIAL
Occurrence	• Most prevalent	• Least prevalent

Causative Agent	• Virus	• Bacteria
		  Hospital-acquired
		    Gram-negative
		    Example: *Staphylococcus aureus*
		  Community acquired
		    Gram-positive
		    Example: *Streptococcus pneumoniae*
		• Oral bacteria

Signs and Symptoms	• Mild symptoms • Cough • Sputum • Mild fever • Dyspnea	• Sudden onset • Coughing, purulent sputum • Fever • Pleuritic chest pain • Dyspnea, tachypnea
Diagnosis	• Patient history • Physical findings • Chest radiographs	• Patient history • Physical findings • Chest radiographs • Sputum sample

Medical Treatment	• Supportive
	  Bed rest
	  Drink fluids
		• Antibiotics

I. GENERAL TYPES[8,9]

A. Community Acquired

• No known predisposing factors; person-to-person transmission.

B. Hospital Acquired (Nosocomial)[10]

• Usually affects debilitated or chronically ill hospitalized patients (hospital intensive care unit, nursing home).

• Most cases are due to aspiration of oropharyngeal secretions into the lungs. Oral bacteria can be released from biofilm into salivary secretions that are then aspirated into the lower respiratory tract to cause pneumonia (aspiration pneumonia).

• Most frequently cultured bacteria from the lungs are gram-negative bacilli and oral bacteria consistent with varieties often found in periodontal pockets.

C. Pneumocystis Pneumonia

• Etiology: *Pneumocystis carinii* (generally considered a protozoan parasite, DNA resembles a fungus).

• Susceptibility is enhanced by chronic debilitating illness and by disease or therapy in which immune mechanisms are impaired (such as in HIV/AIDS).

II. ROLE OF ORAL BACTERIA[11]

Pathogenic bacteria commonly found in the mouth, nose, and throat may produce pneumonia, especially when associated with influenza and:

• As a superinfection following broad-spectrum antibiotic therapy.

• As a complication of chronic obstructive pulmonary disease (COPD).

• After aspiration of gastric contents or tracheostomy.

III. MEDICAL TREATMENT

• *Viral:* supportive treatment of bed rest and fluids.

• *Bacterial:* antibiotic therapy.

IV. DENTAL HYGIENE CARE[12,13]

Control of oral disease and periodontal disease in particular for patients in nursing homes and hospitals will help prevent pathogens from entering the lungs. In addition, dental hygienists practicing in these settings should educate other healthcare workers to reduce risk of nosocomial pneumonia by:

- Maintaining standard precautions.
- Performing daily biofilm control measures on natural teeth and dentures.
- Using an antimicrobial mouth rinse.

■ TUBERCULOSIS (TB)

Tuberculosis is a chronic, infectious, and communicable disease with worldwide public health significance. It is a serious disease that can involve many months and years of lost time during the active states of illness and following convalescence. The incidence has increased in population groups with a high prevalence of HIV infections. Tuberculosis is an AIDS-defining illness.

I. DISEASE DEVELOPMENT[14,15]

A. Etiology

Mycobacterium tuberculosis.

B. Transmission

Tubercle bacilli travel in airborne droplet nuclei from infected saliva or sputum carried during coughing, singing, or sneezing from people with pulmonary or laryngeal tuberculosis.

C. Risk Factors for Exposure

- Degree of exposure: Prolonged close exposure can lead to infection of those in contact.
- Contact in tight living settings such as prisons, shelters, nursing homes, and mental institutions.
- Immunosuppressed persons; HIV/AIDS and other medical risk conditions.

D. Diagnosis

- **Tuberculin Skin Test (Mantoux):** to determine whether a person has been infected. The skin test does not determine clinically active tuberculosis.
- **Chest radiograph, sputum sample culture, and physical examination:** to determine clinically active tuberculosis.

II. DISEASE PROCESS

A. Incubation Period

2 to 10 weeks; latent infection may persist for a lifetime.

B. Medical Treatment

- Multiple antituberculosis drugs: daily for 6 months.

- Drugs used: isoniazid, rifampin, pyrazinamide.
- Drug therapy can produce sputum conversion within several weeks.
- Successful treatment involves rigid patient compliance for 6 months.

C. Multidrug-Resistant Tuberculosis

Treatment that is irregularly taken can lead to the development of resistant bacteria and the redevelopment of disease.

III. DENTAL HYGIENE CARE

A. Patient History Preparation

- Questions for history and symptoms of tuberculosis.
- Medications; length of treatment.

B. Consultation With Physician

- To determine potential for communicability.
- Table 62-3 outlines recommended protocol for dental treatment.

C. Symptoms

Due to extreme communicability of TB, it is imperative that the dental hygienist recognize the symptoms of active disease and follows the procedures listed in Table 62-3 regarding the decision to treat or dismiss the patient.
- **Early:** low-grade fever, weight loss, fatigue, night sweats.
- **Later:** persistent cough, chest pain, hoarseness, hemoptysis (coughing up blood).

D. Oral Manifestations

- Infrequently appears in the oral cavity; most frequently in men.
- Classic lesion: painful, deep, irregular ulcer on dorsum of the tongue.
- May also occur on palate, lips, buccal mucosa, and gingiva.

■ ASTHMA

Asthma is a chronic, inflammatory, respiratory disease consisting of recurrent episodes of dyspnea, coughing, and wheezing and is related to bronchial inflammation and muscle constriction. It is estimated that the average dental practice will have 100 patients with asthma.[16]

▪ TABLE 62-3 DENTAL HYGIENE TREATMENT PROTOCOL FOR PATIENTS WITH TUBERCULOSIS

MEDICAL HISTORY FINDING	DENTAL HYGIENE CARE
Clinically Active Sputum-Positive Tuberculosis	• Do not treat in the dental office (or any outpatient setting). • Urgent care must be performed in a hospital setting (appropriate isolation), with standard procedures (mask, gloves, and gown), engineering controls (ventilation), and filtration masks. • After several weeks on prescribed medication, with physician clearance, patient may be treated as a healthy person.
Past History of Tuberculosis	• Consult with physician to determine current status.
Positive Tuberculin Skin Test	• After consultation with physician to determine absence of disease, dental treatment may be performed. May be placed on prophylactic isoniazid for 6–12 months to prevent clinical disease.
Signs and Symptoms of Tuberculosis	• Do not treat. • Refer to physician for any unexplained dry, nonproductive cough, chest pain, fatigue, fever, dyspnea, or weight loss.

Adapted from Little, J.W., Falace, D.A., Miller, C.S., and Rhodus, N.L.: *Dental Management of the Medically Compromised Patient,* 6th ed. St. Louis, Mosby, 2002, pp. 141–142.

I. CLASSIFICATION

Based on frequency and severity of symptoms and used to determine medical treatment protocols.
- Mild intermittent
- Mild persistent
- Moderate persistent
- Severe persistent

II. ETIOLOGY

The bronchiole lung tissue of patients with asthma is particularly sensitive to a variety of stimuli. The five types of asthma are listed in Box 62-4.

III. PATHOGENESIS OF ATOPIC (ALLERGIC) ASTHMA

Atopic asthma is one type of immunoglobulin E (IgE)–mediated hypersensitivity reaction.

A. Immunoglobulin E (IgE)

- One of the five types of antibodies produced by the body.
- Provides the primary defense against environmental allergens (pollen, tobacco smoke, food substances).

B. Normal Inflammatory Reaction

- IgE breaks down the allergens and removes them from the body.
- Normally, this activity does not produce noticeable symptoms.

C. Asthmatic Hypersensitivity Reaction

- People with asthma are believed to "hyperreact" and produce more IgE antibodies than normal.
- This results in symptoms of asthma: wheezing, coughing, dyspnea.

D. How Do Allergens Trigger Asthma?

Steps in an IgE-Mediated Hypersensitivity Reaction (Figure 62-3).
1. Upon initial exposure to an allergen (dust, pollen), immunoglobulins (IgE) are produced and bind to mast cells (Figure 62-3A).
2. On subsequent exposures, the antigen binds to the IgE on the mast cell (Figure 62-3B).
3. Mast cells release asthma mediators such as histamine, leukotrienes, and prostaglandins (Figure 62-3C).
4. Asthma mediators cause bronchoconstriction, vasodilation, and mucus production, resulting in wheezing, coughing, and dyspnea.

IV. SUMMARY OF IgE-MEDIATED HYPERSENSITIVITY REACTIONS

A. Local Anaphylaxis

- *Allergen binds to mast cell in nasal cavity:* results in allergic rhinitis (hay fever).
- *Allergen binds to mast cell in bronchiole:* results in asthma.

BOX 62-4 The Five Types of Asthma

1. Extrinsic (allergic, atopic)
- Most common type
- Mostly children, young adults are affected
- Triggers from outside the body

  Outdoor: inhaled seasonal allergens (pollen)

  Indoor: dust, mold, animal dander, tobacco smoke

  Occupational: latex

2. Intrinsic (idiosyncratic, nonallergic)
- Triggers from within the body
- Middle-aged adults affected from emotional stress, gastroesophageal acid reflux disease (GERD)
- Common symptom: cough

3. Drug-induced (nonallergic, nonatopic)
- Aspirin
- Nonsteroidal anti-inflammatory drugs (NSAIDS)
- Beta blockers
- Food substances: nuts, shellfish, milk, strawberries, tartrazine (yellow) food dye and color #5

4. Exercise induced
- Exact cause unknown
- Thermal changes during inhalation of cold air provoke mucosal irritation and airway hyperactivity
- Most common in children and young adults

5. Infectious
- Infections in the lungs caused by viruses, bacteria, and fungi result in asthmatic symptoms
- Treatment of the infection improves breathing

Adapted from Little, J.W., Falace, D.A., Miller, C.S., and Rhodus, N.L.: *Dental Management of the Medically Compromised Patient,* 6th ed. St. Louis, Mosby, 2002, pp. 130–131.

B. Systemic Anaphylaxis

- *Allergen (penicillin, bee venom, food substance) binds to mast cells throughout the body:* results in anaphylactic shock.

V. MEDICAL TREATMENT

Types of drugs used in the treatment of asthma.

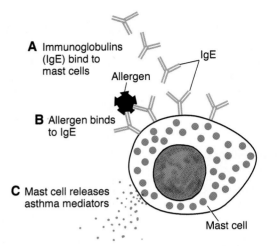

■ FIGURE 62-3 How Do Allergens Trigger Asthma? Steps in an IgE-mediated hypersensitivity reaction. **(A)** Initial exposure. Upon initial exposure to an allergen (dust, pollen), immumoglobulins (IgE) are produced and bind to mast cells. **(B)** Subsequent exposure. On subsequent exposures, allergen binds to IgE on the mast cell. **(C)** Mast cells respond. Mast cells release asthma mediators (histamines, leukotrienes, prostaglandins). These asthma mediators cause bronchoconstriction, vasodilation, and mucus production, resulting in coughing, wheezing, and dyspnea.

1. **Anti-inflammatory agents**
   - *Systemic corticosteroid:* Prednisone
   - *Inhaled corticosteroid:* Beclomethasone (Vanceril®)
   - *Leukotriene modifier:* Montelukast (Singulair®)
   - *Mast cell stabilizer:* Cromolyn (Intal®)
2. **Bronchodilators**
   - *Beta-2 agonist:* Albuterol (Ventolin®), Salmeterol (Serevent®)
   - *Methylxanthine:* Theophylline (Theodore®)
3. **Combined anti-inflammatory and bronchodilator**
   - ADVAIR DISKUS®

VI. ORAL MANIFESTATIONS

- Increase in caries and gingivitis related to decrease in saliva from beta-2 agonist medication.
- Increase in gastroesophageal reflux with use of beta-2 agonists and theophylline contributing to enamel erosion.
- Oral candidiasis may occur with high dosage or frequency of inhaled corticosteroids.

VII. DENTAL HYGIENE CARE[17-19]

Dental hygienists play a leading role in the dental treatment of patients with asthma. Table 62-4 summarizes dental hygiene care before, during, and after treatment.

▪ TABLE 62-4 DENTAL HYGIENE CARE FOR THE PATIENT WITH ASTHMA

TIME	DENTAL HYGIENE CARE

Before Treatment	• Remind the patient to bring inhaler and/or other medications.
	• Assess risk level: Review medical history, frequency and severity of acute episodes, medications, and triggering agents. Questions to ask:
	In the past 2 weeks, how many times have you:
	  a. had problems with coughing, wheezing, shortness of breath, or chest tightness during the day?
	  b. awakened at night from sleep because of coughing or other asthma symptoms?
	  c. awakened in the morning with asthma symptoms?
	  d. had asthma symptoms that did not improve within 15 minutes of using inhaled medication?
	  e. had symptoms while exercising or playing?
	• Evaluate current symptoms: Re-appoint if symptoms are not well-controlled.
	• Ask if any needed medication has been taken.
	• Schedule late morning or late afternoon appointments.
	• Have bronchodilator and oxygen available.
	• Obtain a medical consultation for patients with severe acute asthma or if on corticosteroid to determine necessity of steroid replacement and/or antibiotics to prevent infection.
	• Use bronchodilator as a preventive measure before the appointment.
	• Provide a stress-free environment.

During Treatment	• Prevent triggering a hypersensitive airway by properly placing cotton rolls, fluoride trays, and suction tip. • Use local anesthetic without epinephrine as it contains sulfites that may trigger an attack. • Give fluoride treatment for all patients with asthma especially those using beta-2 agonists. • If asthma attack occurs, stop treatment, rule out foreign body obstruction, initiate emergency procedures. (Table 66-4).
After Treatment	• Home care instructions: advise patient to rinse mouth with water after using inhaler to decrease oral candidiasis. • Analgesic drug of choice is acetaminophen (aspirin or NSAIDs may trigger attack).

Adapted from Steinbacher, D.M. and Glick, M: The Dental Patient With Asthma. An Update and Oral Health Considerations, *J. Am. Dent. Assoc.*, *132*, 1229, September, 2001; Lepore, M., Anolik, R., and Glick, M.: Diseases of the Respiratory Tract, in Greenberg, M.S. and Glick, M., eds.: *Burket's Oral Medicine*, 10th ed. Hamilton, BC Decker Inc., 2002, pp. 354–355; and Little, J.W., Falace, D.A., Miller, C.S., and Rhodus, N.L.: *Dental Management of the Medically Compromised Patient,* 6th ed. St. Louis, Mosby, 2002, pp. 134–136.

A. Emergency Care During an Asthma Attack (Table 66-4).

B. Signs and Symptoms of an Asthma Attack

- Chest tightness, difficulty breathing, sense of suffocation.
- Wheezing.
- Cough.
- Flushed appearance, sweating.
- Confusion due to lack of oxygen.
- Inability to complete a sentence in one breath.

C. Drugs to Avoid

- Aspirin-containing medications.
- Nonsteroidal anti-inflammatory drugs (NSAIDS).
- Narcotics and barbiturates.
- Macrolide antibiotics (such as erythromycin) if patient takes theophylline.
- Sulfite-containing local anesthetic solution.

▪ CHRONIC OBSTRUCTIVE PULMONARY DISEASE (COPD)

The acronym COPD is used to describe pulmonary disorders that obstruct airflow. Two of the most common diseases are chronic bronchitis and emphysema.[20] The primary etiology is use of tobacco and exposure to occupational and environmental pollutants. Motivating a patient with COPD to begin a smoking cessation program can be one of the most rewarding aspects of dental hygiene practice.

I. DEFINITIONS

A. Chronic Bronchitis

Excessive respiratory tract mucus production sufficient to cause a cough with expectoration (coughing up mucus) for at least 3 months of the year for 2 or more years.

- Obstruction caused by small airway and mucus plugging.

- Difficulty breathing present on inspiration (breathing in) and expiration (breathing out).

B. Emphysema

Distension of the air spaces distal to terminal bronchioles due to destruction of alveolar walls (septa).
- Alveolar epithelium is injured and alveolar walls are destroyed, creating large air spaces.
- Difficulty breathing only upon expiration.

II. RISK FACTORS

Poor oral health, especially periodontal involvement, may work in concert with other factors (continuing smoking, environmental pollutants, viral infections, allergy, and/or genetic factors) to promote the progression or exacerbation of COPD.[21]

III. SIGNS AND SYMPTOMS

A. Chronic Bronchitis

- Chronic cough.
- Copious sputum.
- Sedentary, overweight, cyanotic, edematous, breathless, leading to the term "blue bloaters."

B. Emphysema

- Difficulty in breathing upon exertion.
- Minimal, nonproductive cough (dry, no mucus).
- Barrel chest (enlarged chest walls) due to increased use of respiratory chest muscles.
- Weight loss.
- Purses lips to forcibly expel air, leading to the term "pink puffers."

IV. MEDICAL TREATMENT

There is no cure for COPD. Patients are encouraged to stop smoking, have adequate nutrition, drink plenty of water, exercise regularly, and decrease exposure to pollutants. Medical intervention strategies include:
- Pneumonia and influenza vaccine.
- Low-flow oxygen therapy.
- Bronchial dilator therapy.

V. ORAL MANIFESTATIONS

Chronic smokers with COPD have an increased risk of developing:
- Halitosis.
- Nicotine stomatitis.
- Periodontal disease.
- Oral cancer.
- Extrinsic tooth stains.

BOX 62-5 Clinical Signs and Symptoms of Cystic Fibrosis (CF)

Early-stage clinical signs and symptoms of cystic fibrosis
- Persistent cough and wheezing
- Recurrent pneumonia
- Excessive appetite but poor weight gain
- Salty skin or sweat
- Bulky, foul-smelling stools (undigested lipids)

Late-stage clinical signs and symptoms of cystic fibrosis with pulmonary involvement
- Tachypnea (rapid breathing)
- Sustained chronic cough with mucus production with vomiting
- Barrel chest
- Cyanosis and digital (finger) clubbing
- Exertional dyspnea with decreased exercise capacity
- Pneumothorax
- Right heart failure secondary to pulmonary hypertension

Used with permission from: McArdle, W.D., Katch, F.I., and Katch, V.L.: *Exercise Physiology*, 5th ed. Baltimore, Lippincott Williams & Wilkins, 2001, p. 952.

VI. DENTAL HYGIENE CARE

A. Patient History Preparation

- Review history for evidence of concurrent heart disease; take appropriate precautions if heart disease is present.
- Avoid treating if upper respiratory infection is present.
- Treatment may be performed on stable patients with adequate breathing.

B. Clinical Adaptations

- **Appointment length:** may need to modify.
- **Chair positioning:** semi-supine or upright to facilitate breathing.
- **Local anesthesia:** use as usual.
- **Nitrous oxide–oxygen inhalation sedation:** avoid with severe COPD and emphysema.

C. Patient Instruction

- Encourage patient to stop smoking. Smoking cessation strategies are discussed on pages 513 to 515.

Everyday Ethics

It is a beautiful spring day when Lana Thomas arrives for her 3-month preventive maintenance visit. Vicki, the dental hygienist, notices a labored breathing pattern as they walk down the hall to the dental hygiene treatment room. She rechecks the patient history before beginning the intraoral assessment but finds the information unremarkable.

Lana offers that she is taking an OTC product for seasonal allergies but it doesn't seem to be helping with her nasal and chest congestion. The patient also requests that she not be placed so far back in the dental chair because it is difficult for her to breathe. Vicki begins to reconsider her plan to use the ultrasonic scaler given the patient's current condition.

Questions to Consider

1. What baseline information can be obtained and recorded about the patient Ms. Thomas before proceeding?

2. Should a medical consult or clearance be considered since the dental hygiene care plan may need to be adjusted to accommodate the patient's breathing difficulty? If so, who must give consent for this to occur?

3. If treatment must be limited due to the patient's respiratory condition, how should the decision to alter the care plan be made? Explain the rationale.

■ CYSTIC FIBROSIS

Cystic fibrosis is a complex, genetic, life-limiting disorder that involves the pancreas, the liver, and the lungs.[22,23] The disease is progressive and ultimately fatal. With improved, multifaceted healthcare, the average survival has increased in recent years.

I. DISEASE CHARACTERISTICS

- Clinical signs and symptoms of cystic fibrosis are listed in Box 62-5.
- Mucus secretions of the lungs and digestive tissues are a critical feature of cystic fibrosis. The mucus obstructs ducts and passages in the pancreas, liver, and lungs.
- Pulmonary impairment, the most severe of the disease symptoms, leads to chronic airway obstruction and restrictive lung disease (RLD).
- Respiratory failure results from pneumothorax (collapsed lung) and pulmonary hypertension.

II. MEDICAL TREATMENT

Patients should be encouraged to have regular physical activity and to adjust their diet to include enzyme supplements and liquids with high salt intake. Comprehensive care includes:
- Antibiotics.
- Mucus-thinning solution (Pulmozyme®).
- Inhalation solution (Tobramycin®).
- NSAIDS (Ibuprofen®).
- Mucous secretion removal.

III. ORAL MANIFESTATIONS

- Thickening and enlargement of the salivary glands with advanced disease.
- Lower lip may be enlarged, swollen, and dry.
- Halitosis.

 ## Factors To Teach The Patient

- The need for frequent handwashing to help prevent transmission of respiratory disease.

- The need for thorough daily cleaning of toothbrushes to help prevent spread of infections.

- How using a new toothbrush and cleaning dentures/orthodontic appliances after bacterial infections can decrease possibility of re-infection.

- Why elderly patients and those with chronic cardiovascular disease, diabetes, and other immunosuppressed conditions should receive pneumonia vaccine and annual influenza immunization.

■ SUMMARY GUIDELINES FOR DENTAL HYGIENE CARE

Summary guidelines for dental hygiene care for patients with a respiratory disease are shown in Table 62-5.

▪ TABLE 62-5 SUMMARY GUIDELINES FOR DENTAL HYGIENE CARE FOR PATIENTS WITH A RESPIRATORY DISEASE

ITEM	DENTAL HYGIENE CARE
Medical Consultation required when:	• Signs or symptoms suggest respiratory disease. Examples: cough, dyspnea, hemoptysis, sputum, wheeze, chest pain, or positive Mantoux (TB) test. • The clinician is uncertain of the patient's medical status, severity of disease, or level of control. • Patients with systemic conditions have not seen their physician within the past year. • Patients have American Society of Anesthesiologists (ASA) risk status class III or higher (Table 21-1). • Patients have taken corticosteroids within the past 12 months. • Patients are receiving anti-infectives to determine the infectious nature of their disease. • The medications and dosage used are not well known by the patient. • Additional medications, a change in medication to protect the patient's health during dental treatment, or any other special precautions may be needed.
Stress Reduction Protocol: Prevent asthma attack and helpful for patients with COPD	• Short morning appointments. • Avoid precipitating factors.
Chair position	• Semireclined or upright position may make breathing easier.
Anesthesia	• Avoid epinephrine for patients with asthma/COPD. • Be prepared to handle an emergency.
Analgesia	• Avoid aspirin, aspirin-containing analgesics, and other NSAIDS as 10% of patients with asthma have aspirin-induced asthma.
Antibiotics	• Patients with extrinsic asthma may have allergy to antibiotics.
Infection control	• Standard precautions.
Emergency Protocol	• Recognize symptoms of respiratory distress. • Terminate treatment. • Table 66-4.
Use of aerosols	• Ultrasonic, sonic scalers and polishing contraindicated because of aspiration risk.

Adapted from Bricker, S.L., Langlais, R.P., and Miller, C.S.: *Oral Diagnosis, Oral Medicine, and Treatment Planning,* 2nd ed. Hamilton, BC Decker Inc., 2001, pp. 187–191.

REFERENCES

1. Garcia, R.I., Henshaw, M.M., and Krall, E.A.: Relationship Between Periodontal Disease and Systemic Health, *Periodontol. 2000, 25,* 21, 2001.
2. Underwood, J.C.E., Ed.: *General and Systematic Pathology,* 3rd ed. New York, Churchill Livingstone, 2000, pp. 326–328, 344–349.
3. Costerton, J.W., Stewart, P.S., and Greenberg, E.P.: Bacterial Biofilms: A Common Cause of Persistent Infections, *Science, 284,* 1318, May 21, 1999.
4. Lepore, M., Anolik, R., and Glick, M.: Diseases of the Respiratory Tract, in Greenberg, M.S. and Glick, M., eds.: *Burket's Oral Medicine, Diagnosis and Treatment,* 10th ed. Hamilton, BC Decker Inc., 2003, pp. 341–348.
5. Bricker, S.L., Langlais, R.P., and Miller, C.S.: *Oral Diagnosis, Oral Medicine, and Treatment Planning,* 2nd ed. Hamilton, BC Decker Inc., 2002, pp. 165–172.
6. Chin, J., Ed.: *Control of Communicable Diseases Manual,* 17th ed. Washington, D.C., American Public Health Association, 2000, p. 426.
7. Bricker, op. cit., p. 170.
8. Lepore, op. cit., pp. 349–352.
9. Chin, op. cit., pp. 387–398.
10. Scannapieco, F.A.: State of the Art Review: Role of Oral Bacteria in Respiratory Infection, *J. Periodontol., 70,* 793, July, 1999.
11. Chin, op. cit., p. 398.
12. Russell, S.L., Boylan, R.J., Kaslick, R.S., Scannapieco, F.A., and Katz, R.V.: Respiratory Pathogen Colonization of the Dental Plaque of Institutionalized Elders, *Spec. Care Dentist., 19,* 128, May/June, 1999.
13. Yoshino, A., Ebihara, T., Ebihara, S., Fuji, H., and Sasaki, H.: Daily Oral Care and Risk Factors for Pneumonia Among Elderly Nursing Home Patients, *JAMA, 286,* 2235, November 14, 2001.
14. Little, J.W., Falace, D.A., Miller, C.S., and Rhodus, N.L.: *Dental Management of the Medically Compromised Patient,* 6th ed. St. Louis, Mosby, 2002, pp. 136–144.
15. Chin, op. cit., pp. 521–530.
16. Little, op. cit., pp. 130–136.
17. Steinbacher, D.M. and Glick, M: The Dental Patient With Asthma: An Update and Oral Health Considerations, *J. Am. Dent. Assoc., 132,* 1229, September, 2001.
18. Little, op. cit., pp. 134–136.

19. **Lepore**, op. cit., pp. 354–355.
20. **Little**, op. cit., pp. 125–129.
21. **Scannapieco**, F.A. and Ho, A.W.: Potential Associations Between Chronic Respiratory Disease and Periodontal Disease: Analysis of National Health and Nutrition Examination Survey III, *J. Periodontol., 72,* 50, January, 2001.
22. **Bricker**, op. cit., pp. 282–284.
23. **McArdle**, W.D., Katch, F.I., and Katch, V.L.: *Exercise Physiology,* 5th ed. Philadelphia, Lippincott Williams & Wilkins, 2001, p. 952.

SUGGESTED READINGS

Day, M.B.: Managing the Patient With Severe Respiratory Problems, *J. Calif. Dent. Assoc., 28,* 585, August, 2000.

Gurenlian, J.R.: Sinusitis, *Access, 17,* 22, May–June, 2003.

Hatch, C.L., Canaan, T., and Anderson, G.: Pharmacology of the Pulmonary Diseases, *Dent. Clin. North Am., 40,* 521, July, 1996.

Loesche, W.J. and Lopatin, D.E.: Interactions between Periodontal Disease, Medical Diseases and Immunity in the Older Individual, *Periodontol. 2000, 16,* 80, 1998.

Mojon, P.: Oral Health and Respiratory Infection, *J. Can. Dent. Assoc., 68,* 340, June, 2002.

Potera, C.: Forging a Link Between Biofilms and Disease, *Science, 283,* 1837, March 19, 1999.

Scannapieco, F.A.: Relationships Between Periodontal and Respiratory Diseases, in Rose, L.F., Genco, R.J., Cohen, D.W., and Mealey, B.L., eds: *Periodontal Medicine.* Hamilton, B.C. Decker Inc., 2000, pp. 83–97.

Shay, K.: Infectious Complications of Dental and Periodontal Diseases in the Elderly Population, *J. Infect. Dis., 34,* 1215, May, 2002.

Suzuki, J.B. and Delisle, A.L.: Pulmonary Actinomycosis of Periodontal Origin, *J. Periodontol., 55,* 581, October, 1984.

Teng, Y.A., Taylor, G.W., Scannapieco, F., Kinane, D.F., Curtis, M., Beck, J.D., and Kogon, S.: Periodontal Health and Systemic Disorders, *J. Can. Dent. Assoc., 68,* 188, March, 2002.

U.S. Department of Health and Human Services. *Oral Health in America: A Report of the Surgeon General.* Rockville, MD: U.S. Department of Health and Human Services, National Institute of Dental and Craniofacial Research, National Institutes of Health, 2000.

Warren, D.P., Goldschmidt, M.C., Thompson, M.B., Adler-Storthz, K., and Keene, H.J.: The Effects of Toothpastes on the Residual Microbial Contamination of Toothbrushes, *J. Am. Dent. Assoc., 132,* 1241, September, 2001.

Asthma

Meldrum, A.M., Thomson, W.M., Drummond, B.K., and Sears, M.R.: Is Asthma a Risk Factor for Dental Caries? Findings From a Cohort Study, *Caries Res., 35,* 235, July–August, 2001.

Sollecito, T.P. and Tino, G.: Asthma, *Oral Surg. Oral Med. Oral Pathol. Oral Radiol. Endod., 92,* 485, November, 2001.

U.S. Department of Health and Human Services: Key Clinical Activities for Quality Asthma Care: Recommendations of the National Asthma Education and Prevention Program, *MMWR, 52/No. RR-6,* March 28, 2003.

Zhu, J., Hidalgo, H.A., Holmgreen, W.C., Redding, S.W., Hu, J., and Henry, R.J.: Dental Management of Children With Asthma, *Pediatr. Dent., 18,* 363, September/October, 1996.

Chronic Obstructive Pulmonary Disease (COPD)

Hayes, C., Sparrow, D., Cohen, M., Voconas, P.S., and Garcia, R.I.: The Association Between Alveolar Bone Loss and Pulmonary Function: The VA Dental Longitudinal Study, *Ann. Periodontol. 3,* 257, July, 1998.

LaPointe, H.J., Armstrong, J.E., and Larocque, B.: A Clinical Decision Making Framework for the Medically Compromised Patient: Ischemic Heart Disease and Chronic Obstructive Pulmonary Disease, *J. Can. Dent. Assoc., 63,* 510, July–August, 1997.

Cystic Fibrosis

Aps, J.K.M., Van Maele, G.O.G., and Martens, L.C.: Caries Experience and Oral Cleanliness in Cystic Fibrosis Homozygotes and Heterozygotes, *Oral Surg. Oral Med. Oral Pathol. Oral Radiol. Endod., 93,* 560, May, 2002.

Burden, D., Mullally, B., and Sandler, J.: Orthodontic Treatment of Patients with Medical Disorders, *Euro. J. Orthod., 23,* 363, August, 2001.

Influenza

U.S. Department of Health and Human Services: Prevention and Control of Influenza: Part 1, Vaccines, *MMWR, 43/No.RR-9,* 1, May 27, 1994.

Pneumonia

Scannapieco, F.A. and Mylotte, J.M.: Relationships Between Periodontal Disease and Bacterial Pneumonia, *J. Periodontol., 67,* 1114, October, 1996 (Supplement).

Sumi, Y., Miura, H., Sunakawa, M., Michiwaki, Y., and Sakagami, N.: Colonization of Denture Plaque by Respiratory Pathogens in Dependent Elderly, *Gerodontology, 19,* 25, July, 2002.

Tuberculosis

Cleveland, J.L., Gooch, B.F., Bolyard, E.A., Simone, P.M., Mullan, R.J., and Marianos, D.W.: TB Infection Control Recommendations From the CDC, 1994: Considerations for Dentistry, *J. Am. Dent. Assoc., 126,* 593, May, 1995.

Molinari, J.A.: Tuberculosis Infection Control: A Reasonable Approach for Dentistry, *Compend. Dent. Ed. Dent., 16,* 1080, November, 1995.

Phelan, J.A., Jimenez, V., and Tompkins, D.C.: Tuberculosis, *Dent. Clin. North Am., 40,* 327, April, 1996.

Younai, F.S. and Murphy, D.C.: TB and Dentistry, *NY State Dent. J., 63,* 49, January, 1997.

The Patient With a Cardiovascular Disease

Cardiovascular, as the names implies, includes diseases of the heart and blood vessels. Diseases of the heart are the leading causes of death in the United States. Key words and terminology describing the cardiovascular diseases are defined in Box 63-1. Prefixes and suffixes to clarify the terminology are listed on page 1121.

Patients with cardiovascular conditions are encountered frequently in a dental office or clinic and may be from any age group, although the highest incidence is among older people. A heart disease may be present for many years before the symptoms are recognized. The patients seen in the dental office range from those with no obvious symptoms to the nearly disabled.

I. CLASSIFICATION

Classification of the diseases is made on either an anatomic or an etiologic basis. In an anatomic system, diseases of the pericardium, myocardium, endocardium, heart valves, and blood vessels are defined. In an etiologic system, the diseases are named by the cause. The principal causes of heart diseases are infectious agents, atherosclerosis, hypertension, immunologic mechanisms, and congenital anomalies.

II. MAJOR CARDIOVASCULAR DISEASES

The major cardiovascular diseases are congenital heart disease, rheumatic heart disease, infective endocarditis, ischemic heart disease, hypertensive heart disease, and congestive heart failure. Characteristics and symptoms are complex and overlapping. In this chapter, each of the major diseases is described by its principal symptoms and treatments as well as the applications in dental hygiene care.

■ CONGENITAL HEART DISEASES

Anomalies of the anatomic structure of the heart or major blood vessels result following irregularities of development during the first 9 weeks in utero. The fetal heart is completely developed by the ninth week.

Early diagnosis is important because one fourth to one half of the infants born with cardiovascular anomalies require treatment during the first year of life. Treatment usually involves surgical correction.

I. TYPES[1]

Many types of heart defects exist. Those that occur most frequently are the ventricular septal defect, patent ductus arteriosus, atrial septal defect, and transposition of the great vessels.

A diagram of the normal heart is shown in Figure 63-1 to provide a comparison with the anatomic changes that may appear in a defective heart. In the healthy heart, the blood flows in one direction as each chamber contracts, with the valves acting as trap doors that snap shut after each contraction to prevent backflow of blood. The right side of the heart contains deoxygenated blood, and the left side of the heart contains oxygenated blood. The septal wall divides the left and right sides of the heart.

Defects (openings) in the septal wall cause a mixing of oxygenated and deoxygenated blood. Atrial and/or ventricular septal defects result in mixing of the blood from the left and right sides of the heart. Other defects include a passageway between the great arteries and veins, which also causes mixing of oxygenated and deoxygenated blood. The two most common anomalies are described here.

A. Ventricular Septal Defect

In this type of defect, the left and right ventricles exchange blood through an opening in their dividing wall (septum). The oxygenated blood from the lung, which is normally pumped by the left ventricle to the aorta and then to the entire body, can pass across to the right ventricle through the septal defect, as shown in Figure 63-2.

The severity of symptoms is directly related to the specific location and size of the defect. 75% of small defects close without surgical correction.

B. Patent Ductus Arteriosus

A patent ductus arteriosus means the passageway (shunt) is open between the two great arteries that

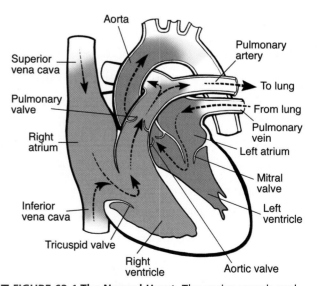

■ **FIGURE 63-1 The Normal Heart.** The major vessels and the location of the tricuspid, pulmonary, aortic, and mitral valves are shown.

BOX 63-1 Key Words: Cardiovascular Disease

Aneurysm: sac formed by the localized dilatation of the wall of an artery, a vein, or the heart.

Angina: a disease marked by spasmodic suffocative attacks.

Angina pectoris: acute pain in the chest from decreased blood supply to the heart muscle.

Anoxia: absence of oxygen in the tissues; may be accompanied by deep respirations, cyanosis, increased pulse rate, and impairment of coordination.

Anticoagulant: a substance that suppresses, delays, or nullifies coagulation of the blood.

Apnea: temporary cessation of breathing.

Arrhythmia: variation from the normal rhythm, especially with reference to the heart.

Arterial blood: oxygenated blood carried by an artery away from the heart to nourish the body tissues.

Asphyxia: a condition in which there is a deficiency of oxygen in the blood and an increase in carbon dioxide.

Atheroma: lipid (cholesterol) deposit on the intima (lining) of an artery; also called atheromatous plaque.

Bradycardia: slowness of heartbeat with slowing of pulse rate to less than 60 per minute.

Cyanosis: bluish discoloration of the skin and mucous membranes caused by excess concentration of reduced hemoglobin in the blood.

Dyspnea: labored or difficult breathing.

Echocardiography: recording of the position and motion of the heart walls and internal structures of the heart and neighboring tissue by the echo obtained from beams of ultrasonic waves directed through the chest wall; used to show valvular and other structural deformities; the record produced is called an echocardiogram.

Edema: abnormal accumulation of fluid in the intercellular spaces of the body.

Electrocardiography: the graphic recording from the body surface of the potential of electric currents generated by the heart as a means of studying the action of the heart muscle; the record produced is called an electrocardiogram (EKG).

Embolism: the sudden blocking of an artery by a clot of foreign material, an embolus, that has been brought to its site of lodgment by the bloodstream; the embolus may be a blood clot (most frequently) or an air bubble, a clump of bacteria, or a fat globule.

Heparin: anticoagulant; prevents platelet agglutination and thrombus formation.

Hypoxia: diminished availability of oxygen to blood tissues.

Infarct: localized area of ischemic necrosis produced by occlusion of the arterial supply or venous drainage of the part.

Ischemia: deficiency of blood to supply oxygen in part resulting from functional constriction or actual obstruction of a blood vessel.

Lumen: the cavity or channel within a tube or tubular organ, such as a blood vessel or the intestine.

Murmur: irregularity of heartbeat caused by a turbulent flow of blood through a valve that has failed to close.

Myocardium: the middle and thickest layer of the heart wall, composed of cardiac muscle.

Occlusion: blockage; state of being closed.

Prolapse: downward displacement.

Sclerosis: induration, hardening.

 Arteriosclerosis: group of diseases characterized by thickening and loss of elasticity of the arterial wall.

Key Words: Cardiovascular Disease, continued

Stenosis: narrowing or contraction of a body passage or opening.

Tachycardia: abnormally rapid heart rate, usually taken to be over 100 beats per minute.

Tetralogy: a group or series of four.

    Tetralogy of Fallot: congenital, cyanotic malformation of the heart that includes pulmonary stenosis, ventricular septal defect, hypertrophy of the right ventricle, and dextroposition of the aorta.

Thrombus: blood clot attached to the intima of a blood vessel; may occlude the lumen; contrast with embolus, which is detached and carried by the bloodstream.

Venous blood: nonoxygenated blood from the tissues; blood pumped from the heart to the lungs for oxygenation.

arise from the heart, namely, the aorta and the pulmonary artery. Normally, the opening is closed during the first few weeks after birth. When the opening does not close, blood from the aorta can pass back to the lungs, as shown in Figure 63-3. The heart compensates in the attempt to provide the body with oxygenated blood and becomes overburdened.

II. ETIOLOGY

Causes are genetic, environmental, or a combination. Many are unknown.

A. Genetic

Heredity is apparent in some types of defects. An example of a chromosomal defect is Down's syndrome, in which congenital heart anomalies occur frequently (page 986).

B. Environmental

Most congenital anomalies originate between the fifth and eighth weeks of fetal life, when the heart is developing.

1. Viral infections (rubella, cytomegalovirus).

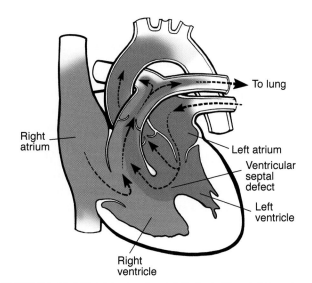

■ **FIGURE 63-2 Ventricular Septal Defect.** The right and left ventricles are connected by an opening that permits oxygenated blood from the left ventricle to shunt across to the right ventricle and then recirculate to the lungs. Compare with Figure 63-1, in which the septum separates the ventricles. (Adapted from Bleck, E.E. and Nagel, D.A.: *Physically Handicapped Children: A Medical Atlas for Teachers.* New York, Grune & Stratton, 1975.)

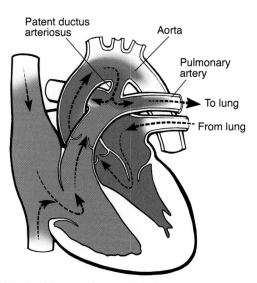

■ **FIGURE 63-3 Patent Ductus Arteriosus.** An open passageway between the aorta and the pulmonary artery permits oxygenated blood from the aorta to pass back into the lungs. Arrows show directions of flow through the patent ductus. Compare with normal anatomy in Figure 63-1. (Adapted from Bleck, E.E. and Nagel, D.A.: *Physically Handicapped Children: A Medical Atlas for Teachers.* New York, Grune & Stratton, 1975.)

2. Drugs.
   a. Chronic maternal alcohol abuse. The fetal alcohol syndrome is described on page 1014.
   b. Thalidomide.

III. PREVENTION

A. Use of rubella vaccine for childhood immunization. Vaccination confers indefinite immunity. Vaccination for women of childbearing age is highly advised for women not vaccinated in childhood. The vaccine should not be given during pregnancy, and not within 3 months of becoming pregnant, because of potential risks to the fetus.

B. No medications used during pregnancy without prior consultation with the physician.

C. Appropriate use of radiologic equipment. A lead apron should be used when oral radiographs are made.

D. Control of tobacco, drug, and alcohol addictions.

E. Genetic counseling.

IV. CLINICAL CONSIDERATIONS

A. Signs and Symptoms of Congenital Heart Disease

General conditions that may be present and that influence patient management are:
1. Easy fatigue.
2. Exertional dyspnea; fainting.
3. Cyanosis of lips and nailbeds.
4. Poor growth and development.
5. Chest deformity.
6. Heart murmurs.
7. Congestive heart failure.

B. Dental Hygiene Concerns

1. *Prevention of Infective Endocarditis.* Defective heart valves are susceptible to endocarditis from bacteremia produced during oral treatments.
2. *Elimination of Oral Disease.* Maintenance of a high level of oral health.

▪ RHEUMATIC HEART DISEASE

Rheumatic heart disease is a complication following rheumatic fever. A rather high percentage of patients with a history of rheumatic fever have permanent heart valve damage. The damaged heart valve, as in congenital heart disease, is susceptible to infective endocarditis.

I. RHEUMATIC FEVER[2,3]

A. Incidence

Approximately 90% of initial attacks occur between ages 5 and 15. The patient is left susceptible to future attacks, which may cause additional damage to previously damaged heart valves. The tendency to recurrence diminishes with age.

B. Etiology

1. The onset of acute rheumatic fever usually appears 2 to 3 weeks after a beta-hemolytic group A streptococcal pharyngeal infection.
2. Rheumatic fever and rheumatic heart disease are believed to be immunologic disorders caused by sensitization to antigens of beta-hemolytic group A streptococci.

C. Prevention

The persistence and severity of the pharyngeal infection are significant factors in whether rheumatic fever follows; therefore, early diagnosis and treatment of streptococcal throat and pharyngeal infections are necessary.

D. Symptoms of Rheumatic Fever

Over a period of several months of low-grade fever, the joints, heart muscles, central nervous system, skin, and subcutaneous tissues become involved. All the following symptoms disappear with recovery except the cardiac valve damage.

1. *Arthritis.* Migratory polyarthritis is present, which may affect more than one joint at a time. The temporomandibular joint is rarely involved.
2. *Carditis.* In a severe case, death may result from heart failure during the acute stage of rheumatic fever, or valvular damage may be sustained with disability. Severity varies, and many patients do not have heart symptoms at the time of the acute illness, some never, and others may have rheumatic heart disease diagnosed later in life without having had evidence of rheumatic fever.

The mitral valve is most commonly affected, followed by the aortic valve (Figure 63-1). Rheumatic carditis is almost always associated with a significant murmur of insufficiency. The damaged valves are susceptible to infection, leading to infective endocarditis.

II. THE COURSE OF RHEUMATIC HEART DISEASE

Many factors influence the outlook after rheumatic fever symptoms subside. Usually, no symptoms persist except the effects of the valvular deformity.

A. Symptoms

1. Stenosis or incompetence of valves; most commonly, the aortic and mitral valves.
2. Heart murmur influenced by the amount of scarring of the valves and myocardium.
3. Cardiac arrhythmias.
4. Late symptoms include shortness of breath, murmur, angina pectoris, epistaxis, elevation of diastolic blood pressure, enlargement of the left ventricle, and increasing signs of congestive cardiac failure.

B. Practice Applications

The significance in dental and dental hygiene practice is the same as that for congenital heart disease.
1. Maintenance of a high level of oral health to prevent a need for treatment of advanced disease.
2. Prevention of infective endocarditis by antibiotic premedication.

■ MITRAL VALVE PROLAPSE

I. DESCRIPTION

The mitral valve is between the left atrium and the left ventricle (Figure 63-1). Oxygenated blood from the lungs passes from the pulmonary vein into the left atrium and on into the left ventricle, where it is pumped through the aortic valve and into the aorta for distribution to the body cells.

When the mitral valve leaflets are damaged, the closure is imperfect, and oxygenated blood can backflow or regurgitate. Mitral valve prolapse is the most common disorder of the valve that causes regurgitation. The mitral valve is prolapsed into the atrium during systole.

II. SYMPTOMS

Most patients with mitral valve prolapse are without symptoms. A small number of cases will have symptoms of palpitations, fatigue, atypical chest pain, and a late systolic murmur.

When there is more severe involvement, an increase in frequency of palpitations and progressive mitral regurgitation is apparent along with a systolic click and murmur. Initial suspicion for diagnosis of valvular heart disease is the recognition of a heart murmur.

III. INDICATIONS FOR PROPHYLACTIC ANTIBIOTIC

Infective endocarditis occurs at a higher incidence in patients with mitral valve prolapse. Patients with mitral valve prolapse with significant regurgitation have been classified as at moderate risk for severe infection and require the AHA Regimen for prophylactic antibiotic. However, mitral valve prolapse without valvular regurgitation does not require prophylactic antibiotic.[4] Figure 7-2 outlines a decision tree for determination of the need for antibiotic prophylaxis. Any patient who presents with a history of mitral valve prolapse should not receive invasive dental procedures, including periodontal probing, exploring, or scaling, until a consultation with the patient's physician determines whether prophylactic antibiotic is indicated prior to treatment.

■ INFECTIVE ENDOCARDITIS[5,6]

Infective endocarditis is a microbial infection of the heart valves or endocardium that is of vital concern in the dental and dental hygiene care of high-risk patients.

A bacteremia, or presence of microorganisms in the bloodstream, is necessary for the development of infective endocarditis. A transitory bacteremia usually is created during invasive dental and dental hygiene treatment when bleeding occurs.

Infective endocarditis is a serious disease, the prognosis of which depends on the degree of cardiac damage, the valves involved, the duration of the infection, and the treatment. Patients are prone to develop heart failure leading to death unless the infection is promptly controlled.

Infective endocarditis is characterized by the formation of vegetations composed of masses of bacteria and blood clots on the heart valves. The vegetations may arise on normal valves but are most likely to occur on previously damaged valves. When bacteremia occurs, the heart valves may become infected, and infective endocarditis can develop.

I. ETIOLOGY

A. Microorganisms

Almost any species of microorganisms may cause infective endocarditis. Streptococci and staphylococci are responsible in most cases, with alpha-hemolytic streptococci being the most prevalent. Because yeast, fungi, and viruses have been implicated, the choice of the name "infective" endocarditis is more inclusive than "bacterial" endocarditis.

B. Risk Factors

1. *Preexisting Cardiac Abnormalities.* Bacteria lodge on the endocardial (valvular) surface during bacteremia.
2. *Prosthetic Heart Valves.* There is an increased number of patients who have had valve

replacement surgery who are susceptible. Patients who have had prosthetic valve replacements have a 3% risk of developing prosthetic valve endocarditis (PVE) with the first year of placement, and each year after the risk is 0.5%.

3. *Intravenous Drug Abuse.* Infected material is injected by contaminated needles directly into the bloodstream. Intravenous drug abusers are at high risk for endocarditis, which can initiate on previously normal valves.

4. *Fenfluramine or Dexfenfluramine Use.* The appetite suppressants commonly called "Fen-phen" have caused valvular disease in approximately 32% of patients who took the drug combination. Any patients who have taken the combination should have an evaluation by a physician prior to invasive dental procedures.

C. Precipitating Factors

1. *Self-induced Bacteremia.* In the oral cavity, self-induced bacteremias may result from eating, bruxing, chewing gum, or any activity that can force bacteria through the wall of a diseased sulcus or pocket. Interdental aids for oral hygiene can also cause self-induced bacteremia. Elimination of gingival inflammation and active periodontal disease should occur before teaching patients how to use interdental aids that promote bleeding.

2. *Infection at Portals of Entry.* Infections at sites where microorganisms may enter the circulating blood provide a constant source of potential infectious microorganisms. In the oral cavity, organisms enter the blood by way of periodontal and gingival pockets, where multitudes of many species of microorganisms are harbored. An open area of infection, such as an ulcer caused by an ill-fitting denture, may also provide a site of entry.

3. *Trauma to Tissues by Iinstrumentation.* Bacteremias are created during general or oral surgery, endodontic procedures, periodontal therapy, scaling, and, particularly, any therapy that causes bleeding.

II. DISEASE PROCESS

A. Bacteremia Initiated

1. Trauma from instrumentation can rupture blood vessels in the gingival sulcus or pocket.

2. Pressure from trauma forces oral microorganisms into the blood. Ease of entry of organisms

directly relates to the severity of trauma and the severity of the gingivitis or periodontitis.

B. Bacterial Implantation

1. Circulating microorganisms attach to a damaged heart valve, prosthetic valve, or other susceptible area. The mitral valve is most often affected.

2. Microorganisms proliferate to form vegetative lesions containing masses of plasma cells, fibrin, and bacteria.

3. Heart valve becomes inflamed; function is diminished.

4. Clumps of microorganisms (emboli) may break off and spread by way of the general circulation; complications result.

C. Clinical Course

1. A small number of patients are symptomatic within 2 days, but usually symptoms appear within 2 weeks. Severe symptoms of fever, loss of appetite and weight loss, weakness, arthralgia, and heart murmurs require hospitalization. Diagnosis is based on symptoms, echocardiography, blood cell count, and positive blood cultures.

2. Emboli can lead to paralysis and chest and other body pains.

3. Complications lead to eventual susceptibility to reinfection with infective endocarditis, congestive heart failure, and cerebrovascular disease.

III. PREVENTION

The three basic areas for attention in dental and dental hygiene care that contribute to the prevention of infective endocarditis are shown in Box 63-2.

A. Patient History

1. *Special Content.* Specific questions should be directed to elicit any history of rheumatic fever and its related symptoms, congenital heart defects, cardiac surgery, presence of prosthetic valves, acquired valvular defects, or previous episode of infective endocarditis.

2. *Consultation With Patient's Physician.* Consultation can be assumed necessary for all patients with a history of rheumatic fever, heart defects, and any other condition suggesting the need for prophylactic antibiotic premedication. Instrumentation, including the use of a probe or explorer during assessment of the patient, must be withheld until the medical status is cleared.

BOX 63-2 Prevention of Infective Endocarditis

- Identification of risk patients
  - Medical and personal history
  - Consultation with physician
- Prophylactic antibiotic coverage during appointments
- Upgrading and maintenance of the patient's oral health
  - Personal: daily dental biofilm removal
  - Professional: supervision, instruction, and motivation through frequent maintenance appointments

---

B. Prophylactic Antibiotic Premedication

1. *Recommended Regimens.* The recommendations of the American Heart Association are outlined on pages 122 to 125.
2. *Objectives of the Recommended Regimen.*
   a. Prevent, or reduce the severity and magnitude of, bacteremia.
   b. Administer antibiotic 1 hour before so the blood level at the time of the actual procedure is adequate to control infection and prevent infective endocarditis. Question the patient at the time of the appointment to ascertain that the antibiotic was taken on schedule. In the patient record, document the name of the antibiotic, time, and dosage that was taken by the patient.

C. Dental Hygiene Care

Maintenance of a high degree of oral health is important to each patient susceptible to infective endocarditis.

1. *Instruction.* Instruction in brushing and flossing at initial appointments should be provided while the patient is under antibiotic coverage.
2. *Sequence of Treatment.* Biofilm removal instruction should precede instrumentation for scaling to bring the tissues to as healthy a state as possible. The more severe the disease, the higher the incidence of bacteremia during and following instrumentation.
3. *Instrumentation.* Reduce the microbial population about the teeth and on the oral mucosa prior to instrumentation by having the patient brush, floss, and rinse thoroughly with an antiseptic mouthrinse.

▪ HYPERTENSION[7]

Hypertension means an abnormal elevation of arterial blood pressure. It has been called the "Silent Killer," as one third of people who have it do not have symptoms. It is a contributing risk factor in many vascular diseases, or it may be a result or an effect of underlying pathologic changes.

Detection of blood pressure for dental and dental hygiene patients has become an essential step in patient assessment prior to treatment. Early detection, with referral for additional diagnosis and treatment when indicated, can prove to be lifesaving for certain people. In addition, knowledge of the health problems of patients is needed so treatment can be safe and free from dangers of emergencies that may arise.

I. ETIOLOGY

A. Primary or Essential Hypertension

1. *Incidence.* Approximately 95% of all hypertension is primary or essential.
2. *Predisposing or Risk Factors.* Combinations of the factors listed are more significant than any one alone.
   a. *Cigarette Smoking.* Risk factors for atherosclerosis are interrelated (page 1046).
   b. *Heredity.*
   c. *Overweight.*
   d. *Race.* The incidence is higher among African Americans than among white Americans, the illness is more severe, and the mortality rate is higher at a younger age.
   e. *Climate.* Hypertension is less common in tropical and semitropical countries.
   f. *Salt.* Particularly in excess in the diet.

g. *Sex.* Men are more affected before age 45; women slightly more than men in later years.

h. *Age.* General increase from birth to age 20; leveling off until 40 years of age; then a slow increase into the older age group.

i. *Environment.* Environmental conditions that increase stress factors.

B. Secondary Hypertension

About 5% of all hypertension is secondary to other underlying medical conditions. In secondary hypertension, usually both systolic and diastolic blood pressures are elevated. Examples of causes are:

1. *Oral Contraceptives.* Severe hypertension from contraceptives is uncommon. Increased hypertension over years of using contraceptives has been shown to be the most common cause of secondary hypertension in women.

2. *Renal Disease.*
   a. Renal artery obstruction.
   b. Pyelonephritis.
   c. Renal failure.

3. *Endocrine Disorders.*
   a. Hyperthyroidism.
   b. Diabetes.
   c. Cushing's Syndrome.
   d. Pheochromocytoma tumor of the adrenal medulla.

II. BLOOD PRESSURE LEVELS

The diastolic blood pressure is the pressure exerted by the blood within the arteries during the total resting resistance after the contraction of the left ventricle.

The systolic blood pressure is the pressure exerted against the arterial walls during the ventricular contraction. It is altered by the cardiac output, resistance of the capillary bed, and volume and viscosity of the blood. Diseases can have an effect on any of these factors, altering the blood pressure.

Procedures for blood pressure determination are described with other vital signs in Chapter 8.

Blood pressure fluctuates, so more than one reading is needed to determine the average level. The blood pressure should be measured two or three times and the average reading entered in the patient's record. When physicians plan treatment for a hypertensive patient, the individual's pattern is usually studied by making at least three determinations on at least two different days.

A. Normal and High Blood Pressure[8]

Table 63-1 shows the normal and high normal readings for blood pressure and the stages of hypertension for adults 18 years and over.

B. Low Blood Pressure

Many healthy people have a normal diastolic pressure under 90 mmHg or even under 80 mmHg, which may be considered "low blood pressure." Such a level is normal for that person, and no clinical problems are evident.

A marked sudden drop in blood pressure is usually associated with an emergency, such as severe blood loss, shock, myocardial infarction, or other medical problems. Immediate attention, in the category of a medical emergency, is indicated. Referral to specific procedures can be found in Table 66-4.

C. Postural Hypotension

Postural or orthostatic hypotension is a condition in which there is a sudden drop in the arterial blood pressure when a person sits up quickly from a supine position or stands up quickly from a sitting position. Postural hypotension is an adverse effect associated with many medications, mostly antihypertensives and antidepressants.

III. CLINICAL SYMPTOMS OF HYPERTENSION

Essential hypertension is frequently recognized only by blood pressure readings. The condition goes unrecognized because of the lack of clinical symptoms.

▪ TABLE 63-1 CLASSIFICATION OF BLOOD PRESSURE FOR ADULTS AGE 18 YEARS OR OLDER		
BLOOD PRESSURE CATEGORY	**SYSTOLIC (mmHg)**	**DIASTOLIC (mmHg)**
Normal	<120	<80
Prehypertension	120–139	80–89
Stage 1 hypertension	140–159	90–99
Stage 2 hypertension	≥160	≥100

Data from *The Seventh Report of the Joint National Committee on Prevention, Detection, Evaluation, and Treatment of High Blood Pressure.* National Institutes of Health, National Heart, Lung, and Blood Institute, Publication 03-5233, May, 2003.)

A. High Blood Pressure

Those who have early symptoms may describe them as:
1. Occipital headaches.
2. Dizziness.
3. Visual disturbances.
4. Weakness.
5. Ringing in the ears.
6. Tingling of the hands and feet.

B. Long-standing Severe Elevation of Blood Pressure

Hypertensive crisis is a life-threatening disorder. The brain, eyes, heart, or kidney may undergo marked changes in function. In the severe state, if any or all of the following are noted, the patient should be referred immediately.
1. Any of the symptoms associated with early symptoms.
2. Mental confusion leading to stupor, coma, convulsions.
3. Blurring of vision; possible loss of sight.
4. Severe dyspnea.
5. Chest pains similar to angina pectoris.

C. Major Sequela

1. Hypertensive heart disease; enlarged heart with eventual cardiac failure.
2. Cerebral vascular accident (stroke, page 929).
3. Hypertensive renal disease.
4. Ischemic heart disease.

D. Malignant Hypertension

Malignant hypertension occurs in approximately 5% of patients who have primary or secondary hyperten-sion. The blood pressure rises rapidly to levels greater than 200 mmHg systolic and 100 mmHg diastolic. Often referred to as a hypertensive crisis, malignant hypertension presents a risk for a cerebrovascular accident (CVA).

IV. TREATMENT

A. Goals

1. *Primary Hypertension.*
   a. Achieve and maintain diastolic pressure level at 90 mmHg or below with minimal adverse effects.
   b. Lower the risk of serious complications and premature death.
2. *Secondary Hypertension.* Surgical or other correction of the cause is needed.

B. Lifestyle Changes (Box 63-3)

1. *Diet.* Salt restriction and weight loss may be all that are needed for the control of mild elevations of blood pressure.
2. *Cigarette Smoking.* All forms of tobacco must be eliminated.
3. *Other Risk Factors.* Factors that contribute to stress and tension must be decreased or mini-mized.

V. HYPERTENSION IN CHILDREN

Children 3 years of age and older need to have blood pressure determinations made at least annually. A variety of blood pressure cuff sizes are available, and other pro-cedural suggestions are described on pages 133 to 134.

When a child between ages 3 and 12 has a diastolic pressure greater than 90 mmHg, or if over age 12, greater than 100 mmHg, further investigation is indicated.

BOX 63-3 Lifestyle Modifications for Hypertension Control and/or Overall Cardiovascular Risk

- Lose weight if overweight.

- Limit alcohol intake to no more than 1 ounce of ethanol per day (24 ounces of beer, 8 ounces of wine, or 2 ounces of 100-proof whiskey).

- Exercise (aerobic) daily.

- Reduce sodium intake to less than 100 mmol per day (2.4 g of sodium or <6 g of sodium chloride).

- Maintain adequate dietary potassium, calcium, and magnesium intake.

- Stop smoking and reduce dietary saturated fat and cholesterol intake for overall cardiovascular health. Reducing fat intake also helps to reduce caloric intake—important for control of weight and type 2 diabetes.

Because hypertension has a familial tendency, determining the pressure levels for children of parents known to have hypertension may reveal important information about the health of the child.

■ HYPERTENSIVE HEART DISEASE[9]

Hypertensive heart disease results from the increased load on the heart because of elevated blood pressure. When the peripheral arterial resistance to the flow of blood pumped from the heart is increased, the blood pressure rises. The heart attempts to maintain its normal output. To cope with the increased workload resulting from the peripheral resistance, muscle fibers are stretched and the heart enlarges.

The effect of hypertension on the heart is at first a thickening of the left ventricle. In later stages, the entire heart is enlarged. This may be discerned by radiographic and medical examination.

Cardiac enlargement has no specific symptoms, but the patient may have symptoms of hypertension, such as headaches, weakness, and others listed on page 1045. When undiagnosed and untreated, the severity increases and left ventricular congestive failure occurs, resulting from the disturbance of cardiac function.

■ ISCHEMIC HEART DISEASE

Ischemic heart disease is the cardiac disability, acute and chronic, that arises from reduction or arrest of blood supply to the myocardium.

The heart muscle (myocardium) is supplied through the coronary arteries, which are branches of the descending aorta. Because of the relationship to the coronary arteries, the disease is often referred to as coronary heart disease or coronary artery disease.

Ischemia means oxygen deprivation in a local area from a reduced passage of fluid into the area. Ischemic heart disease is the result of an imbalance of the oxygen supply and demand of the myocardium, which, in turn, results from a narrowing or blocking of the lumen of the coronary arteries.

I. ETIOLOGY[10]

Other factors may be involved, but the principal cause of the reduction of blood flow to the heart muscle is atherosclerosis of the vessel walls, which narrows the lumen, thus obstructing the flow of blood.

A. Definition of Atherosclerosis

Atherosclerosis is a disease of medium and large arteries in which atheromas deposit on and thicken the intimal layer of the involved blood vessel. An atheroma is a fibro-fatty deposit or plaque containing several lipids, especially cholesterol. With time, the plaques continue to thicken and, eventually, close the vessel (Figure 63-4). Some plaques calcify, whereas others may develop an overlying thrombus.

B. Predisposing Factors for Atherosclerosis

Each of the risk factors listed here is significant alone. When these factors occur in combinations, the risk of atherosclerosis, and therefore of ischemic heart disease, is increased. Prevention depends on educational programs along with early identification of persons at risk.

1. Elevated levels of blood lipids; the result of an increased dietary intake of cholesterol, saturated fat, carbohydrate, especially sucrose, alcohol, and calories.
2. Elevated blood pressure.
3. Cigarette smoking.
4. Diabetes.
5. Obesity.
6. Insufficient physical activity.
7. Increased tensions; emotional stress.
8. Family history. Genetic inheritance can be one factor along with the perpetuation of familial lifestyle habits. Diet, smoking habits, tensions, and tendencies toward lack of exercise are typical examples.

II. MANIFESTATIONS OF ISCHEMIC HEART DISEASE

A. Components

1. Angina pectoris.
2. Myocardial infarction.
3. Congestive heart failure.
4. Sudden death.

B. Treatment

1. *Counseling.* With a brief history of angina pain, the patient is counseled to be reassured that lifestyle changes are necessary but that a productive life can be led.
2. *Lifestyle Changes.* Necessary changes in lifestyle (Box 63-3) are encouraged, notably diet, exercise, and no smoking.
3. *Medications.* A variety of medications may be required depending on individual needs.
4. *Surgery.*
    a. Percutaneous transluminal coronary angioplasty (coronary dilation).

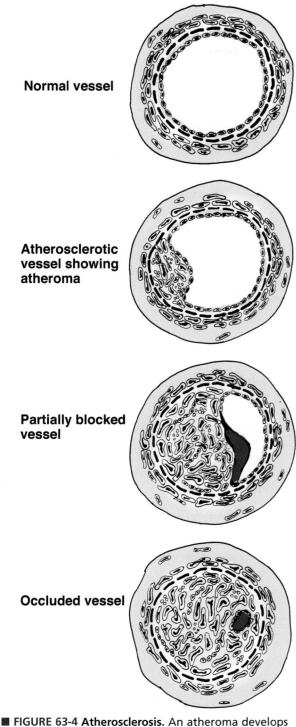

Normal vessel

Atherosclerotic vessel showing atheroma

Partially blocked vessel

Occluded vessel

■ **FIGURE 63-4 Atherosclerosis.** An atheroma develops within the lining of the normal blood vessel. The atheroma is made of a fatty deposit containing cholesterol. At first, the atheroma is small and no symptoms are apparent, but eventually it enlarges and completely blocks the vessel, thus depriving the area served by the vessel of oxygen. (From Arteriosclerosis 1981. Report of the Working Group on Arteriosclerosis of the National Heart, Lung, and Blood Institute, National Institutes of Health, United States Department of Health and Human Services, NIH Publication No. 81–2034, June, 1981.)

b. Coronary bypass for patients with significant obstruction. The purpose is to "jump-pass" over arteries that have been narrowed with atherosclerosis. The beneficial effects are relief from anginal pains, less workload for the heart, and an increase of oxygen and blood supply to the myocardium. Figure 63-5 shows the use of a vein graft and the internal mammary artery for bypasses.

■ ANGINA PECTORIS

Angina pectoris is chest pain, the most common symptom of coronary atherosclerotic heart disease. The pain is described as a heavy, squeezing pressure or tightness in the midchest region. The pain may radiate to the left or right arm and neck or even the mandible. On rare occasion, the pain may be limited to one of these areas and not occur in the chest area at all. The patient may be pale and also experience faintness, sweating, difficulty in breathing, anxiety, or fear. The pain lasts 1 to 5 minutes if precipitating factors are eliminated.

Although other forms of coronary disease may cause similar pain symptoms, approximately 90% of angina attacks are related to coronary artery atherosclerosis.

I. PRECIPITATING FACTORS

A. *Stable angina* may be precipitated by exertion or exercise, emotion, or a heavy meal. In the dental office or clinic, a preventive atmosphere of calmness and quiet can do much to alleviate stress. Stable angina is predictable and consistent in frequency, intensity, and duration.

B. *Unstable angina* occurs without exertion or other precipitating factors. The pain may occur while the patient is at rest, and it may vary in intensity at each attack.

II. TREATMENT

A vasodilator, usually nitroglycerin, is administered sublingually. Basic life support that includes supplemental oxygen is part of the treatment provided in a dental office or clinic.

III. PROCEDURE DURING AN ATTACK IN THE DENTAL OFFICE

A. Terminate Treatment

Stop the dental or dental hygiene procedure. Call for assistance and the emergency kit or cart.

B. Position Patient

Bring seat up to a comfortable position; reassure the patient.

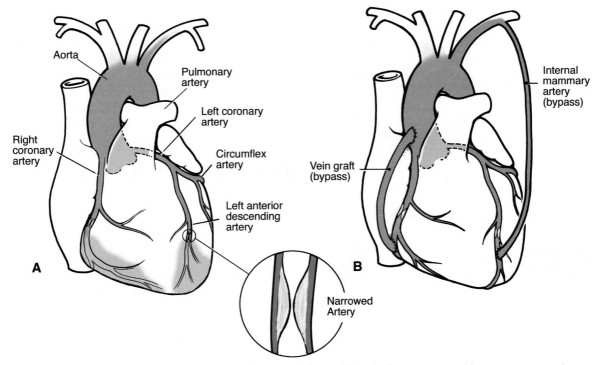

■ **FIGURE 63-5 Coronary Bypass Surgery. (A)** Heart showing infarcted (shaded) areas created by coronary arteries narrowed by atherosclerosis. **(B)** Vein graft from saphenous vein connected with aorta to bypass narrowed area of right coronary artery, and internal mammary artery used to bypass narrowed left anterior descending artery.

C. Administer Vasodilator

Administer nitroglycerin sublingually. Use of the patient's own supply is preferable. Prior to starting procedures of the appointment, the patient's supply should be placed within reach. The patient can be asked when the nitroglycerin was purchased because the potency is lost after 6 months out of a sealed storage container.

Patient with xerostomia may not have sufficient saliva to moisten the nitroglycerin. A few drops of water from the unit syringe can be placed on the tablet under the tongue.

D. Check Patient Response

Give additional vasodilator. Usually, the first tablet relieves the condition within minutes. When it is suspected that the patient's supply may not be fresh and the first tablet has been ineffective, use of a second tablet from the dental office emergency kit may be advisable.

E. Call for Medical Assistance

When the patient does not respond to the second dose of vasodilator, assume the attack to be a myocardial infarction. Oxygen administration may be indicated.

F. Record Vital Signs

1. Use the *Medical Emergency Report,* Figure 66-1.
2. Measure blood pressure, take pulse rate, and count respirations.

G. Observe Recovery

For the patient who recovers without additional medical assistance, allow a rest period before dismissal. Record vital signs again.

IV. SUBSEQUENT DENTAL AND DENTAL HYGIENE APPOINTMENTS

Keep a copy of the *Medical Emergency Report* in the patient's permanent file for reference when planning future appointments.

■ MYOCARDIAL INFARCTION

Myocardial infarction is the most extreme manifestation of ischemic heart disease. It is also called heart attack, coronary occlusion, or coronary thrombosis. It results from a sudden reduction or arrest of coronary blood flow.

The most common artery associated with a myocardial infarction is the anterior descending branch of the left coronary artery. That is also the most common site of advanced atherosclerosis.

I. ETIOLOGY

The immediate cause often is a thrombosis that blocks an artery already narrowed by atherosclerosis. In turn, the blockage creates an area of infarction, which leads to myocardial necrosis of the area. Necrosis of the area can occur within a few hours.

A few patients die immediately or within a few hours. Sudden death may be caused by ventricular fibrillation.

II. SYMPTOMS

A. Pain

1. *Location.* Pain symptoms may start under the sternum, with feelings of indigestion, or in the middle to upper sternum. Pain may last for extended periods, even hours. When the pain is severe, it gives a pressing or crushing heavy sensation and is not relieved by rest or nitroglycerin.
2. *Onset.* The pain may have a sudden onset, sometimes during sleep or following exercise. The pain may be radial, similar to angina pectoris, which extends to the left or right arm, neck, and mandible.

B. Other Symptoms

Cold sweat, weakness and faintness, shortness of breath, nausea, and vomiting may occur. Blood pressure falls below baseline.

III. MANAGEMENT DURING AN ATTACK

A. Terminate Treatment

Sit the patient up for comfortable breathing, give nitroglycerin, and reassure the patient.

B. Summon Medical Assistance

1. When nitroglycerin does not reduce the angina-like pain within 3 minutes, call both a physician and an ambulance with paramedical personnel (Table 66-4).
2. Use *Medical Emergency Report,* Figure 66-1, and record vital signs.
3. Administer oxygen.
4. Apply cardiopulmonary resuscitation if indicated while waiting for medical assistance.
5. Transport to hospital.

IV. TREATMENT AFTER ACUTE SYMPTOMS

A. Medical Supervision

Current medical care for heart attack calls for a shortened rest period with increased activity, in keeping with the strength and progress of the patient. Most patients experience extreme fatigue during their convalescence.

B. Lifestyle Changes

Dietary changes and elimination of smoking and stressful activities, as well as control of diseases that exacerbate ischemic heart disease, are essential. Many patients need considerable education, reassurance, and motivation.

C. Subsequent Appointments

Elective dental and dental hygiene appointments may be postponed 6 months or more until the patient's physician has given consent.

■ CONGESTIVE HEART FAILURE

Heart failure is a syndrome in which an abnormality of cardiac function is responsible for the inability or failure of the heart to pump blood at a rate necessary to meet the needs of the body tissues. Because of the collection of fluids in various body organs and the inability of the heart to empty each chamber with sufficient contractile force, the term congestive heart failure is used.

I. ETIOLOGY

The many causes of heart failure fall into two categories: underlying and precipitating causes.

A. Underlying Causes

Examples of cardiovascular disease that result in heart failure are:
1. Heart valve damage (rheumatic heart disease, congenital heart disease).
2. Myocardial failure as a result of an abnormality of heart muscle or secondary to ischemia.

B. Precipitating Causes

Examples that place an additional load on a chronically burdened myocardium are:
1. *Acute Hypertensive Crisis.* Severe symptoms of headache, mental confusion, dizziness, shortness of breath, and chest pain may predispose to heart failure.
2. *Massive Pulmonary Embolism.* A thrombus may form in a lower extremity of an inactive person with low cardiac output and circulatory stasis. The thrombus may break loose and,

carried by the blood, lodge in the pulmonary artery to cause a pulmonary embolism. Severe dyspnea, cyanosis, congestive failure, and shock result.

3. *Arrhythmia.* After resuscitation of a person with myocardial infarction, ventricular fibrillation, a type of arrhythmia, is the major risk leading to sudden death.

II. CLINICAL MANIFESTATIONS

The clinical manifestations coincide with the parts of the heart involved. Signs and symptoms are different, depending, in general, on whether the left or the right side of the heart or both are affected. The general effects are extreme weakness, fatigue, fear, and anxiety.

A. Left Heart Failure

The left side of the heart receives oxygenated blood from the lungs and pumps the blood into the aorta to the rest of the body. A pathologic condition of the left ventricle or the mitral valve alters output, and causes respiratory difficulty because of the backup of serous fluid into the lungs.

Clinical symptoms are more prominent at night. The patient rests better in a sitting or semi-sitting position with more than one pillow.

1. *Subjective Symptoms*
   a. Weakness, fatigue.
   b. Dyspnea, particularly evident on exertion. Shortness of breath when lying supine, relieved when sitting up.
   c. Cough and expectoration.
   d. Nocturia.
2. *Objective Symptoms*
   a. Pallor; sweating, cold skin.
   b. Breathing obviously difficult.
   c. Diastolic blood pressure increased.
   d. Heart rate rapid.
   e. Anxiety, fear.

B. Right Heart Failure

The right heart receives the venous blood from the vena cava and pumps it to the lungs for oxygenation. Right heart failure shows evidence of systemic venous congestion with peripheral edema. When left heart failure precedes right heart failure, the heart is already congested. Resistance to receiving the venous blood is an additional factor.

1. *Subjective Symptoms*
   a. Weakness, fatigue.
   b. Swelling of the feet and/or ankles. The edema progresses to the thighs and abdomen (ascites) in advanced stages of heart failure.
   c. Cold hands and feet.
2. *Objective Symptoms*
   a. Cyanosis of mucous membranes and nailbeds.
   b. Prominent jugular veins.
   c. Congestion with edema in various organs: enlarged spleen and liver; gastrointestinal distress with nausea and vomiting; central nervous system involvement with headache and irritability.
   d. Anxiety, fear.

III. TREATMENT DURING CHRONIC STAGES

A patient with an appointment in a dental office or clinic may be receiving a variety of medical treatments. These should be revealed by questioning during preparation of histories. Nearly all patients with heart failure complications have the following in their medical treatment plan:

A. Drug Therapy

Physicians may prescribe many different medications for patients with cardiovascular disease. The general types are listed in Table 7-3.

B. Dietary Control

1. Limited sodium intake to alleviate fluid retention.
2. Weight reduction.

C. Limitation of Activity

Activity should be limited depending on the severity of the health problem and the advice of the physician.

IV. EMERGENCY CARE FOR HEART FAILURE AND ACUTE PULMONARY EDEMA

A medical emergency that demands urgent attention may occur anywhere. The patient with heart failure or acute pulmonary edema is usually conscious.

A. Position the patient upright for comfortable breathing (Table 66-4).
B. Administer oxygen.
C. Use the *Medical Emergency Report,* Figure 66-1, and monitor vital signs (blood pressure, respiratory rate, and pulse).
D. Reassure the patient.
E. Obtain medical assistance, including both physician and ambulance.

■ SUDDEN DEATH

Clinical death that occurs within 24 hours after onset of symptoms is known as sudden death, whereas death within 30 seconds is instantaneous death. Biologic death occurs when permanent cellular damage has been done, primarily from lack of adequate oxygen supply. Biologic death takes place when oxygen delivery to the brain is inadequate for 4 to 6 minutes.

I. ETIOLOGY

Nearly all sudden deaths are from a cardiovascular cause, predominantly coronary atherosclerosis. Examples of noncardiac causes are cerebral hemorrhage, drug overdose or toxicity, and pulmonary thromboembolism.

II. MECHANISM OF SUDDEN CARDIOVASCULAR DEATH

A. Definition and Description

Most sudden deaths are caused by ventricular fibrillation. Because of many premature beats in which individual muscle bundles fibrillate or contract independently, the ventricle cannot be refilled. Insufficient blood is pumped into the coronary arteries to supply the myocardium. A severe lack of oxygen to the heart muscles causes ventricular standstill, which is one form of cardiac arrest.

B. Clinical Signs of Death

1. Loss of consciousness.
2. No respiration, no pulse, no blood pressure.
3. Dilated pupils.

III. EMERGENCY CARE

A. Immediate Need: Oxygen

Every second counts; only 4 minutes, or 6 at the most, can elapse before enough brain cells die from lack of oxygen to produce biologic death.

B. Basic Life Support

Details of the procedures are described on pages 1099 to 1100.
1. Provide artificial ventilation.
2. Provide artificial circulation.
3. Provide transportation to a hospital.

■ CARDIAC PACEMAKER

The natural pacemaker, or center where the normal heartbeat is initiated, is the sino-atrial (S-A) node located in the right atrium. From that node, impulses are sent along the muscle walls to stimulate and regulate the contractions of the ventricles, which pump the blood throughout the body.

When the natural pacemaker cells are not able to maintain a reliable rhythm, or when the impulses are interrupted because of heart block, cardiac arrest, various arrhythmias, or other disease conditions, treatment by a cardiologist may include the placement of an artificial pacemaker.

I. DESCRIPTION

A. Definition

A cardiac pacemaker is an electronic stimulator used to send a specified electrical current to the myocardium to control or maintain a minimum heart rate. It may be single chambered (to ventricle or atrium) or dual chambered to sense and pace both heart chambers.

B. Parts and Power

A permanently implanted pacemaker has electrodes inserted transvenously to the endocardium. Less commonly, the leads may go to the pericardium of the external heart wall.

The electrodes are connected to the power source, a plastic- or metal-encased, hermetically sealed pulse generator containing a lithium anode battery. The pulse generator is implanted under the skin in the thorax or upper abdomen. The area selected depends on the individual condition as determined by the cardiologist (Figure 63-6).

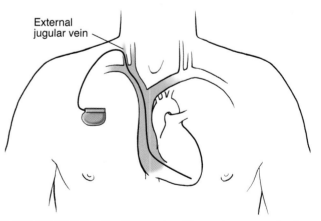

External
jugular vein

■ **FIGURE 63-6 Cardiac Pacemaker.** The pulse generator is implanted under the skin in the thorax or upper abdomen. The lead electrodes may go to the ventricle or to the atrium or both to provide the necessary stimulus for regulation of the heartbeat.

C. Types

Research has provided many advancements in pacemaker technology. Current systems involve rate-responsive or physiologic pacing. Sensors may be alert to muscle or physical activity vibrations, body temperature, or respiration rate. The research will have a significant impact on the future of pacing. The two general types are demand and fixed rate.

1. *Demand.* The demand pacemaker stimulates the heart only when the rate varies from a predetermined norm. By sensing a discrepancy in the electrical signals produced by natural means, the pacemaker sends a signal or stimulus, which regulates the heartbeat.

2. *Fixed Rate.* A preset rate of electrical stimuli is provided independent of the natural heart activity when the natural beat is too slow. Each patient is evaluated for the type of pacemaker that is best for the condition of that individual's heart. The fixed rate is used infrequently.

II. INTERFERENCES AND THEIR EFFECTS

External electromagnetic interferences can stop or alter the function of a pacemaker. Different models of pacemakers and their sensitivities to interference vary. Newer models are made with a special shielding to protect against interference.

Historically, ultrasonic scaling units, electrodesensitizing equipment, pulp testers, electric toothbrushes, electrosurgery machines, certain casting equipment, and the Myomonitor were among the potential sources of interference with a pacemaker in a dental care setting. Dental devices that apply an electric current directly to the patient were considered those most likely to interfere.

The dental environment has been shown to be a source of moderate electromagnetic interference. All dental equipment should be kept in good repair. Electric devices that contact or can contact the patient should be checked for leakage because leakage can be a source of interference. Electrical appliances must be earth-grounded.

The effect of distance has not been sufficiently researched; hence, patients in adjacent dental treatment rooms should be checked before equipment is used.

Although the evidence for interferences in the dental setting is not great, concern must be shown because all pacemakers are not the same.

III. PACEMAKER MALFUNCTION

A. Symptoms

A patient may mention feelings of discomfort. At the same time, the clinician must be aware of possible changes and signs in the event of stopping or altering of a pacemaker.

1. Difficulty in breathing.
2. Dizziness, light-headedness, feelings of faintness, or syncope.
3. Changes in pulse rate.
4. Swelling of legs, ankles, arms, wrists.
5. Chest pain.
6. Prolonged hiccoughing.
7. Muscle twitching.

B. Emergency Procedures

In the event a pacemaker should be turned off, immediate action is needed.

1. Turn off all suspected sources of interference.
2. Call for medical assistance; a defibrillator may be needed.
3. Position the patient for cardiopulmonary resuscitation.
4. Open airway, check for breathing, and begin mouth-to-mouth ventilation. The complete procedure is described on page 1103.
5. Observe the patient. When the heart is forced to assume its rhythm again as a result of artificial circulation, the pacemaker is set into action to resume the generation and regulation of the pulse.

IV. APPOINTMENT GUIDELINES FOR THE PATIENT WITH A PACEMAKER

General procedures for all patients with cardiovascular involvement apply to the patient wearing a pacemaker. In addition, certain adaptations are recommended.

A. Informed Consent

The signature of the patient or the patient's parent or guardian on a formal statement is a necessary protection against any legal liability in the event of complications or undesirable effects. The patient should receive careful instruction in the anticipated procedures and materials used. Dental and dental hygiene records should be accurate and all-inclusive, with a detailed record for each appointment.

B. Patient Histories

The usual health history should be supplemented with information about the type of pacemaker, how long it has been in use, where it is located, the underlying disease condition, and other information pertinent to the patient's safety during dental and dental hygiene appointments. Consultation with the patient's cardiologist is indicated.

C. Prophylactic Antibiotic Premedication

The underlying cardiovascular disease is the basic determinant for the use of antibiotic prophylaxis. Infective endocarditis has occurred in patients with pacemakers.

Antibiotic prophylaxis may be indicated during the first 6 months following placement of a pacemaker. After implantation, the pulse generator and the electrodes are usually covered by endothelium. Although the patient with a pacemaker appears to be at low risk of endocarditis, the dentist and the cardiologist may choose to use antibiotics to cover dental and dental hygiene procedures.

D. Patient Preparation

1. *Chair Position.* Positioning the patient to support breathing and circulation is important. If the patient experiences difficulty in breathing when in the supine position, the chair back should be elevated to reduce stress.

   The patient may experience some discomfort from wire tension or strain at the implant site if the chair is positioned too far back. That depends on the location of the pulse generator. Care must be taken that no pressure is placed over the site of a pacemaker in the patient's chest.
2. *Lead Apron.* Protection of the pulse generator and the lead wires may be indicated. A lead apron can serve to interrupt interferences that may be created by electric devices, including handpieces. A lead apron can be heavy and uncomfortable, however, and therefore may require some consideration.

E. Instrumentation

The use of manual procedures is advisable. Ultrasonic instruments should be avoided.

■ ANTICOAGULANT THERAPY

Anticoagulants are used in the treatment of many cardiovascular diseases to prevent embolus and thrombus formation. A prescribed drug may be continued indefinitely in the patient's life as a preventive measure.

Drugs most commonly used to prevent or delay blood coagulation are heparin (hospital-administered intravenous) and coumarin derivatives. Although precautions are needed to prevent hemorrhage, discontinuing the drug may be more hazardous for the patient than performing dental and dental hygiene therapy with precautions. When extensive surgical procedures are required, the patient may be hospitalized.

I. CLINICAL PROCEDURES

A. Consultation

Information about the patient's prothrombin time is obtained from the physician during an initial consultation. The prothrombin time is a test of the coagulation phase of blood clotting used to monitor therapy with anticoagulants. A therapeutic range of 1 1/2 to 2 1/2 times the normal level is preferred.

B. Treatment Planning[11]

1. *Pretest for Prothrombin Time*
   a. Determine the prothrombin time within 24 hours before an appointment. The patient can have the test made on the day of a dental appointment by preplanning with the physician and the laboratory. Most patients have a routine appointment for monitoring of the blood, and dental appointment dates can be planned to coincide.
   b. Safe level for dental and dental hygiene procedures is considered to be 1 1/2 times the normal, provided precautions are taken during instrumentation and postoperative care.
2. *Quadrant Scaling and Root Planing*
   a. Treat the most healthy quadrant first. The least bleeding will occur.
   b. Teach and emphasize daily dental biofilm control procedures in a series of appointments to prepare the gingival tissue for instrumentation. Healthy, healed tissue does not bleed as readily or as profusely.
   c. Complete treatment, including removal of all calculus and subgingival biofilm and other irritants, is necessary to contribute to the goal of healthy tissue that does not bleed.

C. Local Hemostatic Measures

Instrumentation can be performed for most patients without complication, provided precautions are taken to minimize tissue trauma and control bleeding and not to dismiss the patient until bleeding has stopped.

1. *Pressure.* Pressure with sponges or cotton pellets packed interdentally can aid in control.
2. *Suture.* Sutures may be used to close and adapt the tissue interdentally following deep scaling and root planing.
3. *Periodontal Dressing.* Placement of a dressing is sometimes advisable to provide pressure and protection from trauma that may initiate bleeding. Dressing placement is described on pages 706 to 707.

II. POSTPROCEDURAL INSTRUCTIONS

The practice by oral surgeons of closely observing patients for 6 to 8 hours following a surgical procedure has application following certain dental and dental hygiene procedures for selected patients. At the least, a check that postcare instructions are being followed is advisable.

The patient is advised to avoid vigorous toothbrushing and rinsing for several hours or until the next day. The use of extraoral icepacks may be helpful. General postcare instructions may be found on page 854; for the care of an area with a dressing, see Table 40-1 (page 708).

The use of a soft diet, cool rather than hot foods, and general moderation in activity may be advisable.

Long-term instruction must emphasize the maintenance of gingival health to prevent future bleeding problems.

▪ CARDIAC SURGERY[12]

Cardiac surgery has become widely used. Patients in dental offices and clinics who have had or will have surgery should be identified and need special procedures. Because the patient with a cardiac prosthesis is at risk for infective endocarditis, all possible dental treatment must be completed before the date of cardiac surgery, and preventive measures must be emphasized.

I. PRESURGICAL

Before elective cardiac surgery, the patient should be brought to a state of optimum oral health, with all sources of infection removed. All restorations and other dental procedures must be completed.

Patients requiring cardiac surgery need information and motivation relative to the importance of oral health in eliminating a potential source of infective endocarditis. Vigilance in a preventive program that includes plaque control and self-applied fluorides is essential.

II. POSTSURGICAL

A. Maintenance Appointments

Frequent appointments are necessary for supervision and maintenance.

B. Prophylactic Antibiotic

1. Antibiotic coverage for all dental and dental hygiene procedures for patients with synthetic prostheses is essential. Because of the high susceptibility to infections, a special regimen for high-risk patients may be indicated.

2. Patients with implanted vascular autographs generally do not need antibiotic premedication before dental and dental hygiene appointments. An example of an implanted vascular autograph is the use of a patient's own blood vessel to provide a coronary bypass (Figure 63-5). The saphenous vein and the internal mammary artery are most commonly used.

C. Immunosuppressive Therapy

Principal drugs used for patients with transplants are cyclosporin, azathioprine, and prednisolone to prevent rejection of the transplant. Among the side effects, particularly of cyclosporin, is gingival enlargement.[13] Many

✔ Factors To Teach The Patient

Hypertension Therapy

- Encourage patients who have been diagnosed as hypertensive to continue their prescribed therapy.

Stress Reduction Procedures[14]

- Select an appointment time that is optimum with respect to time of day when the patient is feeling best and may be less fatigued. Most anxious patients prefer a morning appointment.

- Get adequate sleep and rest, and engage in nonfatiguing activities during the 24 hours before the appointment.

- Use premedication as prescribed for sleeping the night before. A sedative may be prescribed to be taken 60 minutes before an appointment or at the dental office, if possible. When taken at home 1 hour before, the patient should not drive a car.

- Allow time to get to the dental office or clinic; bring own reading material, knitting or sewing, or other relaxing activity in the event that waiting is unavoidable.

- Eat breakfast, lunch, or other usual between-meal food and take usual medications on schedule.

- When other family members, especially children, have dental or dental hygiene appointments, do not add to their stress by relaying personal negative feelings.

also receive medication with the nifedipine group, also effective in causing gingival enlargement. Special periodontal care will be needed.

REFERENCES

1. **Burns, D.K.** and Kumar, V.: The Heart, in Kumar, V., Cotran, R.S., and Robbins, S.L.: *Basic Pathology, 7th ed.,* Philadelphia, Saunders, 2003, pp. 388–392.
2. **Burns** and Kumar: op. cit., pp. 375–378.
3. **Little,** J.W., Falace, D.A., Miller C.S., and Rhodus, N.L.: *Dental Management of the Medically Compromised Patient,* 6th ed. St. Louis, Mosby, 2002, pp. 45–46, 57.
4. **Dajani,** A.S., Taubert, K.A., Wilson, W., Bolger, A.F., Bayer, A., Ferrieri, P., Gewitz, M.H., Shulman, S.T., Nouri, S., Newberger, J.W., Hutto, C., Pallasch, T.J., Gage, T.W., Levison, M.E., Peter, G., and Zuccaro, G.: Prevention of Bacterial Endocarditis: Recommendations by the American Heart Association, *Circulation, 96,* 358, July 1, 1997.
5. **Little,** Falace, Miller, and Rhodus: op. cit., pp. 21–27.
6. **Burns** and Kumar: op. cit., pp. 381–383.
7. **Kumar,** V., Cotran, R.S., and Robbins, S.L.: *Basic Pathology,* 7th ed. Philadelphia, W.B. Saunders Co., 2003, pp. 338–340.
8. **United States National Institutes of Health,** National Heart, Lung, and Blood Institute: *The Seventh Report of the Joint National Committee on Prevention, Detection, Evaluation, and Treatment of High Blood Pressure.* National Institutes of Health, National Heart, Lung, and Blood Institute, Publication No. 03-5233, May, 2003.
9. **Burns** and Kumar: op. cit., pp. 372–374.
10. **Little,** Falace, Miller, and Rhodus: op. cit., pp. 79–92.
11. **Little,** Falace, Miller, and Rhodus: op. cit., pp. DM 38–41.
12. **Little,** Falace, Miller, and Rhodus: op. cit., pp. DM 70–71, 504–506.
13. **Thomason,** J.M., Seymour, R.A., Ellis, J.S., Kelly, P.J., Parry, G., Dark, J., and Idle, J.R.: Iatrogenic Gingival Overgrowth in Cardiac Transplantation, *J. Periodontol., 66,* 742, August, 1995.
14. **Malamed,** S.F.: *Handbook of Medical Emergencies in the Dental Office,* 5th ed. St. Louis, Mosby, 2000, pp. 44–48.

SUGGESTED READINGS

Boraz, R.A. and Myers, R.: A National Survey of Dental Protocols for the Patient With a Cardiac Transplant, *Spec. Care Dentist., 10,* 26, January–February, 1990.

Carabello, B.A. and Crawford, F.A.: Valvular Heart Disease, *N. Engl. J. Med., 337,* 32, July 3, 1997.

Carlson-Mann, L.D.: Case Study: Dental Management of a Heart Transplant Patient, *Canad. Dent. Hyg. (Probe), 30,* 77, March/April, 1996.

Hays, G.L., McMahon, J.C., Zimmerman, S.J., Lusk, S.S., and DeVoll, R.E.: Screening for Cardiovascular Disease, *Gen. Dent., 40,* 26, January–February, 1992.

Herman, W.W. and Konzelman, J.L.: Angina: An Update for Dentistry, *J. Am. Dent. Assoc., 127,* 98, January, 1996.

Hollander, J.E.: The Management of Cocaine-Associated Myocardial Ischemia, *N. Engl. J. Med., 333,* 1267, November 9, 1995.

Mueller-Joseph, L.: Cardiovascular Diseases: Implications for Dental Hygiene Care, *DentalHygienistNews, 8,* 5, Number 3, 1995.

Muzyra, B.C. and Glick, M.: The Hypertensive Dental Patient, *J. Am. Dent. Assoc., 128,* 1109, August, 1997.

Roelke, M. and Bernstein, A.D.: Cardiac Pacemakers and Cellular Telephones (Editorial), *N. Engl. J. Med., 336,* 1518, May 22, 1997.

Ross, R.: Atherosclerosis—An Inflammatory Disease, *N. Engl. J. Med., 340,* 115, January 14, 1999.

Sandor, G.K.B., Vasilakos, S.S., and Vasilakos, J.S.: Mitral Valve Prolapse: A Review of the Syndrome With Emphasis on Current Antibiotic Prophylaxis, *J. Can. Dent. Assoc., 57,* 321, April, 1991.

Souliman, S.K. and Christie, J.: Pacemaker Failure Induced by Radiotherapy, *Pace, 17,* 270, March, 1994.

Vongpatanasin, W., Hillis, L.D., and Lange, R.A.: Prosthetic Heart Valves, *N. Engl. J. Med. 335,* 407, August 8, 1996.

Treatment

Biron, C.R.: Antianginal Therapy, *RDH, 15,* 44, October, 1996.

Biron, C.R.: Drug Therapy for Congestive Heart Failure Poses Several Risks During Dental Treatment, *RDH, 16,* 46, February, 1996.

Bittl, J.A.: Advances in Coronary Angioplasty, *N. Engl. J. Med., 335,* 1290, October 24, 1996.

Bypass Angioplasty Revascularization Investigation (BARI) Investigators: Comparison of Coronary Bypass Surgery With Angioplasty in Patients With Multivessel Disease, *N. Engl. J. Med., 335,* 217, July 25, 1996.

Caplan, L.R.: Diagnosis and Treatment of Ischemic Stroke, *JAMA, 266,* 2413, November 6, 1991.

Cowper, T.R.: Pharmacologic Management of the Patient With Disorders of the Cardiovascular System: Infective Carditis, *Dent. Clin. North Am., 40,* 611, July, 1996.

Ganzberg, S.: Cardiovascular Drugs, in *ADA Guide to Dental Therapeutics.* Chicago, ADA Publishing Co., 1998, pp. 295–318.

Kusumoto, F.M. and Goldschlager, N.: Cardiac Pacing, *N. Engl. J. Med., 334,* 99, January 11, 1996.

Parker, J.D. and Parker, J.O.: Nitrate Therapy for Stable Angina Pectoris, *N. Engl. J. Med., 338,* 520, February 19, 1998.

Periodontal Relationships

American Academy of Periodontology, Committee on Research, Science and Therapy: Periodontal Management of Patients With Cardiovascular Diseases, *J. Periodontol., 67,* 627, June, 1996.

Beck, J., Garcia, R., Heiss, G., Vokonas, P.S., and Offenbacher, S.: Periodontal Disease and Cardiovascular Disease, *J. Periodontol., 67,* 1123, October, 1996, Supplement.

Khocht, A. and Schneider, L.C.: Periodontal Management of Gingival Overgrowth in the Heart Transplant Patient: A Case Report, *J. Periodontol., 68,* 1140, November, 1997.

Loesche, W.J.: Periodontal Disease as a Risk Factor for Heart Disease, *Compend. Cont. Educ. Dent., 15,* 976, August, 1994.

Infective Endocarditis

Biancaniello, T.M. and Romero, J.R.: Bacterial Endocarditis After Adjustment of Orthodontic Appliances, *J. Pediatr., 118,* 248, February, 1991.

Doerffel, W., Fietze, I., Baumann, G., and Witt, C.: Severe Prosthetic Valve-Related Endocarditis Following Dental Scaling: A Case Report, *Quintessence Int., 28,* 271, April, 1997.

Duffin, P.R., McGimpsey, J.G., Pallister, M.L., and McGowan, D.A.: Dental Care of Patients Susceptible to Infective Endocarditis, *Br. Dent. J., 173,* 169, September 19, 1992.

Felder, R.S., Nardone, D., and Palac, R.: Prevalence of Predisposing Factors for Endocarditis Among an Elderly Institutionalized Population, *Oral Surg. Oral Med. Oral Pathol., 73,* 30, January, 1992.

Franklin, C.D.: The Aetiology, Epidemiology, Pathogenesis and Changing Pattern of Infective Endocarditis, With a Note on Prophylaxis, *Br. Dent. J., 172,* 369, May 23, 1992.

Knox, K.W. and Hunter, N.: The Role of Oral Bacteria in the Pathogenesis of Infective Endocarditis, *Aust. Dent. J., 36,* 286, August, 1991.

Children

Creighton, J.M.: Dental Care for the Pediatric Cardiac Patient, *J. Can. Dent. Assoc., 58,* 201, March, 1992.

Hallett, K.B., Radford, D.J., and Seow, W.K.: Oral Health of Children With Congenital Cardiac Diseases: A Controlled Study, *Pediatr. Dent., 14,* 224, July/August, 1992.

Liberthson, R.R.: Sudden Death From Cardiac Causes in Children and Young Adults, *N. Engl. J. Med., 334,* 1039, April 18, 1996.

Sinaiko, A.R.: Hypertension in Children, *N. Engl. J. Med., 335,* 1968, December 26, 1996.

Anticoagulant

Carr, M.M. and Mason, R.B.: Dental Management of Anticoagulated Patients, *J. Can. Dent. Assoc., 58,* 838, October, 1992.

Herman, W.W., Konzelman, J.L., and Sutley, S.H.: Current Perspectives on Dental Patients Receiving Coumarin Anticoagulant Therapy, *J. Am. Dent. Assoc., 128,* 327, March, 1997.

Kearon, C. and Hirsh, J.: Management of Anticoagulation Before and After Elective Surgery, *N. Engl. J. Med., 336,* 1506, May 22, 1997.

Martinowitz, U., Mazar, A.L., Taicher, S., Varon, D., Gitel, S.N., Ramot, B., and Rakocz, M.: Dental Extraction for Patients on Oral Anticoagulant Therapy, *Oral Surg. Oral Med. Oral Pathol., 70,* 274, September, 1990.

Meehan, S., Schmidt, M.C., and Mitchell, P.F.: The International Normalized Ratio as a Measure of Anticoagulation: Significance for the Management of the Dental Outpatient, *Spec. Care Dentist., 17,* 94, May/June, 1997.

Pellegrino, S.V. and Berardi, T.R.: Dental Management of Patients on Anticoagulant Therapy, *Gen. Dent., 43,* 351, July–August, 1995.

Steinberg, M.J. and Moores, J.F.: Use of INR to Assess Degree of Anticoagulation in Patients Who Have Dental Procedures, *Oral Surg. Oral Med. Oral Pathol., 80,* 175, August, 1995.

Stern, R., Karlis, V., Kinney, L., and Glickman, R.: Using the International Normalized Ratio to Standardize Prothrombin Time, *J. Am. Dent. Assoc., 128,* 1121, August, 1997.

Terezhalmy, G.T. and Lichtin, A.E.: Antithrombotic, Anticoagulant, and Thrombolytic Agents, *Dent. Clin. North Am., 40,* 649, July, 1996.

The Patient With a Blood Disorder

Lisa B. Stefanou, RDH, MPH

Oral soft tissue changes, lowered resistance to infection, and bleeding tendencies are major factors to be considered for a patient with a blood disorder. Oral manifestations of blood disorders are generally exaggerated in the presence of dental biofilm and local predisposing factors.

Box 64-1 lists and defines terminology used to describe hematologic conditions. Prefixes, suffixes, and other word derivatives to clarify the terminology are listed on page 1121.

■ ORAL FINDINGS SUGGESTIVE OF BLOOD DISORDERS

Early signs of systemic conditions frequently appear in the oral soft tissues. The patient's medical history may not show the existence of a blood disorder, but clinical examination may reveal tissue characteristics suggestive of disease. An important referral for medical examination may lead to diagnosis and treatment of a serious

BOX 64-1 KEY WORDS: Blood Disorders

Anaplasia: loss of structural differentiation with reversion to a more primitive type of cell.

Aplasia: defective development or congenital absence of an organ or tissue.

Coagulation factor: factor essential to normal blood clotting contained within the blood plasma; designated by Roman numerals I to V and VII to XIII; their absence, diminution, or excess may lead to abnormality of clotting.

Differential cell count: record of number of white blood cells, including the determination of the percent of each type of cell present; the "differential" is used in the diagnosis of various blood disorders, infections, and other abnormal conditions of the body.

Ecchymosis: hemorrhagic spot larger than a petechia in the skin or mucous membrane; nonelevated, blue or purplish.

Epistaxis: hemorrhage from the nose.

Erythropoiesis: formation of red blood cells.

Glossitis: inflammation of the tongue.

Glossodynia: pain in the tongue.

Hemarthrosis: blood in a joint cavity.

Hematocrit: volume percentage of erythrocytes (red blood cells) in whole blood.

Hematopoiesis: the formation and development of blood cells, usually in bone marrow.

Hemoglobin: protein in the erythrocyte that transports molecular oxygen to body cells.

> **Oxyhemoglobin:** oxygenated arterial blood; bright red and about 97% saturated with oxygen; venous blood is a darker color and contains only 20% to 70% oxygen.

Hemolysis: rupture of erythrocytes with the release of hemoglobin into the plasma.

Hypoxia: diminished availability of oxygen to body tissues.

> **Diffusion hypoxia:** lack of adequate amounts of oxygen that can result from the rapid diffusion of nitrous oxide molecules from the blood stream into the lungs. Occurs if 100% oxygen is not administered at the conclusion of a nitrous oxide sedation procedure.

Leukocytosis: increase in the total number of leukocytes.

Leukopenia: reduction in total number of leukocytes in the blood; count under 500 per ml.

Lysis: destruction or decomposition, as of a cell, bacterium, or other substance.

Macrocyte: abnormally large red blood cell; contrast with **microcyte,** abnormally small erythrocyte.

Myelocyte: young cell of the granulocyte series; occurs normally in bone marrow; found in circulating blood in certain diseases.

Neutropenia: diminished number of neutrophils (polymorphonuclear leukocytes or PMNs).

Petechia: minute, pinpoint, round, nonraised, purplish-red spot in the skin or mucous membrane, caused by hemorrhage.

Phagocytosis: engulfing of microorganisms and foreign particles by phagocytes, such as macrophages.

Plasma cell: cell in connective tissue converted from B lymphocyte: involved in chronic inflammation and immune response.

Purpura: hemorrhage into the tissues, under the skin, and through the mucous membranes; produces petechiae and ecchymoses.

Thrombocytic purpura: when circulating platelets are decreased.

disease. In addition, the findings of a laboratory blood examination may provide essential information for safe and effective treatment.

Oral soft tissue changes that may occur in patients with blood diseases are not necessarily exclusive to systemic blood disorders. The important thing is to recognize change in a previously healthy patient, or an apparently exaggerated response in a patient being examined at an initial appointment.

Findings that may suggest a blood disorder include the following:

- Gingival bleeding, spontaneously or upon gentle probing.
- History of difficulty in controlling bleeding by usual procedures.
- History of bruising easily, with large ecchymoses.
- Numerous petechiae.
- Marked pallor of the mucous membranes.
- Atrophy of the papillae of the tongue.
- Persistent sore or painful tongue (glossodynia).
- Acute or chronic infections, such as candidiasis, that do not respond to usual treatment.
- Severe ulcerations associated with a lack of response to treatment.
- Exaggerated gingival response to local irritants, sometimes with characteristics of necrotizing ulcerative gingivitis (ulceration, necrosis, bleeding, pseudomembrane).

▪ NORMAL BLOOD[1]

I. COMPOSITION

The blood is composed of 55% plasma fluid and 45% formed elements. The formed elements are categorized by type into *erythrocytes* (red blood cells or corpuscles), *leukocytes* (white blood cells), and *thrombocytes* (platelets). The cell forms and nuclei are shown in Figure 64-1.

The red blood cells compose about 44% and the white blood cells 1% of the 45% total formed elements.

The *hematocrit* is the percentage of packed volume of blood cells, the normal value of which approximates 45%, as shown in Table 64-1. The test for the hematocrit is commonly used in general health evaluations. Table 64-2 contains reference values for blood cells and the names of conditions in which increases or decreases in the normal values occur.

II. ORIGIN

In adults, all blood cells originate in the bone marrow. The erythrocytes and granulocytes pass through a series of transformations from the stem cell (cell of origin), the *hemocytoblast,* and leave the bone marrow as mature cells to enter the circulating blood.

The bone marrow also produces the stem cells for the agranulocytes. The lymphocytes and monocytes leave the bone marrow in immature forms and go to the lymphoid tissues for later maturing. In certain blood diseases and cancers, the immature cell forms predominate.

III. PLASMA

The constituents of the fluid portion of the blood are similar to the fluid constituents of the connective tissue. The plasma is composed 90% of water and 10% of the following:

A. Plasma Proteins

- Albumin (functions to maintain tissue fluid pressure).
- Gamma globulins (circulating antibodies essential in the immune system).
- Beta globulins (transport of hormones, metallic ions, and lipids).
- Fibrinogen and prothrombin (blood clotting).

B. Inorganic Salts

Sodium, potassium, calcium, bicarbonate, chloride.

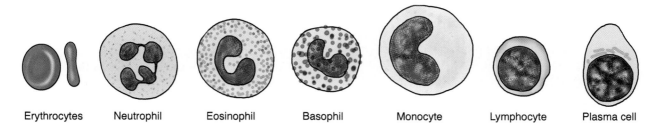

Erythrocytes   Neutrophil   Eosinophil   Basophil   Monocyte   Lymphocyte   Plasma cell

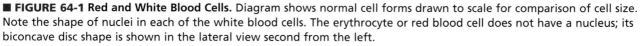

▪ **FIGURE 64-1 Red and White Blood Cells.** Diagram shows normal cell forms drawn to scale for comparison of cell size. Note the shape of nuclei in each of the white blood cells. The erythrocyte or red blood cell does not have a nucleus; its biconcave disc shape is shown in the lateral view second from the left.

▪ TABLE 64-1 TESTS USED FOR BLOOD EVALUATION

TEST	NORMAL RANGE*	CAUSES OF DEVIATIONS
Hemoglobin	**Males: 14–18 g/100 ml** **Females: 12–16 g/100 ml**	**Increased in:** • Polycythemia • Dehydration **Decreased in:** • Anemias • Hemorrhage • Leukemias
Hematocrit (volume of packed red cells)	**Males: 40%–54%** **Females: 37%–47%**	**Increased in:** • Polycythemia • Dehydration **Decreased in:** • Anemias • Hemorrhage • Leukemias
Bleeding time	**Duke: 1–3 1/2 minutes** **Ivy: less than 5 minutes** **Modified Ivy: 2 1/2–10** minutes (Mielke template)	**Prolonged in:** • Disorders of platelet function • Thrombocytopenia • von Willebrand's disease • Leukemias • Aspirin and certain other drug use
Clotting time	Glass tube: 4–8 minutes	**Prolonged in:** • Vitamin K deficiency • Severe hemophilia • Anticoagulant therapy • Liver diseases
Prothrombin time (PT)	11–15 seconds	**Prolonged in:** • Polycythemia vera • Prothrombin deficiency • Anticoagulant therapy • Vitamin K deficiency • Liver diseases • Aspirin use
Partial thromboplastin time (PTT)	68–82 seconds	**Prolonged in:** • Hemophilia A and B • von Willebrand's disease • Anticoagulant therapy

*The normal range varies with the specificity of the technique used. There is also a range variation, depending on the health facility and the laboratory.

C. Gases

Dissolved oxygen, carbon dioxide, and nitrogen.

D. Substances Being Transported

Hormones, nutrients, waste products, enzymes.

IV. RED BLOOD CELLS (ERYTHROCYTES)

A. Description

- Although usually called red blood cells, they are more properly termed corpuscles because they have no nuclei (Figure 64-1).

- Biconcave discs that contain hemoglobin.
- Sensitive and flexible; change shape readily as they pass through small capillaries.

B. Functions

- Transport hemoglobin.
- Carry oxygen to the body cells in the form of oxyhemoglobin.
- Carbon dioxide is transported from the cells.

The hemoglobin is measured in grams (g) per 100 milliliters (ml). Normal values are shown in Table 64-1 and range from 12 to 16 g per 100 ml. The values reflect the anemic state when the hemoglobin is lowered. They also

■ TABLE 64-2 BLOOD CELLS REFERENCE VALUES

CELL TYPE	NORMAL VALUE	CAUSES OF INCREASE	CAUSES OF DECREASE
Red Blood Cells (Erythrocytes)	Males: 4.5–6.0 million per mm^3 Females: 4.3–5.5 million per mm^3	Polycythemia Dehydration	Anemias Leukemias Hemorrhage
Platelets (Thrombocytes)	150,000–400,000 per mm^3 Wintrobe method: 140,000–440,000 per mm^3	Polycythemia vera Chronic myelocytic leukemia Sickle cell anemia Rheumatic fever Hemolytic anemias Bone fractures	Acute severe infections Cirrhosis of the liver Thrombocytopenic purpura Acute leukemias Aplastic anemias Pernicious anemia
White Blood Cells (Leukocytes)	5,000–10,000 per mm^3	Inflammation Overexertion Polycythemia vera Leukemia	Aplastic anemia Granulocytopenia Drug poisoning Thrombocytopenia Radiation Severe infections (HIV/AIDS)
Differential White Cell Count **Granulocytes** 1. Neutrophils	60%–70%	Acute infections Myelogenous leukemia Poisoning Erythroblastosis	Aplastic anemia Granulocytopenia
2. Eosinophils	1%–3%	Allergic diseases Dermatitis Hodgkin's disease Scarlet fever	Aplastic anemia Typhoid fever
3. Basophils	1%	Certain chronic infections	Aplastic anemia
Agranulocytes 1. Lymphocytes	20%–35%	Lymphocytic leukemia Chronic infections Viral diseases	Aplastic anemia Myelogenous leukemia Radiation
2. Monocytes	2%–6%	Monocytic leukemias Tuberculosis Infective endocarditis Hodgkin's disease	Aplastic anemia

reflect pathologic conditions in which the hemoglobin is increased to a level higher than normal.

V. WHITE BLOOD CELLS (LEUKOCYTES)

A. Types of Leukocytes

White blood cells are divided into two general groups, the granulocytes and the agranulocytes. Granulocytes have granules in their cytoplasm, whereas the agranulocytes do not. They are further subdivided as shown here:

1. *Granulocytes:* neutrophils, eosinophils, basophils.
2. *Agranulocytes:* lymphocytes, monocytes.

B. Functions: Amoeboid or Motile

- Able to pass through the walls at the terminal ends of capillaries and into the connective tissue.
- Phagocytic, immunologic, and other functions related to the inflammatory process in the connective tissue.
- Large number of cells migrate into area of injury.
- Neutrophils arrive first and are active in the phagocytosis of foreign material and microorganisms.
- The blood functions as a transport medium for the white cells as they pass to areas in the connective tissue where they are needed.

- Numbers and proportions in the blood maintain a constant level in health, as shown in Table 64-2.
- Differential cell count of the white blood cells is used in the detection and monitoring of diseased states. Increases and decreases of each cell type can be associated with certain conditions.

C. Agranulocytes

1. **Lymphocytes**
   - Small round cell with a round nucleus that nearly fills the cell with a narrow rim of cytoplasm (Figure 64-1).
   - Can move back and forth between the vessels and the extravascular tissues
   - Capable of reverting to blast-like cells.
   - When so transformed, can multiply as immunologic need arises.
2. **Monocytes**
   - Large cell with a bean-shaped or indented nucleus.
   - Actively phagocytic.
   - In connective tissue, monocytes differentiate into macrophages, which are important in immunologic processes.

D. Granulocytes

1. **Neutrophils**
   - Also called polymorphonuclear leukocytes "PMNs" or "polys."
   - Most numerous of all the white blood cells.
   - Nucleus has three to five lobes connected by thin chromatin threads.
   - Cells are round in circulation.
   - In the tissues they are amoeboid and function in phagocytosis. Neutrophils are part of the first line of defense of the body.
2. **Eosinophils**
   - Two-lobed nucleus and larger, coarser granules than those of a neutrophil.
   - Microscopically the cells stain a distinct bright pink; readily recognized.
   - Few in number; increase markedly during allergic conditions.
3. **Basophils**
   - Nucleus is "U" or "S" form.
   - Function is to increase vascular permeability during inflammation so phagocytic cells can pass into the area.

VI. PLATELETS

- Small round or oval formed element without a nucleus.

- They are approximately one fourth the size of a red blood cell.
- Active in the blood clotting mechanism.
- Essential in the maintenance of the integrity of blood capillaries by closing them at a time of injury.
- Participate in clot dissolution after healing.

▪ ANEMIAS

Anemia means a reduction of the hemoglobin concentration, the hematocrit, or the number of red blood cells to a level below that which is normal for the individual. As a result of anemia, oxygen-carrying capacity to the cells is diminished. Oxygen is essential in all body tissues for normal maintenance.

I. CLASSIFICATION BY CAUSE

A. Caused by Blood Loss

1. *Acute.* Blood loss from trauma or disease.
2. *Chronic.* An internal lesion with constant slow bleeding, usually of gastrointestinal or gynecologic origin, can lead to a chronic loss of blood. An *iron deficiency anemia* can result.

B. Caused by Increased Hemolysis

Hemolysis means the destruction of red blood cells. These types of anemias are called "hemolytic anemias" because of the cell destruction.
1. **Hereditary Hemolytic Disorders**
Example: *sickle cell disease,* which belongs to the group of hereditary disorders called the hemoglobinopathies.
2. **Acquired Hemolytic Disorders**
Examples: drugs, infections, and certain physical and chemical agents that may cause red cell destruction. In the category of antibody-mediated anemia, *erythroblastosis fetalis* occurs when a mother is Rh negative and develops antibodies against a fetus that is Rh positive. It is sometimes called hemolytic disease of the newborn.

C. Caused by Diminished Production of Red Blood Cells

A nutritional deficiency or bone marrow failure may be the reason for diminished production.
1. **Nutritional Deficiency**
a. Inadequate dietary choices or inadequate intake.
b. Defective absorption from the gastrointestinal tract. Example: *pernicious anemia,* which results from a B_{12} vitamin absorption deficiency.

c. Increased demand for nutrients.
    Example: *iron deficiency anemia*, which may occur during pregnancy or during a growth spurt.

2. **Bone Marrow Failure**
    Example: *Aplastic anemia* (which can be inherited) can occur without apparent cause or can occur when the bone marrow is injured by medications, radiation, chemotherapy, or infection. In aplastic anemia, a combination occurs of anemia, neutropenia, and thrombocytopenia, which means a quantitative decrease in all cells formed in the bone marrow.

D. Caused by Genetic Blood Disorders[2]

Example: *Thalassemia*. Thalassemias are a diverse group of genetic blood disorders characterized by absent or decreased production of normal hemoglobin.

*   Thalassemia is an inherited condition that typically affects people of Mediterranean, African, Middle Eastern, and Southeast Asian descent.
*   Condition can range in severity from mild to life threatening.
*   The most severe form is called Cooley's anemia.

II. CLINICAL CHARACTERISTICS OF ANEMIA

When a patient's medical history shows the presence of anemia, certain general characteristics may be anticipated for which clinical adaptations may be needed. The general signs and symptoms are:

*   Pale thin skin.
*   Weakness, malaise, easy fatigability.
*   Dyspnea on slight exertion, faintness.
*   Headache, vertigo, tinnitus.
*   Dimness of vision, spots before the eyes.
*   Brittle nails with loss of convexity.

▪ IRON DEFICIENCY ANEMIA

Iron deficiency anemia is a hypochromic microcytic anemia, which means that the hemoglobin is deficient (hypochromic) and the red blood corpuscles are smaller than normal and deficient in hemoglobin (microcytic). In general, it is found more in younger than in older people, and more in females than in males.

I. CAUSES

A. **Malnutrition or malabsorption**
B. **Chronic infection**
C. **Increased body demand for iron over and above the daily intake.** Example: during pregnancy.

D. **Chronic blood loss.** When iron deficiency anemia occurs in men or in postmenopausal women, it usually indicates internal bleeding, and tests are needed to find the source.
    1. Causes of internal bleeding
        *   Gastrointestinal diseases, such as ulcer, cancer.
        *   Drugs, notably aspirin.
        *   Hemorrhoids.
    2. Excessive menstrual flow.
    3. Frequent blood donations.

II. SIGNS AND SYMPTOMS

A. General

*   General weakness, headache, pallor.
*   Fatigue on slight exertion.

B. Oral

*   Pallor of the mucosa and gingiva.
*   Tongue changes: Atrophic glossitis with loss of filiform papillae. In moderate and severe anemia, when the hemoglobin is at 10 or below, the tongue is smooth and shiny. The patient may have burning, painful sensations (glossodynia).
*   Secondary irritations to the thinned, atrophic mucosa may result from smoking, mechanical trauma, or hot, spicy foods.
*   Angular cheilitis.

III. THERAPY

*   Treated with oral ferrous iron tablets.
*   Liquid preparations, which are sometimes used for children, may stain the teeth. Administering the medicine by way of a straw is advised.

▪ MEGALOBLASTIC ANEMIAS[3]

*   Characterized by abnormally large (megalo-) red blood cells, many of which are oval shaped.
*   A megaloblastic anemia can result from a deficiency of either vitamin B_{12} or folate, or both.
*   Two principal types of megaloblastic anemias are *pernicious anemia* and *folate deficiency anemia.*
*   Pernicious anemia is caused by a deficiency of vitamin B_{12}.
*   Folate deficiency anemia is from a deficiency of folate, or folic acid.
*   These two vitamins are essential in red blood cell production in the bone marrow.

I. PERNICIOUS ANEMIA

A. Etiologic Factors

1. Deficiency Vitamin B_{12} can be caused by:
   - Decreased intake (inadequate diet or impaired absorption).
   - Increased requirement (pregnancy, hyperparathyroidism, disseminated cancer).
2. Impaired absorption of B_{12}:
   - Due to deficiency of intrinsic factor. Failure of production of *intrinsic factor (IF)*; a substance created by the stomach parietal cells that is necessary for the absorption of Vitamin B_{12}.
   - Lack of production of *intrinsic factor* is either chronic atrophic gastritis or surgical removal of partial or all of the stomach.

B. Age Characteristics

- Pernicious anemia is primarily a disease of people over 40 years of age.
- Childhood form of the disease: other causes in effect; no gastric abnormality exists. Although more research is needed, the cause may be either that a hereditary inability to produce intrinsic factor exists or the intrinsic factor produced is ineffective.

C. Clinical Findings

1. **General**
   - Fatigue, weakness, tingling, or numbness of fingers and toes.
   - Palpitations, weight loss, and syncope.
2. **Central Nervous System Involvement**
   - Difficulty walking.
   - Lack of coordination.
   - Mental confusion.
3. **Oral Findings**
   - Tongue (atrophic glossitis, burning tongue). Painful and inflamed, flabby, red, smooth, and shiny loss of filiform papillae.
   - Sensitivity to hot or spicy foods.
   - Painful swallowing.
   - Gingiva and mucosa: pale, atrophic similar to vitamin B deficiency.

D. Treatment

- Vitamin B_{12} administered by injection twice weekly until the condition is controlled, and then monthly, indefinitely.
- Diet. Good dietary sources of vitamin B_{12} are meat, kidney, fish, oyster, clams, milk, cheese and eggs. Liver is a rich source and was originally used in therapy before the development of synthetic B_{12}.

II. FOLATE DEFICIENCY ANEMIA[4]

Folate deficiency anemia has the same characteristics as pernicious anemia, except clinically, no neurologic changes are evident.

A. Etiologic Factors

1. **Decreased Intake**
   - Inadequate diet.
   - Impaired absorption.
2. **Increased Requirement**
   - Pregnancy.
   - Disseminated cancer.
   - Certain drugs impair the utilization of folate, for example, cancer chemotherapy drugs.
   - Blocked activation.

B. Dietary Factors: Sources

- Fresh fruits, green leafy vegetables, and cruciferous vegetables (cauliflower, broccoli, and brussel sprouts).
- Liver and kidney.
- Dairy products and whole grain cereals. Vegetables need to be eaten raw or lightly cooked. Only minimal subsistence diets or special diets influenced by such factors as poverty, food fadism, or alcoholism, when the use of alcohol takes precedence over food, are likely to be deficient in folates. Folate deficiency anemia is not uncommon, but it may be more frequently related to malabsorption than to inadequate intake.

C. Fetal Development

- Folic acid deficiency can cause neural tube defects.
- Spina bifida: a severe condition affecting the formation of the nerves of the spinal cord, and resulting in infant paralysis. Spina bifida is described on page 927.

■ SICKLE CELL DISEASE[5]

Sickle cell disease is a hereditary form of hemolytic anemia, resulting from a defective hemoglobin molecule. The name is derived from the crescent or "sickle" shape the erythrocytes assume when they become deoxygenated.

I. DISEASE PROCESS

- Occurs primarily in the African American population and in white populations of Mediterranean origin.

- Testing: Simple blood test, hemoglobin electrophoresis will detect sickle cell disease or sickle cell trait (parental carrier).
- Genetic counseling can play an important role in prevention.
- Detection of the presence of sickle cell disease is possible before birth, so that proper observation and supervision of the infant and young child can be provided.
- Signs and symptoms do not appear until after approximately the sixth month, when hemoglobin has matured.
- Growth and development may be impaired during the early years. Young children are markedly susceptible to communicable diseases and especially to pneumococcal infections. The disease abnormality is in the type and solubility of hemoglobin.
- The defective hemoglobin loses oxygen, and the red blood cells become distorted into sickled shapes (Figure 64-2).
- Increases in fluid viscosity result, and blood stasis occurs, which can lead to thrombosis and infarction.

II. CLINICAL COURSE

A. Severe Hemolytic Anemia

- Adults: chronic hemolytic sickle cell disease can be severe. The hematocrit may range between 18% and 30%.
- Life span of red blood cells normally is from 90 to 120 days, whereas in hemolytic anemia, such as sickle cell anemia, the red blood cell survival rate is about 10 to 15 days.

B. Sickle Cell Crisis

Periodic recurrences of clinical exacerbations of the disease with periods of remission characterize child-

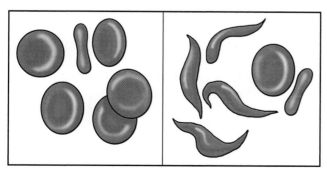

■ **FIGURE 64-2 Sickle Cell Disease.** *Left,* diagrammatic drawing of normal red blood cells. *Right,* sickle shapes of red blood cells of a patient with sickle cell disease.

hood and adolescence. The acute form of the disease is called sickle cell crisis.

1. **Precipitating Factors**
   - Crisis may appear at any time with or without stimuli.
   - Viral or bacterial infections and other systemic diseases.
   - Hypoxia, dehydration, sudden changes in temperature.
   - Physical activity (tissue anoxia), extreme fatigue, acidosis.
   - Stress/anxiety, additional physical burden (pregnancy), trauma.

2. **Clinical Signs and Symptoms**
   - A crisis is characterized by self-limited, reversible, pain episodes involving the extremities, head, back, chest, and abdomen.
   - Infarctions occur in various tissues and organs.
   - Symptoms of seizure, stroke, or coma may develop when nervous system becomes involved.
   - Effects of crisis may be reversible; severe physical conditions can result.
   - Infection or other complications reduce red cell production and there is increased trappings of red cells in the spleen and liver.
   - A crisis can be fatal.
   - High mortality rate in young children may be the result of the effects of crisis or of severe bacterial infections.
   - Children younger than three (3) years of age are at great risk for fatal sepsis and meningitis.

C. Systemic Changes That May Occur

Chronic changes may occur in any organ system at any age.
- Major organ affected: kidney.
- Cardiopulmonary system can result in enlargement of the heart, heart murmurs, and coronary insufficiency.
- Ocular disturbances, even leading to blindness.
- Some patients are susceptible to cerebrovascular accidents with hemiplegia.
- Damage may also occur to the lungs, liver, and spleen.
- Changes that occur in all bones, including the mandible, result from thrombosis with infarction and from infection.

D. Treatment[6]

1. **Preventive Procedures**
   - Use folate supplements daily to cope with increased need by the bone marrow.

- Avoid and/or promptly treat infections; administer pneumococcal polyvalent vaccine to children.
- Obtain genetic counseling for those with sickle cell trait.
- Allogeneic stem-cell transplantation may provide a cure for young patients with symptomatic sickle cell disease.
- Daily penicillin until age six to prevent infection.

2. **Treatment for Disease State**
   - Supportive and palliative treatments include those for specific symptoms during crises.
   - Pain relief and the use of antibiotics for infectious diseases.
   - Oxygen therapy and blood transfusions are not used for routine pain episodes but may have limited selective use.

III. ORAL IMPLICATIONS

A. Radiographic Findings[7,8]

1. Decreased radiodensity; increased osteoporosis.
2. Coarse trabecular pattern appearing as horizontal rows between teeth ("step-ladder"), with large marrow spaces.
3. Significant bone loss in children, indicating the presence of periodontitis.

B. Oral Manifestations

- Generalized pallor of tissues.
- Jaundiced color from liver disease.
- Periodontal involvement has been a cause for sickle cell crisis.[9]
- Periodontal evaluation is likely to reveal pockets, infection, and bleeding.
- Patient requires strict preventive treatment program.

IV. APPOINTMENT MANAGEMENT[10]

- The objective during therapy is to provide care without precipitating a sickle cell crisis. During a sickle cell crisis, treatment should be limited to emergency relief.
- Teach and supervise a comprehensive preventive program to minimize oral infection and control etiologic factors.
- Plan routine care in noncrisis periods; short appointments.
- Prepare or review the comprehensive medical history.
- Use prophylactic antibiotics. For a patient so highly susceptible to infection, antibiotics should be considered routine, because any form of tissue manipulation can create a bacteremia.

- Use local anesthesia without epinephrine.
- Use nitrous oxide–oxygen with greater than 50% oxygen, high flow rate, good ventilation.
- Avoid long complicated dental appointments by maintaining good personal oral health and arranging frequent appointments with the dental hygienist.

▪ POLYCYTHEMIAS

Polycythemia means an increase in the number and concentration of red blood cells above the normal level. Hemoglobin and hematocrit values are raised. The three general categories are relative, primary, and secondary.

I. RELATIVE POLYCYTHEMIA

- Loss of plasma occurs without a corresponding loss of red blood cells.
- The concentration of cells increases and a relative polycythemia results.
- Causes of fluid loss may be such conditions as dehydration, diarrhea, repeated vomiting, sweating, or loss of fluid from burns.
- Other contributing factors may be smoking, hypertension, becoming mildly overweight, and stress, particularly in middle-aged men.

II. POLYCYTHEMIA VERA (PRIMARY POLYCYTHEMIA)[11]

- Results from actual increased red blood cell count and hemoglobin value.
- White cell and platelet counts are elevated.
- Blood viscosity increased, affecting oxygen transport to tissues.

A. Cause

Polycythemia vera is a neoplastic condition resulting from a bone disorder in which the primitive red cells or stem cells proliferate.

B. Oral Signs and Symptoms

1. The tongue, mucous membranes, and gingiva are deep purplish-red.
2. The gingiva are enlarged, with bleeding on slight provocation.
3. Submucosal petechiae, ecchymosis, and hematoma formation.

C. Treatment

1. Chemotherapy or radiation.
2. Phlebotomy, to reduce the total volume, and particularly the red cell volume, of the blood.

D. Dental Hygiene Treatment Considerations

- Frequent maintenance appointments needed to maintain superior health.

III. SECONDARY POLYCYTHEMIA

- Secondary polycythemia is also called erythrocytosis, which means an increase in numbers of red blood cells.
- The increased red cell production can result from hypoxia such as occurs in residents of high altitudes, pulmonary disease, heart disease, and tobacco smoking.
- Bleeding tendencies may be partially controlled with control of gingival irritants.

▪ WHITE BLOOD CELLS

Disorders of the white blood cells may occur because of a decrease (leukopenia) or an increase (leukocytosis) in cell numbers. The types of white blood cells are described in Table 64-2 and illustrated in Figure 64-1.

I. LEUKOPENIA[12]

A decrease in the total number of white blood cells results when cell production cannot keep pace with the turnover rate or when an accelerated rate of removal of cells occurs, as in certain disease states.

A. Conditions in Which Leukopenia Occurs

1. *Specific Infections.* HIV/AIDS, typhoid fever, influenza, malaria, measles (rubeola), and German measles (rubella) are examples.
2. *Disease or Intoxification of the Bone Marrow.* Chronic drug poisoning, radiation, and autoimmune or drug-induced immune reactions may be implicated.

B. Agranulocytosis (malignant neutropenia)

- Rare, serious disease involving the destruction of bone marrow.
- Causes relate to toxicity from drugs and chemicals, antipsychotic drugs, and autoimmune reactions.
- Increased susceptibility to infection; oral ulceration and necrosis of tissue.
- Clinical course of sharp drop in white cells; depression of bone marrow; rapid acute illness leading to death.

II. LEUKOCYTOSIS

- Increase in the number of circulating white blood cells.
- Caused by inflammatory and infectious states, trauma, exertion, and other conditions listed in Table 64-2.
- The most extreme abnormal cause of leukocytosis is leukemia. Leukemias are malignant neoplasms of immature white blood cells. They are characterized by abnormally large numbers of specific types of leukocytes and their precursors located within the circulating blood and bone marrow and infiltrated into other body tissues and organs.

▪ BLEEDING DISORDERS

- Bleeding disorders have in common tendencies to spontaneous bleeding and moderate to excessive bleeding following trauma or a surgical procedure.
- Spontaneous bleeding occurs as small hemorrhages into the skin or mucous membranes and other tissues, and appears as petechiae or purpura.
- Moderate to excessive bleeding or prolonged bleeding may follow dental hygiene therapy, including nonsurgical instrumentation.
- A history or suspicion of a bleeding problem should be fully evaluated before treatment is started.

I. DETECTION

A. Patient's Medical and Dental Histories

1. **Basic Health Questionnaire**
   - Includes items related to bleeding, bruising, blood transfusions (and for what reasons they were needed), blood disorders, familial blood disorders, and previous abnormal bleeding that may have followed past dental or dental hygiene appointments.
2. **Consultation and Follow-up**
   - Follow-up with conversational questioning after "yes-no" answers on a written questionnaire can delve into sufficient detail to determine the need for blood tests before treatment is started.
   - Additional information is also obtained by consultation with the patient's physician.
   - When blood tests have been made in the past but are not recent, new reports are requested.

B. Laboratory Blood Tests

- Selected basic tests are listed in Table 64-1 with their normal values. Additional tests are frequently needed for a thorough evaluation of specific conditions.

- Certain tests may be needed on the same day as treatment because blood values may fluctuate. For example, the patient taking anticoagulants is required to have a prothrombin time determination within 24 hours of appointment. Consulting with the patient's physician in advance is mandatory.

II. TYPES OF BLEEDING DISORDERS

A. Abnormalities of the Blood Capillaries

1. **Characteristics**
   - Vascular fragility is increased; petechial and purpuric hemorrhages in the skin or mucous membranes, including the gingiva.
2. **Conditions Predisposing to Bleeding**
   - Severe infections (septicemias, severe measles, typhoid fever).
   - Drug reactions (sulfonamides, phenacetin).
   - Scurvy or vitamin C deficiency (impaired collagen leads to fragility of vessel wall).

B. Platelet Deficiency or Dysfunction

1. **Thrombocytopenia**
   - A lowered number of platelets may be caused by decreased production in the bone marrow.
   - Bone marrow depression may be an invasive disease, such as leukemia, or deficiencies, such as folate or vitamin B_{12} deficiency anemias.
2. **Platelet Dysfunction**
   - Interference with the blood clotting mechanism leads to a prolonged bleeding time.
   - Defects occur as a result of certain hereditary states, uremia, von Willebrand's disease, and certain drugs such as salicylates (aspirin).

C. Blood Clotting Defects

A possible irregularity or disorder is associated with each of the many clotting factors.
1. **Acquired Disorders**
   - Vitamin K deficiency. Vitamin K is essential for prothrombin synthesis and factors VII, IX, X.
   - Liver disease. Nearly all the clotting factors are produced in the liver. When the liver is not functioning properly, the clotting factors may be altered.
2. **Hereditary Disorders**
   - At least 30 hereditary coagulation disorders exist, each resulting from a deficiency or abnormality of a plasma protein.

- Clinically, signs and symptoms are similar. The following three are described in detail in the next section:
  a. Hemophilia A (factor VIII abnormality).
  b. Hemophilia B (factor IX abnormality).
  c. von Willebrand's disease (von Willebrand factor, which chemically forms a large part of the factor VIII complex, is either too low or does not function properly).

▪ HEMOPHILIAS[13]

The hemophilias are a group of congenital disorders of the blood clotting mechanism.

- The two types of hemophilia are hemophilia A (also called classic hemophilia) and hemophilia B (also called Christmas disease).
- Hemophilia A is the more common. About 85% of people who have hemophilia have this form.
- The most common hereditary disorder of the platelet function is von Willebrand's disease.
- Hemophilias A and B are inherited by males through an X-linked recessive trait carried by females.
- von Willebrand's disease is transmitted by an autosomal co-dominant trait.
- Rarely is a female affected by hemophilias A or B, but von Willebrand's disease occurs in males and females.

I. LEVEL OF CLOTTING FACTOR

- The severity of the disease can be related directly to the level of the clotting factor in the circulating blood.
- Normal concentrations of the clotting factors are between 55% and 150%.
- Patients with severe hemophilia have a clotting factor VIII or IX of less than 1%.
- Spontaneous bleeding into muscles, joints, and soft tissues, and severe, prolonged bleeding after minor trauma.
- Less severe, hemophilia has a clotting factor in the 2% to 5% range. Spontaneous bleeding may be only occasional; gross bleeding occurs after light but definite trauma.
- von Willebrand disease is prolonged bleeding time in the presence of a normal platelet count.

II. EFFECTS AND LONG-TERM COMPLICATIONS

A. Effects of Minor Trauma

Bleeding and bruising from minor trauma vary, depending on the severity of the disease.

B. Hemarthroses

Bleeding into the soft tissue of joints (knees, ankles, elbows) begins in the very young with severe hemophilia. Much swelling, pain, and incapacitation are created.

C. Joint Deformity and Crippling

Permanent joint damage can result, and the patient may need splints, braces, or orthopedic surgery.

D. Intramuscular Hemorrhage

Hemorrhage into the muscles is accompanied by pain and limitation of motion.

E. Oral Bleeding

- Bleeding from the gingiva is common and more extensive when periodontal infection is more severe.
- Because of the fear of bleeding, patients may neglect toothbrushing and flossing; doing so can lead to increased dental biofilm accumulation and inflammation.
- Small children may injure the oral area when they tumble, and severe bleeding can result.

■ DENTAL HYGIENE CARE PLAN

Although prevention and control of bleeding are the main issues when treating a patient with hemophilia, other factors require attention. Patients with hemophilia have many emotional stresses related to the disease, its treatment, and excessive cost. Patients now can take more responsibility for self-care regimens as opposed to previous issues of long hospitalizations and separations from family, friends, and school.

As a result of internal and cerebral hemorrhages a few patients may be multihandicapped, have mental and physical problems, or may be limited intellectually. Suggestions for appointments from Chapter 53 may be useful for the patient who has had hemarthroses and orthopedic treatment.

I. PATIENT HISTORY

- Medical history must include information regarding the type, severity, treatment, medications, and family history of the hemophilia patient.
- Dental history: discussion with the patient to include previous dental care and perceived treatment needs.

II. CONSULTATION WITH PHYSICIAN/HEMATOLOGIST

- Consultation with the physician/hematologist is necessary to obtain complete and accurate information.
- Prophylactic antibiotic premedication is usually required because of the susceptibility to infection in joint prostheses and/or indwelling catheter.
- Many procedures require factor replacement therapy just prior to the dental appointment.

III. CLINICAL PROCEDURES

- Prevention of gingival infection and dental caries is an essential aspect of care for patients with hemophilia.
- Preliminary tissue conditioning can help prevent severe bleeding during instrumentation. Teach daily personal biofilm removal at the initial appointment and reinforce at each session.
- Plan scaling in small segments.

IV. ORAL HYGIENE PROGRAM

- Patients must be encouraged to improve and maintain good oral health. Spontaneous oral bleeding problems can be partially controlled by the elimination of oral infections.
- Meticulous dental biofilm removal must be practiced and repeated. A soft toothbrush is indicated.
- Teach flossing carefully and correctly to prevent cutting the gingiva and inducing proximal bleeding.
- Patients with limited manual dexterity can benefit from special oral hygiene aids described on pages 898 to 901.
- All preventive measures must be age appropriate. Fluoride treatments, sealants, biofilm control, professional dental supervision, and nutritional counseling for caries control.

V. MISCELLANEOUS TREATMENT SUGGESTIONS FOR DENTAL PROFESSIONALS

Analyzing techniques and procedures can help ensure that all excess trauma to the patient is prevented. The same procedures are applied to all patients, but they are more significant with a patient who has a bleeding problem.

  1. *Pain Relief.* Never use aspirin for a patient with a bleeding disorder. The bleeding tendency is greatly increased by a drug-induced platelet dysfunction caused by aspirin.

Everyday Ethics

Just as Dena, the dental hygienist, begins to probe for recording the gingival examination for Mr. Bennett, the patient, the receptionist interrupts to give Dena a medical clearance form that has been faxed from the patient's physician. As Dena reviews the information she understands that the patient has a blood disorder but is unclear as to its extent from the laboratory values in the report. She briefly questions Mr. Bennett about any medical tests and he indicates that he was in the hospital 4 days last month.

As Dena continues the probing she notices considerable bleeding with oozing around the gingival margins.

Questions for Consideration

1. What action, if any, should Dena take to ensure she is performing beneficently on behalf of the patient?

2. It appears that Mr. Bennett has not given sufficient information about his medical condition prior to this maintenance appointment. What obligation does a patient have to update the medical history at each appointment? And what obligation does the professional person have to help the patient understand this obligation?

3. While Dena quietly acknowledges to herself that she used to know the information about bleeding conditions, she is currently uncertain of the meaning of the laboratory values in this patient's report. Ethically, how should this realization be assessed? What is the immediate need? What can be done to prevent such a situation from occurring again in the future?

---

2. *Periodontal Dressing.* After subgingival scaling and planing, a periodontal dressing can provide pressure and adapt the tissue against the teeth as an aid for the prevention of postappointment bleeding.
3. *Frequency of Maintenance Care.* Frequent appointments can aid in keeping the oral tissues in an optimum state of health and help to prevent the need for complex dental treatments.
4. *Rubber Dam* for sealant placement. Because of the importance of a dry clean pit or fissure, a dam is recommended. A thin rubber dam may be

✔ **Factors To Teach The Patient**

- Meticulous oral hygiene techniques to practice daily: toothbrushing, flossing, and other interdental cleaning devices.

- How to self-evaluate the oral cavity for deviations from normal. Any changes should be reported to the dentist and dental hygienist.

- Selection of noncariogenic foods to prevent caries, and knowledge about the diet's relationship to health.

- Avoid use of salicylates (aspirin); control pain with acetaminophen.

more gentle to the oral tissues than a heavy one. The use of a Young's frame may eliminate pressure, especially at the corners of the mouth. Rubber dam clamps can be checked for sharp corners and placed carefully without damage to the gingival tissues.
5. *Film Placement.* Films can cut and press on the mucous membranes. Care in placement must be exercised.
6. *Impressions.* Beading the rims of the trays protects the mucosa from pressure and damage from a hard, possibly rough surface (page 194).
7. *Evacuation.* High-vacuum suction tips may be sharp. Caution in the use of suction is necessary to prevent pulling the sublingual or other mucosal tissues into the suction tip and causing hematomas.
8. *Treatment for Hematoma.* Ice pack application may limit the spread of a hematoma as a temporary measure. Prompt replacement therapy may be needed.

REFERENCES

1. **Young**, B. and Heath, J.: *Wheater's Functional Histology,* 4th ed. London, Churchill & Livingstone, 2000, pp. 46–66.
2. **Al-Wahadni**, A.M., Taani, D.Q., and Al-Omari, M.O.: Dental Diseases in Subjects With B–Thalassemia Major, *Community Dent. Oral Epidemiol., 30,* 418, December, 2002.
3. **Cotran**, R.S., Kumar, V., and Collins, T.: *Robbins' Pathologic Basis of Disease,* 6th ed. Philadelphia, W.B. Saunders Co., 1999, pp. 621–627.

4. **Wardlaw**, G.: *Perspectives in Nutrition,* 4th ed. New York, McGraw Hill Co, 1999, pp. 431–438.

5. **Platt**, A., Eckman, J.R., Beasley, J., and Miller, G.: Treating Sickle Cell Pain: An Update From the Georgia Comprehensive Sickle Cell Center, *J. Emerg. Nurs., 28,* 297, August, 2002.

6. **Walters**, M.C., Patience, M., Leisenring, W., Eckman, J.R., Scott, J.P., Mentzer, W.C., Davies, S.C., Ohene-Frempong, K., Bernaudin, F., Matthews, D.C., Storb, R., and Sullivan, K.M.: Bone Marrow Transplantation for Sickle Cell Disease, *N. Engl. J. Med., 335,* 369, August 8, 1996.

7. **Taylor**, L.B., Nowak, A.J., Giller, R.H., and Casamassimo, P.S.: Sickle Cell Anemia: A Review of the Dental Concerns and a Retrospective Study of Dental and Bony Changes, *Spec. Care Dentist., 15,* 38, January/February, 1995.

8. **Ibsen**, O.A.C., Phelan, J.A., and Vernillo, A.T.: Oral Manifestations of Systemic Diseases, in Ibsen, O.A.C. and Phelan, J.A.: *Oral Pathology for the Dental Hygienist,* 3rd ed. Philadelphia, W.B. Saunders Co., 2000, pp. 360–361.

9. **Rada**, R.E., Bronny, A.T., and Hasiakos, P.S.: Sickle Cell Crisis Precipitated by Periodontal Infection: Report of Two Cases. *J. Am. Dent. Assoc., 114,* 799, June, 1987.

10. **Little**, J.W., Falace, D.A., Miller, C.S., and Rhodus, N.L.: *Dental Management of the Medically Compromised Patient,* 6th ed. St. Louis, Mosby, 2000, p. 379.

11. **Ibsen**, Phelan, and Vernillo: op. cit., pp. 362–364.

12. **Little**, Falace, Miller, and Rhodus: op. cit., pp. 369–370.

13. **Kessler**, C.M.: Coagulation Factor Deficiencies, in Goldman, L. and Bennett, J.C.: *Cecil Textbook of Medicine,* 21st ed. Philadelphia, W.B. Saunders Co., 2000, pp. 1004–1010.

SUGGESTED READINGS

Basi, D.L. and Schmiechen, N.J.: Bleeding and Coagulation Problems in the Dental Patient: Hereditary Disease and Medication-Induced Risks, *Dent. Clin. North Am., 43,* 457, July, 1999.

Brennan, M.T., Sankar, V., Baccaglini, L., Pillemer, S.R., Kingman, A., Nunez, O., Young, N.S., and Atkinson, J.C.: Oral Manifestations in Patients With Aplastic Anemia, *Oral Surg., Oral Med., Oral Pathol., Oral Radiol., Endod., 92,* 503, November, 2001.

Pernu, H.E., Pajari, U.H., and Lanning, M.: The Importance of Regular Dental Treatment in Patients With Cyclic Neutropenia: Follow-up of 2 Cases, *J. Periodontol., 67,* 454, April, 1996.

Toh, B.-H., van Driel, I.R., and Gleeson, P.A.: Pernicious Anemia, *N. Engl. J. Med., 337,* 1441, November 13, 1997.

Sickle Cell Anemia

Arowojolu, M.O. and Savage, K.O.: Alveolar Bone Patterns in Sickle Cell Anemia and Non-sickle Cell Anemia Adolescent Nigerians: A Comparative Study, *J. Periodontol., 68,* 225, March, 1997.

Bunn, H.F.: Pathogenesis and Treatment of Sickle Cell Disease, *N. Engl. J. Med., 337,* 762, September 11, 1997.

Duggal, M.S., Bedi, R., Kinsey, S.E., and Williams, S.A.: The Dental Management of Children With Sickle Cell Disease and Beta-Thalassemia, *Int. J. Paediatr. Dent. , 6,* 227, December, 1996.

Kelleher, M., Bishop, K., and Briggs, P.: Oral Complications Associated With Sickle Cell Anemia, *Oral Med., Oral Pathol., Oral Surg., Oral Radiol., Endod., 82,* 225, August, 1996.

Nathan, D.G.: Search for Improved Therapy of Sickle Cell Anemia (Guest Commentary), *J. Pediatr. Hematol./Oncol., 24,* 700, December, 2002.

Patton, L.L., Brahim, J.S., and Travis, W.D.: Mandibular Osteomyelitis in a Patient With Sickle Cell Anemia: Report of Case, *J. Am. Dent. Assoc., 121,* 602, November, 1990.

Hemophilia/Bleeding Disorder

Federici, A.B., Sacco, R., Stabile, F., Carpenedo, M., Zingaro, E., and Manucci, P.M.: Optimizing Local Therapy During Oral Surgery in Patients With von Willebrand Disease, *Haemophilia, 6,* 71, March, 2000.

Harrington, B.: Primary Dental Care of Patients with Haemophilia [Review], *Haemophilia, 6,* 7, Supplement 1, 2000.

Izumi, Y., Taniguchi, T., Maruyama, Y., and Sueda, T.: Effective Periodontal Treatment in a Patient With Type IIA von Willebrand's Disease: Report of a Case, *J. Periodontol., 70,* 548, May, 1999.

Piot, B., Sigaud-Fiks, M., Huet, P., Fressinaud, E., Trossaert, M., and Mercier, J.: Management of Dental Extractions in Patients With Bleeding Disorders, *Oral Surg., Oral Med., Oral Pathol., Oral Radiol., Endod., 93,* 247, March, 2002.

The Patient With Diabetes Mellitus

Kathryn Ragalis, RDH, MS, DMD

CHAPTER OUTLINE

An effective dental hygiene program is vital for the patient with diabetes mellitus. Signs and symptoms of diabetes can be identified by thorough medical history questions. Clinical assessment can reveal oral changes that are indicative of this systemic disease. Dental professionals may be the first to recognize the warnings and refer the patient for early diagnosis. Early diagnosis and treatment can significantly reduce the life-threatening complications of the disease and improve quality of life.

A patient with diabetes may have a lowered resistance to infections, delayed healing, multiple systemic complications, and is prone to life-threatening emergencies. The presence of infection, including periodontitis, may intensify symptoms and make diabetes more difficult to regulate.

The dental team has a significant responsibility to:
• Recognize signs and symptoms of diabetes to promote early diagnosis.

- Work with the patient and other healthcare professionals to provide instruction and oral care aimed at maintaining health and preventing infections and emergencies.
- Identify and treat acute emergencies.

Modifications in dental and dental hygiene procedures may be indicated. No treatment should be initiated until the state of the diabetes has been confirmed. Key words and abbreviations used in this chapter are found in Box 65-1 and Box 65-2, respectively.

■ DIABETES MELLITUS

I. DEFINITION[1]

A. Diabetes mellitus is a group of metabolic diseases characterized by hyperglycemia. The symptoms of hyperglycemia are listed in Box 65-3.
B. Hyperglycemia results from a defect in insulin secretion, insulin action, or both. There is a relative or absolute lack of insulin or an inadequate function of insulin.
C. Chronic hyperglycemia is associated with long-term damage, dysfunction, and failure of numerous organs.

II. IMPACT

A. Over 6% of the population in the United States is estimated to have diabetes. Approximately a third who have the disease have not yet been diagnosed.
B. As the population ages and with increases in obesity, diabetes becomes more prevalent.
C. Due to the prevalence, cost of treatment, and lost productivity, diabetes is one of the most costly health conditions.

■ INSULIN

I. DEFINITION

Insulin is a hormone produced by the beta cells in the pancreas. It directly or indirectly affects every organ in the body.

II. DESCRIPTION

A. Food is ingested and converted into glucose.
B. Increase in blood glucose level stimulates the pancreas to release insulin into the blood stream.
C. Insulin enables glucose transport into cells to use as energy.
D. Blood glucose level then decreases.

E. Figure 65-1A shows the healthy pancreas and the action of insulin as it is taken up by the body cells.

III. FUNCTIONS

The functions of insulin are listed in Box 65-4. Without insulin, glucose accumulates in the blood, resulting in hyperglycemia. Normal blood glucose levels in healthy individuals usually range from 60–150 mg/dL. In diabetes, levels range much higher.

IV. EFFECTS OF DECREASED INSULIN (TYPE 1 DIABETES)

A. Less glucose is transmitted through cell walls into the cells.
B. Glucose increases in the circulating blood (hyperglycemia) until a threshold is reached and glucose spills over into the urine (glycosuria).
C. Increased glycosuria induces osmotic diuresis with excretion of large amounts of urine (polyuria). Water and electrolytes are lost.
D. Fluid loss signals excessive thirst to the brain (polydipsia).
E. Cells starving for glucose may cause the patient to increase food intake (polyphagia), but weight loss may still occur.
F. Without glucose to use for energy, the body metabolizes fat for energy.
   - End products of fat metabolism are harmful ketones that accumulate in the blood.
   - Ketones are acidic, and when they accumulate, they are usually neutralized in the blood. When the quantity is large, the neutralizing effect is depleted rapidly and an acidic condition (metabolic acidosis) results.
   - Metabolic acidosis leads to diabetic coma (ketoacidosis) if not treated promptly.
G. Figure 65-1B shows changes in pancreas function that occur in type 1 diabetes.

V. EFFECTS OF DECREASED ACTION OF INSULIN (TYPE 2 DIABETES)

A. Insulin production and secretion by the pancreas remains at normal levels
B. Cell surface insulin receptors develop defects, and glucose cannot be transmitted into the cell.
C. Blood glucose level increases as the insulin resistance of the cells increases. This stimulates more insulin to be released.
D. Over time, insulin secretion may also decline and lead to both decrease of insulin in the blood as well as increased insulin resistance of cells.

BOX 65-1 KEY WORDS: Diabetes Mellitus

Beta cells: insulin-producing cells of the islets of Langerhans in the pancreas.

Brittle diabetes: term formerly used to describe very unstable type 1 diabetes; characterized by unexplained oscillation between hypoglycemia and diabetic ketoacidosis.

Casual plasma glucose: blood glucose level at any time of day with no regard to time of eating.

Exocrine: secreting externally via a duct.

Exogenous insulin: insulin from source outside patient.

Gestational diabetes: diabetes that occurs during pregnancy.

Gluconeogenesis: synthesis of glucose from noncarbohydrate sources, such as amino acids and glycerol; can occur in the liver and kidneys when the carbohydrate intake is insufficient to meet the body's needs.

Glycated or glycosylated hemoglobin (HbA1c): the primary assay for assessing long-term glycemic control. Indicates blood glucose levels for the previous 6–8 weeks.

Glycemia: presence of glucose in blood.

Hyperpnea: abnormal increase in depth and rate of respiration.

Hypoglycemia: an abnormally low level of glucose in the blood; opposite of **hyperglycemia,** very high blood glucose.

Insulin: a powerful hormone secreted by the beta cells in the islets of Langerhans of the pancreas; the major fuel-regulating hormone; enters the blood in response to a rise in concentration of blood glucose and is transported immediately to bind with cell surface receptors throughout the body.

Ketoacidosis: diabetic coma; too little insulin; accumulation of ketone bodies in the blood.

Ketone bodies: normal metabolic products of lipid (fat) within the liver; excess production leads to urinary excretion of these acidic chemicals.

Ketonuria: excess concentration of ketone bodies in the urine.

Oral glucose tolerance test: a test of the body's ability to utilize carbohydrates; aid to the diagnosis of diabetes mellitus. After ingestion of a specific amount of glucose solution, the fasting blood glucose rises promptly in a nondiabetic person, then falls to normal within an hour. In diabetes mellitus, the blood glucose rise is greater and the return to normal is prolonged.

Oral hypoglycemic agent: synthetic drug that lowers the blood sugar level; stimulates the synthesis and release of insulin from the beta cells of the islets of Langerhans in the pancreas; used to treat patients with type 2 diabetes mellitus.

Polydipsia: excessive thirst.

Polyphagia: excessive ingestion of food.

Polyuria: excessive excretion of urine.

Postprandial: after a meal.

Pruritus: itching.

Retinopathy: noninflammatory degenerative disease of the retina; called **diabetic retinopathy** when it occurs with diabetes of long standing.

BOX 65-2 Key of Abbreviations: Diabetes Mellitus

A1c (A One C)   Common abbreviation for glycosylated hemoglobin (HbA1c)

EMS   Emergency Medical Service

FPG   Fasting plasma glucose

GDM   Gestational diabetes mellitus

HbA1c   Glycosylated hemoglobin

HDL   High-density lipoprotein

IDDM   Insulin-dependent diabetes mellitus

IFG   Impaired fasting glucose

IGT   Impaired glucose tolerance

LDL   Low-density lipoprotein

NIDDM   Non-insulin-dependent diabetes mellitus

OGTT   Oral glucose tolerance test

PP   Postprandial

SMBG   Self-monitoring of blood glucose

WHO   World Health Organization

E. Figure 65-1C shows the effects of decreased insulin and action of insulin that can occur in type 2 diabetes. Note the defective receptor on the body cell.

VI. INSULIN COMPLICATIONS

Earlier diagnosis, improved treatment, and better informed patient, family, and friends have reduced the occurrence of emergency insulin complications. Constant verbal and visual contact must be maintained with a patient to identify early behavioral and physical changes indicative of a developing crisis.

BOX 65-3 Symptoms of Hyperglycemia

Polyuria

Polydipsia

Weight loss

Polyphagia

Blurred vision

Increased susceptibility to infections

A. Hypoglycemia/Insulin Shock

- Too much insulin (hyperinsulinism), which lowers level of blood glucose (hypoglycemia).
- Hypoglycemia is the emergency more likely to occur in the dental setting.

B. Hyperglycemic Reaction/Diabetic Coma (Ketoacidosis)

- Too little insulin (hypoinsulinism) with increased levels of blood glucose (hyperglycemia).
- Table 65-1 shows a comparison of the characteristics of hyperglycemic and hypoglycemic reactions, along with the respective treatment procedures.

■ DIABETES MELLITUS ETIOLOGIC CLASSIFICATION

In 1997, an international expert committee, organized by the American Diabetes Association, revised the classification of diabetes. The new system is based on the etiology of the disease wherever possible. A comparison of types 1 and 2 diabetes is found in Table 65-2.

I.   TYPE 1 DIABETES

A. Description

Figure 65-1B illustrates changes in type 1 diabetes.
- An absolute insulin deficiency.
- Results from the destruction of the insulin-producing beta cells in the pancreas. The loss of the beta cells is due to either a cell-mediated autoimmune destruction or an unknown etiology and unclear environmental factors.
- Patients are dependent on exogenous insulin to sustain life.
- Prone to ketoacidosis.
- Usually arises in childhood or puberty, but may occur at any age.

B. Former Names

Type I diabetes, insulin-dependent diabetes mellitus (IDDM), juvenile diabetes, juvenile-onset diabetes, ketosis-prone diabetes, brittle diabetes.

II. TYPE 2 DIABETES

A. Description

Figure 65-1C shows changes listed below.
- Pancreatic insulin secretion may be low, normal, or even higher than normal, but the patient exhibits an insulin resistance that impairs the use of insulin.

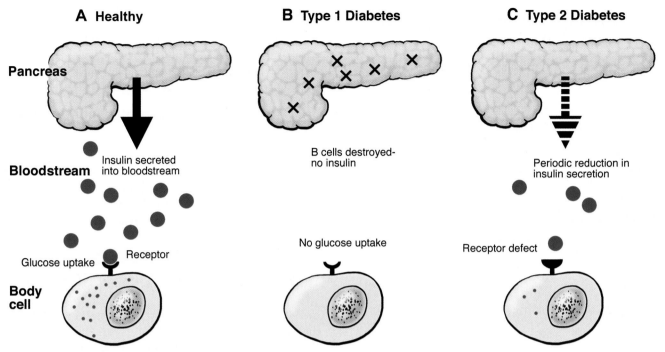

■ **FIGURE 65-1 Pancreas and Action of Insulin on Body Cell in Health, and Type 1 and 2 Diabetes. (A)** Healthy pancreas excretes insulin into bloodstream that enables glucose uptake by body cell. **(B)** Type 1 diabetes shows no insulin produced by pancreas and no glucose uptake by cell. **(C)** Type 2 diabetes shows normal, increased, or decreased insulin production by pancreas and the defective receptor on cell that hampers insulin uptake.

- Patients have insulin resistance with a relative, not absolute, insulin deficiency.
- Insulin resistance is the inability of the peripheral tissues to respond to the insulin that is produced.
- Risk factors for developing this type of diabetes are listed in Box 65-5.
- Onset typical after 30 years of age, but may occur at any age. Incidence has increased dramatically in children and adolescents in recent years, possibly due to increases in sedentary lifestyle and obesity in children.

BOX 65-4 Functions of Insulin

1. Facilitates glucose uptake from blood into tissues, which lowers blood glucose level.

2. Speeds the oxidation of glucose within the cells to use for energy.

3. Speeds the conversion of glucose to glycogen to store in the liver and skeletal muscles and to prevent the conversion of glycogen back to glucose.

4. Facilitates conversion of glucose to fat in adipose tissue.

- Most prevalent type of diabetes, more than 90% of all patients with diabetes.

B. Screening[2]

Type 1 diabetes is usually identified after acute symptoms prompt immediate evaluation. Screening is recommended for type 2 diabetes. Because of the severe complications, screening should be done for those who are asymptomatic. Basic criteria for testing in healthcare setting:

- Age 45 and above, repeated every 3 years.
- Testing should begin earlier and more frequently if patient has any risk factors listed in Box 65-5. This includes testing children and adolescents who are overweight and have other risk factors.

C. Former Names

- Type II diabetes, non-insulin-dependent diabetes mellitus (NIDDM), adult-onset diabetes, maturity-onset diabetes, ketosis-resistant diabetes.

III. GESTATIONAL DIABETES MELLITUS (GDM)

A. Defined as any degree of glucose intolerance with onset or first recognition during pregnancy.

■ TABLE 65-1 COMPARISON OF INSULIN REACTION AND DIABETIC COMA

	HYPOGLYCEMIA/INSULIN SHOCK	DIABETIC COMA/KETOACIDOSIS
History/Predisposing Factors	Too much insulin Too little food: omitted or delayed Excessive exercise Stress	Too little insulin: omission of dose or failure to increase dose when requirements increased Too much food Less exercise than planned Infection, illness of any sort Trauma, drugs, alcohol abuse Stress
Occurrence	More common complication than ketoacidosis, especially with less stable type 1 diabetes	Type I diabetes especially if poorly controlled, unstable
Onset	Sudden	Develops slowly over hours/days
Behavior Changes	Confusion, stupor Drowsy, restless Anxious, irritable, agitated Incoordination, weakness	Any hypoglycemia behavior change
Physical Findings	Skin: moist, sweaty, perspiration Hunger Headache Tremor, shakiness, weakness Pallor Dilated pupils, blurry vision Dizziness, staggering gait	Skin: flushed, dry Abdominal pain Nausea, vomiting Lack of appetite Dry mouth, thirst Fruity smelling breath Increased urination
Vital Signs Temperature: Respiration: Pulse Blood Pressure	Normal or below Normal Fast, irregular Normal or slightly elevated	Elevated when infection Hyperpnea, rapid and labored Acetone or fruity smelling breath Rapid, weak Lowered, person may go into shock
If Left Untreated	Possible convulsions, eventual coma and death	Eventual coma and death
Treatment	GIVE SUGAR to raise blood glucose level (apple juice, cake frosting, glucose tablets) Revival is prompt If unconscious/unresponsive; injection of glucagon or intravenous glucose	Immediate professional care Activate EMS, hospitalize Monitor vital signs Keep patient warm Fluids for conscious patient Insulin injection after medical assessment
Prevention	Smooth regulation of blood sugar and frequent blood glucose monitoring	Smooth regulation of blood sugar and frequent blood glucose monitoring

B. Related to genetics, obesity, and hormones causing insulin resistance usually in third trimester.

C. Occurs in about 4% of pregnancies in the United States.

D. Diagnosis is reclassified 6 or more weeks after pregnancy ends.

E. Insulin adjustment, carefully supervised prenatal care, and improved obstetric practices have lessened much of the potential danger for the mother.

F. Infants are larger; premature births more frequent; incidence of congenital malformations and perinatal death high; lower rate with improved prenatal care.

G. Have tendency to develop type 2 diabetes later in life.

IV. OTHER SPECIFIC TYPES OF DIABETES[1]

Other types of diabetes result from genetic defects, diseases, endocrinopathies, surgery, drugs, malnutrition, infections, and injury.

A. Genetic defects of the beta cell

III. NEPHROPATHY

- Diabetes is a leading cause of renal disease, and the most common cause of end-stage renal disease (ESRD) in the U.S. and Europe. Dialysis or kidney transplant is needed.
- Patients diagnosed with diabetes should be screened for microalbuminuria.

IV. RETINOPATHY

- Diabetes is a leading cause of blindness through the progression of diabetic retinopathy.
- Patients are more likely to have glaucoma and cataracts.

V. CARDIOVASCULAR DISEASE

- Includes cardiovascular disease, peripheral vascular disease, cerebrovascular disease, and hypertension and may lead to myocardial infarction and stroke.
- Due to the excessive risk of coronary heart disease (CHD), aggressive treatment for dyslipidemia (elevated triglyceride and decreased HDL cholesterol levels) is usually recommended.
- Low-dose aspirin therapy is recommended for prevention of cardiovascular disease in patients with type 2 diabetes. Daily aspirin intake increases bleeding time.

VI. AMPUTATION

Diabetes is a major cause of limb amputation (usually foot) from possible complications of neuropathy and vascular disease.

VII. PREGNANCY COMPLICATIONS

Patients with diabetes are at higher risk for spontaneous miscarriages, having babies with birth defects and increased weight.

VIII. PSYCHOSOCIAL

- Complications of diabetes and daily life of patient and those close to patient are significantly affected by diabetes.
- Treatment regimens may be difficult to cope with and lead to emotional and social problems, including depression.
- Make an appropriate referral for professional help, which may improve quality of life and patient's compliance with treatment.

IX. SILENT KILLER

- Average life span is reduced.
- Diabetes and its complications are leading causes of death.

■ MEDICAL TREATMENT AND MODIFICATIONS FOR DIABETES CONTROL

There is no known cure for diabetes. Treatment methods depend on the severity of the disease and on the individual. Consideration must be given to individualized needs related to age, activities, vocation, lifestyle, knowledge, attitudes, personality, culture, emotional and psychological needs, as well as the health status and nutritional and weight issues of the patient.

I. GENERAL PROCEDURES

A. Early diagnosis.
B. Patient education for self-care.
C. Attain the best possible overall health: control hypertension; keep reasonable weight; maintain personal, physical, and psychological health.
D. Maintain tight glycemic control to reduce the complications of diabetes.
E. Receive preventive general physical examinations and specialty examinations on a routine basis to identify effectiveness of treatment and early complications of diabetes.
F. Immediate treatment to manage acute symptoms.
   - Aggressive treatment of infections.
   - Eliminate sources of infection, including oral diseases.
   - Prevent injuries.

II. INSTRUCTION

A. Health Team

- Initial and ongoing individualized education must be provided by the health team.
- Members include physicians, registered nurses, dietitians, pharmacists, mental health professionals, dental professionals, and other specialists, such as endocrinologist, cardiologist, ophthalmologist, and podiatrist.

B. Instructional Materials

- *Books and Journals.* A number of excellent books, professional journals, and other printed materials have been prepared for the patient and for health professionals. Review of these materials can provide the dental team members with greater insight into the background and knowledge of the patient in preparation for oral health instruction.

- *Internet.* An extensive resource for information, support groups, and products that can be helpful to the dental team, patient, family, friends, and other health professionals. Note: care should be used to determine validity of information on some Web sites.

III. EXERCISE

A. An essential part of the treatment program.
B. Contributes to lowering insulin requirements.
C. Lowers the cardiovascular risk factors of obesity, inactivity, and LDL cholesterol level.
D. Many cases of type 2 diabetes can be controlled with weight reduction and exercise alone.

IV. DIET

Diet counseling is basic and planned by the physician, dietitian, and patient. Diet planning is ongoing and based on individual needs and treatment goals. There is no specific diabetic diet. Healthy, well-controlled individuals can have a diet very similar to a healthy person without diabetes. No foods are prohibited but eaten in moderation at observed times.

A. Goals of Nutritional Therapy[6]

- Attain and maintain near-normal blood glucose levels to reduce complications of diabetes.
- Maintain optimal serum lipid levels and blood pressure to reduce risk for vascular disease.
- Modify nutrient intake as appropriate for treatment or prevention of complications, including obesity, dyslipidemia, cardiovascular disease, hypertension, nephropathy.
- Healthy food choices and physical activity to improve overall health.
- Take into consideration personal and cultural preferences, lifestyle, and individual wishes.

B. Fundamentals of Diet

- Diet selection should be based on individual quantitative need and may be identical to an individual without diabetes.
- Proper nutrition is stressed so adequate calories are provided to attain and maintain ideal body weight and health. High fiber, low fat, low cholesterol, and low sodium to reduce risk of vascular and heart disease.

- Amount of carbohydrates consumed monitored and controlled with less regard to source. Foods containing high proportions of sugars should be used sparingly.
- The obese patient benefits with a weight-reduction diet that is more successful if combined with exercise and behavior modification.
- Food lost, as in vomiting, may affect glucose balance.
- Consistent, specific times for medication and food intake to control blood glucose levels. Usually three on-time meals and three interval feedings are followed.

V. HABITS

A. Tobacco

- Patient must avoid all types of tobacco.
- Smoking is a major health hazard for everyone and is especially dangerous for those with diabetes. It increases risk of heart disease, stroke, myocardial infarction, limb amputations, periodontal disease, and numerous other health problems.
- Refer patient to appropriate smoking cessation program (page 513).

B. Alcohol

- Avoid excessive alcohol; alcohol can raise blood pressure and contribute to other health problems (page 1013).

■ MEDICATIONS

I. INSULIN THERAPY

All patients with type 1 diabetes require exogenous insulin for survival. Type 2 patients may need to use insulin for control.

A. Types of Insulin

Insulin is classified as rapid, short, intermediate, or long-acting based on the onset, peak, and duration of action. The types of insulin and range of peak action are found in Table 65-3.

B. Dosage

Depends on the individual.
1. *Objective.* Attain optimum utilization of glucose throughout each 24 hours.
2. *Factors affecting the need for insulin.* Food intake, illness, stress, variations in exercise, or infections.

▪ **TABLE 65-3 TYPES AND ACTION OF INSULIN**

CLASS OF INSULIN	TYPE	PEAK ACTION
Rapid acting	Lispro, aspart	30–90 minutes
Short acting	Regular	2–3 hours
Intermediate acting	NPH Lente	4–10 hours 4–12 hours
Long acting	Ultralente, glargine	12–16 hours

3. *"Sick Day Rules."* Insulin dose is adjusted if there are any factors that are affecting the need for insulin.

C. Methods for Insulin Administration

1. *Subcutaneous injection with syringe.* Injection sites are rotated usually on abdomen, thighs, and upper arm.
2. *Continuous subcutaneous insulin infusion with a battery-operated insulin pump.*
   a. The insulin pump delivers preprogrammed continuous basal rate of insulin and bolus doses when needed.
   b. Offers greater flexibility, smoother control of glycemia, but may increase the risk of hypoglycemia.
   c. The pager size pump can be worn in a pocket or on a belt or waistband, as shown in Figure 65-2.
3. Future modes for insulin administration under experiment include an insulin patch, inhaled insulin, and implantable insulin pumps.

II. ORAL HYPOGLYCEMIC AGENTS

Oral medications are commonly used to treat type 2 diabetes in conjunction with diet, exercise, and possibly the injection of insulin. The medications, listed in Table 65-4, may be used individually or in certain combinations.

▪ PANCREAS TRANSPLANTATION

- Pancreas transplantation can be a successful option for treatment of selected patients.
- Successful transplantation has eliminated the need for exogenous insulin in thousands of type 1 patients.
- Lifelong immunosuppression therapy is required to prevent rejection and the autoimmune process that may destroy the islet cells again.

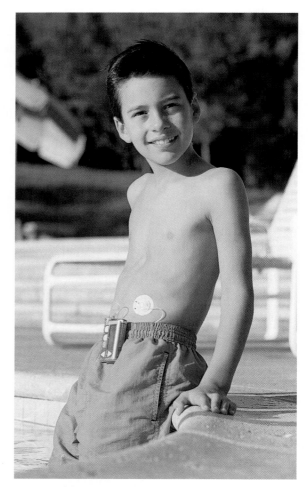

▪ **FIGURE 65-2 Patient Wearing Insulin Pump.** Young boy with active lifestyle wearing an insulin pump. Photo courtesy of Minimed.

- A complete medical history must be confirmed along with any additional recommendations for antibiotic premedication for these patients.
- Pancreatic islet cell transplantation is experimental at this time and holds hope for the future.
- Due to the shortage of donors, an implantable artificial pancreas is under research and development.
- An artificial pancreas consists of three components: a continuous blood glucose monitor, an insulin pump to deliver the appropriate amount, and a control system to complete a closed feedback loop.

▪ BLOOD GLUCOSE TESTING

- Blood glucose testing is used to diagnose diabetes and to monitor blood glucose levels.

■ TABLE 65-4 ORAL HYPOGLYCEMIC AGENTS USED FOR TREATMENT OF TYPE 2 DIABETES

Sulfonylureas	First generation: chloropamide, tolbutamide, tolazamide, acetohexamide Second generation: glyburide, glipizide, glimepiride	-Act by stimulating insulin release by the pancreas -May cause hypoglycemia
Biguanides	Metformin	-Prevents liver glycogen breakdown to glucose -Increases tissue sensitivity to insulin
Alpha-glucosidase Inhibitors	Acarbose	-Slows digestion and glucose uptake into blood
Thiazolidinediones	Rosiglitazone, pioglitazone	-Increases tissue sensitivity to insulin
Meglitinides	Repaglinide, nateglinide	-Lowers blood glucose by increasing insulin release by pancreas -May cause hypoglycemia

- Patients with type 1 diabetes typically do self-monitoring of blood glucose level three or more times per day. Frequency of testing for type 2 patients varies.
- Blood glucose testing can be accomplished in the dental setting to confirm a safe blood glucose level prior to treatment.
- Interpretation of routine tests is in Table 65-5.

I. SELF-ADMINISTERED TESTS

Self-administered glucose tests also may be sent to a laboratory for analysis and comparison of accuracy of patient's technique.

A. Timing of When Blood Sugar Level Is Taken

1. *Fasting Plasma Glucose (FPG):* measurement taken after fasting at least 8 hours.
2. *Postprandial (PP):* measurement taken after consuming a meal.
3. *Casual Plasma Glucose:* measurement taken with no regard for time or food ingestion.

B. Tests

1. Blood Glucose Test
   a. *Test Strip.* Finger prick blood placed on a test strip. Color change of strip is compared to a chart; used at home or in the dental setting.
   b. *Glucose Meter.* Finger prick blood placed on test strip and inserted into the glucose meter; self-monitoring equipment for accurate measurement of blood glucose level; used at home or in the dental setting.
2. Urine Ketone Test
   a. *Objective.* To measure ketones; indicates burning of fat instead of glucose.
   b. *Use.* Used during illness or stress. Performed by patient at home or can be analyzed in lab.

II. LABORATORY TESTS

Glycated Hemoglobin Assay (HbA1c)
- *Objective.* To measure amount of glucose irreversibly bound to a hemoglobin molecule.
- *Use.* Value is proportional to blood glucose status over the half-life of the red blood cell; complements daily monitoring and helps predict risk for developing complications by indicating glycemic control over a 2-3 month period so usually performed every 3 months.
- Along with the FPG, HbA1c has become the measurement of choice for monitoring the treatment of diabetes.
- Also referred to as glycosylated hemoglobin, glycohemoglobin, A1c test.

■ TABLE 65-5 INDIVIDUAL BLOOD GLUCOSE TEST VALUES RELATED TO CONTROL OF DIABETES

	FPG	PP	HbA1c
Healthy, well controlled	<126 mg/dL	<160 mg/dL	<6%
Moderate control	<160 mg/dL	160–200 mg/dL	6%–7%
Uncontrolled	>160 mg/dL	>200 mg/dL	>8%
FPG = fasting plasma glucose; PP = postprandial; HbA1c = glycosylated hemoglobin.			

■ ORAL RELATIONSHIPS

The oral cavity of a patient with diabetes may show unusual susceptibility and marked reactions to injury, infections, and all local irritants. Responses are related to lowered resistance and the delayed healing that are especially prevalent in undiagnosed, uncontrolled, and poorly controlled diabetes. Oral findings may be indicative of undiagnosed diabetes and should be referred for early detection testing.

I. PERIODONTAL INVOLVEMENT[7,8]

Diabetes is a significant risk factor for periodontal infections. Periodontal infections also affect control of blood glucose levels in diabetes. Sudden changes in periodontal status of a patient with diabetes should be immediately referred to the patient's physician for evaluation of diabetes status.

A. Diabetes Effect on Periodontal Disease

- Marked periodontal disease at young age, particularly in patients with type 1 diabetes, and is related to lack of glycemic control. Patients with uncontrolled glucose levels have more severe periodontal disease at younger ages.

- Diabetes acts as a conditioning, modifying, and accelerating factor for disease.
- Inadequate dental biofilm control contributes to more severe tissue response because of decreased resistance.

B. Periodontal Status Effect on Diabetes

- Poorly controlled periodontal health may alter blood glucose levels. Infection affects insulin requirements and may lead to unstable diabetes.
- Treatment of periodontal infection and reduction of periodontal inflammation is associated with a reduction in level of glycosylated hemoglobin (HbA1c).[9]

II. OTHER ORAL FINDINGS

Diabetes does not cause oral disease but may lower resistance and increase susceptibility to the oral findings listed in Table 65-6.

■ DENTAL HYGIENE CARE PLAN

- The control of oral infections is vital. Infection can alter the course and treatment of diabetes.

■ TABLE 65-6 ORAL FINDINGS THAT MAY OCCUR WITH DIABETES

LOCATION	FINDINGS
Gingiva	Increased gingival inflammation
Periodontium	Periodontitis: more frequent, severe, longer duration Attachment loss: more frequent, more extensive Probing depths: more teeth with deep pockets Alveolar bone loss: more Tooth mobility and migration: increased Healing: delayed, increased infection after surgery
Teeth	Poorly controlled diabetes: increased risk of caries related to decreased saliva, diet, and less successful resolution of endodontic therapy related to decreased resistance to infection Well-controlled diabetes: decreased caries related to low sugar, regular eating habits, dental maintenance appointments
Lips	Dry, cracking, angular cheilitis
Saliva	Decreased flow Glucose in sulcular fluid Xerostomia, contributes to opportunistic infection such as oral candidiasis
Mucosa	Edematous, red Oral candidiasis Burning mouth and/or tongue, altered taste Poor tolerance for removable prostheses Delayed healing May have increased occurrence of lichen planus

- Frequent, thorough care, with supervision, is needed and requires the patient's utmost cooperation and motivation.
- The patient with diabetes is prone to life-threatening emergencies.
- The dental team must practice to prevent an emergency, identify early indications of a developing emergency, and act swiftly and appropriately.

I. PATIENT HISTORY

A. Refer for Early Diagnosis

- Questions regarding signs and symptoms of diabetes are basic on any standard medical history questionnaire. Appropriate questions to ask are in Box 65-6.
- If an unexplained positive response is present, the patient is referred to a physician.

B. Medical History

- Supplement the basic medical history with additional questions about diabetes found in Box 65-7 for patients with diabetes.
- Update at each appointment.
- Inquire about recent hypoglycemic reactions: patient who recently had a hypoglycemic reaction may be more likely to have another.
- Identify other health problems, complications of diabetes that may influence dental treatment. Refer to specialist when indicated.
- Ask about exercise and tobacco use; review effect on health.

BOX 65-6 Common Medical History Questions to Screen for Diabetes

1. Have you ever been diagnosed with diabetes?	YES	NO
2. Have any members of your family ever been diagnosed with diabetes?	YES	NO
3. Do you urinate (pass water) more than six times per day?	YES	NO
4. Are you thirsty much of the time?	YES	NO
5. Does your mouth frequently become dry?	YES	NO
6. Have you had any unexplained weight loss?	YES	NO

BOX 65-7 Information to Obtain From Patient With Diabetes

Adherence to treatments prescribed by health team

Medications taken on schedule

Meals and snacks eaten on schedule

Recent history of glycemic control

History of hypoglycemia/hyperglycemia and symptoms experienced

Results of recent blood glucose level testing, including HbA1c

Symptoms suggestive of the complications of diabetes

Medical changes, including other recent illnesses

Current medications, prescribed and over-the-counter, including aspirin

Other vitamins, homeopathic, or herbal supplements used (check side effects)

History of exercise, tobacco use and alcohol use

Stress such as life, psychological, and social changes

Date of most recent physical exam and findings

II. CONSULTATION WITH PHYSICIAN

If unable to obtain complete and accurate information from a patient, or if diabetes is not well controlled, a consultation between dental professional and physician is necessary before any treatment.

III. APPOINTMENT PLANNING

Stress, including that created during a dental or dental hygiene appointment, increases glycemia and a tendency toward acidosis. Appointment planning centers around many factors, including stress prevention.

A. Antibiotic Premedication

- *Well-controlled diabetes.* In general, the patient with well-controlled diabetes is treated the same as the patient without diabetes and requires no premedication related to diabetes.
- *Uncontrolled, unstable diabetes.* Routine dental treatment is deferred until diabetes is stabilized. Only emergency care is given to the uncontrolled patient. Antibiotic premedication may be required due to the reduced ability to resist infection.

B. Time

- Always treat patient on full stomach.
- Avoid peak insulin level noted in Table 65-3.
- Ideal time of appointment varies with individual patient's lifestyle and method of insulin intake.
- Preferred appointment may be morning, soon after the patient's normal breakfast and medication, during the ascending portion of the blood glucose level curve. Note: a patient who eats breakfast at 6 AM does not have a full stomach for a 9 AM appointment.
- Alternative appointment time may be after lunch. Always ask if patient has eaten.

C. Precautions: Prevent/Prepare for Emergency

- Do not keep the patient waiting.
- Do not interfere with the patient's regular meal and between-meal eating schedule.
- Avoid long, stressful procedures; dental and dental hygiene care should be divided into short appointments appropriate to the individual's needs.
- Take additional precautions indicated for the patient with long-term diabetes with complications related to atherosclerosis and other cardiovascular diseases. Needs of the gerodontic patient may be applied.
- Prevent and treat all infections promptly.
- Prepare for diabetic emergency. Keep a tube of cake frosting or a jar of baby apple juice for the conscious patient as part of the office emergency

supplies. These items have a long shelf life and are less likely to be consumed by staff.

D. Emergency

- Recognize any change in patient behavior that signals a diabetic emergency and follow flow chart in Figure 65-3.

IV. CLINICAL PROCEDURES

A. Dental Biofilm Control Instruction

- Due to the impact of diabetes on periodontal health and the effect of oral infection on diabetes status, daily meticulous home care is crucial.
- A biofilm check and individualized self-care measures for biofilm control must be reviewed continuously.

B. Instrumentation

- *Quadrant or Area Scaling.* Complete scaling and root planing reduces the possibility of periodontal abscess formation. Allow several short appointments if needed for stress management.
- *Healing.* Undue trauma to tissues must be avoided to encourage healing without complications.

C. Fluoride Application

- Fluoride treatments, varnishes, and home use of fluoride are encouraged, particularly with xerostomia.
- Methods for daily self-fluoride application are described on page 556.

Everyday Ethics

(?) Ed Smith, a 45-year-old restaurant owner, presents for an appointment with Susan, the dental hygienist. She has treated this patient before but he has not had an appointment for over 2 years. The review of his medical history determines he is overweight, complains of a dry mouth, has excessive thirst, and has not seen his physician in several years. An intraoral exam reveals candidiasis. Susan suggests that he see his physician, but he refuses to even talk about it. He insists that he just wants "clean teeth" for his daughter's upcoming wedding.

Questions for Consideration

1. What options should be considered before treating this patient and how should the patient be informed of the protocol?

2. Given the medical and dental assessment of this patient, would Susan be violating the patient's rights if she denies Mr. Smith's access to dental hygiene care?

3. Describe how each of the core values apply to this scenario.

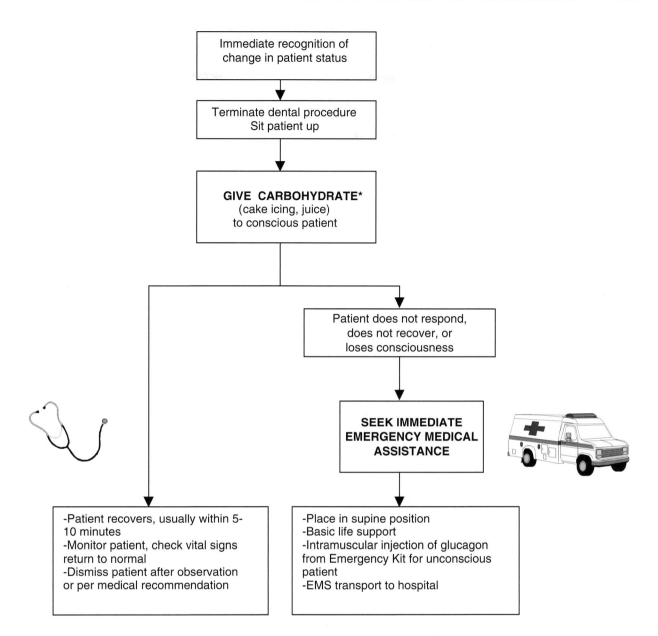

*Carbohydrate can be given for any diabetic emergency. If hypoglycemia (insulin reaction), patient will have rapid recovery. If hyperglycemia (diabetic coma): there will be no improvement, but no worsening of condition. If ketoacidosis or diabetic coma is suspected, seek immediate emergency medical care.

■ **FIGURE 65-3 Diabetic Emergency Action.** Flow chart to show actions to take when patient exhibits signs of diabetic complications.

V. MAINTENANCE PHASE

A. Appointment for supervision and examination on regular 3- to 6-month basis as needed. Calculus should not accumulate. Effectiveness of daily home care must be evaluated.

B. Probe carefully to detect early gingival bleeding and evidence of pocket formation.

C. Assess soft tissue with attention to areas of irritation related to fixed and removable prostheses.

D. Identify any changes that require referral to patient's physician, dietitian, mental health professional, or other specialist.

E. Check for dental biofilm control and review with the patient at each appointment. Gingival health is of major importance. Keep the patient motivated.

✔ Factors To Teach The Patient

FACTORS TO TEACH PATIENTS WITH DIABETES

- Seek regular medical examinations.

- Learn about diabetes. Know status of diabetes, names and doses of medications, including over-the-counter medications, and other changes in medical history.

- Recognize the early warnings of hypoglycemia and hyperglycemia and know how to treat them.

- Control the diabetes and blood sugar level through diet, exercise, medications, and glucose monitoring. This may reduce the long-term, life-threatening complications of diabetes.

- Prevent and treat the complications of diabetes through regular dental care, eye examinations, blood pressure checks, blood tests for cholesterol, lipids, and kidney readings, and self-examination, particularly of feet, for nerve involvement or delayed healing.

- Seek immediate medical attention for any complications.

- Practice a healthy lifestyle, including healthy diet, daily exercise, no tobacco products, avoid alcohol, and attain ideal weight. Offer assistance for smoking cessation, discussed on page 513.

- Review practice of meticulous oral hygiene to prevent dental disease and help control blood sugar levels.

- Reduce stress.

FACTORS TO TEACH PATIENTS NOT DIAGNOSED WITH DIABETES

- Seek regular medical examinations and screening for diabetes.

- Recognize the early warning signs of diabetes and seek medical consult.

- Practice a healthy lifestyle, including healthy diet, daily exercise, no tobacco products, avoid alcohol, and maintain ideal weight. Offer assistance for smoking cessation, discussed on page 513.

- Review practice of meticulous oral hygiene to prevent dental and periodontal disease.

- Reduce stress.

▪ DIABETES INSIPIDUS

Diabetes insipidus should not be confused with diabetes mellitus. Diabetes insipidus is a rare disease characterized by polyuria and polydipsia. It is induced by an antidiuretic hormone defect.

REFERENCES

1. **American Diabetes Association:** Diagnosis and Classification of Diabetes Mellitus, *Diabetes Care,* Supplement 1, January, 2004.
2. **American Diabetes Association:** Screening for Type 2 Diabetes, *Diabetes Care, 27,* S11, Supplement 1, January, 2004.
3. **American Diabetes Association, Diabetes Control and Complications Trial Research Group:** The Effect of Intensive Treatment of Diabetes on the Development and Progression of Long-term Complications of Insulin-Dependent Diabetes Mellitus, *N. Engl. J. Med., 329,* 977, September 30, 1993.
4. **American Diabetes Association, Diabetes Control and Complications Trial Research Group:** Hypoglycemia in the Diabetes Control and Complications Trial, *Diabetes, 46,* 271, February, 1997.
5. **American Diabetes Association:** Implications of the United Kingdom Prospective Diabetes Study, *Diabetes Care, 26,* S28, Supplement 1, January, 2003.
6. **American Diabetes Association:** Nutrition Principles and Recommendations in Diabetes, *Diabetes Care, 27,* S36, Supplement 1, January, 2004.
7. **American Academy of Periodontology, Committee on Research, Science and Therapy:** Position Paper: Diabetes and Periodontal Diseases, *J. Periodontol, 71,* 664, April, 2001.
8. **American Academy of Periodontology, Committee on Research, Science and Therapy:** Periodontal Disease as a Potential Risk Factor for Systemic Diseases, *J. Periodontol., 69,* 841, July, 1998.
9. **Grossi,** S.G., Skrepcinski, F.B., DeCaro, T., Robertson, D.C., Ho, A.W., Dunford, R.G., and Genco, R.J.: Treatment of Periodontal Disease in Diabetics Reduces Glycated Hemoglobin, *J. Periodontol., 68,* 713, August, 1997.

SUGGESTED READINGS

Diabetes Information

American Diabetes Association: Standards of Medical Care in Diabetes Mellitus, *Diabetes Care, 27,* S15, Supplement 1, January, 2004.

Boyle, J.P., Honeycutt, A.A., Venkat Narayan, K.M., Hoerger, T.J., Geiss, L.S., Chen, H., and Thompson, T.J.: Projection of Diabetes Burden Through 2050: Impact of Changing Demography and Disease Prevalence in the U.S., *Diabetes Care, 24,* 1936, November, 2001.

Cooper, D.S. and DeAngelis, C.D.: Diabetes, A JAMA Theme Issue, *JAMA, 287,* 1, May 15, 2002.

Knowler, W.C., Barrett-Conner, E., Fowler, S.E., Hamman, R.F., Lachin, J.M., Walker, E.A., and Nathan, D.M.: Reduction in the Incidence of Type 2 Diabetes With Lifestyle Intervention or Metformin, *N. Engl. J. Med., 346,* 393, February 7, 2002.

Mokdad, A.H., Ford, E.S., Bowman, B.A., Dietz, W.H., Vinicor, F., Bales, V.S., and Marks, J.S.: Prevalence of Obesity, Diabetes, and Obesity-Related Health Risk Factors, 2001, *JAMA, 289,* 76, January 1, 2003.

Mokdad, A.H., Ford, E.S., Bowman, B.A., Nelson, D.E., Engelgau, M.M., Vinicor, F., and Marks, J.S.,: Diabetes Trends in the U.S.: 1990-1998, *Diabetes Care, 23,* 1278, September, 2000.

General Dentistry

Farzad, P., Andersson, L., and Nyberg, J.: Dental Implant Treatment in Diabetic Patients, *Implant Dent., 11,* 262, Fall, 2002.

Fouad, A.F. and Burleson, J.: The Effect of Diabetes Mellitus on Endodontic Treatment Outcome: Data From an Electronic Patient Record, *J. Am. Dent. Assoc., 134,* 43, January, 2003.

Friedlander, A.H., Garrett, N.R., and Norman, D.C.: The Prevalence of Calcified Carotid Artery Atheromas on Panoramic Radiographs of Patients With Type 2 Diabetes Mellitus, *J. Am. Dent. Assoc., 133,* 1516, November, 2002.

Gurenlian, J.R.: Diabetes Mellitus: Overview and Guidelines for Providing Oral Health Care, *Contemp. Oral Hyg., 1,* 14, September, 2001.

Keene, J.R., Kaltman, S.I., and Kaplan, H.M.: Treatment of Patients Who Have Type 1 Diabetes Mellitus, Physiological Misconceptions and Infusion Pump Therapy, *J. Am. Dent. Assoc., 133,* 1088, August, 2002.

Lin, B.P.-J., Taylor, G.W., Allen, D.J., and Ship, J.A.: Dental Caries in Older Adults With Diabetes Mellitus, *Spec. Care Dentist., 19,* 8, January/February, 1999.

Lyle, D.M.: Diabetes Mellitus, *RDH, 23,* 54, March, 2003.

Mattson, J.S. and Cerutis, D.R.: Diabetes Mellitus: A Review of the Literature and Dental Implications, *Compend. Contin. Ed. Dent., 22,* 757, September, 2001.

Silverstein, L.H. and Brown, A.D.: Diabetic Dental Patients: Management of Medical Emergencies, *J. Pract. Hyg., 7,* 11, September/October, 1998

Vernillo, A.T.: Diabetes Mellitus: Relevance to Dental Treatment, *Oral Surg. Oral Med. Oral Pathol. Oral Radiol. Endod., 91,* 263, March, 2001.

Periodontal Findings

AAP Committee on Research, Science and Therapy: Position Paper: Diabetes and Periodontal Diseases, *J. Periodontol, 71,* 664, April, 2000.

Löe, H.: Periodontal Disease: The Sixth Complication of Diabetes Mellitus, *Diabetes Care, 16,* 329, Supplement 1, January, 1993.

Lyle, D.M.: Diabetes: A Risk Factor for Periodontal Diseases, *J. Pract. Hyg., 10,* 11, November/December, 2001.

Matthews, D.C.: The Relationship Between Diabetes and Periodontal Disease, *J. Can. Dent. Assoc., 68,* 161, March, 2002.

Newman, M.G., Takei, H.H., and Carranza, F.A.: *Carranza's Clinical Periodontology,* 9th ed. Philadelphia, W.B. Saunders Co., 2002, pp. 533–536.

Pucher, J.J. and Otomo-Corgel, J.: Periodontal Disease and Systemic Health—Diabetes, *CDA Journal, 30,* 312, April, 2002.

Taylor, G.W.: Bidirectional Interrelationships Between Diabetes and Periodontal Diseases: An Epidemiologic Perspective, *Ann. Periodontol, 6,* 99, December, 2001.

Patient Information Handout

ADA Division of Communications: Diabetes and Oral Health, *J. Am. Dent. Assoc., 133,* 1299, September, 2002.

Artificial and Transplanted Pancreas

Bode, B.W., Sabbah, H.T., Gross, T.M., Fredrickson, L.P., and Davidson, P.C.: Diabetes Management in the New Millennium Using Insulin Pump Therapy, *Diabetes Metab. Res. Rev., 18,* S14, Supplement 1, January–February 2002.

Fioretto, P., Steffes, M.W., Sutherland, D.E.R., Goetz, F.C., and Mauer, M.: Reversal of Lesions of Diabetic Nephropathy After Pancreas Transplantation, *N. Engl. J. Med., 339,* 69, July 9, 1998.

Jaremko, J. and Rorstad, O.: Advances Toward the Implantable Artificial Pancreas for Treatment of Diabetes, *Diabetes Care, 21,* 444, March, 1998.

Porte, D., Baker, L., Bollinger, R.R., Genuth, S., Scharp, D.W., and Sutherland, D.E.R.: Pancreas Transplantation for Patients With Diabetes Mellitus (Technical Review), *Diabetes Care, 15,* 1668, November, 1992.

Prokop, A.: Bioartificial Pancreas: Materials, Devices, Function, and Limitations, *Diabetes Technol Ther., 3,* 431, Fall, 2001.

Emergency Care

Cynthia R. Biron, RDH, EMT, MA

It is relatively easy to be skillful in techniques that are repeated frequently. Emergency care is performed only occasionally and, in instances that involve lifesaving measures, may be performed once in many years. To be prepared for that rare moment is difficult, but the public expects an individual trained in a health profession to be able to act in an emergency. Periodic review of procedures is necessary if application is to be effective.

Emergencies may occur within or in the vicinity of a dental office or clinic. Readiness involves having not only knowledge of proper procedures, but equipment kept in a convenient place. A quick, handy reference of emergency measures, which may be in the form of a posted chart with characteristic symptoms and related treatment, is important.

The information included in this chapter is basic and is presented with no attempt to mention all types of emergencies that may arise, particularly those of complex traumatic injuries. The principal objectives are to list the symptoms and management of the more common emergencies that can occur and to provide a list of the equipment that must be readily available. Other up-to-date references should be kept in the dental office, so that all dental personnel can familiarize themselves with such sources of information. Key words and definitions are provided in Box 66-1.

BOX 66-1 KEY WORDS: Emergencies

Angioneurotic edema: sudden and temporary appearance of large areas of painless swelling in the subcutaneous tissue or submucosa; a symptom related to allergy; also called angioedema.

Arrhythmia: variation from normal rhythm, especially the heartbeat.

Basic life support: the phase of emergency cardiac care that supports the ventilation of a victim of respiratory arrest with rescue breathing and supports the ventilation and circulation of a victim of cardiac arrest with cardiopulmonary resuscitation.

Cannula: a tube for insertion into a duct or cavity.

> **Nasal cannula:** a semicircle of plastic tubing with two plastic tips that fit into the patient's nostrils.

Cardiac arrest: sudden and often unexpected stoppage of heart action; circulation ceases and vital organs are deprived of oxygen.

Crepitation: dry crackling sound, such as that produced by the grating of the ends of a fractured bone.

Cricothyrotomy: incision through the skin and the cricothyroid membrane to secure a patent airway for emergency relief of upper airway obstruction.

Defibrillation: termination of atrial or ventricular fibrillation, usually accomplished by electric shock.

Defibrillator: an apparatus used to produce defibrillation by application of brief electric shock to the heart directly or through electrodes placed on the chest wall.

Dyspnea: labored or difficult breathing; indication of inadequate ventilation or of insufficient oxygen in the circulating blood.

Fibrillation: involuntary muscular contraction caused by spontaneous activation of single muscle cells or fibers.

> **Ventricular fibrillation:** a cardiac arrhythmia marked by fibrillary contractions of the ventricular muscle caused by rapid repetitive excitation of myocardial fibers without coordinated ventricular contraction; a frequent cause of cardiac arrest.

Hypoxemia: deficient oxygenation of the blood; insufficient oxygenation of the blood eventually leads to **hypoxia,** which is diminished oxygen to body tissues.

Kussmaul breathing: loud, slow, labored breathing common to patients in diabetic coma.

Parenteral: not through the alimentary canal; administered by subcutaneous, intramuscular, or intravenous injection.

Rescue breathing: a rescuer delivers a volume of 800 to 1200 mL with each ventilation; the exhaled air contains 16% to 17% oxygen, sufficient for the needs of the victim.

Syncope: temporary loss of consciousness caused by a sudden fall in blood pressure resulting in generalized cerebral ischemia; can have serious consequences, particularly in patients with a cardiovascular disease; commonly referred to as **fainting.**

Trendelenburg's position: the patient is supine with the heart higher than the head on a surface inclined downward about 45°.

Urticaria: vascular reaction of the skin with transient appearance of slightly elevated patches (wheals) that are redder or paler than the surrounding skin; may be accompanied by severe itching; also called hives.

▪ PREVENTION OF EMERGENCIES

I. ATTENTION TO PREVENTION

The best way to prevent an emergency is to employ proper patient assessment techniques, including
   A. Thorough medical history questionnaires.
   B. Documentation of vital signs.
   C. Documentation of findings on Medical Alert Tags.
Wrist or ankle bracelet or necklace that provides information on patient's medical condition. Available from Medic Alert Foundation International, Turlock, CA 95380.
   D. Completion of a physical assessment of the patient.
      Begins with the first interaction with a patient
      1. If by telephone: voice, communication style, attitude.
      2. Visual: gait, physical appearance.
      3. Handwriting on medical history indicates steadiness, ability to communicate, and education.
      4. Extraoral and intraoral examinations.

Having gathered the information from the patient assessment, proper risk management and stress reduction protocols can be incorporated into the patient care plan. Prior to each appointment, the record must be reviewed and updated so that preparatory steps can be taken. Box 66-2 suggests a basic five-point plan for emergency prevention.

Prevention of emergencies requires preparedness, alertness, and anticipation. Some of the procedures that contribute to meeting the requirements are described here.

II. FACTORS CONTRIBUTING TO EMERGENCIES

   A. Increased number of older patients in society with natural teeth and dental diseases that require invasive procedures.
   B. Older patients and many other patients are taking medications that interact adversely with drugs used in dentistry.
   C. More complex dental procedures require longer appointments.
   D. Increased use of drugs in dentistry.
      1. Anesthesia: local, general, conscious sedation.
      2. Tranquilizers.
      3. Pain medications (CNS depressants).
      4. Antibiotics.

BOX 66-2 Five-Point Plan to Prevent Emergencies

1. Use careful, routine patient assessment procedures.

2. Document and update accurate, comprehensive patient records.

3. Implement stress reduction protocols.

4. Recognize early signs of emergency distress.

5. Organize team management plan for emergency preparedness.

▪ PATIENT ASSESSMENT

I. ASSESSMENT FOR ROUTINE TREATMENT

A. First Contact

1. Start with the first interaction with the patient.
2. Note abnormalities of patient's voice on the telephone during appointment scheduling.
3. Assess overall appearance and gait when patient enters the dental office or clinic.
4. Document findings in the patient's chart.

B. Parts of the Assessment

1. Physical assessment (signs and symptoms).
2. Comprehensive medical history.
3. Vital signs.
4. Extraoral and intraoral examination.
5. Comprehensive documentation of findings.

C. Emergency Indicators

Changes in a patient's appearance on the day of an appointment may suggest indicators that encourage preparation for emergencies.

II. THE PATIENT'S MEDICAL HISTORY

A. Update and Document Changes

1. Review at each appointment.
2. Discuss changes with dental team members who are providing treatment for the patient.
3. A comprehensive medical history includes all the items listed in Tables 7-1, 7-2, and 7-3.

B. Use of Medical Alert Box

A "Medical Alert Box" at the top of the inside front page of the patient's record folder should include information that may predispose the patient to medical emergencies. *Confidentiality must be maintained.* Significant items include:

1. Physical conditions that may lead to an emergency.
2. Diseases the patient has or previously had.
3. Medical emergencies the patient experienced previously.
4. Medications the patient has taken within the past 2 years.
5. Allergies and adverse drug reactions.
6. Previous adverse reactions to dental treatments.

III. VITAL SIGNS

Vital signs are essential to assess a patient's overall health status and to evaluate the severity of a medical emergency. A well-prepared dental team takes vital signs routinely, not only during the earliest sign of emergency distress.

A. The Eight Vital Signs

Pulse, blood pressure, respirations, temperature, height, weight, age, and the information from the Medical Alert Tag (bracelet, necklace, anklet) provide essential information for patient care.

B. Baseline Vital Signs

The vital signs taken at a routine appointment are considered baseline. The ranges of vital signs are described in Table 8-1.

C. During Emergency

In a medical emergency the vital signs that are taken are compared to the baseline findings.

1. *"Compensating."* In most medical emergencies, patients will experience a "fight or flight" reaction, during which time they are said to be compensating. The vital signs are elevated above the baseline findings.
2. *"Decompensating."* The vital signs have fallen below baseline, and the patient could be going into a state of shock.
3. *Shock.* A state of lack of perfusion (saturation) of oxygenated blood to all cells of the brain and body. When brain cells are deprived of oxygenated blood, they cease to provide respiratory and circulatory function.

IV. EXTRAORAL AND INTRAORAL EXAMINATIONS

Extraoral and intraoral examinations can provide significant findings that are clues to underlying disease processes that predispose a patient to a medical emergency.

Thorough examinations are an integral part of the prevention of medical emergencies.

A. Extraoral

Blood disorders and endocrine disorders may be discovered from extraoral palpation, skin color changes, abnormalities of the eyes, and asymmetry of the face or neck.

B. Intraoral

Oral manifestations and lesions can be indications of many disease states, such as diabetes, anemia, leukemia, lupus, or AIDS.

V. RECOGNITION OF INCREASED RISK FACTORS

The carefully prepared and regularly updated medical and personal history, with adequate follow-up consultation with the patient's physician for integration of dental and medical care, can prevent many emergencies by alerting dental personnel to the individual patient's needs and idiosyncrasies. Special needs may include:

A. Specific physical conditions that may lead to an emergency, for example, genetic predispositions, seizures, diabetes.
B. Diseases for which the patient is (or has been) under the care of a physician and the type of treatment, including medications.
C. Allergies or drug reactions.

VI. COMPREHENSIVE RECORD KEEPING

All details about the patient, the treatments, reactions, healing, and comments by the patient, provide crucial information should a medical emergency or posttreatment complication occur.

A. Document

1. All medical findings and changes.
2. Treatments provided, including types and amounts of local anesthesia, general anesthesia, and nitrous oxide.
3. Regimens of medications prescribed for patients are crucial information should a medical emergency or a posttreatment complication occur.

B. Consults

Document in the patient's record telephone and written responses of consultations with physicians.

C. New Entries

1. *Response to Treatment.* Document a patient's reactions and responses to treatments, whether they are unremarkable or remarkable.
2. *Previous Appointment Review.* Complete a comprehensive review of previous appointment documentation before providing additional treatment at sequential appointments.
3. *Current Information.* Update information about the patient's health status as an integral part of the prevention of medical emergencies.

▪ STRESS MINIMIZATION

Stress and anxiety are the basis for many of the common emergencies that occur in a dental office or clinic. The office atmosphere and the warmth and sincerity of the personnel can help a patient feel accepted and secure. The apprehension and anxiety that can be associated with dental treatment compounds the risk factors for medical emergencies.

I. RECOGNIZE THE PATIENT WITH STRESS PROBLEMS

A. Apprehensive about any dental appointment.
B. Elderly patients are especially prone to medical emergencies, as they may have cardiovascular diseases that have or have not been diagnosed.
C. Essential medications: certain prescriptions must be taken on schedule or the patient is at risk for an emergency.

II. SUGGESTIONS FOR EFFECTIVE COMMUNICATION

Any patient who is apprehensive or medically predisposed to emergencies should be provided with a stress reduction plan. Reduction of stress includes the development of patient rapport through effective communication between the dental team and the patient.

A. Actively Listen to a Patient's Fears

1. Develop rapport so the patient senses that the listener is empathetic and interested in alleviating the apprehension.
2. Communicate with a patient about fear. A discussion can be very beneficial for emergency prevention.

B. Effects of Fear

Patients who try to repress their fears are more likely to hyperventilate or experience syncopal episodes.

III. REDUCTION OF STRESS

A. Appointment Scheduling[1]

1. *New Patient.* Initial appointment for a new patient used for consultation and assessment will build rapport and provide opportunity to evaluate the level of anxiety. Stress reduction can be built into treatment appointments.
2. *Time of Appointment.* Plan in accord with personal health requirements.
3. *Waiting Time Minimized.* First appointment in the morning prevents building of anxiety by waiting all day for the appointment.
4. *Eating Requirements.* Usual mealtime and previous meal checked to prevent hunger anxiety or hypoglycemia.
5. *Length of Appointment.* Limited to the patient's durability.

B. Medication

1. Premedication when indicated and recommended by the physician and dentist.
2. Pain control during treatment.
3. Patient's own prescriptions. Patients who are subject to emergencies are instructed to bring their own prescribed medicines; for example, the patient with asthma or one who is subject to attacks of angina pectoris.

C. Posttreatment Care

1. Postcare instructions for prevention and/or relief of discomfort.
2. Follow-up telephone call for anxious patient. Organization is a key concept in being prepared for an emergency. Group planning and individual acceptance of responsibility can provide the team with efficiency, composure, and freedom from fear at the time of crisis.

▪ EMERGENCY MATERIALS AND PREPARATION

I. COMMUNICATION: TELEPHONE NUMBERS FOR MEDICAL AID

Telephone numbers should be posted near each extension from which outside calls can be made.

A. Rescue squads with paramedics (fire, police, flying squad, or 911 in many cities in the United States).
B. Ambulance service.
C. Nearest hospital emergency department.

D. Poison information center.
E. Physicians
1. Patient's physician should be listed in the permanent record in a standard, convenient place.
2. Physicians available for emergency calls.

II. EQUIPMENT FOR USE IN AN EMERGENCY

Every dental office or clinic should have an emergency kit or cart,[1,2] and everyone in the office must be familiar with its contents. The kit should be in order, its contents replenished, and outdated materials replaced as needed.

The emergency equipment should be portable and kept in a place readily accessible to all treatment rooms. Materials are plainly marked and kept separate from other office supplies. Materials included are selected to accomplish emergency treatment by current methods.

The items included in the kit imply proper training in their use. A team can work out additions to the list in keeping with their training and abilities. See Table 66-1, Emergency Equipment.

III. CARE OF DRUGS

All dental personnel must be familiar with the emergency drugs maintained in the particular office or clinic. Only specially trained, experienced persons should administer injectable medications. If no one on the team has the proper background and experience, the drugs should not be kept in the office with the emergency supplies.[3]

A. Identification

The purpose and method of administration of each drug should be clearly identified with the container. A compartmentalized clear plastic cabinet or box can be particularly useful for this purpose because the labels and instructions can be seen from the outside and efficient selection can be made. The replacement date must appear clearly on each item with a limited shelf life. When narcotics are included in the list of drugs available for emergencies, storage in a less accessible place than an emergency kit and purchase in small amounts are indicated to prevent them from being stolen easily.

B. Record of Drugs

1. Label each with information about shelf life and due date for replacement. Nitroglycerin, for example, must be changed at 6 months.
2. Check weekly to maintain emergency kit in workable order.
3. Dispose of an outdated narcotic drug in the presence of a witness to prevent question that the drug may have been stolen.

4. A complete record of each available drug is kept. Recorded are the:
a Name of drug.
b. Dosage.
c. Date purchased.
d. Address of source if different from the usual local pharmacy.
e. Each itemized record is signed by the staff member responsible.
f. As each drug is used, a specific entry is made.
g. Expiration dates can be checked at routine intervals.

IV. RECORD OF EMERGENCY

Figure 66-1 shows an example of a form that can be used to record the essential information during an emergency. Such a form can be printed into pads for the convenience of having a carbon copy to place in the patient's permanent record when the original accompanies the patient to a hospital or other medical facility.

A. Purposes

1. Organize data collected during the emergency.
2. Serve as a time reference during the monitoring of vital signs.
3. Prepare a record from which the medical personnel can interpret the patient's condition at the time of transfer from the dental facility.

B. Uses

1. Evaluation for planning dental and dental hygiene appointments so that future emergencies for the patient can be avoided.
2. Provide a reference in the event legal questions arise. A well-kept record can be vital, and each emergency, however insignificant the incident may seem, should be recorded.[4]

V. PRACTICE AND DRILL

A. Staff Instruction

Each member of the clinic or office staff must be thoroughly familiar with the location, purpose, effect, and application of each item of equipment and its source.

B. Assignments

Specific responsibilities must be assigned to each staff member to prevent confusion. Each must know the order of procedures in all types of emergencies, however, and be able to assume any role when needed. Moments count, and there is no time for fumbling or discussion.

▪ TABLE 66-1 EMERGENCY EQUIPMENT

EQUIPMENT	INJECTABLE DRUGS	NONINJECTABLE ITEMS	SUPPLEMENTARY EQUIPMENT
Pocket masks for each clinician	Epinephrine	Oxygen	Pen flashlight
Series E portable oxygen tank	Diphenhydramine	Antiplatelet: aspirin	Stopwatch
Low flow oxygen regulator	Cortisone*	Nifedipine*	Scissors
Nasal cannula	Glucagon*	Respiratory stimulant: ammonia vaporoles	Emesis basin
Simple face mask	Midazolam*	Bronchodilator: albuterol inhaler	Blanket
Nonrebreather mask	Atropine*	Antihypoglycemic for conscious patients: frosting, sugar, glucagon paste	Backboard, 12×24", for patients who cannot be moved to floor for CPR
Bag-valve masks Adult and pedo		Sterile irrigating solution for eyes	Quick-activated cold packs
Demand valve resuscitator		Vasodilator: nitroglycerine tablets, nitrolingual spray	Medical emergency report form and pen on clipboard
Oropharyngeal airways 5 sizes: pedo to adult large		Diphenhydramine tablets	Sterile packages of gauze: 2×2, 4×4
Nasopharyngeal airways 5 sizes: pedo to adult large			Adhesive bandages
Water-soluble lubricant for insertion of nasopharyngeal			Rolled bandage: 1" × 5yd, 2" × 5 yd
Suction tips (tonsil suctions)			Adhesive tape
Sphygmomanometer			Inflatable splints
Blood pressure cuffs: child, adult-regular, adult-large			Pillow
Magill forceps			Cotton pliers
Cricothyrotomy equipment*			Thermometer
Syringes: 2–3 mL luer-lock tip 21-gauge needles			Betadine wipes
I.V. equipment*			Glucose monitor
Automatic external defibrillator			

*Treatment methods that should be administered only by those who have had advanced medical training.

C. Flowchart

Figure 66-2 shows an example of possible distribution of duties when three people are available to attend to the patient. Although a chart can be posted for study, the persons concerned must memorize it. In a real emergency, no one would have time to consult a flowchart.

1. *Advantages*
    a. Organization efficiently uses personnel.
    b. Sharing responsibility relieves pressure.
    c. Duties can be carried out quietly, without excess discussion.
    d. Necessary work gets done without duplication and without omissions.
2. *Preparation.* The preparation of a flowchart and the assignment of all duties related to emergencies should be a result of planning by the whole team.

Medical Emergency Report

Patient's Name: _____   Today's Date: _____

Description of Incident: _____

_____

_____

Time of Onset:		Time EMS Summoned:		Time EMS Arrived:	
Stopwatch:	Clock TIme:	Stopwatch:	Clock TIme:	Stopwatch:	Clock TIme:

Time Patient Released:			Patient Released to:
Stopwatch:	Clock TIme:		

	Finding:	Stopwatch Time:	Finding:	Stopwatch Time:	Finding:	Stopwatch Time:
Blood Pressure	/		/		/	
Pulse:						
Respirations:						
Oxygen Delivery Method:						

Cessation of Breathing	Stopwatch:	Cessation of Pulse	Stopwatch:	CPR Initiated	Stopwatch:

Drugs Administered	Route	Dosage	Stopwatch Time:

▪ **FIGURE 66-1 Medical Emergency Report.** The form is prepared in duplicate. One copy accompanies the patient to the emergency clinic, and the second copy is retained in the patient's dental record file.

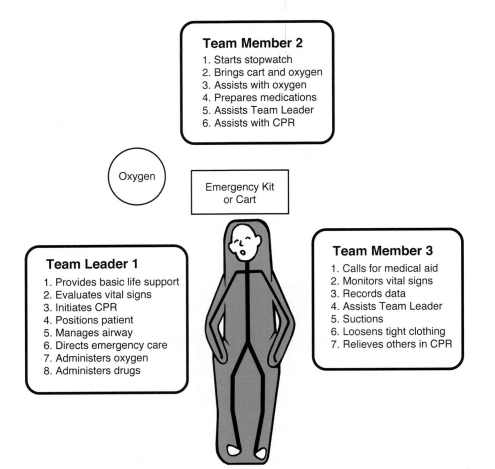

Team Member 2
1. Starts stopwatch
2. Brings cart and oxygen
3. Assists with oxygen
4. Prepares medications
5. Assists Team Leader
6. Assists with CPR

Oxygen

Emergency Kit or Cart

Team Leader 1
1. Provides basic life support
2. Evaluates vital signs
3. Initiates CPR
4. Positions patient
5. Manages airway
6. Directs emergency care
7. Administers oxygen
8. Administers drugs

Team Member 3
1. Calls for medical aid
2. Monitors vital signs
3. Records data
4. Assists Team Leader
5. Suctions
6. Loosens tight clothing
7. Relieves others in CPR

▪ **FIGURE 66-2 Emergency Team Flowchart: Three People.** Suggested distribution of responsibilities to be memorized and practiced by the dental personnel who form the emergency team.

3. *Substitutions.* Because a staff member may be absent from the scene at the time of an emergency, each person should know the duties for all positions so that substitutions can be made and duties doubled with a minimum of discussion and no confusion.

D. Drills

1. Regular reviews and rehearsals for each type of emergency should be conducted, preferably on a "surprise" basis, at least once a month. A specific code call can be used when an intercom or other message system is available.

2. Practice in the use of all procedures, including oxygen administration, resuscitation, and airway maneuvers, as well as of specific positioning of a patient for all emergencies, is indicated.

3. Equipment and materials can be checked at the time of the drill to ensure their availability and that each is in working order. Outdated supplies can be replaced. One staff member should be in charge of the emergency supplies.

4. Keep a record of drills by making a diary of dates and names of those present.

E. New Staff Member

1. Assignment of duties and practice for the new member should be a part of the first working day's orientation.

2. New members must be expected to renew CPR certificates by taking necessary refresher courses within a specified time. Such a procedure is not necessary in a state where a renewal certificate is required for annual licensure.

F. Procedures Manual

A loose-leaf manual, reviewed and updated three or four times each year, can provide a valuable study and work reference. It is particularly useful during the orientation of a new member. The notebook can contain work assignments and checklists for equipment and resources. Direct reference information concerning specific emergencies with their symptoms and initial treatment may be placed in alphabetic order in a specially color-coded section. Members of the team can keep the manual current by bringing references and notes from readings and courses.

■ BASIC LIFE SUPPORT

Sudden cessation of effective respiration and circulation must be treated immediately. Without breathing and heart action, oxygen cannot be carried to the cells and a deficiency occurs quickly. The flowchart in Figure 66-3

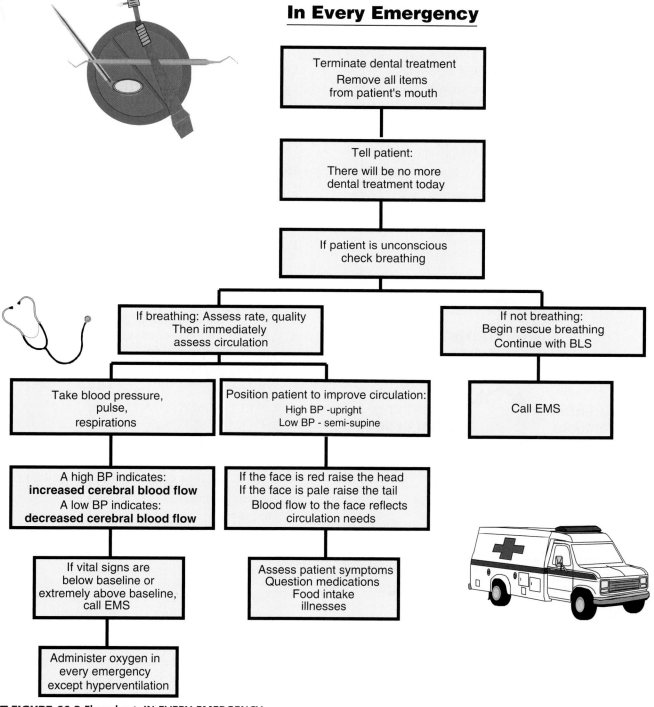

In Every Emergency

Terminate dental treatment
Remove all items
from patient's mouth

Tell patient:
There will be no more
dental treatment today

If patient is unconscious
check breathing

If breathing: Assess rate, quality
Then immediately
assess circulation

If not breathing:
Begin rescue breathing
Continue with BLS

Take blood pressure,
pulse,
respirations

Position patient to improve circulation:
High BP -upright
Low BP - semi-supine

Call EMS

A high BP indicates:
increased cerebral blood flow
A low BP indicates:
decreased cerebral blood flow

If the face is red raise the head
If the face is pale raise the tail
Blood flow to the face reflects
circulation needs

If vital signs are
below baseline or
extremely above baseline,
call EMS

Assess patient symptoms
Question medications
Food intake
illnesses

Administer oxygen in
every emergency
except hyperventilation

■ **FIGURE 66-3 Flowchart: IN EVERY EMERGENCY.**

shows the steps to take in every emergency. *Irreversible brain tissue damage may occur within 4 to 6 minutes in the absence of oxygenated blood. After 6 minutes, brain damage nearly always occurs.*

The cause of collapse, respiratory arrest, or cardiac arrest cannot always be determined at the outset. Survival rates depend on prompt entry into emergency medical service (EMS) for state-of-the-art medical attention. Preliminary assessment of the state of consciousness (response, breathing, and pulse rate) must be made quickly, and the EMS activated promptly. Basic patient care in an emergency is defined by the letters A-B-C-D (Figure 66-4).

It is necessary to keep calm and act promptly, but not hastily. The incorrect procedure may be more harmful than none at all. Each member of the dental team should have participated in courses in emergency procedures and resuscitation techniques while in school and periodically since graduation for refresher, renewal, and updating.

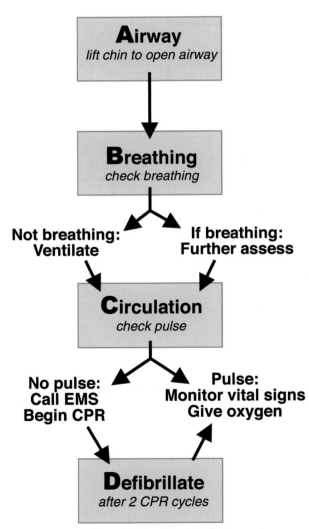

■ **FIGURE 66-4** The A-B-C-D of Basic Life Support.

BOX 66-3 Emergency Care Abbreviations	
ACLS	Advanced Cardiac Life Support
AED	Automated External Defibrillator
AHA	American Heart Association
ALS	Advanced Life Support
BLS	Basic Life Support
BCLS	Basic Cardiac Life Support
CAD	Coronary Artery Disease
CPR	Cardiopulmonary Resuscitation
ECC	Emergency Cardiac Care
ECG	Electrocardiogram
EMD	Emergency Medical Dispatcher
EMS	Emergency Medical Service
EMT	Emergency Medical Technician
EMT-D	Emergency Medical Technician-Defibrillation

This section is intended to provide an outline for reference and review. Abbreviations pertaining to emergency care are listed in Box 66-3. The steps described are carried out in rapid succession.

I. QUICKLY LOWER DENTAL CHAIR (IN DENTAL SETTING)

A. Adjust patient for supine position.
B. Remove a round or wedge-shaped accessory head or shoulder support to permit the head to lie flat and the chin to be raised without resistance.

II. DETERMINE STATE OF CONSCIOUSNESS (FIGURE 66-5)

A. Tap or gently shake the shoulder and shout "Are you OK?" If fractures are suspected, the shake must be light.
B. Unconscious patient does not respond.
C. Call for help. When available, use an alert (buzzer) system of an office or clinic.
D. Start the stopwatch (Figure 66-6).
E. See diagram (Figure 66-4) A-B-C-D of CPR.

Assessment of the Unconscious Patient

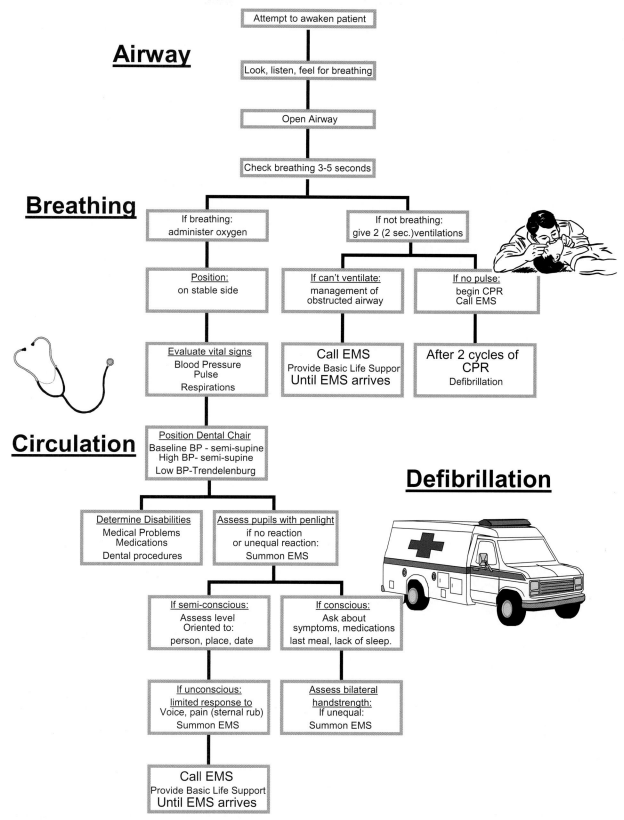

■ **FIGURE 66-5 Assessment of the Unconscious Patient.**

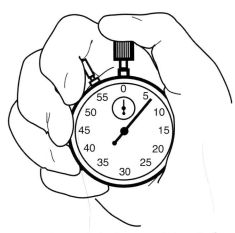

■ **FIGURE 66-6 Stopwatch.** An essential part of every emergency kit. It is turned on at the onset of an emergency and turned off when the EMS takes the patient to the hospital, or when the medical emergency is over. Time is recorded on the *Medical Emergency Report.*

III. OPEN AIRWAY

A. Head Tilt With Chin Lift or Jaw Thrust

1. Place palm of hand on the forehead to apply a backward pressure.
2. Place fingertips (not thumb) of other hand under the chin with light pressure on the mandible to bring the chin up (Figure 66-7).

B. Modified Jaw Thrust

1. Indication. When a neck or spinal injury is suspected, the airway can be opened without extending the neck. DO NOT use head tilt/chin lift maneuver when spinal injury is suspected.
2. Procedure
   a. From over the top of the head, place thumbs on zygomas and grasp angles of the mandible with fingertips.
   b. Lift fingers upward to open airway.
   c. Never tilt the head when spinal injury is suspected.

IV. CHECK BREATHING (3 TO 5 SECONDS)

A. From beside the patient at the shoulder (kneeling if patient is on the floor), place ear over the patient's mouth and nose while looking at the chest.
B. LOOK for chest movement.
C. LISTEN for and FEEL air from the nose and mouth.
   1. If patient is unconscious and breathing, check pulse.
   2. If patient is unconscious with no breathing, say "no breathing" when signaling second rescuer.

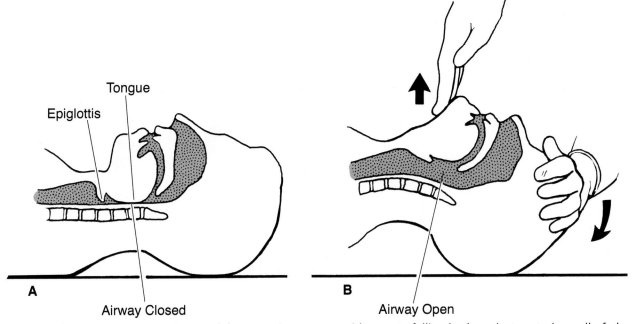

■ **FIGURE 66-7 Chin Lift to Open Airway. (A)** Unconscious person with tongue falling back against posterior wall of pharynx and obstructing the air passage. **(B)** Head is tilted back and chin is lifted by light pressure under the mandible. When neck injury is suspected, a jaw thrust is used. See text for instructions. (After Malamed, S.F.: *Handbook of Medical Emergencies in the Dental Office,* 4th ed. St. Louis, Mosby, 1993, p. 106).

D. When NO breathing:
    1. Place pocket mask or bag mask on patient.
    2. Place thumbs on each side of mask (to obtain seal).
    3. Immediately administer two slow breaths, 2 seconds per breath—chest must rise from ventilation and fall from exhalation between breaths.
    4. **When patient cannot be ventilated,** obstruction is apparent. Proceed to **Airway Obstruction** Management (page 1107).

V. CHECK PULSE

A. Location

1. *Adult.* Carotid pulse in neck (Figure 66-8).
2. *Child* (ages 1 to 8 years). Carotid pulse in neck.
3. *Infant* (younger than 1 year). Brachial pulse of the inner upper arm (Figure 8-4).

B. Determine Need for Cardiopulmonary Resuscitation (CPR)

1. **If pulse present** and patient not breathing, **proceed with rescue breathing.**
2. Give 1 breath every 5 seconds (10–12 breaths per minute).
3. **If NO pulse, proceed with CPR.**

VI. ACTIVATE EMERGENCY MEDICAL SERVICES

Telephone 911 or appropriate number for the given community.

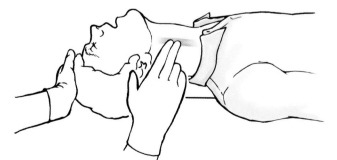

▪ **FIGURE 66-8 Carotid Pulse.** To locate the pulse, two or three fingers are placed on the patient's pharynx. The fingers are then slid down into the groove between the trachea and the neck muscles. With gentle pressure, the pulse can be detected.

▪ RESCUE BREATHING

I. CLEAR THE MOUTH

Turn the patient's head to the side to clear the mouth of mucus, vomitus, and other foreign material. Use suction, gauze, and finger. Dentures should be left in place to provide support unless the dentures are very loose and could cause throat obstruction if displaced.

II. RESCUE BREATHING

A. Place resuscitation mask on patient.
B. Hold with thumbs (on sides of mask) and place fingers on the border of the ramus to obtain a seal.
C. Apply modified jaw thrust to open airway.
D. Deliver two breaths (2 seconds each breath).
E. Rescuer must take in fresh air between each breath, but avoid becoming hyperventilated from taking too many deep breaths.
F. For child or infant, use only enough breath volume for chest to rise and fall.

III. REPEAT THE VENTILATIONS

A. For adult, repeat one ventilation every 5 seconds (12 per minute).
B. For child, repeat one ventilation every 3 seconds (20 per minute).
C. For infant, repeat one ventilation every 3 seconds (20 per minute).
D. Rescue breathing is considered effective when the patient's chest rises with each ventilation.

IV. MAKE A PULSE CHECK EACH MINUTE

A. **If no pulse,** start CPR.
B. **With pulse present,** continue rescue breathing.

▪ EXTERNAL CHEST COMPRESSIONS

There are two mechanisms for blood flow during CPR. One is the principle that rhythmic pressure applied over the lower half of the sternum compresses the heart to produce artificial circulation. The procedure is also called *external cardiac compression.*

The second mechanism involves the intrathoracic pressure, which rises during chest compression. The rise in intrathoracic pressure provides a significant mechanism for movement of blood to the brain. Both cardiac and intrathoracic pressures may be in effect during resuscitation efforts.

Chest compressions are usually accompanied by rescue breathing, but in situations where pocket masks were not available, rescuers have performed chest compressions without mouth to mouth ventilations, and it is believed that the chest compressions alone are better than no CPR at all.[5]

I. POSITION

The patient is in a supine position. When working in a dental chair, lower the chair to its lowest position and support the patient's head as two to three team members drag the patient to the floor by the long axis of the body. The floor provides a solid surface for compression. Most dental chairs bounce during chest compressions, preventing adequate intrathoracic pressure.

II. ADULT OR OLDER CHILD (8 YEARS OR OLDER)

A. Locate Point for Compression

1. Run the middle finger of hand 1 along the lower edge of the rib cage to the notch in the midline.
2. With the middle finger in the notch and the index finger beside it, place the heel of hand 2 next to the index finger on the midline of the sternum.

3. Place the heel of hand 1 on top of hand 2 with the fingers in the same direction. Link and close the fingers.
4. Hold the fingers up so that only the heel of hand 2 is on the sternum (Figure 66-9).

B. Compression

1. Lean forward over the positioned hands, arms straight, until shoulders are directly over the sternum.
2. Use a firm, steady, vertical pressure (not a blow). The sternum moves down 1.5 to 2 inches (Figure 66-9).
3. Release pressure but maintain contact and position of the hands with sternum.
4. Compress at a rate of 100 times per minute.
5. Make the compressions smooth and uninterrupted, with compression and relaxation of equal duration.
6. Use the natural weight of the upper body to prevent pushing from the shoulders or depending on arm strength.
7. As the heart is compressed between the sternum and the spine, blood is forced out of the heart into the circulation.
8. Release of pressure allows blood to flow into the heart.

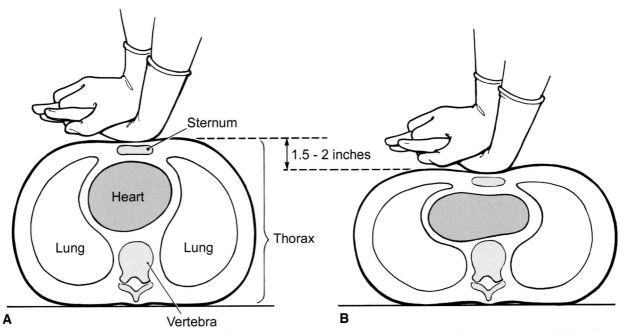

■ FIGURE 66-9 External Chest Compression. (A) Hands in position on the sternum with fingers turned up. **(B)** Application of firm vertical pressure compresses the heart. The sternum should be compressed 1 1/2 to 2 inches and then released. Hands are held in position for the next compression. For an adult, compressions are repeated at a rate of 80 to 100 per minute.

9. Regardless of whether one-man or two-man CPR is being performed, the ratio of chest compressions to ventilations is 15:2. Every four cycles for an unprotected airway (not intubated).

10. When an AED arrives, it is used after two cycles of CPR. See Table 66-2 for a CPR Quick Reference for Healthcare Providers.

III. CHILD (1–8 YEARS OLD)

A. Locate Point for Compression

1. Follow the lower edge of the rib cage to the notch where the sternum and ribs meet.

2. Place the middle finger in the notch with the index finger beside it.

3. Place the heel of the other hand next to the index finger.

B. Compression

1. Use the heel of one hand only; compress to a depth of 1 to 1.5 inches.

2. Release to allow chest to return to normal level.

3. Compress at a rate of 100 per minute, using a smooth, even rhythm.

4. Keep fingers up, off the chest.

▪ TABLE 66-2 CPR QUICK REFERENCE FOR HEALTHCARE PROVIDERS

BREATHING AND COMPRESSIONS	>8-YEAR-OLD CHILD TO ADULT	1- TO 8-YEAR-OLD CHILD	INFANT (<1 YEAR OLD)	NEWBORN
Determine if unconscious				
Open airway	Head tilt-chin lift Jaw thrust if injury	Head tilt-chin lift Jaw thrust if injury	Head tilt-chin lift Jaw thrust if injury	Head tilt-chin lift Jaw thrust if injury
Look, listen, feel for breathing. *If breathing:* recovery position				
If not breathing: immediately give:	Two 2-second breaths	Two 1- to 1.5-second breaths	Two 1- to 1.5-second breaths	Two 1-second breaths
Follow up with:	12 breaths per minute	20 breaths per minute	20 breaths per minute	30–60 breaths per minute
Airway obstruction	Abdominal thrusts	Abdominal thrusts	Back blows or chest thrusts	Back blows or chest thrusts
Circulation	Carotid pulse check	Carotid pulse check	Brachial pulse check	Unbilical pulse check
Compression landmarks	Lower half of sternum	Lower half of sternum	One finger width below mammary line	One finger width below mammary line
Compression technique	Heel of one hand Interlace fingers of other hand and place on top	Heel of just one hand	1 rescuer: 2 fingers 2 rescuers: thumb encircling hands	1 rescuer: 2 fingers 2 rescuers: thumb encircling hands
Compression depth	1 1/2 to 2 inches	1/3 to 1/2 depth of chest	1/3 to 1/2 depth of chest	1/3 depth of chest
Compression rate	100/minute	100/minute	≥100/minute	120/minute 90 compressions: 30 breaths
Compression: ventilation ratio	1 or 2 rescuers: 15:2 if unprotected airway 2 rescuers: 5:1 if patient intubated	1 or 2 rescuers: 5:1	1 or 2 rescuers: 5:1	1 or 2 rescuers: 3:1

IV. INFANT (UP TO 1 YEAR OLD)

A. Locate Point for Compression

1. Place fingers along the sternum, with the index finger just below an imaginary line between the nipples. Lift the index finger. If the fingers are on the xiphoid process, move the fingers closer to the nipples.
2. Use the area under the middle and ring fingers.

B. Compression

1. One rescuer: compress with two fingers
2. Two rescuers: compress with two thumbs and hands encircling body to a depth of one third to one half the depth of the chest; release to allow chest to return to normal after each compression.
3. Compress at a rate of at least 100 per minute, using a smooth rhythm.

V. COORDINATED ACTIVITY FOR CPR

A. Lone Rescuer

1. Provide ventilation and compressions.
2. *Adult Patient*
   a. Use ratio 15 compressions followed by 2 lung inflations.
   b. Compress at the rate of 100 per minute (count "1, 2, 3").
   c. Check carotid pulse after four cycles of compressions and ventilations; continue if no pulse; check pulse regularly.
3. *Child and Infant*
   a. Use a ratio of five compressions with a slight pause for one ventilation.
   b. Compress at the rate of 100 per minute for a child; minimum of 100 for an infant.
   c. Reassess pulse after 10 cycles, and every few minutes.

B. Two Rescuers

1. First person begins airway, breathing, and circulation treatment as has been described.
2. Second person calls for medical assistance and ambulance, then promptly takes over compression.
3. Use coordinated rhythm of one lung inflation after five compressions.
4. The rescuer at the patient's head maintains the open airway, monitors the carotid pulse, and provides rescue breathing.
5. The compressor calls the time for a switch of positions between ventilation and compression.
6. Always finish the cycle with a ventilation and after a pulse check.
7. Start the cycle with a ventilation.

VI. LENGTH OF TREATMENT

A. Signs of recovery: normal skin color returns, patient may gasp or show other sign of breathing, and the body may move or wiggle.
B. Do not stop heart compressions while patient is being transported to the hospital.
C. When circulation and breathing appear to have returned do not leave patient; watch for need to continue resuscitation in case of relapse. Place the patient in the "Recovery Position": Patient is placed on one side with the top leg bent at the hip and knee to form a right angle. The arm closest to the floor is outstretched above the head so that it will stabilize the upper body, while the bent knee stabilizes the lower body.

VII. SEQUELAE

Cardiopulmonary resuscitation must be continued until medical assistance arrives or the patient begins to recover. While the patient is transported to a hospital, resuscitation must continue. For emergencies that do not require hospitalization, the patient can be moved to a couch for rest but must be watched carefully. The cause of the emergency must be determined and additional treatment provided when indicated.

The *Medical Emergency Report* with monitored vital signs should accompany the patient to the medical care facility for reference by the persons assuming responsibility. The carbon copy for the patient's dental files is marked clearly with recommendations for prevention of future emergencies.

VIII. DEFIBRILLATION WITH THE AUTOMATIC EXTERNAL DEFIBRILLATOR (AED)

Patients who are in cardiac arrest have an initial rhythm of ventricular fibrillation (VF), which is an erratic rhythm that is ineffective at producing normal contractile force of the ventricles.

Electrical defibrillation interrupts VF, establishing a normal sinus rhythm. Without defibrillation intervention, VF shifts to asystole (no rhythm) in a matter of minutes. For every minute that defibrillation is delayed, survival from cardiac arrest declines by as much as 10%. Adhesive electrode pads are placed on the patient.

A. AED will advise the rescuer to press the "shock" button to defibrillate the heart, or the AED voice prompt will say, "shock not indicated." (Figure 66-10)

B. The AED analyzes the ECG signals to determine if the patient's heart is in VF, ventricular tachycardia (VT), or pulseless.

C. If the heart has a normal rhythm, the AED will advise the rescuer.

There are many commercial AEDs available for dental offices, physician's offices, airlines, and public health centers. Training on the specific AED purchased is of great importance. Being familiar with the emergency equipment available increases confidence and accuracy in managing any medical emergency. A defibrillator may be used only by dental professionals who are trained in a special program on how to use the defibrillation equipment.

The AED may not be indicated or effective in some situations. Examples are:

1. The patient is less than 8 years old or weighs less than 25 kg.
2. The patient is in or near some type of standing water.
3. The patient has an implanted pacemaker or defibrillator.
4. The patient has a transdermal patch in the place where the electrode pads must be placed.
5. The patient has hair on the area where the electrode pads must be placed and the hair interferes with the adhesion of the pads.
6. The patient is perspiring so much that the skin is too wet for the electrode pads to properly adhere to the skin.

■ AIRWAY OBSTRUCTION

A procedure of subdiaphragmatic abdominal thrusts, the Heimlich maneuver, is recommended for removal of a foreign body obstructing an airway in adults and children.

I. PREVENTION

With thought and planning, care can be exercised to prevent aspiration of objects by a patient during a dental or dental hygiene appointment. A few of the procedures that contribute to safety are as follows:

A. Place the patient in supine position during examination and treatment. The throat is closed (Figure 66-7).

B. Use a rubber dam for all appropriate procedures.

C. Use a length of floss to tie to small objects, such as a rubber dam clamp or a bite block. Floss hangs out from angle of lips.

D. Use low-speed handpiece to prevent splashing or spinning masses of agents into the throat.

E. Have assistant use aspirator for various procedures that involve large pieces of calculus, copious blood clots, excess saliva, excess water for ultrasonic scaling, restorative materials, and other potentially inhalable items.

F. Pay attention to mobile permanent or exfoliating primary teeth that could be inadvertently displaced.

II. RECOGNITION OF AIRWAY OBSTRUCTION

Immediate recognition is essential. Differentiation from other emergencies, such as fainting, heart attack, or stroke, in which a sudden respiratory failure may also occur, may be necessary when no object or material was involved that could have been inhaled.

When no doubt exists that an object has been inhaled, medical aid must be obtained. A radiograph may be needed to confirm the location of a radiopaque object.

A. Signs and Symptoms of Partial Obstruction

1. Air exchange
   a. Poor air exchange with gasping and irregular respirations.
   b. Good air exchange with wheezing and forceful coughing.
2. Patient's face is red or cyanotic.
3. Treat poor air exchange as a complete obstruction.

B. Signs of Complete Obstruction

1. No air exchange with attempts at breathing; no sounds from larynx or pharynx.
2. Patient demonstrates the *universal distress signal* (clutches neck with hand).
3. Cyanosis and unconsciousness follow unless emergency care is provided quickly.

III. OUTLINE OF TREATMENT

An airway must be established within 4 to 6 minutes to prevent possible brain damage from oxygen deficiency. With total obstruction, the patient may become unconscious within a few seconds. Treatment begins with the A-B-C-D of Basic Life Support, unless inhalation of a specific item was observed. When the inspiration is

CPR and AED

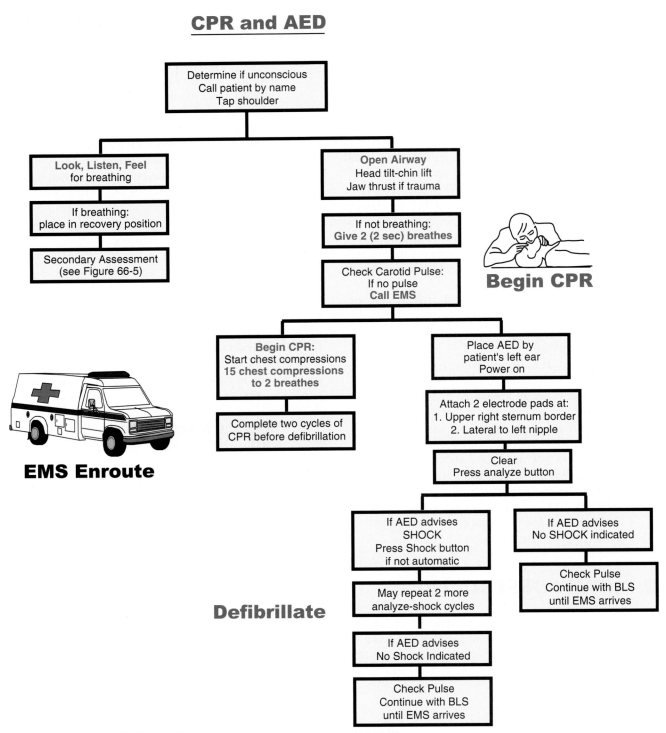

```
                    ┌─────────────────────────┐
                    │  Determine if unconscious│
                    │   Call patient by name   │
                    │      Tap shoulder        │
                    └─────────────────────────┘
```

Look, Listen, Feel
for breathing

If breathing:
place in recovery position

Secondary Assessment
(see Figure 66-5)

Open Airway
Head tilt-chin lift
Jaw thrust if trauma

If not breathing:
Give 2 (2 sec) breathes

Check Carotid Pulse:
If no pulse
Call EMS

Begin CPR

EMS Enroute

Begin CPR:
Start chest compressions
15 chest compressions
to 2 breathes

Complete two cycles of
CPR before defibrillation

Place AED by
patient's left ear
Power on

Attach 2 electrode pads at:
1. Upper right sternum border
2. Lateral to left nipple

Clear
Press analyze button

If AED advises
SHOCK
Press Shock button
if not automatic

If AED advises
No SHOCK indicated

Check Pulse
Continue with BLS
until EMS arrives

May repeat 2 more
analyze-shock cycles

Defibrillate

If AED advises
No Shock Indicated

Check Pulse
Continue with BLS
until EMS arrives

■ **FIGURE 66-10 Defibrillation With the Automatic External Defibrillator.**

known, the rescuer can proceed directly to attempt to dislodge the obstructing object.

A. Conscious Adult Patient

1. With good air exchange, let patient cough.

2. Object may become dislodged; follow up with medical examination.
3. **Foreign Body Airway Obstruction (FBAO)**
4. Patient may become unconscious; proceed for unconscious patient.

B. Unconscious Adult Patient

1. Initiate A-B-C-D of Basic Life Support.
2. When breathing attempt is not successful, readjust airway and attempt again.
3. Activate EMS.
4. Proceed with airway obstruction management.
   a. Foreign body airway obstruction: 5 abdominal thrusts.
   b. Examine mouth for object; apply finger sweep.
   c. Place resuscitation mask; open airway; give two breaths.
   d. Repeat steps a and b until object is expelled.

IV. FOREIGN BODY AIRWAY OBSTRUCTION (FBAO)

Manual thrusts are made to the upper abdomen or, in selected cases, the chest. The abdominal thrust should not be used during pregnancy.

The thrusts are given to provide pressure against the diaphragm that compresses the lungs. In turn, the pressure in the lungs is increased, thereby forcing air through the trachea and perhaps forcing out the obstructing object.

A. Patient Standing or Sitting: Conscious

1. From behind, wrap the arms around the waist of the patient. Make a fist.
2. Hold thumb side of the fist on the patient's upper abdomen above the navel and below the xiphoid. Grab the fist with the other hand.
3. Press the fist into the abdomen with quick upward thrusts until the object is dislodged, or the patient may become unconscious.

B. Patient in Supine Position: Unconscious

1. Open the airway.
2. Stand beside and facing the head of the chair when the patient is in the dental chair. On the floor, a more direct thrust can be applied from astride the patient.
3. Hold the heel of one hand over the upper abdomen, with the other hand on top.
4. Apply 5 quick upward thrusts followed by a finger sweep and several ventilations.
5. If no airway: Repeat abdominal thrusts, finger sweeps, and ventilations.

V. CHEST THRUST

The chest thrust is not used routinely but is recommended only when it is not possible to use the abdominal thrust, such as during pregnancy and for very obese individuals.

A. Patient Standing or Sitting With Clinician Behind

1. From behind, wrap arms around the chest of the patient at level of armpits.
2. Make a fist. Position the thumb side of the fist on the sternum. The thrust definitely should not be made on the ribs or on the xiphoid because fracture is possible.
3. Grasp the fist with the other hand and apply quick backward thrusts.

B. Patient in Supine Position

1. Open the airway.
2. Position hands on the lower sternum in the same position as for external cardiac compression (Figure 66-9).
3. Apply quick downward thrusts.

VI. FINGER SWEEP: UNCONSCIOUS

After each series of 5 abdominal thrusts, an attempt should be made to remove the offending object by examination of the mouth and throat and by using the fingers, gauze, or suction appropriately. Care must be taken not to force the object deeper.

Finger sweeps are not used for children and infants unless the object is visible.

A. Open the Mouth

Lift the tongue and mandible with the thumb and index finger of nondominant hand.

B. Index Finger Sweep

1. Slide the index finger of other hand along the buccal mucosa and deep into the throat to the base of the tongue.
2. Anticipate contact with an object, move slowly, with care not to push the object farther into the throat.
3. Hook the end of the finger under and around to remove the object.

C. Repeat

1. Repeat abdominal thrusts, mouth examination, and finger sweep until object is expelled.
2. Place resuscitation mask, open airway, give two ventilations.

VII. INFANT

A. Conscious

1. If good air exchange, encourage coughing.
2. If poor air exchange or complete obstruction, proceed with airway obstruction management.
3. Hold the infant face down over the forearm, with the head supported in the hand. Head is lower than the body.
4. Apply up to five back blows with the heel of the hand, between the infant's shoulder blades.
5. Turn the infant over by placing the free arm over the back and supporting the infant's head with the hand. Place the infant across the thigh with the infant's head lower than its body.
6. Apply five chest thrusts. The point of pressure is the same as for external cardiac compression in the infant.
7. Repeat back blows and chest thrusts until object is dislodged or infant becomes unconscious.

B. Unconscious

1. Initiate A-B-C-D of Basic Life Support.
2. When breathing attempt is not successful, reposition airway and attempt again.
3. **Activate EMS.**
4. Proceed with airway obstruction management as for conscious infant, with five back blows and five chest thrusts.

5. Examine mouth for object; if visible, use a finger sweep to remove it.
6. Give several ventilations.
7. Repeat steps 3 to 5 until object is expelled.
8. Check airway, breathing, and pulse.

■ OXYGEN ADMINISTRATION

Oxygen is an important agent, useful in most emergencies. High concentration of oxygen is contraindicated for chronic obstructive lung diseases, especially emphysema. Oxygen is also not indicated in the presence of hyperventilation because the patient is receiving increased amounts of oxygen in air inhaled and is in need of carbon dioxide.

The use of oxygen is beneficial in all other emergencies. When the patient is not breathing, *positive pressure oxygen* (also known as demand valve resuscitator) delivery is needed.

I. EQUIPMENT

Oxygen delivery systems with indications, flow rate, and percent oxygen delivered are shown in Table 66-3.

A. Parts

Oxygen resuscitation equipment consists of an oxygen tank, a reducing valve, a flow meter, tubing, mask, and a positive pressure bag. The *E* cylinder, which can provide oxygen for 30 minutes, is the minimum size recommended. Smaller tanks provide

■ TABLE 66-3 OXYGEN DELIVERY SYSTEMS

DEVICE	INDICATIONS	FLOW RATE	OXYGEN DELIVERY
Cannula	For patient who is breathing and needs low levels of oxygen.	2–6 liters per minute	25–40%
Face mask	For patient who is breathing and needs moderate levels of oxygen: • When cannula is not tolerated • When more oxygen is desired • Patient is in shock	8–12 liters per minute	60%
Nonrebreather mask	For patient who is breathing and needs high level of oxygen: • Patient is in shock • When more oxygen is desired	10–15 liters per minute	60–90%
Bag mask	When patient has stopped breathing; bag mask is used instead of mouth-to-mouth resuscitation	10–15 liters per minute	90–100%
Demand valve resuscitation	Positive pressure delivery of oxygen on demand	Used by EMTs or others professionally trained	100%

LAMINATE AND AFFIX TO THE OXYGEN TANK.

too little oxygen for a real emergency, and larger tanks are less portable.

B. Directions

Box 66-4 outlines the steps for operation of an oxygen tank. Clear, readable directions should be permanently attached to the tank. Practice is a definite part of team drills.

II. PATIENT BREATHING: USE SUPPLEMENTAL OXYGEN

A. Apply a full-face clear mask or a nasal cannula.
B. Supplemental oxygen is started at 4 to 6 L per minute.
C. Monitor breathing; if breathing stops, proceed with positive pressure oxygen.

III. PATIENT NOT BREATHING: USE POSITIVE PRESSURE

For persons not trained in the use of the bag-valve-mask or positive pressure delivery, a mouth-to-mask procedure should be used.

A. Apply full-face clear mask; must fit with a tight seal. One dental team member may need to apply pressure to the facemask to maintain a complete seal.
B. Adjust oxygen flow so that the positive pressure bag remains filled.
C. Compress the bag manually at 5-second intervals to provide 12 respirations per minute for an adult. For a child, use 3-second intervals.
D. Watch chest rise and fall. When the chest does not rise and fall, recheck airway for obstruction. Proceed with airway obstruction management.
E. Obtain medical assistance.

▪ SPECIFIC EMERGENCIES

Certain systemic disease conditions and physical injuries require specific treatment during an emergency CPR. In Tables 66-4 and 66-5, the *Emergency Reference Charts*, several conditions are listed with their symptoms and treatment procedures. Some of the same conditions have been described in detail in Section VII of this book.

BOX 66-4 Operation of Oxygen Tank

TO TURN ON:
1. Attach oxygen delivery system to tank.

2. Turn **key** on top of tank in *counter-clockwise direction* to open flow of oxygen.

3. Read **Low Flow Regulator Knob:**
   To increase O$_2$ flow: turn the knob in the direction the arrow indicates. (Many regulators are the opposite of sink faucets and open clockwise instead of counter-clockwise.)

4. Attach oxygen delivery system from patient.

TO TURN OFF:
1. Remove oxygen delivery system from patient.

2. Turn **key** on top of tank in *clockwise direction* to shut off flow of oxygen.

3. Turn the **Low Flow Regulator Knob** to open position to bleed oxygen from the system.

4. After bleeding, gently close the **Low Flow Regulator Knob.**

LAMINATE AND AFFIX TO OXYGEN TANK

■ TABLE 66-4 EMERGENCY REFERENCE CHART: MEDICAL EMERGENCIES

EMERGENCY	SIGNS/SYMPTOMS	PROCEDURE

All Cases		I. Determine consciousness (shake and shout): yell for help
		If patient is unconscious:
		II. Conduct Primary Assessment:
		   A. Airway: open with head tilt-chin lift
		   B. Breathing: (look, listen, feel) if none: **Give 2 breaths**
		   C. Circulation: Check for pulse, if none: Start CPR
		   D. Defibrillate: after 2 cycles of CPR
		If patient is breathing and conscious:
		III. Conduct Secondary Assessment
		   E. Evaluate level of consciousness
		     1. Does patient know own name, location, date
		     2. Use penlight to see if pupils react equally to light
		     3. If conscious: check patient for equal hand strength
		     4. Position according to signs/symptoms
		       If face is red, raise the head
		       If face is pale, raise the tale
		     5. Evaluate heart rate, blood pressure, respirations
		   F. Findings in patient record or medical alert bracelet
		     1. Disabilities, diseases, drugs, baseline vital signs: activate EMS

Respiratory Failure	Labored or weak respirations or cessation of breathing
	Cyanosis or ashen-white with blood loss
	Pupils dilated
	Loss of consciousness
		Position: semi-supine if not breathing; upright if breathing
		Check for and remove foreign material from mouth
		Establish airway
		Rescue breathing:
		  Adult 1 breath every 5 seconds
		  Child (1–8 yrs) 1 breath every 3 seconds
		  Infant (<1 yr) 1 breath every 3 seconds
		Monitor vital signs: blood pressure, pulse, respirations
		Administer oxygen by nonrebreather mask if patient is already breathing

Airway Obstruction	Good air exchange, coughing, wheezing (patient can speak)	Sit patient up Loosen tight collar, belt No treatment; let patient cough
Partial Obstruction	Poor air exchange; noisy breathing; weak, ineffective cough; difficult respirations; gasping (usually patient cannot talk, but makes crowing sounds on taking in air); patient is panicky	Reassure patient Treat for complete obstruction

Complete Obstruction	Gasping with great effort; no noises
	Patient clutches throat
	Unable to speak, breathe, cough
	Cyanosis
	Dilated pupils
		Conscious patient
		  Perform Heimlich maneuver
		  Patient becomes unconscious: proceed for unconsciousness
		Unconscious patient
		  Initiate A-B-C-D of Basic Life Support
		  Unsuccessful breathing attempts: proceed with airway obstruction management
		  Perform Heimlich maneuver: 6–10 thrusts
		  Examine mouth: apply finger sweep
		  Open airway: give 2 ventilations
		  Repeat manual thrusts and finger sweep until object is expelled
		  Try rescue breathing again
		Obtain medical assistance

(continued)

■ TABLE 66-4 EMERGENCY REFERENCE CHART: MEDICAL EMERGENCIES (Continued)

EMERGENCY	SIGNS/SYMPTOMS	PROCEDURE
Hyperventilation Syndrome	Light-headedness, giddiness Anxiety, confusion Dizziness Overbreathing (25–30 respirations per minute) Feelings of suffocation Deep respirations Palpitations (heart pounds) Tingling or numbness in the extremities	Terminate oral procedure Remove rubber dam and objects from mouth Position upright Immediately tell patient: "There will be no more dental treatment today" Loosen tight collar Reassure patient Explain overbreathing; request that each breath be held to a count of 10. Ask patient to breath deeply (7–10 per minute) into a paper bag adapted closely over nose and mouth. Never use a bag for a patient with diabetes or patients exhibiting signs of diabetic coma, e.g., fruity breath odor, Kussmaul breathing, lethargy, dry skin. **Carbon dioxide is indicated, NOT oxygen**
Heart Failure	Difficult or labored breathing Pulmonary congestion with cough and difficulty breathing May cough up pink sputum Rapid, weak pulse Dilated pupils May have chest pain	Place patient in upright position Urgent medical assistance needed Make patient comfortable: cover with blanket Administer oxygen by nonrebreather mask Reassure patient
Cardiac Arrest	Skin: ashen gray, cold, clammy No pulse No heart sounds No respirations Eyes fixed, with dilated pupils; no constriction with light Unconscious	Position: supine Basic life support Check oral cavity for debris or vomitus; leave dentures in place for a seal **Begin cardiopulmonary resuscitation: minutes count**
Asthma Attack	Difficulty breathing, wheezing, (extreme cases—silence, indicating little to no air exchange) Cyanosis Dilated pupils Confusion due to lack of oxygen Chest pressure Sweating	Position patient upright with arms up and supported forward Assist with patient's own bronchodilator Administer supplemental oxygen by nasal cannula Epinephrine if patient decompensates Supplemental cortisone to patients who are or have been on corticosteroid therapy Basic life support—may need demand valve resuscitator if patient experiences respiratory depression **Activate EMS**
Syncope (Fainting)	Pale gray face, anxiety Dilated pupils Weakness, giddiness, dizziness, faintness, nausea Profuse cold perspiration Rapid pulse at first, followed by slow pulse Shallow breathing Drop in blood pressure Loss of consciousness	Position: Trendelenburg Loosen tight collar, belt Place cold, damp towel on forehead Crush ammonia vaporole under patient's nose Keep warm (blanket) Monitor vital signs: blood pressure, pulse, respirations Keep airway open Administer oxygen by nasal cannula Keep in supine position 10 minutes after recovery to prevent nausea and dizziness Reassure patient, especially during recovery

(continued)

■ TABLE 66-4 EMERGENCY REFERENCE CHART: MEDICAL EMERGENCIES (Continued)

EMERGENCY	SIGNS/SYMPTOMS	PROCEDURE
Shock	Skin: pale, moist, clammy Rapid, shallow breathing Low blood pressure Weakness and/or restless- ness Nausea, vomiting Thirst, if shock is from bleeding Eventual unconsciousness if untreated	Position: Trendelenburg Keep quiet and warm Monitor vital signs: blood pressure, respirations, pulse Keep airway open Administer oxygen by nonrebreather bag **Summon medical assistance**
Stroke (Cerebrovascular Accident)	*Premonitory* Dizziness, vertigo Transient paresthesia or weakness Transient speech defects *Serious* Headache (with cerebral hemorrhage) Breathing labored, deep, slow Chills Paralysis one side of body Nausea, vomiting Convulsions Loss of consciousness (slow or sudden onset)	**Conscious patient** Turn patient on paralyzed side; semi-upright Loosen clothing about the throat Reassure patient; keep calm, quiet Monitor vital signs: blood pressure, pulse, respirations Administer oxygen by nasal cannula Clear airway; suction vomitus because the throat muscles may be paralyzed **Seek medical assistance promptly** **Unconscious patient** Position: supine Basic life support Cardiopulmonary resuscitation if indicated
Cardiovascular Diseases	Symptoms vary depending on cause	**For all patients** Be calm and reassure patient Keep patient warm and quiet; restrict effort Always administer oxygen when there is chest pain Call for medical assistance
Angina Pectoris	Sudden crushing, paroxys- mal pain in substernal area Pain may radiate to shoul- der, neck, arms Pallor, faintness Shallow breathing Anxiety, fear	Position: upright, as patient requests, for comfortable breathing Place nitroglycerin sublingually only when the blood pressure is at or above baseline Administer oxygen by nasal cannula Reassure patient Without prompt relief after a second nitroglycerin, treat as a myocardial infarction
Myocardial Infarction (Heart Attack)	Sudden pain similar to angina pectoris, which may radiate, but of longer duration Pallor; cold, clammy skin Cyanosis Nausea Breathing difficulty Marked weakness Anxiety, fear Possible loss of consciousness	Position: with head up for comfortable breathing Symptoms are not relieved with nitroglycerin Monitor vital signs: blood pressure, pulse, respirations Administer oxygen by nonrebreather bag Alleviate anxiety; reassure **Call for medical assistance for transfer to hospital**

(continued)

■ TABLE 66-4 EMERGENCY REFERENCE CHART: MEDICAL EMERGENCIES (Continued)

EMERGENCY	SIGNS/SYMPTOMS	PROCEDURE
Adrenal Crisis (Cortisol Mental Deficiency)	Anxious, stressed Confusion Pain in abdomen, back, legs Muscle weakness Extreme fatigue Nausea, vomiting Lowered blood pressure Elevated pulse Loss of consciousness Coma	**Conscious patient** Terminate oral procedure Call for help and emergency kit Place patient in supine position with legs slightly raised Request telephone call for medical assistance Administer oxygen by nonrebreather mask Monitor blood pressure and pulse Place patient on stable side with legs slightly raised **Unconscious patient** Basic life support Try ammonia vaporole when cause is undecided Administer oxygen **Summon medical assistance** **Transport to hospital**
Insulin Reaction (Hyperinsulinism, hypoglycemia)	Sudden onset Skin: moist, cold, pale Confused, nervous, anxious Bounding pulse Salivation Normal to shallow respirations Convulsions (late)	**Conscious patient** Administer oral sugar (cubes, apple juice, candy, or frosting) Observe patient for 1 hour before dismissal Determine time since previous meal, and arrange next appointment following food intake **Unconscious patient** Basic life support Position: supine Maintain airway Administer oxygen by nonrebreather bag Monitor vital signs **Summon medical assistance** Administer intramuscular glucagon or intravenous glucose
Diabetic Coma (Ketoacidosis) (Hyperglycemia)	Slow onset Skin: flushed and dry Breath: fruity odor Dry mouth, thirst Low blood pressure Weak, rapid pulse Exaggerated respirations (Kussmaul breathing) Coma	**Conscious patient** Terminate oral procedure Obtain medical care; hospitalization indicated Keep patient warm Administer oxygen by nasal cannula **Unconscious patient** Basic life support Position: supine **Urgent medical assistance needed**
Epileptic Seizure 1. Generalized tonic-clonic	Anxiety or depression Pale, may become cyanotic Muscular contractions Loss of consciousness	Position supine: Do not attempt to move from dental chair Make safe by placing movable equipment out of reach Do not force anything between the teeth; a soft towel or large sponges may be placed while mouth is open Open airway; monitor vital signs Administer oxygen by nasal cannula Allow patient to sleep during postconvulsive stage Do not dismiss the patient if unaccompanied
2. Generalized absence	Brief loss of consciousness Fixed posture Rhythmic twitching of eyelids, eyebrows, or head May be pale	Take objects from patient's hands to prevent their being dropped

(continued)

■ TABLE 66-4 EMERGENCY REFERENCE CHART: MEDICAL EMERGENCIES (Continued)

EMERGENCY	SIGNS/SYMPTOMS	PROCEDURE

Allergic Reaction
1. Delayed
	Skin
	  Erythema (rash)
	  Urticaria (wheals, itching)
	  Angioedema (localized
	    swelling of mucous
	    membranes, lips, larynx,
	    pharynx)
	Respiration
	  Distress, dyspnea
	  Wheezing
	  Extension of angioedema
	    to larynx: may have
	    obstruction from swelling
	    of vocal apparatus
		Skin
		  Administer antihistamine
		Respiration
		  Position: upright
		  Administer oxygen by nasal cannula
		  Epinephrine
		Airway obstruction
		Position: supine
		Airway maintenance
		Epinephrine
		Summon medical assistance

2. Immediate
   Anaphylaxis
   (Anaphylactic
   shock)
	Skin
	Urticaria (wheals, itching)
	Flushing
	Nausea, abdominal cramps,
	  vomiting, diarrhea
	Angioedema
	  Swelling of lips,
	    membranes, eyelids
	  Laryngeal edema with
	    difficult swallowing
	Respiration distress
	  Cough, wheezing
	  Dyspnea
	  Airway obstruction
	  Cyanosis
	Cardiovascular collapse
	  Profound drop in blood
	    pressure
	  Rapid, weak pulse
	  Palpitations
	  Dilation of pupils
	  Loss of consciousness
	    (sudden)
	  Cardiac arrest
		Rapid treatment needed (epinephrine)
		Position: supine (except when dyspnea predominates)
		Administer oxygen by nonrebreather mask
		Basic life support
		Monitor vital signs
		Cardiopulmonary resuscitation
		Summon medical assistance; transfer to hospital

Local Anesthesia **Reactions** 1. Psychogenic	Reaction to injection, not the anesthetic Syncope Hyperventilation syndrome	Page 1113 (syncope) Page 1113 (hyperventilation)

2. Allergic
   (very rare)
	Anaphylactic shock
	Allergic skin and mucous
	  membrane reactions
	Allergic bronchial asthma
	  attack
		See earlier in this table

(continued)

■ TABLE 66-4 EMERGENCY REFERENCE CHART: MEDICAL EMERGENCIES (Continued)

EMERGENCY	SIGNS/SYMPTOMS	PROCEDURE

3. Toxic Overdose	Effects of intravascular injection rather than increased quantity of drug are more common
	Stimulation phase
	  Anxious, restless, apprehensive, confused
	  Rapid pulse and respirations
	  Elevated blood pressure
	  Tremors
	  Convulsions
	Depressive phase
	  Follows stimulation phase
	  Drowsiness, lethargy
	  Shock-like symptoms: pallor, sweating
	  Rapid, weak pulse and respirations
	  Drop in blood pressure
	  Respiratory depression or respiratory arrest
	Unconsciousness
		Mild reaction
		  Stop injection
		  Position: supine
		  Loosen tight clothing
		  Reassure patient
		  Monitor blood pressure, heart rate, respirations
		  Administer oxygen by nasal cannula
		Summon medical assistance
		
		Severe reaction
		  Basic life support: maintain airway
		  Administer oxygen by nonrebreather mask
		  Continue to monitor vital signs
		  Cardiopulmonary resuscitation
		  Administration of anticonvulsant

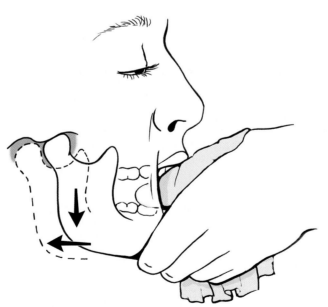

■ **FIGURE 66-11 Treatment for a Dislocated Mandible.** With thumbs wrapped in toweling and placed on the buccal cusps of the mandibular teeth, the fingers are curved under the body of the mandible. The jaw is pressed down and back with the thumbs while pulling up and forward with the fingers to permit the condyle to pass over the articular eminence into its normal position in the glenoid fossa. As the jaw slips into place, the thumbs must be moved quickly aside.

■ TABLE 66-5 EMERGENCY REFERENCE CHART: TRAUMATIC INJURIES

EMERGENCY	SIGNS/SYMPTOMS	PROCEDURE
Hemorrhage	Prolonged bleeding Spurting blood: artery Oozing blood: vein	Compression over bleeding area a. Apply gauze pack with direct pressure b. Bandage pack into place firmly where possible c. Elevate injury above the heart if possible Severe bleeding: digital pressure on pressure point of supplying vessel Watch for shock symptoms
	Bleeding from tooth socket	Pack with folded gauze; do not dab Have patient bite down firmly If bleeding does not stop, instruct patient to gently bite down on a damp tea bag and hold in place for 10 minutes Do not rinse
	Bleeding of an extremity	Elevate the part: support with pillows or substitute Apply tourniquet only when limb is amputated, mangled, or crushed
	Nosebleed	Tell patient to breathe through mouth Apply cold application to nose Press nostril on bleeding side for a few minutes Advise patient not to blow the nose for an hour or more If bleeding does not stop, wet cotton rolls with water and lubricate with water-soluble lubricant Pack nostril Instruct patient to breathe through the mouth Leave packing in place until medical assistance is available to the patient
Burns 1. First-degree	Skin reddened Swelling Pain	*First- and Second-Degree Burns* Do not give food or liquids; anticipate nausea Be alert for signs of shock
2. Second-degree (partial thickness)	Skin reddened, blisters Swelling Wet surface Pain (more than third degree) Heightened sensitivity to touch	Do not apply ointment, grease, or bicarbonate of soda Immerse in cool water to relieve pain; do not apply ice Gently clean with a mild antiseptic Dress lightly with a dry sterile bandage Elevate burned part **Obtain medical assistance**
3. Third-degree (full thickness)	Leathery look Insensitive to touch	Request medical assistance and transport system Treat for shock Basic life support: maintain airway Check for other injuries Wrap in clean sheet; transport
4. Chemical burn	Reddened, discolored	Immediate, copious irrigation with water for 1/2 hour Check directions on container from which the chemical came for antidote or other advice Burn caused by an acid may be rinsed with bicarbonate of soda, burn caused by alkali may be rinsed in weak acid such as acetic (vinegar) **Medical assistance needed**

(continued)

■ TABLE 66-5 EMERGENCY REFERENCE CHART: TRAUMATIC INJURIES (Continued)

EMERGENCY	SIGNS/SYMPTOMS	PROCEDURE
Internal Poisoning	Signs of corrosive burn around or in oral cavity Evidence of empty container or information from patient Nausea, vomiting, cramps	Be calm and supportive Basic life support: airway maintenance Artificial ventilation (inhaled poison) Record vital signs **Call Poison Control Center**
		Conscious patient Dilute poison in the stomach with 1 or 2 glasses of water or milk Induce vomiting by giving 1 tablespoon of syrup of Ipecac followed by 1 to 2 glasses of water Do not induce vomiting if caustic, corrosive, or petroleum products have been ingested Avoid nonspecific and questionably effective antidotes, stimulants, sedatives, or other agents, which may do more harm **Obtain medical assistance**
Foreign Body in Eye	Tears Blinking	Wash hands Ask patient to look down Bring upper lid down over lower lid for a moment; move it upward Turn down lower lid and examine: if particle is visible, remove with moistened cotton applicator Use eye cup: wash out eye with plain water When unsuccessful, seek medical attention: prevent patient from rubbing eye by placing gauze pack over eye and stabilizing with adhesive tape
Chemical Solution in Eye	Tears Stinging	Irrigate promptly with copious amounts of water Turn head so water flows away from inner aspect of the eye; continue for 15–20 minutes
Dislocated Jaw	Mouth is open: patient is unable to close	Stand in front of seated patient Wrap thumbs in towels and place on occlusal surfaces of mandibular posterior teeth Curve fingers and place under body of the mandible Press down and back with thumbs, and at same time pull up and forward with fingers (Figure 66-11) As joint slips into place, quickly move thumbs outward Place bandage around head to support jaw
Facial Fracture	Pain, swelling Ecchymoses Deformity, limitation of movement Crepitation on manipulation Zygoma fracture: depression of cheek Mandibular fracture: abnormal occlusion	Place patient on side Basic life support Support with bandage around face, under chin, and tied on the top of the head (Barton) **Seek prompt transport to emergency care facility**
Tooth Forcibly Displaced (avulsed tooth)	Swelling, bruises, or other signs of trauma depending on the type of accident	Instruct patient or parent to hold the tooth by the crown, and avoid touching the root(s) If the tooth is dirty, rinse it gently in cool water, but do not scrub it or remove tissue fragments from its root surface Keep the tooth moist by placing it in water or a wet cloth Bring the tooth and the patient to dental office or clinic *immediately* The longer the time lapse between avulsion and replantation, the poorer the prognosis

Everyday Ethics

A 12-year-old male patient has just received local anesthesia in the dentist's operatory. Suddenly the boy begins to have a generalized seizure. You assist with the team dental office protocol for medical emergencies, and within 1 minute the seizure is over and the patient is conscious with no other effects or symptoms. The dentist continues treatment as if nothing happened. There is no documentation in the patient's record of the seizure episode, and nothing is said to the boy's parents.

Questions for Consideration

1. What should you say to the dentist?

2. Would you ask him if you could add the documentation to the patient record?

3. Should you get the chart and add the documentation without his consent, as you assisted in the management of the medical emergency?

4. Would you tell the dentist that you are not comfortable with his unethical behavior in this situation?

Factors To Teach The Patient

Stress Minimization to Prevent Emergencies

- Take medication prescribed by dentist at times indicated on the prescription.

- Schedule appointments when there is no waiting, first appointment of the morning or afternoon.

- Eat breakfast before morning appointment, or lunch before afternoon appointment.

- If patient has prescription medications for emergency episodes, bring those medications to the dental office on the day of appointment. Examples: nitroglycerine tablets for angina, asthma inhaler, glucagon for hypoglycemia.

REFERENCES

1. **Meiller.** T.F., Wynn, R.L., McMullin, A.M., Biron, C., and Crossley, H.L.: *Dental Office Medical Emergencies,* 2nd ed. Hudson, Ohio, Lexi-Comp, 2000, pp. 6-9.
2. **Hass**, D.A.: Overview of Emergency Drugs, *Dent. Clin. North Am.,* 46, 815, October, 2002.
3. **Malamed**, S.F.: *Handbook of Medical Emergencies in the Dental Office,* 5th ed. St. St. Louis, Mosby, 2000, pp. 93-103.
4. **Stapleton**, E.R.: *BLS for Healthcare Providers.* Dallas, American Heart Association, 2001.
5. **Hallstrom**, A., Cobb, L., Johnson, E., and Copass, M.: Cardiopulmonary Resuscitation By Chest Compression Alone or With Mouth-to-mouth Ventilation, *N. Engl. J. Med.,* 342, 1546, May 25, 2000.

SUGGESTED READINGS

Preparation

ADA Council on Scientific Affairs: Office emergencies and emergency kits, *J. Am. Dent. Assoc., 133,* 364, March, 2002.

Garfunkel, A., Galili, D., Findler, M., Zusman, S.P., Malamed, S.F., Elad, S., Kaufman, E.: Chest pains in the dental environment. *Refuat Hapeh Vehashinayim., 19,* 51, January, 2002.

Levin, J.: The use of automatic defibrillators in the dental office, *Va Dent. J., 76,* 38, October–December, 1999.

Malamed, S.F.: Medical emergencies in dentistry. *Refuat Hapeh Vehashinayim., 19,* 6, January, 2002.

Miller, C.H.: Creating the position of office safety, *Dent. Assist., 71,* 10, March–April, 2002.

Nunn, P.: Medical emergencies in the oral health care setting, *J. Dent. Hyg., 74,* 136; quiz 152, Spring, 2000.

Children

Agostini, F.G., Flaitz, C.M., Hicks, M.J.: Dental emergencies in a university-based pediatric dentistry postgraduate outpatient clinic: a retrospective study. *ASDC J. Dent. Child., 68,* 316, 2001.

Al-Jundi, S.H.: Dental emergencies presenting to a dental teaching hospital due to complications from traumatic dental injuries. *Dent Traumatol., 18,* 181, 2002.

McTigue, D.J.: Diagnosis and management of dental injuries in children, *Pediatr. Clin. North Am., 47,* 1067, 2000.

Milzman, D.P., Milzman, B.I.: Focused care of pediatric patients in the dental office, *Dent. Clin. North Am., 43,* 527, July, 1999.

Rosenberg, M.B. and Phero J.C.: Resuscitation of the pediatric patient, *Dent. Clin. North Am., 39,* 663, July, 1995.

Shusterman, S.: Emergency management of oral trauma in children, *Curr. Opin. Pediatr., 9,* 242, June, 1997.

Sullivan, D.D.: Brushing up on dental emergencies: initial care for fractures, luxations, and avulsions, *JAAPA, 15,* 48, 2002.

Villasenor, A.: Aspiration of gauze pressure-pack following a dental extraction: a case report, *Pediatr. Dent., 21,* 135, March–April, 1999.

Wilson, S., Farrell, K., Griffen, A., Coury, D.: Conscious sedation experiences in graduate pediatric dentistry programs, *Pediatr. Dent., 23,* 307, 2001.

Wilson, S., Smith, G.A., Preisch, J., Casamassimo, P.S.: Epidemiology of dental trauma treated in an urban pediatric emergency department, *Pediatr. Emerg. Care., 13,* 12, February, 1997.

Prefixes, Suffixes, and Combining Forms

A

a-, an- absence, lack, without, e.g. *a*morphous
ab- from, away, e.g. *ab*normal
ad- (change d to c, f, g, p, s, or t before words beginning with those consonants) to, toward, e.g. *ad*hesion, *ac*cretion
adeno- gland, e.g. *adeno*fibroma
-algia pain, e.g. neur*algia*
ambi- all (both) sides, round, e.g. *ambi*dexterity
amelo- enamel, e.g. *amelo*genesis
amphi-, ampho- on both sides, double, e.g. *ampho*diplopia
ana- up, excessive, again, e.g. *ana*bolism
andro- masculine, male, e.g. *andro*gen
angio- vessel, e.g. *angio*ma
ante- before, e.g. *ante*febrile
anti- against, e.g. *anti*dote
aqu-, aqua- water, e.g. *aqu*eous
arthro-, arth- joints, e.g. *arth*ritis
-ase denotes an enzyme, e.g. dextrin*ase*
-asthenia weakness, e.g. my*asthenia* gravis
auto-, aut- self, e.g. *auto*transplant

B

bi- two, twice, double, e.g. *bi*furcation
bio-, bi- life, living, e.g. *bio*psy
-blast formative cell, e.g. osteo*blast*
-brachy- short, e.g. *brachy*dactylic
brady- slow, e.g. *brady*cardia
bucc- cheek, e.g. *bucc*inator

C

calc- stone, calcium, lime, e.g. *calc*ification
cardio-, cardi- heart, e.g. *cardio*vascular
cata- down, against, e.g. *cata*bolism
-cele swelling, protrusion, hernia, e.g. meningo*cele*
cephalo-, cephal- head, e.g. *cephal*ometry
cerebro-, cerebr- brain, e.g. *cerebr*al palsy
cheilo-, cheil- lip, e.g. *cheil*itis
chloro-, chlor- pale green, e.g. *chloro*phyll
chromo-, chromat- color, pigmentation, e.g. *chromo*genic
-cidal killing, e.g. bacteri*cidal*
-clast break up, divide into parts, e.g. osteo*clast*
-clus- shut, e.g. oc*clus*ion

co-, com-, con-, cor- with, together, e.g. *co*ngenital
coll- glue, e.g. *coll*oid
contra- opposite, e.g. *contra*lateral
cryo, cry- cold, freezing, e.g. *cryo*therapy
cuti- skin, e.g. *cuti*cle
cyan- blue, e.g. *cyan*otic
-cyto-, -cyt- cell, e.g., leuko*cyte*

D

-dactyl, dactylo- fingers, e.g. *dactyl*edema
de- down, away from, separation, e.g. *de*calcification
denti-, dent- tooth, e.g. *dent*ition
-derm-, derma- skin, e.g. hypo*derm*ic
dextr-, dextro- right, toward right, e.g. *dextro*cardia
di- twice, two, e.g. *di*plopia
dia- (drop *a* before words beginning with a vowel) through, apart, e.g. *dia*phragm
dis- separation, opposite, taking apart, e.g. *dis*infect
disto-, dist- posterior, distant from center, e.g. *disto*buccal
-drome course, e.g. syn*drome*
dur- hard, e.g. in*dur*ation
dys- bad, ill, difficult, e.g. *dys*trophy

E

ecto-, ect- without, outer side, e.g. *ecto*derm
-ectomy surgical removal, e.g. gingiv*ectomy*
-emia (-aemia) blood condition, e.g. bacter*emia*
en- in, on, into, e.g. *en*demic
encephal-, encephalo- brain, e.g. *encephalo*meningitis
endo- inside, e.g. *endo*dontics
entero-, enter- intestine, e.g. *entero*toxin
epi- upon, after, in addition, e.g. *epi*dermis
erythro-, eryth- red, e.g. *eryth*ema
esthesio-, esthesia (-aesthesia) sensation, perception, e.g. an*esthesia*
ex- beyond, from, out of, e.g. *ex*udate
extra- outside of, beyond the scope of, e.g. *extra*cellular

F

faci- face, e.g. *faci*al
-facient causes or brings about, e.g. rube*facient*
-ferent carry, bear, e.g. af*ferent*
fibro-, fibr- fibers, fibrous tissue, e.g. *fibro*blast
fract- break, e.g. *fract*ional

G

galacto-, galact- milk, e.g. *galact*ose
gastro-, gastr- stomach, e.g. *gastr*itis
-gen- produced, e.g. glyco*gen*
genio- chin, lower jaw, e.g. *genio*plasty
germ- bud, early growth, e.g. *germ*inal
gero- old age, e.g. *gero*dontics
glosso-, gloss- tongue, e.g. *gloss*itis
gluco-, gluc- glucose e.g. *gluc*oneogenesis
glyco-, glyc- sweet, e.g. *glyc*erin
gnatho-, gnath- jaw, e.g. *gnath*odynamometer
-gnosis knowledge, e.g. pro*gnosis*
-gram, -graph write, draw, e.g. radio*graph*ic
gran- grain, particle, e.g. *gran*uloma
gyn-, gyne-, gynec- woman, e.g. *gynec*ology

H

hemi- half, e.g. *hemi*section
hemo- (haemo-) blood, e.g. *hemo*rrhage
hepato-, hepat- liver, e.g. *hepat*itis
hetero-, heter- other, different, e.g. *hetero*geneous
histo-, hist- tissue, e.g. *hist*ology
homo-, homeo- like, similar, e.g. *homeo*stasis
hydro-, hydr- water, e.g. *hydro*cephalic
hygro-, hygr- moisture, e.g. *hygro*phobia
hyper- abnormal, excessive, e.g. *hyper*trophy
hypno-, hypn- sleep, e.g. *hypn*otic
hypo-, hyp- deficiency, lack, below, e.g. *hypo*tonic
hystero-, hyster- uterus or hysteria, e.g. *hyster*ectomy

I

-ia state or condition, e.g. glycosur*ia*
iatro- relation to medicine, a physician, dentist, or other health professional, e.g. *iatro*genic
-ic of, pertaining to, e.g. gastr*ic*
idio- one's own, separate, distinct, e.g. *idio*pathic
in- not, without, e.g. *in*activate
infra- beneath, below, e.g. *infra*orbital
inter- between, among, e.g. *inter*cellular
intra- within, into, e.g. *intra*oral
ischo-, isch- suppression, stoppage, e.g. *isch*emia
iso- equality, similarity, e.g. *iso*tonic
-ist one who practices, holds certain principles, e.g. hygien*ist*
-itis inflammation, e.g. dermat*itis*

J

-ject- throw, e.g. in*ject*ion
juxta- next to, near, e.g. *juxta*position

K

karyo-, kary- nucleus of a cell, e.g. *karyo*lysis
kerato-, kerat- horny, keratinized tissue, e.g. *kerat*inization
kin- move, e.g. *kin*etic

L

labio- lip, e.g. *labio*version
lacto-, lact- milk, e.g. *lact*ation
laryngo-, laryn- larynx, e.g. *laryn*gitis
later- side, e.g. *later*oversion
leuko-, leuk- white, e.g. *leuk*oplakia
linguo, lingu- tongue, e.g. *lingu*al
lipo-, lip- fat, fatty, e.g. *lip*oma
-logy doctrine, science, e.g. periodont*ology*
lympho-, lymph- lymph, e.g. *lymph*angioma
-lysin, -lysis, -lytic dissolving, destructive, e.g. hemo*lysis*

M

macro-, macr- enlargement, elongated part, e.g. *macr*odontia
mal- bad, ill, e.g. *mal*nutrition
mast-, mastro- breast, e.g. *mast*ectomy
-megalo-, -megal- large, great, e.g. *megalo*blast
melano- dark-colored, relating to melanin, e.g. *melano*genesis
meningo-, mening- meninges, e.g. *mening*itis
meno- month, e.g. *meno*pause
mes-, medi, mesio- middle, intermediate, e.g. *meso*derm
meta-, met- over, beyond, transformation, e.g. *meta*bolism
metro-, metra- uterus, e.g. *metro*fibroma
-metry measure, e.g. cephalo*metry*
micro-, micr- small, e.g. *micro*organism
mono- one, single, e.g. *mono*saccharide
morpho-, morph- form, shape, e.g. *morph*ology
muco-, muc- relating to mucous membrane, e.g. *muco*gingival
myel-, myelo- bone marrow, spinal cord, e.g. *myelo*blast
mylo- molar teeth or posterior portion of mandible, e.g. *mylo*hyoid
myo-, my- muscle, e.g. *myo*cardium

N

naso- nose, e.g. *naso*palatine
necr- death, e.g. *necr*otic
neo-, ne- new, recent, e.g. *neo*plasm
nephro-, nephr- kidneys, e.g. *nephr*itis
neuro-, neuri-, neur- pertaining to nerves, e.g. *neur*asthenia
nucleo-, nucle- pertaining to nucleus, e.g. *nucleo*protein

O

ob- (change b to c before words beginning with c) against, toward, e.g. *oc*clusion
odonto-, odont- tooth, e.g. *odont*algia
-oid like, resembling, e.g. ameb*oid*
-olig-, oligo- a few, a little, e.g. *oligo*dontia
-oma swelling, tumor, e.g. lip*oma*
-opia, -opy sight, eye defect, e.g. my*opia*
oro- mouth, oral, e.g. *oro*nasal
ortho-, orth- straight, normal, e.g. *ortho*dontics
-osis condition, state, e.g. cyan*osis*
osteo-, oste- bone, e.g. *osteo*porosis
oto-, ot- ear, e.g. *oto*plasty
-ous full of, having, e.g. aque*ous*
ovi-, ovo-, ovu- egg, e.g. *ovu*lation

P

pan- all, every, general, e.g. *pan*acea
para- beyond, beside, near, e.g. *para*site
patho-, path- disease, e.g. *patho*gnomonic
pedia-, pedo- (paedo-) child, e.g. *pedo*dontics
-penia deficiency, e.g. leuko*penia*
per- throughout, completely, e.g. *per*cussion
peri- around, near, e.g. *peri*apical
phago- to eat, e.g. *phago*cytic
-phile, -phil- loving, e.g. hemo*phil*ia
phlebo-, phleb- vein, e.g. *phleb*itis
-phobe, -phobia fear, dread, e.g. photo*phobia*
pilo- hair, e.g. *pilo*erection
-plas- mold, shape, e.g. gingivo*plas*ty
plasmo-, plasm- form, e.g. cyto*plasm*
-plegia, -plexy paralysis, stroke, e.g. hemi*plegia*
pleo- more, e.g. *pleo*morphism
-pnea (-pnoea) breathing, e.g. dys*pnea*
pneumo- air, lung, e.g. *pneumo*thorax
-poiesis, -poietic production, e.g. erythro*poietic*
poly- many, much, e.g. *poly*saccharide
pont- bridge, e.g. *pont*ic
poro-, -por- opening, pore, duct, e.g. *por*ous
post- behind, after, e.g. *post*natal
pre- before, in front of, e.g. *pre*maxilla
pro- before, in front of, e.g. *pro*gnathic
proprio- one's own, e.g. *proprio*ceptive
proto- first, e.g. *proto*plasm
pseudo- false, deceptive, e.g. *pseudo*membrane
psycho-, psych- mind, mental processes, e.g. *psycho*somatic
pulmo- lung, e.g. *pulmo*nary
pur- pus, e.g. *pur*ulent
pyo- pus, e.g. *pyo*rrhea
pyro- fever, heat, e.g. *pyro*genic

R

re- back, again, e.g. *re*gurgitate
-renal kidney, e.g. ad*renal*
retro- back, backward, behind, e.g. *retro*molar
-rhage breaking, bursting forth, profuse flow, e.g. hemor*rhage*
-rhea (-rhoea) flow, discharge, e.g. pyor*rhea*
rhino-, rhin- nose, e.g. *rhin*itis
rube- red, e.g. *rube*facient

S

sarco- flesh, muscle, e.g. *sarco*ma
sclero- hard, e.g. *sclero*derma
-scopy examination, inspection, e.g. micro*scopy*
semi- half, partly, e.g. *semi*permeable
sero- serum, serous, e.g. *sero*purulent
sial-, sialo- saliva, e.g. *sialo*graphy
somat-, somato-, -some body, e.g. chromo*some*
-squam- scale, e.g. des*quam*ative
stomat- mouth, e.g. *stomat*itis
sub- beneath, under, deficient, e.g. *sub*acute
super- above, upon, excessive, e.g. *super*numerary tooth
syn- with, together, e.g. *syn*drome

T

tachy- swift, e.g. *tachy*cardia
tact- touch, e.g. *tact*ile
tera-, terato- monster, malformed fetus, e.g. *terato*genic
thermo- heat, e.g. *thermo*phile
thrombo-, thromb- clot, coagulation, e.g. *thromb*in
-thym-, thymo- mind, soul, emotions, e.g. dys*thym*ia
trans- beyond, through, across, e.g. *trans*plantation
tropho-, trophic nutrition, nourishment, e.g., hyper*trophic*
-tropic turning toward, changing, e.g. hydro*tropic*

U

-ule diminutive, small, e.g. tub*ule*
-uria urine, e.g. glucos*uria*

V

vaso- blood vessels, e.g. *vaso*dilation
vita- life, e.g. *vita*min

X

xero- dry, e.g. *xero*stomia

American Dental Hygienists' Association Code of Ethics for Dental Hygienists

1. PREAMBLE

As dental hygienists, we are a community of professionals devoted to the prevention of disease and the promotion and improvement of the public's health. We are preventive oral health professionals who provide educational, clinical, and therapeutic services to the public. We strive to live meaningful, productive, satisfying lives that simultaneously serve us, our profession, our society, and the world. Our actions, behaviors, and attitudes are consistent with our commitment to public service. We endorse and incorporate the Code into our daily lives.

2. PURPOSE

The purpose of a professional code of ethics is to achieve high levels of ethical consciousness, decision making, and practice by the members of the profession. Specific objectives of the Dental Hygiene Code of Ethics are:

- To increase our professional and ethical consciousness and sense of ethical responsibility.
- To lead us to recognize ethical issues and choices and to guide us in making more informed ethical decisions.
- To establish a standard for professional judgment and conduct.
- To provide a statement of the ethical behavior the public can expect from us.

The Dental Hygiene Code of Ethics is meant to influence us throughout our careers. It stimulates our continuing study of ethical issues and challenges us to explore our ethical responsibilities. The Code establishes concise standards of behavior to guide the public's expectations of our profession and supports existing dental hygiene practice, laws, and regulations. By holding ourselves accountable to meeting the standards stated in the Code, we enhance the public's trust on which our professional privilege and status are founded.

3. KEY CONCEPTS

Our beliefs, principles, values, and ethics are concepts reflected in the Code. They are the essential elements of our comprehensive and definitive code of ethics and are interrelated and mutually dependent.

4. BASIC BELIEFS

We recognize the importance of the following beliefs that guide our practice and provide context for our ethics:
- The services we provide contribute to the health and well-being of society.
- Our education and licensure qualify us to serve the public by preventing and treating oral disease and helping individuals achieve and maintain optimal health.
- Individuals have intrinsic worth, are responsible for their own health, and are entitled to make choices regarding their health.
- Dental hygiene care is an essential component of overall healthcare, and we function interdependently with other healthcare providers.
- All people should have access to healthcare, including oral healthcare.
- We are individually responsible for our actions and the quality of care we provide.

5. FUNDAMENTAL PRINCIPLES

These fundamental principles, universal concepts, and general laws of conduct provide the foundation for our ethics.

Universality

The principle of universality assumes that if one individual judges an action to be right or wrong in a given situation, other people considering the same action in the same situation would make the same judgment.

Complementarity

The principle of complementarity assumes the existence of an obligation to justice and basic human rights. It requires us to act toward others in the same way they would act toward us if roles were reversed. In all relationships, it means considering the values and perspectives of others before making decisions or taking actions affecting them.

Ethics

Ethics are the general standards of right and wrong that guide behavior within society. As generally accepted actions, they can be judged by determining the extent to which they promote good and minimize harm. Ethics compel us to engage in health promotion/disease prevention activities.

Community

This principle expresses our concern for the bond between individuals, the community, and society in general. It leads us to preserve natural resources and inspires us to show concern for the global environment.

Responsibility

Responsibility is central to our ethics. We recognize that there are guidelines for making ethical choices and accept responsibility for knowing and applying them. We accept the consequences of our actions or the failure to act and are willing to make ethical choices and publicly affirm them.

6. CORE VALUES

We acknowledge these values as general for our choices and actions.

Individual Autonomy and Respect for Human Beings

People have the right to be treated with respect. They have the right to informed consent prior to treatment, and they have the right to full disclosure of all relevant information so that they can make informed choices about their care.

Confidentiality

We respect the confidentiality of client information and relationships as a demonstration of the value we place on individual autonomy. We acknowledge our obligation to justify any violation of a confidence.

Societal Trust

We value client trust and understand that public trust in our profession is based on our actions and behavior.

Nonmaleficence

We accept our fundamental obligation to provide services in a manner that protects all clients and minimizes harm to them and others involved in their treatment.

Beneficence

We have a primary role in promoting the well-being of individuals and the public by engaging in health promotion/disease prevention activities.

Justice and Fairness

We value justice and support the fair and equitable distribution of healthcare resources. We believe all people should have access to high-quality, affordable oral healthcare.

Veracity

We accept the obligation to tell the truth and assume that others will do the same. We value self-knowledge and seek truth and honesty in all relationships.

7. STANDARDS OF PROFESSIONAL RESPONSIBILITY

We are obligated to practice our profession in a manner that supports our purpose, beliefs, and values in accordance with the fundamental principles that support our ethics. We acknowledge the following responsibilities:

To Ourselves as Individuals . . .

- Avoid self-deception, and continually strive for knowledge and personal growth.
- Establish and maintain a lifestyle that supports optimal health.
- Create a safe work environment.
- Assert our own interests in ways that are fair and equitable.
- Seek the advice and counsel of others when challenged with ethical dilemmas.
- Have realistic expectations of ourselves and recognize our limitations.

To Ourselves as Professionals . . .

- Enhance professional competencies through continuous learning in order to practice according to high standards of care.

Canadian Dental Hygienists' Association Code of Ethics

PREAMBLE

Dental hygienists believe that oral health is an integral part of a person's overall health, well-being, and quality of life. The profession of dental hygiene is devoted to promoting optimal oral health for all. Dental hygiene has an identified body of knowledge and a distinctive expertise which dental hygienists use to serve the needs of their clients and promote the public good.

The Code of Ethics sets down the ethical principles and ethical practice standards of the dental hygiene profession. The **principles** express the broad ideals to which dental hygienists aspire and which guide them in their practice. The **standards** provide more specific direction for conduct. They are more precise and prescriptive as to what a given principle requires under particular circumstances. Clients, colleagues, and the public in general can reasonably expect dental hygienists to be guided by, and to be accountable under, the principles and standards articulated in this Code.

The purpose of the Code of Ethics is to
- Elaborate the ethical principles and standards by which dental hygienists are guided and under which they are accountable.
- Serve as a resource for education, reflection, self-evaluation, and peer review.
- Educate the public about the ethical principles and standards of the profession.
- Promote accountability.

The Code of Ethics is a public document that augments and complements the relevant laws and regulations under which dental hygienists practise. By elaborating on the profession's ethical principles and standards, the Code promotes accountability and worthiness of the public's trust.

The Code of Ethics applies to dental hygienists and dental hygiene students in all practice settings, including, but not limited to, private practice, institutions, research, education, administration, community health, and industry.

Interpretation and application of the Code in specific circumstances requires individual judgment. Several aids are appended to the Code to assist in this.

SUMMARY OF THE MAIN PRINCIPLES IN THE CODE

The fundamental principle underlying this Code is that the dental hygienist's primary responsibility is to the client, whether the client is an individual or a community.

Principle I: Beneficence

Beneficence involves caring about and acting to promote the good of another. Dental hygienists use their knowledge and skills to assist clients to achieve and maintain optimal oral health and to promote fair and reasonable access to quality oral health services.

Principle II: Autonomy

Autonomy pertains to the right to make one's own choices. By communicating relevant information openly and truthfully, dental hygienists assist clients to make informed choices and to participate actively in achieving and maintaining their optimal oral health.

Principle III: Privacy and Confidentiality

Privacy pertains to the individual's right to decide the conditions under which others will be permitted access to his or her personal life or information. Confidentiality is the duty to hold secret any information acquired in the professional relationship. Dental hygienists respect the privacy of clients and hold in confidence information disclosed to them, subject to certain narrowly defined exceptions.

Principle IV: Accountability

Accountability pertains to the acceptance of responsibility for one's actions and omissions in light of relevant principles, standards, laws, and regulations and the potential to self-evaluate and to be evaluated accordingly. Dental hygienists practise competently in conformity with relevant principles, standards, laws, and regulations and accept responsibility for their behaviour and decisions in the professional context.

Principle V: Professionalism

Professionalism is the commitment to use and advance professional knowledge and skills to serve the client and the public good. Dental hygienists express their professional commitment individually in their practice and communally through their professional associations and regulatory bodies.

PRINCIPLE I: BENEFICENCE

Beneficence involves caring about and acting to promote the good of another. Dental hygienists use their knowledge and skills to assist clients to achieve and maintain optimal oral health and to promote fair and reasonable access to quality oral health services.

Standards for Principle I

Dental hygienists:

1a. provide services to their clients in a caring and respectful manner, in recognition of the inherent dignity of human beings;

1b. provide services to their clients with respect for their individual needs and values and life circumstances;

1c. provide services fairly and without discrimination, in recognition of fundamental human rights;

1d. put the needs, values, and interests of their clients first and avoid exploiting their clients for personal gain;

1e. seek to improve the quality of care and advance knowledge in the field of oral health through such activities as quality assurance, research, education, and advocacy in the public arena.

PRINCIPLE II: AUTONOMY

Autonomy pertains to the right to make one's own choices. By communicating relevant information openly and truthfully, dental hygienists assist clients to make informed choices and to participate actively in achieving and maintaining their optimal oral health.

Standards for Principle II

Dental hygienists:

2a. actively involve clients in their oral health care and promote informed choice by communicating relevant information openly, truthfully, and sensitively in recognition of the client's needs, values, and capacity to understand;

2b. in the case of clients who lack the capacity for informed choice, actively involve and promote informed choice on the part of the client's substitute decision-makers, involving the client to the extent of the client's capacity;

2c. honour the client's informed choices, including refusal of treatment, and regard informed choice as a precondition of treatment;

2d. do not rely upon coercion or manipulative tactics in assisting the client to make informed choices;

2e. recommend or provide only those services they believe are necessary for the client's oral health or as consistent with the client's informed choice.

Note: Critical elements of informed choice include disclosure (i.e., revealing pertinent information, including risks and benefits); willingness (i.e., the choice is not coerced or manipulated); and capacity (i.e., the cognitive capacity to understand and process the relevant information). "Informed choice" encompasses what is sometimes referred to as "informed consent."

PRINCIPLE III: PRIVACY AND CONFIDENTIALITY

Privacy pertains to the individual's right to decide the conditions under which others will be permitted access to his or her personal life or information. Confidentiality is the duty to hold secret any information acquired in the professional relationship. Dental hygienists respect the privacy of clients and hold in confidence information disclosed to them, subject to certain narrowly defined exceptions.

Standards for Principle III

Dental hygienists:

3a. demonstrate regard for the privacy of their clients;

3b. hold confidential any information acquired in the professional relationship and do not use or disclose it to others without the client's express consent, except:

3b.i   as required by law

3b.ii as required by the policy of the practice environment (e.g., quality assurance)

3b.iii in an emergency situation

3b.iv in cases where disclosure is necessary to prevent serious harm to others

3b.v   to the guardian or substitute decision-maker of a client in these cases, disclose to others only as much information as is necessary to accomplish the purpose for the disclosure;

3c. may infer the client's consent for disclosure to others directly involved in delivering and administering services to the client, provided there is no reason to believe the client would not give express consent if asked;

3d. obtain the client's express consent to use or share information about the client for the purpose of teaching or research;

3e. inform their clients in advance of treatment about how they will use or share their information, in particular about any uses or sharing that may occur without the client's express consent;

3f. promote practices, policies, and information systems that are designed to respect client privacy and confidentiality.

PRINCIPLE IV: ACCOUNTABILITY

Accountability pertains to the acceptance of responsibility for one's actions and omissions in light of relevant principles, standards, laws, and regulations and the potential to self-evaluate and to be evaluated accordingly. Dental hygienists practise competently in conformity with relevant principles, standards, laws and regulations, and accept responsibility for their behaviour and decisions in the professional context.

Standards for Principle IV

Dental hygienists:

4a. accept responsibility for knowing and acting consistently with the principles, standards, laws, and regulations under which they are accountable;

4b. accept responsibility for providing safe, quality, competent care, including, but not limited to, addressing issues in the practice environment within their capacity that may hinder or impede the provision of such care;

4c. take appropriate action to ensure first and foremost the client's safety and quality of care when they suspect unethical or incompetent care;

4d. practise within the bounds of their competence, scope of practice, and personal and/or professional limitations, and refer clients requiring care outside these bounds;

4e. inform the dental hygiene regulatory body when an injury, dependency, infection, condition, or any other serious incapacity has immediately affected, or may affect over time, their continuing ability to practise safely and competently;

4f. promote workplace practices and policies that facilitate professional practice in accordance with the principles, standards, laws, and regulations under which they are accountable.

PRINCIPLE V: PROFESSIONALISM

Professionalism is the commitment to use and advance professional knowledge and skills to serve the client and the public good. Dental hygienists express their professional commitment individually in their practice and communally through their professional associations and regulatory bodies.

Standards for Principle V

Dental hygienists:

5a. uphold the principles and standards of the profession before clients, colleagues, and others;

5b. maintain and advance their knowledge and skills in dental hygiene through continuing education and the quality of the care they provide through ongoing self-evaluation and quality assurance;

5c. advance general knowledge and skills in the field of oral health by supporting, participating in, or conducting ethically approved research;

5d. participate in professional activities such as meetings, committee work, peer review, and participation in public forums to promote oral health;

5e. participate in mentoring, education, and dissemination of knowledge and skills in oral health care;

5f. support the work of their professional associations and regulatory bodies to promote oral health and professional practice;

5g. inform potential employers about the principles, standards, laws, and regulations to which they are accountable and determine whether employment conditions facilitate professional practice accordingly;

5h. collaborate with colleagues in a cooperative, constructive, and respectful manner toward the primary end of providing safe, competent, fair, quality care to clients;

5i. communicate the nature and costs of professional services fairly and accurately.

ETHICAL CHALLENGES/PROBLEMS

No code of ethics can be expected to resolve definitively all ethical challenges or problems that may arise in practice. The analysis below is intended to help dental hygienists understand the nature of ethical challenges or problems and thereby better resolve them.

Ethical challenges or problems faced by practising dental hygienists tend to fall into the categories of ethical violations, ethical dilemmas, and ethical distress.

Ethical violations: when dental hygienists fail to meet or neglect their specific ethical responsibilities as expressed in the Code's standards. An example would be a dental hygienist who recommends unnecessary treatment in order to achieve personal gain at the expense of the client.

Ethical dilemmas: when one or more ethical principles conflict either with other ethical principle(s) or with self-interest(s) and no apparent course of action will satisfy both sides of the dilemma. An example would be a client with a hip prosthesis who may refuse to be premedicated prior to receiving invasive dental treatment. In this case, the principle of autonomy conflicts with the principle of beneficence.

Ethical distress: when dental hygienists experience constraints or limitations in relation to which they are or feel powerless and which compromise their ability to practise in full accordance with their professional principles or standards. An example would be a dental hygienist who is expected by the employer to complete dental hygiene treatment in a length of time insufficient to render quality care or to provide an acceptable level of infection control.

This Code is a useful guide in helping dental hygienists to identify, work through, and put into words ethical issues in light of their responsibilities as articulated in the Code's principles and standards, and to decide on an ethically responsible course of action. It is important to realize that some challenges or problems are perceived to be primarily ethical in nature when, in fact, they arise less from conflicting principles than from poor communication or lack of information. Reflecting on a perceived challenge or problem in light of the Code can help determine to what extent the problem or challenge is truly rooted in conflicting ethical principles, and to what extent it can be resolved by improved communication or by new information.

The Code provides clear direction for avoiding ethical violations. When a course of action is mandated by a standard in the Code or by a principle where there exists no opposing principle, ethical conduct requires that course of action.

In the case of ethical dilemmas and ethical distress, the Code cannot always provide a clear direction. The resolution of dilemmas often depends on the specific circumstances of the case in question. Total satisfaction by all parties involved may not be achieved. Resolution may also depend on which opposing ethical principle is considered to be more important, a matter on which reasonable people may disagree. Ethical distress often arises in situations where the dental hygienist is significantly limited by factors beyond his or her immediate control that may not be resolvable in the specific context.

In all cases, dental hygienists are accountable for how they conduct themselves in professional practice. Even in situations of ethical dilemma or distress where the Code does not prescribe a specific course of action, the hygienist can be expected to give account of his or her chosen action in light of the principles and standards expressed in the Code. Ultimately, dental hygienists must reconcile their actions with their consciences in caring for clients.

REPORTING SUSPECTED INCOMPETENCE OR UNETHICAL CONDUCT

The first consideration of the dental hygienist who suspects incompetence or unethical conduct in colleagues or associates is the welfare of present clients and/or potential harm to future clients. Adherence to the following guidelines could be helpful:

1. First, confirm the facts of the situation.
2. Ensure you are familiar with existing protocols in the practice setting for reporting incidents, incompetence, or unethical care, and follow those protocols.
3. Document and report issues that cannot be resolved within the practice setting and report to the appropriate authority or regulatory body.

The dental hygienist who attempts to protect clients threatened by incompetent or unethical conduct should not be placed in jeopardy (e.g., loss of employment). Colleagues and professional organizations are morally obligated to support dental hygienists who fulfill their ethical obligations under the Code.

DECISION-PROCEDURE

Guidance Regarding the Process for Resolving Ethical Challenges

Ethical problems or challenges arise in a variety of contexts and require thoughtful analysis and careful judgment. The following guide may be useful to assist dental hygienists faced with an ethical challenge, recognizing that other stakeholders may need to be involved in resolving the matter. Talking with or getting advice from others at any step on the way to a decision can be very helpful.

1. Identify in a preliminary way the nature of the challenge or problem. What is the issue? What kind of issue is it? What ethical principles are at stake?
2. Become suitably informed and gather information (e.g., talk to others to find out the facts; research relevant policy statements) relevant to the challenge or problem, including:
   a. Factual information about the situation. What has happened? What is the sequence of events?
   b. Applicable policies, laws, or regulations. Does a workplace policy address the issue? What does the Code say? What does law or regulation say?

c. Who are the relevant stakeholders? How do they view the situation?

3. Clarify and elaborate the challenge or problem after getting this information. Now that you are better informed, What is the issue? What ethical principles are at stake? What stakeholders need to be consulted or involved in resolving the challenge or problem?

4. Identify various options for actions, recognizing that the best option may not be obvious at first and realizing it may require creativity or imagination.

5. Assess the various options in light of applicable policy, law, or regulation, being as clear as possible in your mind of the pluses and minuses of each option as assessed in this light.

6. Decide on a course of action, mindful of how you would justify or defend your decision in light of the applicable policy, law, or regulation, if you are called to account.

7. Implement your decision as thoughtfully and sensitively as possible, communicating a willingness to explain or justify the reasons for taking it.

8. Assess the consequences of your decision. Evaluate the process you used to arrive at the decision and the decision itself in light of those consequences. Did things turn out as you thought they would? Would you do the same thing again? What went wrong? Or, what went right?

In all of this, bear in mind that reasonable people can disagree about what is the right thing to do when faced with an ethical challenge or problem. If you cannot be certain whether you have made the right decision, you can at least have some assurance that you came to your decision in a responsible way. The test for this is whether you are able to defend your decision in light of relevant laws, principles, and regulations and to defend the process by which you came to your decision. Reference to the above guidelines will help in this.

In addition, there is a very rich literature on ethics that can be very helpful for thinking through ethical challenges and problems in dental hygiene or for ongoing professional education and development.

Dental hygienists may also find it useful to familiarize themselves with various ethical theories, which tend to guide or orient ethical thinking along different lines. The main ethical theories current today are briefly described below:

- DEONTOLOGY guides ethical thinking in terms of duties and rights, which the philosopher Immanuel Kant grounds in the fundamental imperative to act in relation to others according to principles that apply universally to all people, and that one would also wish for others to apply in their actions in relation to oneself.

- UTILITARIANISM guides ethical thinking in terms of harms and benefits, which the philosopher J.S. Mill grounds in the fundamental imperative to promote the greatest good for the greatest number.

- The ETHIC OF CARE guides ethical thinking in terms of preserving and enhancing relationships and service to others. This theory derives from the work of Carol Gilligan, who found in her research that this style of ethical thinking tends to be more associated with females than with males.

- VIRTUE ETHICS guides ethical thinking in terms of habits of acting and assesses actions in terms of virtues and vices of character. This theory derives from the work of the philosopher Aristotle, who emphasized that ethics cannot be reduced to rules or formulas and held that the person of good character (the "good man") is the ultimate standard of right and wrong and should be emulated by others as a role model.

- FEMINIST ETHICS guides ethical thinking in terms of sensitivity to the power or political dimension of human interaction. The philosopher Susan Sherwin grounds feminist ethics in the allegiance to those who are oppressed, vulnerable, or disadvantaged and the imperative to improve their situation.

This is by no means a complete listing of ethical theories, nor is the richness of these theories captured in the condensed descriptions given. Moreover, considerable controversy exists not only among these theories but also among adherents of each theory.

REFERENCES

Canadian Dental Hygienists Association: "Dental Hygiene: Client's Bill of Rights." Ottawa: CDHA, October 2001
———: Code of Ethics. Ottawa: CDHA, July 1997
College of Dental Hygienists of Ontario: Code of Ethics. Toronto: CDHO, 1996
College of Dental Hygienists of British Columbia: Code of Ethics. Victoria: CDHBC, March 1, 1995
Canadian Dental Association: Code of Ethics. Ottawa: CDA, August 1991
American Dental Hygienists Association: Code of Ethics for Dental Hygienists. Chicago: ADHA, 1995
Canadian Dental Assistants Association: CDAA Code of Ethics. Ottawa: CDAA, 2000
Canadian Medical Association: Code of Ethics of the Canadian Medical Association. Ottawa: CMA, 1997
Canadian Nurses Association: Code of Ethics for Registered Nurses. Ottawa: CNA, March 1997

Guidelines for Infection Control in Dental Health-Care Settings—2003

RECOMMENDATIONS

Each recommendation is categorized on the basis of existing scientific data, theoretical rationale, and applicability. Rankings are based on the system used by CDC and the Healthcare Infection Control Practices Advisory Committee (HICPAC) to categorize recommendations:

Category IA. Strongly recommended for implementation and strongly supported by well-designed experimental, clinical, or epidemiologic studies.

Category IB. Strongly recommended for implementation and supported by experimental, clinical, or epidemiologic studies and a strong theoretical rationale.

Category IC. Required for implementation as mandated by federal or state regulation or standard. When IC is used, a second rating can be included to provide the basis of existing scientific data, theoretical rationale, and applicability. Because of state differences, the reader should not assume that the absence of a IC implies the absence of state regulations.

Category II. Suggested for implementation and supported by suggestive clinical or epidemiologic studies or a theoretical rationale.

Unresolved issue. No recommendation. Insufficient evidence or no consensus regarding efficacy exists.

I. PERSONNEL HEALTH ELEMENTS OF AN INFECTION-CONTROL PROGRAM

A. General Recommendations

1. Develop a written health program for DHCP that includes policies, procedures, and guidelines for education and training; immunizations; exposure prevention and postexposure management; medical conditions, work-related illness, and associated work restrictions; contact dermatitis and latex hypersensitivity; and maintenance of records, data management, and confidentiality (IB) (5,16–18,22).

2. Establish referral arrangements with qualified health-care professionals to ensure prompt and appropriate provision of preventive services, occupationally related medical services, and postexposure management with medical follow-up (IB, IC) (5,13,19,22).

B. Education and Training

1. Provide DHCP 1) on initial employment, 2) when new tasks or procedures affect the employee's occupational exposure, and 3) at a minimum, annually, with education and training regarding occupational exposure to potentially infectious agents and infection-control procedures/protocols appropriate for and specific to their assigned duties (IB, IC) (5,11,13, 14,16,19,22).

2. Provide educational information appropriate in content and vocabulary to the educational level, literacy, and language of DHCP (IB, IC) (5,13).

C. Immunization Programs

1. Develop a written comprehensive policy regarding immunizing DHCP, including a list of all required and recommended immunizations (IB) (5,17,18).

2. Refer DHCP to a prearranged qualified health-care professional or to their own health-care professional to receive all appropriate immunizations based on the latest recommendations as well as their medical history and risk for occupational exposure (IB) (5,17).

D. Exposure Prevention and Postexposure Management

1. Develop a comprehensive postexposure management and medical follow-up program (IB, IC) (5,13,14,19).

a. Include policies and procedures for prompt reporting, evaluation, counseling, treatment, and medical follow-up of occupational exposures.

b. Establish mechanisms for referral to a qualified health-care professional for medical evaluation and follow-up.

c. Conduct a baseline TST, preferably by using a two-step test, for all DHCP who might have contact with persons with suspected or confirmed infectious TB, regardless of the risk classification of the setting (IB) (20).

E. Medical Conditions, Work-Related Illness, and Work Restrictions

1. Develop and have readily available to all DHCP comprehensive written policies regarding work restriction and exclusion that include a statement of authority defining who can implement such policies (IB) (5,22).

2. Develop policies for work restriction and exclusion that encourage DHCP to seek appropriate preventive and curative care and report their illnesses, medical conditions, or treatments that can render them more susceptible to opportunistic infection or exposures; do not penalize DHCP with loss of wages, benefits, or job status (IB) (5,22).

3. Develop policies and procedures for evaluation, diagnosis, and management of DHCP with suspected or known occupational contact dermatitis (IB) (32).

4. Seek definitive diagnosis by a qualified health-care professional for any DHCP with suspected latex allergy to carefully determine its specific etiology and appropriate treatment as well as work restrictions and accommodations (IB) (32).

F. Records Maintenance, Data Management, and Confidentiality

1. Establish and maintain confidential medical records (e.g., immunization records and documentation of tests received as a result of occupational exposure) for all DHCP (IB, IC) (5,13).

2. Ensure that the practice complies with all applicable federal, state, and local laws regarding medical recordkeeping and confidentiality (IC) (13,34).

II. PREVENTING TRANSMISSION OF BLOODBORNE PATHOGENS

A. HBV Vaccination

1. Offer the HBV vaccination series to all DHCP with potential occupational exposure to blood or other potentially infectious material (IA, IC) (2,13,14,19).

2. Always follow U.S. Public Health Service/CDC recommendations for hepatitis B vaccination, serologic testing, follow-up, and booster dosing (IA, IC) (13,14,19).

3. Test DHCP for anti-HBs 1–2 months after completion of the 3-dose vaccination series (IA, IC) (14,19).

4. DHCP should complete a second 3-dose vaccine series or be evaluated to determine if they are HBsAg-positive if no antibody response occurs to the primary vaccine series (IA, IC) (14,19).

5. Retest for anti-HBs at the completion of the second vaccine series. If no response to the second 3-dose series occurs, nonresponders should be tested for HBsAg (IC) (14,19).

6. Counsel nonresponders to vaccination who are HBsAg-negative regarding their susceptibility to HBV infection and precautions to take (IA, IC) (14,19).

7. Provide employees appropriate education regarding the risks of HBV transmission and the availability of the vaccine. Employees who decline the vaccination should sign a declination form to be kept on file with the employer (IC) (13).

B. Preventing Exposures to Blood and OPIM

1. General recommendations
    a. Use standard precautions (OSHA's bloodborne pathogen standard retains the term universal precautions) for all patient encounters (IA, IC) (11,13,19,53).
    b. Consider sharp items (e.g., needles, scalers, burs, lab knives, and wires) that are contaminated with patient blood and saliva as potentially infective and establish engineering controls and work practices to prevent injuries (IB, IC) (6,13,113).
    c. Implement a written, comprehensive program designed to minimize and manage DHCP exposures to blood and body fluids (IB, IC). (13,14,19,97).

2. Engineering and work-practice controls
   a. Identify, evaluate, and select devices with engineered safety features at least annually and as they become available on the market (e.g., safer anesthetic syringes, blunt suture needle, retractable scalpel, or needleless IV systems) (IC) *(13,97,110–112)*.
   b. Place used disposable syringes and needles, scalpel blades, and other sharp items in appropriate puncture-resistant containers located as close as feasible to the area in which the items are used (IA, IC) *(2,7,13,19,113, 115)*.
   c. Do not recap used needles by using both hands or any other technique that involves directing the point of a needle toward any part of the body. Do not bend, break, or remove needles before disposal (IA, IC) *(2,7,8,13,97,113)*.
   d. Use either a one-handed scoop technique or a mechanical device designed for holding the needle cap when recapping needles (e.g., between multiple injections and before removing from a nondisposable aspirating syringe) (IA, IC) *(2,7,8,13,14,113)*.
3. Postexposure management and prophylaxis
   a. Follow CDC recommendations after percutaneous, mucous membrane, or nonintact skin exposure to blood or other potentially infectious material (IA, IC) *(13,14,19)*.

III. HAND HYGIENE

A. General Considerations

1. Perform hand hygiene with either a nonantimicrobial or antimicrobial soap and water when hands are visibly dirty or contaminated with blood or other potentially infectious material. If hands are not visibly soiled, an alcohol-based hand rub can also be used. Follow the manufacturer's instructions (IA) *(123)*.
2. Indications for hand hygiene include
   a. when hands are visibly soiled (IA, IC);
   b. after bare-handed touching of inanimate objects likely to be contaminated by blood, saliva, or respiratory secretions (IA, IC);
   c. before and after treating each patient (IB);
   d. before donning gloves (IB); and
   e. immediately after removing gloves (IB, IC) *(7–9,11,13,113,120–123,125,126,138)*.
3. For oral surgical procedures, perform surgical hand antisepsis before donning sterile surgeon's gloves. Follow the manufacturer's instructions by

using either an antimicrobial soap and water, or soap and water followed by drying hands and application of an alcohol-based surgical hand-scrub product with persistent activity (IB) *(121–123,127–133,144,145)*.
4. Store liquid hand-care products in either disposable closed containers or closed containers that can be washed and dried before refilling. Do not add soap or lotion to (i.e., top off) a partially empty dispenser (IA) *(9,120,122,149,150)*.

B. Special Considerations for Hand Hygiene and Glove Use

1. Use hand lotions to prevent skin dryness associated with handwashing (IA) *(153,154)*.
2. Consider the compatibility of lotion and antiseptic products and the effect of petroleum or other oil emollients on the integrity of gloves during product selection and glove use (IB) *(2,14,122,155)*.
3. Keep fingernails short with smooth, filed edges to allow thorough cleaning and prevent glove tears (II) *(122,123,156)*.
4. Do not wear artificial fingernails or extenders when having direct contact with patients at high risk (e.g., those in intensive care units or operating rooms) (IA) *(123,157–160)*.
5. Use of artificial fingernails is usually not recommended (II) *(157–160)*.
6. Do not wear hand or nail jewelry if it makes donning gloves more difficult or compromises the fit and integrity of the glove (II) *(123,142, 143)*.

IV. PPE

A. Masks, Protective Eyewear, and Face Shields

1. Wear a surgical mask and eye protection with solid side shields or a face shield to protect mucous membranes of the eyes, nose, and mouth during procedures likely to generate splashing or spattering of blood or other body fluids (IB, IC) *(1,2,7,8,11,13,137)*.
2. Change masks between patients or during patient treatment if the mask becomes wet (IB) *(2)*.
3. Clean with soap and water, or if visibly soiled, clean and disinfect reusable facial protective equipment (e.g., clinician and patient protective eyewear or face shields) between patients (II) *(2)*.

B. Protective Clothing

1. Wear protective clothing (e.g., reusable or disposable gown, laboratory coat, or uniform) that covers personal clothing and skin (e.g., forearms) likely to be soiled with blood, saliva, or OPIM (IB, IC) (7,8,11,13,137).

2. Change protective clothing if visibly soiled (134); change immediately or as soon as feasible if penetrated by blood or other potentially infectious fluids (IB, IC) (13).

3. Remove barrier protection, including gloves, mask, eyewear, and gown before departing work area (e.g., dental patient care, instrument processing, or laboratory areas) (IC) (13).

C. Gloves

1. Wear medical gloves when a potential exists for contacting blood, saliva, OPIM, or mucous membranes (IB, IC) (1,2,7,8,13).

2. Wear a new pair of medical gloves for each patient, remove them promptly after use, and wash hands immediately to avoid transfer of microorganisms to other patients or environments (IB) (1,7,8,123).

3. Remove gloves that are torn, cut, or punctured as soon as feasible and wash hands before regloving (IB, IC) (13,210,211).

4. Do not wash surgeon's or patient examination gloves before use or wash, disinfect, or sterilize gloves for reuse (IB, IC) (13,138,177,212,213).

5. Ensure that appropriate gloves in the correct size are readily accessible (IC) (13).

6. Use appropriate gloves (e.g., puncture- and chemical-resistant utility gloves) when cleaning instruments and performing housekeeping tasks involving contact with blood or OPIM (IB, IC) (7,13,15).

7. Consult with glove manufacturers regarding the chemical compatibility of glove material and dental materials used (II).

D. Sterile Surgeon's Gloves and Double Gloving During Oral Surgical Procedures

1. Wear sterile surgeon's gloves when performing oral surgical procedures (IB) (2,8,137).

2. No recommendation is offered regarding the effectiveness of wearing two pairs of gloves to prevent disease transmission during oral surgical procedures. The majority of studies among HCP and DHCP have demonstrated a lower frequency of inner glove perforation and visible blood on the surgeon's hands when double gloves are worn; however, the effectiveness of wearing two pairs of gloves in preventing disease transmission has not been demonstrated (Unresolved issue).

V. CONTACT DERMATITIS AND LATEX HYPERSENSITIVITY

A. General Recommendations

1. Educate DHCP regarding the signs, symptoms, and diagnoses of skin reactions associated with frequent hand hygiene and glove use (IB) (5,31,32).

2. Screen all patients for latex allergy (e.g., take health history and refer for medical consultation when latex allergy is suspected) (IB) (32).

3. Ensure a latex-safe environment for patients and DHCP with latex allergy (IB) (32).

4. Have emergency treatment kits with latex-free products available at all times (II) (32).

VI. STERILIZATION AND DISINFECTION OF PATIENT-CARE ITEMS

A. General Recommendations

1. Use only FDA-cleared medical devices for sterilization and follow the manufacturer's instructions for correct use (IB) (248).

2. Clean and heat-sterilize critical dental instruments before each use (IA) (2,137,243,244, 246,249,407).

3. Clean and heat-sterilize semicritical items before each use (IB) (2,249,260,407).

4. Allow packages to dry in the sterilizer before they are handled to avoid contamination (IB) (247).

5. Use of heat-stable semicritical alternatives is encouraged (IB) (2).

6. Reprocess heat-sensitive critical and semicritical instruments by using FDA-cleared sterilant/high-level disinfectants or an FDA-cleared low-temperature sterilization method (e.g., ethylene oxide). Follow manufacturer's instructions for use of chemical sterilants/high-level disinfectants (IB) (243).

7. Single-use disposable instruments are acceptable alternatives if they are used only once and disposed of correctly (IB, IC) (243,383).

8. Do not use liquid chemical sterilants/high-level disinfectants for environmental surface disinfection or as holding solutions (IB, IC) (243,245).

9. Ensure that noncritical patient-care items are barrier-protected or cleaned, or if visibly soiled, cleaned and disinfected after each use with an

EPA-registered hospital disinfectant. If visibly contaminated with blood, use an EPA-registered hospital disinfectant with a tuberculocidal claim (i.e., intermediate level) (IB) (2,243,244).

10. Inform DHCP of all OSHA guidelines for exposure to chemical agents used for disinfection and sterilization. Using this report, identify areas and tasks that have potential for exposure (IC) (15).

B. Instrument Processing Area

1. Designate a central processing area. Divide the instrument processing area, physically or, at a minimum, spatially into distinct areas for 1) receiving, cleaning, and decontamination; 2) preparation and packaging; 3) sterilization; and 4) storage. Do not store instruments in an area where contaminated instruments are held or cleaned (II) (173,247,248).

2. Train DHCP to employ work practices that prevent contamination of clean areas (II).

C. Receiving, Cleaning, and Decontamination Work Area

1. Minimize handling of loose contaminated instruments during transport to the instrument processing area. Use work-practice controls (e.g., carry instruments in a covered container) to minimize exposure potential (II). Clean all visible blood and other contamination from dental instruments and devices before sterilization or disinfection procedures (IA) (243,249–252).

2. Use automated cleaning equipment (e.g., ultrasonic cleaner or washer-disinfector) to remove debris to improve cleaning effectiveness and decrease worker exposure to blood (IB) (2,253).

3. Use work-practice controls that minimize contact with sharp instruments if manual cleaning is necessary (e.g., long-handled brush) (IC) (14).

4. Wear puncture- and chemical-resistant/heavy-duty utility gloves for instrument cleaning and decontamination procedures (IB) (7).

5. Wear appropriate PPE (e.g., mask, protective eyewear, and gown) when splashing or spraying is anticipated during cleaning (IC) (13).

D. Preparation and Packaging

1. Use an internal chemical indicator in each package. If the internal indicator cannot be seen from outside the package, also use an external indicator (II) (243,254,257).

2. Use a container system or wrapping compatible with the type of sterilization process used and

that has received FDA clearance (IB) (243,247, 256).

3. Before sterilization of critical and semicritical instruments, inspect instruments for cleanliness, then wrap or place them in containers designed to maintain sterility during storage (e.g., cassettes and organizing trays) (IA) (2,247,255,256).

E. Sterilization of Unwrapped Instruments

1. Clean and dry instruments before the unwrapped sterilization cycle (IB) (248).

2. Use mechanical and chemical indicators for each unwrapped sterilization cycle (i.e., place an internal chemical indicator among the instruments or items to be sterilized) (IB) (243,258).

3. Allow unwrapped instruments to dry and cool in the sterilizer before they are handled to avoid contamination and thermal injury (II) (260).

4. Semicritical instruments that will be used immediately or within a short time can be sterilized unwrapped on a tray or in a container system, provided that the instruments are handled aseptically during removal from the sterilizer and transport to the point of use (II).

5. Critical instruments intended for immediate reuse can be sterilized unwrapped if the instruments are maintained sterile during removal from the sterilizer and transport to the point of use (e.g., transported in a sterile covered container) (IB) (258).

6. Do not sterilize implantable devices unwrapped (IB) (243,247).

7. Do not store critical instruments unwrapped (IB) (248).

F. Sterilization Monitoring

1. Use mechanical, chemical, and biological monitors according to the manufacturer's instructions to ensure the effectiveness of the sterilization process (IB) (248,278,279).

2. Monitor each load with mechanical (e.g., time, temperature, and pressure) and chemical indicators (II) (243,248).

3. Place a chemical indicator on the inside of each package. If the internal indicator is not visible from the outside, also place an exterior chemical indicator on the package (II) (243,254,257).

4. Place items/packages correctly and loosely into the sterilizer so as not to impede penetration of the sterilant (IB) (243).

5. Do not use instrument packs if mechanical or chemical indicators indicate inadequate processing (IB) (243,247,248).

6. Monitor sterilizers at least weekly by using a biological indicator with a matching control (i.e., biological indicator and control from same lot number) (IB) (2,9,243,247,278,279).

7. Use a biological indicator for every sterilizer load that contains an implantable device. Verify results before using the implantable device, whenever possible (IB) (243,248).

8. The following are recommended in the case of a positive spore test:
   a. Remove the sterilizer from service and review sterilization procedures (e.g., work practices and use of mechanical and chemical indicators) to determine whether operator error could be responsible (II) (8).
   b. Retest the sterilizer by using biological, mechanical, and chemical indicators after correcting any identified procedural problems (II).
   c. If the repeat spore test is negative, and mechanical and chemical indicators are within normal limits, put the sterilizer back in service (II) (9,243).

9. The following are recommended if the repeat spore test is positive:
   a. Do not use the sterilizer until it has been inspected or repaired or the exact reason for the positive test has been determined (II) (9,243).
   b. Recall, to the extent possible, and reprocess all items processed since the last negative spore test (II) (9,243,283).
   c. Before placing the sterilizer back in service, rechallenge the sterilizer with biological indicator tests in three consecutive empty chamber sterilization cycles after the cause of the sterilizer failure has been determined and corrected (II) (9,243,283).

10. Maintain sterilization records (i.e., mechanical, chemical, and biological) in compliance with state and local regulations (IB) (243).

G. Storage Area for Sterilized Items and Clean Dental Supplies

1. Implement practices on the basis of date- or event-related shelf-life for storage of wrapped, sterilized instruments and devices (IB) (243, 284).

2. Even for event-related packaging, at a minimum, place the date of sterilization, and if multiple sterilizers are used in the facility, the sterilizer used, on the outside of the packaging material to facilitate the retrieval of processed items in the event of a sterilization failure (IB) (243,247).

3. Examine wrapped packages of sterilized instruments before opening them to ensure the barrier wrap has not been compromised during storage (II) (243,284).

4. Reclean, repack, and resterilize any instrument package that has been compromised (II).

5. Store sterile items and dental supplies in covered or closed cabinets, if possible (II) (285).

VII. ENVIRONMENTAL INFECTION CONTROL

A. General Recommendations

1. Follow the manufacturers' instructions for correct use of cleaning and EPA-registered hospital disinfecting products (IB, IC) (243–245).

2. Do not use liquid chemical sterilants/high-level disinfectants for disinfection of environmental surfaces (clinical contact or housekeeping) (IB, IC) (243–245).

3. Use PPE, as appropriate, when cleaning and disinfecting environmental surfaces. Such equipment might include gloves (e.g., puncture- and chemical-resistant utility), protective clothing (e.g., gown, jacket, or lab coat), and protective eyewear/face shield, and mask (IC) (13,15).

B. Clinical Contact Surfaces

1. Use surface barriers to protect clinical contact surfaces, particularly those that are difficult to clean (e.g., switches on dental chairs) and change surface barriers between patients (II) (1,2,260, 288).

2. Clean and disinfect clinical contact surfaces that are not barrier-protected, by using an EPA-registered hospital disinfectant with a low- (i.e., HIV and HBV label claims) to intermediate-level (i.e., tuberculocidal claim) activity after each patient. Use an intermediate-level disinfectant if visibly contaminated with blood (IB) (2,243,244).

C. Housekeeping Surfaces

1. Clean housekeeping surfaces (e.g., floors, walls, and sinks) with a detergent and water or an EPA-registered hospital disinfectant/detergent on a routine basis, depending on the nature of the surface and type and degree of contamination, and as appropriate, based on the location in the facility, and when visibly soiled (IB) (243,244).

2. Clean mops and cloths after use and allow to dry before reuse; or use single-use, disposable mop heads or cloths (II) (243,244).

3. Prepare fresh cleaning or EPA-registered disinfecting solutions daily and as instructed by the manufacturer (II) (243,244).

4. Clean walls, blinds, and window curtains in patient-care areas when they are visibly dusty or soiled (II) (*9,244*).

D. Spills of Blood and Body Substances

1. Clean spills of blood or OPIM and decontaminate surface with an EPA-registered hospital disinfectant with low-level (i.e., HBV and HIV label claims) to intermediate-level (i.e., tuberculocidal claim) activity, depending on size of spill and surface porosity (IB, IC) (*13,113*).

E. Carpet and Cloth Furnishings

1. Avoid using carpeting and cloth-upholstered furnishings in dental operatories, laboratories, and instrument processing areas (II) (*9,293–295*).

F. Regulated Medical Waste

1. General Recommendations
   a. Develop a medical waste management program. Disposal of regulated medical waste must follow federal, state, and local regulations (IC) (*13,301*).
   b. Ensure that DHCP who handle and dispose of regulated medical waste are trained in appropriate handling and disposal methods and are informed of the possible health and safety hazards (IC) (*13*).
2. Management of Regulated Medical Waste in Dental Health-Care Facilities
   a. Use a color-coded or labeled container that prevents leakage (e.g., biohazard bag) to contain nonsharp regulated medical waste (IC) (*13*).
   b. Place sharp items (e.g., needles, scalpel blades, orthodontic bands, broken metal instruments, and burs) in an appropriate sharps container (e.g., puncture resistant, color-coded, and leakproof). Close container immediately before removal or replacement to prevent spillage or protrusion of contents during handling, storage, transport, or shipping (IC) (*2,8,13,113,115*).
   c. Pour blood, suctioned fluids, or other liquid waste carefully into a drain connected to a sanitary sewer system, if local sewage discharge requirements are met and the state has declared this an acceptable method of disposal. Wear appropriate PPE while performing this task (IC) (*7,9,13*).

VIII. DENTAL UNIT WATERLINES, BIOFILM, AND WATER QUALITY

A. General Recommendations

1. Use water that meets EPA regulatory standards for drinking water (i.e., ≤500 CFU/mL of heterotrophic water bacteria) for routine dental treatment output water (IB, IC) (*341,342*).
2. Consult with the dental unit manufacturer for appropriate methods and equipment to maintain the recommended quality of dental water (II) (*339*).
3. Follow recommendations for monitoring water quality provided by the manufacturer of the unit or waterline treatment product (II).
4. Discharge water and air for a minimum of 20–30 seconds after each patient, from any device connected to the dental water system that enters the patient's mouth (e.g., handpieces, ultrasonic scalers, and air/water syringes) (II) (*2,311,344*).
5. Consult with the dental unit manufacturer on the need for periodic maintenance of antiretraction mechanisms (IB) (*2,311*).

B. Boil-Water Advisories

1. The following apply while a boil-water advisory is in effect:
   a. Do not deliver water from the public water system to the patient through the dental operative unit, ultrasonic scaler, or other dental equipment that uses the public water system (IB, IC) (*341,342,346,349,350*).
   b. Do not use water from the public water system for dental treatment, patient rinsing, or handwashing (IB, IC) (*341,342,346,349, 350*).
   c. For handwashing, use antimicrobial-containing products that do not require water for use (e.g., alcohol-based hand rubs). If hands are visibly contaminated, use bottled water, if available, and soap for handwashing or an antiseptic towelette (IB, IC) (*13,122*).
2. The following apply when the boil-water advisory is cancelled:
   a. Follow guidance given by the local water utility regarding adequate flushing of waterlines. If no guidance is provided, flush dental waterlines and faucets for 1–5 minutes before using for patient care (IC) (*244,346, 351,352*).
   b. Disinfect dental waterlines as recommended by the dental unit manufacturer (II).

IX. SPECIAL CONSIDERATIONS

A. Dental Handpieces and Other Devices Attached to Air and Waterlines

1. Clean and heat-sterilize handpieces and other intraoral instruments that can be removed from the air and waterlines of dental units between patients (IB, IC) (2,246,275,356,357,360,407).
2. Follow the manufacturer's instructions for cleaning, lubrication, and sterilization of handpieces and other intraoral instruments that can be removed from the air and waterlines of dental units (IB) (361–363).
3. Do not surface-disinfect, use liquid chemical sterilants, or ethylene oxide on handpieces and other intraoral instruments that can be removed from the air and waterlines of dental units (IC) (2,246,250,275).
4. Do not advise patients to close their lips tightly around the tip of the saliva ejector to evacuate oral fluids (II) (364–366).

B. Dental Radiology

1. Wear gloves when exposing radiographs and handling contaminated film packets. Use other PPE (e.g., protective eyewear, mask, and gown) as appropriate if spattering of blood or other body fluids is likely (IA, IC) (11,13).
2. Use heat-tolerant or disposable intraoral devices whenever possible (e.g., film-holding and positioning devices). Clean and heat-sterilize heat-tolerant devices between patients. At a minimum, high-level disinfect semicritical heat-sensitive devices, according to manufacturer's instructions (IB) (243).
3. Transport and handle exposed radiographs in an aseptic manner to prevent contamination of developing equipment (II).
4. The following apply for digital radiography sensors:
   a. Use FDA-cleared barriers (IB) (243).
   b. Clean and heat-sterilize, or high-level disinfect, between patients, barrier-protected semicritical items. If the item cannot tolerate these procedures, then, at a minimum, protect with an FDA-cleared barrier and clean and disinfect with an EPA-registered hospital disinfectant with intermediate-level (i.e., tuberculocidal claim) activity, between patients. Consult with the manufacturer for methods of disinfection and sterilization of digital radiology sensors and

for protection of associated computer hardware (IB) (243).

C. Aseptic Technique for Parenteral Medications

1. Do not administer medication from a syringe to multiple patients, even if the needle on the syringe is changed (IA) (378).
2. Use single-dose vials for parenteral medications when possible (II) (376,377).
3. Do not combine the leftover contents of single-use vials for later use (IA) (376,377).
4. The following apply if multidose vials are used:
   a. Cleanse the access diaphragm with 70% alcohol before inserting a device into the vial (IA) (380,381).
   b. Use a sterile device to access a multiple-dose vial and avoid touching the access diaphragm. Both the needle and syringe used to access the multidose vial should be sterile. Do not reuse a syringe even if the needle is changed (IA) (380,381).
   c. Keep multidose vials away from the immediate patient treatment area to prevent inadvertent contamination by spray or spatter (II).
   d. Discard the multidose vial if sterility is compromised (IA) (380,381).
5. Use fluid infusion and administration sets (i.e., IV bags, tubings, and connections) for one patient only and dispose of appropriately (IB) (378).

D. Single-Use (Disposable) Devices

1. Use single-use devices for one patient only and dispose of them appropriately (IC) (383).

E. Preprocedural Mouthrinses

1. No recommendation is offered regarding use of preprocedural antimicrobial mouthrinses to prevent clinical infections among DHCP or patients. Although studies have demonstrated that a preprocedural antimicrobial rinse (e.g., chlorhexidine gluconate, essential oils, or povidone-iodine) can reduce the level of oral microorganisms in aerosols and spatter generated during routine dental procedures and can decrease the number of microorganisms introduced in the patient's bloodstream during invasive dental procedures (391–399), the scientific evidence is inconclusive that using these rinses prevents clinical infections among DHCP or patients (see discussion, Preprocedural Mouthrinses) (Unresolved issue).

F. Oral Surgical Procedures

1. The following apply when performing oral surgical procedures:
   a. Perform surgical hand antisepsis by using an antimicrobial product (e.g., antimicrobial soap and water, or soap and water followed by alcohol-based hand scrub with persistent activity) before donning sterile surgeon's gloves (IB) (127–132,137).
   b. Use sterile surgeon's gloves (IB) (2,7,121, 123,137).
   c. Use sterile saline or sterile water as a coolant/irrigatant when performing oral surgical procedures. Use devices specifically designed for delivering sterile irrigating fluids (e.g., bulb syringe, single-use disposable products, and sterilizable tubing) (IB) (2,121).

G. Handling of Biopsy Specimens

1. During transport, place biopsy specimens in a sturdy, leakproof container labeled with the biohazard symbol (IC) (2,13,14).
2. If a biopsy specimen container is visibly contaminated, clean and disinfect the outside of a container or place it in an impervious bag labeled with the biohazard symbol, (IC) (2,13).

H. Handling of Extracted Teeth

1. Dispose of extracted teeth as regulated medical waste unless returned to the patient (IC) (13,14).
2. Do not dispose of extracted teeth containing amalgam in regulated medical waste intended for incineration (II).
3. Clean and place extracted teeth in a leakproof container, labeled with a biohazard symbol, and maintain hydration for transport to educational institutions or a dental laboratory (IC) (13,14).
4. Heat-sterilize teeth that do not contain amalgam before they are used for educational purposes (IB) (403,405,406).

I. Dental Laboratory

1. Use PPE when handling items received in the laboratory until they have been decontaminated (IA, IC) (2,7,11,13,113).
2. Before they are handled in the laboratory, clean, disinfect, and rinse all dental prostheses and prosthodontic materials (e.g., impressions, bite registrations, occlusal rims, and extracted teeth) by using an EPA-registered hospital disinfectant having at least an intermediate-level

(i.e., tuberculocidal claim) activity (IB) (2,249,252,407).
3. Consult with manufacturers regarding the stability of specific materials (e.g., impression materials) relative to disinfection procedures (II).
4. Include specific information regarding disinfection techniques used (e.g., solution used and duration), when laboratory cases are sent off-site and on their return (II) (2,407,409).
5. Clean and heat-sterilize heat-tolerant items used in the mouth (e.g., metal impression trays and face-bow forks) (IB) (2,407).
6. Follow manufacturers' instructions for cleaning and sterilizing or disinfecting items that become contaminated but do not normally contact the patient (e.g., burs, polishing points, rag wheels, articulators, case pans, and lathes). If manufacturer instructions are unavailable, clean and heat-sterilize heat-tolerant items or clean and disinfect with an EPA-registered hospital disinfectant with low-level (HIV, HBV effectiveness claim) to intermediate-level (tuberculocidal claim) activity, depending on the degree of contamination (II).

J. Laser/Electrosurgery Plumes/ Surgical Smoke

1. No recommendation is offered regarding practices to reduce DHCP exposure to laser plumes/surgical smoke when using lasers in dental practice. Practices to reduce HCP exposure to laser plumes/surgical smoke have been suggested, including use of a) standard precautions (e.g., high-filtration surgical masks and possibly full face shields) (437); b) central room suction units with in-line filters to collect particulate matter from minimal plumes; and c) dedicated mechanical smoke exhaust systems with a high-efficiency filter to remove substantial amounts of laser-plume particles. The effect of the exposure (e.g., disease transmission or adverse respiratory effects) on DHCP from dental applications of lasers has not been adequately evaluated (see previous discussion, Laser/Electrosurgery Plumes or Surgical Smoke) (Unresolved issue).

K. Mycobacterium tuberculosis

1. General Recommendations
   a. Educate all DHCP regarding the recognition of signs, symptoms, and transmission of TB (IB) (20,21).
   b. Conduct a baseline TST, preferably by using a two-step test, for all DHCP who might have contact with persons with suspected or

confirmed active TB, regardless of the risk classification of the setting (IB) (*20*).

c. Assess each patient for a history of TB as well as symptoms indicative of TB and document on the medical history form (IB) (*20,21*).

d. Follow CDC recommendations for 1) developing, maintaining, and implementing a written TB infection-control plan; 2) managing a patient with suspected or active TB; 3) completing a community risk-assessment to guide employee TSTs and follow-up; and 4) managing DHCP with TB disease (IB) (*2,21*).

2. The following apply for patients known or suspected to have active TB:

a. Evaluate the patient away from other patients and DHCP. When not being evaluated, the patient should wear a surgical mask or be instructed to cover mouth and nose when coughing or sneezing (IB) (*20,21*).

b. Defer elective dental treatment until the patient is noninfectious (IB) (*20,21*).

c. Refer patients requiring urgent dental treatment to a previously identified facility with TB engineering controls and a respiratory protection program (IB) (*20,21*).

L. Creutzfeldt-Jakob Disease (CJD) and Other Prion Diseases

1. No recommendation is offered regarding use of special precautions in addition to standard precautions when treating known CJD or vCJD patients. Potential infectivity of oral tissues in CJD or vCJD patients is an unresolved issue. Scientific data indicate the risk, if any, of sporadic CJD transmission during dental and oral surgical procedures is low to nil. Until additional information exists regarding the transmissibility of CJD or vCJD during dental procedures, special precautions in addition to standard precautions might be indicated when treating known CJD or vCJD patients; a list of such precautions is provided for consideration without recommendation (see Creutzfeldt-Jakob Disease and Other Prion Diseases) (Unresolved issue).

M. Program Evaluation

1. Establish routine evaluation of the infection-control program, including evaluation of performance indicators, at an established frequency (II) (*470-471*).

INFECTION-CONTROL INTERNET RESOURCES

Advisory Committee on Immunization Practices
http://www.cdc.gov/nip/ACIP/default.htm

American Dental Association
http://www.ada.org

American Institute of Architects Academy of Architecture for Health
http://www.aahaia.org

American Society of Heating, Refrigeration, Air-conditioning Engineers
http://www.ashrae.org

Association for Professionals in Infection Control and Epidemiology, Inc.
http://www.apic.org/resc/guidlist.cfm

CDC, Division of Healthcare Quality Promotion
http://www.cdc.gov/ncidod/hip

CDC, Division of Oral Health, Infection Control
http://www.cdc.gov/OralHealth/infectioncontrol/index.htm

CDC, *Morbidity and Mortality Weekly Report*
http://www.cdc.gov/mmwr

CDC, NIOSH
http://www.cdc.gov/niosh/homepage.html

CDC Recommends, Prevention Guidelines System
http://www.phppo.cdc.gov/cdcRecommends/AdvSearchV.asp

EPA, Antimicrobial Chemicals
http://www.epa.gov/oppad001/chemregindex.htm

FDA
http://www.fda.gov

Immunization Action Coalition
http://www.immunize.org/acip

Infectious Diseases Society of America
http://www.idsociety.org/PG/toc.htm

OSHA, Dentistry, Bloodborne Pathogens
http://www.osha.gov/SLTC/dentistry/index.html
http://www.osha.gov/SLTC/bloodbornepathogens/index.html

Organization for Safety and Asepsis Procedures
http://www.osap.org

Society for Healthcare Epidemiology of America, Inc., Position Papers
http://www.shea-online.org/PositionPapers.html

Acknowledgement
The Division of Oral Health thanks the working group as well as CDC and other federal and external reviewers for their efforts in developing and reviewing drafts of this report and acknowledges that all opinions of the reviewers might not be reflected in all of the recommendations.

REFERENCES

1. CDC. Recommended infection-control practices for dentistry. MMWR 1986;35:237–42.

2. CDC. Recommended infection-control practices for dentistry, 1993. MMWR 1993;42(No. RR-8).

3. US Census Bureau. Statistical Abstract of the United States: 2001. Washington, DC: US Census Bureau, 2001. Available at http://www.census.gov/prod/www/statistical-abstract-02.html.

4. Health Resources and Services Administration, Bureau of Health Professions. United States health workforce personnel factbook. Rockville, MD: US Department of Health and Human Services, Health Resources and Services Administration, 2000.

5. Bolyard EA, Tablan OC, Williams WW, Pearson ML, Shapiro CN, Deitchman SD, Hospital Infection Control Practices Advisory Committee. Guideline for infection control in health care personnel, 1998. Am J Infect Control 1998;26:289–354.

6. Greene VW. Microbiological contamination control in hospitals. 1. Perspectives. Hospitals 1969;43:78–88.

7. CDC. Perspectives in disease prevention and health promotion update: universal precautions for prevention of transmission of human immunodeficiency virus, hepatitis B virus, and other bloodborne pathogens in health-care settings. MMWR 1988;38:377–82, 387–8.

8. CDC. Guidelines for prevention of transmission of human immunodeficiency virus and hepatitis B virus to health-care and public-safety workers: a response to P.L. 100-607 The Health Omnibus Programs Extension Act of 1988. MMWR 1989;38(suppl No. 6S).

9. Garner JS, Favero MS. CDC guideline for handwashing and hospital environmental control, 1985. Infect Control 1986;7:231–43.

10. CDC. Recommendations for prevention of HIV transmission in health-care settings. MMWR 1987;36(suppl No. 2S).

11. Garner JS, Hospital Infection Control Practices Advisory Committee. Guideline for isolation precautions in hospitals. Infect Control Hosp Epidemiol 1996;17:53–80.

12. Chiarello LA, Bartley J. Prevention of blood exposure in health-care personnel. Semin Infect Control 2001;1:30–43.

13. US Department of Labor, Occupational Safety and Health Administration. 29 CFR Part 1910.1030. Occupational exposure to bloodborne pathogens; needlesticks and other sharps injuries; final rule. Federal Register 2001;66:5317–25. As amended from and includes 29 CFR Part 1910.1030. Occupational exposure to bloodborne pathogens; final rule. Federal Register 1991;56:64174–82. Available at http://www.osha.gov/SLTC/dentistry/index.html.

14. US Department of Labor, Occupational Safety and Health Administration. OSHA instruction: enforcement procedures for the occupational exposure to bloodborne pathogens. Washington, DC: US Department of Labor, Occupational Safety and Health Administration, 2001; directive no. CPL 2-2.69.

15. US Department of Labor, Occupational Safety and Health Administration. 29 CFR 1910.1200. Hazard communication. Federal Register 1994;59:17479.

16. Gershon RR, Karkashian CD, Grosch JW, et al. Hospital safety climate and its relationship with safe work practices and workplace exposure incidents. Am J Infect Control 2000;28:211–21.

17. CDC. Immunization of health-care workers: recommendations of the Advisory Committee on Immunization Practices (ACIP) and the Hospital Infection Control Practices Advisory Committee (HICPAC). MMWR 1997;46(No. RR-18).

18. Association for Professionals in Infection Control and Epidemiology. APIC position paper: immunization. Am J Infect Control 1999;27:52–3.

19. CDC. Updated U.S. Public Health Service guidelines for the management of occupational exposures to HBV, HCV, and HIV and recommendations for postexposure prophylaxis. MMWR 2001;50(No. RR-11).

20. CDC. Guidelines for preventing the transmission of *Mycobacterium tuberculosis* in health-care facilities, 1994. MMWR 1994;43(No. RR-13).

21. Cleveland JL, Gooch BF, Bolyard EA, Simone PM, Mullan RJ, Marianos DW. TB infection control recommendations from the CDC, 1994: considerations for dentistry. J Am Dent Assoc 1995;126:593–9.

22. Herwaldt LA, Pottinger JM, Carter CD, Barr BA, Miller ED. Exposure workups. Infect Control Hosp Epidemiol 1997;18:850–71.

23. Nash KD. How infection control procedures are affecting dental practice today. J Am Dent Assoc 1992;123:67–73.

24. Berky ZT, Luciano WJ, James WD. Latex glove allergy: a survey of the US Army Dental Corps. JAMA 1992;268:2695–7.

25. Bubak ME, Reed CE, Fransway AF, et al. Allergic reactions to latex among health-care workers. Mayo Clin Proc 1992;67:1075–9.

26. Fisher AA. Allergic contact reactions in health personnel. J Allergy Clin Immunol 1992;90:729–38.

27. Smart ER, Macleod RI, Lawrence CM. Allergic reactions to rubber gloves in dental patients: report of three cases. Br Dent J 1992;172:445–7.

28. Yassin MS, Lierl MB, Fischer TJ, O'Brien K, Cross J, Steinmetz C. Latex allergy in hospital employees. Ann Allergy 1994;72:245–9.

29. Zaza S, Reeder JM, Charles LE, Jarvis WR. Latex sensitivity among perioperative nurses. AORN J 1994;60:806–12.

30. Hunt LW, Fransway AF, Reed CE, et al. An epidemic of occupational allergy to latex involving health care workers. J Occup Environ Med 1995;37:1204–9.

31. American Dental Association Council on Scientific Affairs. The dental team and latex hypersensitivity. J Am Dent Assoc 1999;130:257–64.

32. CDC. National Institute for Occupational Safety and Health. NIOSH Alert: preventing allergic reactions to natural rubber latex in the workplace. Cincinnati, OH: US Department of Health and Human Services, Public Health Service, CDC, National Institute for Occupational Safety and Health, 1997.

33. Terezhalmy GT, Molinari JA. Personal protective equipment and barrier techniques. In: Cottone JA, Terezhalmy GT, Molinari JA, eds. Practical infection control in dentisty. 2nd ed. Baltimore, MD: Williams & Wilkins, 1996:136–45.

34. US Department of Health and Human Services, Office of the Secretary, Office for Civil Rights. 45 CFR Parts 160 and 164. Standards for privacy of individually identifiable health information; final rule. Federal Register 2000;65:82462–829.

35. Occupational Safety and Health Administration. Access to medical and exposure records. Washington, DC: US Department of Labor, Occupational Safety and Health Administration, 2001. OSHA publication no. 3110.

36. Mast EE, Alter MJ. Prevention of hepatitis B virus infection among health-care workers. In: Ellis RW, ed. Hepatitis B vaccines in clinical practice. New York, NY: Marcel Dekker, 1993:295–307.

37. Beltrami EM, Williams IT, Shapiro CN, Chamberland ME. Risk and management of blood-borne infections in health care workers. Clin Microbiol Rev 2000;13:385–407.

38. Werner BG, Grady GF. Accidental hepatitis-B-surface-antigen-positive inoculations: use of e antigen to estimate infectivity. Ann Intern Med 1982;97:367–9.

39. Bond WW, Petersen NJ, Favero MS. Viral hepatitis B: aspects of environmental control. Health Lab Sci 1977;14:235–52.

40. Garibaldi RA, Hatch FE, Bisno AL, Hatch MH, Gregg MB. Non-parenteral serum hepatitis: report of an outbreak. JAMA 1972;220:963–6.

41. Rosenberg JL, Jones DP, Lipitz LR, Kirsner JB. Viral hepatitis: an occupational hazard to surgeons. JAMA 1973;223:395–400.

42. Callender ME, White YS, Williams R. Hepatitis B virus infection in medical and health care personnel. Br Med J 1982;284:324–6.

43. Chaudhuri AK, Follett EA. Hepatitis B virus infection in medical and health care personnel [Letter]. Br Med J 1982;284:1408.

44. Bond WW, Favero MS, Petersen NJ, Gravelle CR, Ebert JW, Maynard JE. Survival of hepatitis B virus after drying and storage for one week [Letter]. Lancet 1981;1:550–1.

45. Francis DP, Favero MS, Maynard JE. Transmission of hepatitis B virus [Review]. Semin Liver Dis 1981;1:27–32.

46. Favero MS, Maynard JE, Petersen NJ, et al. Hepatitis-B antigen on environmental surfaces [Letter]. Lancet 1973;2:1455.

47. Lauer JL, VanDrunen NA, Washburn JW, Balfour HH Jr. Transmission of hepatitis B virus in clinical laboratory areas. J Infect Dis 1979;140:513–6.

48. Hennekens CH. Hemodialysis-associated hepatitis: an outbreak among hospital personnel. JAMA 1973;225:407–8.

49. Garibaldi RA, Forrest JN, Bryan JA, Hanson BF, Dismukes WE. Hemodialysis-associated hepatitis. JAMA 1973;225:384–9.

50. Snydman DR, Bryan JA, Macon EJ, Gregg MB. Hemodialysis-associated hepatitis: a report of an epidemic with further evidence on mechanisms of transmission. Am J Epidemiol 1976;104:563–70.

51. Shapiro CN. Occupational risk of infection with hepatitis B and hepatitis C virus. Surg Clin North Am 1995;75:1047–56.

52. Cleveland JL, Siew C, Lockwood SA, Gruninger SE, Gooch BF, Shapiro CN. Hepatitis B vaccination and infection among U.S. dentists, 1983–1992. J Am Dent Assoc 1996;127:1385–90.

53. CDC. Recommendations for preventing transmission of human immunodeficiency virus and hepatitis B virus to patients during exposure-prone invasive procedures. MMWR 1991;40(No. RR-8).

54. Chamberland ME. HIV transmission from health care worker to patient: what is the risk [Letter]? Ann Intern Med 1992;116:871–3.

55. Robert LM, Chamberland ME, Cleveland JL, et al. Investigation of patients of health care workers infected with HIV: the Centers for Disease Control and Prevention database. Ann Intern Med 1995;122:653–7.

56. CDC. Investigations of persons treated by HIV-infected health-care workers—United States. MMWR 1993;42:329–31, 37.

57. Siew C, Chang SB, Gruninger SE, Verrusio AC, Neidle EA. Self-reported percutaneous injuries in dentists: implications for HBV, HIV, transmission risk. J Am Dent Assoc 1992;123:36–44.

58. Ahtone J, Goodman RA. Hepatitis B and dental personnel: transmission to patients and prevention issues. J Am Dent Assoc 1983;106:219–22.

59. Hadler SC, Sorley DL, Acree KH, et al. An outbreak of hepatitis B in a dental practice. Ann Intern Med 1981;95:133–8.

60. CDC. Epidemiologic notes and reports: hepatitis B among dental patients—Indiana. MMWR 1985;34:73–5.

61. Levin ML, Maddrey WC, Wands JR, Mendeloff AL. Hepatitis B transmission by dentists. JAMA 1974;228:1139–40.

62. Rimland D, Parkin WE, Miller GB Jr, Schrack WD. Hepatitis B outbreak traced to an oral surgeon. N Engl J Med 1977;296:953–8.

63. Goodwin D, Fannin SL, McCracken BB. An oral surgeon-related hepatitis-B outbreak. California Morbidity 1976;14:1.

64. Reingold AL, Kane MA, Murphy BL, Checko P, Francis DP, Maynard JE. Transmission of hepatitis B by an oral surgeon. J Infect Dis 1982;145:262–8.

65. Goodman RA, Ahtone JL, Finton RJ. Hepatitis B transmission from dental personnel to patients: unfinished business. Ann Intern Med 1982;96:119.

66. Shaw FE Jr, Barrett CL, Hamm R, et al. Lethal outbreak of hepatitis B in a dental practice. JAMA 1986;255:3260–4.

67. CDC. Epidemiologic notes and reports: outbreak of hepatitis B associated with an oral surgeon—New Hampshire. MMWR 1987;36:132–3.

68. US Department of Labor, Occupational Safety and Health Administration. 29 CFR Part 1910.1030. Occupational exposure to bloodborne pathogens; final rule. Federal Register 1991;56:64004–182.

69. CDC. Hepatitis B virus: a comprehensive strategy for eliminating transmission in the United States through universal childhood vaccination: recommendations of the Immunization Practices Advisory Committee (ACIP). MMWR 1991;40(No. RR-13).

70. Polish LB, Gallagher M, Fields HA, Hadler SC. Delta hepatitis: molecular biology and clinical and epidemiological features. Clin Microbiol Rev 1993;6:211–29.

71. Alter MJ. The epidemiology of acute and chronic hepatitis C. Clin Liver Dis 1997;1:559–68.

72. Puro V, Petrosillo N, Ippolito G. Risk of hepatitis C seroconversion after occupational exposures in health care workers: Italian Study Group on Occupational Risk of HIV and Other Bloodborne Infections. Am J Infect Control 1995;23:273–7.

73. Lanphear BP, Linnemann CC Jr, Cannon CG, DeRonde MM, Pendy L, Kerley LM. Hepatitis C virus infection in healthcare workers: risk of exposure and infection. Infect Control Hosp Epidemiol 1994;15:745–50.

74. Mitsui T, Iwano K, Masuko K, et al. Hepatitis C virus infection in medical personnel after needlestick accident. Hepatology 1992;16:1109–14.

75. Sartori M, La Terra G, Aglietta M, Manzin A, Navino C, Verzetti G. Transmission of hepatitis C via blood splash into conjunctiva. Scand J Infect Dis 1993;25:270–1.

76. Ippolito G, Puro V, De Carli G. The risk of occupational human immunodeficiency virus in health care workers: Italian Multicenter Study, The Italian Study Group on Occupational Risk of HIV Infection. Arch Intern Med 1993;153:1451–8.

77. Beltrami EM, Kozak A, Williams IT, et al. Transmission of HIV and hepatitis C virus from a nursing home patient to a health care worker. Am J Infect Control. 2003;31:168–75.

78. Cooper BW, Krusell A, Tilton RC, Goodwin R, Levitz RE. Seroprevalence of antibodies to hepatitis C virus in high-risk hospital personnel. Infect Control Hosp Epidemiol 1992;13:82–5.

79. Panlilio AL, Shapiro CN, Schable CA, et al. Serosurvey of human immunodeficiency virus, hepatitis B virus, and hepatitis C virus infection among hospital-based surgeons. Serosurvey Study Group. J Am Coll Surg 1995;180:16–24.

80. Polish LB, Tong MJ, Co RL, Coleman PJ, Alter MJ. Risk factors for hepatitis C virus infection among health care personnel in a community hospital. Am J Infect Control 1993;21:196–200.

81. Shapiro CN, Tokars JI, Chamberland ME, American Academy of Orthopaedic Surgeons Serosurvey Study Committee. Use of the hepatitis-B vaccine and infection with hepatitis B and C among orthopaedic surgeons. J Bone Joint Surg Am 1996;78:1791–800.

82. Gerberding JL. Incidence and prevalence of human immunodeficiency virus, hepatitis B virus, hepatitis C virus, and cytomegalovirus among health care personnel at risk for blood exposure: final report from a longitudinal study. J Infect Dis 1994;170:1410–7.

83. Klein RS, Freeman K, Taylor PE, Stevens CE. Occupational risk for hepatitis C virus infection among New York City dentists. Lancet 1991;338:1539–42.

84. Thomas DL, Gruninger SE, Siew C, Joy ED, Quinn TC. Occupational risk of hepatitis C infections among general dentists and oral surgeons in North America. Am J Med 1996;100:41–5.

85. Cleveland JL, Gooch BF, Shearer BG, Lyerla RL. Risk and prevention of hepatitis C virus infection: implications for dentistry. J Am Dent Assoc 1999;130:641–7.

86. Gruninger SE, Siew C, Azzolin KL, Meyer DM. Update of hepatitis C infection among dental professionals [Abstract 1825]. J Dent Res 2001;80:264.

87. Esteban JI, Gomez J, Martell M, et al. Transmission of hepatitis C virus by a cardiac surgeon. N Engl J Med 1996;334:555–60.

88. Duckworth GJ, Heptonstall J, Aitken C. Transmission of hepatitis C virus from a surgeon to a patient: the Incident Control Team. Commun Dis Public Health 1999;2:188–92.

89. Ross RS, Viazov S, Gross T, Hofmann F, Seipp HM, Roggendorf M. Brief report: transmission of hepatitis C virus from a patient to an anesthesiology assistant to five patients. N Engl J Med 2000;343:1851–4.

90. Cody SH, Nainan OV, Garfein RS, et al. Hepatitis C virus transmission from an anesthesiologist to a patient. Arch Intern Med 2002;162:345–50.

91. Do AN, Ciesielski CA, Metler RP, Hammett TA, Li J, Fleming PL. Occupationally acquired human immunodeficiency virus (HIV) infection: national case surveillance data during 20 years of the HIV epidemic in the United States. Infect Control Hosp Epidemiol 2003;24:86–96.

92. Ciesielski C, Marianos D, Ou CY, et al. Transmission of human immunodeficiency virus in a dental practice. Ann Intern Med 1992;116:798–805.

93. CDC. Investigations of patients who have been treated by HIV-infected health-care workers—United States. MMWR 1993;42: 329–31, 337.

94. Bell DM. Occupational risk of human immunodeficiency virus infection in healthcare workers: an overview. Am J Med 1997;102(5B):9–15.

95. Cardo DM, Culver DH, Ciesielski CA, et al, Centers for Disease Control and Prevention Needlestick Surveillance Group. A case-control study of HIV seroconversion in health care workers after percutaneous exposure. N Engl J Med 1997;337:1485–90.

96. Beltrami EM. The risk and prevention of occupational human immunodeficiency virus infection. Semin Infect Control 2001;1:2–18.

97. CDC. National Institute for Occupational Safety and Health. NIOSH alert: Preventing needlestick injuries in health care settings. Cincinnati, OH: US Department of Health and Human Services, Public Health Service, CDC, National Institute for Occupational Safety and Health, 1999.

98. Klein RS, Phelan JA, Freeman K, et al. Low occupational risk of human immunodeficiency virus infection among dental professionals. N Engl J Med 1988;318:86–90.

99. Gruninger SE, Siew C, Chang SB, et al. Human immunodeficiency virus type I: infection among dentists. J Am Dent Assoc 1992;123:59–64.

100. Siew C, Gruninger SE, Miaw CL, Neidle EA. Percutaneous injuries in practicing dentists: a prospective study using a 20-day diary. J Am Dent Assoc 1995;126:1227–34.

101. Cleveland JL, Lockwood SA, Gooch BF, et al. Percutaneous injuries in dentistry: an observational study. J Am Dent Assoc 1995;126:745–51.

102. Ramos-Gomez F, Ellison J, Greenspan D, Bird W, Lowe S, Gerberding JL. Accidental exposures to blood and body fluids

among health care workers in dental teaching clinics: a prospective study. J Am Dent Assoc 1997;128:1253–61.

103. Cleveland JL, Gooch BF, Lockwood SA. Occupational blood exposure in dentistry: a decade in review. Infect Control Hosp Epidemiol 1997;18:717–21.

104. Gooch BF, Siew C, Cleveland JL, Gruninger SE, Lockwood SA, Joy ED. Occupational blood exposure and HIV infection among oral and maxillofacial surgeons. Oral Surg Oral Med Oral Pathol Oral Radiol Endod 1998;85:128–34.

105. Gooch BF, Cardo DM, Marcus R, et al. Percutaneous exposures to HIV–infected blood among dental workers enrolled in the CDC needlestick study. J Am Dent Assoc 1995;126:1237–42.

106. Younai FS, Murphy DC, Kotelchuck D. Occupational exposures to blood in a dental teaching environment: results of a ten-year surveillance study. J Dent Educ 2001;65:436–8.

107. Carlton JE, Dodson TB, Cleveland JL, Lockwood SA. Percutaneous injuries during oral and maxillofacial surgery procedures. J Oral Maxillofac Surg 1997;55:553–6.

108. Harte J, Davis R, Plamondon T, Richardson B. The influence of dental unit design on percutaneous injury. J Am Dent Assoc 1998;129:1725–31.

109. US Department of Labor, Occupational Health and Safety Administration. 29 CFR Part 1910. Occupational exposure to bloodborne pathogens; needlesticks and other sharps injuries, final rule. Federal Register 2001;66:5325.

110. CDC. Evaluation of safety devices for preventing percutaneous injuries among health-care workers during phlebotomy procedures—Minneapolis-St. Paul, New York City, and San Francisco, 1993–1995. MMWR 1997;46:21–5.

111. CDC. Evaluation of blunt suture needles in preventing percutaneous injuries among health-care workers during gynecologic surgical procedures—New York City, March 1993–June 1994. MMWR 1997;46:25–9.

112. Mendelson MH, Lin-Chen BY, Solomon R, Bailey E, Kogan G, Goldbold J. Evaluation of a safety resheathable winged steel needle for prevention of percutaneous injuries associated with intravascular-access procedures among healthcare workers. Infect Control Hosp Epidemiol 2003;24:105–12.

113. CDC. Recommendations for prevention of HIV transmission in health-care settings. MMWR 1987;36(No. S2).

114. CDC. Guidelines for prevention of transmission of human immunodeficiency virus and hepatitis B virus to health-care and public-safety workers: a response to P.L. 100-607. The Health Omnibus Programs Extension Act of 1988. MMWR 1989;38(No. S6).

115. CDC. National Institute for Occupational Safety and Health. Selecting, evaluating, and using sharps disposal containers. Cincinnati, OH: US Department of Health and Human Services, Public Health Service, CDC, National Institute for Occupational Safety and Health, 1998. DHHS publication no. (NIOSH) 97-111.

116. CDC. Public Health Service statement on management of occupational exposure to human immunodeficiency virus, including considerations regarding zidovudine postexposure use. MMWR 1990;39 (No. RR-1).

117. CDC. Notice to readers update: provisional Public Health Service recommendations for chemoprophylaxis after occupational exposure to HIV. MMWR 1996;45:468–72.

118. CDC. Public Health Service guidelines for the management of health-care worker exposures to HIV and recommendations for postexposure prophylaxis. MMWR 1998;47(No. RR-7).

119. CDC. Recommendations for prevention and control of hepatitis C virus (HCV) infection and HCV-related chronic disease. MMWR 1998;47(No. RR-19).

120. Steere AC, Mallison GF. Handwashing practices for the prevention of nosocomial infections. Ann Intern Med 1975;83:683–90.

121. Garner JS. CDC guideline for prevention of surgical wound infections, 1985. Supersedes guideline for prevention of surgical wound infections published in 1982. (Originally published in November 1985). Revised. Infect Control 1986;7:193–200.

122. Larson EL. APIC guideline for hand washing and hand antisepsis in health-care settings. Am J Infect Control 1995;23:251–69.

123. CDC. Guideline for hand hygiene in health-care settings: recommendations of the Healthcare Infection Control Practices Advisory Committee and the HICPAC/SHEA/APIC/IDSA Hand Hygiene Task Force. MMWR 2002;51(No. RR-16).

124. Casewell M, Phillips I. Hands as route of transmission for *Klebsiella* species. Br Med J 1977;2:1315–7.

125. Larson EL, Early E, Cloonan P, Sugrue S, Parides M. An organizational climate intervention associated with increased handwashing and decreased nosocomial infections. Behav Med 2000;26:14–22.

126. Pittet D, Hugonnet S, Harbarth S, et al. Effectiveness of a hospital-wide programme to improve compliance with hand hygiene. Lancet 2000;356:1307–12.

127. Price PB. New studies in surgical bacteriology and surgical technique. JAMA 1938;111:1993–6.

128. Dewar NE, Gravens DL. Effectiveness of septisol antiseptic foam as a surgical scrub agent. Appl Microbiol 1973;26:544–9.

129. Lowbury EJ, Lilly HA. Disinfection of the hands of surgeons and nurses. Br Med J 1960;1445–50.

130. Rotter M. Hand washing and hand disinfection. In: Mayhall CG, ed. Hospital epidemiology and infection control. 2nd ed. Philadelphia, PA: Lippincott Williams & Wilkins, 1999:1339–55.

131. Widmer AF. Replace hand washing with use of a waterless alcohol hand rub? Clin Infect Dis 2000;31:136–43.

132. Larson EL, Butz AM, Gullette DL, Laughon BA. Alcohol for surgical scrubbing? Infect Control Hosp Epidemiol 1990;11:139–43.

133. Faoagali J, Fong J, George N, Mahoney P, O'Rouke V. Comparison of the immediate, residual, and cumulative antibacterial effects of Novaderm R,* Novascrub R,* Betadine Surgical Scrub, Hibiclens, and liquid soap. Am J Infect Control 1995;23:337–43.

134. Association of Perioperative Registered Nurses. Recommended practices for sterilization in the practice setting. In: Fogg D, Parker N, Shevlin D, eds. 2002 standards, recommended practices, and guidelines. Denver, CO: AORN, 2002:333–42.

135. US Department Of Health and Human Services, Food and Drug Administration. Tentative final monograph for healthcare antiseptic drug products; proposed rule. Federal Register 1994;59:31441–52.

136. Larson E. A causal link between handwashing and risk of infection? Examination of the evidence. Infect Control.1988;9:28–36.

137. Mangram AJ, Horan TC, Pearson ML, Silver LC, Jarvis WR, Hospital Infection Control Practices Advisory Committee. Guideline for prevention of surgical site infection, 1999. Infect Control Hosp Epidemiol 1999;20:250–78.

138. Doebbeling BN, Pfaller MA, Houston AK, Wenzel RP. Removal of nosocomial pathogens from the contaminated glove. Ann Intern Med 1988;109:394–8.

139. Kabara JJ, Brady MB. Contamination of bar soaps under "in-use" conditions. J Environ Pathol Toxicol Oncol 1984;5:1–14.

140. Ojajärvi J. The importance of soap selection for routine hand hygiene in hospital. J Hyg (Lond) 1981;86:275–83.

141. Larson E, Leyden JJ, McGinley KJ, Grove GL, Talbot GH. Physiologic and microbiologic changes in skin related to frequent handwashing. Infect Control 1986;7:59–63.

142. Larson E. Handwashing: it's essential—even when you use gloves. Am J Nurs 1989;89:934–9.

143. Field EA, McGowan P, Pearce PK, Martin MV. Rings and watches: should they be removed prior to operative dental procedures? J Dent 1996;24:65–9.

144. Hobson DW, Woller W, Anderson L, Guthery E. Development and evaluation of a new alcohol-based surgical hand scrub formulation with persistent antimicrobial characteristics and brushless application. Am J Infect Control 1998;26:507–12.

145. Mulberry G, Snyder AT, Heilman J, Pyrek J, Stahl J. Evaluation of a waterless, scrubless chlorhexidine gluconate/ethanol surgical scrub for antimicrobial efficacy. Am J Infect Control 2001;29:377–82.

146. Association of Perioperative Registered Nurses. Recommended practices for surgical hand scrubs. In: Fogg D, Parker N, eds. 2003 standards, recommended practices, and guidelines. Denver, CO: AORN, Inc., 2003:277–80.

147. Larson E, Killien M. Factors influencing handwashing behavior of patient care personnel. Am J Infect Control 1982;10:93–9.

148. Zimakoff J, Kjelsberg AB, Larson SO, Holstein B. A multicenter questionnaire investigation of attitudes toward hand hygiene, assessed by the staff in fifteen hospitals in Denmark and Norway. Am J Infect Control 1992;20:58–64.

149. Grohskopf LA, Roth VR, Feikin DR, et al. *Serratia liquefaciens* bloodstream infections from contamination of epoetin alfa at a hemodialysis center. N Engl J Med 2001;344:1491–7.

150. Archibald LK, Corl A, Shah B, et al. *Serratia marcescens* outbreak associated with extrinsic contamination of 1% chlorxylenol soap. Infect Control Hosp Epidemiol 1997;18:704–9.

151. Larson EL, Norton Hughes CA, Pyrak JD, Sparks SM, Cagatay EU, Bartkus JM. Changes in bacterial flora associated with skin damage on hands of health care personnel. Am J Infect Control 1998;26:513–21.

152. Ojajärvi J, Mäkelä P, Rantasalo I. Failure of hand disinfection with frequent hand washing: a need for prolonged field studies. J Hyg (Lond) 1977;79:107–19.

153. Berndt U, Wigger-Alberti W, Gabard B, Elsner P. Efficacy of a barrier cream and its vehicle as protective measures against occupational irritant contact dermatitis. Contact Dermatitis 2000;42:77–80.

154. McCormick RD, Buchman TL, Maki DG. Double-blind, randomized trial of scheduled use of a novel barrier cream and an oil-containing lotion for protecting the hands of health care workers. Am J Infect Control 2000;28:302–10.

155. Larson E, Anderson JK, Baxendale L, Bobo L. Effects of a protective foam on scrubbing and gloving. Am J Infect Control 1993;21:297–301.

156. McGinley KJ, Larson EL, Leyden JJ. Composition and density of microflora in the subungual space of the hand. J Clin Microbiol 1988;26:950–3.

157. Pottinger J, Burns S, Manske C. Bacterial carriage by artificial versus natural nails. Am J Infect Control 1989;17:340–4.

158. McNeil SA, Foster CL, Hedderwick SA, Kauffman CA. Effect of hand cleansing with antimicrobial soap or alcohol-based gel on microbial colonization of artificial fingernails worn by health care workers. Clin Infect Dis 2001;32:367–72.

159. Rubin DM. Prosthetic fingernails in the OR: a research study. AORN J 1988;47:944–5.

160. Hedderwick SA, McNeil SA, Lyons MJ, Kauffman CA. Pathogenic organisms associated with artificial fingernails worn by healthcare workers. Infect Control Hosp Epidemiol 2000;21:505–9.

161. Passaro DJ, Waring L, Armstrong R, et al. Postoperative *Serratia marcescens* wound infections traced to an out-of-hospital source. J Infect Dis 1997;175:992–5.

162. Foca M, Jakob K, Whittier S, et al. Endemic *Pseudomonas aeruginosa* infection in a neonatal intensive care unit. N Engl J Med 2000;343:695–700.

163. Parry MF, Grant B, Yukna M, et al. Candida osteomyelitis and diskitis after spinal surgery: an outbreak that implicates artificial nail use. Clin Infect Dis 2001;32:352–7.

164. Moolenaar RL, Crutcher M, San Joaquin VH, et al. A prolonged outbreak of *Pseudomonas aeruginosa* in a neonatal intensive care unit: did staff fingernails play a role in disease transmission? Infect Control Hosp Epidemiol 2000;21:80–5.

165. Baumgardner CA, Maragos CS, Walz J, Larson E. Effects of nail polish on microbial growth of fingernails: dispelling sacred cows. AORN J 1993;58:84–8.

166. Wynd CA, Samstag DE, Lapp AM. Bacterial carriage on the fingernails of OR nurses. AORN J 1994;60:796, 799–805.

167. Lowbury EJ. Aseptic methods in the operating suite. Lancet 1968;1:705–9.

168. Hoffman PN, Cooke EM, McCarville MR, Emmerson AM. Micro-organisms isolated from skin under wedding rings worn by hospital staff. Br Med J 1985;290:206–7.

169. Jacobson G, Thiele JE, McCune JH, Farrell LD. Handwashing: ring-wearing and number of microorganisms. Nurs Res 1985;34:186–8.

170. Trick WE, Vernon MO, Hayes RA, et al. Impact of ring wearing on hand contamination and comparison of hand hygiene agents in a hospital. Clin Infect Dis 2003;36:1383–90.

171. Salisbury DM, Hutfilz P, Treen LM, Bollin GE, Gautam S. The effect of rings on microbial load of health care workers' hands. Am J Infect Control 1997;25:24–7.

172. Cochran MA, Miller CH, Sheldrake MS. The efficacy of the rubber dam as a barrier to the spread of microorganisms during dental treatment. J Am Dent Assoc 1989;119:141–4.

173. Miller CH, Palenik DJ. Aseptic techniques [Chapter 10]. In: Miller CH, Palenik DJ, eds. Infection control and management of hazardous materials for the dental team. 2nd ed. St. Louis, MO: Mosby, 1998.

174. CDC. National Institute for Occupational Safety and Health. TB respiratory protection program in health care facilities: administrator's guide. Cincinnati, OH: US Department of Health and Human Services, Public Health Service, CDC, National Institute for Occupational Safety and Health, 1999. DHHS publication no. (NIOSH) 99-143.

175. US Department of Labor, Occupational Safety and Health Administration. OSHA 29 CFR 1910.139. Respiratory protection for *M. tuberculosis*. Federal Register 1998;49:442–9.

176. CDC. National Institute for Occupational Safety and Health. NIOSH guide to the selection and use of particulate respirators certified under 42 CFR 84. Cincinnati, OH: US Department of Health and Human Services, Public Health Service, CDC, National Institute for Occupational Safety and Health, 1996. DHHS publication no. (NIOSH) 96-101.

177. DeGroot-Kosolcharoen J, Jones JM. Permeability of latex and vinyl gloves to water and blood. Am J Infect Control 1989;17:196–201.

178. Korniewicz DM, Laughon BE, Butz A, Larson E. Integrity of vinyl and latex procedure gloves. Nurs Res 1989;38:144–6.

179. Olsen RJ, Lynch P, Coyle MB, Cummings J, Bokete T, Stamm WE. Examination gloves as barriers to hand contamination in clinical practice. JAMA 1993;270:350–3.

180. Murray CA, Burke FJ, McHugh S. An assessment of the incidence of punctures in latex and non-latex dental examination gloves in routine clinical practice. Br Dent J 2001;190:377–80.

181. Burke FJ, Baggett FJ, Lomax AM. Assessment of the risk of glove puncture during oral surgery procedures. Oral Surg Oral Med Oral Pathol Oral Radiol Endod 1996;82:18–21.

182. Burke FJ, Wilson NH. The incidence of undiagnosed punctures in non-sterile gloves. Br Dent J 1990;168:67–71.

183. Nikawa H, Hamada T, Tamamoto M, Abekura H. Perforation and proteinaceous contamination of dental gloves during prosthodontic treatments. Int J Prosthodont 1994;7:559–66.

184. Nikawa H, Hamada T, Tamamoto M, Abekura H, Murata H. Perforation of dental gloves during prosthodontic treatments as assessed by the conductivity and water inflation tests. Int J Prosthodont 1996;9:362–6.

185. Avery CM, Hjort A, Walsh S, Johnson PA. Glove perforation during surgical extraction of wisdom teeth. Oral Surg Oral Med Oral Pathol Oral Radiol Endod 1998;86:23–5.

186. Otis LL, Cottone JA. Prevalence of perforations in disposable latex gloves during routine dental treatment. J Am Dent Assoc 1989;118:321–4.

187. Kotilainen HR, Brinker JP, Avato JL, Gantz NM. Latex and vinyl examination gloves. Quality control procedures and implications for health care workers. Arch Intern Med 1989;149:2749–53.

188. Food and Drug Administration. Glove powder report. Rockville, MD: US Department of Health and Human Services, Food and Drug Administration, 1997. Available at http://www.fda.gov/cdrh/glvpwd.html.

189. Morgan DJ, Adams D. Permeability studies on protective gloves used in dental practice. Br Dent J 1989;166:11–3.

190. Albin MS, Bunegin L, Duke ES, Ritter RR, Page CP. Anatomy of a defective barrier: sequential glove leak detection in a surgical and dental environment. Crit Care Med 1992;20:170–84.

191. Merchant VA, Molinari JA, Pickett T. Microbial penetration of gloves following usage in routine dental procedures. Am J Dent 1992;5:95–6.

192. Pitten FA, Herdemann G, Kramer A. The integrity of latex gloves in clinical dental practice. Infection 2000;28:388–92.

193. Jamal A, Wilkinson S. The mechanical and microbiological integrity of surgical gloves. ANZ J Surg 2003;73:140–3.

194. Korniewicz DM, El-Masri MM, Broyles JM, Martin CD, O'Connell KP. A laboratory-based study to assess the performance of surgical gloves. AORN J 2003;77:772–9.

195. Schwimmer A, Massoumi M, Barr CE. Efficacy of double gloving to prevent inner glove perforation during outpatient oral surgical procedures. J Am Dent Assoc 1994;125:196–8.

196. Patton LL, Campbell TL, Evers SP. Prevalence of glove perforations during double-gloving for dental procedures. Gen Dent 1995;43:22–6.

197. Gerberding JL, Littell C, Tarkington A, Brown A, Schecter WP. Risk of exposure of surgical personnel to patients' blood during surgery at San Francisco General Hospital. N Engl J Med 1990;322:1788–93.

198. Klein RC, Party E, Gershey EL. Virus penetration of examination gloves. Biotechniques 1990;9:196–9.

199. Mellstrom GA, Lindberg M, Boman A. Permeation and destructive effects of disinfectants on protective gloves. Contact Dermatitis 1992;26:163–70.

200. Jordan SL, Stowers MF, Trawick EG, Theis AB. Glutaraldehyde permeation: choosing the proper glove. Am J Infect Control 1996;24:67–9.

201. Cappuccio WR, Lees PS, Breysse PN, Margolick JB. Evaluation of integrity of gloves used in a flow cytometry laboratory. Infect Control Hosp Epidemiol 1997;18:423–5.

202. Monticello MV, Gaber DJ. Glove resistance to permeation by a 7.5% hydrogen peroxide sterilizing and disinfecting solution. Am J Infect Control 1999;27:364–6.

203. Baumann MA, Rath B, Fischer JH, Iffland R. The permeability of dental procedure and examination gloves by an alcohol based disinfectant. Dent Mater 2000;16:139–44.

204. Ready MA, Schuster GS, Wilson JT, Hanes CM. Effects of dental medicants on examination glove permeability. J Prosthet Dent 1989;61:499–503.

205. Richards JM, Sydiskis RJ, Davidson WM, Josell SD, Lavine DS. Permeability of latex gloves after contact with dental materials. Am J Orthod Dentofacial Orthop 1993;104:224–9.

206. Andersson T, Bruze M, Bjorkner B. In vivo testing of the protection of gloves against acrylates in dentin-bonding systems on patients with known contact allergy to acrylates. Contact Dermatitis 1999;41:254–9.

207. Reitz CD, Clark NP. The setting of vinyl polysiloxane and condensation silicone putties when mixed with gloved hands. J Am Dent Assoc 1988;116:371–5.

208. Kahn RL, Donovan TE, Chee WW. Interaction of gloves and rubber dam with a poly (vinyl siloxane) impression material: a screening test. Int J Prosthodont 1989;2:342–6.

209. Matis BA, Valadez D, Valadez E. The effect of the use of dental gloves on mixing vinyl polysiloxane putties. J Prosthodont 1997;6:189–92.

210. Wright JG, McGeer AJ, Chyatte D, Ransohoff DF. Mechanisms of glove tears and sharp injuries among surgical personnel. JAMA 1991;266:1668–71.

211. Dodds RD, Guy PJ, Peacock AM, Duffy SR, Barker SG, Thomas MH. Surgical glove perforation. Br J Surg 1988;75:966–8.

212. Adams D, Bagg J, Limaye M, Parsons K, Absi EG. A clinical evaluation of glove washing and re-use in dental practice. J Hosp Infect 1992;20:153–62.

213. Martin MV, Dunn HM, Field EA, et al. A physical and microbiological evaluation of the re-use of non-sterile gloves. Br Dent J 1988;165:321–4.

214. US Department of Health and Human Services, Food and Drug Administration. 21 CFR Part 800. Medical devices; patient examination and surgeon's gloves. Adulteration, final rule. Federal Register 1990;55:51254–8.

215. Giglio JA, Roland RW, Laskin DM, Grenevicki L. The use of sterile versus nonsterile gloves during out-patient exodontia. Quintessence Int 1993;24:543–5.

216. Cheung LK, Chow LK, Tsang MH, Tung LK. An evaluation of complications following dental extractions using either sterile or clean gloves. Int J Oral Maxillofac Surg 2001;30:550–4.

217. Gani JS, Anseline PF, Bissett RL. Efficacy of double versus single gloving in protecting the operating team. Aust N Z J Surg 1990;60:171–5.

218. Short LJ, Bell DM. Risk of occupational infection with blood-borne pathogens in operating and delivery room settings. Am J Infect Control 1993;21:343–50.

219. Tokars JI, Culver DH, Mendelson MH, et al. Skin and mucous membrane contacts with blood during surgical procedures: risk and prevention. Infect Control Hosp Epidemiol 1995;16:703–11.

220. Tanner J, Parkinson H. Double gloving to reduce surgical cross-infection (Cochrane Review). The Cochrane Library 2003;(Issue 2):1–32.

221. Webb JM, Pentlow BD. Double gloving and surgical technique. Ann R Coll Surg Engl 1993;75:291–2.

222. Watts D, Tassler PL, Dellon AL. The effect of double gloving on cutaneous sensibility, skin compliance and suture identification. Contemp Surg 1994;44:289–92.

223. Wilson SJ, Sellu D, Uy A, Jaffer MA. Subjective effects of double gloves on surgical performance. Ann R Coll Surg Engl 1996;78:20–2.

224. Food and Drug Administration. Guidance for industry and FDA: medical glove guidance manual [Draft guidance]. Rockville, MD: US Department of Health and Human Services, Food and Drug Administration, 1999. Available at http://www.fda.gov/cdrh/dsma/135.html#_Toc458914315.

225. Dillard SF, Hefflin B, Kaczmarek RG, Petsonk EL, Gross TP. Health effects associated with medical glove use. AORN J 2002;76:88–96.

226. Hamann CP, Turjanmaa K, Rietschel R, et al. Natural rubber latex hypersensitivity: incidence and prevalence of type I allergy in the dental professional. J Am Dent Assoc 1998;129:43–54.

227. Siew C, Hamann C, Gruninger SE, Rodgers P, Sullivan KM. Type I Latex Allergic Reactions among Dental Professionals, 1996–2001. J Dent Res 2003;82(Special Issue):1718.

228. Saary MJ, Kanani A, Alghadeer H, Holness DL, Tarlo SM. Changes in rates of natural rubber latex sensitivity among dental school students and staff members after changes in latex gloves. J Allergy Clin Immunol 2002;109:131–5.

229. Hunt LW, Kelkar P, Reed CE, Yunginger JW. Management of occupational allergy to natural rubber latex in a medical center: the importance of quantitative latex allergen measurement and objective follow-up. J Allergy Clin Immunol 2002;110(suppl 2):S96–106.

230. Turjanmaa K, Kanto M, Kautiainen H, Reunala T, Palosuo T. Long-term outcome of 160 adult patients with natural rubber latex allergy. J Allergy Clin Immunol 2002;110(suppl 2):S70–4.

231. Heilman DK, Jones RT, Swanson MC, Yunginger JW. A prospective, controlled study showing that rubber gloves are the major contributor to latex aeroallergen levels in the operating room. J Allergy Clin Immunol 1996;98:325–30.

232. Baur X, Jager D. Airborne antigens from latex gloves. Lancet 1990;335:912.

233. Turjanmaa K, Reunala T, Alenius H, Brummer-Korvenkontio H, Palosuo T. Allergens in latex surgical gloves and glove powder. Lancet 1990;336:1588.

234. Baur X, Chen Z, Allmers H. Can a threshold limit value for natural rubber latex airborne allergens be defined? J Allergy Clin Immunol 1998;101:24–7.

235. Trape M, Schenck P, Warren A. Latex gloves use and symptoms in health care workers 1 year after implementation of a policy restricting the use of powdered gloves. Am J Infect Control 2000;28:352–8.

236. Allmers H, Brehler R, Chen Z, Raulf-Heimsoth M, Fels H, Baur X. Reduction of latex aeroallergens and latex-specific IgE antibodies in sensitized workers after removal of powdered natural rubber latex gloves in a hospital. Allergy Clin Immunol 1998;102:841–6.

237. Tarlo SM, Sussman G, Contala A, Swanson MC. Control of airborne latex by use of powder-free latex gloves. J Allergy Clin Immunol 1994;93:985–9.

238. Swanson MC, Bubak ME, Hunt LW, Yunginger JW, Warner MA, Reed CE. Quantification of occupational latex aeroallergens in a medical center. J Allergy Clin Immunol 1994;94:445–551.

239. Hermesch CB, Spackman GK, Dodge WW, Salazar A. Effect of powder-free latex examination glove use on airborne powder levels in a dental school clinic. J Dent Educ 1999;63:814–20.

240. Miller CH. Infection control strategies for the dental office [Chapter 29]. In: Ciancio SG, ed. ADA guide to dental therapeutics. 2nd ed. Chicago, IL: ADA Publishing, 2000:543–58.

241. Primeau MN, Adkinson NF Jr, Hamilton RG. Natural rubber pharmaceutical vial closures release latex allergens that produce skin reactions. J Allergy Clin Immunol 2001;107:958–62.

242. Spaulding EH. Chemical disinfection of medical and surgical materials [Chapter 32]. In: Lawrence CA, Block SS, eds.

Disinfection, sterilization and preservation. Philadelphia, PA: Lea & Febiger, 1968: 517–31.

243. CDC. Guideline for disinfection and sterilization in healthcare facilities: recommendations of CDC and the Healthcare Infection Control Practices Advisory Committee (HICPAC). MMWR (in press).

244. CDC. Guidelines for environmental infection control in health-care facilities: recommendations of CDC and the Healthcare Infection Control Practices Advisory Committee (HICPAC). MMWR 2003;52(No. RR-10).

245. US Environmental Protection Agency. 40 CFR Parts 152, 156, and 158. Exemption of certain pesticide substances from federal insecticide, fungicide, and rodenticide act requirements. Amended 1996. Federal Register 1996;61:8876–9.

246. Food and Drug Administration. Dental handpiece sterilization [Letter]. Rockville, MD: US Department of Health and Human Services, Food and Drug Administration, 1992.

247. Association for the Advancement of Medical Instrumentation, American National Standards Institute. Steam sterilization and sterility assurance in health care facilities. ANSI/AAMI ST46-2002. Arlington, VA: Association for the Advancement of Medical Instrumentation, 2002.

248. Association for the Advancement of Medical Instrumentation, American National Standards Institute. Steam sterilization and sterility assurance using table-top sterilizers in office-based, ambulatory-care medical, surgical, and dental facilities. ANSI/AAMI ST40-1998. Arlington, VA: Association for the Advancement of Medical Instrumentation, 1998.

249. Favero MS, Bond WW. Chemical disinfection of medical and surgical material [Chapter 43]. In: Block SS, ed. Disinfection, sterilization and preservation. 5th ed. Philadelphia, PA: Lippincott Williams & Wilkins, 2001:881–917.

250. Parker HH 4th, Johnson RB. Effectiveness of ethylene oxide for sterilization of dental handpieces. J Dent 1995;23:113–5.

251. Alfa MJ, Olson N, Degagne P, Hizon R. New low temperature sterilization technologies: microbicidal activity and clinical efficacy [Chapter 9]. In: Rutala WA, ed. Disinfection, sterilization, and antisepsis in health-care. Champlain, NY: Polyscience Publications, 1998:67–78.

252. Rutala WA, Weber DJ. Clinical effectiveness of low-temperature sterilization technologies. Infect Control Hosp Epidemiol 1998;19:798–804.

253. Miller CH, Tan CM, Beiswanger MA, Gaines DJ, Setcos JC, Palenik CJ. Cleaning dental instruments: measuring the effectiveness of an instrument washer/disinfector. Am J Dent 2000;13:39–43.

254. Association for the Advancement of Medical Instrumentation. Chemical indicators—guidance for the selection, use, and interpretation of results. AAMI Technical Information Report No. 25. Arlington, VA: Association for the Advancement of Medical Instrumentation, 1999.

255. Ninemeier J. Central service technical manual. 5th ed. Chicago, IL: International Association of Healthcare Central Service Materiel Management, 1998.

256. Rutala WA, Weber DJ. Choosing a sterilization wrap for surgical packs. Infect Control Today 2000;4:64, 70.

257. Association for the Advancement of Medical Instrumentation, American National Standards Institute. Good hospital practice: steam sterilization and sterility assurance. ANSI/AAMI ST46-1993. Arlington, VA: Association for the Advancement of Medical Instrumentation, 1993.

258. Association for the Advancement of Medical Instrumentation, American National Standards Institute. Flash sterilization: steam sterilization of patient care items for immediate use. ANSI/AAMI

ST37-1996. Arlington, VA: Association for the Advancement of Medical Instrumentation, 1996.

259. Association for the Advancement of Medical Instrumentation, American National Standards Institute. Ethylene oxide sterilization in health care facilities: safety and effectiveness. ANSI/AAMI ST41-1999. Arlington, VA: Association for the Advancement of Medical Instrumentation, 1999.

260. Miller CH, Palenik CJ. Sterilization, disinfection, and asepsis in dentistry [Chapter 53]. In: Block SS, ed. 5th ed. Disinfection, sterilization, and preservation. Philadelphia, PA: Lippincott Williams & Wilkins, 2001:1049–68.

261. Joslyn LJ. Sterilization by heat [Chapter 36]. In: Block SS, ed. 5th ed. Disinfection, sterilization, and preservation. Philadelphia, PA: Lippincott Williams & Wilkins, 2001:695–728.

262. Rutala WA, Weber DJ, Chappell KJ. Patient injury from flash-sterilized instruments. Infect Control Hosp Epidemiol 1999;20:458.

263. Bond WW. Biological indicators for a liquid chemical sterilizer: a solution to the instrument reprocessing problem? Infect Control Hosp Epidemiol 1993;14:309–12.

264. Stingeni L, Lapomarda V, Lisi P. Occupational hand dermatitis in hospital environments. Contact Dermatitis 1995;33:172–6.

265. Ashdown BC, Stricof DD, May ML, Sherman SJ, Carmody RF. Hydrogen peroxide poisoning causing brain infarction: neuroimaging findings. Am J Roentgenol 1998;170:1653–5.

266. Ballantyne B. Toxicology of glutaraldehyde: review of studies and human health effects. Danbury, CT: Union Carbide, 1995.

267. CDC. National Institute for Occupational Safety and Health. Glutaraldehyde: occupational hazards in hospitals. Cincinnati, OH: US Department of Health and Human Services, Public Health Service, CDC, National Institute for Occupational Safety and Health, 2001. DHHS publication no. (NIOSH) 2001-115.

268. CDC. Epidemiologic notes and reports: symptoms of irritation associated with exposure to glutaraldehyde—Colorado. MMWR 1987;36:190–1.

269. Lehman PA, Franz TJ, Guin JD. Penetration of glutaraldehyde through glove material: tactylon versus natural rubber latex. Contact Dermatitis 1994;30:176–7.

270. Hamann CP, Rodgers PA, Sullivan K. Allergic contact dermatitis in dental professionals: effective diagnosis and treatment. J Am Dent Assoc 2003;134:185–94.

271. Association for the Advancement of Medical Instrumentation, American National Standards Institute. Safe use and handling of glutaraldehyde-based products in health care facilities. ANSI/AAMI ST58-1996. Arlington, VA: Association for the Advancement of Medical Instrumentation, 1996.

272. Fisher AA. Ethylene oxide dermatitis. Cutis 1984;34:20, 22, 24.

273. Jay WM, Swift TR, Hull DS. Possible relationship of ethylene oxide exposure to cataract formation. Am J Ophthalmol 1982;93:727–32.

274. US Department of Labor, Occupational Safety and Health Administration. Review of the ethylene oxide standard. Federal Register 2000;65:35127–8.

275. Pratt LH, Smith DG, Thornton RH, Simmons JB, Depta BB, Johnson RB. The effectiveness of two sterilization methods when different precleaning techniques are employed. J Dent 1999;27:247–8.

276. US Department of Health and Human Services, Food and Drug Administration. 21 CFR Part 872.6730. Dental devices; endodontic dry heat sterilizer; final rule. Federal Register 1997;62:2903.

277. Favero MS. Current issues in hospital hygiene and sterilization technology. J Infect Control (Asia Pacific Edition) 1998;1:8–10.

278. Greene WW. Control of sterilization process [Chapter 22]. In: Russell AD, Hugo WB, Ayliffe GA, eds. Principles and practice of disinfection, preservation, and sterilization. Oxford, England: Blackwell Scientific Publications, 1992:605–24.

279. Favero MS. Developing indicators for sterilization [Chapter 13]. In: Rutala W, ed. Disinfection, sterilization, and antisepsis in health care. Washington, DC: Association for Professionals in Infection Control and Epidemiology, Inc., 1998:119–32.

280. Maki DG, Hassemer CA. Flash sterilization: carefully measured haste. Infect Control 1987;8:307–10.

281. Andres MT, Tejerina JM, Fierro JF. Reliability of biologic indicators in a mail-return sterilization-monitoring service: a review of 3 years. Quintessence Int 1995;26:865–70.

282. Miller CH, Sheldrake MA. The ability of biological indicators to detect sterilization failures. Am J Dent 1994;7:95–7.

283. Association of Operating Room Nurses. AORN standards and recommended practices for perioperative nursing. Denver, CO: AORN, 1987.

284. Mayworm D. Sterile shelf life and expiration dating. J Hosp Supply Process Distrib 1984;2:32–5.

285. Cardo DM, Sehulster LM. Central sterile supply [Chapter 65]. In: Mayhall CG, ed. Hospital Epidemiology and Infection Control. 2nd ed. Philadelphia, PA: Lippincott Williams & Wilkins, 1999:1023–30.

286. Maki DG, Alvarado CJ, Hassemer CA, Zilz MA. Relation of the inanimate hospital environment to endemic nosocomial infection. N Engl J Med 1982;307:1562–6.

287. Danforth D, Nicolle LE, Hume K, Alfieri N, Sims H. Nosocomial infections on nursing units with floors cleaned with a disinfectant compared with detergent. J Hosp Infect 1987;10:229–35.

288. Crawford JJ. Clinical asepsis in dentistry. Mesquite, TX: Oral Medicine Press, 1987.

289. Food and Drug Administration. Design control guidance for medical device manufacturers. Rockville, MD: US Department of Health and Human Services, Food and Drug Administration, 1997.

290. Fauerbach LL, Janelle JW. Practical applications in infection control [Chapter 45]. In: Block SS, ed. 5th ed. Disinfection, sterilization, and preservation. Philadelphia, PA: Lippincott Williams & Wilkins, 2001:935–44.

291. Martin LS, McDougal JS, Loskoski SL. Disinfection and inactivation of the human T lymphotrophic virus type III/lymphadenopathy-associated virus. J Infect Dis 1985;152:400–3.

292. Bloomfield SF, Smith-Burchnell CA, Dalgleish AG. Evaluation of hypochlorite-releasing disinfectants against the human immunodeficiency virus (HIV). J Hosp Infect 1990;15:273–8.

293. Gerson SL, Parker P, Jacobs MR, Creger R, Lazarus HM. Aspergillosis due to carpet contamination. Infect Control Hosp Epidemiol 1994;15:221–3.

294. Suzuki A, Namba Y, Matsuura M, Horisawa A. Bacterial contamination of floors and other surfaces in operating rooms: a five-year survey. J Hyg (Lond) 1984;93:559–66.

295. Skoutelis AT, Westenfelder GO, Beckerdite M, Phair JP. Hospital carpeting and epidemiology of *Clostridium difficile*. Am J Infect Control 1994;22:212–7.

296. Rutala WA, Odette RL, Samsa GP. Management of infectious waste by US hospitals. JAMA 1989;262:1635–40.

297. CDC. Perspectives in disease prevention and health promotion. Summary of the Agency for Toxic Substances and Disease Registry report to Congress: the public health implications of medical waste. MMWR 1990;39:822–4.

298. Palenik CJ. Managing regulated waste in dental environments. J Contemp Dent Pract 2003;4:76.

299. Rutala WA, Mayhall CG. Medical waste. Infect Control Hosp Edidemiol 1992;13:38–48.

300. Greene R, State and Territorial Association on Alternate Treatment Technologies. Technical assistance manual: state regulatory oversight of medical waste treatment technologies. 2nd ed. Washington, DC: US Environmental Protection Agency, 1994. Available at http://www.epa.gov/epaoswer/other/medical/mwpdfs/ta/1.pdf.

301. US Environmental Protection Agency. 40 CFR Part 60. Standards of performance for new stationary sources and emission guidelines for existing sources: hospital/medical/infectious waste incinerators; final rule. Federal Register 1997;62:48347–91.

302. Slade JS, Pike EB, Eglin RP, Colbourne JS, Kurtz JB. The survival of human immunodeficiency virus in water, sewage, and sea water. Water Sci Tech 1989;21:55–9.

303. Walker JT, Bradshaw DJ, Bennett AM, Fulford MR, Martin MV, Marsh PD. Microbial biofilm formation and contamination of dental-unit water systems in general dental practice. Appl Environ Microbiol 2000;66:3363–7.

304. Schulze-Robbecke R, Feldmann C, Fischeder R, Janning B, Exner M, Wahl G. Dental units: an environmental study of sources of potentially pathogenic mycobacteria. Tuber Lung Dis 1995;76:318–23.

305. Barbeau J, Tanguay R, Faucher E, et al. Multiparametric analysis of waterline contamination in dental units. Appl Environ Microbiol 1996;62:3954–9.

306. Atlas RM, Williams JF, Huntington MK. *Legionella* contamination of dental-unit waters. Appl Environ Microbiol 1995;61:1208–13.

307. Kelstrup J, Funder-Nielsen T, Theilade J. Microbial aggregate contamination of water lines in dental equipment and its control. Acta Pathol Microbiol Scand [B] 1977;85:177–83.

308. Challacombe SJ, Fernandes LL. Detecting *Legionella pneumophila* in water systems: a comparison of various dental units. J Am Dent Assoc 1995;126:603–8.

309. Mayo JA, Oertling KM, Andrieu SC. Bacterial biofilm: a source of contamination in dental air-water syringes. Clin Prev Dent 1990;12:13–20.

310. Scheid RC, Kim CK, Bright JS, Whitely MS, Rosen S. Reduction of microbes in handpieces by flushing before use. J Am Dent Assoc 1982;105:658–60.

311. Bagga BS, Murphy RA, Anderson AW, Punwani I. Contamination of dental unit cooling water with oral microorganisms and its prevention. J Am Dent Assoc 1984;109:712–6.

312. Martin MV. The significance of the bacterial contamination of dental unit water systems. Br Dent J 1987;163:152–4.

313. Pankhurst CL, Philpott-Howard JN, Hewitt JH, Casewell MW. The efficacy of chlorination and filtration in the control and eradication of *Legionella* from dental chair water systems. J Hosp Infect 1990;16:9–18.

314. Mills SE, Lauderdale PW, Mayhew RB. Reduction of microbial contamination in dental units with povidone-iodine 10%. J Am Dent Assoc 1986;113:280–4.

315. Williams JF, Johnston AM, Johnson B, Huntington MK, Mackenzie CD. Microbial contamination of dental unit waterlines: prevalence, intensity and microbiological characteristics. J Am Dent Assoc 1993;124:59–65.

316. Mills SE. The dental unit waterline controversy: defusing the myths, defining the solutions. J Am Dent Assoc 2000;131:1427–41.

317. Jones F, Bartlett CL. Infections associated with whirlpools and spas. Soc Appl Bacteriol Symp Ser 1985;14:61S–6S.

318. Hollyoak V, Allison D, Summers J. *Pseudomonas aeruginosa* wound infection associated with a nursing home's whirlpool bath. Commun Dis Rep CDR Rev 1995;5:R100–2.

319. Begg N, O'Mahony M, Penny P, Richardson EA, Basavaraj DS. *Mycobacterium chelonei* associated with a hospital hydrotherapy pool. Community Med 1986;8:348–50.

320. Laussucq S, Baltch AL, Smith RP, et al. Nosocomial *Mycobacterium fortuitum* colonization from a contaminated ice machine. Am Rev Respir Dis 1988;138:891–4.

321. Struelens MJ, Rost F, Deplano A, et al. *Pseudomonas aeruginosa* and *Enterobacteriaceae* bacteremia after biliary endoscopy: an outbreak investigation using DNA macrorestriction analysis. Am J Med 1993;95:489–98.

322. Kuritsky JN, Bullen MG, Broome CV, Silcox VA, Good RC, Wallace RJ Jr. Sternal wound infections and endocarditis due to organisms of the *Mycobacterium fortuitum* complex. Ann Intern Med 1983;98:938–9.

323. Bolan G, Reingold AL, Carson LA, et al. Infections with *Mycobacterium chelonei* in patients receiving dialysis and using processed hemodialyzers. J Infect Dis 1985;152:1013–9.

324. Lessing MP, Walker MM. Fatal pulmonary infection due to *Mycobacterium fortuitum*. J Clin Pathol 1993;46:271–2.

325. Arnow PM, Chou T, Weil D, Shapiro EN, Kretzschmar C. Nosocomial Legionnaires' disease caused by aerosolized tap water from respiratory devices. J Infect Dis 1982;146:460–7.

326. Breiman RF, Fields BS, Sanden GN, Volmer L, Meier A, Spika JS. Association of shower use with Legionnaires' disease: possible role of amoebae. JAMA 1990;263:2924–6.

327. Garbe PL, Davis BJ, Weisfeld JS, et al. Nosocomial Legionnaires' disease: epidemiologic demonstration of cooling towers as a source. JAMA 1985;254:521–4.

328. Fallon RJ, Rowbotham TJ. Microbiological investigations into an outbreak of Pontiac fever due to *Legionella micdadei* associated with use of a whirlpool. J Clin Pathol 1990;43:479–83.

329. Rose CS, Martyny JW, Newman LS, et al. "Lifeguard lung": endemic granulomatous pneumonitis in an indoor swimming pool. Am J Public Health 1998;88:1795–1800.

330. CDC. Epidemiologic notes and reports: Legionnaires' disease outbreak associated with a grocery store mist machine—Louisiana, 1989. MMWR 1990;39:108–10.

331. Jacobs RL, Thorner RE, Holcomb JR, Schwietz LA, Jacobs FO. Hypersensitivity pneumonitis caused by *Cladosporium* in an enclosed hot-tub area. Ann Intern Med 1986;105:204–6.

332. Clark A. Bacterial colonization of dental units and the nasal flora of dental personnel. Proc Roy Soc Med 1974;67:1269–70.

333. Fotos PG, Westfall HN, Snyder IS, Miller RW, Mutchler BM. Prevalence of *Legionella*-specific IgG and IgM antibody in a dental clinic population. J Dent Res 1985;64:1382–5.

334. Reinthaler FF, Mascher F, Stunzner D. Serological examinations for antibodies against *Legionella* species in dental personnel. J Dent Res 1988;67:942–3.

335. Putnins EE, Di Giovanni D, Bhullar AS. Dental unit waterline contamination and its possible implications during periodontal surgery. J Periodontol 2001;72:393–400.

336. United States Pharmacopeial Convention. Sterile water for irrigation. In: United States Pharmacopeial Convention. United States pharmacopeia and national formulary. USP 24–NF 19. Rockville, MD: United States Pharmacopeial Convention, 1997:1753.

337. Milton DK, Wypij D, Kriebel D, Walters MD, Hammond SK, Evans JS. Endotoxin exposure-response in a fiberglass manufacturing facility. Am J Ind Med 1996;29:3–13.

338. Santiago JI. Microbial contamination of dental unit waterlines: short and long term effects of flushing. Gen Dent 1994;42:528–35.

339. Shearer BG. Biofilm and the dental office. J Am Dent Assoc 1996;127:181–9.

340. Association for the Advancement of Medical Instrumentation, American National Standards Institute. Hemodialysis systems. ANSI/AAMI RD5-1992. Arlington, VA: Association for the Advancement of Medical Instrumentation, 1993.

341. US Environmental Protection Agency. National primary drinking water regulations, 1999: list of contaminants. Washington DC: US Environmental Protection Agency, 1999. Available at http://www.epa.gov/safewater/mcl.html.

342. American Public Health Association, American Water Works Association, Water Environment Foundation. In: Eaton AD, Clesceri LS, Greenberg AE, eds. Standard methods for the examination of water and wastewater. Washington, DC: American Public Health Association, 1999.

343. Williams HN, Johnson A, Kelley JI, et al. Bacterial contamination of the water supply in newly installed dental units. Quintessence Int 1995;26:331–7.

344. Scheid RC, Rosen S, Beck FM. Reduction of CFUs in high-speed handpiece water lines over time. Clin Prev Dent 1990;12:9–12.

345. Williams HN, Kelley J, Folineo D, Williams GC, Hawley CL, Sibiski J. Assessing microbial contamination in clean water dental units and compliance with disinfection protocol. J Am Dent Assoc 1994;125:1205–11.

346. CDC, Working Group on Waterborne Cryptosporidiosis. Cryptosporidium and water: a public health handbook. Atlanta, GA: US Department of Health and Human Services, Public Health Service, CDC, 1997.

347. MacKenzie WR, Hoxie NJ, Proctor ME, et al. A massive outbreak in Milwaukee of cryptosporidium infection transmitted through the public water supply. N Engl J Med 1994;331:161–7.

348. Kaminski JC. Cryptosporidium and the public water supply. N Engl J Med 1994;331:1529–30.

349. CDC. Assessing the public health threat associated with waterborne cryptosporidiosis: report of a workshop. MMWR 1995;44(No. RR-6).

350. CDC. Surveillance for waterborne-disease outbreaks—United States, 1993–1994. MMWR 1996;45(No. SS-1).

351. Office of Water, US Environmental Protection Agency. Lead and copper rule: summary of revisions. EPA 815–R–99–020. Washington DC: US Environmental Protection Agency, 2000.

352. US Environmental Protection Agency. 65 CFR Parts 141 and 142. National primary drinking water regulations for lead and copper, final rule. Federal Register 2000;1949–2015.

353. Gooch B, Marianos D, Ciesielski C, et al. Lack of evidence for patient-to-patient transmission of HIV in a dental practice. J Am Dent Assoc 1993;124:38–44.

354. Crawford JJ, Broderius C. Control of cross-infection risks in the dental operatory: prevention of water retraction by bur cooling spray systems. J Am Dent Assoc 1988;116:685–7.

355. Mills SE, Kuehne JC, Bradley DV Jr. Bacteriological analysis of high-speed handpiece turbines. J Am Dent Assoc 1993;124:59–62.

356. Lewis DL, Arens M, Appleton SS, et al. Cross-contamination potential with dental equipment. Lancet 1992;340:1252–4.

357. Lewis DL, Boe RK. Cross-infection risks associated with current procedures for using high-speed dental handpieces. J Clin Microbiol 1992;30:401–6.

358. Checchi L, Montebugnoli L, Samaritani S. Contamination of the turbine air chamber: a risk of cross infection. J Clin Periodontol 1998;25:607–11.

359. Epstein JB, Rea G, Sibau L, Sherlock CH, Le ND. Assessing viral retention and elimination in rotary dental instruments. J Am Dent Assoc 1995;126:87–92.

360. Kolstad RA. How well does the chemiclave sterilize handpieces? J Am Dent Assoc 1998;129:985–91.

361. Kuehne JS, Cohen ME, Monroe SB. Performance and durability of autoclavable high-speed dental handpieces. NDRI-PR 92-03. Bethesda, MD: Naval Dental Research Institute, 1992.

362. Andersen HK, Fiehn NE, Larsen T. Effect of steam sterilization inside the turbine chambers of dental turbines. Oral Surg Oral Med Oral Pathol Oral Radiol Endod 1999;87:184–8.

363. Leonard DL, Charlton DG. Performance of high-speed dental handpieces subjected to simulated clinical use and sterilization. J Am Dent Assoc 1999;130:1301–11.

364. Barbeau J, ten Bokum L, Gauthier C, Prevost AP. Cross-contamination potential of saliva ejectors used in dentistry. J Hosp Infect 1998;40:303–11.

365. Mann GL, Campbell TL, Crawford JJ. Backflow in low-volume suction lines: the impact of pressure changes. J Am Dent Assoc 1996;127:611–5.

366. Watson CM, Whitehouse RL. Possibility of cross-contamination between dental patients by means of the saliva ejector. J Am Dent Assoc 1993;124:77–80.

367. Glass BJ, Terezhalmy GT. Infection control in dental radiology [Chapter 15]. In: Cottone JA, Terezhalamy GT, Molinari JA, eds. Practical infection control in dentisty. 2nd ed. Baltimore. MD: Williams & Wilkins, 1996:229–38.

368. Haring JI, Jansen L. Infection control and the dental radiographer. In: Haring JI, Jansen L, eds. Dental radiography: principles and techniques. Philadelphia, PA: WB Saunders Co., 2000:194–204.

369. Hignett M, Claman P. High rates of perforation are found in endovaginal ultrasound probe covers before and after oocyte retrieval for in vitro fertilization-embryo transfer. J Assist Reprod Genet 1995;12:606–9.

370. Fritz S, Hust MH, Ochs C, Gratwohl I, Staiger M, Braun B. Use of a latex cover sheath for transesophageal echocardiography (TEE) instead of regular disinfection of the echoscope? Clin Cardiol 1993;16:737–40.

371. Milki AA, Fisch JD. Vaginal ultrasound probe cover leakage: implications for patient care. Fertil Steril 1998;69:409–11.

372. Storment JM, Monga M, Blanco JD. Ineffectiveness of latex condoms in preventing contamination of the transvaginal ultrasound transducer head. South Med J 1997;90:206–8.

373. Amis S, Ruddy M, Kibbler CC, Economides DL, MacLean AB. Assessment of condoms as probe covers for transvaginal sonography. J Clin Ultrasound 2000;28:295–8.

374. Rooks VJ, Yancey MK, Elg SA, Brueske L. Comparison of probe sheaths for endovaginal sonography. Obstet Gynecol 1996;87:27–9.

375. Hokett SD, Honey JR, Ruiz F, Baisden MK, Hoen MM. Assessing the effectiveness of direct digital radiography barrier sheaths and finger cots. J Am Dent Assoc 2000;131:463–7.

376. ASHP Council on Professional Affairs. ASHP guidelines on quality assurance for pharmacy-prepared sterile products. Am J Health Syst Pharm 2000;57:1150–69.

377. Green KA, Mustachi B, Schoer K, Moro D, Blend R, McGeer A. Gadolinium-based MR contrast media: potential for growth of microbial contaminants when single vials are used for multiple patients. Am J Roentgenol 1995;165:669–71.

378. American Society of Anesthesiologists. Recommendations for infection control for the practice of anesthesiology. 2nd ed. Park Ridge, IL: American Society of Anesthesiologists, 1999.

379. Henry B, Plante-Jenkins C, Ostrowska K. An outbreak of *Serratia marcescens* associated with the anesthetic agent propofol. Am J Infect Control 2001;29:312–5.

380. Plott RT, Wagner RF Jr, Tyring SK. Iatrogenic contamination of multidose vials in simulated use: A reassessment of current patient injection technique. Arch Dermatol 1990;126:1441–4.

381. Arrington ME, Gabbert KC, Mazgaj PW, Wolf MT. Multidose vial contamination in anesthesia. AANA J 1990;58:462–6.

382. CDC. Recommendations for preventing transmission of infections among chronic hemodialysis patients. MMWR 2001;50(No. RR-5).

383. Food and Drug Administration. Labeling recommendations for single-use devices reprocessed by third parties and hospitals;

final guidance for industry and FDA. Rockville, MD: US Department of Health and Human Services, Food and Drug Administration, 2001.

384. Villasenor A, Hill SD, Seale NS. Comparison of two ultrasonic cleaning units for deterioration of cutting edges and debris removal on dental burs. Pediatr Dent 1992;14:326–30.

385. Rapisarda E, Bonaccorso A, Tripi TR, Condorelli GG. Effect of sterilization on the cutting efficiency of rotary nickel-titanium endodontic files. Oral Surg Oral Med Oral Pathol Oral Radiol Endod 1999;88:343–7.

386. Filho IB, Esberard RM, Leonardo R, del Rio CE. Microscopic evaluation of three endodontic files pre- and postinstrumentation. J Endodontics 1998;24:461–4.

387. Silvaggio J, Hicks ML. Effect of heat sterilization on the torsional properties of rotary nickel-titanium endodontic files. J Endod 1997;23:731–4.

388. Kazemi RB, Stenman E, Spangberg LS. The endodontic file is a disposable instrument. J Endod 1995;21:451–5.

389. Dajani AS, Bisno AL, Chung KJ, et al. Prevention of bacterial endocarditis: recommendations by the American Heart Association. JAMA 1990;264:2919–22.

390. Pallasch TJ, Slots J. Antibiotic prophylaxis and the medically compromised patient. Periodontol 2000 1996;10:107–38.

391. Litsky BY, Mascis JD, Litsky W. Use of an antimicrobial mouthwash to minimize the bacterial aerosol contamination generated by the high-speed drill. Oral Surg Oral Med Oral Pathol 1970;29:25–30.

392. Mohammed CI, Monserrate V. Preoperative oral rinsing as a means of reducing air contamination during use of air turbine handpieces. Oral Surg Oral Med Oral Pathol 1970;29:291–4.

393. Wyler D, Miller RL, Micik RE. Efficacy of self-administered preoperative oral hygiene procedures in reducing the concentration of bacteria in aerosols generated during dental procedures. J Dent Res 1971;50:509.

394. Muir KF, Ross PW, MacPhee IT, Holbrook WP, Kowolik MJ. Reduction of microbial contamination from ultrasonic scalers. Br Dent J 1978;145:76–8.

395. Fine DH, Mendieta C, Barnett ML, et al. Efficacy of preprocedural rinsing with an antiseptic in reducing viable bacteria in dental aerosols. J Periodontol 1992;63:821–4.

396. Fine DH, Furgang D, Korik I, Olshan A, Barnett ML, Vincent JW. Reduction of viable bacteria in dental aerosols by preprocedural rinsing with an antiseptic mouthrinse. Am J Dent 1993;6:219–21.

397. Fine DH, Yip J, Furgang D, Barnett ML, Olshan AM, Vincent J. Reducing bacteria in dental aerosols: pre-procedural use of an antiseptic mouth rinse. J Am Dent Assoc 1993;124:56–8.

398. Logothetis DD, Martinez-Welles JM. Reducing bacterial aerosol contamination with a chlorhexidine gluconate pre-rinse. J Am Dent Assoc 1995;126:1634–9.

399. Klyn SL, Cummings DE, Richardson BW, Davis RD. Reduction of bacteria-containing spray produced during ultrasonic scaling. Gen Dent 2001;49:648–52.

400. Brown AR, Papasian CJ, Shultz P, Theisen FC, Shultz RE. Bacteremia and intraoral suture removal: can an antimicrobial rinse help? J Am Dent Assoc 1998;129:1455–61.

401. Lockhart PB. An analysis of bacteremias during dental extractions: A double-blind, placebo-controlled study of chlorhexidine. Arch Intern Med 1996;156:513–20.

402. Dajani AS, Bisno AL, Chung KJ, et al. Prevention of bacterial endocarditis: recommendations by the American Heart Association. JAMA 1997;277:1794–1801.

403. Tate WH, White RR. Disinfection of human teeth for educational purposes. J Dent Educ 1991;55:583–5.

404. Pantera EA Jr, Zambon JJ, Shih-Levine M. Indirect immunofluorescence for the detection of *Bacteroides* species in human dental pulp. J Endod 1988;14:218–23.

405. Pantera EA Jr, Schuster GS. Sterilization of extracted human teeth. J Dent Educ 1990;54:283–5.

406. Parsell DE, Stewart BM, Barker JR, Nick TG, Karns L, Johnson RB. The effect of steam sterilization on the physical properties and perceived cutting characteristics of extracted teeth. J Dent Educ 1998;62;260–3.

407. American Dental Association's Council on Scientific Affairs and Council on Dental Practice. Infection control recommendations for the dental office and the dental laboratory. J Am Dent Assoc 1996;127:672–80.

408. Dental Laboratory Relationship Working Group, Organization for Safety and Asepsis Procedures (OSAP). Laboratory asepsis position paper. Annapolis, MD: OSAP Foundation, 1998. Available at http://www.osap.org/issues/pages/position/LAB.pdf.

409. Kugel G, Perry RD, Ferrari M, Lalicata P. Disinfection and communication practices: a survey of U. S. dental laboratories. J Am Dent Assoc 2000;131:786–92.

410. US Department of Transportation. 49 CFR 173.196 infectious substances (etiologic agents) 173.197 regulated medical waste. Available at http://www.access.gpo.gov/nara/cfr/waisidx_02/49cfr173_02.html.

411. Chau VB, Saunders TR, Pimsler M, Elfring DR. In-depth disinfection of acrylic resins. J Prosthet Dent 1995;74:309–13.

412. Powell GL, Runnells RD, Saxon BA, Whisenant BK. The presence and identification of organisms transmitted to dental laboratories. J Prosthet Dent 1990;64:235–7.

413. Giblin J, Podesta R, White J. Dimensional stability of impression materials immersed in an iodophor disinfectant. Int J Prosthodont 1990;3:72–7.

414. Plummer KD, Wakefield CW. Practical infection control in dental laboratories. Gen Dent 1994;42:545–8.

415. Merchant VA. Infection control in the dental laboratory equipment [Chapter 16]. In: Cottone JA, Terezhalamy GT, Molinari JA, eds. Practical infection control in dentistry. 2nd ed. Baltimore, MD: Williams & Wilkins, 1996:239–54.

416. Molinari J. Dental. In: Association for Professionals in Infection Control and Epidemiology, Inc. (APIC). APIC text of infection control and epidemiology. Washington, DC: Association for Professionals in Infection Control and Epidemiology, Inc, 2002.

417. Sofou A, Larsen T, Fiehn NE, Owall B. Contamination level of alginate impressions arriving at a dental laboratory. Clin Oral Invest 2002;6:161–5.

418. McNeill MR, Coulter WA, Hussey DL. Disinfection of irreversible hydrocolloid impressions: a comparative study. Int J Prosthodont 1992;5:563–7.

419. Gerhardt DE, Sydiskis RJ. Impression materials and virus. J Am Dent Assoc 1991;122:51–4.

420. Leung RL, Schonfeld SE. Gypsum casts as a potential source of microbial cross-contamination. J Prosthet Dent 1983;49:210–1.

421. Huizing KL, Palenik CJ, Setcos JC, Sheldrake MA, Miller, CH. Method of evaluating the antimicrobial abilities of disinfectant-containing gypsum products. QDT Yearbook 1994;17:172–6.

422. Verran J, Kossar S, McCord JF. Microbiological study of selected risk areas in dental technology laboratories. J Dent 1996;24:77–80.

423. CDC. National Institute for Occupational Safety and Health. NIOSH Health Hazard Evaluation and Technical Assistance Report. Cincinnati, OH: US Department of Health and Human Services, Public Health Service, CDC, National Institute for Occupational Safety and Health, 1988. HETA 85-136-1932.

424. CDC. National Institute for Occupational Safety and Health. NIOSH Health Hazard Evaluation and Technical Assistance Report. Cincinnati, OH: US Department of Health and Human Services, Public Health Service, CDC, National Institute for Occupational Safety and Health, 1990. HETA 88-101-2008.

425. CDC. National Institute for Occupational Safety and Health. Control of smoke from laser/electric surgical procedures. Cincinnati, OH: US Department of Health and Human Services, Public Health Service, CDC, National Institute for Occupational Safety and Health, 1996. DHHS publication no. (NIOSH) 96-128.

426. Taravella MJ, Weinberg A, Blackburn P, May M. Do intact viral particles survive excimer laser ablation? Arch Ophthalmol 1997;115:1028–30.

427. Hagen KB, Kettering JD, Aprecio RM, Beltran F, Maloney RK. Lack of virus transmission by the excimer laser plume. Am J Ophthalmol 1997;124:206–11.

428. Kunachak S, Sithisarn P, Kulapaditharom B. Are laryngeal papilloma virus-infected cells viable in the plume derived from a continuous mode carbon dioxide laser, and are they infectious? A preliminary report on one laser mode. J Laryng Otol 1996;110:1031–3.

429. Hughes PS, Hughes AP. Absence of human papillomavirus DNA in the plume of erbium: YAG laser-treated warts. J Am Acad Dermatol 1998;38:426–8.

430. Garden JM, O'Banion MK, Shelnitz LS, et al. Papillomavirus in the vapor of carbon dioxide laser-treated verrucae. JAMA 1988;259: 1199–1202.

431. Sawchuk WS, Weber PJ, Lowry DR, Dzubow LM. Infectious papillomavirus in the vapor of warts treated with carbon dioxide laser or electrocoagulation: detection and protection. J Am Acad Dermatol 1989;21:41–9.

432. Baggish MS, Poiesz BJ, Joret D, Williamson P, Rafai A. Presence of human immunodeficiency virus DNA in laser smoke. Lasers Surg Med 1991;11:197–203.

433. Capizzi PJ, Clay RP, Battey MJ. Microbiologic activity in laser resurfacing plume and debris. Lasers Surg Med 1998;23:172–4.

434. McKinley IB Jr, Ludlow MO. Hazards of laser smoke during endodontic therapy. J Endod 1994;20:558–9.

435. Favero MS, Bolyard EA. Microbiologic considerations. Disinfection and sterilization strategies and the potential for airborne transmission of bloodborne pathogens. Surg Clin North Am 1995;75:1071–89.

436. Association of Operating Room Nurses. Recommended practices for laser safety in the practice setting. In: Fogg D, ed. Standards, recommended practices and guidelines. Denver, CO: AORN, 2003.

437. Streifel AJ. Recognizing IAQ risk and implementing an IAQ program. In: Hansen W, ed. A guide to managing indoor air quality in health care organizations. Oakbrook Terrace, IL: Joint Commission on Accreditation of Healthcare Organizations Publishers, 1997.

438. US Department of Labor, Occupational Safety and Health Administration. Safety and health topics: laser/electrosurgery plume. Washington DC: US Department of Labor, Occupational Safety and Health Administration, 2003. Available at http://www.osha-slc.gov/SLTC/laserelectrosurgeryplume.

439. American Thoracic Society, CDC. Diagnostic standards and classification of tuberculosis in adults and children. Am J Respir Crit Care Med 2000;161:1376–95.

440. Wells WF. Aerodynamics of droplet nuclei [Chapter 3]. In: Wells WF, ed. Airborne contagion and air hygiene: an ecological study of droplet infections. Cambridge, MA: Harvard University Press, 1955.

441. CDC. Prevention and treatment of tuberculosis among patients infected with human immunodeficiency virus: principles of therapy and revised recommendations. MMWR 1998;47(No. RR-20).

442. Smith WH, Davies D, Mason KD, Onions JP. Intraoral and pulmonary tuberculosis following dental treatment. Lancet 1982;1:842–4.

443. CDC. Self-reported tuberculin skin testing among Indian Health Service and Bureau of Prisons Dentists, 1993. MMWR 1994;43:209–11.

444. Mikitka D, Mills SE, Dazey SE, Gabriel ME. Tuberculosis infection in US Air Force dentists. Am J Dent 1995;8:33–6.

445. CDC. World Health Organization consultation on public health issues related to bovine spongiform encephalopathy and the emergence of a new variant of Creutzfeldt-Jakob Disease. MMWR 1996;45:295–6.

446. CDC. Surveillance for Creutzfeldt-Jakob disease—United States. MMWR 1996;45:665–8.

447. Johnson RT, Gibbs CJ Jr. Creutzfeldt-Jakob disease and related transmissible spongiform encephalopathies. N Engl J Med 1998;339:1994–2004.

448. CDC. New variant CJD: fact sheet. Atlanta, GA: US Department of Health and Human Services, Public Health Service, CDC, 2003. Available at http://www.cdc.gov/ncidod/diseases/cjd/cjd_fact_sheet.htm.

449. Will RG, Ironside JW, Zeidler M, et al. A new variant of Creutzfeldt-Jakob disease in the UK. Lancet 1996;347:921–5.

450. Bruce ME, Will RG, Ironside JW, et al. Transmission to mice indicate that 'new variant' CJD is caused by the BSE agent. Nature 1997;389:498–501.

451. Collinge J, Sidle KC, Meads J, Ironside J, Hill AF. Molecular analysis of prion strain variation and the aetiology of 'new variant' CJD. Nature 1996;383:685–90.

452. World Health Organization. Bovine spongiform encephalopathy (BSE). Fact Sheet No. 113. Geneva, Switzerland: World Health Organization, 2002. Available at http://www.who.int/mediacentre/factsheets/fs113/en/.

453. CDC. Probable variant Creutzfeldt-Jakob disease in a U.S. resident—Florida, 2002. MMWR 2002;51:927–9.

454. Hill AF, Butterworth RJ, Joiner S, et al. Investigation of variant Creutzfeldt-Jakob disease and other human prion diseases with tonsil biopsy specimens. Lancet 1999;353:183–9.

455. Brown P, Gibbs CJ Jr, Rodgers-Johnson P, et al. Human spongiform encephalopathy: the National Institutes of Health series of 300 cases of experimentally transmitted disease. Ann Neurol 1994;35:513–29.

456. Brown P. Environmental causes of human spongiform encephalopathy [Chapter 8]. In: Baker HF, Baker HF, eds. Prion diseases. Totowa, NJ: Humana Press Inc, 1996:139–54.

457. Carp RI. Transmission of scrapie by oral route: effect of gingival scarification. Lancet 1982;1:170–1.

458. Ingrosso L, Pisani F, Pocchiari M. Transmission of the 263K scrapie strain by the dental route. J Gen Virol 1999;80:3043–7.

459. Bernoulli C, Siegfried J, Baumgartner G, et al. Danger of accidental person-to-person transmission of Creutzfeldt-Jakob disease by surgery. Lancet 1977;1:478–9.

460. Brown P, Gajdusek DC, Gibbs CJ Jr, Asher DM. Potential epidemic of Creutzfeldt-Jakob disease from human growth hormone therapy. N Engl J Med 1985;313:728–31.

461. CDC. Fatal degenerative neurologic disease in patients who received pituitary-derived human growth hormone. MMWR 1985;34:359–60, 365–6.

462. Duffy P, Wolf J, Collins G, DeVoe AG, Streeten B, Cowen D. Possible person-to-person transmission of Creutzfeldt-Jakob disease. N Engl J Med 1974;290:692–3.

463. CDC. Epidemiologic notes and reports: rapidly progressive dementia in a patient who received a cadaveric dura mater graft. MMWR 1987;36:49–50, 55.

464. Thadani V, Penar PL, Partington J, et al. Creutzfeldt-Jakob disease probably acquired from a cadaveric dura mater graft: case report. J Neurosurg 1988;69:766–9.

465. Kondo K, Kuroiwa Y. A case control study of Creutzfeldt-Jakob disease: association with physical injuries. Ann Neurol 1982;11:377–81.

466. Van Duijn CM, Delasnerie-Laupretre N, Masullo C, et al, and European Union (EU) Collaborative Study Group of Creutzfeldt-Jacob disease (CJD). Case-control study of risk factors of Creutzfeldt-Jakob disease in Europe during 1993–95. Lancet 1998;351:1081–5.

467. Collins S, Law MG, Fletcher A, Boyd A, Kaldor J, Masters CL. Surgical treatment and risk of sporadic Creutzfeldt-Jakob disease: a case-control study. Lancet 1999;353:693–7.

468. Blanquet-Grossard F, Sazdovitch V, Jean A, et al. Prion protein is not detectable in dental pulp from patients with Creutzfeldt-Jakob disease. J Dent Res 2000;79:700.

469. World Health Organization. Infection control guidelines for transmissible spongiform encephalopathies: report of a WHO consultation, Geneva, Switzerland, 23–26 March 1999. Geneva, Switzerland: World Health Organization, 2000. Available at http://www.who.int/emc-documents/tse/whocdscsraph2003c.html.

470. Institute of Medicine, Committee on Quality of Health Care in America. Kohn LT, Corrigan JM, Donadlson MS, eds. To err is human: building a safe health system. Washington, DC: National Academy Press, 1999.

471. CDC. Framework for program evaluation in public health. MMWR 1999;48(No. RR-11).

Reprinted from **Centers for Disease Control and Prevention**: Guidelines for Infection Control in Dental Health-Care Settings—2003, *MMWR*, 52, 1-61, December, 2003.

APPENDIX IV

Average Measurements of Human Teeth

■ TABLE A-1 AVERAGE MEASUREMENTS OF THE PRIMARY TEETH (IN MILLIMETERS)

		OVERALL LENGTH	LENGTH OF CROWN	LENGTH OF ROOT	WIDTH OF CROWN (MESIAL-DISTAL AT WIDEST POINT)
Maxillary	Central Incisor	16.0	6.0	10.0	6.5
	Lateral Incisor	15.8	5.6	11.4	5.1
	Canine	19.0	6.5	13.5	7.0
	First Molar	15.2	5.1	10.0	7.3
	Second Molar	17.5	5.7	11.7	8.2
Mandibular	Central Incisor	14.0	5.0	9.0	4.2
	Lateral Incisor	15.0	5.2	10.0	4.1
	Canine	17.5	6.0	11.5	5.0
	First Molar	15.8	6.0	9.8	7.7
	Second Molar	18.8	5.5	11.3	9.9

(From Black, G.V.: *Descriptive Anatomy of the Human Teeth,* 4th ed. Philadelphia, The S.S. White Dental Manufacturing Company, 1897, according to Ash, M.M.: *Wheeler's Dental Anatomy, Physiology, and Occlusion,* 7th ed. Philadelphia, W.B. Saunders, Co., 1993, p. 58.)

■ TABLE A-2 AVERAGE MEASUREMENTS OF THE PERMANENT TEETH (IN MILLIMETERS)

		OVERALL LENGTH	LENGTH OF CROWN	LENGTH OF ROOT	WIDTH OF CROWN (MESIAL-DISTAL AT WIDEST POINT)
Maxillary	Central Incisor	23.5	10.5	13.0	8.5
	Lateral Incisor	22.0	9.9	13.0	6.5
	Canine	27.0	10.0	17.0	7.5
	First Premolar	22.5	8.5	14.0	7.0
	Second Premolar	22.5	8.5	14.0	7.0
	First Molar	B* L 19.5 20.5	7.5	B L 12 13	10.0
	Second Molar	B L 17.0 19.0	7.0	B L 11 12	9.0
	Third Molar	17.5	6.5	11.0	8.5
Mandibular	Central Incisor	21.5	9.0	12.5	5.0
	Lateral Incisor	23.5	9.5	14.0	5.5
	Canine	27.0	11.0	16.0	7.0
	First Premolar	22.5	8.5	14.0	7.0
	Second Premolar	22.5	8.0	14.5	7.0
	First Molar	21.5	7.5	14.0	11.0
	Second Molar	20.0	7.0	13.0	10.5
	Third Molar	18.0	7.0	11.0	10.0

*B = Buccal measurement; L = Lingual measurement
(From Ash, M.M.: *Wheeler's Dental Anatomy, Physiology, and Occlusion,* 7th ed. Philadelphia, W.B. Saunders Co., 1993, p. 15.)

Index

Page numbers followed by b indicate box; those followed by t indicate table. Pages numbers in *italics* indicate figure.

A

Abfraction
  in dentin hypersensitivity, 714, *715*
  pain associated with, 719t
Abrasion
  definition of, 727b, 743b
  gingiva, 403b
  tooth, *268*, 268–269
    definition of, 403b, 421
    in older persons, 830
    from toothbrushing, 421–422
Abrasive, definition of, 727b
Abrasive agents, for polishing, 730–732
  application of, 731
  calcium carbonate, 731
  characteristics of, 730–731
  commercial preparations, 732
  diamond particles, 732
  emery (corundum), 731
  preparation of, 732
  pumice, 731
  rouge (Jeweler's Rouge), 731
  Silex (silicon dioxide), 731
Abrasive discs, definition of, 743b
Abrasive system, definition of, 544b
Abscess (*See also* Periodontal abscess)
  definition of, 690b
  from partial scaling, 650
Absence seizure, 969b, 971
Absorbed dose, definition of, 151b
Abstinence
  from alcohol, 1016
  definition of, 1011b
Abuse (*See also* Child abuse; Family abuse and neglect)
  definition of, 961, 1011b
  physical
    behavioral indicators of, 962t
    conditions that mimic, 962t
    definition of, 961t
    of elderly, 963
  psychological
    behavioral indicators of, 962t
    definition of, 961t
    of elderly, 964
  sexual
    behavioral indicators of, 962t
    definition of, 961t
    of elderly, 964
    signs of, 963
  signs of alcohol, 1012
Abutment, 470, 470b, *471*
Accessibility
  instrumentation and, 627
  scaling and, 654
Accessibility standards, definition of, 884b
Accessory root canal, definition of, 261b
Acellular, definition of, 291b
Acid etchant, definition of, 570b
Acid etching, in sealant application, 571, 573t, 575
Acid production, in dental caries, 394
Acidic foods, dentin hypersensitivity and, 712, 720–721
Acidogenic, definition of, 544b
Acidogenic bacteria
  definition of, 394b
  in dental caries, 393

Acidulated phosphate fluoride (APF), 553, 554t
Acne rosacea, definition of, 1011b
Acne vulgaris, 814b, 817
Acoustic turbulence, definition of, 660
Acquired pellicle, 289–290, 292t
  formation of, 289–290
  significance of, 290
  types of, 290
Activation (*See* Stroke (instrument))
Active immunity, definition of, 19b
Acute, definition of, 690b, 1022b
Acute primary herpetic gingivostomatitis, definition of, 961b
ADA (American Dental Association), 65b
Adaptation (instrument), 623–624
  characteristics of well-adapted, 623
  definition of, 611b
  problem areas for, 623–624
  relation to tooth, 623, *623*
  for scaling, 656, *657*, 658
  in ultrasonic or sonic scaling, *667*, 667–668
Adaptive functioning, 981–982
Addiction (*See also* Alcoholism)
  definition of, 1011b
  drug, definition of, 502b, 1011b
  nicotine, 506–508
ADHA (American Dental Hygienists' Association), 4b (*See also* American Dental Hygienists' Association (ADHA))
Adherence, definition of, 758b
ADLs (activities of daily living), 352b, 353, 355t
Adolescence
  definition of, 814b
  dental biofilm control during, 818–819
  dental caries during, 817
  dental hygiene care during, 817–819
  dietary considerations during, 815–816, 819
  fluoride application during, 819
  patient teaching during, 819
  periodontal disease during, 817
  periodontitis during, 817
  personal factors in, 816–817
  physical development, 815
  psychosocial development, 815, 816t
  pubertal changes, 814–815
  stages of, 813–814
Adrenal crisis, 1115t
Adsorption, definition of, 291b
Adult speech aid prosthesis, definition of, 804b
Advanced directives, 767t
Advocacy
  about tobacco use, 516–517
  dental hygienist role, 5b
Aerobe, definition of, 291b
Aerosol
  definition of, 19b
  microbial, 19b
Aerosol production, 22–23
  in air-powder polishing, 737–738
  in polishing, 727
Aerosol spray, topical anesthesia, 606
Affect, definition of, 994b
Affective learning, definition of, 376b
Age
  biological, 826
  chronological, 825–826
  classification by function, 826–827
  disease and, 827

    functional, 826–827
    psychological, 826b
Ageism, definition of, 826b
Aging
  alcoholism and, 828
  Alzheimer's disease, 829, 829t
  changes associated with, 827–828
  definition of, 826b
  dental hygiene care for older persons, 831–833
    assessment, 831–832
    dental biofilm control, 832–833
    extraoral and intraoral examination, 832
    medications, 832
    preventive care plan, 832
  dietary considerations, 833–835
    dietary habits, 833–834
    dietary needs, 834–835
    patient teaching, 835
  medication use in older persons, 832
  oral findings in, 829–831
    biofilm formation, 833
    dentin hypersensitivity, 714, 716
    periodontium, 831
    soft tissues, 830
    teeth, 830–831
  osteoporosis, 828–829
  patient teaching, 833, 834t, 835
  prophylactic premedication in older persons, 832
  visual impairment and, 952
Agitation, definition of, 994b
Agranulocytes, 1061–1062, 1061t
Agranulocytosis, 1067
AI (adequate intake), definition of, 521b, 522
Air application, instruments for, 225
Air-powder polisher, definition of, 727b
Air-powder polishing, 737–739, *738*
  contraindications for, 739
  description, 737
  precautions for, 737–738
  for restorations, 739, 739t
  technique for, 737
  uses of, 737
Air syringe, compressed, 225
Airborne infection, 22–23
  aerosol production, 22–23
  dust-borne organisms, 22
  prevention of transmission, 23
Airway, in basic life support, 1100, *1100, 1102,
  1102*
Airway obstruction, 1107–1110, *1109,* 1112t
  complete, 1107, 1112t
  partial, 1107, 1112t
  prevention of, 1107
  recognition of, 1107
  treatment
    chest thrust, 1109
    conscious patient, 1108
    finger sweep, 1109
    foreign body, 1109
    for infant, 1110
    unconscious patient, 1109
AIs, 522
Akinesia, definition of, 923b
ALARA Concept, 151
Alcohol
  blood alcohol concentration, 1013
  metabolism of, 1012–1013